ENDOCRINE SURGERY SECOND EDITION

ENDOCRINE SURGERY SECOND EDITION

Edited by

Demetrius Pertsemlidis, MD FACS
The Bradley H. Jack Professor of Surgery
Icahn School of Medicine at Mount Sinai
New York, New York, USA

William B. Inabnet III, MD FACS
Chairman, Department of Surgery
Mount Sinai Beth Israel
Eugene W. Friedman Professor of Surgery
Icahn School of Medicine at Mount Sinai
New York, New York, USA

Michel Gagner, MD FRCSC, FACS, FASMBS
Clinical Professor of Surgery
Herbert Wertheim School of Medicine
Florida International University
Miami, Florida, USA
and
Senior Consultant
Hôpital du Sacré-Cœur
Montreal, Quebec, Canada

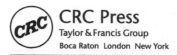

CRC Press
Taylor & Francis Group
Boca Raton London New York

CRC Press is an imprint of the
Taylor & Francis Group, an **informa** business

CRC Press
Taylor & Francis Group
6000 Broken Sound Parkway NW, Suite 300
Boca Raton, FL 33487-2742

First issued in paperback 2020

Version Date: 20170301

ISBN 13: 978-0-367-57346-1 (pbk)
ISBN 13: 978-1-4822-5959-9 (hbk)

Library of Congress Cataloging-in-Publication Data

Names: Pertsemlidis, Demetrius, 1929- editor. | Inabnet, William B., III, editor. | Gagner, Michel, editor.
Title: Endocrine surgery / [edited by] Demetrius Pertsemlidis, William B. Inabnet III, Michel Gagner.
Other titles: Endocrine surgery (Schwartz)
Description: Second edition. | Boca Raton : CRC Press, [2016] | Includes bibliographical references and index.
Identifiers: LCCN 2016021845| ISBN 9781482259599 (pack : alk. paper) | ISBN 9781482259605 (ebook PDF) | ISBN 9781498715966 (ebook Vitalsource)
Subjects: | MESH: Endocrine System Diseases--surgery | Endocrine Surgical Procedures--methods
Classification: LCC RD599 | NLM WK 148 | DDC 617.4/4--dc23
LC record available at https://lccn.loc.gov/2016021845

Visit the Taylor & Francis Web site at
http://www.taylorandfrancis.com

and the CRC Press Web site at
http://www.crcpress.com

To Lois, my wife, sons Alexander and David, and grandchildren Sarah, Helen, and William.
In gratitude to Bradley H. Jack, philanthropist and friend, whose endowment has allowed continuation of my clinical and academic work.

Demetrius Pertsemlidis

To my wife, Kathleen, and children, Frances and William, whose unconditional support is a true blessing. And to my patients, who consistently put their genuine trust in me to shepherd them to improved health.

William B. Inabnet III

For France, who is always there, and sons Xavier, Guillaume, and Maxime

Michel Gagner

Contents

Foreword

Today's endocrine surgery is based on the ongoing efforts and contributions of many clinicians and scientists. The early luminaries in surgery, Billroth, Kocher, and Halsted, made important contributions not only to the technical development and performance of operative procedures on endocrine glands but also to the understanding of the pathophysiology of the underlying diseases and of the resulting effects of surgery. In 1902, Bayliss and Starling first discovered that a chemical messenger from one tissue could be transported in the bloodstream to affect the function of a different tissue or organ. Bayliss coined the term "hormone" to categorize this action of secretin. The subsequent identification of other hormones such as insulin by Banting and Best and gastrin by Gregory illustrate the profound impact that endocrinology and endocrine surgery have had on the course of medicine and the care of patients. Endocrinology has always been a dynamic field but now more than ever the pace of discovery and depth of understanding of the cellular and physiologic processes in this field has rapidly accelerated. This is especially true since the publication of the first edition of *Endocrine Surgery*.

Endocrine surgery is now a well recognized subspecialty with advanced training programs that develop the required expertise to deal with the technical and, most importantly, the intellectual aspects of the field. The complexities involved in the diagnosis, management, and treatment options of endocrine surgical disease necessitate a multidisciplinary approach to produce a comprehensive, up-to-date clinically relevant textbook, Drs. Pertsemlides, Inabnet, and Gagner have assembled a nationally and internationally recognized group of authors from the diverse fields that impact the care and management of the endocrine surgical patient. The depth of knowledge and experience of these experts in endocrinology, pathology, radiology, basic science, surgery and surgical subspecialties provides useful approaches for the reader in all areas of endocrine surgical disease. It emphasizes that a skilled team is needed to deal with the multi-faceted aspects of these problems if the best results are to be obtained. Drs. Pertsemlides, Inabnet, and Gagner have provided a clear and integrated presentation of the clinical signs and symptoms, diagnostic laboratory tests, imaging findings and methods of localization, medical and surgical treatment options and the steps involved in the operative procedures for both benign and malignant disease. By emphasizing the multispecialty aspects of endocrine surgery, the reader not only strengthens their knowledge and understanding in their area of interest but also becomes conversant in the scope of expertise that is the purview of their colleagues.

This textbook brings together much new information and knowledge that has expanded the understanding of endocrine and metabolic surgical disease. From the molecular biology that underpins these diseases to the newest technologies and techniques that are being applied to the diagnosis, imaging and treatment of endocrine problems, the text provides a very functional source of valuable information. This edition will serve as the go to reference for Endocrine Surgery. It has much to offer physicians, endocrinologists, endocrine surgery fellows, residents and students, and non-clinicians with research interests in the field. It elucidates the standard approaches to current endocrine surgical problems but also looks forward to developing techniques of endoscopic and robotic surgery. As specialization in medicine increases, it is very useful to have a comprehensive text that deals with all aspects of a field even though one's interest may be limited to a particular area of that field. I feel that anyone who deals with an endocrine surgical patient will find many areas of interest in this second edition of *Surgical Endocrinology*. I am sure that readers of this text will not be disappointed and will find a vast array of useful information in dealing with the clinical aspects of endocrine surgical disease.

Dr. Richard A. Prinz, MD, FACS
Vice Chairman of Surgery
North Shore University Health System
and
Clinical Professor of Surgery
The University of Chicago Pritzker School of Medicine

Preface

This second edition of *Endocrine Surgery* provides the standard reference source for clinicians and scientists, house staff, and students. The textbook is contemporary, up to date, and complete, with its contents ranging from morphology and physiology to molecular and genetic aspects of endocrine diseases. An online version of the entire book is also available.

All chapters have been updated, extensively revised, or entirely rewritten. In addition, a new section on metabolic surgery, which includes four chapters, has been added.

The authors and their educational institutions come from across the world, making this book of universal relevance. The geographical locations are in North and South America, Europe, the Far East, the Near East, and Australia.

The goal of this book is to enhance the day-to-day practice of medical and surgical endocrinologists by including modern applications for the care of adults and, to some extent, adolescents and children as well.

Prominent contributing leaders in endocrinology and endocrine surgery and the well-known publishing house of CRC Press/Taylor & Francis Group have created this global anthology, which merits recognition by educational institutions and libraries, as well as by individual readers.

Our table of contents spans 10 parts and accommodates 57 chapters. The first two parts are devoted to pituitary, pulmonary, and thymic endocrine neoplasms. Parts 3 and 4 are dedicated to the thyroid and parathyroids. Eleven chapters on the adrenal glands and seven on the pancreas constitute Parts 5 and 6. Part 7 is a single but long contribution entitled "Inherited Syndromes," and the chapter title is "Multiple Endocrine Neoplasias." Nine chapters comprise Part 8, "Gastroenteropancreatic System." The new Part 9 is a constellation of four important chapters, including one on pancreas transplantation, and all welcome new additions to this edition. Finally, and looking to the future, the last single chapter, and Part 10, is entitled "Robotic Endocrine Surgery."

Demetrius Pertsemlidis
William B. Inabnet III
Michel Gagner
New York

Landmarks in endocrinology and endocrine surgery

DEMETRIUS PERTSEMLIDIS

Endocrinology and endocrine surgery have advanced rapidly and rightfully gained stately recognition in the academic environment and the world of medicine. The first biochemical assay for a hormone, secretin, was achieved at the beginning of the last century [1]. In 1946, Ulf van Euler, a catecholamine physiologist at the Karolinska Institute in Sweden, discovered that norepinephrine had the properties of a neurotransmitter. In 1970, he shared the Nobel Prize with Sir Bernard Katz of Great Britain and Julius Axelrod of the United States for the recognition of adrenergic neurotransmitter function [2,3].

In 1954, Paul Wermer described the inherited constellation of pituitary, parathyroid, and pancreatic islet cell neoplasia and named it "familial adenomatosis of the endocrine glands", later defined as MEN 1. In 1961, John Sipple described the association of thyroid carcinoma and pheochromocytoma, later termed Sipple syndrome, or MEN 2 [4].

In 1956, vanillylmandelic acid (VMA), a urinary metabolite of catecholamines, was discovered by M.D. Armstrong; a second urinary metabolite, metanephrine, was discovered the following year by J. Axelrod. Until the early 1950s, about one-half of pheochromocytomas were discovered at autopsy. These biochemical discoveries have permitted early detection with high accuracy (up to 95%) and low surgical mortality (close to zero) in the past four decades [2].

In the 1960s, Rosalyn Yalow and Solomon Berson, then at the Bronx Veterans Administration Medical Center and later faculty members of the Mount Sinai Hospital in New York, developed radioimmunoassay (RIA) to identify and characterize peptides, hormones, and amines. Solomon Berson died prematurely, before the Nobel Prize was given to Dr Yalow in 1977. RIA and later immunohistochemistry revolutionized endocrinology and endocrine surgery through better diagnosis and surgical skills [2,3].

MOLECULAR BIOLOGY

In the 1930s, macromolecules and their crystalline properties were studied using the technique of ultracentrifugation. In the 1950s, Linus Pauling (Nobel Prize 1954) discovered the three-dimensional structure of proteins, and the double helix of the DNA molecule was described by James Watson and Francis Crick (Nobel Prize laureates in 1962) [4,5].

By the 1980s, the landscapes of endocrinology and endocrine surgery benefited from the rapid scientific advances of molecular biology.

MOLECULAR ENDOCRINOLOGY

Molecular and cellular endocrinology emerged in 1974, encompassing genetic, epigenetic, biochemical, molecular endocrine, and cell regulation. Hormones, neurotransmitters, interaction with receptors, intracellular signaling, hormone-regulated genes, gene structure or endocrine functions, and multiple endocrine neoplasia were integrated into molecular endocrinology. Concepts and techniques borrowed from molecular biology significantly expanded the field [6].

Autoimmune diseases, type I diabetes mellitus, autoimmune thyroid diseases, and genetic diseases all stemmed from deficiencies of hormones, binding proteins, or steroid enzymatic biosynthesis. Hormone resistance caused by mutations in the gene for hormone receptors; resistance to insulin, thyroid hormone, androgen, and vitamin D; and glucocorticoid resistance are included in molecular endocrinology [6].

THE HUMAN GENOME

The Human Genome Project was launched in 1990, with the first "rough draft" of the genome completed in 2000, and final sequence mapping completed in 2003 [7–9]. The completed human genome and advances in molecular biology added better understanding of molecular physiology and diseases in all areas of medicine and endocrinology [5].

The 3.2 billion base pairs of DNA per haploid genome contain 22 autosomes and the X and Y sex chromosomes, coding for roughly 21,000 genes, which are transcribed into RNA, which is then translated into more than 250,000 proteins. The human genome contains 21,000 genes. Each chromosome contains many genes, the source of physical and functional units and heredity. Genes are located in specific sequences of bases that encode the transition to proteins, performers of the function of life. Interestingly, genes make up only 1.5% of DNA. The remaining DNA consists of sequences—some repetitive and most not completely understood—that are transcribed into RNA but do not make proteins. A large portion of this noncoding DNA has biochemical activity, including regulating gene expression, organizing chromosomal architecture, and controlling epigenetic inheritance.

From prediction to reality, studies of the genome have led to diagnosis and treatment of diseases.

EPIGENETIC SILENCING

Classical genetics cannot explain the entire spectrum of cancers [10]. There is no genetic explanation for how monozygotic twins with identical DNA can have different phenotypes and different susceptibilities to a disease. Epigenetic changes such as DNA methylation and histone modification can alter patterns of gene expression without changes in the underlying DNA sequence.

The best-known epigenetic inactivation (silencing) is through DNA methylation of tumor suppression genes, and plays a critical role in controlling gene activity and architecture of the nucleus. Epigenetic silencing has been observed in many cancers: breast, lung, prostate, kidney, glioma, esophagus, stomach, liver, ovaries, leukemia, and lymphoma. Unlike mutations, DNA methylation is reversible. Hypermethylated tumor suppressor genes can be reactivated with drugs. Demethylating agents, however, have not shown successful clinical antitumor activity.

MICRORNAS

MicroRNAs (miRNAs) are 19- to 23-nucleotide-long noncoding RNAs that post-transcriptionally regulate gene expression by interacting with messenger RNAs, triggering degradation or translational repression [11–14]. They are involved in nearly every physiologic process, are critical to development, and play a significant role in cancer initiation and progression.

MiRNAs have been shown to regulate gene expression in metabolically active tissues, including the endocrine pancreas, liver, and adipose tissue; their expression has been implicated in the development of the endocrine pancreas and may regulate the progression of diabetes and metabolic syndrome. In the pancreas, miR-375 has been implicated in islet cell viability and function, with perturbations of intracellular levels of miR-375 having significant effects on glucose metabolism [11,12]. In the liver, miR-122 has been shown to be critical for normal lipid metabolism [13]. Specific patterns of tumor and serum miRNA expression have been associated with different types of thyroid tumors, including anaplastic, follicular, and papillary thyroid carcinomas, with variation in the sequence of a single miRNA associated with a familiar risk for papillary thyroid carcinoma (PTC) [14].

Thus, both variation in miRNA sequence and differences in miRNA expression add molecular tools to the diagnostic, prognostic, and therapeutic armamentarium of endocrinology.

MOLECULAR ISOTOPIC IMAGING

Somatostatin is an anterior pituitary hormone and a regulatory peptide with receptors (somatostatin receptor (SSTR)) in numerous organs: the brain, thyroid, pancreas, gastrointestinal system, spleen, and kidney [15–19]. Somatostatin has a short half-life (3–4 minutes) and is susceptible to quick enzymatic degradation.

Somatostatin suppresses the secretion of hormones of numerous glands and has been used to treat diseases with hormonal hypersecretion by inhibiting adenylyl cyclase simultaneously with hormone binding.

[111]Indium-DTPA (diethylenetriamine pentaacetic acid)-octreotide and [90]Yttrium octreotide have been the most commonly used with somatostatin analog. ^{111}In-DTPA-octreotide has a high affinity to somatostatin receptor type II (SSTR2).

Carcinoid tumors show higher sensitivity when octreotide is labeled with [111]Indium compared with ^{123}I-MIBG (methyl-iodo-benzylguanidine). ^{111}In-octreotide is less sensitive in detecting pheochromocytoma (originating from the adrenal medulla or extra-adrenal) and medullary thyroid cancer.

[90]Y-octreotide is very sensitive (80%–100%) in detecting carcinoid tumors. The sensitivity for gastrinoma is 60%–90% and for insulinoma is limited to 50%, due to low affinity and small tumor size.

In the search for better nuclear medicine molecular imaging for insulinoma, exendin-4, an analog of glucagon-like peptide (GLP-1), was discovered. Exendin-4 offers the highest affinity to the radiotracers [111]Indium and [68]Gallium, and strong conjugation with abundant receptors in pancreatic β-cells.

In recent years, peptide ligands DOTA, DOTATOC, and DOTANOC have been discovered to form complexes with the following metal tracers: [111]In, ^{68}Ga, ^{64}Cu, ^{90}Y, and [177]Lu. DOTA (1,4,7,10-tetraazacyclododecane-1,4,7,10-tetraacetic acid), DOTATOC (phenylalanine replaced by tyrosine at molecule position 3), and DOTANOC (DOTA-1-NaI-octreotide) have chemical purity and high affinity to neuroendocrine tumors. The phenylalanine replacement by tyrosine at position 3 in the molecule increases hydrophilia and offers stronger conjugation with SSTR2 in somatostatin-avid tumors.

^{68}Ga-DOTA-PET, a recent introduction for clinical research use, markedly improved nuclear medicine molecular imaging, especially in neuroendocrine tumors. The sensitivity of 97% and specificity of 92% reached an accuracy up to 96%. It has been a landmark discovery in neuroendocrinology.

Several therapeutic radiopharmaceuticals have been used in small nonrandomized trials, including

[111]In-pentareotide, ^{90}Y-DOTA-lanreotide, ^{90}Y-DOTATOC, ^{177}Lu-DOTATATE, ^{90}Y-DOTANOC, ^{90}Y-DTPA-D-Glu[1]-minigastrin, ^{177}Lu-AMBA, ^{90}Y-DOTAGA-substance P, and ^{131}I-MIBG.

ENDOCRINE AND METABOLIC SURGERY

Metabolism and metabolic surgery have been ingredients of endocrinology and endocrine surgery [4,11]. The terms encompass changes in biosynthesis, enzymatic and biologic degradation, biochemical interactions, and energy storage.

The surgical interventions for endocrine disorders include modulation of hormones causing a physiologic or pathologic metabolic effect. Common disorders encompass thyrotoxicosis, hypothyroidism, goiter, pituitary and adrenal diseases, obesity, and diabetes mellitus and hyperlipidemia.

In recent years, the horizon of metabolic surgery has been expanded to integrate bariatric procedures for obesity, type II diabetes mellitus, post-gastric bypass nonpancreatogenous hyperinsulinemia, and nesidioblastosis in MEN 1 patients with diffuse multicentric insulinomas or hyperplasia/hypertrophy of the entire pancreas.

The enormities of endocrinology and metabolism have created complexities that at times make it difficult to distinguish malfunctions from diseases.

THE ENDOCRINE PATIENT

The patient expressing hormonal hypersecretion, or suspected endocrinopathy, is initially directed to an endocrinologist by the clinician. The history, clinical findings, and family background are recorded in detail. Biochemical testing starts with a basal and, if needed, stimulated hormonal hypersecretion or antigenic profile in both functioning and silent neuroendocrine neoplasia.

Traditional imaging with ultrasound, computed helical tomography, and magnetic resonance are standard noninvasive, radioactive instruments.

Before exposure of a patient to nuclear medicine procedures, it is mandatory to explain in practical terms the events, the approximate times, and the instruments to be used. The patient preparation should include information about diet, hydration, medication needed or restricted, and the rationale for these requirements. The radiation risk must be explained to the patient in writing, and that possible consequences may occur over a long time period. The distinction between diagnostic and therapeutic radiopharmaceuticals should be clarified before the consent is signed.

The final interpretation of the results should be explained by placing them into clinical context. Interference with performance of the instruments or interpretation of the results should be revealed to the patient.

Genetic testing and counseling is essential for the patient if the family heredity is known, or in young patients with an unknown family link or skipped generations.

Every patient's case is reviewed by the multidisciplinary committee, where the discussions usually reach a maximum of indications and choice of procedures.

Current instruments, surgical techniques (endoscopy, laparoscopy, and robotic), molecular biochemistry, isotopic imaging, and genetic and genomic advancements offer unique diagnostic and therapeutic outcomes.

CHANGES THAT IMPROVED OUTCOMES IN ADRENALECTOMIES

Preoperative pharmacologic vasodilatation

It is common practice to start ambulatory preoperative adrenergic blockade for 4–6 weeks, expecting expansion of the circulating blood volume [20–22]. The described oral dose is usually designed to control the blood pressure, heart rate and rhythm, sweating, and metabolic activity under conditions without stress.

Physical trauma or emotional stress will most likely cause hypertensive or arrhythmic crisis due to insufficiency of drug concentration in the ambulatory state.

Phenoxybenzamine, a long-acting ($t\frac{1}{2} = 2$–3 hours), nonselective oral α-adrenergic blocker is given orally three times a day (preferably every 6 hours) to a total dose of 40–100 mg/day. After α-adrenergic blockade, a β-blocker (metoprolol or atenolol) or calcium channel blocker (nicardipine) is added.

Plasma and erythrocyte volumes in pheochromocytoma have been proven to be within the normal range [20,21]. Preoperative attempts to create pharmacologic expansion of the circulating volume do not prevent cardiovascular intraoperative crises or hypotension after removal of pheochromocytoma [22]. The optimal time for volume restoration with isotonic crystalloid (rarely blood) is immediately after tumor removal.

Unknown duality of the adrenergic system

We strictly separated paragangliomas from adrenomedullary pheochromocytomas in the adrenergic system. Common embryologic ancestry from the neural crest, secretion of norepinephrine, and potential production of ectopic hormones are the only similarities.

Paraganglioma patients are younger, the tumors are derived from sympathetic ganglia, genetics differ completely, tumor multiplicity is 30%, malignancy is more prominent, and the association with other neoplastic syndromes is not distinguishable. As a result, the preoperative radiologic detection, molecular imaging, intraoperative dissection, and postoperative surveillance are more difficult.

Choice of adrenergic blockers

We have always used only intraoperative continuous intravenous short-acting α-1 blocker (phentolamine) and short-acting β-1 antiarrhythmic blocker (esmolol).

When phentolamine was no longer manufactured, we substituted the calcium channel blocker (nicardipine).

Long-acting adrenergic blockers are not suitable in the operating theater. They block the catecholamine receptors partially or completely, rendering them ineffective. Substitution of effective adrenergic blockers with less effective antihypertensive medications is a mistake. We have routinely stopped the long-acting adrenergic blockers the day before surgery and started intravenous short-acting blockade for 24 hours in a monitored bed.

The preoperative initiation of the continuous intravenous adrenergic blockade offers a high degree of receptor affinity and allows preparation of the appropriate concentration for controlling the intraoperative crisis.

Experience in pheochromocytoma and adrenocortical neoplasia

We, Demetrius and David Pertsemlidis, performed 245 consecutive operations (87 laparoscopic) in 225 patients with pheochromocytomas (30 paragangliomas); there was zero surgical mortality over a period of 4½ decades in a single institution.

Early on, we created programmatic canons and applied them strictly by preparing a well-organized pharmacologic environment, working with highly skilled anesthesiologists, selecting an appropriate surgical approach conforming to tumor size or anatomic location, and continuing close monitoring during immediate postsurgical recovery, until normo-volemia is restored.

One hundred fifty adrenocortical neoplasms were treated by laparoscopy or open traditional methods: Cushing's adenomas, adrenocorticotropic hormone (ACTH)-dependent hypercortisolism, adrenocortical carcinoma, aldosteronoma, nonfunctioning adrenocortical adenomas, and metastases to adrenals. R0 resection margins are essential to avoid recurrent Cushing's hypercortisolism or tumor, if there is a millimeter fraction of cortex left behind. Restoration of function in the suppressed contralateral adrenal, following unilateral adrenalectomy for Cushing's adenoma, may be as long as 6 months.

REFERENCES

1. Bayliss WM, Starling EH. The mechanism of pancreatic secretion. *J Physiol* 1902;28:323–53.
2. Pertsemlidis DS. *Pheochromocytoma: Textbook of Endocrine Surgery*. 2nd ed. Abingdon, UK: CRC Press, Taylor & Francis Group.
3. Yalow R, Berson S. Philadelphia: Chemical Heritage Foundation, 2010.
4. Becker KL, Nylen ES, Snider RH Jr. *Endocrinology and the Endocrine Patient: Principles and Practice of Endocrinology and Metabolism*. 3rd ed. Philadelphia: Lippincott Williams & Wilkins, 2002.
5. Leder P, Clayton DA, Rubenstein E, eds. *Molecular Medicine, Introduction*. New York: Scientific American, 1994.
6. Weintraub BD, ed. *Molecular Endocrinology: Basic Concepts and Clinical Correlations*. New York: Raven Press, 1994.
7. Thompson EB. The impact of genomics and proteomics on endocrinology. *Endocr Rev* 2002;23:366–8.
8. Dattani MT, Martinez-Barbera JP. The future of genomic endocrinology. *Front Endocrinol* 2011;2:1–2.
9. Collins FS, Green ED, Guttmacher AE, Guyer MS. A vision for the future of genomics research. *Nature* 2003;422:836–47.
10. Esteller M. Epigenetics in cancer. *N Engl J Med* 2008;358:1148–59.
11. Latreille M, Herrmanns K, Renwick N et al. miR-375 gene dosage in pancreatic β-cells: Implications for regulation of β-cell mass and biomarker development. *J Mol Med (Berl)* 2015;93(10):1159–69.
12. Poy MN, Eliasson L, Krutzfeldt J et al. A pancreatic islet-specific microRNA regulates insulin secretion. *Nature* 2004;432:226–30.
13. Wen J, Friedman JR. miR-122 regulates hepatic lipid metabolism and tumor suppression. *J Clin Invest* 2012;122(8):2773–6.
14. Mancikova V, Castelblanco E, Pineiro-Yanez E et al. MicroRNA deep-sequencing reveals master regulators of follicular and papillary thyroid tumors. *Mod Pathol* 2015;28:748–57.
15. Al-Nahhas A, Win Z, Szyszko T et al. Gallium-68 PET: A new frontier in receptor cancer imaging. *Anticancer Res* 2007;27:4088–94.
16. Advance Online Publication. *Nature Reviews Endocrinology*. Macmillan Publishers Limited, 2011; 106. www.nature.com/nrendon.
17. Antunes P, Ginj M, Zhang H et al. Are radiogallium-labelled DOTA-conjugated somatostatin analogues superior to those labelled with other radiometals? *Eur J Nucl Med Mol Imaging* 2007;34:982–93.
18. Poeppel TD, Binse I, Petersenn S et al. ^{68}Ga-DOTATOC versus ^{68}Ga-DOTATATE PET/CT in functional imaging of neuroendocrine tumors. *J Nucl Med* 2011;52:1864.
19. Gabriel M, Decristoforo C, Kendler D et al. PET with ^{68}Ga-DOTA-Tyr^3: Comparison of 3 imaging modalities: PET, SPECT, CT. *J Nucl Med* 2007;48;508–18.
20. Johns VJ, Brunjes S. Pheochromocytoma. *Am J Cardiol* 1962;9:120–5.
21. Sjoerdsma A, Waldman TA, Cooperman LH, Hammond WG. Pheochromocytoma: Current concepts of diagnosis and treatment; combined clinical staff conference at the National Institutes of Health. *Am Intern Med* 1996;65:1302–6.
22. Newell KA, Prinz RA, Brooks MH et al. Plasma catecholamines changes during excision of pheochromocytoma. *Surgery* 1988;104:1064–73.

Contributors

David H. Adams MD
Department of Cardiothoracic Surgery
Icahn School of Medicine at Mount Sinai
New York, New York

David C. Aron MD MS
Department of Medicine
Case Western Reserve University School of Medicine
and
Center for Quality Improvement Research
Louis Stokes Department of Veterans Affairs
Medical Center
Cleveland, Ohio

Alexandria Atuahene MD
Division of Endocrinology, Diabetes and Bone Diseases
Icahn School of Medicine at Mount Sinai
New York, New York

Yamil Castillo Beauchamp MD
Medical Pavilion
San Juan, Puerto Rico

Christopher A. Behr MD
Feinstein Institute for Medical Research
Hofstra-North Shore LIJ School of Medicine
Cohen Children's Medical Center
Manhasset, New York

Eren Berber MD
Center for Endocrine Surgery
Cleveland Clinic Lerner College of Medicine
Case Western Reserve University School of Medicine
Cleveland, Ohio

Yaniv Berger MD
Department of Investigative Medicine
Imperial College London
London, United Kingdom

Stephen R. Bloom DSc MD FMedSci FHEA FRSB FRCP FRCPath FRS
North West London Pathology Consortium
Division of Diabetes, Endocrinology and Metabolism
Imperial College London
London, United Kingdom

Angela L. Carrelli MD
Division of Endocrinology
Columbia University College of Physicians
and Surgeons
New York, New York

Sally E. Carty MD FACS
Division of Endocrine Surgery
Department of Surgery
University of Pittsburgh
Pittsburgh, Pennsylvania

Charvi A. Cassano MD
Department of Pathology
Icahn School of Medicine at Mount Sinai
New York, New York

Javier G. Castillo MD
Department of Cardiothoracic Surgery
Icahn School of Medicine at Mount Sinai
New York, New York

Terry F. Davies MB BS MD FRCP FACE
Division of Endocrinology, Diabetes and
Bone Diseases
Icahn School of Medicine at Mount Sinai
Mount Sinai Beth Israel
New York, New York

Reade De Leacy MBBS FRANZCR
Department of Radiology
Icahn School of Medicine at Mount Sinai
New York, New York

Elizabeth G. Demicco MD PhD
Department of Pathology
Icahn School of Medicine at Mount Sinai
New York, New York

Celia M. Divino MD FACS
Department of Surgery
Icahn School of Medicine at Mount Sinai
New York, New York

Stephen E. Dolgin MD FACS
Department of Pediatric Surgery
Hofstra-North Shore Long Island Jewish School of Medicine
Cohen Children's Medical Center
New Hyde Park, New York

Amish H. Doshi MD
Department of Radiology and Neurosurgery
Icahn School of Medicine at Mount Sinai
New York, New York

Stephen Farrell MBBS FRACS
St. Vincent's and Austin
Teaching Hospitals
University of Melbourne
Royal Children's Hospital
Melbourne, Australia

Raja Flores MD
Department of Thoracic Surgery
Icahn School of Medicine at Mount Sinai
New York, New York

Sander Florman MD FACS
Recanati/Miller Transplantation Institute
Mount Sinai Hospital
New York, New York

Michel Gagner MD FRCSC FACS FASMBS
Herbert Wertheim School of Medicine
Florida International University
Miami, Florida
and
Hôpital du Sacré-Cœur
Montreal, Quebec, Canada

Gillian M. Goddard MD
Division of Endocrinology
Icahn School of Medicine at Mount Sinai
New York, New York

Dani O. Gonzalez MD
Department of Surgery
Icahn School of Medicine at Mount Sinai
New York, New York

John R. Gosney MB ChB
Department of Cellular Pathology
Royal Liverpool University Hospital
Liverpool, United Kingdom

Richard S. Haber MD
Division of Endocrinology, Metabolism and Bone Diseases
Icahn School of Medicine at Mount Sinai
New York, New York

G. Kenneth Haines III MD
Department of Pathology
Icahn School of Medicine at Mount Sinai
New York, New York

Per Hellman MD
Department of Surgical Sciences
University Hospital
Uppsala, Sweden

Daniel Herron MD FACS
Department of Surgery
Icahn School of Medicine at Mount Sinai
New York, New York

O. Joe Hines MD
Department of Surgery
David Geffen School of Medicine at UCLA
Los Angeles, California

Chenchan Huang MD
Department of Radiology
Icahn School of Medicine at Mount Sinai
New York, New York

William B. Inabnet III MD FACS
Department of Surgery
Mount Sinai Beth Israel
Icahn School of Medicine at Mount Sinai
New York, New York

Leslie James BA
Department of Thoracic Surgery
The Icahn School of Medicine at Mount Sinai
New York, New York

Bernard Khoo MD
ENETS Centre for Excellence
Royal Free London NHS Foundation Trust
London, United Kingdom

Lale Kostakoglu MD MPH
Department of Radiology Nuclear Medicine
Icahn School of Medicine at Mount Sinai
New York, New York

Daniel M. Labow MD FACS
Division of Surgical Oncology
Icahn School of Medicine at Mount Sinai
New York, New York

Blandine Laferrère MD
Department of Medicine
Columbia University College of Physicians and
Surgeons
New York, New York

Cho Rok Lee MD
Department of Surgery
Yonsei University College of Medicine
Seoul, Korea

Safet Lekperic MD
Department of Radiology
Icahn School of Medicine at Mount Sinai
New York, New York

Alice C. Levine MD
Division of Endocrinology, Metabolism and
Bone Diseases
Icahn School of Medicine at Mount Sinai
New York, New York

James Y. Lim MD
Division of Surgical Oncology
Oregon Health Sciences University
Portland, Oregon

Wendy S. Liu MBBS
Department of Surgery—Head and Neck
Surgery
School of Medicine
University of Western Sydney
Campbelltown, Australia

Masha J. Livhits MD
Section of Endocrine Surgery
UCLA David Geffen School of Medicine
Los Angeles, California

Grace Lo MD
Department of Radiology
Icahn School of Medicine at Mount Sinai
New York, New York

Robert A. Lookstein MD
Department of Radiology
Icahn School of Medicine at Mount Sinai
New York, New York

Nir Lubezky MD
Recanati/Miller Transplantation Institute
Mount Sinai Hospital
New York, New York

Josef Machac MD
Department of Nuclear Medicine, Radiology
Icahn School of Medicine at Mount Sinai
New York, New York

Marcus M. Malek MD FAAP
University of Pittsburgh School of Medicine
Children's Hospital of Pittsburgh of UPMC
Pittsburgh, Pennsylvania

Spyridoula Maraka MD
Division of Endocrinology, Diabetes, Metabolism,
and Nutrition
Mayo Clinic
Rochester, Minnesota

Justin R. Mascitelli MD
Department of Neurosurgery
Icahn School of Medicine at Mount Sinai
New York, New York

Gabriele Materazzi MD
Department of Surgery
University of Pisa
Pisa, Italy

Kelly L. McCoy MD FACS
Division of Endocrine Surgery
Department of Surgery
University of Pittsburgh
Pittsburgh, Pennsylvania

James J. McGinty MD FACS
Department of Surgery
Icahn School of Medicine at Mount Sinai
Mount Sinai St. Luke's and Mount Sinai Roosevelt Hospitals
New York, New York

Paolo Miccoli MD
Department of Surgery
University of Pisa
Pisa, Italy

Richard Nakache MD
Division of General Surgery
Tel-Aviv Medical Center
Affiliated with the Sackler Faculty of Medicine
Tel-Aviv University
Tel-Aviv, Israel

Kee-Hyun Nam MD
Department of Surgery
Yonsei University College of Medicine
Seoul, Korea

Salem I. Noureldine MD
Department of Otolaryngology—Head and
Neck Surgery
Johns Hopkins University School of Medicine
Baltimore, Maryland

Kjell Öberg MD PhD
Department of Endocrine Oncology
Uppsala University Hospital
Uppsala, Sweden

Alexis K. Okoh MD
Center for Endocrine Surgery
Cleveland Clinic Lerner College of Medicine
Case Western Reserve University School of Medicine
Cleveland, Ohio

Michael Olausson MD
Department of Transplantation Surgery
Sahlgrenska University Hospital
Göteborg, Sweden

Randall P. Owen MD MS FACS
Department of Surgery
Icahn School of Medicine at Mount Sinai
New York, New York

Aman B. Patel MD
Department of Neurosurgery
Massachusetts General Hospital
Harvard Medical School
Boston, Massachusetts

Vivek V. Patil MD
Department of Interventional Radiology
Icahn School of Medicine at Mount Sinai
New York, New York

Puneet S. Pawha MD
Department of Radiology
Icahn School of Medicine at Mount Sinai
New York, New York

Nancy D. Perrier MD FACS
Department of Surgical Endocrinology
University of Texas MD Anderson Cancer Center
Houston, Texas

David S. Pertsemlidis MD FACS
Department of Surgery
Icahn School of Medicine at Mount Sinai
Morristown Medical Center
Morristown, New Jersey

Demetrius Pertsemlidis MD FACS
The Bradley H. Jack Professor of Surgery
Department of Surgery
Icahn School of Medicine at Mount Sinai
New York, New York

Susan C. Pitt MD MPHS
Brigham and Women's Hospital
Department of Surgery
Boston, Massachusetts

Kalmon D. Post MD
Departments of Neurosurgery and Medicine
Icahn School of Medicine at Mount Sinai
New York, New York

Minerva Angelica Romero Arenas MD MPH
Department of Endocrine Surgery
University of Texas
MD Anderson Cancer Center
Houston, Texas

Daniel Ruan MD
Norman Parathyroid Center
Tampa, Florida

Christopher A. Sarkiss MD resident
Department of Neurosurgery
Icahn School of Medicine at Mount Sinai
New York, New York

Mark Sawicki MD
Department of Surgery
University of California, Los Angeles
Los Angeles, California

Myron E. Schwartz MD FACS
Recanati/Miller Transplantation Institute
Mount Sinai Hospital
New York, New York

Ashok R. Shaha MD FACS
Department of Oncology—Head and
Neck Surgery
Memorial Sloan-Kettering Cancer Center
New York, New York

Daniel Shouhed MD
Department of Surgery
Cedars Sinai Medical Center
Los Angeles, California

Raj K. Shrivastava MD
Department of Neurosurgery in Otolaryngology
Icahn School of Medicine at Mount Sinai
New York, New York

Shonni J. Silverberg MD
Division of Endocrinology
Columbia University College of Physicians
and Surgeons
New York, New York

William L. Simpson Jr. MD
Department of Radiology
Icahn School of Medicine at Mount Sinai
New York, New York

Peter Stålberg MD
Department of Surgical Sciences
University Hospital
Uppsala, Sweden

Alexander Stark MD
Department of Surgery
David Geffen School of Medicine at UCLA
Los Angeles, California

Ashley Stewart MD
University of Texas MD Anderson Cancer Center
Houston, Texas

Constantine A. Stratakis MD D(med)Sci
Section on Endocrinology and Genetics
Program on Developmental Endocrinology
and Genetics
Eunice Kennedy Shriver National Institute of Child
Health and Human Development
National Institutes of Health
Bethesda, Maryland

Arnold H. Szporn MD
Department of Pathology
Icahn School of Medicine at Mount Sinai
New York, New York

Parissa Tabrizian MD
Recanati/Miller Transplantation Institute
Mount Sinai Hospital
New York, New York

Tricia Tan MD
Department of Investigative Medicine
Division of Diabetes, Endocrinology and
Metabolism
Imperial College
London, United Kingdom

Ralph P. Tufano MD MBA FACS
Department of Otolaryngology—Head and Neck
Surgery
Johns Hopkins University School of Medicine
Baltimore, Maryland

Daniel M. Tuvin MD
Division of Surgical Oncology
Icahn School of Medicine at Mount Sinai
New York, New York

Adrian Vella MD
Division of Endocrinology, Diabetes, Metabolism,
and Nutrition
Mayo Clinic
Rochester, Minnesota

James P. Villamere MD FRCSC
Department of Surgery
Icahn School of Medicine at Mount Sinai
Mount Sinai St. Luke's and Mount Sinai Roosevelt
Hospitals
New York, New York

Bo Wängberg MD
Department of Surgery
Sahlgrenska University Hospital
Göteborg, Sweden

Richard R.P. Warner MD
Division of Gastrointestinal Surgery
Center for Carcinoid and Neuroendocrine Tumors
Icahn School of Medicine at Mount Sinai
New York, New York

Eric J. Wilck MD
Department of Radiology
Icahn School of Medicine at Mount Sinai
New York, New York

Andrea Wolf MD
Department of Thoracic Surgery
Icahn School of Medicine at Mount Sinai
New York, New York

Michael W. Yeh MD FACS
Section of Endocrine Surgery
UCLA David Geffen School of Medicine
Los Angeles, California

Linwah Yip MD
Department of Surgery
University of Pittsburgh
Pittsburgh, Pennsylvania

Hongfa Zhu MD
Department of Pathology
Icahn School of Medicine at Mount Sinai
New York, New York

Mihail Zilbermint MD
Department of Pediatric Endocrinology and Genetics
National Institutes of Health
Bethesda, Maryland

and

Division of Endocrinology, Diabetes, and Metabolism
Johns Hopkins University School of Medicine
Baltimore, Maryland

Pituitary Gland

Selective sampling of petrosal veins

JUSTIN R. MASCITELLI AND AMAN B. PATEL

INTRODUCTIONS AND RATIONALE

Cushing's syndrome (CS) describes the signs and symptoms that are secondary to persistent hypercortisolemia, including stigmata of hypertension, diabetes, truncal obesity, osteopenia, bruising, abdominal striae, moon facies, generalized malaise, fatigue, and emotional lability. Cushing's disease (CD) is restricted to hypercortisolemia secondary to an adrenocorticotropic hormone (ACTH)-secreting pituitary adenoma. CD accounts for approximately 70% of adult cases of CS [1]. The prompt identification and treatment of CD is paramount since CD left untreated can carry a high morbidity and mortality. Untreated CD has a 5-year survival rate of only 50% [2].

The differentiation of CD from CS secondary to an ectopic ACTH-producing tumor generally relies on a number of different biochemical tests, especially when MRI does not definitively demonstrate a pituitary adenoma as the cause. The three most commonly used tests to diagnose hypercortisolism are urinary free cortisol (UFC), low-dose dexamethasone suppression tests (DSTs), and midnight serum cortisol or late-night salivary cortisol, but these tests carry variable sensitivity and specificity. Tests to further differentiate CD and CS include serum ACTH, high-dose DST, corticotropin-releasing hormone (CRH) or desmopressin stimulation testing, and MRI of the brain [3]. The high-dose DST has been reported to have a sensitivity of only 80% [4]. MRI has been reported to have a false-negative rate of up to 50% [5]. This accuracy may be improved by using techniques such as dynamic contrast spin echo (DC-SE) and volume-interpolated three-dimensional spoiled gradient echo (VI-SGE) MR sequences [6], as well as 3 T MRI [7].

Inferior petrosal sinus sampling (IPSS) was first reported in 1981 to differentiate CD and CS due to an ectopic ACTH-producing tumor [8]. IPSS with CRH stimulation is currently considered to be the gold standard in diagnosing CD when all other methods have failed, with sensitivity and specificity rates in the range of 96% and 100%, respectively [9]. Although IPSS was traditionally advocated for all cases with negative imaging [10], it is currently considered in selected cases with hypercortisolemia when both laboratory and radiographic tests fail to make the diagnosis with a high degree of certainty or in cases of persistent hypercortisolemia after hypophysectomy if not previously performed [11,12]. In these cases, a preoperative positive MRI scan may have represented a nonsecreting pituitary adenoma.

The rationale for IPSS is that a large proportion of the venous drainage of the pituitary gland is via the IPSs, allowing for analysis of blood samples uncontaminated from other sources. Therefore, in CD the concentration of ACTH is expected to be higher in the IPS draining the hemihypophysis bearing the tumor than in the contralateral IPS or in the peripheral blood [10,13]. CRH is released from the paraventricular nucleus of the hypothalamus into the hypophyseal portal system and stimulates the release of ACTH from the anterior pituitary. CRH stimulation has long been known to increase sensitivity and specificity of IPSS [10].

ANATOMY AND SAMPLING TECHNIQUE

Venous sampling must be obtained from a source that represents the venous drainage of the pituitary gland. The venous drainage of the pituitary gland is via the cavernous sinus. The cavernous sinus then usually drains into the IPSs, superior petrosal sinuses (SPSs), and basilar venous plexus. These all have variable drainage courses into the internal jugular vein (IJV) and paraspinal venous plexus. There are as many as four intercavernous venous connections (the largest of which is the basilar plexus located along the dorsum sellae). Despite these connections, pituitary venous drainage is unilateral under normal circumstances [14,15]. Therefore, bilateral simultaneous sampling is required to evaluate the side of possible pituitary microadenoma. The IPSs are usually the best sites to obtain venous samples from, since they usually capture a large portion of the cavernous sinus drainage from their respective side.

It is important to ensure that the patient is hypercortisolemic at the time of IPSS; otherwise, the test may yield a false-negative result. Midnight salivary cortisol the night before the procedure [16] and 24-hour urinary cortisol the day before (our protocol), and same-day analysis of the samples, offer assurance.

Anticoagulation

Venous thrombosis of the IPS, cavernous sinus, basilar venous plexus, or IJV is an undesired event that can potentially have severe consequences. Therefore, systemic anticoagulation is maintained during the procedure [10] with a bolus of 4000 units of intravenous heparin followed by 1000 units intravenously every hour thereafter. Alternatively, the dosage of heparin can be titrated to maintain an activated clotting time (ACT) of greater than 200. At the minimum, the catheters will be in place for 30 minutes, and in cases of difficult catheterization, it is not unusual to have a catheter in place for a longer period of time.

Jugular vein catheterization

Bilateral venous access is established by the standard transfemoral approach. On one side, a 5 French (Fr.) sheath is placed, so that concomitant peripheral venous sampling can be obtained during the procedure. A 4 Fr. sheath is placed into the contralateral femoral vein. The IJVs and, subsequently, the IPSs are catheterized with 4 Fr. catheters. The catheter used should have a 20°–30° angled tip, followed by a 2 cm straight segment. Occasionally, a different angle or shape may be necessary depending upon the specific anatomy. When sampling, each side should be accessed with the respective IPS to match sampling sides and catheters [10].

On the left, the junction of the innominate vein and the superior vena cava (SVC) is relatively large. Once the catheter is aimed in the correct direction, a hydrophilic-coated guidewire should allow easy passage from the SVC to the left subclavian vein. Catheterization of the left IJV can be challenging, usually because of a valve located at the thoracic inlet. Getting the wire to enter the IJV is usually a matter of chance with repetitive prodding during various phases of respiration. A forceful contrast injection into the subclavian vein will often show the location of various inflow veins as

stumps, due to the venous valve system, which can then be used as guides.

Accessing the right IJV is usually more straightforward than the left, as the course is relatively straight. There can be variations that make the catheterization more difficult, but access can usually be achieved with a small amount of searching. The valve is usually not as much of a problem on the left.

Inferior petrosal sinus catheterization

The venous drainage of the skull base is variable [17], making entry of the IPSs into the jugular system more difficult to find. In fact, advancing the catheter into the IPS is often the most challenging aspect of the procedure. The most common site of IPS entrance is at the apex of the jugular/sigmoid sinus curve and is typically located anterior and medial. Careful probing with a hydrophilic guidewire aimed in the appropriate direction will allow one to the find the IPS. Occasionally, a contrast injection will be needed to identify the location of the IPS. Once the guidewire is positioned in the IPS, the catheter can be passed into the distal aspect of the IPS. Once the catheter is within the IPS, anteroposterior (AP) and lateral venograms are performed to confirm the position and to assess the venous drainage. With good positioning, retrograde filling of both cavernous sinuses, the contralateral IPS and basilar venous plexus, is commonly seen (Figures 1.1 and 1.2). Occasionally, the IPS will be too small for a 4 Fr. catheter, in which case a microcatheter and microwire can be used.

Normal AP

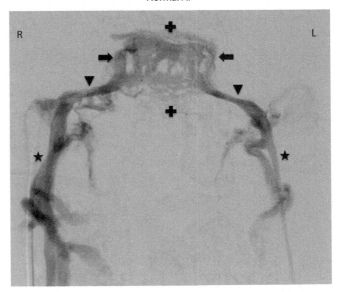

Figure 1.1 Right IPS injection, AP view. Normal symmetric IPSs. Note that the right-sided injection opacifies the bilateral IPSs (arrowheads), the bilateral cavernous sinuses (arrows), the intercavernous sinus (plus signs), and the bilateral IJVs (stars). The catheter is well positioned in the right IPS (arrowhead). Note that the IPS arises medially from the IJV.

Normal lateral

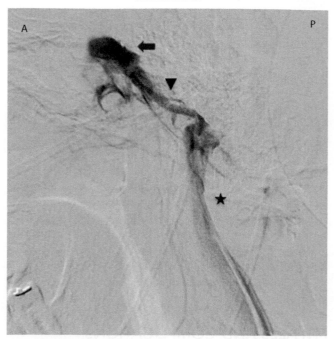

Figure 1.2 Right IPS injection, lateral view. Lateral venogram in the same patient as shown in Figure 1.1. The cavernous sinus (arrow), IPS (arrowhead), and IJV (star) can be seen well. Note that the IPS arises anteriorly from the IJV.

Plexiform IPS

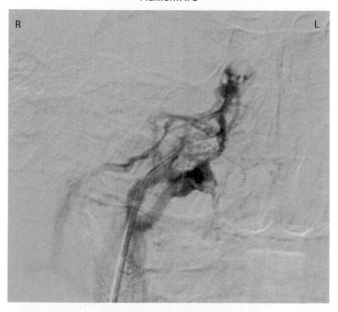

Figure 1.3 Right IPS plexus injection, AP view. This injection reveals a plexus of veins representing the right IJV, which could make catheterization difficult and decrease the accuracy of the test. Options include sampling from the right IJV or attempting to place a microcatheter into one of the smaller plexiform veins. There is risk of obtaining a false-negative result.

There are some variable anatomical patterns to consider. Small venous channels originating in the cerebellopontomedullary angle can infrequently drain into the IPS. Additionally, small bridging veins can also be found connecting the IPS with the transverse pontine vein, the vein of the pontomedullary sulcus, or the lateral medullary vein near the jugular bulb [18]. The anterior condylar vein is an important tributary vein that can dilute the sample if the catheter is not positioned distal to its junction with the IPS [19]. Occasionally, the IPS drains into the IJV as a plexus of veins, leading to difficult catheterization and reduced accuracy of the test (Figure 1.3). Even less commonly, the IPS drains directly into the vertebral venous plexus and does not connect to the IJV, which could potentially lead to false-negative results [9]. There also may be an absent IJV (Figure 1.4) that precludes lateralization. In addition, it is possible to have an abnormally located junction between the IPS and the IJV (Figure 1.5) that, if not appreciated, may make catheterization of the IPS difficult and possibly even dangerous due to repetitive unsuccessful attempts via the normal anatomic configuration.

Anomalous venous anatomy can make catheterization of the IPS difficult for even the most skilled practitioners. If difficulty is encountered, the interventionalist should suspect a duplicated IJV or anomalous drainage of the IPS. In these circumstances, venography of the other IPS would invariably fill across the midline, clearly demonstrating the contralateral IPS. It is then possible to locate the exact entry point of the IPS into the opposite IJV. In the most difficult cases,

No IJV

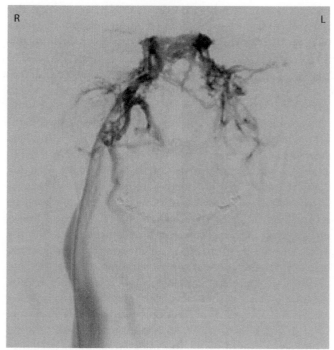

Figure 1.4 Right IPS injection, AP view. This injection reveals complete absence of the left IJV after many attempts at catheterization on the left. Although testing can be performed from the right IPS and compared with peripheral blood, this variant precludes tumor lateralization.

Abnormal IPS-IJV junction

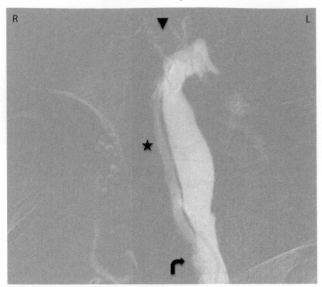

Figure 1.5 Left IJV injection, oblique view. This injection reveals that the IPS (arrowhead) enters the IJV in the mid-cervical region (curved arrow), which is a rare variant of this anatomy. There is a small vein (star) that lies anterior and slightly medial to the IJV that connects the IPS to the IJV. If this variable anatomy is not appreciated, catheterization of the IPS will be impossible and potentially dangerous due to persistent attempts to catheterize via the normal anatomic configuration.

it is necessary to catheterize the arterial system, select the internal carotid artery, and perform a standard angiogram to locate the cavernous sinuses and visualize their drainage.

Venous sampling procedure

After the catheters are in position bilaterally, baseline samples are taken from each IPS catheter and the peripheral 5 Fr. sheath simultaneously. One must take care to place samples in the appropriate specimen tubes. For ACTH analysis, samples are placed in the same tubes used for complete blood counts (usually "lavender top") and kept on ice. Prolactin and growth hormone samples are placed in serum chemistry (usually "red top") tubes. These are guidelines, and for each institution, prior contact with the appropriate laboratory should be made for confirmation of these instructions and coordination of handling.

After the baseline samples are collected, challenge or stimulation testing should be performed. This is most commonly performed for the workup of CS. For ACTH testing, CRH or Acthrel (ovine CRH) is administered in a 1 µg/kg (up to a maximum of 100 µg) intravenous bolus peripherally. After administration, samples are obtained simultaneously from IPSs and peripheral blood at 2, 5, 10, and 15 minutes. These samples are then placed in the appropriate tubes, labeled, placed on ice, and then sent to the laboratory for the appropriate analysis.

After the samples have been obtained, the IPS catheters are removed, heparin is reversed using protamine, and the sheaths are withdrawn. Pressure is applied to the femoral veins for approximately 10 minutes or until hemostasis is obtained. The patient is then observed for 2 hours with the head of the bed flat and then discharged.

A ratio between IPS and peripheral ACTH concentrations of 2:1 or greater at baseline or 3:1 after administration of CRH has been classically considered a positive test and indicative of CD. In addition, a ratio of 1.4:1 or greater in the detected ACTH concentration of one IPS versus the other can suggest the laterality of the tumor [10]. It has been reported that prolactin measurement during IPSS can improve the accuracy of IPSS [20]. A baseline ratio of prolactin IPS to peripheral of 1.8 or more suggests successful catheterization of the IPS. In addition, ratios of prolactin-normalized ACTH IPS to peripheral can then be used to differentiate between a pituitary and ectopic source of ACTH. Prolactin measurement has not been used at our institution.

PITFALLS AND COMPLICATIONS

Pitfalls

The false-negative rate has been reported as 1%–10% [9]. Doppman et al. reviewed the venograms of patients in a large series of surgically proven CD and negative MRI and found that all patients with false-negative results had either hypoplastic or plexiform IPS ipsilateral to the adenoma [21]. Another explanation for a false-negative result is a potential additional drainage through the portal sinuses, ascending through the pituitary stalk into the hypothalamus. Sampling errors may also occur secondary to dilution of pituitary blood from nonpituitary sources secondary to extensive anastomoses between the IPS and the basilar venous plexus, retrograde drainage of the SPSs, or misplaced catheters [22]. Presampling visualization of anatomical variants may give an indication of the possibility of a false-negative result. However, even when venograms show correct position of the catheter, there is no definitive proof of correct sampling of pituitary blood from both IPSs.

Additionally, the ability for IPSS to lateralize the tumor is not as good as its ability to identify the pituitary as the overall source of hypercortisolemia. A recent analysis of more than 500 patients found IPSS to have a positive predictive value of 69% in its ability to lateralize the tumor [23]. Asymmetric IPSs or the complete absence of one IPS can confuse or preclude lateralization.

The high frequency of incidentalomas raises the questions of the reliability of an abnormal MRI to confirm CD [24]. If transphenoidal surgery is performed based upon the endocrine data and an abnormal MRI and an ACTH-staining tumor is not found, we also then perform IPSS, if not previously performed.

Complications

IPSS is a safe and reliable procedure, but it is nonetheless an invasive test and should be used with caution. Although extremely rare, brainstem vascular damage and transient or permanent neurological deficit can occur [25–28]. In most cases, however, IPSS causes only minor complications, such as groin hematomas, vasovagal reaction, or transient ear discomfort. Due to vascular fragility and hypercoagulability of patients with CS, heparin should be given to prevent thrombotic events. Injury to the vascular wall with subsequent thrombosis is the presumed cause of venous thromboembolism after IPSS [29,30]. Although severe adverse events are rare, IPSS should be performed only in specialized referral centers, where safety of the procedure is a high standard. IPSS is acceptable when imaging fails to demonstrate a well-defined lesion or when biochemical or clinical findings are inconsistent with CD [11].

The Mount Sinai Hospital experience

At Mount Sinai Hospital, from 2001 to 2007, the major complication rate was reported to be 1 in 44 (2.3%) [27]. This patient sustained a brainstem stroke from the procedure. From 2007 to 2014, 76 additional IPSS procedures were performed and there were no additional major complications. Therefore, the major complication rate at Mount Sinai from 2001 to 2014 was 1 in 120 (0.8%). Additionally, at Mount Sinai, from 1987 to 2005, the false-negative rate was reported to be 2 in 105 (1.9%) and there were no false positives (0%) [11]. Furthermore, in the 1987–2005 cohort, lateralization was only possible in 66% of patients.

CONCLUSIONS

Bilateral IPSS with CRH stimulation is the procedure of choice in confirming the diagnosis of CD. It should be considered in cases when the laboratory tests are discordant with MRI of the brain or when a patient remains hypercortisolemic following transphenoidal surgery. IPSS is safe and accurate, but it is important to remember that rare and serious complications such as brainstem strokes can occur.

ACKNOWLEDGMENT

We would like to acknowledge the previous authors of this chapter including Scott Meyer, Dave Johnson, and Chirag Gandhi.

REFERENCES

1. Nieman LK, Ilias I. Evaluation and treatment of Cushing's syndrome. *Am J Med* 2005;118(12):1340–6.
2. Clayton RN et al. Mortality and morbidity in Cushing's disease over 50 years in Stoke-on-Trent, UK: Audit and meta-analysis of literature. *J Clin Endocrinol Metab* 2011;96(3):632–42.
3. Vilar L et al. Pitfalls in the diagnosis of Cushing's syndrome. *Arq Bras Endocrinol Metabol* 2007;51(8):1207.
4. Meier CA, Biller BM. Clinical and biochemical evaluation of Cushing's syndrome. *Endocrinol Metab Clin North Am* 1997;26:741–62.
5. Tabarin A et al. Comparative evaluation of conventional and dynamic magnetic resonance imaging of the pituitary gland for the diagnosis of Cushing's disease. *Clin Endocrinol (Oxf)* 1998;49(3):293–300.
6. Kasaliwal R et al. Volume interpolated 3D-spoiled gradient echo sequence is better than dynamic contrast spin echo sequence for MRI detection of corticotropin secreting pituitary microadenomas. *Clin Endocrinol (Oxf)* 2013;78(6):825–30.
7. Erickson D et al. 3 Tesla magnetic resonance imaging with and without corticotropin releasing hormone stimulation for the detection of microadenomas in Cushing's syndrome. *Clin Endocrinol (Oxf)* 2010;72(6):793–9.
8. Findling JW et al. Selective venous sampling for ACTH in Cushing's syndrome: Differentiation between Cushing disease and the ectopic ACTH syndrome. *Ann Intern Med* 1981;94(5):647–52.
9. Deipolyi AR, Hirsch JA, Oklu R. Bilateral inferior petrosal sinus sampling. *Neurointerv Surg* 2012;4(3):215–8.
10. Oldfield EH et al. Petrosal sinus sampling with and without corticotropin-releasing hormone for the differential diagnosis of Cushing's syndrome. *N Engl J Med* 1991;325(13):897–905.
11. Jehle S et al. Selective use of bilateral inferior petrosal sinus sampling in patients with adrenocorticotropin-dependent Cushing's syndrome prior to transsphenoidal surgery. *J Clin Endocrinol Metab* 2008;93(12):4624–32.
12. Tomycz ND, Horowitz MB. Inferior petrosal sinus sampling in the diagnosis of sellar neuropathology. *Neurosurg Clin N Am* 2009;20(3):361–7.
13. Corrigan DF et al. Selective venous sampling to differentiate ectopic ACTH secretion from pituitary Cushing's syndrome. *N Engl J Med* 1977;296(15):861–2.
14. Doppman JL et al. Petrosal sinus sampling for Cushing syndrome: Anatomical and technical considerations. Work in progress. *Radiology* 1984;150(1):99–103.
15. Aquini MG, Marrone AC, Schneider FL. Intercavernous venous communications in the human skull base. *Skull Base Surg* 1994;4:145.
16. Deipolyi AR, Alexander B, Rho J, Hirsch JA, Oklu R. Bilateral inferior petrosal sinus sampling using desmopressin or corticotropic-releasing hormone: A single-center experience. *J Neurointerv Surg* 2015;7:690–3.
17. Huang YP, Wolf BS, Antin SP, Okudera T. The veins of the posterior fossa—Anterior or petrosal draining group. *Am J Roentgenol Radium Ther Nucl Med* 1968;104:36–56.

18. Matsushima T, Rhoton AL Jr, de Oliveira E, Peace D. Microsurgical anatomy of the veins of the posterior fossa. *J Neurosurg* 1983;59:63–105.

19. Miller DL, Doppman JL. Petrosal sinus sampling: Technique and rationale. *Radiology* 1991;178(37):e47.

20. Sharma ST, Nieman LK. Is prolactin measurement of value during inferior petrosal sinus sampling in patients with adrenocorticotropic hormone-dependent Cushing's syndrome? *J Endocrinol Invest* 2013;36(11):1112–6.

21. Doppman JL et al. The hypoplastic inferior petrosal sinus: A potential source of false-negative results in petrosal sampling for Cushing's disease. *J Clin Endocrinol Metab* 1999;84(2):533–40.

22. Doppman JL et al. Basilar venous plexus of the posterior fossa: A potential source of error in petrosal sinus sampling. *Radiology* 1985;155(2):375–8.

23. Wind JJ et al. The lateralization accuracy of inferior petrosal sinus sampling in 501 patients with Cushing's disease. *J Clin Endocrinol Metab* 2013;98(6):2285–93.

24. Freda PU et al. Pituitary incidentaloma: An endocrine society clinical practice guideline. *J Clin Endocrinol Metab* 2011;96(4):894–904.

25. Lefournier V et al. One transient neurological complication (sixth nerve palsy) in 166 consecutive inferior petrosal sinus samplings for the etiological diagnosis of Cushing's syndrome. *J Clin Endocrinol Metab* 1999;84(9):3401–2.

26. Bonelli FS et al. Venous subarachnoid hemorrhage after inferior petrosal sinus sampling for adrenocorticotropic hormone. *AJNR Am J Neuroradiol* 1999;20(2):306–7.

27. Gandhi CD, et al. Neurologic complications of inferior petrosal sinus sampling. *AJNR Am J Neuroradiol* 2008;29(4):760–5.

28. Sturrock ND, Jeffcoate WJ. A neurological complication of inferior petrosal sinus sampling during investigation for Cushing's disease: A case report. *J Neurol Neurosurg Psychiatry* 1997;62(5):527–8.

29. Díez JJ, Iglesias P. Complications of inferior petrosal sinus sampling for the etiological diagnosis of Cushing's syndrome. *J Endocrinol Invest* 2002;25(2):195–6.

30. Obuobie K et al. Venous thrombo-embolism following inferior petrosal sinus sampling in Cushing's disease. *J Endocrinol Invest* 2000;23(8):542–4.

Pituitary tumors and their management

CHRISTOPHER A. SARKISS, RAJ K. SHRIVASTAVA, AND KALMON D. POST

INTRODUCTION TO THE HYPOTHALAMIC–PITUITARY UNIT

The anterior pituitary gland is under predominantly stimulatory control by the hypothalamus. The function of the normal pituitary gland depends on the integrity of the hypothalamus, the portal circulation, and the pituitary stalk. Portal vessels originate in a capillary bed in the median eminence and extend through long portal vessels into the pituitary stalk and to the adenohypophysis. The pituitary hormones adrenocorticotropic hormone (ACTH), growth hormone (GH), prolactin, thyroid-stimulating hormone (TSH), luteinizing hormone (LH), and follicle-stimulating hormone (FSH) are controlled by the hypothalamic hormones corticotropin-releasing factor (CRF), dopamine (aka prolactin inhibitory factor [PIF]), thyroid-releasing hormone (TRH), and gonadotropin-releasing hormone (Gn-RH), respectively. This is efficiently accomplished via a portal vascular system connecting the hypothalamus with the anterior pituitary gland. These hypothalamic releasing factors are then under negative feedback control from the end-organ products, i.e., adrenal gland products, thyroid hormone, etc., thereby completing the axis loop [1]. The predominant net hypothalamic regulatory influence is stimulatory for all pituitary hormones except prolactin, which is under dominant inhibitory control [2]. Any interruption or compression of the network of portal vessels as a result of pressure or invasion by any perisellar mass can alter the delivery of these hypothalamic factors to the anterior pituitary and cause impairment in its function.

The anterior pituitary gland is responsible for the secretion and regulation of a variety of peptide hormones and regulating factors. Tumors originating in the anterior pituitary gland may therefore produce excess quantities of a particular peptide hormone. Pituitary adenomas are benign monoclonal tumors that arise from the cells comprising the anterior pituitary gland. They account for approximately 15% of all intracranial tumors. When a pituitary adenoma secretes one or more hormones, the resulting adenoma is classified as a functioning or secretory adenoma. Tumors without hormonal activity are logically classified as nonfunctioning or nonsecretory adenomas. In this chapter, we briefly review the different types of functioning pituitary tumors. To this end, we first review the hypothalamic–pituitary organ axis to help understand the diagnosis and treatment of patients with functioning pituitary tumors.

Anterior pituitary gland adenomas are identified pathologically both by their *in vivo* endocrine activity and by their *in vitro* immunohistochemical staining characteristics. The advent of immunohistochemical staining for the various peptide hormones has revealed the fact that many adenomas once thought to be nonsecretory actually secrete endocrinologically inactive peptides [3]. The alpha-subunit, which has no known systemic effects, is one of the commonly found peptides.

Adenomas may be further subdivided into micro- or macroadenomas based upon size [4] (Figure 2.1). Tumors less than 1 cm in diamter are considered microadenomas and are predictably located solely within the sella turcica. They characteristically do not invade neighboring structures such as the sphenoid and cavernous sinuses. Macroadenomas, by definition greater than 1 cm, typically enlarge the sella turcica and frequently invade neighboring structures (Figure 2.2). Microadenomas usually are discovered either incidentally or because of an endocrinopathy,

whereas macroadenomas present with compressive effects of the tumor, i.e., bitemporal hemianopsia, as well as endocrinopathy. The endocrinopathy may be one of either oversecretion or undersecretion.

The evaluation of a patient with a suspected functioning pituitary tumor will be discussed in relation to each tumor type; however, because of the protean and often subtle manifestations of these endocrinopathies, a detailed history and physical examination are mandatory in guiding the rest of the workup. Subtle changes in hair growth, skin texture or color, and body mass may be the only heralds of early endocrine dysfunction. MRI technology has dramatically changed the radiographic evaluation of pituitary adenomas. MRI with and without gadolinium enhancement is now considered the study of choice in evaluating patients with suspected pituitary abnormalities [5–8]. The normal pituitary gland will enhance within 5 minutes of contrast

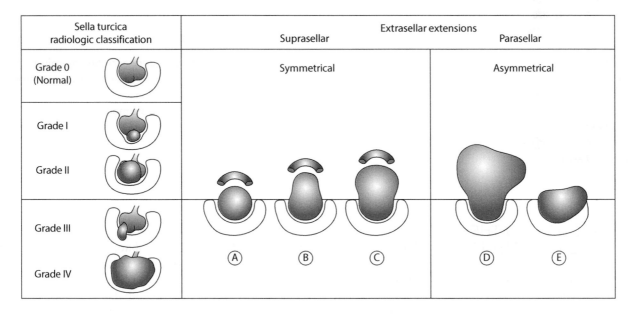

Figure 2.1 Radiograpic/imaging classfication of pituitary adenomas. Grades I and II are enclosed adenomas. Grades III and IV are invasive adenomas. Extensions A, B, C are directly suprasellar, while D is asymmetric intracranial and E is asymmetric into the cavernous sinus. (Adapted from Post K, Shrivastava R. Functioning pituitary tumors. In: Rengachary S, Ellenbogen R, eds., *Principles of Neurosurgery*. New York: Elsevier Mosby, 2005:603–20.)

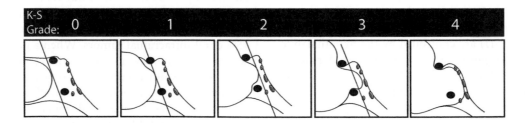

Figure 2.2 Knosp-Steiner classification scheme: Grade 0, no invasion, the lesion does not reach the medical aspect of the CCA; Grade 1, invasion extending to, but not past, the intercarotid line; Grade 2, invassion extending to, but not past, the lateral aspect of the CCA; Grade 3, invasion past the lateral aspect of the CCA but not completely filling the CS; and Grade 4, completely filling the CS both medial and lateral to the CCA. (Adapted with permission from Lippincott Williams and Wilkins/Wolters Kluwer Health: *Neurosurgery*. Knosp et al.: Pituitary adenomas with invasion of the cavernous sinus space: a magnetic resonance imaging classification compared with surgical findings. *Neurosurgery* 33(4):610–618, copyright 1993.)

administration, leaving the adenoma hypointense compared with the surrounding pituitary (Figures 2.3 through 2.5). If the study is performed more than 5 minutes after contrast administration, the tumor will appear enhanced while the normal gland will appear unenhanced. It is therefore necessary that the neuroradiologist indicate the timing of the study in relation to contrast enhancement. Findings on high-resolution MRI studies are highly sensitive, with a 60%–70% sensitivity on unenhanced studies and increasing by 10% on postcontrast studies. CT scans are helpful in evaluating bony changes in the sella and surrounding structures, but they are much less sensitive than MRI in detecting small adenomas [9–12]. All patients with pituitary adenomas ought to undergo detailed visual field testing; however, this is most important in those patients with macroadenomas.

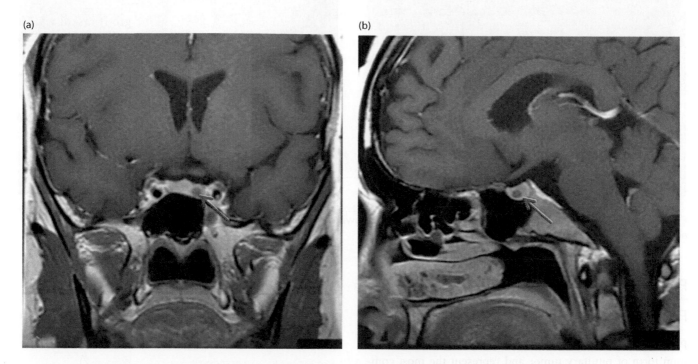

Figure 2.3 Coronal **(a)** and sagittal **(b)** post contrast MRI showing a non-functioning microadenoma.

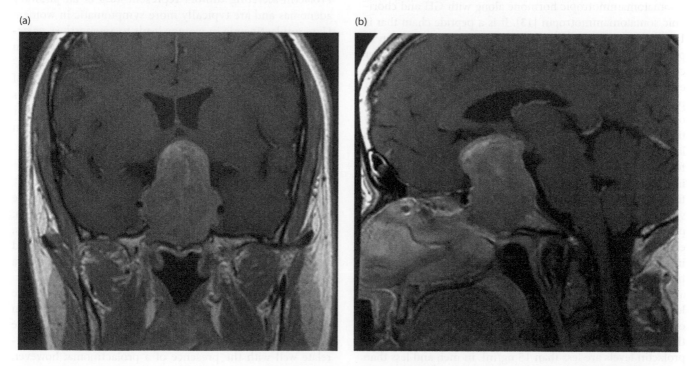

Figure 2.4 Coronal **(a)** and sagittal **(b)** post contrast MRI showing a large sellar–suprasellar non-functioning pituitary adenoma that is abutting both the right and left cavernous sinus.

(a)

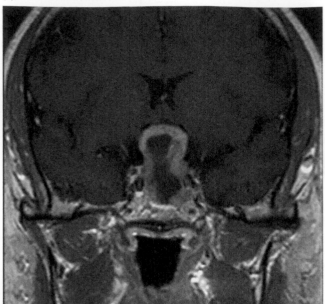

(b)

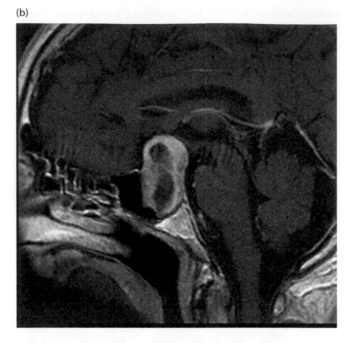

Figure 2.5 Coronal **(a)** and sagittal **(b)** post contrast MRI showing a large sellar–suprasellar non-functioning pituitary adenoma that has a solid and cystic portion.

PITUITARY TUMORS AND NEUROSURGERY

Prolactin-secreting adenomas

Prolactin-secreting pituitary adenomas are the most common form of pituitary tumor and represent the most common cause of hyperprolactinemia. Prolactin is classified as a somatomammotropic hormone along with GH and chorionic somatomammotropin [13]. It is a peptide chain that is 198 amino acids long, necessary for the normal lactation in postpartum women. Prolactin levels begin to rise shortly after conception and reach levels of 150–200 ng/mL at term; however, it is not until the postpartum decline in estrogen is complete that lactation may occur. Stimulation of tactile receptors on the nipple and areola of the breast leads to prolactin secretion that in the postpartum estrogen-primed breast results in lactation. Hyperprolactinemia disrupts normal reproductive function by altering the pulsatile gonadotropin secretion, interfering with sex steroid feedback at the level of the hypothalamus, and inhibiting gonadal steroidogenesis. TRH and vasoactive intestinal peptide (VIP) both appear to have minor prolactin-releasing activity, although their significance is presently unclear. Although the above stimuli lead to increases in prolactin secretion, the overwhelming control of prolactin release is inhibitory in nature, via dopamine. Dopamine, also known as a PIF, is released by the hypothalamus and leads to a decrease in prolactin secretion. As mentioned earlier, this inhibitory control becomes vitally important in the medical management of prolactinomas [14,15]. Normal prolactin levels are less than 15 ng/mL in men and less than 20 ng/mL in nonpregnant women. Causes of hyperprolactinemia other than a pituitary adenoma include pregnancy, stress, hypoglycemia, renal failure, hypothyroidism, and phenothiazine-like medications. These, as well as several other etiologies, must be considered prior to a detailed investigation of a patient's pituitary gland [16].

SIGNS AND SYMPTOMS

Prolactin-secreting tumors represent 40% of all pituitary adenomas and are typically more symptomatic in women. Hyperprolactinemia in women leads to amenorrhea, galactorrhea, and osteoporosis, while in men it may result in diminished sexual drive and impotence, or it may be asymptomatic. The menstrual disturbances are present in 93% of premenopausal women with prolactinomas. Because of this difference, men are not usually diagnosed until the tumor has reached a size sufficient to cause compressive effects on neighboring structures [17].

DIAGNOSIS

Random measurements of the serum prolactin level are reliable to establish the diagnosis of hyperprolactinemia. In the absence of the other above-mentioned disorders, investigation of the pituitary gland is necessary. This should begin with an MRI with contrast, which often discloses a pituitary macroadenoma. Hyperprolactinemia in the presence of a macroadenoma does not mean *a priori* that the tumor is a prolactinoma. The degree of prolactin elevation is believed to be directly related to the functionality of the tumor. Serum prolactin levels greater than 250 ng/mL correlate well with the presence of a prolactinoma; however, milder elevations may be due to stalk compression leading to interference with the inhibitory effects of dopamine [18].

TREATMENT

The dopamine agonists bromocriptine and cabergoline have fundamentally changed the treatment of symptomatic prolactinomas [19–33]. Other than selected indications, dopamine agonist therapy has virtually replaced trans-sphenoidal resection as the therapy of choice. They directly stimulate the dopamine receptors located on lactotrophs (prolactin-secreting cells). Response to medical therapy can be dramatic. Prolactin levels begin to decrease in a matter of hours following the first dose, and tumor size

often diminishes within a few days. Patients with visual field deficits may begin to improve after a few days of treatment. Other than a rapidly deteriorating visual or neurological function, there are virtually no contraindications to an initial trial of dopamine agonist therapy. Follow-up with periodic serum prolactin measurements and imaging studies of the sella is necessary to ensure that therapy is effective. In approximately 66% of patients, tumor size will be reduced by as much as 75%, with the best response seen in patients with large tumors [22] (Figure 2.6). Endocrine

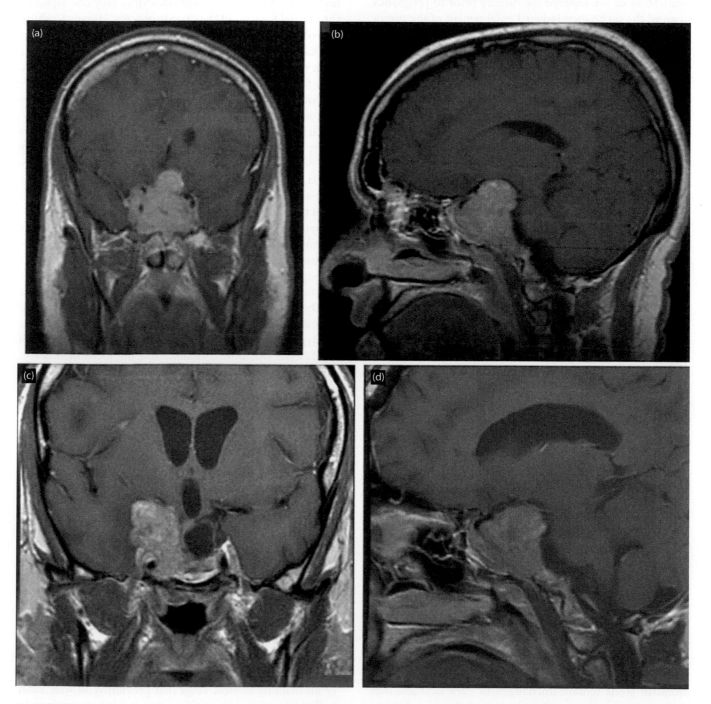

Figure 2.6 Coronal (a) and sagittal (b) post contrast MRI showing a large sellar–suprasellar prolactinoma pre medical therapy and coronal (c) and sagittal (d) post contrast MRI 3 months after initiating medical therapy with significant decrease in left side of the tumor.

functions often return to normal with establishment of cyclic menses in women and return of libido in men. Many previously infertile women have, in fact, been able to conceive while on bromocriptine therapy. The side effects, if present, usually consist of nausea, vomiting, headache, and dizziness, which do not occur as frequently with cabergoline therapy [34]. There are no known teratogenic effects from dopamine agonists, and they are therefore safe during pregnancy [35]. Women with tumors larger than 12 mm who wish to conceive either must remain on the medication or are referred for surgery prior to pregnancy to avoid the pregnancy-induced enlargement of the tumor and its secondary neurological symptoms. For women with tumors less than 12 mm, there is a less than 1% risk of neurological dysfunction [36]. A recently published systematic review has shown that cabergoline carries fewer side effects and is more effective in normalizing serum prolactin levels, thereby surpassing bromocriptine as the first choice in treatment of prolactinomas [34,37].

Since dopamine agonists are not tumoricidal, it is said that tumor re-expansion will occur when therapy is stopped [38]. There is, however, a subset of patients in which neither discontinuation of therapy nor microdosage leads to a return of symptoms [22,39]. Since there is no way of knowing which patients will have a continued need for medical therapy, it is prudent to stop therapy every few years and determine if there is a current need for treatment [40]. There now exists newer nonergot dopamine agonists, such as CV 502-205, which has shown promise in a once-daily administration.

The indications for surgery in patients with prolactinomas are for those who either are completely intolerant or show minimal response to medical therapy, as well as for patients with a severe or worsening visual field deficit. Surgery is also recommended for those patients who do not show a response after 3 months of medical therapy [41], those who desire pregnancy and prefer not to continue medication, and those on certain psychotropic medications where dopaminergic drugs are contraindicated.

The role of radiation therapy in prolactinomas is limited. Primary radiation therapy is reserved for elderly or debilitated patients who have large tumors and who are not helped by medical therapy. Radiation therapy is mostly used as an adjunctive to surgery in those patients with residual tumor who are unresponsive to medical therapy.

The role of pretreatment with bromocriptine prior to surgery to "shrink" the tumor has been suggested to increase the cure rate [42,43]. Since long-term treatment with bromocriptine has been associated with tumor fibrosis, if surgery is indicated, it is best performed within a year of therapy [44,45].

There exists a subset of patients with so-called asymptomatic microprolactinomas whose tumor size and serum prolactin levels remain unchanged or even decrease over many years in follow-up. For this population, regular surveillance without treatment may be sufficient [46,47]. It still remains to be determined whether there are any beneficial effects to normalizing prolactin levels in this population [48,49]. However, if hyperprolactinemia leads to amenorrhea, treatment is advised even if pregnancy is no longer a concern to prevent osteoporosis.

Growth hormone-secreting adenomas (acromegaly)

Acromegaly or gigantism results from the hypersecretion of GH. The term *acromegaly*, derived from the Greek *akron* (extremity) and *megale* (large), describes only one aspect of the clinical features of the disease process. Harvey Cushing is credited with relating the overproduction of GH from a pituitary source [50]. GH is a polypeptide, 191 amino acids long, normally produced and released by the somatotropic cells found in the anterior pituitary in response to hypothalamic GH-releasing factor (GRF) [51]. Somatostatin is a 14-amino acid cyclic peptide-releasing factor that inhibits GH release [52]. Three or four bursts of GH secretions occur per day, punctuating a basal state of minimal activity [53]. Sleep, physical exertion or stress, hyper- and hypoglycemia, and a variety of pharmacologic agents can also precipitate GH release. Circulating GH results in the secretion from the liver of a family of peptides called somatomedins. Somatomedin-C (insulin-like growth factor 1 [IGF-1]) is the most familiar somatomedin measured. These secondary hormones, in turn, produce a variety of anabolic effects throughout the body and mediate the effects of GH at the end-organ level. Unlike GH, the somatomedins do not exhibit significant diurnal variation in serum levels, and therefore may be a better means of evaluating patients [54].

Hypersecretion of GH can result from a number of conditions. The most common, and the focus of this section, is a pituitary adenoma. GH may also be produced by ectopic adenomas derived from remnants of the embryonic pituitary diverticulum or from tumors of the breast, lung, or ovary [55]. Acromegaly may rarely be caused be excessive production of GRF by a hypothalamic tumor or from peripheral sources, such as carcinoid tumors of the abdomen [56].

SIGNS AND SYMPTOMS

Acromegaly affects males and females equally in the fifth decade [57]. The effects of chronically elevated GH are gradual and will result in gigantism in a child whose epiphyseal plates have not yet closed or in classic acromegalic features in an adult. Typically, there is an insidious coarsening of the facial features and an increase in the soft tissues. A significant number of patients present not because of somatic disturbances, but because of local compressive effects of the pituitary tumor. The somatic changes may be so insidious as to go unnoticed until old photographs are used for comparison. Classically, patients first note an increase in shoe size or an inability to wear rings that previously fit well. Later in the disease process, patients may develop visceromegaly, arthralgias, nerve entrapment syndromes, hyperhydrosis, prognathism, and acrochordon (skin tags) (Figure 2.7).

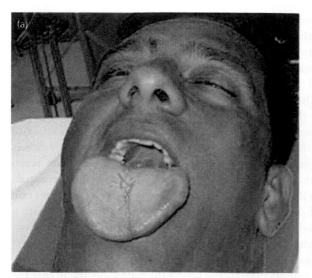
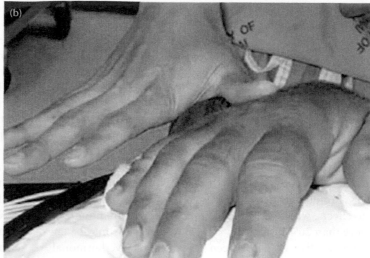

Figure 2.7 Patient demonstrating acromegalic features with soft tissue swelling causing **(a)** enlargement of the nose, macroglossia and **(b)** enlargement of hands compared to a healthy adult female hand.

The development of skin tags is interesting and deserves some comment because of its relationship to potentially malignant colonic polyps. It has been noted in several studies that as many as 46% of patients will have colonic polyps, of which more than 50% are adenomatous [58]. Some studies have also shown that the incidence of true colon carcinoma in acromegalics may be higher than in the general population. Because of this relationship, it has been recommended that acromegalic patients older than 50 years, patients with more than a 10-year history of acromegaly, or patients with more than three skin tags should have careful screening for colonic disease [59].

DIAGNOSIS

The laboratory diagnosis of acromegaly is hampered by the normally wide daily variations in serum GH levels. In fact, the daily bursts of secretion are maintained even in the presence of oversecretion of GH from an adenoma. Unlike the other secretory adenomas, static measurements of serum GH are therefore unreliable in establishing the diagnosis of acromegaly. Normal basal GH levels are generally below 1 ng/mL, with several secretory bursts seen throughout the day [60]. In acromegaly, the basal level is often elevated to levels above 5 ng/mL, although some patients may have normal basal levels with elevations only during the daily secretory burst.

Fortunately, IGF-1 (somatomedin-C) levels not only are even throughout the day, but also are consistently elevated in acromegaly. Static measurements of IGF-1 are an effective and reliable method for confirming the diagnosis of acromegaly [61,62]. Additionally, a glucose tolerance test can be performed. Normally, GH is suppressed to levels below 1 ng/mL 2 hours after an oral glucose load (75 g). Failure of this normal suppression is consistent with hypersecretion of GH. In addition, infusions of either GRF or TRH will lead to increased GH in affected individuals but not in normal subjects.

Once a patient is confirmed as having a hypersecretory state, the goal is to discover the source. The overwhelming majority of patients will have an anterior pituitary adenoma, and therefore the radiographic workup should begin with a contrast MRI. Only in the few cases where no pituitary mass is demonstrated should a search be made for ectopic sources of GH. When discovered on MRI, about 25% are microadenomas and 75% are macroadenomas. In studies done by our team, the typical latency of diagnosis can be 8 years.

TREATMENT

The effects of untreated acromegaly can eventually be fatal. Patients will develop cardiac failure, diabetes, disfigurement, and possibly blindness, leading to a markedly shortened life expectancy [63]. The goal of treatment, therefore, is the safe and rapid reduction of GH levels, elimination of any mass effect, and preservation of normal hormonal balance. The type of treatment must be judged by its ability to normalize GH levels and thereby to eliminate the development of the various metabolic derangements associated with hypersecretory states. The criteria for successful treatment of acromegaly are controversial. The accepted postoperative levels of GH that are indicative of a remission have declined in recent years. The current standard for clinical remission is a postoperative GH level of <1 ng/mL with a normal IGF-1 level [64]. GH levels may return to normal in hours or days, but it has been our experience that IGF-1 levels may take weeks or months to normalize. Also, a return to normal oral glucose tolerance test (OGTT) is required. Postoperative adjuvant therapy should be reserved for patients that do not meet these criteria.

Trans-sphenoidal resection remains the primary treatment modality for acromegaly. Successful resection results in a rapid reduction in GH levels, and can be achieved with very low morbidity and mortality, even in older patients [4,65–70]. In addition, the preservation of pituitary function has been reported to be as high as 95%, avoiding the need for lifelong hormone replacement. For larger tumors not amenable to curative resection, surgery still plays a significant role in reducing tumor load prior to any adjuvant therapy.

While trans-sphenoidal resection of pituitary adenomas is a safe and well-tolerated procedure, there are still many patients who are not surgical candidates. In those cases, medical therapy and radiotherapy have therapeutic importance. The medical treatment of acromegalics has undergone considerable change in the past 10–15 years. Medical therapy that included estrogens, chlorpromazine, and antiserotonergic agents, had met with only limited success. Bromocriptine therapy, then used for its dopaminergic effects, was able to reduce GH levels to 5–10 ng/mL in more than 20% of patients [71–75]. Cabergoline may be far more effective, as it has been shown to achieve hormonal control in 15%–40% of patients [34,76,77]. Most patients did achieve some relief of their somatic symptomatology, with reduced soft tissue swelling and decreased perspiration, even though GH levels were still elevated. The dosages necessary to achieve these effects are much higher than the dosages needed to control a prolactinoma, and the consequent incidence of side effects and drug intolerance is much higher.

Since somatostatin naturally suppresses GH production, the ideal medication would be somatostatin; however, this would require multiple administrations each day for life because of somatostain's short half-life (2 minutes). A somatostatin analogue named octreotide has a longer half-life and has been shown to be very effective [78–86]. It must be administered three times each day as a subcutaneous injection or as a continuous subcutaneous infusion. The most common side effects reported include diarrhea and cholelithiasis [87], and the incidence of these side effects increases the longer the drug is administered. Some recent studies have shown dramatic reductions in GH levels and moderate tumor shrinkage. The perioperative period may be significantly improved by using octreotide for 3–4 months preoperatively. The soft tissue changes in the tongue and throat may lessen the risks of anesthesia. Long-acting Sandostatin analogs are used now far more effectively, administered by deep intramuscular injection once each month. A long-term study spanning 9 years demonstrated that approximately 70% of patients treated with long-acting octreotide had normal IGF-1 levels and GH levels of <2.5 µg/L [88]. Moreover, a multicenter trial investigating the effect of long-acting lanreotide demonstrated a 62.9% rate of clinically significant tumor volume reduction (≥20%) with significant improvements in GH and IGF-1 levels, as well as quality of life [89]. Additionally, a study comparing pasireotide, a multi-receptor-targeted somatostatin analogue, and octreotide demonstrated greater biochemical control (GH < 2.5 µg/L and normal IGF-1) with pasireotide [90]. Recently, GH receptor antagonists such as pegvisomant (Somavert) given 15–20 mg daily have been shown to reduce production of IGF-1, with normalization of values in up to 63% of patients, with up to 90% radiographic stability or

decrease in size of tumors after treatment, thereby halting the symptoms of acromegaly. In addition, it has a high safety profile with a reported low incidence of tumor size increase, elevated liver enzymes, and injection site reactions seen [91,92].

The only other treatment option for patients is radiation therapy. Not only is this treatment fraught with difficulties, but it has not been shown to be uniformly effective [93]. Many patients will have persistently elevated GH levels for years following radiation therapy and may never reach normal levels, resulting in delayed or incomplete remission [94]. There is an approximate 60%–65% remission rate (IGF-1 normalization) with radiotherapy, combined with a 30%–35% pituitary hormone deficiency rate, and therefore, it should only be employed in postsurgical patients not tolerating medical therapy or in patients with recurrent, aggressive tumors [34,95]. The longer the follow-up, the higher the rate of recurrence and hypopituitarism.

Glycoprotein-secreting adenomas (TSH, FSH, LH)

The glycoprotein hormones produced in the mammalian pituitary gland are TSH, LH, and FSH. Although these hormones are clearly related structurally, their roles are markedly different. TSH, as its name implies, regulates the metabolic rate via thyroid hormones, while the gonadotropic hormones LH and FSH are responsible for sexual maturation and play pivotal roles in reproduction. Structurally, all three are composed of a common alpha-subunit bonded to a beta-subunit that is unique to each hormone.

A number of laboratory advances have changed our understanding of glycoprotein-secreting adenomas. Two in particular were the development of specific immunohistochemical techniques for looking at tumor specimens and the improved techniques of measuring hormone and subunit levels in vivo. It has always been taught that glycoprotein-secreting adenomas represent a very small percentage of all pituitary tumors (approximately 1%). These improved techniques are revealing that many so-called "nonfunctioning" adenomas have evidence of glycoprotein production by immunohistochemical staining and serum radioimmunoassay techniques.

SIGNS AND SYMPTOMS

Except for TSH-secreting tumors, which may present as hyperthyroidism, the glycoprotein-secreting adenomas do not produce any specific clinical syndrome. Consequentially, these adenomas are not diagnosed until they produce compressive effects with visual change or hypopituitarism. This unfortunately means that many of these tumors will grow to a size and extent that precludes any curative resection.

Hyperthyroidism caused by a TSH adenoma differs significantly from Graves' disease, for which it is very often mistaken [96,97]. The typical features of Graves' disease, including ophthalmopathy, pretibial edema, female preponderance, and serum thyroid-stimulating immunoglobin, are lacking in hyperthyroidism of pituitary origin. While these differences are not usually enough to make a clear distinction, they should raise questions as to the accuracy of the diagnosis of Graves' disease. Of note is a rare inherited disorder (autosomal dominant) designated as "selective pituitary resistance to thyroid hormone," in which the normal feedback effect of thyroid hormone upon TSH secretion is defective. This leads to TSH hypersecretion and continued production of active thyroid hormone, resulting in clinical hyperthyroidism. The TSH levels increase with TRH simulation, and this disorder is often associated with deaf–mutism, stippled epiphyses, and goiter, distinguishing it from a pituitary adenoma.

DIAGNOSIS

As mentioned above, these tumors do not typically present with symptoms of hormone hypersecretion. As a result, the determination that a pituitary tumor is secreting one of the glycoproteins is usually made after the tumor itself is discovered. Each of the hormones is composed of an alpha and beta subunit. Although the alpha-subunit is the same for all three hormones, the beta-subunit is specific to each type. We are currently only able to measure serum intact hormone levels (alpha + beta), or alpha-subunit levels alone. The measurement of beta-subunit levels is possible, but is only available in some research laboratories. We have learned that not all patients will have an elevated intact hormone level, and some may in fact have low intact hormone levels with evidence of hormone production seen on pathologic examinations [98]. Fortunately, alpha-subunit levels are elevated consistently in these tumors, decrease after successful treatment, and rise with tumor recurrence, although 22% of truly nonfunctional adenomas will have an associated alpha-subunit association [99,100]. Even with this small false-positive rate, alpha-subunit measurements serve as reliable guides to tumor therapy and recurrence. Ultrasensitive assays for TSH measurement have led to faster discoveries of hyperthyroid states with inappropriate TSH secretion, thereby lending a clue to investigate for a potential TSHoma [101].

As with all other pituitary adenomas, MRI with contrast has replaced all other imaging modalities for evaluation of tumor anatomy. Specific to glycoprotein-secreting adenomas is the tendency to be larger and involve adjacent structures more often [102]. Aside from this, there is no way to distinguish these adenomas from any other pituitary adenoma based on radiographic studies alone.

TREATMENT

The treatment of patients with glycoprotein-secreting adeomas is often difficult. Because of the delay in clinical presentation, these tumors usually have suprasellar extension and involvement of the cavernous sinuses, lowering the chances for a surgical cure. Trans-sphenoidal resection is necessary for tissue diagnosis as well as decompression of the optic chiasm. Most patients have adequate symptomatic relief postoperatively; however, surgery is very often combined with radiotherapy or adjuvant medical therapy. Since the response of the tumor to radiation has not been impressive, the indications for it remain controversial [103]. Trials with a somatostatin analogue and bromocritpine in the treatment of these tumors have met with some success, but not as much as in the treatment of acromegaly and prolactinomas, respectively [104]. At our institution, these patients are managed with trans-sphenoidal adenomectomy, followed by radiation therapy if residual tumor is seen on postoperative scans and enlarges on follow-up. If the postoperative studies suggest a "cure," they are repeated every 12 months. A recent study of 70 patients demonstrated a 75% rate of normalized thyroid function, with an approximate 60% rate of normalized pituitary imaging and hormone profile. In those patients in whom surgery was unsuccessful, radiotherapy and somatostatin analogues were used to control hyperthyroidism and tumor growth [101].

ACTH-secreting adenomas (Cushing's disease)

Cushing's syndrome was first described by Harvey Cushing in 1912. Cushing's syndrome is a condition of hypercortisolemia from any source, while the term *Cushing's disease* refers exclusively to an ACTH-secreting pituitary adenoma. Cushing's disease, more than any other pituitary tumor, remains the most diagnostically and therapeutically challenging. Hypercortisolemia can cause a myriad of clinically significant problems. In general, patients tend to feel poorly and have diffuse muscle weakness and pain, emotional lability, and profound fatigue. The presence of cortisol-induced or accelerated atherosclerosis, hypertension, diabetes, osteoporosis, obesity, susceptibility to infections, and perhaps peptic ulcer disease and thrombosis provides compelling evidence to identify the diagnosis.

The usefulness of standard radiologic imaging in Cushing's disease has been either negative or nonspecifically (thereby misleadingly) positive [105–113]. More recent advances in high-resolution 3 T MRI with contrast may change this [114,115].

Most cases of hypercortisolemia seen in the adult population are caused by microadenomas of the anterior pituitary gland [116]. Other sources that are less common include ectopic overproduction of ACTH [117,118] or corticotropin-releasing hormone (CRH) [119,120]; benign or malignant adrenal tumors; iatrogenic or exogenous hypercortisolemia; and alcoholic, depressive, or obese "pseudo-Cushing's" states. The presence of neural tissue within an adenoma and either a distinct adenoma or diffuse or nodular hyperplasia may support the concept that pituitary Cushing's disease is actually a heterogeneous disorder [112,121].

The implications of this pathological finding are important in the clinical management. Primary pituitary Cushing's (with a single adenoma) might be curable by selective adenomectomy. Hyperplasia (perhaps from central overstimulation of the pituitary) might best be treated by complete hypophysectomy or medication aimed at modulating that stimulation [122]. Intermediate-lobe Cushing's, on the other hand, may be responsive to bromocriptine or pasireotide, a medication that normally has no effect in other types of Cushing's [123].

SIGNS AND SYMPTOMS

There is a female preponderance with a median age of approximately 40 years. All patients present clinically with varying degrees of hypercortisolemia. Typically, patients will have truncal obesity, hypertension, easy bruisability, abdominal striae, and plethoric or moon facies. Because of this impressive clinical picture, patients generally present early in terms of tumor growth, making detection and identification of a source challenging (Figure 2.8).

DIAGNOSIS

The diagnosis of Cushing's disease is linked to the complex endocrine pathway involved with ACTH action. ACTH, stimulated by CRH, increases the production and secretion of cortisol from the adrenal cortex. There is a normal diurnal pattern to cortisol release, with the highest level seen in the morning and lowest seen in the evening. Cortisol negatively feeds back to reduce ACTH secretion. Circulating levels of cortisol or its urinary metabolites are used for diagnosis.

While Cushing's syndrome is easy to recognize clinically, its etiology is difficult to determine. Various diagnostic protocols have been developed; however, no main paradigm has emerged [116,117,124–137]. Measurements of midnight salivary cortisol, plasma, and urinary cortisol and its derivatives, basally and in response to dexamethasone or metyrapone, as well as determination of plasma ACTH, may suggest a primary adrenal, pituitary, or ectopic neoplastic source of disease [132,138,139]. If these data are equivocal, CRH measurements [119,120,128,140] and CRH stimulation testing with measurement of ACTH or cortisol [115,125,126,130,131,136], peripherally or in the bilateral venous effluent from the petrosal sinuses [129,133,135,137], are now frequently employed to provide additional biochemical evidence for the diagnosis of Cushing's disease in the clear state of hypercortisolemia.

Once it has been determined that a patient has a pituitary source of ACTH hypersecretion (Cushing's disease), it can be extremely difficult to identify the pituitary source. Since most ACTH-producing adenomas are small, their radiographic detection is difficult at best. Improvements in MRI with contrast have identified many microadenomas that would be radiographically invisible. Because many cases have no evidence of tumor on MRI, the technique of petrosal sinus sampling has been developed to confirm the diagnosis and guide the surgical resection (Figures 2.9 through 2.11). The rationale behind this technique, described in detail elsewhere, is straightforward [135]. Patients with Cushing's disease should have high (or inappropriately high) levels of ACTH production coming directly from the pituitary gland [129], and the levels may lateralize [135–137] to the side containing the adenoma. Comparison of pituitary to peripheral ACTH levels should demonstrate a gradient.

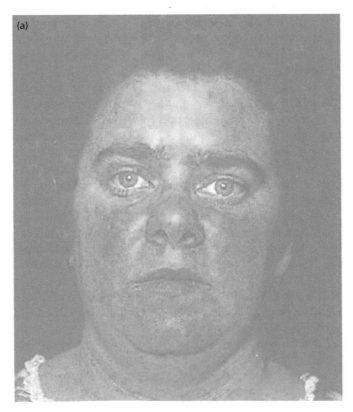
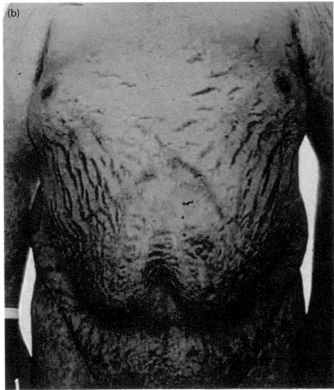

Figure 2.8 Patient demonstrating cushingoid changes with facial fullness **(a)** and central obesity along with atrophic red striae **(b)**.

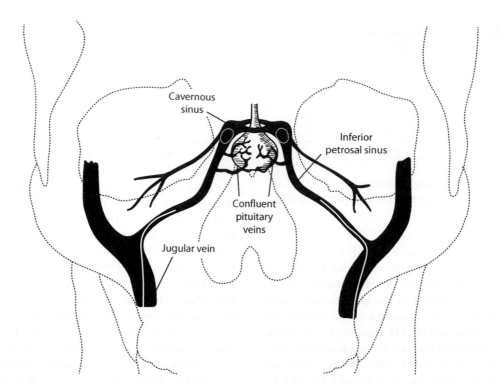

Figure 2.9 Catheter placement for bilateral simultaneous blood sampling of the inferior petrosal sinuses. Confluent pituitary veins empty laterally into the cavernous sinuses, which drain into the inferior petrosal sinuses. (Adapted from Oldfield EH et al. *N Engl J Med* 1985;312:101.)

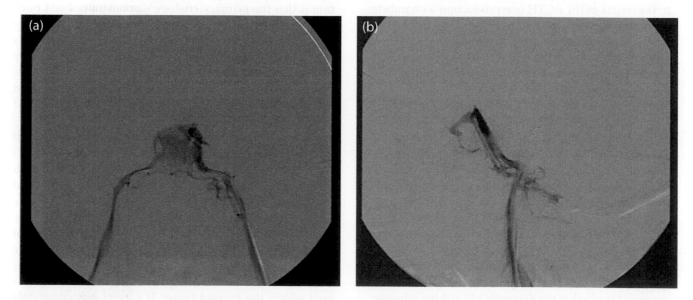

Figure 2.10 Angiogram of bilateral inferior petrosal sinus AP **(a)** and lateral **(b)** view venogram.

Those with ectopic ACTH secretion whose pituitary glands are suppressed should have neither an elevated pituitary-to-peripheral gradient nor a difference between sides. Patients without a discrete pituitary tumor (i.e., with hyperplasia of the corticotrophs) may have an increased central level of ACTH that is equal in blood from both sides of the gland. Some have advocated petrosal sinus sampling in all patients with ACTH-dependent disease, either to supplement or to supplant the conventional methods for establishing the

etiology of the hypercortisolism [125,133,138]. Published series indicate that the usefulness and reliability of this technique may be variable.

In Mampalam et al.'s series [111], 39 of 116 subjects (34%) had selective venous sampling of ACTH. A gradient of inferior petrosal sinus to peripheral was seen in 36. Of these 36, 31 (86%) were found to have adenomas. In three patients without a significant gradient, two had adenomas. Nine percent had false localization as to the site

Inferior petrosal sinus sampling with CRH stimulation

		ACTH (pg/mL)		
		Peripheral	Right IPS	Left IPS
Time (minutes)	0	29	60	449
	2	30	323	5809
	5	56	992	8733
	10	119	305	4936
	15	130	947	3225

Figure 2.11 Positive IPSS results noting a greater than 2–3 fold step up from peripheral to central sampling. IPS, inferior petrosal sinus.

of the adenoma. In Ludecke's series [134], 6 of 19 (31%) had incorrect lateralization of the adenoma by inferior petrosal sinus sampling. Ludecke recommended intraoperative measurement of ACTH in the perpituitary blood as a means of lateralizing the adenoma. A recent series of 501 patients with confirmed ACTH adenomas underwent sampling, which demonstrated a 98% confirmation rate. Increased accuracy was seen with left-sided lateralization and consistent lateralization prior to and after CRH administration [141]. In our institution, we use the technique in the following situations:

1. Patients with clear hypercortisolemia but doubt exists as to the source of the ACTH overproduction with unhelpful radiographic studies.
2. Patients with laboratory data clearly pointing to the pituitary gland but with normal radiographic studies. A petrosal sinus-directed hemihypophysectomy is done if an adenoma is not seen at surgery.
3. Young patients, especially women, for whom preservation of fertility is an important consideration and whose radiological studies are not grossly abnormal. Even when the lab studies clearly indicate pituitary-dependent disease, we routinely study these patients to try to lateralize the tumor. If nothing is found at the time of surgery, hemihypophysectomy on the side with the higher CRH-stimulated ACTH levels would then be done. However, there is a 40% incidence of incorrect lateralization.
4. Patients who have not been cured following transsphenoidal surgery. In these patients, the question to be answered is whether the diagnosis of Cushing's disease was truly correct.

In the most skilled hands, this sampling of venous effluent from the petrosal sinuses appears to be reliable and safe, although there is a 1.5% incidence of complications, some of which can be very serious, such as posterior reversible encephalopathy syndrome (PRES) [142].

TREATMENT

The treatment of Cushing's disease has advanced by the development of microsurgical transsphenoidal surgery. Successful surgery can cause reversal of hypercortisolism and eventual return of normal pituitary cortitroph function.

Most cases of Cushing's disease are caused by isolated adenomas of the anterior gland. The treatment of choice for Cushing's disease is transsphenoidal surgery with either selective adenomectomy or partial or hemihypophysectomy [108–112,143,144]. For those patients with very large tumors, surgery followed by conventional radiation therapy would be indicated and, very rarely, adrenalectomy. The surgical treatment paradigm remains controversial. The cure rate for this illness in all series remains under 90%. The surgical options for initial intervention include visual exploration of the gland, with removal of abnormal tissue [111], petrosal sinus-directed hemihypophysectomy [110], and total hypophysectomy [145]. Complications arise because incidental adenomas or small inhomogeneities in the gland are common, and the surgeon may be guided toward an abnormal part of the gland that is not responsible for the disease. Recurrence rates from 4% to 14% have been reported [108,110–112,144,146]. Many of these patients have been re-explored. According to Nakane et al. [112], verification of all pituitary adenomas was done by reoperation, during which time no corticotroph cell hyperplasia was found. It was concluded that late recurrence of Cushing's disease may follow adenomectomy due to regrowth of adenoma cells not removed from peritumoral tissue during the original surgery. The alternative explanation is that the primary etiology was not an isolated pituitary tumor but rather overstimulation; thus, as remaining pituitary tissue continues to be overstimulated, relapse is inevitable. In Friedman et al.'s study [147] of the efficacy of repeat surgery for recurrent Cushing's disease, the incidence of remission of hypercortisolism was highest if an adenoma was identified at surgery and the patient received selective adenomectomy.

Patients who are not cured by selective resection fall into several groups: (1) those with invasive adenomas, (2) those with unidentified microadenomas, (3) those with corticotroph hyperplasia without a discrete adenoma, and (4) those with ectopic secretion of ACTH or CRH. Those with lateral invasive extension will not be cured by any surgical procedure, and therefore hypophysectomy is not a consideration. Patients with microadenomas that are unidentified preoperatively are often cured by partial or total hypophysectomy; the microadenomas may be discovered within the excised tissue. If surgery has completely removed the tumor, the patient will be hypocorticsolemic for 6–12 months. Patients who are eucortisolemic immediately postoperatively have a high incidence of recurrence [148,149]. A study of 55 patients demonstrated that an ACTH level of >20 ng/L perioperatively is predictive of recurrence [150].

While transsphenoidal resection remains the primary procedure of choice, it does not obtain a 100% success rate. There are other treatment modalities available for use as adjuvants for those cases in which initial or repeat surgical therapy has failed.

Stereotactic radiation has been used alone or in combination with surgery for the treatment of Cushing's disease [151,152]; reports on its efficacy vary from 50% to 70% [153]. Because of the length of time needed to effect a cure and because of the high incidence of hypopituitarism, we currently suggest that radiation therapy be used only when pituitary surgery has failed and when medical therapy is not completely effective.

The medical therapies for Cushing's disease currently only address the symptomatic effects of the disease process rather than treat the underlying tumor pathology. These therapies primarily block ACTH or cortisol production at its end stage rather than treat the release process. Ketoconazole, a potent antifungal agent, inhibits adrenal steroidogenesis by blocking the 11beta-hydroxylase (and other enzymes involved in both cortisol and testosterone production as well). It is generally well tolerated, although sedation is a potential side effect. It is difficult to titrate the dose to achieve eucortisolemia. Often, the aim is to achieve complete adrenal suppression, at which time supplemental steroid treatment is begun [154,155]. Because several steps in steroid production are halted, effects on cholesterol, vitamin D, mineralocorticoid, and estrogen and androgen production need to be evaluated more closely before ketoconazole's use on a long-term basis should be recommended. We often use this drug if there is to be a delay between diagnosis and treatment, or if precise etiological diagnosis is in doubt (depression versus mild Cushing's) and some interim treatment is desirable. A newer agent on the market is Op'DDD (Lysodren), which is an adrenolytic agent, destroying the adrenocortical tissue and thereby initiating a "chemical adrenalectomy." It has been shown to decrease cortisol production in up to 80% of Cushing's patients [156]. Moreover, mifepristone (RU 486), which targets the glucocorticoid receptor, has also been shown to decrease the peripheral effects of cortisol, such as weight gain and insulin resistance, through the recently published SEISMIC study [157]. Pasireotide, the first pituitary-targeted treatment for Cushing's disease, is a new multi-receptor-targeted somatostatin analogue with high affinity for the D5 receptor, in addition to the D1 and D2 receptors. It is effective in the treatment of Cushing's disease due to the fact that corticotroph adenomas have been shown to have high expression of the D5 receptor [34,158,159]. A short-term, Phase II study of 29 patients demonstrated a 17% normalization and 76% reduction in urinary free cortisol levels after a 15-day treatment of 600 μg of subcutaneous pasireotide twice daily [160]. The major side effects include hyperglycemia, nausea, and diarrhea [158]. A multicenter Phase III trial of 162 patients further demonstrated that pasireotide led to a 20% normalization and 50% reduction in urinary free cortisol levels, with the effects being seen in the first 2 months of treatment. In addition to the observed effects on urinary free cortisol, decreased tumor volume, as well as quality of life, weight, and blood pressure improvements, was also demonstrated [161].

Figure 2.12 Visual field examination of a patient with a pituitary adenoma causing a bitemporal hemianoptic field defect.

Nonfunctioning adenomas

Whereas functioning adenomas require immediate treatment, nonfunctioning adenomas in asymptomatic patients may be managed by clinical observation. These patients should at first obtain yearly MRI surveillance, which can then be spaced to every 2–3 years if there is no growth of tumor [162]. Factors such as growth of tumor or the onset of neurologic symptoms, especially visual changes, necessitate close monitoring and referral for neurosurgical evaluation (Figure 2.12).

BRIEF HISTORY OF PITUITARY SURGERY AND THE EMERGING ROLE OF THE ENDOSCOPIC APPROACH TO PITUITARY TUMORS

The evolution of the field of pituitary surgery has made great advances over the past century. The first reports of pituitary surgery take us back to the days of Sir Victor Horsley in 1889, when he achieved the first transcranial pituitary surgery, and the days of Canton and Paul in 1893, who used a transcranial, temporal approach to pituitary resection [163,164]. In 1907, the first, albeit unsuccessful, attempt at transsphenoidal resection was conducted by Schloffer, namely due to the lack of proper imaging studies, which would not be remedied until the introduction of pneumoencephalography by Dandy in 1919 [165,166].

Over the next 20 years, Cushing and Hirsch popularized the sublabial and transnasal approaches, respectively, with Dr. Cushing achieving a noteworthy 5.6% mortality rate [167–169]. With Cushing's decision to solely implement the transcranial approach in 1929, the transsphenoidal approach was deserted by most practicing neurosurgeons until its resurgence in the midhalf of the twentieth century due to the discovery of new imaging modalities, namely, fluoroscopy by Guiot in 1958 and the surgical microscope by Hardy in 1967 [170–172]. The next advancement in the field occurred in the 1970s with the use of the endoscope in assistance to microscopic pituitary resection, allowing for much greater visualization, which eventually led to the development of pure endoscopic pituitary resection in the

1990s led by teams of neurosurgeons and head and neck surgeons [173–178].

Transsphenoidal surgery is unique in neurosurgery in that the operating surgical corridor is narrow, limiting the surgeon's view. In addition, during tumor removal only a fraction of the tumor can be visualized, which makes the confirmation of complete tumor removal often difficult. The indications for the use of endoscopic transsphenoidal surgery are essentially the same as for the standard approach. Endoscopic surgery through use of the short focal length offers the advantages of enhanced illumination and a wider angle of viewing than the microscope. The tumor morphology often dictates the approach in each case. Tumors with extensive suprasellar extension may require a craniotomy rather than a transsphenoidal resection. In addition to a detailed history, physical, and endocrinological workup, the use of high-resolution MRI with and without contrast is imperative before surgery. Special coronal sella windows help delineate the sella anatomy, especially the location of the carotid arteries and the optic chiasm. The extent of sphenoid sinus pneumatization is also important when planning the appropriate surgical approach. Many endoscopic surgeons also favor high-resolution computed tomography of the sphenoid and sella to better assess the bony anatomy of the sphenoid.

The operative technique employed in endoscopic transsphenoidal surgery varies with the instrumentation used. While a variety of techniques have been described, almost all approaches utilize the 3.7 mm 0°, 30°, or 70° endoscope. The angled endoscopes provide oblique views into the sinuses and lateral walls of the sphenoid and sella. A smaller 2.7 mm endoscope is also available for use in children or in patients with small nares. As in all endoscopes, the smaller size reduces the optical resolution and illumination (Figures 2.13 and 2.14).

In order for a purely endoscopic technique to be adopted as the gold standard method of pituitary resection, it must first be regarded as adequate and safe as the microscopic approach to resection, and second, it must demonstrate increased advantages while minimizing any complications.

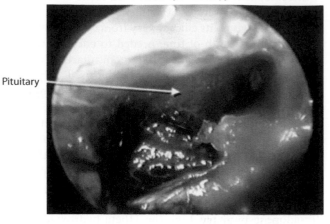

Figure 2.14 Pituitary fossa visualized via endoscopy.

Several case series over the past few years have demonstrated comparable, if not greater, efficacy of the endoscopic technique to that of the microscopic route of pituitary resection with decreased rates of complication [179–182]. Moreover, a meta-analysis of 821 patients conducted by Tabaee et al. bodes favorably for the endoscopic approach when compared with historical data in achieving gross tumor resection and improved endocrinological outcomes of hormone-secreting tumors, with similar rates of cerebrospinal fluid (CSF) leak and permanent diabetes insipidus complications [183]. Conversely, a meta-analysis of 24 endoscopic and 22 microscopic datasets of 5643 patients from 1990 to 2011, conducted by Ammirati et al. [184], investigated the extent of tumor removal and evaluated the following complications: CSF leak, meningitis, vascular injury, visual deficits, diabetes insipidus, hypopituitarism, and cranial nerve injury. The only significant difference that they found was a greater incidence of vascular injury with the endoscopic method, possibly due to the absence of three-dimensional depth perception with this approach ($p < 0.0001$).

The limitations of endoscopic transsphenoidal surgery are a lack of stereoscopic depth perception and limited visualization when bleeding is encountered. It is these authors' belief that in the hands of an experienced microscopic surgeon, the microscopic approach is as successful in the removal of pituitary tumors as the endoscopic approach, with fewer complication rates. However, endoscopic assistance is sometimes employed in tumors with far lateral or suprasellar extent.

A WORD ON THE ROLE OF RADIATION

In addition to the mentions of radiation therapy given above, stereotactic radiosurgery can also be used in the treatment of medically and surgically refractory pituitary tumors. In a series of 418 patients published by Sheehan et al., Gamma Knife radiosurgery achieved up to 90% tumor control and approximately 50% biochemical remission, with a median time to remission of approximately 49 months [185]. Further

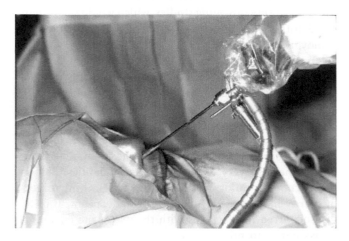

Figure 2.13 Transnasal transsphenoidal surgery with endoscope.

study is needed to investigate the potential side effects of radiosurgery, such as visual deficits and long-term outcomes over a long follow-up period. Some studies have demonstrated approximately 85%–90% tumor control between a 5- and 10-year follow-up period [186–188]. A peer review by Starke et al., encompassing 731 patients, describes a tumor control rate with radiotherapy ranging from 66% to 100% and an endocrine remission rate ranging from 17% to 100% [189]. Endocrine remission rates are highest in Cushing's disease and lowest in prolactinomas [190].

PITUITARY TUMORS AND PATHOLOGIC MARKERS

While most pituitary tumors remain benign, it would be helpful to identify biomarkers obtained at the time of pathologic examination that would predict malignant behavior of tumors. Various markers ranging from oncogenes to tumor suppressor genes to growth factors to cell adhesion and angiogenic factors to chromosomal alterations have been studied. Of these, fibroblast growth factor receptor 4 (FGFR4); matrix metalloproteinases (MMPs), specifically MMPs 2 and 9; pituitary tumor transforming gene (PTTG); Ki-67; p53; and deletions in chromosome 11 have been identified in some studies to predict aggressive behavior [191–197]. Further study is indicated to determine the extent that these and other biomarkers can predict malignant behavior among pituitary adenomas.

CONCLUSION

Patients with functioning pituitary adenomas pose very different management problems and decisions than do patients with nonfunctioning adenomas. The unique pathology of each tumor requires careful history and physical examinations, coupled with a detailed endocrinological workup. Therapy employed should include not only surgery but also the current best-indicated medical or radiation therapy that is specific to the presentation of the individual patient. The recent advances in endoscopic and minimally invasive transsphenoidal surgery will continue to reduce the already low morbidity and enhance the high efficacy achieved through microsurgical resection. Meticulous follow-up with the potential aid of tumor markers is crucial in maintaining tumor control and treating possible tumor recurrence.

REFERENCES

1. Reichlin S. Anatomical and physiological basis of hypothalamic-pituitary regulation. In: Post KD, Jackson IMD, Reichlin S, eds., *The Pituitary Adenoma*. New York: Plenum, 1980:3–28.
2. Klibanksi A. Nonsecreting pituitary tumors. *Endocrinol Metab Clin North Am* 1987;16:793–804.
3. Hardy J. Transsphenoidal microsurgery of the normal and pathological pituitary. *Clin Neurosurg* 1969;16:185–217.
4. Hardy J, Somma M. Acromegaly: Surgical treatment by transsphenoidal microsurgical removal of the pituitary adenoma. In: Tindall GT, Collins WF, eds., *Clinical Management of Pituitary Disorders*. New York: Raven Press, 1979:209–17.
5. Litt AW, Kricheff II. Magnetic resonance imaging of pituitary tumors. In: Cooper PR, ed., *Contemporary Diagnosis and Management of Pituitary Adenomas*. Chicago: American Association of Neurologic Surgeons, 1991:1–19.
6. Macpherson P, Hadley DM, Teasdale E et al. Pituitary microadenomas: Does gadolinium enhance their demonstration? *Neuroradiology* 1989;31:293–8.
7. Kulkarni MV, Lee KF, McArdle CB et al. 1.5T MR imaging of pituitary microadenomas: Technical considerations and CT correlation. *AJNR Am J Neuroradiol* 1988;9:5–11.
8. Doppman JL, Frank JA, Dwyer AJ et al. Gadolinium DTPA enhanced MR imaging of ACTH-secreting microadenomas of the pituitary gland. *J Comput Assist Tomogr* 1988;12:728–35.
9. Marcovitz S, Wee R, Chan J et al. The diagnostic accuracy of preoperative CT scanning in the evaluation of pituitary ACTH-secreting adenomas. *AJR Am J Roentgenol* 1987;149:803–6.
10. Marcovitz S, Wee R, Chan J et al. Diagnostic accuracy of preoperative scanning of pituitary prolactinomas. *AJNR Am J Neuroradiol* 1988;9:13–7.
11. Marcovitz S, Wee R, Chan J et al. Diagnostic accuracy of preoperative CT scanning of pituitary somatotroph adenomas. *AJNR Am J Neuroradiol* 1988;9:19–22.
12. Davis PC, Hoffman JC Jr, Tindall GT et al. Prolactin-secreting pituitary microadenomas: Inaccuracy of high-resolution CT imaging. *AJR Am J Roentgenol* 1985;144:151–6.
13. Frantz AG. Prolactin. *N Engl J Med* 1978;298:201–7.
14. Jaquet P, Guibout M, Lucioni J et al. Hypothalamopituitary regulation of prolactin in hypersecreting prolactinoma. In: Robyn C, Harter M, eds., *Progress in Prolactin, Physiology and Pathology*. New York: Elsevier-North Holland Biochemical Press, 1978:371–82.
15. Boyd AE III, Reichlin S. Neural control of prolactin secretion in man. *Psychoneuroendocrinology* 1978;3:113–30.
16. Kleinberg DL, Noel GL, Frantz AG. Galactorrhea: A study of 235 cases including 48 with pituitary tumors. *N Engl J Med* 1977;296:589–600.
17. Goodman RH, Molitch MD, Post KD, Jackson IMD. Prolactin secreting adenomas in the male. In: Post KD, Jackson IMD, Reichlin S, eds., *The Pituitary Adenoma*. New York: Plenum Press, 1980:91–108.
18. Melmed S, Casanueva FF, Hoffman AR et al. Diagnosis and treatment of hyperprolactinemia: An Endocrine Society clinical practice guideline. *J Clin Endocrinol Metab* 2011;96:273–88.

19. Thorner MO, McNeilly AS, Hagan C, Besser GM. Long-term treatment of galactorrhea and hypogonadism with bromocriptine. *Br Med J* 1974;2:419–22.

20. Vance ML, Evans WS, Thorner MO. Bromocriptine. *Ann Intern Med* 1984;100:78–91.

21. Zarate A, Canales ES, Cano C, Pilonieta CJ. Follow-up of patients with prolactinomas after discontinuation of long-term therapy with bromocriptine. *Acta Endocrinol (Copenh)* 1983;104:139–42.

22. Molitch ME, Elton RL, Blackwell RE et al. Bromocriptine as primary therapy for prolactin-secreting macroadenomas: Results of a prospective multicenter study. *J Clin Endocrinol Metab* 1985;60:698–705.

23. Thorner MO, Martin WH, Rogol AD et al. Rapid regression of pituitary prolactinomas during bromocriptine treatment. *J Clin Endocrinol Metab* 1980;51:438–45.

24. Tindall GT, Kovacs K, Horvath E et al. Human prolactin-producing adenomas and bromocriptine: A histological, immunocytochemical, ultrastructural, and morphometric study. *J Clin Endocrinol Metab* 1982;55:1178–83.

25. Barrow DL, Tindall GT, Kovacs K et al. Clinical and pathological effects of bromocriptine on prolactin-secreting and other pituitary tumors. *J Neurosurg* 1984;60:1–7.

26. Barrow DL, Mizuno J, Tindall GT. Management of prolactinomas associated with very high serum prolactin levels. *J Neurosurg* 1988;68:554–8.

27. Molitch ME, Reichlin S. Hyperprolactinemic disorders. *Dis Mon* 1982;28:1–58.

28. Reichlin S. The prolactinoma problem. *N Engl J Med* 1979;300:313–5.

29. Thorner MO, Schran HF, Evans WS et al. A broad spectrum of prolactin suppression by bromocriptine in hyperprolactinemic women: A study of serum prolactin and bromocriptine levels after acute and chronic administration of bromocriptine. *J Clin Endocrinol Metab* 1980;50:1026–33.

30. Thorner MO, Edwards CRW, Charlesworth M et al. Pregnancy in patients presenting with hyperprolactinemia. *Br Med J* 1979;2:771–4.

31. Tindall GT, Barrow DL, Tindall SC. Current management of pituitary tumors, II. *Contemp Neurosurg* 1988;10:1–6.

32. Vance ML, Cragun JR, Reimnitz C et al. CV 205-502 treatment of hyperprolactinemia. *J Clin Endocrinol Metab* 1989;68:336–9.

33. Wang C, Lam KSL, Ma JTC et al. Long-term treatment of hyperprolactinaemia with bromocriptine: Effect of drug withdrawal. *Clin Endocrinol (Oxf)* 1987;27:363–71.

34. Biller BMK, Colao A, Petersenn S, Bonert VS, Boscaro M. Prolactinoma. Cushing's disease and acromegaly: Debating the role of medical therapy for secretory pituitary adenomas. *BMC Endocr Disord* 2010;10:1–14.

35. Maiter D, Primeau V. 2012 update in the treatment of prolactinomas. *Ann Endocrinol (Paris)* 2012;73:90–8.

36. Molitch ME. Pregnancy and the hyperprolactinemic woman. *N Engl Med* 1985;312:1364–70.

37. dos Santos Nunes V, Dib El R, Boguszewski CL, Nogueira CR. Cabergoline versus bromocriptine in the treatment of hyperprolactinemia: A systematic review of randomized controlled trials and meta-analysis. *Pituitary* 2011;14:259–65.

38. Thorner MO, Perryman RL, Rogol AD et al. Rapid changes of prolactinoma volume after withdrawal and reinstitution of bromocriptine. *J Clin Endocrinol Metab* 1981;53:480–3.

39. Liuzzi A, Dallabonzana D, Oppizzi G et al. Low doses of dopamine agonists in the long-term treatment of macroprolactinomas. *N Engl J Med* 1985;313:656–9.

40. Kleinberg DL, Boyd AE III, Wardlaw S et al. Pergolide for the treatment of pituitary tumors secreting prolactin or growth hormone. *N Engl J Med* 1983;309:704–9.

41. Post KD. Surgical approaches to the treatment of prolactinomas. In: Olefsky JM, Robbins RJ, eds., *Prolactinomas: Practical Diagnosis and Management*. New York: Churchill Livingstone, 1986:159–94.

42. Fahlbusch R, Buchfelder M, Schrell U. Short-term preoperative treatment of macroprolactinomas by dopamine agonists. *J Neurosurg* 1987;67:807–15.

43. Hubbard JL, Scheithauer BW, Abboud CF, Laws ER Jr. Prolactin-secreting ademonas: The preoperative response to bromocriptine treatment and surgical outcome. *J Neurosurg* 1987;67:816–21.

44. Landolt AM, Osterwalder V. Perivascular fibrosis in prolactinomas: Is it increased by bromocriptine? *J Clin Endocrinol Metab* 1984;58:1179–83.

45. Landolt AM, Keller PJ, Froesch ER et al. Bromocriptine: Does it jeopardize the result of later surgery for prolactinomas? *Lancet* 1982;2:657.

46. Weiss MH, Teal J, Gott P et al. Natural history of microprolactinomas: Six-year follow-up. *Neurosurgery* 1983;12:180–3.

47. Sisam DA, Sheehan JP, Sheeler LR. The natural history of untreated microprolactinoma. *Fertil Steril* 1987;48:67–71.

48. Klibanski A, Greenspan SL. Increase in bone mass after treatment of hyperprolactinemic amenorrhea. *N Engl J Med* 1986;315:542–6.

49. Klibanski A, Biller BMK, Rosenthal DI, Schoenfeld DA, Saxe V. Effects of prolactin and estrogen deficiency in amenorrheic bone loss. *J Clin Endocrinol Metab* 1988;67:124–30.

50. Cushing H. Partial hypophysectomy for acromegaly with remarks on the function of the hypophysis. *Ann Surg* 1909;50:1002–17.

51. Lewis UJ, Singh RN, Tutwiler GF, Sigel MB, Vanderlaan EF, Vanderlaan WP. Human growth hormone: A complex of proteins. *Recent Prog Horm Res* 1980;36:477–508.

52. Reichlin S. Somatostatin. *N Engl J Med* 1983;309:1495–501.

53. Vance ML, Kaiser DL, Evans WS et al. Pulsatile growth hormone secretion in normal man during a continuous 24-hour infusion of human growth hormone releasing factor (1-40): Evidence for intermittent somatostatin secretion. *J Clin Invest* 1985;75:1584–90.

54. Van Wyk JJ. The somatomedins: Biological actions and physiologic control mechanisms. In: Li CH, ed., *Growth Factors.* New York: Academic Press, 1984:81–125.

55. Frohman LA, Szabo M, Berelowitz, Stachura ME. Partial purification and characterization of a peptide with growth hormone-releasing activity from extra-pituitary tumors in patients with acromegaly. *J Clin Invest* 1980;65:43–54.

56. Melmed S, Ziel FH, Braunstein GD, Downs T, Frohman LA. Medical management of acromegaly due to ectopic production of growth hormone-releasing hormone by a carcinoid tumor. *J Clin Endocrinol Metab* 1988;67:395–9.

57. Melmed S. Acromegaly. *N Engl J Med* 1990;322:966–77.

58. Klein I, Parveen G, Van Thiel DH. Colonic polyps in patients with acromegaly. *Ann Intern Med* 1982;97:27–30.

59. Leavitt J, Klein I, Kendricks F, Gavaler J, Van-Thiel DH. Skin tags: A cutaneous marker for colonic polyps. *Ann Intern Med* 1983;98:928–30.

60. Thorner MO, Vance ML. Growth hormone, 1988. *J Clin Invest* 1988;82:745–7.

61. Clemmons DR, Van Wyk JJ, Ridgway EC, Kliman B, Kjellberg RN, Underwood LE. Evaluation of acromegaly by radioimmunoassay of somatomedin-C. *N Engl J Med* 1979;301:1138–42.

62. Barkan AI, Beitins IZ, Kelch RP. Plasma insulin-like growth factor-1/somatomedin-C in acromegaly: Correlation with the degree of growth hormone hypersecretion. *J Clin Endocrinol Metab* 1988;67:69–73.

63. Wright AD, Hill DM, Lowy C, Fraser TR. Mortality in acromegaly. *Q J Med* 1970;39:1–16.

64. Melded, S, Casanueva FF, Cavagnini F et al. Consensus guidelines for acromegaly. *J Clin Endocrinol Metab* 2002;87:4045–58.

65. Ross DA, Wilson CB. Results of transsphenoidal microsurgery for growth hormone-secreting pituitary adenomas in a series of 214 patients. *J Neurosurg* 1988;78:854–67.

66. Grisoli F, Leclercq T, Jaquet P et al. Transsphenoidal surgery for acromegaly—Long term results in 100 patients. *Surg Neurol* 1986;25:513–9.

67. Serri O, Somma M, Comtois R et al. Acromegaly: Biochemical assessment of cure after long-term follow-up of transsphenoidal selective adenomectomy. *J Clin Endorinol Metab* 1985;61:1185–9.

68. Roelfsema F, van Dulken H, Frolich M. Long-term results of transsphenoidal pituitary microsurgery in 60 acromegalic patients. *Clin Endocrinol (Oxf)* 1985;23:555–65.

69. Ludecke DK, Saeger W, William T. Effectiveness of microsurgery in acromegaly: Study of 210 cases. *Period Biol* 1983;85:59–66.

70. Laws ER Jr, Randall RV, Abboud CF. Surgical treatment of acromegaly: Results in 140 patients. In: Givens J, ed., *Hormone-Secreting Pituitary Tumors.* Chicago: Year Book Medical Publishers, 1982:225–8.

71. Liuzzi A, Chiodini PG, Botalla A, Cremascoli G, Muller EE, Silvestrini F. Decreased plasma growth hormone (GH) levels in acromegalics following CB 154 (2-Br-alpha-ergocriptine) administration. *J Clin Endocrinol Metab* 1974;38:910–2.

72. Lindholm J, Riishede J, Verstergaard S, Hummer L, Faber O, Hagen C. No effect of bromocriptine in acromegaly: A controlled trial. *N Engl J Med* 1981;304:1450–4.

73. Wass JAH, Thorner MO, Morris DV et al. Long-term treatment of acromegaly with bromocriptine. *Br Med J* 1977;1:875–8.

74. Bell P, Atkinson AB, Hadden DR et al. Bromocriptine reduces growth hormone in acromegaly. *Arch Intern Med* 1986;146:1145–9.

75. Besser GM, Wass JAH, Thorner MO. Acromegaly results of long-term treatment with bromocriptine. *Acta Endocrinol Suppl (Copenh)* 1978;88(Suppl 216):187–98.

76. Abs R, Verhelst J, Maiter D et al. Cabergoline in the treatment of acromegaly: A study in 64 patients. *J Clin Endocrinol Metab* 1998;83:374–8.

77. Cozzi R, Attanasio R, Barausse M et al. Cabergoline in acromegaly: A renewed role for dopamine agonist treatment? *Eur J Endocrinol* 1998;139:516–21.

78. Lamberts SWJ, Zweens M, Verschoor L, del Pozo E. A comparison among the growth hormone-lowering effects in acromegaly of the somatostatin analog SMS 201-995, bromocriptine, and the combination of both drugs. *J Clin Endocrinol Metab* 1986;63:16–9.

79. Halse J, Harris AG, Kvistborg A et al. A randomized study of SMS 201-995 versus bromocriptine treatment in acromegaly: Clinical and biochemical effects. *J Clin Endocrinol Metab* 1990;70:1254–61.

80. Chiodini PG, Cozi R, Dallabonzana D et al. Medical treatment of acromegaly with SMS 201-995, a somatostatin analog: A comparison with bromocriptine. *J Clin Endocrinol Metab* 1987;64:447–53.

81. Lamberts SW. The role of somatostatin in the regulation of anterior pituitary hormone secretion and the use of its analogs in the treatment of human pituitary tumors. *Endocr Rev* 1988;9:417–36.

82. Kohler PO. Treatment of pituitary adenomas. *N Engl J Med* 1987;317:45–6.

83. Lamberts SWJ, Uitterlinden P, Verschoor L, van Dongen KJ, del Pozo E. Long-term treatment of acromegaly with the somatostatin analogue SMS 201-995. *N Engl J Med* 1985;313:1576–80.

84. Comi RJ, Gorden P. The response of serum growth hormone levels to the long-acting somatostatin analog SMS 201-995 in acromegaly. *J Clin Endocrinol Metab* 1987;64:37–42.

85. Barnard LB, Grantham WG, Lambewrton P, O'Dorsio TM, Jackson IMD. Treatment of resistant acromegaly with long-acting somatostatin analogue (SMS 201-995). *Ann Intern Med* 1986;105:856–61.

86. Harris AG, Prestele H, Herold K et al. Long-term efficacy of Sandostatin (SMS 201-995, octreotide) in 178 acromegalic patients: Results from the International Multicentre Acromegaly Study Group. In: Lamberts SWJ, ed., *Sandostatin in the Treatment of Acromegaly*. New York: Springer-Verlag, 1988:117–25.

87. Ho KY, Weissberger AJ, Marbach P, Lazarus L. Therapeutic efficacy of the somatostatin analog SMS 201-995 (octreotide) in acromegaly: Effects of dose and frequency and long-term safety. *Ann Intern Med* 1990;112:173–81.

88. Cozzi R, Montini M, Attanasio R et al. Primary treatment of acromegaly with octreotide LAR: A long-term (up to 9 years) prospective study of its efficacy in the control of disease activity and tumor shrinkage. *J Clin Endocrinol Metab* 2006;91:1397–403.

89. Caron PJ, Bevan JS, Petersenn S et al. Tumor shrinkage with lanreotide autogel 120 mg as primary therapy in acromegaly: Results of a prospective multicenter trial. *J Clin Endocrinol Metab* 2014;99:1282–90.

90. Colao A, Bronstein MD, Freda P et al. Pasireotide versus octreotide in acromegaly: A head-to-head superiority study. *J Clin Endocrinol Metab* 2014;99:791–9.

91. Trainer PJ, Drake WM, Katznelson L et al. Treatment of acromegaly with the growth hormone-receptor antagonist pegvisomant. *N Engl J Med* 2000;342:1171–7.

92. van der Lely AJ, Biller BMK, Brue T et al. Long-term safety of pegvisomant in patients with acromegaly: Comprehensive review of 1288 subjects in ACROSTUDY. *J Clin Endocrinol Metab* 2012;97:1589–97.

93. Snyder PJ, Fowble BF, Schatz NJ, Savino PJ, Gennarelli TA. Hypopituitarism following radiation therapy of pituitary adenomas. *Am J Med* 1986;81:457–62.

94. Eastman RC, Gorden P, Roth J. Conventional supervoltage irradiation is an effective treatment for acromegaly. *J Clin Endocrinol Metab* 1979;48:931–40.

95. Lee C, Vance ML, Xu Z et al. Stereotactic radiosurgery for acromegaly. *J Clin Endocrinol Metab* 2014;99:1273–81.

96. Smallridge RC. Thyrotropin-secreting pituitary tumors. *Endocrinol Metab Clin North Am* 1987;16:765–92.

97. Smallridge RC, Smith CE. Hyperthyroidism due to thyrotropin-secreting pituitary tumors: Diagnostic and therapeutic consideration. *Arch Intern Med* 1983;143:503–7.

98. Snyder PJ, Johnson J, Muzyka R. Abnormal secretion of glycoprotein alpha-subunit and follicle stimulating hormone (FSH) beta-subunit in men with pituitary adenomas and FSH hypersecretion. *J Clin Endocrinol Metab* 1980;51:579–84.

99. Oppenheim DS, Kana AR, Sangha JS, Klibanski A. Prevalence of alpha-subunit hypersecretion in patients with pituitary tumors: Clinically nonfunctioning and somatotroph adenomas. *J Clin Endocrinol Metab* 1990;70:859–64.

100. Kourides IA, Weintraub BD, Rosen SW, Ridgway EC, Kilman B, Maloof F. Secretion of alpha subunit of glycoprotein hormones by pituitary adenomas. *J Clin Endocrinol Metab* 1976;43:97–106.

101. Malchiodi E, Profka E, Ferrante E et al. Thyrotropin-secreting pituitary adenomas: Outcome of pituitary surgery and irradiation. *J Clin Endocrinol Metab* 2014;99:2069–76.

102. Snyder PJ. Gonadotroph cell adenomas of the pituitary. *Endocr Rev* 1985;6:552–63.

103. Ebersold MJ, Quast LM, Laws ER Jr, Scheithauer B, Randall RV. Long-term results in transsphenoidal removal of nonfunctioning pituitary adenomas. *J Neurosurg* 1986;64:713–9.

104. Comi RJ, Gesundheit N, Murray L, Gorden P, Weintraub BD. Response of thyrotropin-secreting pituitary adenomas to a long-acting somatostatin analogue. *N Engl J Med* 1987;317:12–7.

105. Burch W. Cushing's disease, a review. *Arch Intern Med* 1985;145:1106–11.

106. Burrow GN, Wortzman G, Rewcastle NB et al. Microadenomas of the pituitary and abnormal sellar tomograms in an unselected autopsy series. *N Engl J Med* 1981;304:156–8.

107. Chandler WF, Schteingart DE, Lloyd RV et al. Surgical treatment of Cushing's disease. *J Neurosurg* 1987;66:204–12.

108. Fahlbusch R, Buchfelder M, Muller OA. Transsphenoidal surgery for Cushing's disease. *J R Soc Med* 1986;79:262–9.

109. Guilhaume B, Bertagna X, Thomsen M et al. Transsphenoidal pituitary surgery for the treatment of Cushing's disease: Results in 64 patients and long term follow-up studies. *J Clin Endocrinol Metab* 1988;66:1056–64.

110. Hardy J. Cushing's disease: 50 years later. *Can J Neurol Sci* 1982;2:375–80.

111. Mampalam TJ, Tyrell JB, Wilson CB. Transsphenoidal microsurgery for Cushing's disease. *Ann Intern Med* 1988;109:487–93.

112. Nakane R, Kuwayama A, Watanabe M et al. Long-term results of transsphenoidal adenomectomy in patients with Cushing's disease. *Neurosurgery* 1987;21:218–22.

113. Dwyer AJ, Frank JA, Doppman JL et al. Pituitary adenomas in patients with Cushing's disease: Initial experience with Gd-DTPA-enhanced MR imaging. *Neuroradiology* 1987;163:421–6.

114. Newton DR, Dillon WP, Normal D et al. Gd-DTPA-enhanced MR imaging of pituitary adenomas. *AJNR Am J Neuroradiol* 1989;10:949–54.

115. Saris SC, Patronas NJ, Doppman JL et al. Cushing's syndrome: Pituitary CT scanning. *Radiology* 1987;162:775–7.

116. Orth DN. The old and new in Cushing's syndrome. *N Engl J Med* 1984;310:649–51.

117. Case records of MGH. Case 53-1981. *N Engl J Med* 1981;305:1637–43.

118. Suda T, Kondo M, Totani R et al. Ectopic adreno-corticotropin syndrome caused by lung cancer that responded to corticotropin-releasing hormone. *J Clin Endocrinol Metab* 1986;63:1047–51.

119. Case records of MGH. Case 52-1987. *N Engl J Med* 1987;317:1648–58.

120. Schteingart DE, Lloyd RV, Akil H et al. Cushing's syndrome secondary to ectopic corticotropin-releasing hormone adrenocorticotropin secretion. *J Clin Endocrinol Metab* 1986;63:770–5.

121. Lloyd RV, Chandler WF, McKeever PE, Schteingart DE. The spectrum of ACTH-producing pituitary lesions. *Am J Surg Pathol* 1986;10:618–26.

122. Post KD, Habas JE. Cushing's disease. In: Samii M, ed., *Surgery of the Sellar Region and Paranasal Sinuses*. Berlin: Springer-Verlag, 1991:294–301.

123. Reith P, Monnot EA, Bathija PJ. Prolonged suppression of a corticotropin-producing bronchial carcinoid by oral bromocriptine. *Ann Intern Med* 1987;147:989–91.

124. Nieman LK, Chrousos GP, Oldfield EH et al. The ovine corticotropin-releasing hormone stimulation test and the dexamethasone suppression test in the differential diagnosis of Cushing's syndrome. *Ann Intern Med* 1986;105:862–7.

125. Chrousos GP, Sculte HM, Oldfield EH et al. The corticotropin-releasing factor stimulation test. *N Engl J Med* 1984;310:622–6.

126. Chrousos GP, Schuermeyer TH, Doppman JL et al. Clinical applications of corticotropin-releasing factor. *Ann Intern Med* 1985;102:344–58.

127. Crapo L. Cushing's syndrome: A review of diagnostic tests. *Metabolism* 1979;28:955–77.

128. Cunnah D, Jessop DS, Besser GM, Rees LH. Measurement of circulating-releasing factor in man. *J Endocrinol* 1987;113:1123–31.

129. Findling JW, Aron DC, Tyrell JB et al. Selective venous sampling for ACTH in Cushing's syndrome. *Ann Intern Med* 1981;94:641–52.

130. Fukata J, Nakai Y, Imura H et al. Human corticotropin-releasing hormone test in normal subjects and patients with hypothalamic, pituitary or adrenocortical disorders. *Endocrinol Jpn* 1988;35:491–502.

131. Hermus AR, Pieters GF, Pesman GJ et al. The corticotropin-releasing hormone test versus the high dose dexamethasone test in the differential diagnosis of Cushing's syndrome. *Lancet* 1986;2:540–3.

132. Howlett TA, Drury PL, Perry L et al. Diagnosis and management of ACTH-dependent Cushing's syndrome: Comparison of the features in ectopic and pituitary ACTH production. *Clin Endocrinol (Oxf)* 1986;24:699–713.

133. Landolt AM, Valvanis A, Girard J, Eberle AN. Corticotropin-releasing factor test used with bilateral, simultaneous inferior petrosal sinus blood-sampling for the diagnosis of pituitary-dependent Cushing's disease. *Clin Endocrinol (Oxf)* 1986;25:687–96.

134. Ludecke DK. Intraoperative measurement of adrenocorticotrophic hormone in peripituitary blood in Cushing's disease. *Neurosurgery* 1989;24:201–5.

135. Oldfield EH, Chrousos GP, Schulte HM et al. Preoperative lateralization of ACTH-secreting pituitary microadenomas by bilateral and simultaneous inferior petrosal venous sinus sampling. *N Engl J Med* 1985;312:98–103.

136. Schrell U, Fahlbusch R, Buchfelder M et al. Corticotropin-releasing hormone stimulation test before and after transsphenoidal selective microadenomectomy in 30 patients with Cushing's disease. *J Clin Endocrinol Metab* 1987;64:1150–9.

137. Zovickian J, Oldfield EH, Doppman JL et al. Usefulness of inferior petrosal sinus venous endocrine markers in Cushing's disease. *J Neurosurg* 1988;68:205–10.

138. Findling JW, Tyrell JB. Occult ectopic secretion of corticotropin. *Am J Med* 1986;146:929–33.

139. Elamin MB, Murad MH, Mullan R et al. Accuracy of diagnostic tests for Cushing's syndrome: A systematic review and metaanalyses. *J Clin Endocrinol Metab* 2008;93:1553–62.

140. Carey RM, Varma SK, Drake CR et al. Ectopic secretion of corticotripin-releasing factor as a cause of Cushing's syndrome. *N Engl J Med* 1984;311:13–20.

141. Wind JJ, Lonser RR, Nieman LK, DeVroom HL, Chang R, Oldfield EH. The lateralization accuracy of inferior petrosal sinus sampling in 501 patients with Cushing's disease. *J Clin Endocrinol Metab* 2013;98:2285–93.

142. Jehle S, Walsh JE, Freda PU, Post KD. Selective use of bilateral inferior petrosal sinus sampling in patients with adrenocorticotropin-dependent Cushing's syndrome prior to transsphenoidal surgery. *J Clin Endocrinol Metab* 2008;93:4624–32.

143. Boggan JE, Tyrell JB, Wilson CB. Transsphenoidal microsurgical management of Cushing's disease: A report of 100 cases. *J Neurosurg* 1983;59:195–200.

144. Tindall GT, Herring CJ, Clark RV et al. Cushing's disease: Results of transsphenoidal microsurgery with emphasis on surgical failures. *J Neurosurg* 1990;72:363–9.

145. Krieger DT. Physiopathology of Cushing's disease. *Endocr Rev* 1983;4:22–43.

146. Salassa RM, Laws ER, Carpenter PC. Cushing's disease—50 years later. *Trans Am Clin Climatol Assoc* 1982;94:122–9.

147. Friedman RB, Oldfield EH, Nieman LK et al. Repeat transsphenoidal surgery for Cushing's disease. *J Neurosurg* 1989;71:520–7.

148. Fitzgerald PA, Aron DC, Findling JW et al. Cushing's disease: Transient secondary adrenal insufficiency after selective removal of pituitary microadenomas; evidence for a pituitary origin. *J Clin Endocrinol Metab* 1982;54:413–22.

149. Derome PJ, Delalande O, Visot A, Jedynac CP, Dupuy M. Short and long term results after trans-sphenoidal surgery for Cushing's disease; incidence of recurrences. In: Landolt AM, ed., *Progress in Pituitary Adenoma Research*. London: Pergamon Press, 1988:375–9.

150. Abdelmannan D, Chaiban J, Selman WR, Arafah BM. Recurrences of ACTH-secreting adenomas after pituitary adenomectomy can be accurately predicted by perioperative measurements of plasma ACTH levels. *J Clin Endocrinol Metab* 2013;98:1458–65.

151. Degerblad M, Rahn T, Bergstrand G, Thoren M. Long-term results of stereotactic radiosurgery to the pituitary gland in Cushing's disease. *Acta Endocrinol (Copenh)* 1986;112:310–4.

152. Sandler LM, Richards NT, Carr DH et al. Long term follow-up of patients with Cushing's disease treated by interstitial irradiation. *J Clin Endocrinol Metab* 1987;65:441–7.

153. Biller BM, Grossman PM, Stewart PM. Treatment of adrenocorticotropin-dependent Cushing's syndrome: A consensus statement. *J Clin Endocrinol Metab* 2008;93:2454–62.

154. Loli P, Berselli ME, Tagliaferri M. Use of ketoconazole in the treatment of Cushing's syndrome. *J Clin Endocrinol Metab* 1986;63:1365–71.

155. Sonino N. The use of ketoconazole as an inhibitor of steroid production. *N Engl J Med* 1987;317:812–8.

156. Baudry C, Coste J, Bou Khalil R et al. Efficiency and tolerance of mitotane in Cushing's disease in 76 patients from a single center. *Eur J Endocrinol* 2012;16:473–81.

157. Fleseriu M, Biller BM, Findling JW, Molitch ME, Schteingart DE, Gross C; on behalf of the SEISMIC Study Investigators. Mifepristone, a glucocorticoid receptor antagonist, produces clinical and metabolic benefits in patients with Cushing's syndrome. *J Clin Endocrinol Metab* 2012;97:2039–49.

158. Colao A, Boscaro M, Ferone D, Casanueva FF. Managing Cushing's disease: The state of the art. *Endocrine* 2014;47:9–20.

159. van der Pas R, de Herder WW, Hofland LJ, Feelders RA. Recent developments in drug therapy for Cushing's disease. *Drugs* 2013;73:907–18.

160. Boscaro M, Ludlam WH, Atkinson B et al. Treatment of pituitary dependent Cushing's disease with the multi-receptor ligand somatostatin analog pasire-otide (SOM230): A multi-center, phase II trial. *J Clin Endocrinol Metab* 2009;94:115–22.

161. Colao A, Petersenn S, Newell-Price J et al. A 12-month phase 3 study of pasireotide in Cushing's disease. *N Engl J Med* 2012;366:914–24.

162. Freda PU, Beckers AM, Katznelson L et al. Pituitary incidentaloma: An Endocrine Society clinical practice guideline. *J Clin Endocrinol Metab* 2011;96:894–904.

163. Horsley V. On the technique of operations on the central nervous system. *BMJ* 1906;2:411–23.

164. Canton R, Paul F. Notes of a case of acromegaly treated by operation. *BMJ* 1893;2:1421.

165. Schloffer H. Erfolgreiche Operation eines Hypophysentumors auf nasalem Wege. *Wien Klin Wochenschr* 1907;20:621–4.

166. Gandhi CD, Christiano LD, Eloy JA, Prestigiacomo CJ, Post KD. The historical evolution of trans-sphenoidal surgery: Facilitation by technological advances. *Neurosurg Focus* 2009;27:E8.

167. Cushing H. *Clinical States Produced by Disorders of the Hypophysis Cerebri, in the Pituitary Body and Its Disorders*. Philadelphia: JB Lippincott, 1912.

168. Hirsch O. Demonstration eines nach einer neuen method operiten hypophysentumors. *Verh Dtsch Ges Chir* 1910;39:51–6.

169. Henderson W. The pituitary adenomata. A follow-up study of the surgical results in 338 cases (Dr. Harvey Cushing's series). *Br J Surg* 1939;26:811–921.

170. Rosegay H. Cushing's legacy to transsphenoidal surgery. *J Neurosurg* 1981;54:448–54.

171. Guiot G, Rougerie J, Brion S et al. L'utilisation des amplificateurs de brillance en neuro-radiol-ogie et dans la chirurgie stereotaxique. *Ann Chir* 1958;34:689–95.

172. Hardy J. Surgery of the pituitary gland, using the open transsphenoidal approach. Comparative study of 2 technical methods. *Ann Chir* 1967;21:1011.

173. Apuzzo MLJ, Heifetz M, Weiss MH, Kurze T. Neurosurgical endoscopy using the side-viewing telescope. Technical note. *J Neurosurg* 1977;16:398–400.

174. Bushe KA, Halves E. Modified technique in trans-sphenoidal operations of pituitary adenomas. *Acta Neurochir (Wien)* 1978;41:163–75.

175. Cappabianca P, Alfieri A, de Divitiis E. Endoscopic endonasal transsphenoidal approach to the sella: Towards functional endoscopic pituitary surgery (FEPS). *Minim Invasive Neurosurg* 1998;41:66–73.

176. Jankowski R, Auque J, Simon C, Marchal JC, Hepner H, Wayoff M. Endoscopic pituitary tumor surgery. *Laryngoscope* 1992;102:198–202.

177. Jho HD, Carrau R. Endoscopy assisted transsphenoidal surgery for pituitary adenoma. Technical note. *Acta Neurochir (Wien)* 1996;138:1416–25.

178. Sethi DS, Pillay PK. Endoscopic management of lesions of the sella turcica. *J Laryngol Otol* 1995;109:956–62.

179. Cho DY, Liau WR. Comparison of endonasal endoscopic surgery and sublabial microsurgery for prolactinomas. *Surg Neurol* 2002;58:371–5.

180. Kabil MS, Eby JB, Shahinian HK. Fully endoscopic endonasal vs. transseptal transsphenoidal pituitary surgery. *Minim Invasive Neurosurg* 2005;48:348–54.

181. White DR, Sonnenburg RE, Ewend MG, Senior BA. Safety of minimally invasive pituitary surgery (MIPS) compared with a traditional approach. *Laryngoscope* 2004;114:1945–8.

182. O'Malley BW Jr, Grady MS, Gabel BC et al. Comparison of endoscopic and microscopic removal of pituitary adenomas: Single-surgeon experience and the learning curve. *Neurosurg Focus* 2008;25:E10.

183. Tabaee A, Anand VK, Barron Y et al. Endoscopic pituitary surgery: A systematic review and meta-analysis. *J Neurosurg* 2009;111:545–54.

184. Ammirati M, Wei L, Ciric I. Short-term outcome of endoscopic versus microscopic pituitary adenoma surgery: A systematic review and meta-analysis. *J Neurol Neurosurg Psychiatry* 2013;84:843–9.

185. Sheehan JP, Pouratian N, Steiner L et al. Gamma Knife surgery for pituitary adenomas: Factors related to radiological and endocrine outcomes. *J Neurosurg* 2011;114:303–9.

186. Gopalan R, Schlesinger D, Vance ML et al. Long-term outcomes after Gamma Knife radiosurgery for patients with a nonfunctioning pituitary adenoma. *Neurosurgery* 2011;69:284–93.

187. Park K-J, Kano H, Parry PV et al. Long-term outcomes after Gamma Knife stereotactic radiosurgery for nonfunctional pituitary adenomas. *Neurosurgery* 2011;69:1188–99.

188. Loeffler JS, Shih HA. Radiation therapy in the management of pituitary adenomas. *J Clin Endocrinol Metab* 2011;96:1992–2003.

189. Starke RM, Williams BJ, Vance ML, Sheehan JP. Radiation therapy and stereotactic radiosurgery for the treatment of Cushing's disease: An evidence-based review. *Curr Opin Endocrinol Diabetes Obes* 2010;17:356–64.

190. Ding D, Starke RM, Sheehan JP. Treatment paradigms for pituitary adenomas: Defining the roles of radiosurgery and radiation therapy. *J Neurooncol* 2014;117:445–57.

191. Ezzat S, Asa SL, Couldwell WT et al. The prevalence of pituitary adenomas: A systematic review. *Cancer* 2004;101:613–9.

192. Morita K, Takano K, Yasufuku-Takano J et al. Expression of pituitary tumour-derived, N-terminally truncated isoform of fibroblast growth factor receptor 4 (ptd-FGFR4) correlates with tumour invasiveness but not with G-protein α subunit (gsp) mutation in human GH-secreting pituitary adenomas. *Clin Endocrinol* 2008;68:435–41.

193. Gong J, Zhao Y, Abdel-Fattah R et al. Matrix metalloproteinase-9, a potential biological marker in invasive pituitary adenomas. *Pituitary* 2008;11:37–48.

194. Liu W, Matsumoto Y, Okada M et al. Matrix metalloproteinase 2 and 9 expression correlated with cavernous sinus invasion of pituitary adenomas. *J Med Investigation* 2005;52:151–8.

195. Wierinckx A, Roche M, Raverot G et al. Integrated genomic profiling identifies loss of chromosome 11p impacting transcriptomic activity in aggressive pituitary PRL tumors. *Brain Pathol* 2011;21:533–43.

196. Filippella M, Galland F, Kujas M et al. Pituitary tumour transforming gene (PTTG) expression correlates with the proliferative activity and recurrence status of pituitary adenomas: A clinical and immunohistochemical study. *Clinl Endocrinol* 2006;65:536–43.

197. Mete O, Ezzat S, Asa SL. Biomarkers of aggressive pituitary adenomas. *J Mol Endocrinol* 2012;49:R69–78.

198. Post K, Shrivastava R. Functioning pituitary tumors. In: Rengachary S, Ellenbogen R, eds., *Principles of Neurosurgery*. New York: Elsevier Mosby, 2005:603–20.

199. Knosp E, Steiner E, Kitz K, Matula C. Pituitary adenomas with invasion of the cavernous sinus space: A magnetic resonance imaging classification compared with surgical findings. *Neurosurgery* 1993;33(4):610–18. Adapted with permission from Lippincott Williams & Wilkins/Wolters Kluwer Health: Neurosurgery.

200. Oldfield EH, Chrousos GP, Schulte HM et al. Preoperative lateralization of ACTH-secreting pituitary adenomas by bilateral and simultaneous inferior petrosal sinus sampling. *N Engl J Med* 1985;312:101.

The Endocrine, Lung, and Thymus

PART 2

The Endocrine, Lung, and Thymus

3

Physiology and pathophysiology of pulmonary neuroendocrine cells

JOHN R. GOSNEY

INTRODUCTION

The defining feature of neuroendocrine cells is secretion of amine or peptide hormones that regulate local physiological processes [1]. They act in concert with systemic neural and endocrine control systems and have features of both neurons and endocrine cells, hence their name. Whether scattered as individual cells within epithelia, as in the airways or gut, or aggregated into larger structures, such as the pancreatic islets, neuroendocrine cells are characterized by their morphological uniformity and high degree of organization. Their ultrastructural hallmark is the *neurosecretory* or *dense core* vesicles (DCVs) (Figure 3.1) that store and release their secretory products. Components of these and other secretory vesicles, together with a variety of membrane proteins and enzymes, endow neuroendocrine cells with a characteristic antigenic profile. Their integration with and contribution to the regulation of physiological processes are by a mode of local secretion known as *paracrine* [1–5].

Pulmonary neuroendocrine cells (PNCs) constitute the pulmonary component of this *diffuse neuroendocrine system* (DNS). In healthy, adult human lungs, PNCs are distributed from the trachea to the alveoli, but are most numerous in bronchi and bronchioles [6–8]. The vast majority of human PNCs are solitary (Figure 3.2), and it is unlikely that the highly organized, innervated, corpuscular aggregates of PNCs known as *neuroepithelial bodies* (NEBs) [9], which are so frequent in lower species [10], are ever found in human lungs. It is probable that clusters of PNCs develop in human lungs only when pulmonary tissues are growing and differentiating, typically in fetal lungs, or when pulmonary

tissues are damaged and there is a need for regeneration and repair, processes in which they appear to play a crucial role [1].

Solitary human PNCs (Figure 3.2) rest on the the basal lamina of the respiratory epithelium and vary considerably in shape, but are often columnar or triangular with a broad base. Dendrite-like cytoplasmic processes extend from the apex of the cell toward the lumen of the airway, or insinuate between adjacent cells [10,11]. In human lungs, clusters of these cells appear to comprise closely apposed solitary cells without the highly organized "organoid" structure of true NEBs.

IDENTIFICATION

Although PNCs have been often referred to as "clear cells" because of their lucent cytoplasm [12], they are difficult to detect in a section stained with hematoxylin and eosin. Early studies of them, therefore, had to rely on capricious histochemical techniques, and it was not until the advent of more specific and reliable immunochemical markers of neuroendocrine differentiation that the characteristics of PNCs became precisely defined [1]. Of these antigens, neuron-specific enolase (NSE), protein gene product (PGP) 9.5, and chromogranin have been most widely used in the identification of PNCs. In contrast to seeking these neuroendocrine antigens in the diagnosis of neuroendocrine tumors of the lung, where they are neither sensitive nor specific enough to be of diagnostic utility, they are extremely reliable when used to identify normal or proliferating PNCs outside the context of neoplasia.

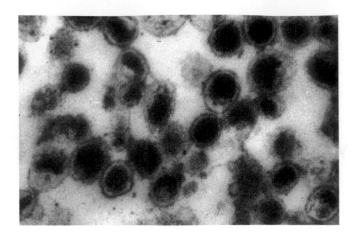

Figure 3.1 The characteristic neurosecretory vesicles or DCVs that are the ultrastructural hallmark of cells of the DNS.

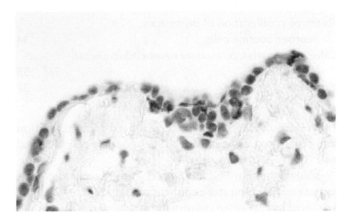

Figure 3.2 Solitary neuroendocrine cells, immunolabeled for chromogranin, in the epithelium of a small airway in a normal human lung. Their fine, arborizing cytoplasmic processes that insinuate between adjacent cells are characteristic.

SECRETORY PRODUCTS

Numerous peptides and amines have been localized to PNCs of different species [13], but those established by repeated demonstration in human lungs are gastrin-releasing peptide (GRP) (the mammalian analog of amphibian bombesin) [14], calcitonin (CT) [15], CT gene-related peptide [16], and the amine serotonin (5-hydroxytryptamine [5HT]) [17]. In healthy human lungs, about two-thirds of PNCs contain GRP and most of the rest CT [6].

ULTRASTRUCTURE

In common with all cells of the DNS, the *neurosecretory (dense core) vesicle* (Figure 3.1) is the ultrastructural hallmark of PNCs [10]. These are spherical structures varying in size from about 100 to 180 nm. They have an electron-dense core separated from a limiting membrane by a clear "halo." The ultrastructure of PNCs is not otherwise particularly

unique [10,18]. Their nuclei are spherical or ovoid, basal or suprabasal, and sometimes indented. The Golgi apparatus is supranuclear, both smooth and rough endoplasmic reticulum are present, and free ribosomes are plentiful. Moderate numbers of mitochondria are found. Intermediate filaments are usually abundant and typically aggregated in sheaves. Microvilli are present on the apical surface, and desmosomes, tight junctions, and junctional complexes bind PNCs to their neighbors.

FUNCTION

The functions of PNCs continue to be debated. Evidence for a chemoreceptive role for NEBs in lower species such as the rabbit is overwhelming [4], but there is little hard evidence for such a function in human lungs, and that linking increased numbers of human PNCs to hypoxia *per se* is unconvincing. They are known to express opioid receptors [19], and it has been recently suggested [20] that human PNCs might be chemosensitive to volatile chemicals in inspired air. Most data, however, particularly from studies of PNCs during fetal pulmonary development and in human lungs affected by naturally occurring pulmonary disease, support the idea that they have a central role in regulating the development, repair, and regeneration of human pulmonary tissues [1,5,21–23].

Evidence for a central role for PNCs in human fetal pulmonary growth is strong. Their prevalence at this time of life has been noted repeatedly, and numbers of GRP-containing PNCs, as well as levels of GRP itself, its mRNA, and its receptor, are markedly elevated during the canalicular period of pulmonary development [24–26]. Not only is GRP powerfully trophic to human bronchial epithelial cells *in vitro* [27], but it stimulates fetal pulmonary growth and maturation *in vivo* and in organ culture in murine and rhesus monkey fetuses [28–30].

REACTIVE PROLIFERATION OF PULMONARY NEUROENDOCRINE CELLS

The only other context in which PNCs are as numerous as in fetal lungs is when they proliferate in lungs subject to injury (Figure 3.3). Most conditions in which this has been described involve inflammatory injury or, less often, some other form of pulmonary damage [1,22,31] (Table 3.1). The initial response of PNCs to pulmonary injury takes the form of an essentially linear proliferation along the basal lamina of the airway (Figure 3.4), at which stage the predominance of GRP as the major secretory product of human PNCs is reversed so that CT is most prevalent. This probably explains the hypercalcitoninemia and hypercalcitoninuria identifiable in patients with inflammatory pulmonary diseases like acute bronchitis, pneumonia, and tuberculosis [32].

If injury persists or is recurrent, a more disorderly pattern of proliferation emerges in which PNCs gather up within the epithelium to form nodular aggregates of cells that form

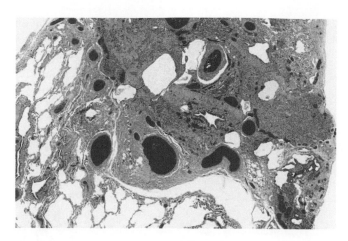

Figure 3.3 Reactive proliferation of neuroendocrine cells in a lung damaged by bronchiectasis and scarring. Note how the proliferating cells are confined to the damaged lung (top and right).

Table 3.1 Conditions in which increased numbers of PNCs have been described

Asthma
Pneumonia
Pulmonary fibrosis
Bronchiectasis
Cystic fibrosis
Chronic obstructive pulmonary disease
In tissue around pulmonary tumors
Eosinophilic granuloma
Plexogenic pulmonary arteriopathy
Mechanical ventilation with oxygen
Beronchopulmonary dysplasia
Wilson–Mikity syndrome
Brainstem injury due to birth asphyxia
Sudden infant death syndrome

Source: Adapted from Gosney JR. *Pulmonary Endocrine Pathology: Endocrine Cells and Endocrine Tumours of the Lung.* Oxford: Butterworth-Heinemann, 1992; Gosney JR. *Microsc Res Tech* 1997;37:107–13.

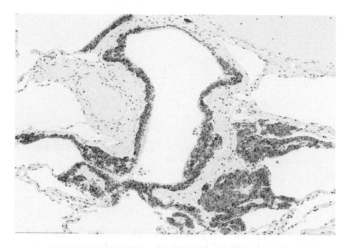

Figure 3.4 Early reactive proliferation of neuroendocrine cells, immunolabeled for chromogranin, in a lung affected by acute bronchitis with focal bronchopneumonia. The cells form generally linear rows along the basal lamina of the airways, but do not invade the parenchyma.

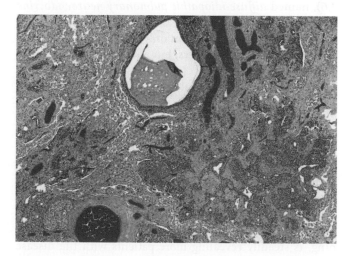

Figure 3.5 Infiltration of proliferating neuroendocrine cells into the damaged parenchyma around a small airway in a lung affected by chronic suppurative inflammation and scarring to form a *tumorlet*. Note the conspicuous fibrous stroma and irregular pattern of infiltration.

irregular masses that may protrude into the lumen of the airway. Sometimes, this process exceptionally results in the development of the small, locally invasive, 2–3 mm diameter aggregates of PNCs known as *tumorlets* [33]. These are characterized by their conspicuously fibrotic stroma and irregular, infiltrative edge (Figure 3.5) and are due to the growth of PNCs across the basement lamina into the adjacent parenchyma. They are typically seen in lungs damaged by bronchiectasis or containing chronically suppurating abscesses or fungus balls. At this stage of the proliferative process, there is a further change in the secretory products of PNCs, with aberrant peptides like adrenocorticotropic hormone (ACTH), growth hormone, vasoactive intestinal polypeptide (VIP), and human chorionic gonadotrophin (HCG) becoming detectable [34,35].

DIFFUSE IDIOPATHIC PULMONARY NEUROENDOCRINE CELL HYPERPLASIA

The proliferation described above, even to the extent of the development of tumorlets with their aberrant peptides, is considered reactive, although clearly it has elements of structural and functional disorder. This belief is based on the fact that even the most florid proliferation of PNCs in injured lungs never results in the development of neuroendocrine tumors, a view supported by studies that reveal fundamental genetic differences between tumorlets and carcinoid tumors [36]. In the early 1990s, however, a condition characterized by diffuse proliferation of PNCs, including linear rows, nodular aggregates, and tumorlets, but in intimate association with peripheral

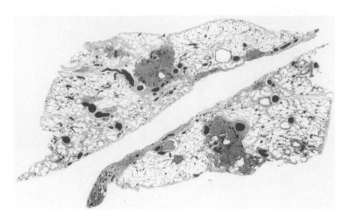

Figure 3.6 A pulmonary wedge biopsy showing the typical features of DIPNECH in which zones of proliferating neuroendocrine cells infiltrate the parenchyma of otherwise normal lung.

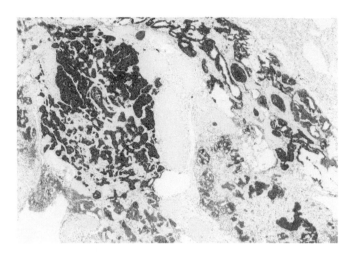

Figure 3.7 Florid proliferation of neuroendocrine cells, immunolabeled for chromogranin, spreading through the parenchyma in a lung affected by DIPNECH.

carcinoids, was described [37–39]. This condition (Figure 3.6), named *diffuse idiopathic pulmonary neuroendocrine cell hyperplasia* (DIPNECH), differs crucially from reactive proliferation of PNCs not only in its association with peripheral carcinoid tumors, but also because it does not arise in the context of the chronic, destructive pulmonary injury that underlies the late stages of reactive PNC proliferation [37–41].

Originally considered rare, DIPNECH is clearly more common than formerly believed. Its slow-burning time course and the nonspecificity of its clinical and radiological manifestations account for its previous underdiagnosis, with scrutiny of the older literature uncovering descriptions of what are clearly cases of the condition [42–46]. Increasing appreciation of DIPNECH, together with improvements in the resolving power of computerized tomographic scanning, is steadily revealing more patients with the disease [31,40,47–49].

Diffuse idiopathic PNC hyperplasia typically arises in middle-aged women [37–40,48]. They are usually never or light smokers with a long history of mild, gradually increasing cough and breathlessness, although many cases come to light incidentally on thoracic imaging for other reasons. Typically, this reveals the combination of mosaicism, due to air trapping caused by obstruction of small airways, and nodules of varying size. Pulmonary function tests reveal an obstructive or mixed obstructive/restrictive pattern. DIPNECH is characterized by slow progression over many years, and the mainstay of management is regular review and reimaging, sometimes with steroids to reduce breathlessness, and with excision of any emerging lesion that has features to suggest it might be a carcinoid. Chemotherapy has been used occasionally [37], but is probably inappropriate and excessive. Occasionally, the disability has become disabling to the point of requiring pulmonary transplantation [50].

DIPNECH is characterized by the proliferation of PNCs forming lesions ranging from small intraepithelial groups

to large, irregular nodules, papillary processes, and tumorlets, the process often extending into the parenchyma of the lung (Figure 3.7). Its features are similar to reactive proliferation of PNCs, and it appears to be associated with the same increase in the variety of their secretory products [51], but it is usually more florid and, as mentioned above, accompanied in about half of cases by *bona fide* carcinoid tumors (Figure 3.8). In this regard, it is of interest that there appear to be differences in the kinetics of the proliferating cells between PNCs proliferating as a reaction to pulmonary injury and those proliferating in DIPNECH [52]. For example, expression of Ki67, a commonly used index of cell proliferation, is detectable in PNCs at all stages of proliferation in DIPNECH, but is not demonstrable at any stage in PNCs undergoing reactive proliferation, even in

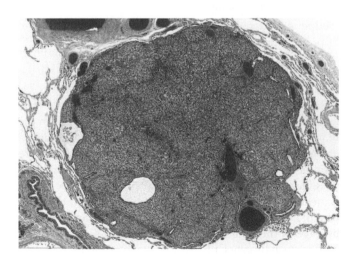

Figure 3.8 A small, typical carcinoid tumor arising in a lung affected by DIPNECH. Note the mild peribronchiolar chronic inflammation and fibrosis around the adjacent airway, bottom left. This is a common, but not universal, finding in DIPNECH.

Table 3.2 Essential differences between reactive proliferation of PNCs and DIPNECH

Characteristic	Reactive proliferation	DIPNECH
Age and sex	No prevalence	Women in fourth to sixth decades
Presentation	That of causative disease	Mild, chronic cough and breathlessness
Imaging	That of causative disease	Mosaicism due to air trapping; nodules
Morphology of proliferation of PNCs	Small intramucosal aggregates and tumorlets, often subtle	Florid, often occlusion of airways and conspicuous involvement of parenchyma
Pattern of proliferation	Confined to zones of disease	Diffuse, often bilateral
Other pathology	That of causative disease	Mild, chronic inflammation and fibrosis of small airways
Cell kinetcs	Ki67 and p53 protein not detected	Ki67 expression at all stages; p53 overexpression by tumorlets
Development of carcinoid tumors	Never	In about half of cases

tumorlets. Similarly, most tumorlets in DIPNECH, but not those in reactive proliferation, overexpress p53 protein. In addition, p16 protein is demonstrable at much earlier stages of proliferation in DIPNECH than in reactively proliferating PNCs. This evidence of earlier and more vigorous activity in DIPNECH in comparison with reactive proliferation of PNCs suggests that the processes are fundamentally different.

Although by definition the diagnosis of DIPNECH requires the surrounding lung to be normal [49], many cases are characterized by mild, chronic inflammation and fibrosis in and around bronchioles (Figure 3.8), and it is possible that this contributes to the clinical and radiological features. It is sometimes argued that this process might actually be the *cause* of DIPNECH, but this is unlikely. The damage to the lung that provokes reactive proliferation of PNCs is usually gross, typically with heavy, chronic inflammation, often suppurative. Additionally, this does not explain the tendency of DIPNECH to generate carcinoids, which do not emerge from reactive proliferation of PNCs. It is more likely that these mild inflammatory and fibrotic changes around airways are a *consequence* of amine or

peptide products, or of transforming growth factor (TGF)-beta acting locally following their release from the proliferating cells [37,39,40,50,53].

Interestingly, the neuroendocrine tumors that arise from DIPNECH are always carcinoids (Figure 3.7). Rarely, they are atypical [40], but the more aggressive types of neuroendocrine tumor, large cell and small cell neuroendocrine carcinomas, never develop in this context.

The essential differences between reactive proliferation of PNCs and DIPNECH are shown in Table 3.2.

REFERENCES

1. Gosney JR. *Pulmonary Endocrine Pathology: Endocrine Cells and Endocrine Tumours of the Lung.* Oxford: Butterworth-Heinemann, 1992.
2. Feyrter F. *Uber Diffuse Endokrine Epitheliale Organe.* Leipzig: J.A. Barth, 1938.
3. Pearse AGE. The cytochemistry and ultrastructure of polypeptide hormone-producing cells of the APUD series and the embryologic, physiologic and pathologic implications of the concept. *J Histochem Cytochem* 1969;17:303–13.
4. Van Lommel A, Bolle T, Fannes W, Lauweryns JM. The pulmonary neuroendocrine system: The past decade. *Arch Histol Cytol* 1999;62:1–6.
5. Linnoila RI. Functional facets of the pulmonary neuroendocrine system. *Lab Invest* 2006;86:425–44.
6. Gosney JR, Sissons MCJ, Allibone RO. Neuroendocrine cell populations in normal human lungs: A quantitative study. *Thorax* 1988;43:878–82.
7. Gosney JR. Neuroendocrine cell populations in postnatal human lungs: Minimal variation from childhood to old age. *Anat Rec* 1993;236:177–80.
8. Boers JE, den Brok JLM, Koudstaal J, Arends JW, Thunnissen BJM. Number and proliferation of neuroendocrine cells in normal human airway epithelium. *Am J Resp Crit Care Med* 1996;154:758–63.
9. Lauweryns JM, Cokelaere M, Theunynck P. Neuroepithelial bodies in the respiratory mucosa of various mammals: A light optical, ultrastructural and histochemical investigation. *Zeitschrift Zellforsch Mikrosk Anat* 1972;135:569–92.
10. Sorokin SP, Hoyt RF. Neuropeithelial bodies and solitary small granule cells. In: Massaro D, ed., *Lung Cell Biology.* New York: Marcel Dekker, 1989:191–344.
11. Weichselbaum M, Sparrow MP, Hamilton EJ, Thompson PJ, Knight DA. A confocal microscopic study of solitary pulmonary neuroendocrine cells in human airway epithelium. *Resp Res* 2005;6:115–25.
12. Frohlich F. Die helle Zelle der Bronchialschleimhaut und ihre Beziehungen zum Problem der Chemoreceptoren. *Frankfurt Zeitschrift Pathol* 1949;60:517–59.
13. Polak J, Becker KL, Becker E et al. Lung endocrine cell markers, peptides and amines. *Anat Rec* 1993;236:169–71.

14. Wharton J, Polak JM, Bloom SR et al. Bombesin-like immunoreactivity in the lung. *Nature* 1978;273:769–70.

15. Becker KL, Monaghan KG, Silva OL. Immunocytochemical localization of calcitonin in Kulchitsky cells of human lung. *Arch Pathol Lab Med* 1980;104:196–8.

16. Johnson DE, Wobken JD. Calcitonin gene-related peptide immunoreactivity in airway epithelial cells of the human fetus and infant. *Cell Tissue Res* 1987;250:579–83.

17. Lauweryns JM, de Bock V, Verhofstad AAJ, Steinbusch HWM. Immuno-histochemical localization of serotonin in intrapulmonary neuroepithelial bodies. *Cell Tissue Res* 1982;226:215–23.

18. Scheuermann DW. Morphology and cytochemistry of the endocrine epithelial system in the lung. *Int Rev Cytol* 1987;106:35–88.

19. Krajnik M, Jassem E, Sobanski P. Opioid receptor bronchial tree: Current science. *Curr Opin Support Palliat Care* 2014;8:191–9.

20. Gu X, Karp PH, Brody SL et al. Chemosensory functions for pulmonary neuroendocrine cells. *Am J Respir Cell Mol Biol* 2014;50:637–46.

21. Cutz E, Gillan JE, Perrin DG. Pulmonary neuroendocrine cell system: An overview of cell biology and pathology with emphasis on pediatric lung disease. *Persp Ped Pathol* 1985;18:32–70.

22. Gosney JR. Pulmonary neuroendocrine cell system in pediatric and adult lung disease. *Microsc Res Tech* 1997;37:107–13.

23. Reynolds SD, Giangreco A, Power JHT, Stripp BR. Neuroepithelial bodies of pulmonary airways serve as a reservoir of progenitor cells capable of epithelial regeneration. *Am J Pathol* 2000;156:269–78.

24. Wang D, Yeger H, Cutz E. Expression of gastrin-releasing peptide receptor gene in developing lung. *Am J Resp Cell Mol Biol* 1996;14:409–16.

25. Spindel ER, Sunday ME, Hofler H, Wolfe HJ, Habener JF, Chin WW. Transient elevation of mRNAs encoding gastrin-releasing peptide (GRP), a putative pulmonary growth factor, in human fetal lung. *J Clin Invest* 1987;80:1172–9.

26. Sunday ME, Hua J, Dai HB, Nusrat A, Torday JS. Bombesin increases fetal lung growth and maturation in utero and in organ culture. *Am J Resp Cell Mol Biol* 1990;3:199–205.

27. Siegfried JM, Guentert PJ, Gaither AL. Effects of bombesin and gastrin-releasing peptide on human bronchial epithelial cells from a series of donors: Individual variation and modulation by bombesin analogs. *Anat Rec* 1993;236:241–7.

28. Sunday ME, Hua J, Reyes B, Masui H, Torday JS. Anti-bombesin monoclonal antibodies modulate fetal mouse lung growth and maturation in utero and in organ cultures. *Anat Rec* 1993;236:25–32.

29. Aguayo SM, Schuyler WE, Murtagh JJ, Roman J. Regulation of lung branching morphogenesis by bombesin-like peptides and neutral endopeptidase. *Am J Resp Cell Mol Biol* 1994;19:635–42.

30. Li K, Nagalla SR, Spindel ER. A rhesus monkey model to characterize the role of gastrin-releasing peptide (GRP) in lung development. *J Clin Invest* 1994;94:1605–15.

31. Gosney JR. Neuroendocrine tumors and other neuroendocrine proliferations of the lung. In Hasleton P, Flieder DB, eds., *Spencer's Pathology of the Lung*. 6th ed. Cambridge: Cambridge University Press, 2013:1151–85.

32. Becker KL, Nash D, Silva OL, Snider RH, Moore CF. Increased serum and urinary calcitonin levels in patients with pulmonary disease. *Chest* 1981;79:211–6.

33. Whitwell F. Tumourlets of the lung. *J Pathol Bacteriol* 1955;70:529–41.

34. Gosney J, Green ART, Taylor W. Appropriate and inappropriate neuroendocrine products in pulmonary tumourlets. *Thorax* 1990;45:679–83.

35. Tsutsumi Y, Osamura RY, Watanabe K, Yanaihara N. Immunohistochemical studies on gastrin-releasing peptide and adrenocorticotropic hormone-containing cells in the human lung. *Lab Invest* 1993;48:623–32.

36. Finkelstein SD, Hasegawa T, Colby T, Yousem SA. 11q13 allelic imbalance discriminates pulmonary carcinoids from tumourlets. *Am J Pathol* 1999;155:633–40.

37. Aguayo SM, Miller YE, Waldron JAJ et al. Brief report: Idiopathic diffuse hyperplasia of pulmonary neuroendocrine cells and airways disease. *N Engl J Med* 1992;327:1285–8.

38. Armas OA, White DA, Erlandson RA, Rosai J. Diffuse idiopathic neuroendocrine cell proliferation presenting as interstitial lung disease. *Am J Surg Pathol* 1995;19:963–70.

39. Miller RR, Muller NL. Neuroendocrine cell hyperplasia and obliterative bronchiolitis in patients with peripheral carcinoid tumors. *Am J Surg Pathol* 1995;19:653–8.

40. Davies SJ, Gosney JR, Hansell DM et al. Diffuse idiopathic pulmonary neuroendocrine cell hyperplasia: An under-recognised spectrum of disease. *Thorax* 2007;62:248–52.

41. Lee JS, Brown KK, Cool C, Lynch DA. Diffuse pulmonary neuroendocrine cell hyperplasia: Radiologic and clinical features. *J Comput Assist Tomogr* 2002;26:180–4.

42. Felton WL, Liebow AA, Lindskog GE. Peripheral and multiple bronchial adenomas. *Cancer* 1953;6:555–67.

43. McDowell EM, Sorokin SP, Hoyt RF, Trump BF. An unusual bronchial carcinoid tumor. Light and electron microscopy. *Hum Pathol* 1981;12:338–48.

44. Miller MA, Mark GJ, Kanarek D. Multiple peripheral pulmonary carcinoids and tumorlets of carcinoid type, with restrictive and obstructive lung disease. *Am J Med* 1978;65:373–8.

45. Skinner C, Ewen SWB. Carcinoid lung: Diffuse pulmonary infiltration by a multifocal bronchial carcinoid. *Thorax* 1976;31:212–9.

46. Sorokin SP, Hoyt RF, McDowell EM. An unusual bronchial carcinoid tumor analyzed by conjunctive staining. *Hum Pathol* 1981;12:302–13.

47. Adams H, Brack T, Kestenholz P, Vogt P, Steinert HC, Russi EW. Diffuse idiopathic pulmonary neuroendocrine cell hyperplasia causing severe airway obstruction in a patient with a carcinoid tumor. *Respiration* 2006;73:690–3.

48. Nassar AA, Jaroszewski DE, Helmers RA, Colby TV, Patel BV, Mookadam F. Diffuse idiopathic neuroendocrine cell hyperplasia: A systematic overview. *Am J Respir Crit Care Med* 2011;184:8–16.

49. Gosney JR, Travis WD. Diffuse idiopathic pulmonary neuroendocrine cell hyperplasia. In Travis WD, Brambilla E, Muller-Hermelink HK, Harris CC, eds. *Pathology and Genetics: Tumours of the Lung, Pleura, Thymus and Heart.* Lyon: IARC Press, 2004:76–7.

50. Sheerin N, Harrison NK, Sheppard MN, Hansell DM, Yacoub M, Clark TJ. Obliterative bronchiolitis caused by multiple tumourlets and microcarcinoids successfully treated by single lung transplantation. *Thorax* 1995;50:207–9.

51. Oba H, Nishida K, Takeuchi S et al. Diffuse idiopathic pulmonary neuroendocrine cell hyperplasia with a central and peripheral carcinoid and multiple tumorlets: A case report emphasizing the role of neuropeptide hormones and human gonadotropin-alpha. *Endocr Pathol* 2013;24:220–8.

52. Gosney JR, Williams IJ, Dodson AR, Foster CS. Morphology and antigen expression profile of pulmonary neuroendocrine cells in reactive proliferations and diffuse idiopathic pulmonary neuroendocrine cell hyperplasia (DIPNECH). *Histopathology* 2011;59:751–62.

53. Sartelet H, Decaussin M, Devouassoux G et al. Expression of vascular endothelial growth factor (VEGF) and its receptors (VEGF-R1 (Flt-1) and VEGF-R2 (KDR/Flk-1)) in tumorlets and in neuroendocrine cell hyperplasia of the lung. *Hum Pathol* 2004;35:1210–7.

4

Bronchopulmonary and thymic carcinoids; other endocrine tumors

LESLIE JAMES, ANDREA WOLF, AND RAJA FLORES

THE LUNG AS AN ENDOCRINE ORGAN

The lung plays an essential role in facilitating the transfer of gases between inspired air and circulation, maintaining concentrations of oxygen and carbon dioxide within plasma and tissues within the narrow range that is compatible with life. In addition to its role in gas exchange, the lung has a number of important metabolic functions. For example, surfactant is manufactured in the lung for local use in increasing pulmonary compliance and preventing atelectasis. The lung also produces and metabolizes derivatives of arachidonic acid, prostaglandins, and leukotrienes [1]. The pulmonary vasculature metabolizes substances produced locally and distally, most importantly the conversion of angiotensin I to angiotensin II by angiotensin-converting enzyme in the pulmonary endothelium [1]. Hormones that are produced via metabolism in the lung, such as angiotensin II, function as chemical messengers and exert their effects on other tissues, effecting the role of the lung as an endocrine organ [1,2]. The pulmonary endocrine system is comprised of a diverse population of cells located throughout the epithelium of the tracheobronchial tree and alveolar spaces [1].

CLASSIFICATION OF PULMONARY NEUROENDOCRINE TUMORS

In addition to effecting endocrine activity, cells within the pulmonary endocrine system have the potential transform into neoplasms. Pulmonary neoplasms may display a broad range of endocrine differentiation with varying clinical consequences. For example, some pulmonary tumors may demonstrate enough aberrant hormone secretion to produce a physiologic response that does not respond to normal negative feedback. Other pulmonary tumors have imperceptible endocrine differentiation, such as morphologically nonendocrine squamous and adenocarcinomas that express hormones [3]. Neuroendocrine tumors (NETs) of the lung are a distinct subset of lung cancers characterized by varying degrees of neuroendocrine morphologic, immunohistochemical, and ultrastructural features [4]. This category includes a wide spectrum of tumor types: low-grade typical carcinoid (TC), intermediate-grade atypical carcinoid (AC), and two high-grade tumors, large cell neuroendocrine carcinoma (LCNEC) and small cell lung carcinoma (SCLC) [2]. Accurate classification of NETs has immense prognostic significance. The grade of malignancy, with impact of worsening prognosis, increases in the following order: (1) TC,

(2) AC, and (3) LCNEC or SCLC [2]. LCNEC and SCLC portend a similar poor prognosis for patients with these types of tumors.

The World Health Organization (WHO) recommends the carcinoid nomenclature over terms such as *well-differentiated neuroendocrine carcinoma* because it provides continuity with established terminology familiar to clinicians [5]. In the 2004 WHO classification, TC and AC are categorized together under the heading of carcinoid tumors, LCNEC is a subtype of large cell carcinoma, and SCLC is in an independent category. Clinically, AC tumors behave similar to SCLC in terms of progression and prognosis.

The annual age-adjusted incidence of NETs in the United States in 2004 was 5.25 cases/100,000 persons, and the prevalence was 35/100,000 persons over the 24-year period between 1974 and 2003 in a large Surveillance, Epidemiology, and End Results (SEER) study [6], making these neoplasms significantly more common than esophageal, gastric, pancreatic, and hepatobiliary cancers [7].

CARCINOID TUMORS

Carcinoid tumors account for 1%–2% of invasive lung malignancies [8]. TCs represent 80%–90% of pulmonary carcinoids and are most frequently diagnosed in the fifth and sixth decades of life, but can occur at any age [9]. ACs are the rarest of lung NETs. Comprising approximately 10% of all carcinoids, they account for only 0.1%–0.2% of lung cancers [8].

Presentation, gross pathology, and histopathology

TC is defined as a tumor 0.5 cm or larger with carcinoid morphology and less than two mitoses per 2 mm high-power field (hpf), and lacking necrosis. A TC smaller than 0.5 cm is termed a "carcinoid tumorlet." AC encompass those neoplasms with carcinoid morphology and 2–10 mitoses per 2 mm hpf and/or the presence of necrosis. The necrosis is often characterized as punctate. Carcinoids can develop in the central or peripheral lung, with up to 40% presenting peripherally [10].

TCs present as well-demarcated but unencapsulated tumors. They are solitary endobronchial polyps, homogenous in texture and appearance, yellow or red-brown in color, and commonly between 2 and 5 cm in diameter at diagnosis. TC tumors usually reveal growth beneath cartilaginous plates. The epithelium overlying these tumors may be normal or show squamous metaplasia, but not dysplasia. These tumors have an indolent growth pattern that occurs over the course of many years. TC is characterized by a well-developed architecture, and the most common pattern of growth is insular, with relatively solid masses of cells neatly separated by fibrovascular stroma. Trabecular and acinar patterns of growth occasionally, but less commonly, occur. Papillary, spindle-cell, and clear-cell lesions are rare, and seen most often in peripheral tumors. Cells are uniform in size and shape, with an abundant cytoplasm that stains pale eosinophilic. The nuclei are small and centrally located, with a round or oval appearance [11].

AC typically presents in patients who are a decade older than those who develop TC, but causes similar symptoms and signs (which may include cough or wheeze, if endobronchial). Relative to TC tumors, ACs are often larger, more invasive, and more peripherally located [12]. ACs typically cause similar symptoms and signs to TC tumors, which may include cough or wheeze, if endobronchial. Broadly, AC is defined as any carcinoid tumor displaying mitotic activity, nuclear pleomorphism, and hyperchromasia or increased cellularity with architectural disorganization or necrosis. While some of these histopathological features are less useful in determining AC behavior, the loss of architectural organization and central necrosis of cell groups are recognized as diagnostic features of paramount importance. Crowding of cells is accompanied by palisading, and central necrosis is seen. Cellular pleomorphism is often a feature and sometimes accompanied by nuclei that are increased in size, elongated, and hyperchromatic [13].

Clinical and radiographic presentation

Central carcinoid tumors often present with signs and symptoms related to airway obstruction, including cough, recurrent pneumonia, wheezing, and hemoptysis. Many patients are treated for prolonged periods for asthma or infection. Any adult who presents with unilateral new wheeze should not be diagnosed with asthma without further investigation (imaging or bronchoscopy). Peripheral carcinoid tumors are usually discovered incidentally in patients without symptoms.

Several endocrine syndromes may be seen in patients with bronchopulmonary carcinoid tumors. Adrenocorticotropic hormone (ACTH) has been extensively studied as a secretory product of pulmonary tumors, and is occasionally produced by carcinoid tumors [13]. Cushing syndrome, which results from prolonged exposure to cortisol, occurs in approximately 4% of patients with bronchopulmonary carcinoid tumors. Bronchial carcinoids account for the most common source of ectopic ACTH production, and confirmed diagnosis of Cushing syndrome warrants a search for such a tumor. Carcinoids that result in Cushing syndrome are usually peripherally located, and approximately 80% are TC [14]. In most patients, the syndrome resolves after resection. Carcinoid syndrome, characterized by episodic flushing and diarrhea, is rare in patients with bronchopulmonary carcinoid tumors, occurring in less than 1% of patients at presentation and in less than 5% during the subsequent course. True carcinoid syndrome is almost exclusively seen in patients with liver metastases [14].

Approximately 70% of carcinoid tumors present as central tumors, defined as visible by bronchoscopy. Most are located in segmental bronchi, specifically within the right middle lobe and lingula. Carcinoid tumors are rarely located in the central airways. Central carcinoid lesions do not have a distinctive radiographic appearance, but atelectasis and postobstructive pneumonia/pneumonitis are often visible. Central carcinoids are predominantly TC. Node enlargement is less common in central carcinoids; however, it may be difficult to distinguish reactive lymphadenopathy that develops in response to postobstructive pneumonia from malignancy-containing nodes. Peripheral carcinoid tumors generally appear as sharply demarcated, round, homogenous masses situated deeply within the parenchyma. Approximately one-third of peripheral carcinoid tumors are AC, and are more likely to metastasize to the hilar or mediastinal lymph nodes. Computed tomography (CT) with intravenous (IV) contrast may elucidate hilar anatomy and lymphadenopathy, and in the setting of a peripheral carcinoid that should not prompt postobstructive pneumonia, adenopathy is more likely to represent lymph node metastases [15].

Surgery

Surgical resection is recommended for isolated pulmonary carcinoids, regardless of location, from tracheobronchial to the lung periphery. The prognosis for resection of TC is quite good, with 82% 10-year survival in Wilkins's series of a 50-year experience at the Massachusetts General Hospital [16], as well as in a modern Australian series [17]. Most surgeons advocate a parenchymal-sparing approach when possible, which may mandate sleeve resection (bronchus, carina, or even trachea) to preserve lung for tumors that are central. Peripheral carcinoids can be managed with sublobar resection, including segmentectomy or wedge resection, with good results, as supported by a recent SEER database evaluation of 3270 pulmonary carcinoid patients, in which sublobar resection compared well to lobectomy when assessed for noninferiority in multivariable analysis [18].

SMALL CELL LUNG CARCINOMA

SCLC occurs predominantly in the seventh and eighth decades of life and represents <20% of all lung cancers. SCLC represents a higher proportion of lung cancers developing in patients less than 40 years of age. While SCLC is more common in men than in women, the size of the difference in incidence between the sexes has diminished in recent years [19].

Presentation, gross pathology, and histopathology

Most SCLCs arise in major bronchi as invasive, partly necrotic, grey-white masses. Symptoms and signs are commonly due to growth of these lesions, their metastases, or in approximately 10% of patients, the effects of ectopic hormone production [20].

SLCL is sometimes referred to as "oat cell carcinoma" because the neoplastic cells resemble oat grains. The cells appear round or somewhat fusiform, with an extremely high nuclear-to-cytoplasmic ratio. In most cases, the cytoplasm is nearly imperceptible. The nucleus contains uniformly dispersed fine or stippled "salt and pepper" chromatin, and inconspicuous nucleoli. Nucleoli may be obscured when nuclei are particularly hyperchromatic. Mitoses are generally abundant, but they may also be partially obscured by hyperchromasia. Cells may coalesce around blood vessels, forming a "pseudorosette." "Cushing" phenomenon, the distortion of groups of cells that coalesce and smear, and necrosis are both characteristic of SCLC [20]. SCLC may be associated with various paraneoplastic syndromes, including hyponatremia due to the syndrome of inappropriate antidiuretic hormone (SIADH), Cushing syndrome due to ectopic ACTH production, and Eaton–Lambert syndrome due to autoantibodies affecting the voltage-gated calcium channels in the presynaptic membranes of the neuromuscular junction.

Clinical and radiographic presentation

Although most patients presenting with SCLC have metastases at the time of presentation, symptoms are most often due to local effects of growth of the primary tumor, such as cough, dyspnea, pain, hemoptysis, and respiratory infection. Most patients with SCLC present with bulky hilar or mediastinal lymphadenopathy [20]. The primary tumor is usually central, and peripheral tumors are distinctly rare. As SCLCs are highly metabolically active and metastasis is common, fluorodeoxy-glucose positron emission tomography (PET)-CT is indicated to diagnose nodal or distant metastases for staging [15]. Given the propensity toward brain metastasis, brain magnetic resonance imaging (MRI) or CT of the head with and without IV contrast (for patients who cannot undergo MRI) is necessary to evaluate the brain due to limitations of PET-CT in diagnosing brain metastasis. Unlike non-small cell lung cancer (NSCLC), SCLC is staged as limited (confined to the ipsilateral hemithorax and regional nodes that may be included in a standard radiation port) or extensive (distant metastatic disease or contralateral hilar or supraclavicular nodal involvement).

Surgery

Historically, SCLC is considered a nonoperative disease. Early randomized studies suggested no benefit to surgery over radiation or chemotherapy alone. The Medical Research Council trial published in 1973 evaluated patients with SCLC involving the bronchus, and complete resection was performed in only 34 of 71 (48%) patients [21]. The Lung Cancer Study Group, Eastern Cooperative Oncology Group, and European Organization for Research and Treatment of Cancer published an intergroup trial in 1994, which randomized patients with limited SCLC who had responded to five cycles of chemotherapy (cyclophosphamide, doxorubicin, and vincristine) to surgery or no surgery, but again, these included only patients who had bronchoscopically visible disease. While most of the surgical patients (54 of 70, 77%) underwent complete resection, 35 (50%) of surgical patients had clinical ipsilateral mediastinal nodal disease (N2), 24 (34%) had pathologic N2 disease, and 12 (17%) were unresectable at the time of surgery [22]. Neither of these studies demonstrating lack of benefit of surgery in "limited" SCLC included patients with early SCLC as defined by modern-day staging techniques, including PET-CT, brain MRI, and endobronchial ultrasound (EBUS) or mediastinoscopy for nodal evaluation.

Resection should be considered for early-stage SCLC. Early-stage SCLC comprises a small proportion of an already rare entity. Ten to fifteen percent of lung cancers are SCLC, and only 3%–7% of these patients present with limited-stage disease, as concluded in a SEER database study of all patients diagnosed with lung cancer between 1988 and 2005 and followed for at least 3 months [23]. Resection offers benefit for tumors that prove to be combined or mixed SCLC/NSCLC (10%–30% of SCLC cases). Additionally, resection offers the best local control in limited disease. The same SEER database analysis [23] found lobectomy alone (47% 5-year overall survival) to be superior to radiation therapy (17% 5-year overall survival), which was significant on a multivariable analysis (hazard ratio [HR] = 0.56; 95% confidence interval [CI] 0.41–0.76). Other studies have demonstrated similar survival for lobectomy in limited-stage SCLC [24]. The National Comprehensive Cancer Network currently recommends lobectomy with mediastinal nodal sampling or dissection for patients with disease equivalent to clinical NSCLC stage I disease (small tumors, no nodal involvement, and no metastases), to be followed by adjuvant chemotherapy, even if nodes are pathologically negative [25]. Patients treated with complete resection should be considered for prophylactic whole brain irradiation following adjuvant chemotherapy if performance status and neurocognitive function are not impaired, given the high propensity of SCLC to metastasize to the brain.

LARGE CELL NEUROENDOCRINE CARCINOMA

LCNEC of the lung is a relatively uncommon and aggressive subset of NSCLC. LCNEC was first reported in 1991 as a separate category of pulmonary NETs [26]. The prognosis of patients with LCNEC is poorer than expected for stage-matched patients with NSCLC and similar to that of those with SCLC. Reported 5-year survival rates for LCNEC range between 15% and 60% [27].

Presentation, gross pathology, and histopathology

LCNEC is characterized by a population of large cells with abundant cytoplasm and distinct cytoplasmic membranes [21]. LCNEC tumors have cells that are at least three times the size of those in SCLC, with an organoid growth pattern, cellular palisading or rosette-like areas, a high mitotic rate, and a variably granular chromatin pattern [28]. Mitotic activity is the most important criterion to establish tumor type. LCNECs are not generally associated with paraneoplastic syndromes, although paraneoplastic syndromes and ectopic hormone production have been observed and occasionally reported [29]. Endocrine differentiation can be detected by electron microscopy or immunohistochemistry [30].

Clinical and radiographic presentation

LCNEC generally presents as a peripheral tumor, in contrast to the central carcinoid and SCLC sites [30]. As a result, patients with LCNEC are usually asymptomatic. On CT imaging, LCNECs often manifest as a well-defined and lobulated nodule or mass, similar to other rapidly growing lesions, such as peripheral SCLC, poorly differentiated adenocarcinomas, and squamous cell carcinomas [30].

THYMIC CARCINOIDS

Thymic neuroendocrine tumors (TNETs) are rare and account for approximately 2%–5% of all thymic tumors [31]. In the 2004 WHO classification, TNETs are included in the thymic carcinoma group, and are classified into four entities in two major histopathologic types: well-differentiated neuroendocrine carcinomas (also called typical and AC) and poorly differentiated neuroendocrine carcinomas (small cell carcinoma and LCNEC) [32]. Nearly 50% of these tumors can be accompanied by endocrine manifestations, either from ectopic ACTH production or from other hormone production related to associated endocrine tumors if accompanied by multiple endocrine neoplasia type 1 (MEN-1) [32]. Up to 25% of patients with a thymic NET also have MEN-1, and among patients with MEN-1, 3%–8% may develop a thymic NET [31]. Nearly all cases of NET associated with MEN-1 occur in male smokers [31]. The peak incidence of NET is in the fifth decade [32].

TNETs closely resemble well-differentiated AC tumors of the lung in their histologic appearance and behavior [31]. The clinical behavior of a TNET correlates with the degree of histologic differentiation [31]. One-third of patients are asymptomatic, and the lesions may be discovered incidentally during imaging surveillance in MEN-1 patients. Distant metastases are often present at the time of diagnosis [31]. Symptoms may result from displacement or compression of mediastinal structures, associated endocrinopathies, or distant metastases. Symptoms vary according to the extent of the disease, and may include cough, dyspnea, chest pain, superior vena cava syndrome, and hoarseness due to recurrent laryngeal nerve involvement [33]. Endocrinopathy due to ectopic hormonal hypersecretion may involve ACTH (Cushing syndrome in 10% of patients) or growth hormone-releasing hormone (causing acromegaly and hypertrophic osteoarthropathy) [33].

Diagnosis of a TNET may be made on plain-film chest X-ray or CT. Somatostatin receptor scintigraphy (octreotide scan) may be used in selected cases, particularly those with ectopic hormone production [33]. PET-CT may often effect false-negative results (as tumors may be hormonally, but not metabolically, active). PET-CT may demonstrate avidity in more aggressive tumors, suggesting high proliferation rate, or if performed with gallium-DOTATATE [33]. Contrast-enhanced CT or MRI is recommended to detect possible invasion of nearby mediastinal structures. Diagnosis is confirmed pathologically, ideally with histologic exam and immunohistochemical neuroendocrine marker detection. While fine-needle aspirate or core needle biopsy may be adequate, biopsy may require anterior mediastinotomy or mediastinoscopy (Chamberlain procedure) or even excision via sternotomy, thoracoscopy, or thoracotomy [33].

Whenever feasible, a localized TNET without metastasis should be managed with radical surgical resection [33]. Due to high rates of recurrence, ongoing surveillance is required indefinitely for patients postoperatively [33]. High rates of local recurrence portend poor prognosis in this aggressive tumor. Patients with low-grade TNETs demonstrate 5- and 10-year survival rates of 50% and 9%, respectively. The 5-year survival for patients with high-grade TNETs is zero. Locally advanced or metastatic disease is best managed with multidisciplinary treatment as indicated (with some combination of chemotherapy, surgery, and radiation). Resection of the primary tumor along with resectable mediastinal structures, if involved, is performed. For large tumors, median sternotomy with or without extension into an anterior thoracotomy ("hemiclamshell" incision) is appropriate [33]. Induction chemotherapy followed by surgical resection, if there is good response, is considered even for metastatic TNET, although chemotherapy regimens demonstrate little impact in this disease. Radioresponsiveness of these tumors is likewise quite poor. TNET may metastasize to the mediastinal lymph nodes or to distant sites (bone, liver, and skin) in 30%–40% patients [33]. Symptomatic metastatic disease confined to the liver may be treated with embolization, radiofrequency ablation, or radioembolization. External beam radiation may be considered for brain and bone metastases, particularly if symptomatic [33].

CONCLUSION

The lung serves vital endocrine functions in addition to its role as a filter and site of gas exchange. Endocrine cells within the lung may transform into neoplasms, and neoplasms that develop in the lung may impart a host of hormone-related effects. NETs of the lung vary in aggressiveness from the well-behaved TC, associated with favorable prognosis, to the often metastatic small cell carcinoma and large cell NETs associated with low rates of long-term survival. TNETs are rare and are often associated with other endocrinopathies, including MEN-1. Management of pulmonary NETs and TNETs depends on the tumor biology and extent of disease, but regardless, a thorough understanding of the endocrine, metabolic, and pathologic characteristics of these entities is mandated for treating these patients.

REFERENCES

1. Gosney JR. *Pulmonary Endocrine Pathology: Endocrine Cells and Endocrine Tumors of the Lung.* Oxford: Butterworth-Heinemann, 1992:1.
2. Asamura H, Kameya T, Matsuno Y et al. Neuroendocrine neoplasms of the lung: A prognostic spectrum. *J Clin Oncol* 2006;24:72.
3. Gosney JR. *Pulmonary Endocrine Pathology: Endocrine Cells and Endocrine Tumors of the Lung.* Oxford: Butterworth-Heinemann, 1992:83.
4. Beasley MB, Brambilla E, Travis WD. The 2004 World Health Organization classification of lung tumors. *Semin Roentgenol* 2005;40:90.
5. Travis WD, Brambilla E, Muller-Hermelink HK, Harris CC, eds. *Pathology and Genetics of Tumours of the Lung, Pleura, Thymus and Heart.* Lyon: International Agency for Research on Cancer, 2004.
6. Yao JC, Phan A, Dagohoy C et al. One hundred years after "carcinoid": Epidemiology of and prognostic factors for neuroendocrine tumors in 35,825 cases in the United States. *J Clin Oncol* 2008;26:3063–72.
7. Filosso PL, Guerrera F, Evangelista A et al. Prognostic model of survival for typical bronchial carcinoid tumours: Analysis of 1109 patients on behalf of the European Society of Thoracic Surgeons (ESTS) Neuroendocrine Tumours Working Group. *Eur J Cardiothorac Surg* 2015;48:441–7.
8. Travis WB. Pathology and diagnosis of neuroendocrine tumors: Lung neuroendocrine. *Thorac Surg Clin* 2014;24:257.
9. Meisinger QC, Klein JS, Butnor KJ, Gentchos G, Leavitt BJ. CT features of peripheral pulmonary carcinoid tumors. *AJR Am J Roentgenol* 2011;197:1073.
10. Travis WB. Pathology and diagnosis of neuroendocrine tumors: Lung neuroendocrine. *Thorac Surg Clin* 2014;24:258.
11. Gosney JR. *Pulmonary Endocrine Pathology: Endocrine Cells and Endocrine Tumors of the Lung.* Oxford: Butterworth-Heinemann, 1992:111.
12. Gosney JR. *Pulmonary Endocrine Pathology: Endocrine Cells and Endocrine Tumors of the Lung.* Oxford: Butterworth-Heinemann, 1992:110.
13. Gosney JR. *Pulmonary Endocrine Pathology: Endocrine Cells and Endocrine Tumors of the Lung.* Oxford: Butterworth-Heinemann, 1992:116.
14. Detterbeck FC. Clinical presentation and evaluation of neuroendocrine tumors of the lung. *Thorac Surg Clin* 2014;24:267.
15. Detterbeck FC. Clinical presentation and evaluation of neuroendocrine tumors of the lung. *Thorac Surg Clin* 2014;24:269.
16. Wilkins EW Jr, Grillo HC, Moncure AC et al. Changing times in surgical management of bronchopulmonary carcinoid tumor. *Ann Thorac Surg* 1984;38:339–44.

17. Cao C, Yan TD, Kennedy C et al. Bronchopulmonary carcinoid tumors: long-term outcomes after resection. *Ann Thorac Surg* 2011;91:339–43.
18. Fox M, Van Berkel V, Bousamra M 2nd et al. Surgical management of pulmonary carcinoid tumors: Sublobar resection versus lobectomy. *Am J Surg* 2013;205:200–8.
19. Gosney JR. *Pulmonary Endocrine Pathology: Endocrine Cells and Endocrine Tumors of the Lung.* Oxford: Butterworth-Heinemann, 1992:117.
20. Gosney JR. *Pulmonary Endocrine Pathology: Endocrine Cells and Endocrine Tumors of the Lung.* Oxford: Butterworth-Heinemann, 1992:119.
21. Fox W, Scadding JG. Medical Research Council comparative trial of surgery and radiotherapy for primary treatment of small-celled or oat-celled carcinoma of bronchus. Ten-year follow-up. *Lancet* 1973;2:63–5.
22. Lad T, Piantadosi S, Thomas P et al. A prospective randomized trial to determine the benefit of surgical resection of residual disease following response of small cell lung cancer to combination chemotherapy. *Chest* 1994;106:320S–323S.
23. Varlotto JM, Recht A, Flickinger JC et al. Lobectomy leads to optimal survival in early-stage small cell lung cancer: A retrospective analysis. *J Thorac Cardiovasc Surg* 2011;142:538–46.
24. Vallieres E, Shepherd FA, Crowley J et al. The IASLC lung cancer staging project: Proposals regarding the relevance of TNM in the pathologic staging of small cell lung cancer in the forthcoming (seventh) edition of the TNM classification for lung cancer. *J Thorac Oncol* 2009;4:1049–59.
25. NCCN. Guidelines. In: http://www.nccn.org/professionals/physician_gls/pdf/scic.pdf; 2013.
26. Sakurai H, Maeshima A, Watanabe S et al. Grade of stromal invasion in small adenocarcinoma of the lung: histopathological minimal invasion and prognosis. *Am J Surg Pathol* 2004;28:198–206.
27. Sakurai H. Large-cell neuroendocrine carcinoma of the lung: Surgical management. *Thorac Surg Clin* 2014;24:305.
28. Battafarano RJ. Large cell neuroendocrine carcinoma: An aggressive form of non–small cell lung cancer. *J Thorac Cardiovasc Surg* 2005;130:166.
29. Detterbeck FC. Clinical presentation and evaluation of neuroendocrine tumors of the lung. *Thorac Surg Clin* 2014;24:268.
30. Sakurai H. Large-cell neuroendocrine carcinoma of the lung: Surgical management. *Thorac Surg Clin* 2014;24:306.
31. Lausi PO, Refai M, Filosso PH et al. Thymic neuroendocrine tumors. *Thorac Surg Clin* 2014;24:327.
32. Filosso PL, Yao X, Ahmad U et al. Outcome of primary neuroendocrine tumors of the thymus: A joint analysis of the International Thymic Malignancy Interest Group and the European Society of Thoracic Surgeons databases. *J Thorac Cardiovasc Surg* 2015;149:103.
33. Lausi PO, Refai M, Filosso PH et al. Thymic neuroendocrine tumors. *Thorac Surg Clin* 2014;24:328.

BIBLIOGRAPHY

Asamura H, Kameya T, Matsuno Y et al. Neuroendocrine neoplasms of the lung: A prognostic spectrum. *J Clin Oncol* 2006;24:70–6.

Battafarano RJ, Fernandez FG, Ritter J et al. Large cell neuroendocrine carcinoma: An aggressive form of non–small cell lung cancer. *J Thorac Cardiovasc Surg* 2005;130:166–72.

Detterbeck FC. Clinical presentation and evaluation of neuroendocrine tumors of the lung. *Thorac Surg Clin* 2014;24:267–76.

Ferone D, Albertelli M. Ectopic Cushing and other paraneoplastic syndromes in thoracic neuroendocrine tumors. *Thorac Surg Clin* 2014;24:277–83.

Filosso PL, Yao X, Ahmad U et al. Outcome of primary neuroendocrine tumors of the thymus: A joint analysis of the International Thymic Malignancy Interest Group and the European Society of Thoracic Surgeons databases. *J Thorac Cardiovasc Surg* 2015;149:103–9.

Filosso PL, Guerrera F, Evangelista A et al. Prognostic model of survival for typical bronchial carcinoid tumours: Analysis of 1109 patients on behalf of the European Society of Thoracic Surgeons (ESTS) Neuroendocrine Tumours Working Group. *Eur J Cardiothorac Surg* 2015;48:441–7.

Gosney JR. *Pulmonary Endocrine Pathology: Endocrine Cells and Endocrine Tumors of the Lung.* Oxford: Butterworth-Heinemann, 1992.

Lausi PO, Refai M, Filosso PL et al. Thymic neuroendocrine tumors. *Thorac Surg Clin* 2014;24:327–32.

Travis WD, Brambilla E, Muller-Hermelink HK, Harris CC, eds. *Pathology and Genetics of Tumours of the Lung, Pleura, Thymus and Heart.* Lyon: International Agency for Research on Cancer, 2004.

Travis WD. Pathology and diagnosis of neuroendocrine tumors: Lung neuroendocrine. *Thorac Surg Clin* 2014;24:257–66.

World Health Organization. World cancer report 2014. Geneva: World Health Organization, 2014: chapter 5.1.

PART 3

Thyroid

Physiology and testing of thyroid function

TERRY F. DAVIES

INTRODUCTION

The safe patient for surgery is the euthyroid patient. Although urgent surgery on unstable thyroid patients can produce good results, it is everyone's experience that the risk of surgery is increased in those who are dysthyroid. It is therefore critical to the surgeon that the patient about to undergo surgery has as normal thyroid function as possible. Hence, an understanding of thyroid physiology and thyroid function testing is a great asset to every surgeon and especially an endocrine surgeon.

The normal thyroid gland is under the control of the pituitary thyroid-stimulating hormone (TSH) (Figure 5.1). Understanding this relationship is the key to understanding thyroid physiology. The pituitary gland controls the output of thyroid hormones via TSH. The thyroid hormones then exert their influence via a classical loop at the level of the hypothalamus and pituitary, to suppress the release of TSH-releasing hormone (TRH) and TSH. Hence, knowing the patient has a normal amount of easily measured serum TSH is often the only "comfort information" a surgeon will find necessary for reassurance.

THYROID HORMONE SYNTHESIS

Thyroid hormones are necessary for the essential metabolism of almost all cells; their excessive or diminished levels have a marked influence on cell function. Thyroid hormone synthesis is localized to the thyroid follicular cells and takes place on the surface of the thyroglobulin (Tg) molecule; thyroxine (T4) and a small amount of diiodothyronine (T3) are subsequently released from the basal side of these cells into the circulation at the same time as Tg is released (https://www.youtube.com/watch?v=uCjpGlnCjeA). However, most T3 is obtained from T4 by 5′-deiodinase enzymes, found in peripheral tissues (Table 5.1, Figure 5.2). This process of deiodination is essential since T4 is biologically inactive; T3 is the true thyroid hormone that binds to a thyroid hormone receptor (TR). Any interruption in the hypothalamic–pituitary–thyroid axis, or any deficiency (e.g., in the availability of iodide), will cause problems with thyroid hormone availability.

ROLE OF IODIDE

Iodide is essential for the production of thyroid hormones; it has been estimated that 100–150 µg of iodine a day is required. This mostly comes from the diet, especially with the introduction of the iodination of salt, bread, and milk, giving total intakes of approximately 300–700 µg/day. Inorganic iodine is transported into the thyroid cells by an iodide transporter, which acts like a pump exchanging iodide for sodium (the sodium iodide symporter, or NIS). This transporter is under the control of TSH. However, NIS is not confined to the thyroid gland; it is also present in salivary glands, gastric mucosa, and mammary glands [1].

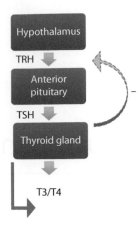

Figure 5.1 Pituitary–thyroid axis. This diagram illustrates the positive influence of the hypothalamus via TRH and the negative influence of thyroid hormone on the pituitary. Thyroid hormone also has some inhibitory influence on TRH.

These sites are often seen on high-dose whole-body radio-iodine scans used in the investigation of thyroid cancer. The physiological role of these extrathyroidal iodide pumps remains unclear.

Total intake of iodine is of particular concern for pregnant women because of the increased turnover of iodide in pregnancy. However, iodine deficiency remains a major health problem only in those parts of the world where the diet is poor in iodine and where there has been no iodization of salt [2]. Severe iodine deficiency may lead to reduced thyroid hormone synthesis and thus to chronic hypothyroidism. This reduces the negative feedback at the pituitary and hypothalamus, resulting in a rise in TSH output. With continuing failure of thyroid hormone feedback, there will be a persistently increased TSH level, which will lead the TSH to induce the development of thyroid nodules, causing multinodular goiters seen so commonly in the developing world. The World Health Organization (WHO) and others have exerted considerable effort to combat iodine deficiency with its consequences to the children of hypothyroid mothers. The effects include not only overt cretinism caused by lack of maternal thyroid hormone during critical periods of brain formation, but also markedly reduced intelligence in large numbers of the population where maternal iodine deficiency is less severe [3], and similar outcomes have been seen in women with pathological thyroid failure and inadequate thyroid hormone replacement [4]. This has been, and continues to be, a major public health problem.

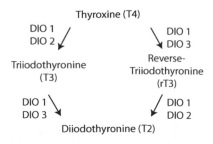

Figure 5.2 Thyroid hormone degradation. The degradation of T4 and T3 and reverse T3 (rT3) is illustrated under the influence of the different deiodinase (DIO) enzymes D1, D2, and D3.

THYROGLOBULIN

With a dimeric molecular weight of 660,000 kDa, Tg is the second largest gene in the human genome. It is the major secretion of the thyroid follicular cell and is exported through the apical membrane to be stored as colloid in the center of the follicle (Figure 5.3). Prior to storage and

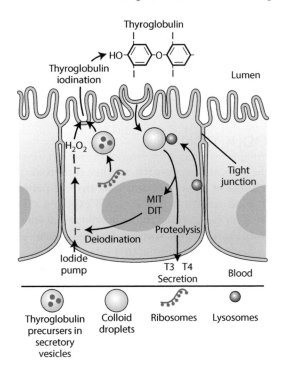

Figure 5.3 Tg and iodide transport through the thyroid cell. Thyroid hormones are formed on the surface of the Tg molecule.

Table 5.1 Deiodinase enzymes

	Type I	Type II	Type III
Location	Liver, kidney, thyroid	CNS, pituitary, placenta, brown	Placenta, CNS, skin
Substrate	rT3 > sulfated thyronines > T4 > T3	T4 > rT3 > T3	T4 ≥ rT3
PTU	Inhibits	No effect	No effect
Selenium	Present	Absent	Absent
Km for T4	High	Low	Low

Note: PTU = propyl thiouracil; Km = affinity.

at the apical membrane, iodination of Tg occurs, forming the thyroid hormones. Under TSH stimulation, Tg loaded with thyroid hormones is withdrawn from the colloid and taken into the thyroid cell by endocytosis, forming colloid droplets within the cell cytoplasm. These droplets fuse with lysosomes, leading to degradation of Tg and release of thyroid hormones. The complex is then transported to the basal membrane, where thyroid hormones and Tg are released into the circulation, once again under the influence of TSH. Any released iodide is largely recycled within the cell.

THYROID HORMONE CONSTRUCTION

Thyroid hormones are synthesized from iodide, under the control of TSH, in reactions that occur on the backbone of Tg using a highly effective and immunogenic enzyme called thyroid peroxidase (TPO). Synthesis takes place at specific iodination sites on Tg and consists of binding of iodide to specific tyrosyl residues to form iodotyrosyls, which are then coupled to form iodothyronines. T4 results from the combination of two diiodotyrosines (DITs, or T2), and T3 results from the union of monoiodotyrosine (MIT, or T1) and one DIT. Only in cases of iodine deficiency is more thyroidal T3 made than T4. As described earlier, the thyroid hormone-loaded Tg is then stored in the colloid of the thyroid follicle. TSH induces this synthesis of thyroid hormones and also induces synthesis of Tg itself. Colloidal Tg is taken back into the thyroid cell and exported at its base into the bloodstream (Figure 5.3). It is easy to see that in addition to disease of the thyroid, interruption in the pituitary TSH control of the thyroid or a shortage of iodide may compromise the synthetic ability of the thyroid cell.

RELEASE AND METABOLISM OF THYROID HORMONES

Pituitary TSH induces the resorption of stored and iodinated Tg from the colloid and also its transportation from the apical to the basal surface of the thyroid follicular cell (Figure 5.3). During this transport, T4 and a smaller amount of T3 are released from the Tg molecule and then released into the circulation. Hence, thyroid hormone levels are a balance between the amount released by the thyroid gland and the amount circulating in the tissues, especially the liver and kidney. Most thyroid hormone released from the thyroid gland is T4, and this undergoes peripheral deiodination to T3, as described earlier (Figure 5.2). Peripheral deiodination of T4 is best understood by considering T4 as a prohormone and T3 as the active hormone. The T4 is converted to T3 by a widely available family of enzymes called the 5′-deiodinases (Table 5.1). T3, therefore, is mainly produced from T4 in the tissues, where it is then available for action. Recent data indicate that an intrathyroidal deiodinase enzyme can also influence the ratio of T4 to T3 released by the gland. In addition, T3 may be inactivated by further deiodination and the

formation of sulfate conjugates, or by the generation of acetic acid analogs. Similarly, the production of inactive reverse T3 also helps regulate circulating T3 levels.

MECHANISM OF ACTION OF THYROID HORMONES

Thyroid hormones act on nearly every cell in the body. They increase the basal metabolic rate, affect protein synthesis, help regulate bone growth and maturation of the nervous system, and increase the body's sensitivity to catecholamines. The thyroid hormones are, therefore, essential for proper development and differentiation of all cells of the human body. These hormones also regulate protein, fat, and carbohydrate metabolism, affecting how cells use energy. In addition, many physiological and pathological influences affect thyroid hormone synthesis.

Unbound, free T4, and free T3 cross the cell membrane; the T4 is deiodinated to T3; and all the T3 then binds to intracellular T3 receptors, which are located in the cell nucleus and act as transcription factors in a complex network of influences on the genes that regulate cell growth, differentiation, and energy release, among other actions (Figure 5.4) [5]. Four T3 nuclear receptors have been well characterized and designated α1, α2, β1, and β2 isoforms. The β2 receptors are unique to the pituitary gland and central to the phenomenon of TSH suppression by thyroid hormone feedback. The other isoforms are widely distributed, and their varying proportions help explain the different influences of thyroid hormone on multiple tissues. Knocking out these receptors in the mouse has provided important information on thyroid hormone action. For example, the α1 receptor is thought to be important in the influence of thyroid hormone on the heart. In addition, mutations in the thyroid hormone β receptors have helped explain the rare syndrome of thyroid hormone resistance, which may vary from mildly abnormal thyroid function tests to reduced growth and mental retardation, as well as hypothyroidism [6].

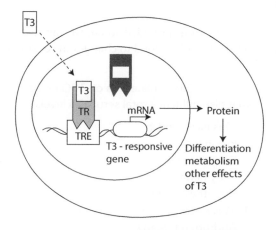

Figure 5.4 Thyroid hormone action. T3 binds to its nuclear receptor (TR), which binds to a thyroid hormone response element (TRE) to influence the activity of RNA polymerase on a T3-responsive gene.

SERUM BINDING OF THYROID HORMONES

It is critically important to understand that thyroid hormones circulate in the blood in two forms—bound and free. Thyroid hormones are bound primarily to serum thyroxine-binding globulin (TBG), but also to other circulating liver proteins, such as transthyretin (TTR), lipoproteins, and albumin. This binding is noncovalent and reversible, but only 0.03% of T4 and 0.3% of T3 is unbound and available as free thyroid hormone (called free T4 and free T3). These free levels are reached by equilibration following changes in the levels of thyroid hormone or binding proteins. All measurements of thyroid hormone must therefore be identified as measurements of serum total or free hormone. Lastly, because much more of T4 than T3 binds to serum protein, the half-life of T4 is much longer (7 days) than that of T3 (1 day), and so serum T3 levels are subject to much more rapid changes than those of T4.

Many factors influence the concentration of TBG, to which 80% of T4 is bound (Table 5.2). For example, estrogen increases TBG levels by enhancing synthesis and altering TBG glycosylation in such a way that the half-life of TBG is prolonged, and therefore more T4 is bound up and total T4 increases. Recent data remind us that even oral contraceptive pills may result in an increase in TBG significant enough such that T4 supplementation may need to be increased in hypothyroid patients. Because there are many influences on the level of thyroid-binding proteins, the measurement of total T4 and total T3 levels must be corrected for the level of serum-binding protein. This results in the expression of T4-to-TBG ratios in varying forms, and hence the increasing preference by physicians for direct or indirect measurements of free T4 [7].

THYROID FUNCTION TESTING

Pituitary–thyroid axis and the response of serum TSH to changes in thyroid hormone levels

From the explanations provided so far, we can deduce that serum TSH levels will respond to changes in serum thyroid

Table 5.2 Some influences on TBG levels that also influence total serum T4 levels

TBG is increased in
    Pregnancy
    Estrogen therapy
    Early hepatitis
    Hypothyroidism
TBG is decreased in
    Androgen therapy
    Hyperthyroidism
    Liver failure
    Renal failure

hormone levels (Figure 5.1). An increased T4 level will lead to increased T3 levels within the TSH-secreting cells of the anterior pituitary after 5′-deiodination by Type II deiodinase. The T3 will then bind to an α2 intracellular TR, which acts as a transcription factor, and the complex will then bind to a thyroid response element (TRE) in the 5′ region of the TSH-β gene. This binding acts in a negative manner, suppressing gene transcription and leading to decreased TSH synthesis and release. A similar phenomenon is employed to control TRH release in the hypothalamus. At the opposite extreme, a lack of T4 will mean less T3 available to bind to its receptor and fewer complexes binding to the TREs. Hence, less negative regulation will lead to increased TSH synthesis and release. This so-called "feedback control" has allowed the measurement of serum TSH levels to be developed as the most sensitive and useful thyroid function test, with suppressed TSH levels indicating hyperthyroidism and raised TSH levels as evidence of hypothyroidism. Nevertheless, any changes in serum TSH should always be confirmed with thyroid hormone measurements.

Measurement of serum TSH

The wide availability of rapid and highly sensitive immunoassays for the measurement of serum TSH has transformed thyroid function testing into a logical area of understanding and greatly reduced the need for additional T4 and T3 testing in the majority of patients with normal TSH results. Today, TSH assays have a sensitivity of <0.01 μU/mL and are able to detect a change well before T4 or T3 changes can be determined. Hence, these TSH assays allow the clear diagnosis of even mild thyroid dysfunction, which we define as an abnormal TSH level with normal T4 and T3 levels. In the absence of obvious pituitary disease, the serum TSH will increase in thyroid failure (>4.0 μU/mL) and be markedly decreased in the presence of an overactive thyroid gland (>0.1 μU/mL). The former may be confirmed with a free T4 assay, and the latter with both free T4 and T3 assays. However, as discussed, mild thyroid disease may present with only changes in TSH, while thyroid hormone levels remain within the normal range (also called subclinical disease).

Total T4 and free T4

The measurement of total T4 remains the easiest thyroid function test to perform and is still an important part of our investigative armamentarium. It is essential to try to confirm a high TSH with a measurement indicating a low T4 level since this allows the distinction between mild (normal T4) and significant (low T4) thyroid failure. However, the disadvantage of total T4 measurement is that a correction must be applied for the level of serum-binding proteins. This can be made in a variety of ways, including the direct measurement of TBG. More commonly, a free T4 measurement may be derived directly from increasingly popular binding tests now available on many automatic analyzers or by the classical dialysis method. The latter, however, is an expensive technique and should be reserved for very extreme situations when TBG is very high or very low, causing the derived methods of estimating free T4 to be unreliable [7].

Total T3 and free T3

After serum TSH measurement, serum T3 levels can be a useful confirmation of an overactive thyroid gland. Less T3 is bound to the serum-binding proteins than T4, and therefore the measurement of total T3 is not as greatly affected by changes in protein binding, as is total T4. However, it remains helpful to know that there are no major binding protein changes when the total T3 level is abnormal, although in practice, free T3 levels are not often needed and the assays are less satisfactory.

Radioiodine scanning versus sonography

The scanning of the thyroid gland using radioiodine (either 125I or 131I) has been largely superseded by real-time sonography performed most efficiently by the physician or surgeon, rather than by a technician. When the serum TSH is suppressed, a thyroid nodule or multinodular gland must have active nodular tissue ("hot") secreting thyroid hormone causing the TSH suppression. When the TSH is normal, the gland is most likely to harbor predominantly underactive nodules ("cold"), with the euthyroid state maintained by the remaining normal tissue. Sonography gives the identification and sizing of thyroid nodules in a manner far superior to any scanning procedure. The major uses of radioiodine scanning today, therefore, are to confirm the presence of a hot nodule and to detect small residual thyroid cancer metastases after total thyroidectomy. In contrast, 24-hour radioiodine uptake measurements remain frequently used to differentiate chemical hyperthyroidism secondary to thyroiditis (no uptake due to cellular destruction) from hyperthyroidism caused by Graves' disease (normal or increased uptake induced by thyroid-stimulating antibodies).

Measuring serum thyroglobulin

Most thyroid diseases cause an increase in serum Tg levels, making it an unreliable measurement of thyroid dysfunction. However, the thyroid gland is the major source of serum Tg, and therefore the measurement of serum Tg has become a clinically useful test for the presence of residual thyroid tissue. This is particularly valuable in the follow-up of patients with thyroid cancer who have been treated by total thyroidectomy followed by radioiodine ablation to remove the presence of all residual thyroid tissue. Under such circumstances, the persistence or development of serum Tg indicates the persistence of residual thyroid tissue. Furthermore, if the serum Tg rises while the patient is receiving thyroid hormone replacement (maintaining a low TSH level), then this is indicative of metastatic disease. In addition, significant residual metastatic disease can be stimulated to secrete Tg in thyroid cancer patients using recombinant human TSH ("Thyrogen") [8]. This can be performed while the patient remains on thyroid hormone suppression, avoiding the unpleasant prolonged withdrawal of thyroid hormone in order to raise endogenous TSH, which is needed for Tg stimulation.

Thyroid autoantibody testing

Thyroid antibody testing does not help the assessment of thyroid function. Such tests are used only in the diagnosis and prediction of autoimmune thyroid disease (Graves' disease and Hashimoto's thyroiditis). The most commonly measured thyroid antibodies are those to the enzyme thyroid peroxidase (anti-TPO) and to Tg (anti-Tg) that are easily measured by enzyme-linked immunoabsorbent assay or competitive binding assays [9]. The measurement of anti-TPO and anti-Tg is complicated by the presence of such antibodies in up to 20% of the normal population. However, these antibodies are usually present in very high titers in patients with Hashimoto's thyroiditis and often in patients with Graves' disease. Another commonly measured antibody, found mostly in patients with Graves' disease, is the cause of hyperthyroidism: the thyroid-stimulating antibodies that bind to and stimulate the TSH receptor [10]. These are antibodies to the TSH receptor and can be easily measured by using competition with radio-labeled TSH for binding to soluble TSH receptors. Only rarely, such as in pregnancy, are biological assays for thyroid-stimulating activity needed. These assays can be performed using thyroid cells or model cells transfected with the TSH receptor. Some 15% of patients with Hashimoto's thyroiditis may have TSH receptor antibodies, usually of the type that block the TSH receptor rather than stimulate it.

SICK EUTHYROID SYNDROME

Despite "normal" thyroid function, total T3 and T4 levels are decreased in the presence of severe and chronic illness, leading to the concept of the sick euthyroid syndrome [11]. There are many reasons for the fall in T3 and T4 levels in this situation, which often first presents with a low T3 and only later with a fall in T4. The half-life of T3 is much shorter than that of T4, and it is bound to binding proteins with much lower affinity than T4, explaining why serum T3 levels change so much more quickly than serum T4 levels. There is also a metabolic block in very sick patients, shifting 5′-deiodination to the production of inactive reverse T3 (Figure 5.5). Hence, a fall in T3 is the dramatic expression of a metabolic problem, exacerbated by an increased distribution space between sick cells, and a fall in effective TSH levels or changes in TSH glycosylation, which reduces its bioactivity. In practice, immunoassayed TSH levels can be quite variable and often marginally increased. Later, particularly as the serum protein levels fall because of inadequate hepatic production, there follows a marked fall in serum T4 levels, which often predicts a poor outlook for the patient.

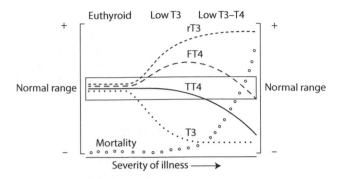

Figure 5.5 Sick euthyroid syndrome. A rapidly rising mortality rate accompanies the fall in serum total T4 and free T3 values. The TSH value is unreliable in such patients because there is often a toxic influence on pituitary function (pseudohypopituitary function). (Adapted from Nicoloff JT. Abnormal measurements in nonendocrine illness. In: Hurst JW, ed., *Medicine for the Practicing Physician*. Butterworth-Heineman, Oxford, 1991, p. 574.)

During these changes in total T3 and T4 levels, the concentration of free hormone levels may remain normal. However, all results may be found depending on the speed of the metabolic changes, with which the free hormone levels have to equilibrate. The presence of true thyroid disease during this phenomenon requires considerable expertise to assess.

URGENT SURGICAL ASSESSMENT OF THYROID FUNCTION

Most medical centers can now provide rapid thyroid function test results within a matter of hours. TSH, FT4, and even T3 levels can all be obtained by automatic analyzers, allowing an early assessment of thyroid function in any situation. Only rarely is thyroid dysfunction sufficient to delay urgent surgery, but elective procedures should await the return to euthyroidism. The physician and the anesthesiologist will work with the surgical team to achieve this aim. The dangers of surgery in an uncontrolled hyperthyroid patient include increased cardiac risk, particularly in an elderly patient, and the occurrence of severely exacerbated hyperthyroidism after surgery ("thyroid storm") [12].

REFERENCES

1. Portulano C, Paroder-Belenitsky M, Carrasco N. The Na+ /I– symporter (NIS): Mechanism and medical impact. *Endocr Rev* 2014;35(1):106–49.
2. Zimmermann MB, Boelaert K. Iodine deficiency and thyroid disorders. *Lancet Diabetes Endocrinol* 2015;3:286–95.
3. Zimmermann MB. Nutrition: Are mild maternal iodine deficiency and child IQ linked? *Nat Rev Endocrinol* 2013;9(9):505–6.
4. Haddow JE, Palomaki BS, Allan WC et al. Maternal thyroid deficiency during pregnancy and subsequent neuropsychological development of the child. *N Engl J Med* 1999;341(8):549–55.
5. Brent GA. Mechanisms of thyroid hormone action. *J Clin Invest* 2012;122(9):3035–43.
6. Dumitrescu AM, Refetoff S. The syndromes of reduced sensitivity to thyroid hormone. *Biochim Biophys Acta* 2013;1830(7):3987–4003.
7. Thienpont LM, Van Utyfanghe K, Poppe K, Velkiniers B. Determination of free thyroid hormones. Best practice & research. *Clin Endocrinol Metab* 2013;27(5):689–700.
8. Evans C, Tennant S, Perros P. Thyroglobulin in differentiated thyroid cancer. *Clin Chim Acta* 2015;444:310–7.
9. Balucan FS, Morshed SA, Davies TF. Thyroid autoantibodies in pregnancy: Their role, regulation and clinical relevance. *J Thyroid Res* 2013;2013:182472.
10. Morshed SA, Latif R, Davies TF. Delineating the autoimmune mechanisms in Graves' disease. *Immunol Res* 2012;54(1–3):191–203.
11. Farwell AP. Nonthyroidal illness syndrome. *Curr Opin Endocrinol Diabetes Obes* 2013;20(5):478–84.
12. Chiha M, Samarasinghe S, Kabaker AS. Thyroid storm: An updated review. *J Intensive Care Med* 2015;30(3):131–40.
13. Nicoloff JT. Abnormal measurements in nonendocrine illness. In: Hurst JW, ed., *Medicine for the Practicing Physician*. Butterworth-Heineman, Oxford, 1991, p. 574.

6

Thyroid disease: Cytopathology and surgical pathology aspects

CHARVI A. CASSANO, ARNOLD H. SZPORN, AND G. KENNETH HAINES III

DEVELOPMENTAL ANOMALIES

Thyroglossal duct cyst

The medial portion of the thyroid derives from the median anlage, forming a thyroglossal duct extending from the foramen cecum in the midline of the posterior tongue, descending into the neck. Thyroid tissue may remain anywhere along this path, or fail to descend at all, giving rise to ectopic thyroid tissue or gland. Persistence of the thyroglossal duct may give rise to a visible or palpable cyst [1]. Rarely, a malignancy develops within the cyst. This is most commonly papillary thyroid carcinoma (PTC), and may be associated with a synchronous lesion in the thyroid and with lymph node metastases [2,3].

When clinically evident, cysts range from 1 to 4 cm in diameter, and are filled with brown serous fluid or purulent material. The cyst is usually lined by a mixture of squamous and respiratory-type epithelium, although the lining may be absent in inflamed cysts. Thyroid tissue should be identified within the cyst wall (Figure 6.1).

INFLAMMATORY AND HYPERPLASTIC PROCESSES

Granulomatous thyroiditis

Subacute (granulomatous and De Quervain) thyroiditis may develop rapidly after a viral infection. The diagnosis is usually made on clinical grounds, noting a symmetrically enlarged, firm, and tender thyroid. Most cases respond well to a course of corticosteroids, without necessitating a biopsy. Nodules may develop, leading to a biopsy to exclude malignancy. Pathologic findings vary with the stage of disease. The initial acute neutrophilic inflammation involving thyroid follicles gives way to chronic and granulomatous inflammation [4].

Lymphocytic (Hashimoto) thyroiditis

Hashimoto thyroiditis (HT) is a common autoimmune disease, characterized by autoantibodies (antithyroglobulin and antithyroid microsomal) and chronic inflammation

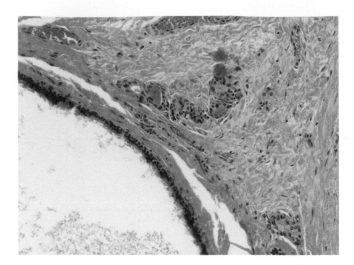

Figure 6.1 Thyroglossal duct cyst. This intact cyst is lined by respiratory-type epithelium. Inflamed cysts may have a squamous lining or be replaced by granulation tissue. Atrophic thyroid tissue is evident within the fibrous cyst wall. H&E, 20×.

with variable destruction of thyroid follicles [5]. The disease occurs over a wide age range, predominantly in females, with a 5–10:1 female-to-male ratio. Some patients may have another coexisting autoimmune disease [6]. In early stages of the disease, patients may present with evidence of hyperparathyroidism, as thyroid hormone is released from damaged follicles. With progressive loss of thyroid parenchyma, hypothyroidism ensues in the majority of patients.

Fine-needle aspiration yields abundant lymphocytes interspersed with large follicular epithelial cells with abundant pink granular cytoplasm (Hürthle cells) and scant colloid [7]. A paucicellular aspirate may suggest a fibrous variant of HT, Riedel thyroiditis (see below), or another process.

In cases that are surgically excised, the thyroid is symmetrically enlarged, weighing up to 200 g. Serial sectioning of the gland shows preservation or enhancement of the normal lobular pattern.

Histologically, a dense lymphocytic or lymphoplasmacytic infiltrate is the most striking feature. Prominent germinal centers are often present. Many follicles are atrophic, with flattened epithelium, while others are lined by large eosinophilic (Hürthle or oncocytic) cells [8] (Figure 6.2a and b). Stromal fibrosis varies from minimal to extensive, the latter designated as the fibrous variant of HT.

Not all cases of histologic "lymphocytic thyroiditis" are HT. Hence, clinical and laboratory correlation (screening for antithyroid antibodies) is required for a definitive diagnosis. A subset of cases resembling the fibrous variant of HT have subsequently been reclassified as manifestations of a localized or systemic immunoglobulin G4 (IgG4)-related sclerosing disease. While there is histologic overlap, the IgG4-related process occurs in a younger age group, has a lower female-to-male ratio, and has more interfollicular fibrosis than non-IgG4-related cases [9].

(a)
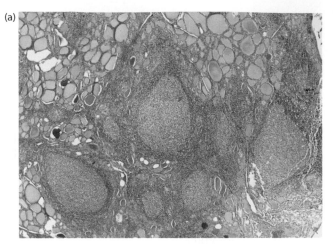

(b)
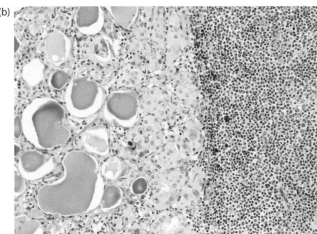

Figure 6.2 Lymphocytic thyroiditis. (a) Large areas of the thyroid parenchyma are replaced by lymphocytes with prominent germinal centers. H&E, 4×. (b) Residual thyroid follicular epithelium characteristically undergoes an oxyphilic metaplasia. Note the large cells with abundant pink cytoplasm adjacent to the lymphocytic infiltrate. H&E, 20×.

The question of whether patients with HT are at increased risk for thyroid cancer has been debated for years. Most studies show HT patients are at increased risk for lymphoma or PTC [10,11].

Riedel thyroiditis

Riedel thyroiditis (invasive fibrous thyroiditis) is a rare, presumably autoimmune disease that may develop *de novo* in some, following a diagnosis of HT or Graves' disease. In the Mayo Clinic series, most patients were female (mean age 42), with a significant smoking history [12]. This entity is now recognized as being closely related to, if not within, the spectrum of IgG4-related sclerosing diseases [13,14].

Histologically, the fibrosis is dense, often keloid-like. In contrast to the fibrous variant of HT, Riedel thyroiditis obliterates the normal lobular architecture of the thyroid, and extends into extrathyroidal soft tissue. The inflammatory infiltrate is variable, consisting of lymphocytes and plasma cells and scattered eosinophils. An obliterative phlebitis may also be seen. The identification of large numbers of IgG4+ plasma cells and a high IgG4-to-IgG ratio by immunohistochemistry is supportive of an IgG4-related process.

Graves' disease (diffuse hyperplasia)

Graves' disease is the most common cause of hyperthyroidism in the United States. It is an autoimmune disorder characterized by the development of antibodies to the thyroid-stimulating hormone receptor (TSHR) on follicular epithelial cells. Rather than causing an immune-mediated destruction of the follicles, binding of these antibodies activates the receptor, leading to an increase in thyroid hormone production and secretion, as well as to a proliferation of the follicular epithelial cells. In addition to signs of hyperthyroidism, many patients present with visual disturbances, sometimes with notable exopthalmos, due to deposition of proteoglycans and a variable inflammatory infiltrate in retro-orbital soft tissue.

Sheets of follicular epithelial cells with eccentric nuclei and often a perinuclear vacuole ("flame cell") are the typical finding on fine-needle aspiration. In surgically excised cases, the thyroid is diffusely and symmetrically enlarged, with minimal nodularity. Cut sections show beefy red parenchyma, contrasting with the pale appearance typical of HT. Histologically, untreated cases show crowded follicles with irregular papillary infolding, lined by tall columnar epithelial cells with pink to amphophilic cytoplasm. The colloid is variable in amount, with prominent peripheral scalloping in patients with active disease. There is a variable lymphoplasmacellular infiltrate with minimal fibrosis. This typical histology may be altered by presurgical therapy. Propylthiouracil or similar agents reduce the scalloping of colloid (indicating decreased release of thyroid hormone), and the lining follicular epithelial cells become cuboidal or flattened, reflecting an inactive state. Treatment with radioactive iodine often induces marked cytologic atypia, with follicular epithelial cells containing large, hyperchromatic nuclei and prominent nucleoli [15,16] (Figure 6.3).

Distinct nodularity in the setting of Graves' disease raises the possibility of a coexisting malignancy. PTC, and particularly the aggressive subtypes of PTC, arises with increased frequency in these patients [17,18].

Simple and multinodular goiter

Enlargement of the thyroid (goiter) is a common condition, with an incidence inversely related to local levels of daily iodine intake, as well as method of detection (palpation vs. ultrasound). Nodular thyroid disease is often reported to be present in 20%–40% of the population in iodine-deficient areas, but may reach up to 80% of the areas of Southeast Asia and Central and Latin America [19,20]. Simple goiter is most common in premenopausal women. When found in the pediatric population, the possibility of a dyshormonogenetic goiter or underlying Cowden syndrome should

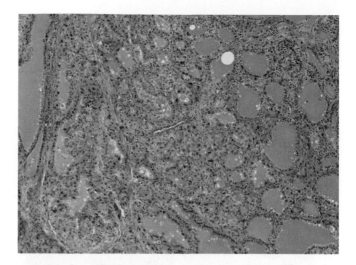

Figure 6.3 In active cases of Graves' disease, the thyroid follicles are lined by columnar cells with abundant cytoplasm. The scalloped edges of the colloid in multiple follicles indicate active resorption and secretion of thyroid hormone. Note the scattered follicular epithelial cells with large, hyperchromatic nuclei—an indication of prior treatment. H&E, 20×.

be considered [21–23]. Most cases show multiple nodules within the thyroid. These develop through repeated cycles of follicular hyperplasia with compromise of local vascular flow and subsequent involution [24]. The thyroid enlargement is often asymptomatic, but may become symptomatic due to compression of adjacent structures. Most patients are euthyroid, but a proportion present with hyper- (toxic goiter) or, rarely, hypothyroidism.

One concern in managing patients with multinodular goiter is the possible development of malignancy. Occult malignancy has been reported in 10%–35% of cases, with both follicular and papillary carcinomas described [25–27]. This is not surprising, as molecular and genetic techniques have shown that a proportion of these "hyperplastic" nodules are monoclonal proliferations. This histologic overlap is reflected in the variable terminology applied to these lesions, such as "adenomatous nodular hyperplasia." As a generalization, features favoring a hyperplastic process include the multiple, poorly encapsulated nodules with a macrofollicular architecture (Figure 6.4a and b). In contrast, a single encapsulated nodule with a solid, trabecular, or microfollicular architecture, composed of cells distinctly different from those outside the nodule, is regarded as neoplastic (Figure 6.4c).

NEOPLASTIC PROCESSES

Follicle-derived epithelial lesions: follicular vs. papillary

Primary neoplasms arising in the thyroid can be derived from follicular epithelial cells, parafollicular C-cells, or stromal cells. For those of follicular origin, the first major

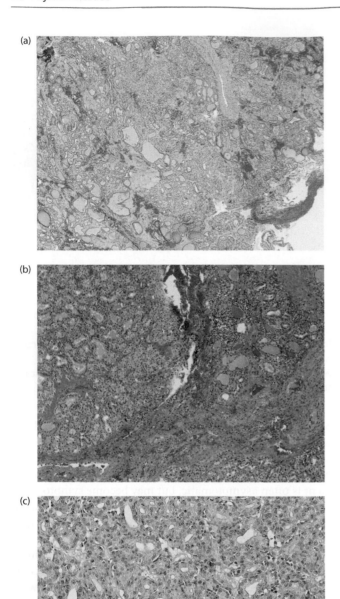

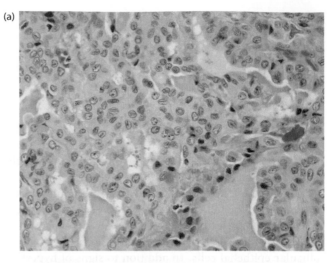

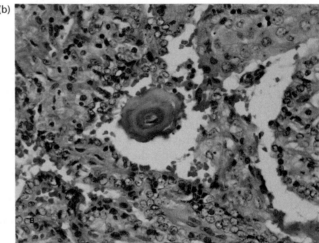

Figure 6.5 Papillary vs. follicular lesions. **(a)** The classic nuclear features of PTC include irregular or elongated, overlapped, pale (hypochromic) nuclei with distinct longitudinal grooves. Note the pseudoinclusion in the center of the field. H&E, 40×. **(b)** Laminated calcifications (psammoma bodies) are a helpful clue to the diagnosis of PTC. H&E, 40×.

Figure 6.4 Follicular lesions: hyperplasia vs. neoplasia. **(a)** Follicles are described as being macro-, normo-, or microfollicular based on comparison with those in normal thyroid tissue. This example of multinodular hyperplasia demonstrates a spectrum of follicle sizes. Note that there is no clear demarcation of the lesion, a feature favoring hyperplasia over neoplasia. H&E, 4×. **(b)** Two thyroid nodules are seen on the left and bottom of the figure. Note that the cytologic features of the follicular lining cells are identical to those outside of the nodules (right side). H&E, 10×. **(c)** Thyroid nodules composed of enlarged epithelial cells arranged in a microfollicular pattern are more likely to represent a neoplastic process. The presence of a single nodule with a distinct fibrous capsule would further support neoplasia. H&E, 20×.

division is between a papillary neoplasm (PTC) and other tumors. Despite the name, the defining characteristic of a PTC lies in its distinctive nuclear features, rather than its architecture. PTC typically shows enlarged, overlapped, hypochromatic nuclei with nuclear membrane irregularities (nuclear grooves and pseudoinclusions) (Figure 6.5a). Concentric calcifications (psammoma bodies) are frequently identified (Figure 6.5b).

Thyroid cytology

Cytologic evaluation has become a routine component of the workup of a thyroid mass. In order to improve the consistency of cytologic interpretation, and to derive standardized outcome data to provide actionable information for patient management, The Bethesda System for Reporting Thyroid Cytopathology (TBSRTC) has been

Table 6.1 Simplified version of the Bethesda system for classifying thyroid lesions

Bethesda category	Risk of malignancy
I. Nondiagnostic	<5%
II. Benign	<5%
III. Lesion of undetermined significance	5%–15%
IV. (Suspicious for) follicular neoplasm	15%–30%
V. Suspicious for malignancy	60%–75%
VI. Malignant	>95%

Note: Each category includes additional clinical information, ranging from a treatment recommendation to subtype of tumor. Standardization of diagnostic criteria and terminology will allow better comparison of performance and outcomes data across institutions.

widely adopted 28,29]. This system contains six broad categories, ranging from I (nondiagnostic or unsatisfactory) to VI (malignant). Each category denotes a certain risk of malignancy and is linked to a patient management suggestion (Table 6.1).

Papillary thyroid carcinoma

PTC is the most common endocrine malignancy, with an incidence currently estimated at 12.5 per 100,000 people [30]. PTC is associated with a number of familial syndromes, including MEN2A, familial adenomatous polyposis (FAP), familial nonmedullary thyroid carcinoma, and Carney complex. It is a well-known side effect of radiation exposure, and occurs more frequently in the setting of HT and Graves' disease [11,17].

Somatic mutations and gene rearrangements are commonly identified in PTC. The RET/PTC rearrangement is seen in a quarter of adult cases, half of pediatric cases, and three-quarters of radiation-induced cases. BRAF mutations, particularly the V600E point mutation, are seen in up to 70% of cases [31,32].

PTC can appear grossly as a single nodule or be multifocal. Whether multifocal tumors represent independent primary tumors or intrathyroidal metastasis is controversial, but may have implications for treatment, depending on the number and size of the lesions [33]. The tumor may be solid or cystic, well circumscribed or infiltrative, with or without calcifications.

Fine-needle aspiration often yields a definitive diagnosis preoperatively with enlarged, oval to irregular nuclei with longitudinal grooves, pale powdery chromatin, and intranuclear pseudoinclusions. The tumor cells may be arranged in papillae, syncytial, or swirling monolayers. Psammoma bodies (laminated calcifications) and multinucleated giant cells may be present.

PAPILLARY THYROID CARCINOMA, CLASSIC VARIANT

The typical (i.e., classic variant) case of PTC shows branching fibrovascular cores lined by a single layer of enlarged

(a)
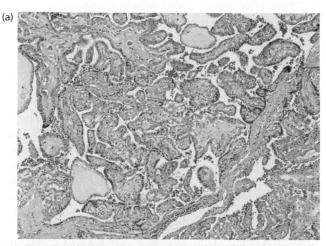

(b)
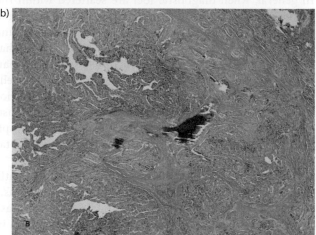

Figure 6.6 PTC: Classic variant. (a) The classic variant of PTC is characterized by complex branching fibrovascular cores lined by low columnar epithelial cells with overlapped, hypochromic grooved nuclei. H&E, 10×. (b) PTC may appear grossly as a fibrotic or calcified nodule within the thyroid. Note the dense eosinophilic fibrous stroma with purple areas of dystrophic calcification. H&E, 4×.

cuboidal to columnar epithelial cells, with ovoid pale or empty ("Orphan Annie" eye) nuclei with longitudinal grooves and occasional pseudoinclusions (apparent invaginations of cytoplasm caused by the irregular nuclear contour) (Figure 6.6a). Concentrically laminated calcifications (psammoma bodies) are often present. Reactive multinucleated giant cells are commonly identified. The tumor may induce a dense fibrotic stromal reaction with dystrophic calcification and ossification (Figure 6.6b). Not infrequently, in addition to the papillary architecture, a portion of the tumor maintains a follicular architecture. Tumors with classic PTC nuclear features and an exclusively follicular architecture (follicular variant of PTC) will be discussed below. The classic variant of PTC may be solid or cystic, encapsulated by a thin fibrous pseudocapsule, or be infiltrative into surrounding thyroid parenchyma. PTC is often multifocal within the thyroid. Whether this represents intrathyroidal metastasis or the development of independent tumors may be difficult to discern [33].

PAPILLARY THYROID CARCINOMA, OTHER VARIANTS

At least a dozen variants of PTC have been described, many having unique genetic or molecular features or significant clinical implications. The most common, *follicular variant of PTC* may be difficult to distinguish from a benign process (nodular hyperplasia or follicular adenoma). The tumor is composed entirely or predominantly of elongated or irregular follicles containing dense eosinophilic "bubble gum" colloid, often with prominent peripheral scalloping (Figure 6.7a). The nuclei are often more rounded than in the classic variant and nuclear pseudoinclusions are rare. Diagnostic nuclear changes may be present only focally within a large nodule, leading to inconsistent reporting of the tumor size. In general, when diagnostic foci are scattered within the nodule, the entire nodule is considered to be a carcinoma. A single focus may be considered to be a microcarcinoma arising within a pre-existing adenoma [34]. Tumors that are encapsulated may represent a different disease than those with an infiltrative pattern. Encapsulated or well-circumscribed tumors generally have an indolent behavior and have RAS, rather than BRAF, mutations. In contrast, invasive tumors often have metastasized to regional lymph nodes and commonly demonstrate the BRAF V600E mutation typical of classic PTC [35,36].

Tall cell variant of PTC is an aggressive tumor, frequently with extrathyroidal extension and lymph node metastasis at time of diagnosis. BRAF V600E and TERT (telomerase reverse transcriptase) promoter mutations are common in this subtype. The tumor most often has a papillary architecture, but may be trabecular or have a follicular pattern. Histopathologic criteria for diagnosing this variant have been inconsistent among publications, with most studies using a height-to-width ratio of 2:1 or 3:1, and a variable proportion (as low as 10%) of tumor showing this feature [37–39] (Figure 6.7b).

Columnar cell variant may be seen as a circumscribed lesion in younger patients, or as an infiltrative tumor, commonly with extrathyroidal extension and metastatic disease in older patients. In contrast to the central nucleus and granular eosinophilic cytoplasm of the tall cell variant, the columnar cell variant shows pseudostratified nuclei with supra- or subnuclear cytoplasmic vacuoles [40] (Figure 6.7c).

The *diffuse sclerosing PTC variant* is another aggressive subtype. As the name implies, the former shows diffuse involvement of the thyroid and extrathyroidal soft tissue with a papillary and follicular tumor with extensive squamous metaplasia and frequent psammoma bodies, in a prominent fibrotic lymphocyte-rich stroma, sometimes resembling Reidel's thyroiditis. RET/PTC1, RET/PTC3, and BRAF V600E mutations or rearrangements are commonly identified in this tumor [41,42].

Other variants of PTC recognized by the World Health Organization include clear cell, cribriform-morular, hobnail, macrofollicular, oncocytic, solid, and Warthin-like.

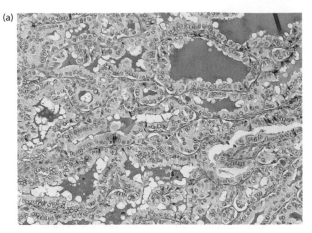

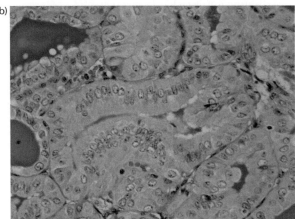

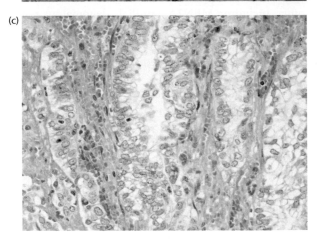

Figure 6.7 PTC: Other variants. **(a)** The follicular variant may closely resemble a follicular neoplasm. Elongated follicles with dense, eosinophilic "bubble gum" colloid with scalloping may be a clue, but recognition of characteristic PTC nuclear features is required for a definitive diagnosis. H&E, 20×. **(b)** The tall cell variant is defined by tumor cells with a height-to-width ratio of 3:1, occupying at least 10% of the tumor. This variant is biologically aggressive, with frequent extrathyroidal disease at time of diagnosis. H&E, 40×. **(c)** Columnar cell variant. While the tall cell variant of PTC is also columnar, this designation is reserved for tumors with nuclear pseudostratification and cytoplasmic vacuoles. H&E, 40×.

Each variant has unique histopathology and molecular or clinical findings [43–45].

Hyalinizing trabecular tumor

Hyalinizing trabecular tumor is an interesting tumor that initially was categorized as a form of PTC due to identical nuclear features. This tumor arises as a well-circumscribed solid nodule. Histologically, the tumor consists of elongated eosinophilic cells with PTC-like nuclei, arranged in trabeculi with hyalinized stroma (Figure 6.8a and b). RET/PTC1 rearrangements have been identified in some cases, but no RAS or BRAF mutations have been reported. The tumor has a unique membranous staining pattern with immunostains for the proliferation marker ki-67. The overwhelming majority of these tumors have followed a benign clinical course, although a few metastasized to regional lymph nodes [46,47].

Follicular neoplasms

FOLLICULAR ADENOMA

Follicular adenoma is the most common neoplasm of the thyroid, and it may arise in association with prior radiation or iodine deficiency, as part of an inherited syndrome (Cowden disease, Carney complex, or Pendred syndrome), or sporadically. The lesions are generally solitary, averaging 3 cm in diameter. The lesion is, by definition, encapsulated with a distinct fibrous capsule (Figure 6.9a). The histologic architecture is variable, with micro-, normo-, or macrofollicular, trabecular, and diffuse (sheet-like) patterns (Figure 6.9b). The distinction from a hyperplastic nodule has been discussed above. In contrast to hyperplastic lesions, the architecture and cytology within the nodule tends to be discrete from that seen elsewhere in the thyroid. As in many endocrine organs, nuclear pleomorphism may be seen and does not denote malignant potential. The distinction from

(a)
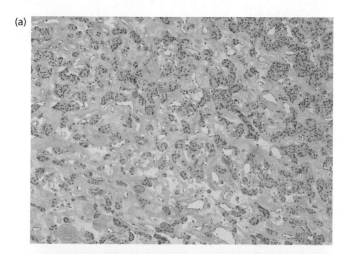

(b)
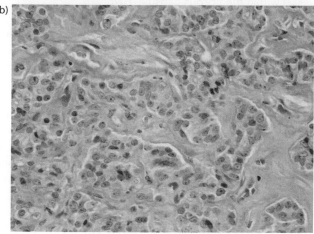

Figure 6.8 Hyalinizing trabecular tumor. (a) Solid cords or trabeculae are interspersed within a dense eosinophilic glassy (hyalinized) stroma. H&E, 10×. (b) Higher magnification shows characteristic PTC nuclear features, including pale powdery chromatin and nuclear grooves. Immunohistochemistry with the proliferation marker, ki-67, shows a unique membranous staining pattern. H&E, 40×.

(a)
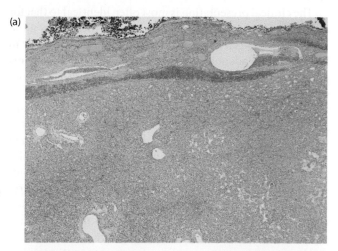

(b)
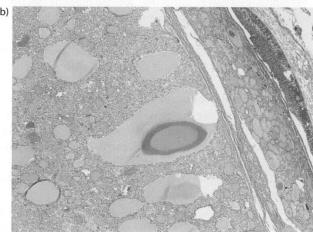

Figure 6.9 Follicular adenoma. (a) This follicular adenoma (bottom) is separated from the adjacent non-neoplastic thyroid tissue (top) by a thin fibrous capsule. H&E, 4×. (b) The follicles in this nodule range from micro- to macrofollicular. The presence of a complete fibrous capsule surrounding the nodule distinguishes this follicular adenoma from a hyperplastic nodule. H&E, 4×.

the follicular variant of papillary carcinoma depends on the identification of characteristic nuclear features of PTC, as discussed above. Immunohistochemical stains may be useful in difficult cases. Diffuse staining with cytokeratin CK19, HMB1-1, and galectin-3 favors PTC over a follicular neoplasm [48]. BRAF mutations and RET/PTC rearrangements are not a feature of follicular adenoma, rather suggesting a diagnosis of PTC. In contrast, point mutations in NRAS and HRAS are more likely to be found in follicular adenomas.

FOLLICULAR CARCINOMA

Follicular carcinoma is less common than PTC, accounting for 10%–20% of thyroid cancers. Women in their 40s and 50s are most commonly affected. Risk factors for follicular carcinoma include radiation exposure and iodine deficiency. Up to 15% of cases arise in a familial setting, such as FAP, Carney complex, or Cowden syndrome [49,50].

The clinical presentation is most often identical to that for follicular adenomas, with a painless mass measuring up to 10 cm. Mutations in RAS, PIK3CA, or PTEN genes occur in both follicular adenomas and carcinomas. Rearrangements or translocations involving the PPARγ and PAX8 genes occur in about one-fifth of cases.

Grossly, minimally invasive carcinomas are indistinguishable from adenomas. Cytologic examination is not useful in this distinction. Rather, histologic examination of the entire tumor capsule (to identify full-thickness capsular penetration or lymphovascular invasion) is necessary for correct classification (Figure 6.10a and b). As these features are often focal, intraoperative (frozen section) consultation is problematic, but may provide clinically important information in select cases [51].

Despite extensive sampling for permanent sections, some cases have equivocal features (indefinite capsular or vascular invasion and questionable PTC nuclear features). Such cases have been designated as thyroid (follicular or well-differentiated) tumors of uncertain malignant potential [52].

Widely invasive follicular carcinomas are easier to recognize preoperatively by ultrasound and intraoperatively on gross examination and frozen section analysis. These tumors often lack a capsule and extend irregularly into adjacent thyroid parenchyma or extrathyroidal tissue.

Upon microscopic evaluation, these tumors show the same spectrum of cytologic and architectural features as follicular adenomas. Definitions of capsular and vascular invasion have evolved over time, with significant interobserver variability in the interpretation of follicular lesions [53]. Criteria are becoming more standardized. For example, in order to diagnose vascular invasion, the vessel must have a distinct wall and be located within or beyond the tumor capsule. The tumor must protrude into the lumen or be attached to the wall and be covered by endothelium and thrombin. For encapsulated or well-circumscribed follicular carcinomas, the identification of vascular invasion

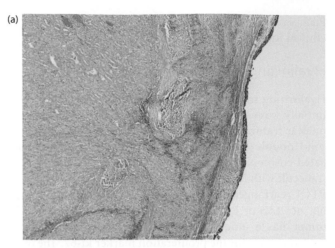

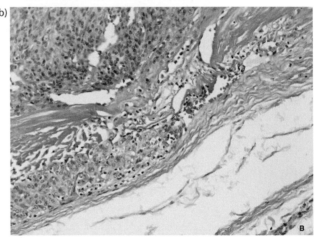

Figure 6.10 Follicular thyroid carcinoma. (a) The fibrous capsule is breached (lower right side), as this follicular carcinoma spills into adjacent thyroid parenchyma. H&E, 4×. (b) This follicular carcinoma has invaded into a blood vessel within the fibrous capsule. H&E, 20×.

carries more prognostic significance than capsular invasion alone. Cases with extensive (four or more vessels) vascular invasion have a worse prognosis than those with lesser degrees of angioinvasion [54].

One subgroup of follicular carcinoma is composed of large polygonal cells with abundant eosinophilic granular cytoplasm and a round nucleus with prominent nucleolus (Figure 6.11). These tumors, previously categorized as Hürthle cell carcinomas and felt to be more aggressive than other follicular carcinomas, are currently classified as an oncocytic variant of follicular carcinoma [55–57].

Poorly differentiated thyroid carcinoma

Poorly differentiated carcinomas of the thyroid occupy an intermediate position between the common papillary and follicular carcinomas (well differentiated) and anaplastic thyroid carcinoma (see the next section). These are rare tumors, accounting for less than 2% of thyroid carcinomas in the United States. They can occur in any age group, but most commonly affect women over 50 years of age. These

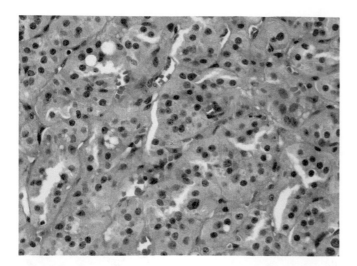

Figure 6.11 The oncocytic variant of follicular carcinoma (formerly known as Hürthle cell carcinoma) is characterized by large cells with abundant granular eosinophilic cytoplasm and a round nucleus with a prominent nucleolus. Criteria for malignancy (i.e., full-thickness capsular invasion or lymphovascular invasion) are the same as those for other follicular carcinomas. H&E, 40×.

tumors have nested (insular), trabecular, and solid growth patterns; absence of PTC nuclear features; and a high mitotic rate (>3 mf/10 hpf), convoluted nuclei, or necrosis (Turin criteria) [58,59] (Figure 6.12a and b). Similar criteria have been used to define a poorly differentiated category of oncocytic tumors [60]. With or without oncocytic features, they are aggressive neoplasms, with frequent distant metastasis and a high 10-year mortality rate. CTNNB1, RAS, and TP53 mutations may be found, but BRAF mutations have not been described in these tumors.

Anaplastic thyroid carcinoma

Undifferentiated or anaplastic thyroid carcinoma is a rare highly aggressive malignancy, accounting for less than 2% of thyroid carcinomas. Most patients present with sudden rapid growth of a pre-existing long-standing thyroid lesion, most often nodular hyperplasia. The bulky tumor often grossly extends into adjacent tissues and metastasizes to lymph nodes and distant sites. There are a number of histologic variants of anaplastic carcinoma, most consisting of pleomorphic, markedly atypical spindled, epithelioid, or giant cells [61] (Figure 6.13a–c). Frequent mitotic figures, abundant necrosis, and extensive lymphovascular and extrathyroidal extension are common. A hypocellular variant exists that may be mistaken for Riedel thyroiditis. This variant may be recognized based on the identification of rare cells with nuclear hyperchromasia. Foci of residual papillary, follicular, or medullary carcinoma may be seen. In such cases, similar mutations may be found in both differentiated and anaplastic portions of the tumor. Most cases of anaplastic thyroid carcinoma demonstrate nuclear staining for p53 and β-catenin.

(a)

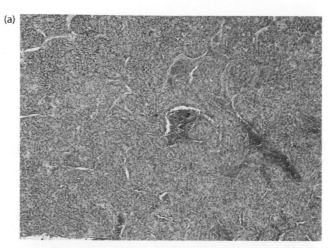

(b)

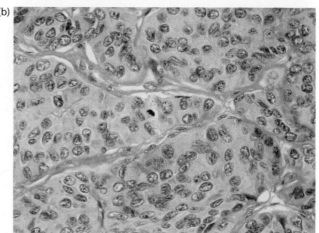

Figure 6.12 Poorly differentiated thyroid carcinoma. (a) This cellular tumor is composed of anastomosing trabeculae and nests of atypical cells. Only a suggestion of follicle formation can be seen. H&E, 10×. (b) The Turin criteria for poorly differentiated thyroid carcinoma include high mitotic activity; insular, trabecular, or solid growth patterns; irregular nuclei; and necrosis. A mitotic figure is evident in this example with an insular growth pattern. H&E, 40×.

Medullary thyroid carcinoma

Medullary thyroid carcinoma accounts for 5%–10% of all thyroid cancers. Up to a quarter of cases are hereditary MEN2 comprising 2a, 2b, and familial MTC, characterized by mutations in the RET proto-oncogene [62,63]. These often present in children or young adults. Sporadic cases occur in an older age group (50–60 years old). Excluding familial cases identified by screening or prophylactic thyroidectomy, the tumor often presents as a painless nodule (or multiple nodules in familial cases). Lymph node metastases are found in about one-half of patients, with distant metastasis seen in a fifth. The tumor is arranged in sheets, nests, or trabeculae. The tumor cells may be clear, eosinophilic, or amphophylic, with round nuclei and "salt and pepper" chromatin (Figure 6.14a and b). Amyloid deposits are often seen in the stroma. The tumor stains for calcitonin,

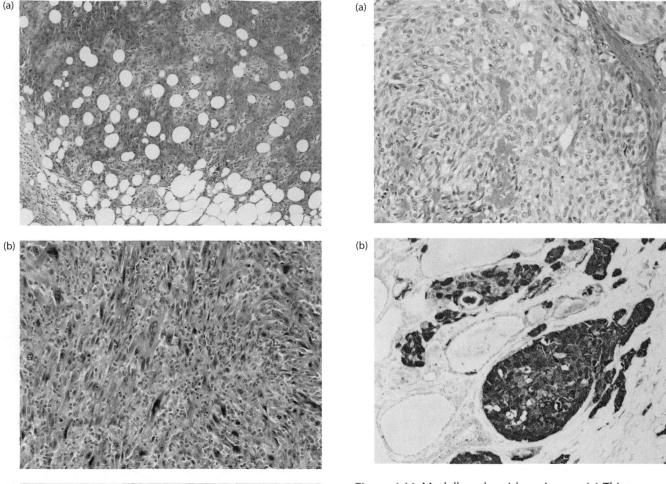

Figure 6.13 Anaplastic thyroid carcinoma. **(a)** Anaplastic thyroid carcinoma can demonstrate a variety of appearances. This example shows an epithelioid tumor widely invasive into extrathyroidal adipose tissue. H&E, 4×. **(b)** This example shows features of an undifferentiated pleomorphic sarcoma. The spindle cells have markedly atypical hyperchromatic nuclei. H&E, 20×. **(c)** This anaplastic carcinoma is composed of sheets of round mononuclear and multinucleated tumor giant cells. H&E, 20×.

Figure 6.14 Medullary thyroid carcinoma. **(a)** This tumor is composed of large nests of round to spindle-shaped cells. Note the dense eosinophilic deposits of amyloid in the stroma. H&E, 20×. **(b)** Medullary thyroid carcinoma infiltrating within thyroid parenchyma. The tumor shows strong staining for calcitonin (illustrated), as well as for neuroendocrine markers and CEA. Note staining of isolated C-cells within the non-neoplastic follicles. In familial cases, clusters of C-cells can be identified by immunohistochemistry. Calcitonin immunostain, 20×.

plasma antigens, (1) synaptophysin, (2) chromogranin A, (3) neuron-specific enolase, (4) pancreatic polypeptide, (5) alpha and beta subunits of human chorionic gonadotrophin, (6) pancreostatin, (7) thyroid transcription factor (TTF)-1, and carcinoembryonic antigen (CEA). The neuroendocrine (except CEA) antigenicity profile plays a significant role in the diagnosis and localization of functioning and also the hormonally inactive neoplasms. Antigenicity also affects the coexistence of ligands for isotopic imaging (low antigenicity is preferable).

C-cells are not identifiable in normal thyroids on routine hematoxylin and eosin (H&E)-stained slides, but may be detected by immunohistochemistry using antibodies against calcitonin. In familial settings, an increase in the number of C-cells may be identified as precursor lesions for the development of medullary carcinoma. These precursors are divided into categories of *C-cell hyperplasia* (clusters of

<50 C-cells) and *neoplastic C-cell hyperplasia* (clusters of >50 C-cells). Differences in clinicopathologic features may be identified based on the specific underlying germline mutation [64].

REFERENCES

1. Wei S, LiVolsi VA, Baloch ZW. Pathology of thyroglossal duct: An institutional experience. *Endocr Pathol* 2015;26:75–9.
2. Rossi ED, Martini M, Straccia P et al. Thyroglossal duct cyst cancer most likely arises from a thyroid gland remnant. *Virchows Arch* 2014;465:67–72.
3. Pellegriti G, Lumera G, Malandrino P et al. Thyroid cancer in thyroglossal duct cysts requires a specific approach due to its unpredictable extension. *J Clin Endocrinol Metab* 2013;98:458–65.
4. Mordes DA, Brachtel EF. Cytopathology of subacute thyroiditis. *Diagn Cytopathol* 2012;40:433–4.
5. Cauuregli P, De Remigis A, Rose NR. Hashimoto thyroiditis: Clinical and diagnostic criteria. *Autoimmun Rev* 2014;13:391–7.
6. Ahmed R, Al-Shaikh S, Akhtar M. Hashimoto thyroiditis: A century later. *Adv Anat Pathol* 2012;19:181–6.
7. Shandanwale SS, Gore CR, Bamanikar SA et al. Cytomorphologic spectrum of Hashimoto's thyroiditis and its clinical correlation: A retrospective study of 52 patients. *Cytojournal* 2014;11:9.
8. Thompson LD. Chronic lymphocytic thyroiditis (Hashimoto thyroiditis). *Ear Nose Throat J* 2014;93:152–3.
9. Li Y, Zhou G, Ozaki T et al. Distinct histopathological features of Hashimoto's thyroiditis with respect to IgG4-related disease. *Mod Pathol* 2012;25:1086–97.
10. Noureldine SI, Tufano RP. Association of Hashimoto's thyroiditis and thyroid cancer. *Curr Opin Oncol* 2015;27:21–5.
11. Zhang Y, Dai J, Wu T et al. The study of the coexistence of Hashimoto's thyroiditis with papillary thyroid carcinoma. *J Cancer Res Clin Oncol* 2014;140:1021–6.
12. Fatourechi MM, Hay ID, McIver B et al. Invasive fibrous thyroiditis (Riedel thyroiditis): The Mayo Clinic experience, 1976–2008. *Thyroid* 2011;21:765–72.
13. Cameselle-Teijeiro J, Ladra MJ, Abdulkader I et al. Increased lymphangiogenesis in Riedel thyroiditis (immunoglobulin G4-related thyroid disease). *Virchows Arch* 2014;465:359–64.
14. Pusztaszeri M, Triponez F, Pache JC et al. Riedel's thyroiditis with increased IgG4 plasma cells: Evidence for an underlying IgG4 related sclerosing disease? *Thyroid* 2012;22:964–8.
15. Thompson LD. Diffuse hyperplasia of the thyroid gland (Graves' disease). *Ear Nose Throat J* 2007;86:666–7.
16. Perez-Montiel MD, Suster S. The spectrum of histologic changes in thyroid hyperplasia: A clinicopathologic study of 300 cases. *Hum Pathol* 2008;39:1080–7.
17. Wei S, Baloch ZW, LiVolsi VA. Thyroid carcinoma in patients with Graves' disease: An institutional experience. *Thyroid* 2012;22:964–8.
18. Boutzios G, Vasileiadis I, Zapanti E et al. Higher incidence of tall cell variant of papillary thyroid carcinoma in Graves' disease. *Thyroid* 2014;24:347–54.
19. Krohn K, Fuhrer D, Bayer Y et al. Molecular pathogenesis of euthyroid and toxic multinodular goiter. *Endocr Rev* 2005;26:504–24.
20. Vanderpump MPJ. The epidemiology of thyroid disease. *Br Med Bull* 2011;99:39–51.
21. Thompson L. Dyshormonogenetic goiter of the thyroid gland. *Ear Nose Throat J* 2005;84:200.
22. Deshpande AH, Bobhate SK. Cytological features of dyshormonogenetic goiter: Case report and review of the literature. *Diagn Cytopathol* 2005;33:252–4.
23. Hall JE, Abdollahian DJ, Sinard RJ. Thyroid disease associated with Cowden syndrome: A meta-analysis. *Head Neck* 2013;35:1189–94.
24. Taylor S. The evolution of nodular goiter. *J Clin Endocrinol Metab* 1953;13:1232.
25. Nixon IJ, Simo R. The neoplastic goitre. *Curr Opin Otolaryngol Head Neck Surg* 2013;21:143–9.
26. Erden ES, Babayigit C, Davran R et al. Papillary thyroid carcinoma with lung metastasis arising from dyshormonogenetic goiter: A case report. *Case Rep Med* 2013;2013:813167.
27. Chertok Shacham E, Ishay A, Irit E, Pohlenz J, Tenenbaum-Rakover Y. Minimally invasive follicular carcinoma developed in dyshormonogenetic multinodular goiter due to thyroid peroxidase gene mutation. *Thyroid* 2012;22:542–6.
28. Cibas ES, Ali SZ. The Bethesda System for Reporting Thyroid Cytopathology. *Am J Clin Pathol* 2009;132:658–65.
29. Colllins J, Rossi ED, Chandra A et al. Terminology and nomenclature schemes for reporting thyroid cytopathology: An overview. *Semin Diagn Pathol* 2015;32:258–63.
30. Morris LGT, Sikora AG, Tosteson TD et al. The increasing incidence of thyroid cancer: The influence of access to care. *Thyroid* 2013;23:885–91.
31. Liu X, Yan K, Lin X et al. The association between $BRAF^{V600E}$ mutation and pathological features in PTC. *Eur Arch Otorhinolaryngol* 2014;271:3041–52.
32. Yip L, Nikiforova MN, Yoo JY et al. Tumor genotype determines phenotype and disease outcomes in thyroid cancer: A study of 1510 patients. *Ann Surg* 2015;262:519–25.
33. Iacobone M, Jansson S, Barczynski M et al. Multifocal papillary thyroid carcinoma—A consensus report of the European Society of Endocrine Surgeons (ESES). *Langenbecks Arch Surg* 2014;399:141–54.
34. Mete O, Asa SL. Pitfalls in the diagnosis of follicular epithelial proliferations of the thyroid. *Adv Anat Pathol* 2012;19:363–73.

35. Ganly I, Wang L, Tuttle RM et al. Invasion rather than nuclear features correlates with outcome in encapsulated follicular tumors: Further evidence for the reclassification of the encapsulated papillary thyroid carcinoma follicular variant. *Hum Pathol* 2015;46:657–64.

36. Xu B, Ghossein R. Encapsulated thyroid carcinoma of follicular origin. *Endocr Pathol* 2015;26:191–9.

37. Axelsson TA, Hrafnkelsson J, Olafsdottir EJ et al. Tall cell variant of papillary thyroid carcinoma: A population based study in Iceland. *Thyroid* 2015;25:216–20.

38. Dettmer MS, Schmitt A, Steinert H et al. Tall cell papillary thyroid carcinoma: New diagnostic criteria and mutations in *BRAF* and *TERT*. *Endocr Relat Cancer* 2015;22:419–29.

39. Ganly I, Ibrahimpasic T, Rivera M et al. Prognostic implications of papillary thyroid carcinoma with tall-cell features. *Thyroid* 2014;24:662–70.

40. Chen JH, Faquin WC, Lloyd RV et al. Clinicopathological and molecular characterization of nine cases of columnar cell variant of papillary thyroid carcinoma. *Mod Pathol* 2011;24:739–49.

41. Joung JY, Kim TH, Jeong DJ et al. Diffuse sclerosing variant of papillary thyroid carcinoma: Major genetic alterations and prognostic implications. *Histopathology* 2016;69:45–53.

42. Pillai S, Gopalan V, Smith RA et al. Diffuse sclerosing variant of papillary thyroid carcinoma—An update of its clinicopathological features and molecular biology. *Crit Rev Oncol Hematol* 2015;94:64–73.

43. Pradhan D, Sharma A, Mohanty SK. Cribriform-morular variant of papillary thyroid carcinoma. *Pathol Res Pract* 2015;211:712–6.

44. Lubitz CC, Economopoulos KP, Pawlak AC et al. Hobnail variant of papillary thyroid carcinoma: An institutional case series and molecular profile. *Thyroid* 2014;24:958–65.

45. Yeo M-K, Bae JS, Oh WJ et al. Macrofollicular variant of papillary thyroid carcinoma with extensive lymph node metastases. *Endocr Pathol* 2014;25:265–72.

46. Hirokawa M, Carney JA, Ohtsuki Y. Hyalinizing trabecular adenoma and papillary carcinoma of the thyroid gland express different cytokeratin patterns. *Am J Surg Pathol* 2000;24:877–81.

47. Carney JA, Hirokawa M, LLoyd RV et al. Hyalinizing trabecular tumors of the thyroid gland are almost all benign. *Am J Surg Pathol* 2008;32:1877–89.

48. Saleh HA, Jin B, Barnwell J et al. Utility of immuno-histochemical markers in differentiating benign from malignant follicular-derived thyroid nodules. *Diagn Pathol* 2010;5:9.

49. Nosé V. Familial thyroid cancer: A review. *Mod Pathol* 2011;24:S19–33.

50. Camelelle-Teijeiro J, Fachal C, Cabezas-Agricola JM et al. Thyroid pathology findings in Cowden syndrome: A clue for the diagnosis of the PTEN hamartoma tumor syndrome. *Am J Clin Pathol* 2015;144:322–8.

51. Posillico SE, Wilhelm SM, McHenry CR. The utility of frozen section examination for determining the extent of thyroidectomy in patients with a thyroid nodule and atypia/follicular lesion of undetermined significance. *Am J Surg* 2015;209:552–6.

52. Nechifor-Boila A, Borda A, Sassolas G et al. Thyroid tumors of uncertain malignant potential: Morphologic and immunohistochemical analysis of 29 cases. *Pathol Res Pract* 2015;211:320–5.

53. Cipriani NA, Nagar S, Kaplan SP et al. Follicular thyroid carcinoma: How have histologic diagnoses changed in the last half-century and what are the prognostic implications? *Thyroid* 2015;25:1209–16.

54. Xu B, Wang L, Tuttle RM et al. Prognostic impact of extent of vascular invasion in low-grade encapsulated follicular cell-derived thyroid carcinomas: A clinicopathologic study of 278 cases. *Hum Pathol* 2015;46:1789–98.

55. Petric R, Gazic B, Besic N. Prognostic factors for disease-specific survival in 108 patients with Hürtle cell thyroid carcinoma: A single-institution experience. *BMC Cancer* 2014;14:777.

56. Xu B, Ghossein R. Encapsulated thyroid carcinoma of follicular cell origin. *Endocr Pathol* 2015;26:191–9.

57. Wei S, LiVolsi VA, Montone KT et al. PTEN and TP53 mutations in oncocytic follicular carcinoma. *Endocr Pathol* 2015;26:365–9.

58. Hod R, Bachar G, Sternov Y et al. Insular thyroid carcinoma: A retrospective clinicopathologic study. *Am J Otolaryngol* 2013;34:292–5.

59. Volante M, Collini P, Nikiforov YE et al. Poorly differentiated thyroid carcinoma: The Turin proposal for the use of uniform diagnostic criteria and an algorithmic diagnostic approach. *Am J Surg Pathol* 2007;31:1256–64.

60. Bai S, Baloch ZW, Samulski TD et al. Poorly differentiated oncocytic (Hürtle cell) follicular carcinoma: An institutional experience. *Endocr Pathol* 2015;26:164–9.

61. Talbott I, Wakely PE Jr. Undifferentiated (anaplastic) thyroid carcinoma: Practical immunohistochemistry and cytologic look-alikes. *Semin Diagn Pathol* 2015;32:305–10.

62. Pusztaszeri MP, Bongiovanni M, Faquin WC. Update on the cytologic and molecular features of medullary thyroid carcinoma. *Adv Anat Pathol* 2014;21:26–35.

63. Chernock RD, Hagemann IS. Molecular pathology of hereditary and sporadic medullary thyroid carcinomas. *Am J Clin Pathol* 2015;143:768–77.

64. Abi-Raad R, Virk RK, Dinauer CA et al. C-cell neoplasia in asymptomatic carriers of RET mutation in extracellular cysteine-rich and intracellular tyrosine kinase domain. *Hum Pathol* 2015;46:1121–28.

7

Thyroid ultrasound imaging

CHENCHAN HUANG, AMISH H. DOSHI, SAFET LEKPERIC, AND GRACE LO

INTRODUCTION

Ultrasound (US) is an imaging modality that is frequently used to evaluate the thyroid gland. It is an accessible and cost-effective tool providing an opportunity to visualize the gland and surrounding tissues for pathology. US allows for resolution of small structures, and therefore provides the ability to screen the thyroid for lesions as small as 2 mm. It is also used to assess surrounding anatomical structures, including the cervical lymph nodes, muscles, and vessels. Routine imaging is performed while the patient is in the supine position. Scanning of the neck takes place from the lower border of the neck to the level of soft tissues just above the sternal notch [1]. Some of the disadvantages of this modality include high dependence on operator and inferior resolution of adenopathy compared with cross-sectional imaging [2].

THYROID GLAND

Normal appearance

Covered by hyperechoic skin, hypoechoic thin strap muscles anteriorly, and hypoechoic sternocleidomastoid muscles anterolaterally, the thyroid is a very superficial gland within the lower neck (infrahyoid compartment) that is easily accessible to US imaging. The thyroid is a bilobed structure whose lobes rest on either side of the trachea; a thin lip of thyroid tissue known as the isthmus attaches these lobes to one another anteriorly at the lower third of the gland (Figure 7.1). Just posterolateral to the thyroid lobes are circular hypoechoic vessels: carotid arteries and further lateral internal jugular veins. Just posteriorly, the longus colli muscles may also be visualized. Posteriorly on transverse imaging, the esophagus can frequently be seen behind the left lobe of the thyroid adjacent to the trachea [1].

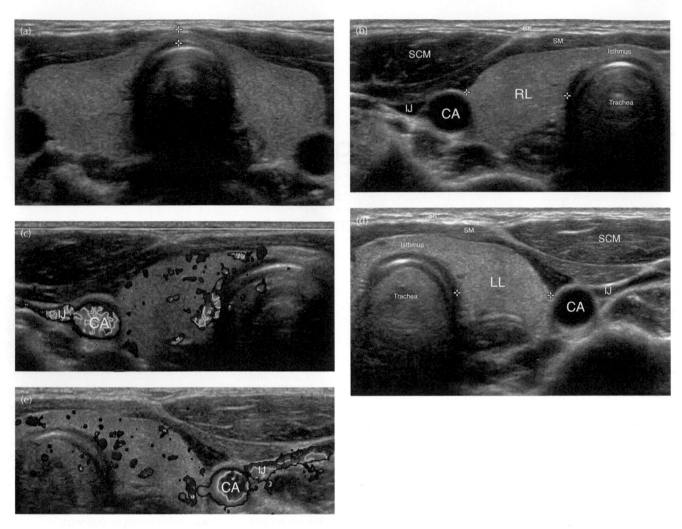

Figure 7.1 Normal thyroid. **(a)** Transverse view of the thyroid lobe shows a normal isthmus indicated by the cursors. **(b)** Transverse view of the right thyroid lobe shows a normal right thyroid lobe (RL) immediately posterior to skin (SK) and strap muscles (SM), and adjacent to lateral neck structures such as the sternocleidomastoid (SCM), internal jugular vein (IJ), and common carotid artery (CA). Just medially adjacent to the right thyroid lobe is the trachea with the overlying isthmus. **(c)** Transverse view of the right thyroid lobe with color Doppler showing normal vascularity of the right thyroid lobe and blood flow through the right common carotid artery and right internal jugular vein. **(d)** Transverse view of the left thyroid lobe (LL) with comparative symmetrical structures. **(e)** Transverse view of the left thyroid lobe with color Doppler showing vascularity of the left thyroid lobe and blood flow through the left common carotid artery and left internal jugular vein.

Ultrasound imaging

The normal thyroid gland is evaluated in the transverse (horizontal) and longitudinal planes. The gland measures 4–6 cm in craniocaudal direction and 1–2 cm in the anteroposterior and transverse dimensions. The isthmus usually measures less than 3 mm in the anteroposterior dimension [3]. A normal thyroid gland usually appears as a homogenously uniform structure with a medium- to high-level echogenicity that is hyperechoic to adjacent muscles (Figure 7.2). The thyroid gland is covered by a thin thyroid capsule, a hyperechoic structure. Occasionally, an additional thyroid lobe known as the pyramidal lobe will be visualized, attaching superiorly to the isthmus (Figure 7.3).

The vascular supply to the thyroid gland can be identified on US as hypoechoic structures with internal color on color Doppler imaging. This includes the superior and inferior thyroid veins and arteries found along the posterior surface of the thyroid.

ULTRASOUND PHYSICS

Ultrasonography is a form of medical imaging utilizing high-frequency sound waves that are magnitudes higher than the audible range. For example, the human ears detect sound frequencies between 20 HZ and 20 kHZ, whereas the sound frequencies employed by US imaging range from 1 to 20 MHZ.

Sound waves are mechanical waves that are generated by an external force that increases pressure. In this case, the US transducers work by changing electrical energy to mechanical energy by changing the shape of PZT (piezoelectric material) located near the tip of the transducer when current is applied [3].

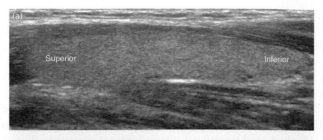

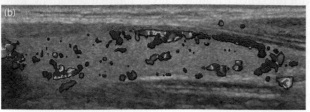

Figure 7.2 Normal thyroid. **(a)** Longitudinal view of either the right or left thyroid lobe. **(b)** Longitudinal view of either the right or left thyroid lobe, with color Doppler showing normal vascularity of the thyroid.

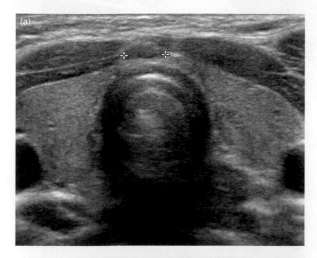

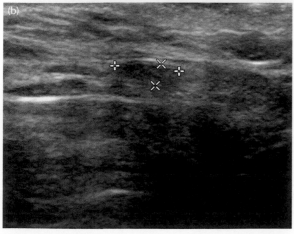

Figure 7.3 Pyramidal lobe. **(a and b)** Transverse and longitudinal views of this pediatric patient demonstrate a small, subcentimeter, well-demarcated, elongated isoechoic structure extending from the isthmus and coursing superiorly, thought to represent pyramidal lobe.

As this mechanical pressure wave travels through a medium, it subsequently exerts pressure in the neighboring medium with resulting pressure change. This cycle continues, and a longitudinal wave is thus generated. The medium and pressure itself do not move. They simply oscillate.

The US waves ultimately result in the following four forms: reflection, absorption, refraction, and scatter [4]. Through these processes, the intensity of sounds waves becomes attenuated. Due to attenuation, signal from deeper structures is lower. To compensate, machine settings are manually adjusted to artificially increase the strength of signal returning from deeper structures, a function called "time gain compensation" [3].

However, in the abnormal thyroid gland, subtle tissue heterogeneity will lead to attenuation differences, which will ultimately result in differences in grayscales, allowing display of thyroid parenchyma heterogeneity and nodules and cysts. In the thyroid gland, due to its lack of air or bone, as we can encounter in abdominal imaging, scatter and absorption play more integral roles in its imaging appearance, relative to reflection and refraction.

There are three main types of US transducers: curvilinear, linear, and phased array. In general, linear transducers are high-frequency transducers, and the higher the frequency, the higher the resolution, while sacrificing depth penetration. Since thyroid gland is a very superficially located small organ, a high-frequency linear transducer is the tool of choice. However, a curvilinear transducer can be helpful in evaluating the enlarged thyroid or thyroid tissue extending into the thoracic inlet. It may also be useful in patients with a larger body habitus or greater soft tissue thickness in the neck region.

Thyromegaly

An enlarged thyroid gland, otherwise known as thyromegaly, is generally considered when the transverse diameter exceeds 2 cm, when the parenchyma extends anterior to the carotids, or if the isthmus is thicker than a few millimeters [5,6]. Goiter is swelling of the neck associated with thyromegaly, usually secondary to abnormal thyroid gland function.

THYROID CONGENTIAL ABNORMALITIES

Thyroid aplasia, hypoplasia, and ectopia

Congenital abnormalities of the thyroid include thyroid aplasia, thyroid hypoplasia, and ectopic thyroid. Thyroid aplasia and hypoplasia are easily evaluated by US, as evidenced by no to little normal thyroid tissue identified in the anterior neck. Occasionally, a unilaterally hypoplastic thyroid lobe will result in hypertrophy of the contralateral lobe.

Ectopic thyroid tissue is not easily evaluated by US and is generally diagnosed with a nuclear medicine I-131 scan, which can easily survey the entire body for ectopic thyroid tissue. When present, ectopic thyroid tissue is most commonly seen between the foramen cecum in the tongue and the epiglottis, otherwise called a lingual thyroid. This entity is seen in approximately 1 in 10,000 healthy individuals [5]. Ectopic thyroid sites also include sublingual, paralaryngeal, intratracheal, and infrasternal [5].

Thyroglossal cysts

Thyroglossal cysts are the most common congenital cysts of the neck. Patients most often present in childhood or young adulthood. During embryogenesis, the thyroid migrates from the foramen cecum in the tongue to the lower neck, leaving an epithelial tract called a thyroglossal duct, which normally involutes by the eighth week of fetal life. In approximately 5% of cases, the thyroglossal duct may retain thyroid cells, which give rise to thyroglossal duct cysts [5]. Thyroglossal duct cysts are often treated by complete excision.

These cysts are typically located midline between the thyroid gland and the hyoid bone, although the more caudad the cyst is located, the more likely it is to be lateral to the midline. Only 20% occur above the hyoid [5]. Sonography is excellent for the initial evaluation of these cysts. On US, these thyroglossal duct cysts usually appear as cystic lesions containing diffuse internal low-level echoes, which represents proteinaceous material secreted by its lining (Figure 7.4). Thyroglossal duct cysts can also be secondarily infected or bleed, in which case they would appear more complex, often with thickened irregular walls or internal septations. Rarely are the cysts simple. Solid components should not be seen within thyroglossal duct cysts and, when present, should suggest the presence of ectopic thyroid tissue or thyroglossal duct carcinoma [7].

THYROID PARENCHYMAL DISEASES

There is a range of inflammatory and immune conditions that affect the thyroid, most commonly subacute thyroiditis, Hashimoto's thyroiditis, and Graves' disease.

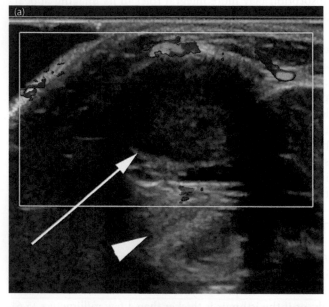

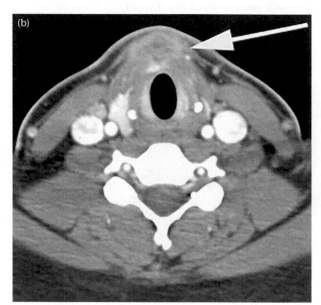

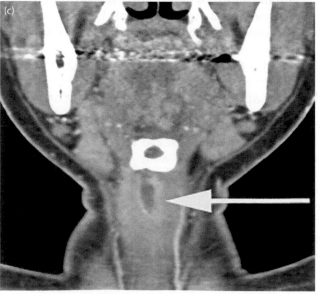

Figure 7.4 Thyroglossal duct cyst. **(a)** Longitudinal US of this pediatric patient demonstrates a large, avascular, well-defined lesion (arrow) with posterior acoustic enhancement (arrowhead), compatible with a cyst. It has homogeneous internal low-level echogenicity, which suggests a complex cyst with proteinacous or hemorrhagic material. **(b and c)** Axial and coronal postcontrast CT images of this cyst demonstrate its characteristic location in the midline along the expected course, from the foramen cecum to the thyroid bed, and clinch the diagnoses for a thyroglossal duct cyst.

Hashimoto's disease

Hashimoto's disease, or chronic autoimmue lymphocytic thyroiditis, is the most common cause of hypothyroidism in the United States, with a peak incidence between ages 40 and 60. It is also the most common inflammatory condition of the thyroid gland and most common cause of goiter [8]. The condition occurs much more commonly in women than men, and it often coexists with other autoimmune diseases, including Sjogren's syndrome, lupus, rheumatoid arthritis, fibrosing mediastinitis, sclerosing cholangitis, and pernicious anemia.

Hashimoto's disease is thought to be caused by autoantibodies to thyroid proteins, including thyroid peroxidase and thyroglobulin. The gland is infiltrated with lymphocytes and plasma cells, and a fibrotic reaction takes place. Initially, the patient may be euthyroid but generally becomes hypothyroid, as the thyroid is destroyed and eventually fails. As the condition is caused by autoantibodies, the diagnosis of this condition can therefore be made serologically.

On US, the gland is usually normal to enlarged in size and is hypoechoic in echotexture. The thyroid may be a more heterogenous than normal homogenous echotexture of the thyroid, which reflects underlying histologic changes as the gland is infiltrated by lymphocytes. Fibrous strands within the thyroid are echogenic and may result in a multilobulated or micronodular appearance (Figure 7.5). The gland is often markedly hypervascular, although flow may be variable [6]. Nodules may form with Hashimoto's disease, which may be benign or malignant. At the late stage of this disease, the gland becomes atrophic and diffusely hypoechoic, similar to the strap muscles in echogenicity [6]. Often, cervical lymphadenopthy is found adjacent to the lower poles of both lobes and may be a helpful diagnostic clue [9].

Thyroid lymphoma is an uncommon entity but is most frequently seen in patients with a history of Hashimoto's thyroiditis. Clinically, these patients usually present with a rapidly enlarging thyroid gland. On US, there is generally a markedly hypoechoic, poorly marginated solid mass with enhanced through transmission in a background of chronic thyroiditis [9]. Diagnosis should be made with fine-needle aspiration (FNA) biopsy.

Graves' disease

Graves' disease, also known as diffuse toxic goiter, is the most common cause of hyperthyroidism. It is an autoimmune disorder in which thyroid-stimulating immunoglobulins stimulate the function of thyroid-stimulating hormone, causing hyperthyroidism. As in Hashimoto's thyroiditis, this disorder can also usually be diagnosed with serologic testing.

The role of US is limited in the diagnosis of Graves' disease, as the disorder can usually be diagnosed serologically and its sonographic findings are highly nonspecific. However, careful evaluation for nodules should be performed, as there

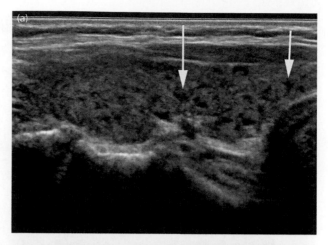

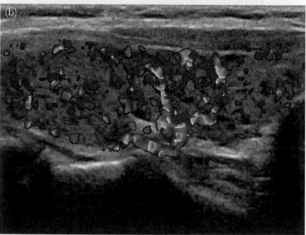

Figure 7.5 Hashimoto's thyroiditis. **(a and b)** Longitudinal view demonstrates a diffusely hypoechoic gland with heterogeneous micronodular pattern (arrows point to the hypoechoic micronodules). Corresponding color Doppler image demonstrates diffusely increased vascularity. Note that vascularity varies with different stages of Hashimoto's thyroiditis, but is typically less than that of Graves' disease.

is suggestion that there is an increased incidence of thyroid cancer in patients with Graves' disease [10].

In Graves' disease, the thyroid is often enlarged, with decreased echogenicity. The thyroid is occasionally heterogenous in nature. The thyroid demonstrates markedly increased vascularity [6] (Figure 7.6). A specific entity known as "thyroid inferno" is associated with Graves' disease. With this condition, there is a distinct pattern consisting of multiple small areas of increased parenchymal flow diffusely throughout the thyroid [11]. The color Doppler flow should demonstrate pulsatile flow when sampled.

Subacute granulomatous thyroiditis

Subacute granulomatous thyroiditis, also called de Quervain's thyroiditis, is thought to be caused by a viral illness and is the most common cause of a painful thyroid [12]. It occurs more often in women, usually in the age range of 30–50 years [8]. The thyroiditis is often preceded

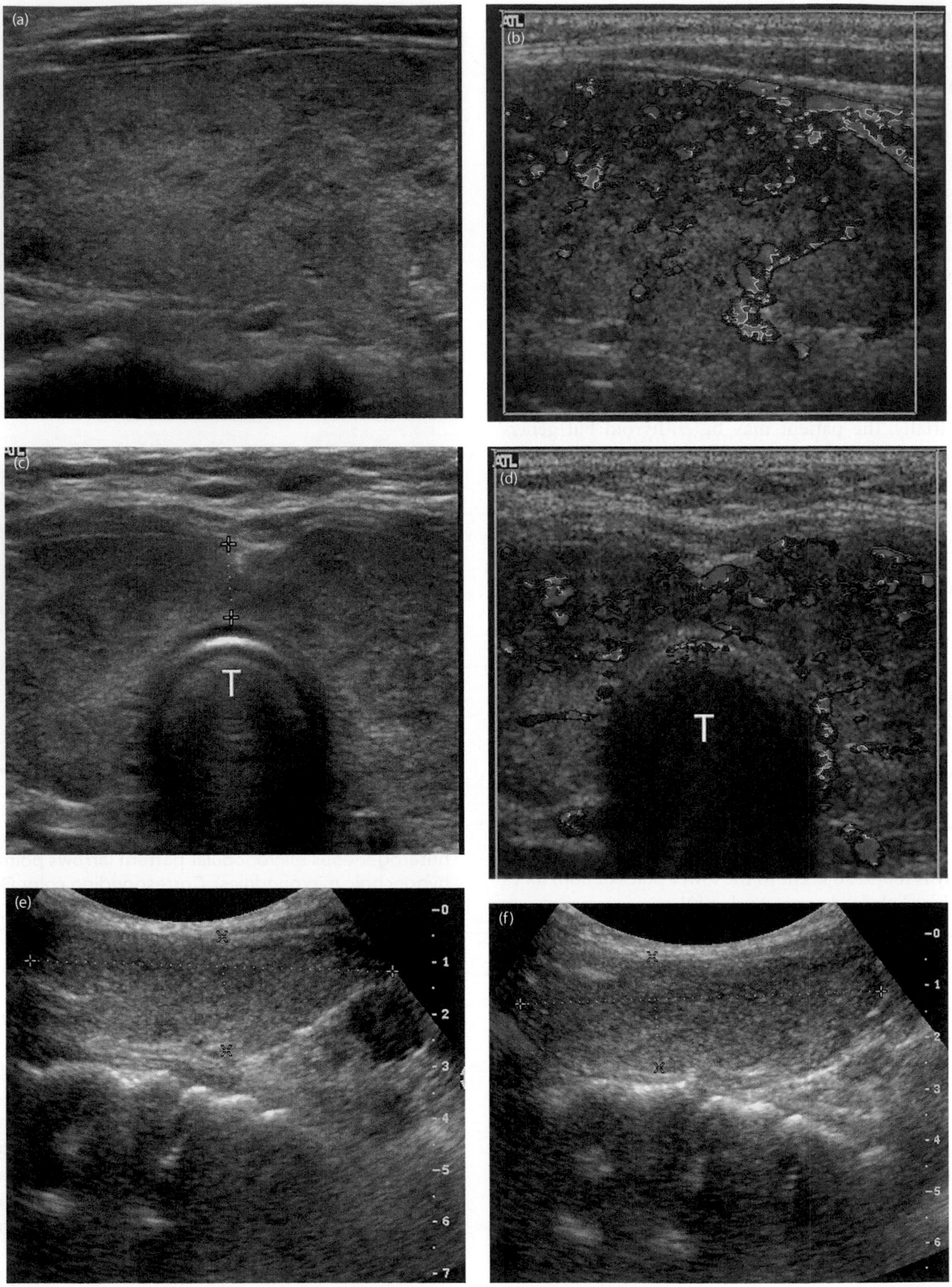

Figure 7.6 Graves' disease. **(a and b)** Longitudinal view shows a diffusely enlarged thyroid gland with heterogeneous echotexture and diffuse hypervascularity in this patient with known Graves' disease. **(c and d)** Transverse view shows a thickened isthmus (calipers) measuring 61 mm with corresponding hypervascularity. T, trachea. **(e and f)** A curvilinear transducer had to be used to capture the entirety of each enlarged thyroid lobe. The right thyroid lobe (calipers) measures 7 cm (cranial–caudal dimension) × 2.2 cm (anterior–posterior dimension). The left thyroid lobe (calipers) also measures 7 cm (cranial–caudal dimension) × 2.2 cm (anterior–posterior dimension). Note that by switching from a linear transducer to a curvilinear transducer, the US images lose spatial resolution, and consequently, the thyroid lobes look less heterogeneous in echotexture.

by an upper respiratory tract infection and results in an enlarged, painful thyroid that is commonly accompanied by fever. The entire gland may be involved, although there may also be focal involvement of the thyroid. Transient hyperthyroidism may be seen in the initial stages of this disease secondary to rapid follicle destruction, leading to a release of preformed thyroid hormone stores, although this is often followed by transient hypothyroidism until the thyroid recovers and hormone production begins again. The condition is most often diagnosed clinically and is self-limiting.

US can be helpful with the initial diagnosis of the condition, as well as with interval follow-up during the months-long course of this condition. On US, the thyroid may have a poorly marginated area or areas of decreased echogenicity in the involved regions of the thyroid. Blood flow to these hypoechoic regions usually demonstrates little to no vascular flow on color Doppler interrogation [6,9]. Importantly, the US features of malignancy, such as microcalcifications, are absent. Follow-up US can be useful to demonstrate regression or resolution of these lesions in subacute granulomatous thyroiditis [13,14]. FNA biopsy can be helpful for troubleshooting these lesions.

THYROID NODULES

Thyroid nodules occur very frequently, with a higher female predominance, and increase with age. As many as 50% of the population has one or more nodules [15], with only 3%–7% of nodules being palpable. US is an important tool in the workup of thyroid nodules because 5%–15% of thyroid nodules harbor malignancy [16]. Thyroid nodules generally do not cause symptoms. The vast majority of thyroid nodules are detected on imaging performed for evaluation of unrelated medical problems, such as chest computed tomography (CT) or carotid artery US. Although malignancy rate is low and mortality of thyroid cancers is excellent, clinicians are obligated to exclude malignancy in these incidentalomas. Consequently, high-resolution thyroid US, being widely available and noninvasive, is often the next step for nodule characterization.

The main goal of thyroid US imaging is to detect and characterize nodules. Thyroid nodules can demonstrate a variety of US features that can help the clinician determine the likelihood of benignity or malignancy. These features can also help include or exclude nodules for FNA or biopsy [17].

Benign thyroid nodules

Sixty to seventy percent of biopsied thyroid nodules are benign and most commonly represent benign follicular nodules or thyroiditis [18]. Benign nodules encompass focal nodular hyperplasia, follicular adenomas, colloid cysts, nodular goiter, and nodules of Graves' disease [19].

Focal nodular hyperplasia or nodular hyperplastic nodules have variable echogenicities compared with the background thyroid parenchyma. They typically have cystic centers. If the cystic centers enlarge and contain inspissated colloid, which can be seen as a comet tail artifact on US, this can confirm the diagnosis of a colloid cyst. The comet tail artifact is specific for the diagnosis of a colloid cyst. It is a grayscale artifact manifest as multiple parallel equidistant brightly echogenic lines distal to the imaging target. It is caused by the brightly echogenic colloid crystals suspended within a colloid cyst (Figure 7.7). Follicular adenomas typically account for 5%–10% of benign nodules. They are well-marginated solid nodules with a thin uniform hypoechoic rim.

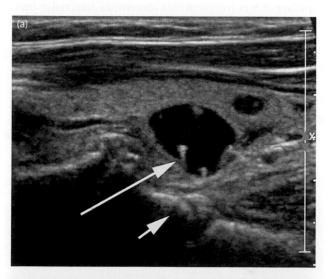

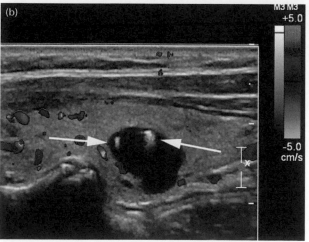

Figure 7.7 Colloid cyst. (a) Longitudinal image of the left thyroid lobe demonstrates a cyst containing several small, brightly echogenic foci with a posterior comet tail artifact (long arrow), which manifest as multiple parallel, equidistant, brightly echogenic lines distal to the imaging target, and represent suspended colloid crystals. A comet tail artifact is specific for a colloid cyst. Also note the posterior acoustic enhancement of this cyst (short arrow). (b) Color Doppler image of the same colloid cyst demonstrates it is an avascular cyst, rather than a markedly hypoechoic solid nodule. An additional comet tail artifact is noted (arrows).

Malignant thyroid nodules

Only 3%–7% of fine-needle biopsied nodules are malignant or suspicious for malignancy on cytopathology, with approximately 95% of those with malignancy suspicion being actual cancers. The majority of thyroid cancers consist of papillary cancer (85%), with follicular cancer making up 10% and the remaining 3% consisting of Hurthle cell or oxyphil tumors [20].

PAPILLARY THYROID CANCER

Papillary cancers have a great prognosis, with a 20-year survival rate of 90%–95% [15]. Some autopsy series show that papillary cancer fragments are sometimes detected in previously asymptomatic patients. The classic US feature consists of a solid hypoechoic mass with microcalcifications (usually 1 mm or less) (Figure 7.8) The microcalcifications result from calcium deposits in psamomma bodies.

FOLLICULAR THYROID CANCER

Follicular cell cancer (CA) can look identical to follicular adenomas on imaging, and even FNA cytology cannot distinguish these two. Contrary to papillary cancer, follicular cancers are often isoechoic or even hyperechoic and without microcalcifications. Surgery and histology analysis are required to look for vascular and capsular invasion to exclude follicular cell CA.

MEDULLARY THYROID CANCER

Medullary thyroid cancer makes up about 5% of thyroid cancers [3]. They are derived from parafollicular cells that secrete calcitonin; therefore, serum calcitonin can be used as a tumor marker. Their US appearance is usually a hypoechoic solid nodule (often markedly hypoechoic) with microcalcifications or macrocalcifications (including rim calcifications) (Figure 7.9). These lesions can be difficult to distinguish from those of the differentiated papillary thyroid cancers [1,18]. However, they are more aggressive than papillary thyroid cancer, and are resistant to chemotherapy or radiation therapy. Medullary cancer is of intermediate aggressiveness with 10-year survival rate of 75% [18]. They are 80% sporadic and 20% associated with multiple endocrine neoplasia (MEN) type 2.

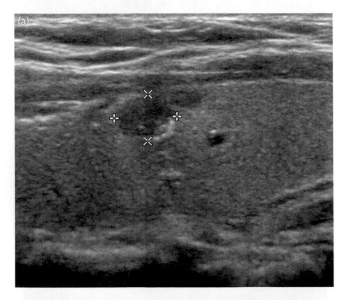

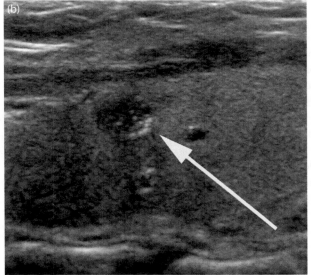

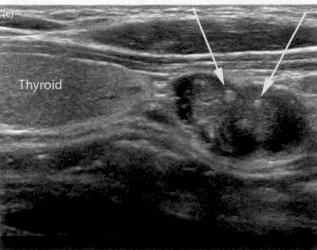

Figure 7.8 Papillary CA with lymph node metastasis. **(a and b)** Grayscale US image demonstrates a subcentimeter hypoechoic nodule (calipers) with multiple punctuate echogenic foci that represent microcalcifications (arrow). Microcalcifications are too small to cause posterior acoustic shadowing, as seen in macrocalcifications. **(c)** Adjacent to the thyroid gland, grayscale US of this same patient demonstrates a mildly enlarged (short axis 1.1 cm) cervical lymph node with an irregular lobulated border and similar-appearing microcalcifications (arrows). Both the thyroid nodule and lymph node were biopsied, and yielded papillary cancer with a metastatic lymph node.

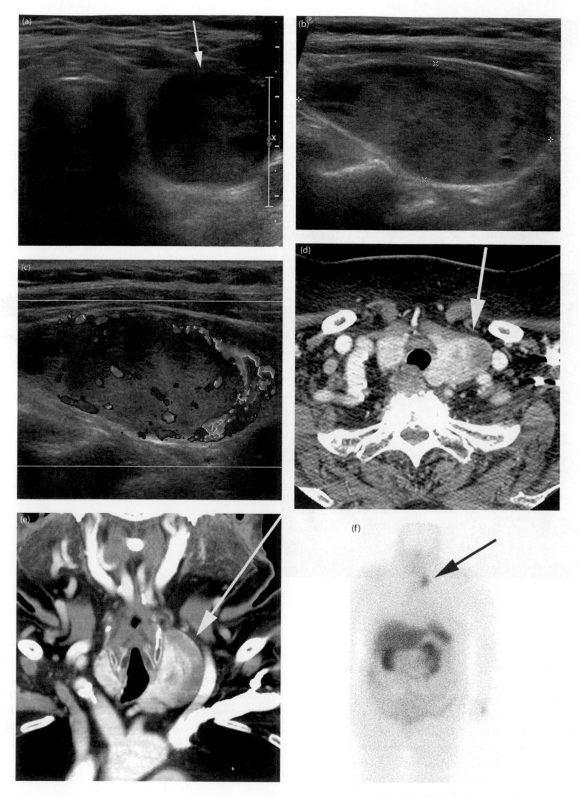

Figure 7.9 Medullary CA. **(a and b)** Transverse and longitudinal thyroid US images of an 83-year-old female patient demonstrate a solitary large (5.1 × 2.4 cm) heterogeneous mass within the left thyroid lobe (arrow and calipers). **(c)** Color Doppler image of this mass demonstrates internal vascularity. Biopsy yielded medullary cancer. **(d and e)** Axial and coronal CT images of the thyroid gland demonstrate a large heterogenous mass within the left lobe (arrows). No metastatic lymph node was present. **(f and g)** Whole body INDIUM-111 OCTREOTIDE scan and axial single-photon emission computed tomography (SPECT) CT images demonstrate an octreotide-avid lesion (arrow) consistent with medullary cancer. No distant metastasis was detected. This was a sporadic case. Consider familial syndromes (i.e., MEN2A and 2B) in young patients or multifocal tumors.

(*Continued*)

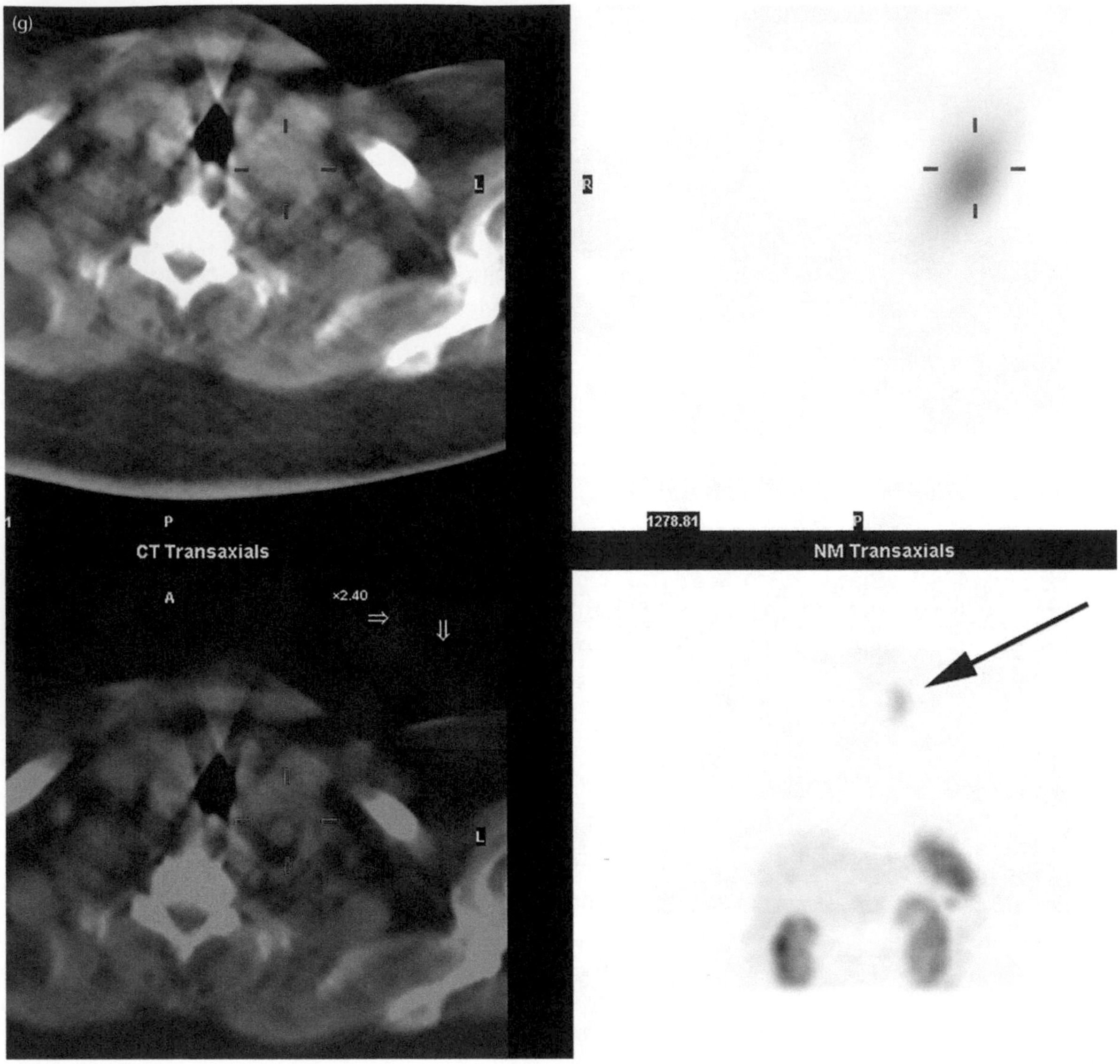

Figure 7.9 (Continued) Medullary CA.

ANAPLASTIC THYROID CANCER

Anaplastic thyroid cancer is the most aggressive type of thyroid cancer. It makes up 1%–3% of all thyroid cancers but carries a dismal prognosis, with median survival of 3–5 months after diagnosis [21]. It is rarely seen in patients younger than 60 years old [3]. It usually appears as a large, solid, hypoechoic mass with lymph node invasion upon initial diagnosis. Due to its large size, cross-imaging studies such as CT or MRI are recommended after biopsy to assess for adjacent vascular and lymph node invasion.

Ultrasound features of benign and malignant thyroid nodules

Although there are many US imaging features associated with benign or malignant lesion, it is often very difficult to definitively diagnose a thyroid nodule based on US appearance. Many of the US characteristics overlap between benign and malignant thyroid nodules. From a practical point of view, it is not necessary to precisely diagnose which nodule is diseased. Rather, it is important to identify suspicious nodules and recommend biopsies to exclude malignancy. In the setting of high-resolution US imaging, there are a number of features that should be examined on a routine basis.

SIZE

There is overall consensus that nodule size does not correlate with risk of malignancy [22,23]. However, when faced with incidental thyroid nodules, there are several guidelines that take nodule size into consideration when recommending biopsies (Table 7.1). From a practical point, with the prevalence of small thyroid nodules, FNA or biopsy of every subcentimeter indeterminate nodule would lead to excessive biopsies and strain medical

Table 7.1 Indications for thyroid nodule biopsy

- Solid and hypoechoic nodule >1 cm
- Nodule of any size with US findings suggestive of extracapsular growth or metastatic cervical lymph nodes
- Nodule of any size in a high-risk patient (see chart for high-risk patient)
- Nodule of diameter <10 mm along with two or more suspicious US criteria

FNA Biopsy of Multinodular Glands

- It is rarely necessary to biopsy more than two nodules when they are selected on the basis of previously described criteria
- If a radioisotope scan is available, do not biopsy hot areas
- In the presence of suspicious cervical lymphadenopathy, FNA biopsy of both the lymph node and suspicious nodule(s) is essential

Source: Adapted from Gharib H et al. *J Endocrinol Invest* 2010; 33(5):287–91.

Table 7.2 High-risk factors

- History of thyroid cancer in one or more first-degree relatives
- History of external beam radiation as a child
- Exposure to ionizing radiation in childhood or adolescence
- Prior hemithyroidectomy with discovery of thyroid cancer, ^{18}F-fluorodeoxyglucose avidity on positron emission tomography scanning
- MEN2 syndrome, FMTC (familial medullary thyroid cancer), or elevated calcitonin (>100 pg = mL)

Source: Adapted from Chan BK et al. *J Ultrasound Med* 2003; 22(10):1083–90.

resources. Additionally, since the majority of thyroid cancers are papillary and follicular cancers, which carry an excellent prognosis [15], some believe that early diagnosis of subcentimeter cancers may not yield clinical benefit [24]. On the other hand, if a patient were to be a high-risk patient (Table 7.2), size criteria are often removed, and a suspicious nodule of any size should be biopsied [20,23] (Table 7.2).

ECHOGENICITY

The majority of thyroid malignancies are found in hypoechoic nodules. However, many benign nodules are also hypoechoic. These types of nodules are less echogenic than the surrounding thyroid parenchyma, while "markedly hypoechoic" means that the nodule is less echogenic than the cervical strap muscles [22]. While the typical hypoechoic nodules with microcalcification are usually found to be papillary thyroid cancers, the rare follicular cancers can appear isoechoic or even hyperechoic, without calcifications [20].

CALCIFICATIONS

Microcalcifications represent calcium deposits within the psamomma bodies of papillary cancer, and are a specific but not sensitive feature, present in only 20%–50% of papillary cancers. In recent years, peripheral rim calcifications (Figure 7.10) and coarse calcifications (also called macrocalcifications) have also been recognized as suspicious features (Table 7.3). These macrocalcifications represent dystrophic calcifications related to tissue necrosis, and can be seen in the setting of multinodular goiter or malignancy (Figure 7.11) [15,25].

Shadowing is a US feature that occurs when the US wave is attenuated by high-density material along a single path, such as with coarse calcifications. Twinkling can be seen in the setting of smaller calcifications. It appears as an area of rapidly changing colors on Doppler US (Figure 7.12) [17,26]. It is more sensitive than shadowing in allowing one to diagnose small calcifications.

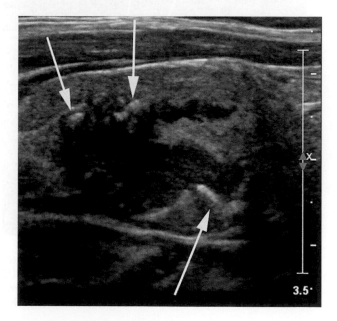

Figure 7.10 Peripheral calcifications. US shows a nodule with an irregular border and peripheral bright calcifications (arrows).

Table 7.3 Suspicious features of thyroid nodules

- Microcalcifications
- Hypoechoic
- Increased nodular vascularity
- Infiltrative margins
- Taller than wide

Source: Adapted from American Thyroid Association (ATA) Guidelines Taskforce on Thyroid Nodules and Differentiated Thyroid Cancer, Cooper DS, Doherty GM et al. *Thyroid* 2009;19(11):1167–214.

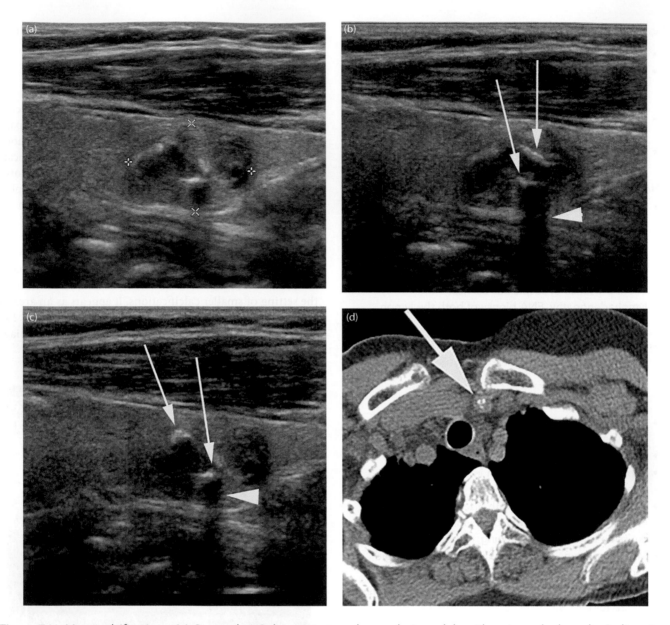

Figure 7.11 Macrocalcifications. **(a)** Grayscale US demonstrates a hypoechoic nodule with an irregular boarder (calipers) and multiple chunky echogenic foci. **(b and c)** Additional US images demonstrate that the chunky echogenic foci (long arrows) have associated posterior acoustic shadowing (arrowhead), compatible with macrocalcifications, also called coarse calcifications. **(d)** An axial chest CT image at the level of the thyroid gland confirms the macrocalcifications seen on US.

MARGIN

Irregular margin is fairly sensitive but not specific. Many benign and malignant nodules can have irregular margins.

HALO

This is the complete ring of thin uniform peripheral pseudo-capsule made of compressed normal thyroid tissue, fibrous tissue, and chronic inflammatory infiltrates (Figure 7.13). This is specific for a benign nodule; however, it is not very sensitive. Recent literature also suggests that up to 10%–24% of papillary cancers can have either a complete or incomplete halo (Figure 7.14) [15].

VASCULARITY

Intranodular hypervascularity has been suggested to be a sign of malignancy. Peripheral hypervascularity may be a sign of focal thyroiditis, although a minority of malignancies may also have peripheral hypervascularity [18]. Studies have shown that papillary cancers tend to have some degree of vascularity, either central or peripheral. Therefore, a completely avascular nodule is very likely benign [25].

TALLER THAN WIDE

In similar fashion to suspicious or malignant breast lesions, the taller than wider sign is fairly specific for malignancy. This describes a nodule as having an anterior–posterior

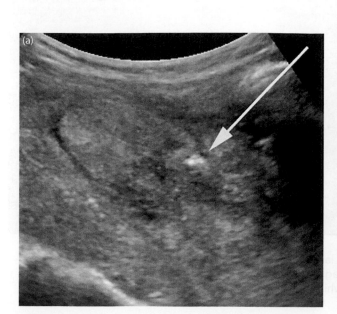

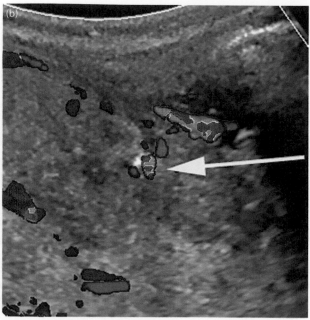

Figure 7.12 Twinkle artifact. **(a)** Grayscale US image demonstrates a small, brightly echogenic focus (arrow). **(b)** Color Doppler image of this echogenic focus demonstrates a "twinkling artifact" (arrow), which is an area of rapidly changing colors. Twinkling artifact is a sensitive sign for small calcifications.

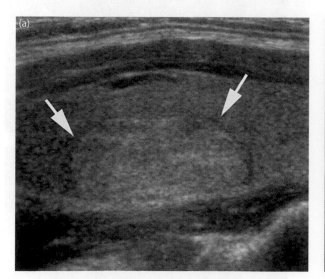

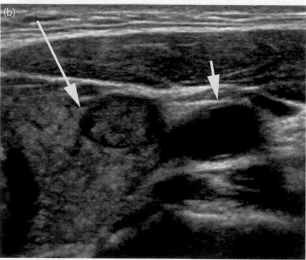

Figure 7.13 Adenoma with halo. **(a)** Longitudinal view demonstrates a homogeneously mildly hyperechoic and well-demarcated nodule with a complete hypoechoic rim (arrows). **(b)** Transverse view of the thyroid demonstrates a homogeneously mildly hypoechoic, well-demarcated nodule with a complete hypoechoic halo (long arrow). The anechoic carotid artery is seen laterally (short arrow). These findings are specific but not sensitive for adenomas.

diameter that is larger than the transverse or horizontal diameter (Figure 7.15). This is thought to be due to the centrifugal growth tendency of tumors at a nonuniform rate in all directions [15,22].

SOLID

Entirely cystic masses with a classic thin rim and posterior acoustic enhancement are definitely benign. However, both benign and malignant nodules can be solid or partially solid.

Posterior acoustic enhancement is an important and useful artifact to diagnose whether a mass is solid versus cystic. It manifests as increased echogenicity distal to the posterior wall of an anechoic nodule. Fluid within a cyst allows for transmission of sound waves and therefore has little attenuation. This leads to increased echogenicity posterior to the

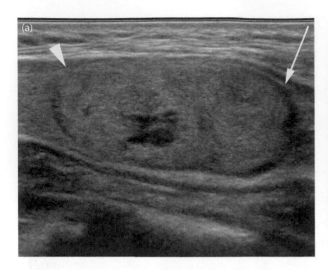

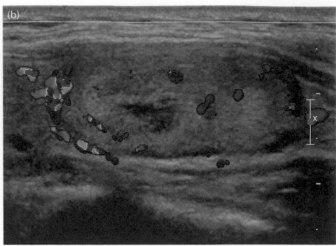

Figure 7.14 Papillar CA with incomplete halo. **(a)** US shows a large solid nodule with a small cystic center and an incomplete hypoechoic halo (arrow). Note arrowhead points to a region without a hypoechoic halo. **(b)** Color Doppler image demonstrates internal vascularity. Patient underwent FNA, which yielded papillary CA, follicular variant.

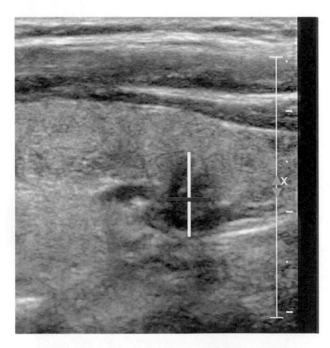

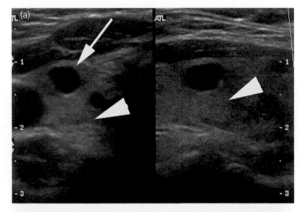

Figure 7.15 Taller than wide. Transverse grayscale US image of the thyroid demonstrates a hypoechoic nodule that is longer in the anterior–posterior dimension (white line) compared with the transverse dimension (red line).

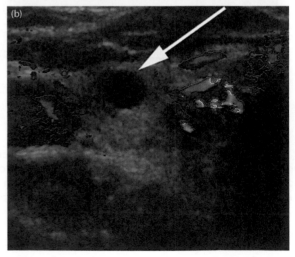

cysts (Figure 7.16). In contrast, the solid thyroid parenchymal tissue will attenuate sound and lead to decreased echogenicity behind the nodule.

SOLITARY

The overall chance of having malignancy in a patient with multiple discrete nodules is the same as that for a person with a solitary nodule. Therefore, this feature does not have correlation with either benign or malignant disease. The exception is when there are multiple similar-sized nodules

Figure 7.16 Simple cyst. **(a)** Transverse and longitudinal US images demonstrate an anechoic lesion (arrow) with a sharp border and posterior acoustic enhancement (arrowhead). These findings are compatible with a benign simple cyst. **(b)** Color Doppler image of this lesion (arrow) demonstrates lack of internal vascularity, confirming it is a cyst and not a vascular structure.

(a)

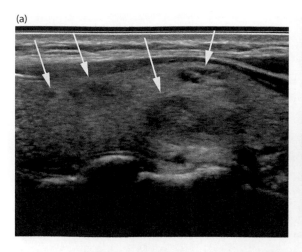

(b)

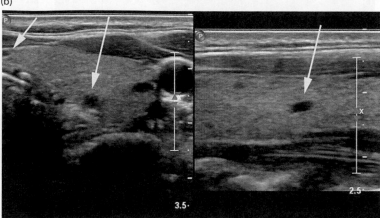

Figure 7.17 Multinodular goiter. **(a and b)** Grayscale US shows multiple nodules (arrows) of similar sizes in two different patients.

without normal intervening parenchyma, as seen in the case of multinodular goiter, which is benign (Figures 7.17 and 7.18). In the event of multiple thyroid nodules, FNA should be based on suspicious US features [23].

Unfortunately, no single US feature listed above is both sensitive and specific for malignant nodules. Furthermore, the classic suspicious features of microcalcifications and irregular margins have been found to be absent in many proven malignant nodules. Several guidelines have been established to help select indeterminate or suspicious nodules for biopsy. On average, a malignant thyroid nodule often demonstrates two or three suspicious US features. On the other hand, although infrequent, there are two benign sonographic features of thyroid nodules that are exempted from biopsies: a purely cystic appearance and a spongiform appearance. The spongiform appearance is defined as an aggregation of multiple microcystic components in more than 50% of the nodule volume, and resembles a water-filled sponge [20].

Evaluation of US features of nodules should be taken in the context of patients who are at higher risk for developing thyroid malignancy. This is defined by the American Thyroid Association (Table 7.2) [20].

LYMPH NODES

The thyroid gland has cervical lymph nodes that drain either side of the gland known as juxtavisceral nodes. These nodes are part of the anterior cervical nodal group located in the tracheoesophageal groove. The most superior portions of these nodes sit directly posterior to the thyroid lobes [27].

When imaging the thyroid gland, cervical lymph nodes will be present around the carotid artery and jugular vein laterally and are deep to muscle. On sonography, the nodes appear hypoechoic peripherally and hyperechoic centrally due to the presence of a fatty hilum. Benign lymph nodes are generally oval in shape (Figure 7.19). The normal cervical lymph node size varies with

neck region, age, and sex, yet generally has an upper limit of 8 mm in maximal short axial diameter [28]. Features that are concerning for malignancy within a lymph node include round morphology, loss of visualization of the echogenic fatty hilum, central liquefaction secondary to necrosis, and large size (Figure 7.20) [29]. Papillary carcinoma and medullary carcinoma of the thyroid involvement of lymph nodes can result in microcalcifications and be cystic within lymph nodes [30].

Abnormal cervical lymph nodes should always warrant further investigation with biopsy. Typically, biopsies of both the suspicious thyroid nodule and the abnormal lymph node are performed at the same time. Signs of an abnormal lymph node include size greater than 1 cm in short axis, loss of fatty hila, cortical thickening with a rounded appearance, and altered vascularity throughout the node instead of central hilar vessels. Reactive lymph nodes may also have this appearance. Therefore, in the absence of active head and neck infection or inflammation, lymph nodes with abnormal features should warrant further evaluation.

PITFALLS OF ULTRASOUND IMAGING OF THE THYROID

1. While thyroid cancers are often found in dominant nodules in the setting of multiple thyroid nodules, one-third of thyroid cancers are found in nondominant thyroid nodules [24]. If one only selects the largest nodule for biopsy, up to 33% of cancers can be missed. It is therefore important to examine additional US features of each nodule carefully.
2. Microcalcifications (often 1–2 mm) and colloid both appear as punctate echogenic foci without shadowing, and can therefore be mistaken for each other. It is important to examine carefully for the presence of ring-down artifact present in colloid nodules.
3. While uncommon, the cystic variant of papillary cancers exists, and can lead one to mistake it as a complex

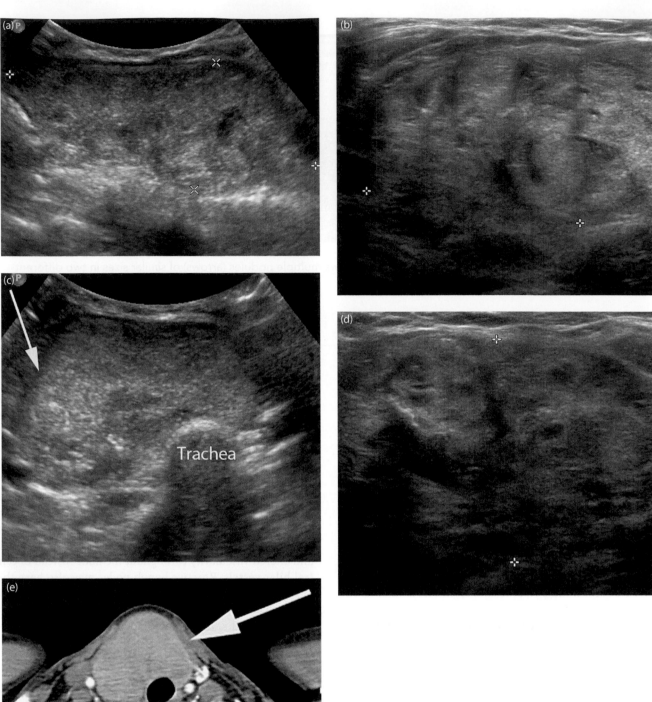

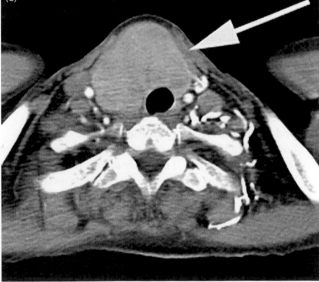

Figure 7.18 Goiter. **(a)** Longitudinal and **(b and c)** transverse grayscale US images of the right thyroid lobe demonstrate a heterogeneous and markedly enlarged right lobe, measuring 8.7 cm (cranial–caudal dimension) × 3.6 cm (anterior–posterior dimension) × 3.3 cm (transverse). **(d)** Transverse view demonstrates a markedly thickened isthmus (calipers), measuring 3.3 cm. **(e)** Postcontrast axial CT image demonstrates enlarged right thyroid lobe and isthmus.

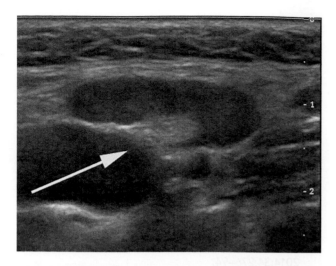

Figure 7.19 Normal vs. abnormal lymph node. Longitudinal image of a normal cervical lymph node. Its benign characteristics include oval shape, measuring less than 1 cm in short axis, and an echogenic fatty hilum (arrow).

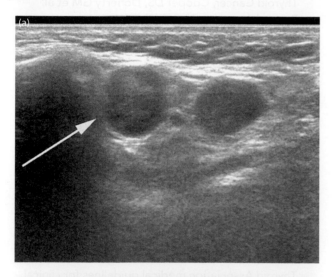

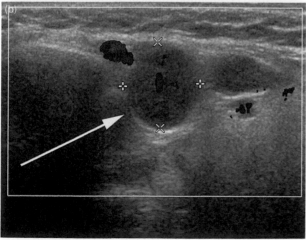

Figure 7.20 Normal vs. abnormal lymph node. **(a and b)** Grayscale and color Doppler images demonstrate an abnormal lymph node (arrow). Suspicious features include a rounded shape (instead of oval) and loss of fatty hilum.

cyst. However, there still would be vascularity in the wall or papillary projections of the cystic papillary cancers. It is therefore important to put color flow onto every nodule [15].

4. Metastasis to the cervical region in proximity to the thyroid gland can be mistaken as thyroid nodules. Typically, these nodules are not completely within the thyroid parenchyma. Therefore, one needs to consider the possibility of metastasis in the absence of a complete rim of normal thyroid nodule parenchyma. The additional maneuver of real-time examining if the nodule in question and the thyroid parenchyma move in the same direction while the patient swallows can help to establish the origin of the nodule in question.

5. Lastly, a diffusely hypervascular infiltrative thyroid cancer can be mistaken as a benign process such as Graves' disease. Careful examination for adjacent nodal metastasis and residual areas of normal parenchyma can alarm the clinician for the possibility of an infiltrative cancer.

ADVANCED THYROID ULTRASOUND IMAGING TECHNIQUES

There are two advanced techniques related to US imaging of thyroid nodules: elastography and contrast-enhanced ultrasonography (CEUS) [31]. Combined with conventional US, CEUS and elastography can improve sensitivity as well as specificity in identifying malignant thyroid nodules from benign ones.

Elastography is a fairly new noninvasive technique in thyroid nodule imaging. It has been integrated into breast and liver imaging. It is introduced to thyroid US to help distinguish benign from malignant nodules and thereby decrease unnecessary biopsies. It is based on the principle that malignant nodules tend to be stiffer than surrounding thyroid parenchyma, while benign nodules tend to be softer. A common technique is to lightly and repetitively tap the skin overlying the nodule, with the region of interest placed onto the nodule and surrounding thyroid parenchyma. A stiffer nodule will be more difficult to deform than a softer one. Compressibility of a nodule is referred to as "strain." Dedicated software can then calculate how much strain each pixel has and assign shades of colors accordingly, typically with a color scale ranging from red (areas of greatest strain or softest component) to blue (areas of no strain or stiffest component). While there have been some studies supporting the role of elastography [23,32,33], there are also studies demonstrating opposite results [34]. For example, a large research study by Moon et al. published in *Radiology* demonstrated that elastography, whether alone or in combination with grayscale US, is not a useful tool in selecting nodules for biopsy when compared with grayscale US features alone [35]. Additionally, one needs to factor in additional scanning time and cost of dedicated software when considering adapting US elastography as an adjunct technique. The role of elastography continues to wait for validation until further extensive multicentric studies based on postsurgery histopathology results become available [36,37].

Contrast-enhanced ultrasonography is another new imaging modality. A contrast agent needs to be injected intravenously. A well-known contrast agent called SonoVue (Bracco, Milan, Italy) is composed of stabilized sulfur hexafluoride microbubbles surrounded by a phospholipid shell. The microbubbles do not get absorbed by blood, and therefore appear hyperechoic on US images. The contrast agent has not been approved by the Food and Drug Administration (FDA) yet, but has been in use in Europe and Asia. It is based on the principle that malignant thyroid nodules tend to enhance less. Specific enhancement patterns have been described for benign and malignant nodules. There is also still ongoing debate regarding its clinical utility [31,38–42].

REFERENCES

1. Loevner LA, Kaplan SL, Cunnane ME, Moonis G. Cross-sectional imaging of the thyroid gland. *Neuroimaging Clin N Am* 2008;18(3):445–61.
2. Loevner LA. Imaging of the thyroid gland [review]. *Semin Ultrasound CT MR* 1996;17(6):539–62.
3. Middleton WD, Kurtz AB, Hertzberg BS. *Ultrasound: The Requisites.* 2nd ed. St. Louis, MO: Mosby, 2003:Chapter 10, 229–262.
4. Bushberg JT, Seibert JA, Leidholdt EM Jr, Boone JM. *The Essential Physics of Medical Imaging.* 3rd North American ed. Philadelphia: Lippincott Williams & Wilkins, 2011.
5. William WD, Kurtz AB, Hertzberg BS. *Ultrasound: The Requisites.* 2nd ed. St. Louis, MO: Mosby, 2003.
6. Sholosh B, Borhani AA. Thyroid ultrasound part 1: Technique and diffuse disease. *Radiol Clin North Am* 2011;49(3):391–416.
7. Kutuya N, Kurosaki Y. Sonographic assessment of thyroglossal duct cysts in children. *J Ultrasound Med* 2008;27(8):1211–9.
8. Slatosky J, Shipton B, Wahba H. Thyroiditis: Differential diagnosis and management. *Am Fam Physician* 2000;61(4):1047–52, 1054.
9. Serres-Creixams X, Castells-Fuste I, Pruna-Comella X, Yetano-Laguna V, Garriga-Farriol V, Gallardo-Agromayor E. Paratracheal lymph nodes: A new sonographic finding in autoimmune thyroiditis. *J Clin Ultrasound* 2008;36(7):418–21.
10. Sheth S. Role of ultrasonography in thyroid disease. *Otolaryngol Clin North Am* 2010;43(2):239–55.
11. Ralls PW, Mayekawa DS, Lee KP et al. Color-flow Doppler sonography in Graves disease: "Thyroid inferno." *AJR Am J Roentgenol* 1988;150(4):781–4.
12. Dayan CM, Daniels GH. Chronic autoimmune thyroiditis. *N Engl J Med* 1996;335(2):99–107.
13. Tokuda Y, Kasagi K, Iida Y et al. Sonography of subacute thyroiditis: Changes in the findings during the course of the disease. *J Clin Ultrasound* 1990;18(1):21–6.
14. Park SY, Kim EK, Kim MJ et al. Ultrasonographic characteristics of subacute granulomatous thyroiditis. *Korean J Radiol* 2006;7(4):229–34.
15. Hoang JK, Lee WK, Lee M, Johnson D, Farrell S. US features of thyroid malignancy: Pearls and pitfalls. *Radiographics* 2007;27:847–65.
16. Matthey-Gie ML, Walsh SM, O'Neill AC et al. Ultrasound predictors of malignancy in indeterminate thyroid nodules. *Ir J Med Sci* 2014;183:633–7.
17. Feldman MK, Blackwood MS. US artifacts. *Radiographics* 2009;29:1179–89.
18. Nachiappan AC, Metwalli ZA, Hailey BS, Patel RA, Ostrowski ML, Wynne DM. The thyroid: Review of imaging features and biopsy techniques with radiologic-pathologic correlation. *Radiographics* 2014;34:276–94.
19. Hegedus L. Clinical practice. The thyroid nodule. *N Engl J Med* 2004;351(17):1764–71.
20. American Thyroid Association (ATA) Guidelines Taskforce on Thyroid Nodules and Differentiated Thyroid Cancer, Cooper DS, Doherty GM et al. Revised American Thyroid Association management guidelines for patients with thyroid nodules and differentiated thyroid cancer. *Thyroid* 2009;19(11):1167–214.
21. Suh HJ, Moon HJ, Kwak JY, Choi JS, Kim EK. Anaplastic thyroid cancer: Ultrasonographic findings and the role of ultrasonography-guided fine needle aspiration biopsy. *Yonsei Med J* 2013;54(6):1400–6.
22. Kim EK, Park CS, Chung WY et al. New sonographic criteria for recommending fine-needle aspiration biopsy of nonpalpable solid nodules of the thyroid. *AJR Am J Roentgenol* 2002;178(3):687–91.
23. Gharib H, Papini E, Paschke R et al. American Association of Clinical Endocrinologists, Associazione Medici Endocrinologi, and European Thyroid Association medical guidelines for clinical practice for the diagnosis and management of thyroid nodules: Executive summary of recommendations. *J Endocrinol Invest* 2010;33(5):287–91.
24. Frates MC, Benson CB, Charboneau JW et al. Management of thyroid nodules detected at US: Society of Radiologists in Ultrasound consensus conference statement. *Radiology* 2005;237(3):794–800.
25. Chan BK, Desser TS, McDougall IR, Weigel RJ, Jeffrey RB Jr. Common and uncommon sonographic features of papillary thyroid carcinoma. *J Ultrasound Med* 2003;22(10):1083–90.
26. Hassani H, Brasseur A, Raynal G et al. Twinkling artifact on Doppler US: Clinical presentations. *J Radiol* 2010;91(5 Pt 1):539–42.
27. Som PM. Lymph nodes of the neck. *Radiology* 1987;165(3):593–600.
28. Ying M, Ahuja A. Sonography of neck lymph nodes. Part I: Normal lymph nodes [review]. *Clin Radiol* 2003;58(5):351–8.

29. Sakai F, Kiyono K, Sone S et al. Ultrasonic evaluation of cervical metastatic lymphadenopathy. *J Ultrasound Med* 1988;7:305–10.

30. Ahuja AT, Chow L, Chick W, King W, Metreweli C. Metastatic cervical nodes in papillary carcinoma of the thyroid: Ultrasound and histological correlation. *Clin Radiol* 1995;50:229–331.

31. Deng J, Zhou P, Tian SM, Zhang L, Li JL, Qian Y. Comparison of diagnostic efficacy of contrast-enhanced ultrasound, acoustic radiation force impulse imaging, and their combined use in differentiating focal solid thyroid nodules. *PLoS One* 2014;9(3):e90674.

32. Akcay MA, Semiz-Oysu A, Ahiskali R, Aribal E. The value of ultrasound elastography in differentiation of malignancy in thyroid nodules. *Clin Imaging* 2014;38(2):100–3.

33. Sun J, Cai J, Wang X. Real-time ultrasound elastography for differentiation of benign and malignant thyroid nodules: A meta-analysis. *J Ultrasound Med* 2014;33(3):495–502.

34. Rivo-Vazquez A, Rodriguez-Lorenzo A, Rivo-Vazquez JE et al. The use of ultrasound elastography in the assessment of malignancy risk in thyroid nodules and multinodular goitres. *Clin Endocrinol (Oxf)* 79(6):887–91.

35. Moon HJ, Sung JM, Kim E-K, Yoon JH, Youk JH, Kwak JY. Diagnostic performance of gray-scale US and elastography in solid thyroid nodules. *Radiology* 2012;262:1002–13.

36. Cantisani V, Lodise P, Grazhdani H et al. Ultrasound elastography in the evaluation of thyroid pathology. Current status. *Eur J Radiol* 2014;83(3):420–8.

37. Kwak JY, Kim EK. Ultrasound elastography for thyroid nodules: Recent advances. *Ultrasonography* 2014;33(2):75–82.

38. Li F, Luo H. Comparative study of thyroid puncture biopsy guided by contrast-enhanced ultrasonography and conventional ultrasound. *Exp Ther Med* 2013;5(5):1381–4.

39. Ma JJ, Ding H, Xu BH et al. Diagnostic performances of various gray-scale, color Doppler, and contrast-enhanced ultrasonography findings in predicting malignant thyroid nodules. *Thyroid* 2014;24(2):355–63.

40. Zheng XJ, Zhang YK, Zhao CY et al. Diagnosis of thyroid space-occupying lesions using real-time contrast-enhanced ultrasonography with sulphur hexafluoride microbubbles. *Zhonghua Er Bi Yan Hou Tou Jing Wai Ke Za Zhi* 2009;44(4):277–81.

41. Zhang B, Jiang YX, Liu JB et al. Utility of contrast-enhanced ultrasound for evaluation of thyroid nodules. *Thyroid* 2010;20(1):51–7.

42. Giusti M, Orlandi D, Melle G et al. Is there a real diagnostic impact of elastosonography and contrast-enhanced ultrasonography in the management of thyroid nodules? *J Zhejiang Univ Sci B* 2013;14(3):195–206.

8

Thyroid radionuclide imaging and therapy in thyroid cancer

JOSEF MACHAC

INTRODUCTION

This review discusses radionuclide imaging of the thyroid gland to help in distinguishing malignant from benign thyroid nodules, followed by a discussion of radioiodine diagnostic imaging after thyroidectomy and in follow-up of thyroid cancer, and then by a review of therapy of thyroid cancer with radioiodine, using traditional as well as some promising new approaches.

DIAGNOSTIC IMAGING OF THE THYROID

Radiotracers

The use of radioactive isotopes and analogs of elemental nonradioactive iodine, iodine-123, iodine-131, iodine-124, and technetium-99m (Tc-99m) pertechnetate, takes advantage of their mimicking its physiological handling by thyroid tissue and the rest of the body. Radioactive iodine

(RAI), just like nonradioactive dietary iodine, is consumed orally and absorbed through the intestinal tract [1], from where it is transported to the thyroid and other organs: the kidneys, salivary glands, gastric mucosa, sweat glands, and mammary glands. Most of salivary gland uptake is secreted into saliva and is again reabsorbed from the gastrointestinal tract. The excretion of radioiodine is mainly by glomerular filtration [1], and is inversely related to thyroid uptake [2]. Radioiodine is also excreted in sweat, and cleared by the mammary glands, especially during lactation [3]. The placenta transports radioiodine across the placenta [4]. During gestation, there is an increasing amount of radioiodine uptake in the thyroid after the 14th week.

Iodine-123, with a half-life of 13.3 hours, decays with principal gamma emission of 159 keV energy, and is imaged 4 hours after oral ingestion. Iodine-123 is also used in some centers for whole body imaging of thyroid cancer. Tc-99m, with a half-life of 6.02 hours and principal gamma energy of 140 keV, is inexpensive and readily available as a starting point for other Tc-99m-based radiotracers in routine nuclear medicine imaging. Tc-99m pertechnetate, a +7 anionic form of Tc-99m combined with four oxygen atoms, has a net valence of −1 and shows biologic behavior similar to that of iodide. Following intravenous administration, it is trapped in the thyroid gland in the same manner as iodide [5]. Unlike iodide, Tc-99m pertechnetate does not undergo organification, and washes out of the thyroid gland after 30 minutes. Imaging of the thyroid gland is done usually at 20–30 minutes after injection [6].

Tc-99m pertechnetate also crosses the placental barrier and delivers radiation to the fetus, and is contraindicated in pregnancy [7,8]. Tc-99m pertechnetate is excreted in human breast milk [9]. The length of time required to interrupt nursing ranges from 12 to 48 hours, but 24 hours is considered sufficient [10]. Tc-99m pertechnetate is eliminated in urine and in feces [11], in addition to radioactive decay.

Iodine-131, with a half-life of 8 days, decays by beta and gamma emissions. The principal gamma decay has a mean energy of 364 keV [12]. It is the high-energy beta emissions that produce the high ionization potential of iodine-131, which, together with the long physical half-life, leads to higher exposure to the thyroid gland and the whole body than iodine-123 when used diagnostically, an unwanted side effect, but which is used for desired therapeutic purposes in hyperthyroidism or in thyroid cancer.

The suggested oral dose of I-131 for measurement of intact thyroid uptake is small, 6–10 µCi (0.22–0.37 MBq). Iodine-131 is rarely used today for imaging of the intact thyroid gland due to its inferior imaging characteristics compared with I-123 or Tc-99m pertechnetate and high radiation exposure to the thyroid gland from the usual scanning dose of 100 µCi (3.7 MBq), except for occasional imaging of suspected substernal thyroid gland, due to the need for several days' clearance from the mediastinal and cardiac blood pool. Iodine-131 continues to be used for whole body imaging for thyroid cancer, using activities of 1–5 mCi (37–185 MBq), where imaging of local and peripheral metastatic disease is enhanced by several days of background activity clearance, and where radiation exposure to the thyroid gland is no longer a concern.

Cyclotron-produced iodine-124 has a half-life of 4.2 days, and decays with either electron capture (70% of the time), resulting in a high-energy gamma ray emission, or positron decay (about 23% of the time), which allows positron emission tomography (PET) imaging, with enhanced resolution and quantification capability. Like I-131, it also has a relatively high radiation exposure due to its positron emission and long half-life [13].

Individuals with so-called "iodine allergy" are almost never allergic to RAI, a condition that is necessarily extremely rare, since iodide is essential for the production of thyroid hormone and widely abundant in table salt and many other foods.

Intact thyroid gland imaging

The role of radionuclide thyroid imaging in the evaluation of a thyroid nodule is primarily to determine if the nodule is functional (warm), hyperfunctional (hot), or hypofunctional (cold). In the past, radionuclide thyroid imaging was used to assist in the differentiation between benign and potentially malignant nodules. More recently, such patients are routinely evaluated with ultrasound (US) imaging and, if needed, fine-needle aspiration (FNA) [14]. An appreciable number of patients still undergo functional thyroid imaging. A patient with a thyroid nodule and an inconclusive US may have undergone multiple attempts in FNA without success. Patients are still routinely referred for radionuclide in the setting of hyperthyroidism and a palpable or US-detected thyroid nodule or multiple nodules, to distinguish a single toxic nodule (Figure 8.1) or multiple autonomous toxic nodules (Figure 8.2), responsible for the hyperthyroid state, in which case an FNA is not necessary, as a hyperfunctioning nodule is rarely malignant, from a hypofunctional and therefore potentially malignant nodule [15]. In the presence of multiple nodules and a low thyroid-stimulating hormone (TSH), each nodule needs to be evaluated for its functional status, and correlated with the US. If one or more nodules are suspicious or inconclusive, an FNA is indicated [15].

Hypofunctional nodules, as seen in Figure 8.3, are more likely to be malignant than nodules that are warm or hot, with an incidence of 20%–35% for being malignant. Patients with a history of childhood irradiation of the neck are particularly at risk of malignancy [15], as well as those of male gender and extremes of age. According to one study, in a multinodular goiter with a predominant hypofunctional nodule or a hypofunctional nodule that is increasing in size in the presence of two or more thyroid nodules larger than 1–1.5 cm, the rate of malignant nodules is similar to the rate of 8%–10% in patients with solitary cold nodules [16]. Hypofunctional nodules are sometimes incidentally found in the setting of preparation for radioiodine therapy for Graves' disease (Figure 8.3).

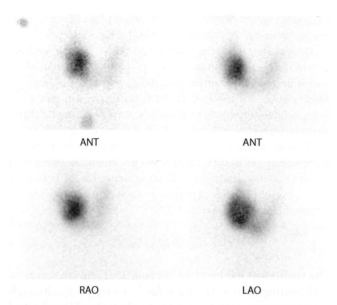

ANT   ANT

RAO   LAO

Figure 8.1 Autonomous toxic nodule. I-123 scan in a 55-year-old female who presented with hyperthyroidism and a palpable thyroid nodule. The 24-hour RAI thyroid uptake was 29%. The thyroid scan shows increased uptake in the right thyroid lobe, with suppression of uptake in the rest of the thyroid gland, compatible with a toxic thyroid nodule. ANT, anterior.

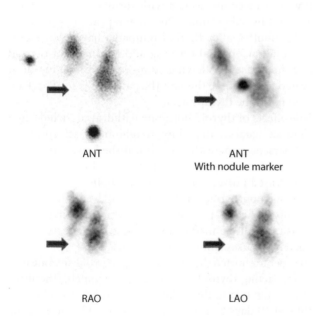

ANT   ANT
                       With nodule marker

RAO   LAO

Figure 8.2 Toxic multinodular goiter. I-123 scan in a 67-year-old female with mild hyperthyroidism in the presence of a multinodular goiter with three larger nodules. The patient was referred for thyroid imaging to help guide biopsies of any suspicious nodules. The 24-hour RAI thyroid uptake was 30%. The scan shows multiple hyperfunctional nodules, with suppressed or hypofunctional areas in the rest of the gland, corresponding to several hypofunctional nodules, the most prominent of which, occupying the lower half of the right lobe and the isthmus, is marked with a marker dot (arrow).

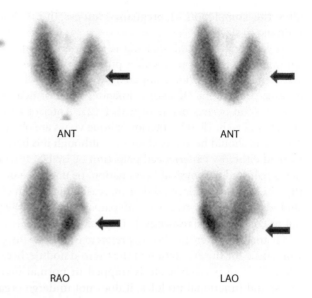

ANT   ANT

RAO   LAO

Figure 8.3 Thyroid cancer in a patient with Graves' disease. A 54-year-old man presented with 10 months of shortness of breath, palpitations, loose stools, and feeling hot, diagnosed as hyperthyroidism due to Graves' disease. After initial treatment with methimazole, and switching to propylthiouracil and a beta blocker due to liver side effects, followed by relief of symptoms, the patient was referred for RAI therapy. The 24-hour RAI thyroid uptake was 68%. A Tc-99m pertechnetate thyroid scan shows uniform uptake in an enlarged thyroid gland, consistent with Graves' disease, plus a hypofunctional palpable nodule in the midlateral aspect of the left lobe. The planned RAI therapy for Graves' disease was deferred, and the patient was referred for US, which confirmed a 3 cm nodule with suspicious calcifications. FNA confirmed papillary thyroid carcinoma. A total thyroidectomy revealed a 3.2 cm papillary thyroid carcinoma, follicular variant, in the left lobe, with lymphovascular invasion and local capsular invasion.

Hyperthyroidism may also occur in the setting of a nodular gland due to subacute thyroiditis, in which case the thyroid uptake is usually very low, preventing useful evaluation of nodules with radionuclide imaging.

Although thyroid nodules occur less commonly in children than in adults [17], some studies suggest that thyroid malignancy is more common in children who have them, with a rate of 15%–20% [18], while others suggest it is similar to the frequency found in adults [11]. The recommended diagnostic approach to pediatric thyroid nodules is similar to that in adults [15], with initial evaluation by US and, if necessary, an FNA. Some pediatric endocrinologists, though, are more reluctant to biopsy suspicious nodules in children, preferring to perform a radionuclide scan first.

The evaluation of thyroid nodules in pregnant women with radionuclide imaging is contraindicated, and US evaluation is routinely used. In women with a suppressed TSH and a detectable nodule or nodules, radionuclide imaging and FNA of nonfunctional nodule(s) can be deferred until after the completion of pregnancy, unless the nodule is growing in size [15].

Thyroid radionuclide imaging is best performed with a gamma camera equipped with a pinhole collimator, which yields the best resolution compared with imaging with parallel-hole collimators. Diagnostic imaging is performed either with Tc-99m pertechnetate or with I-123. Anterior and left (LAO) and right (RAO) anterior oblique views are obtained. The gland should be assessed for size, although it is best performed either by experienced palpation or by US. If a nodule is palpated on physical examination, or if an area on the thyroid scan shows decreased or increased uptake, an effort should be made to correlate it with palpation with the help of hot or cold markers, respectively (Figure 8.2).

Historically, there has been a preference for I-123 imaging when used for the evaluation of the thyroid nodule, because while Tc-99m pertechnetate is trapped in normal thyroid tissue and functional nodules, it does not undergo organification, with potential mismatch between the two tracers. However, in 316 patients, Kusic et al. [19] compared Tc-99m pertechnetate and I-123 imaging in the same patients and found a significant difference only for a few patients. A difference involving thyroid carcinoma was rare.

Whole body radioiodine imaging

Whole body radioiodine imaging is used following total or near-total thyroidectomy prior to ablation of thyroid remnants and treatment of residual disease, in posttherapy imaging, at 6–12 months' follow-up after ablation therapy, as part of surveillance, and in patients with known or suspected metastatic disease, with the intent of treating radioiodine-avid disease with I-131.

PATIENT PREPARATION

In order to compensate for the lower avidity of thyroid cancer for radioiodine compared with normal thyroid tissue, patients are prepared by either withdrawal from thyroid hormone therapy or the use of recombinant human TSH (rhTSH). In addition, patients should undergo 2 weeks of low-iodine diet. If it is determined that the patient needs I-131 treatment, the low-iodine diet and withholding of thyroid hormone should be continued until after the treatment is completed. Care must be taken to determine if a woman is pregnant prior to the administration of RAI for either diagnostic or therapeutic purposes, as I-131 is concentrated in the fetal thyroid [15].

The aim of a low-iodine diet is to decrease the amount of iodine intake (and excretion) to below 50 μg/day, preferably 30–50 μg/day, compared with a normal average that is several times that rate [20]. The details of a low-iodine diet are discussed elsewhere [21], but include avoidance of all seafood; iodized salt and all foods prepared with iodized salt; dairy products; egg yolks; commercially baked products containing salt, dairy products, and eggs; and foods containing artificial red dyes. Allowed foods consist of food prepared from fresh produce, including all fresh or frozen fruits and vegetables; unprocessed meats; potatoes; plain rice and plain pasta; spices free of salt; and any vegetable cooking oil.

Drugs that interfere with radioiodine uptake include perchlorate, thiocyanate, and pertechnetate; inorganic iodide and organic iodine-containing preparations, such as Lugol's solution; SSKI; vitamin and mineral supplements; kelp; iodide-containing antitussives; topical iodine tincture; amiodarone; contrast dye; and antithyroid drugs [22].

Routine testing of urine iodine is not required, unless compliance with diet is unknown. One can check the patient's iodine status by collecting urine for 24 hours for iodide excretion loads of greater than 50 μg/day as evidence of insufficient preparation [1,22].

TSH STIMULATION: THYROID HORMONE WITHDRAWAL

The traditional method of achieving TSH stimulation is by withholding thyroid hormone for 2–3 weeks [15], although sometimes requiring 4–6 weeks. The TSH should be checked and should rise to or above 30 μU/L before proceeding with diagnostic RAI imaging or therapy [23]. A large thyroid remnant may produce enough amount of thyroid hormone to prevent the TSH from rising sufficiently. After documenting a large remnant with RAI diagnostic imaging, one may proceed to ablate it with a modest dose of 30 mCi (1110 MBq) of I-131 first, as treatment with a higher dose of I-131 may produce painful thyroiditis, while treatment of thyroid cancer metastases with insufficient TSH elevation would be suboptimal. One may repeat the procedure in 6–12 months, after thyroid remnants have been eliminated, to allow optimal imaging and treatment of thyroid cancer metastases. Following completion of imaging or, if indicated, radioiodine therapy, the patient is placed back on thyroid hormone therapy again.

Side effects of thyroid hormone withdrawal include cold intolerance; coarse, dry skin; weight increase; constipation; hoarseness; paresthesias; diminished sweating; signs of slow movement; periorbital puffiness; slow ankle jerks; and decreased pulses [23,24]. The metabolism or excretion of patients' nonthyroid medications may be altered, which is of importance in patients with multiple medical problems using multiple medications. These side effects can be avoided if one uses stimulation with rhTSH.

In order to shorten the period of hypothyroidism, one may use short-acting thyroid hormone T3 (Cytomel). The usual dose is 25 μg, two to three times a day. The Cytomel is discontinued 10 days to 2 weeks prior to the radioiodine scan. Thyroid hormone withdrawal, with or without the interim use of T3, can achieve adequate TSH levels in 90% of patients [25]. Cytomel can be used after surgery until initial RAI imaging and ablation therapy is achieved, or between imaging and therapy, if the treatment must be postponed by a few weeks. Cytomel is usually not given when restarting thyroid [15].

USE OF RECOMBINANT TSH STIMULATION

Advances in biotechnology led to the introduction of rhTSH (Thyrogen). The recommended procedure consists of two 0.9 mg rhTSH doses injected 24 hours apart, on day 1 and day 2, followed by 2–4 mCi (74–148 MBq) of I-131 on day 3, and by imaging on day 5 [24]. In a phase II study [24], the mean serum level of TSH was 132 mU/L 24 hours after the second injection of rhTSH, compared with101 mU/L after thyroid hormone withdrawal. The findings on I-131 scans were concordant in 66% of positive scans; the post-withdrawal scans were superior in 29% of positive scans, and the post rhTSH studies were superior in 5% of positive scans. The fractional uptake of I-131 was not as high with rhTSH as that after withdrawal. The maximal level of thyroglobulin (Tg) was achieved 48–72 hours after the second rhTSH injection. The sensitivity and specificity of Tg at a level of 3 ng/mL were 72% and 95% after rhTSH injection, similar to thyroid hormone withdrawal. Thus, the combination of radionuclide imaging and Tg level measurement after rhTSH was equivalent to withdrawal from thyroid hormone. Similar results were found in a phase III study, in 229 patients. The difference was not statistically significant. Tg measurement of 2 ng/mL or greater was detected in 22% while on thyroid hormone therapy, in 52% after rhTSH stimulation, and in 56% after thyroid hormone withdrawal when tumor was limited to the thyroid bed; in 80% while on thyroid hormone therapy and in 100% after rhTSH stimulation; and in 100% of patients with metastatic disease [26]. This plus a second phase III study showed that scans with rhTSH failed to detect remnant or cancer localized to the thyroid bed in 16% (20/124) of patients detected by a withdrawal scan. The scan with rhTSH failed to detect metastatic disease in 24% (9/38) of patients detected after withdrawal. Post-rhTSH stimulation Tg levels greater than 2.5 ng/mL detected metastatic disease in all patients with metastases [27]. Thus, the diagnostic sensitivity of RAI imaging is similar for regional neck metastatic disease with both methods. There is still consensus to use thyroid hormone withdrawal for known or suspected peripheral metastatic disease, unless hormone withdrawal is contraindicated [15].

Side effects of rhTSH include nausea (10.5%), vomiting (2.1%), headache (7.3%), asthenia (3.4%), chills (1.0%), fever (1.0%), flu symptoms (1.0%), dizziness (1.6%), and paresthesias (1.6%) [24].

POSTTHYROIDECTOMY WHOLE BODY RADIOIODINE IMAGING

The purpose of postthyroidectomy radioiodine imaging is to assist in initial staging for prognostication and follow-up management strategy, in preparation for radio-iodine thyroid remnant ablation and treatment of residual or metastatic disease. The patient who has undergone a complete thyroidectomy usually still has a small amount of thyroid remnant tissue (Figure 8.4). Occasionally, the remnant may be large, making the detection of nearby uptake within locoregional lymph nodes difficult [28], and the TSH level may remain insufficiently elevated even after hormone withdrawal. If the thyroidectomy is known to be incomplete, one may image the thyroid with Tc-99m

pertechnetate, I-123, or I-131 to assess the size of the remnant, measure the uptake, and administer a small ablation dose, e.g., 30 mCi (1110 MBq) of I-131, to avoid painful thyroiditis with a larger dose. The patient is reevaluated at 6–12 months, with the intent of treating the metastatic disease [15] (Figure 8.4).

The dose of I-131 used for whole body imaging is limited to 1–5 mCi (37–185 MBq) after thyroid hormone withdrawal and 2–4 mCi (74–148 MBq) after rhTSH, to address concerns about "stunning" effects with higher doses [29]. A whole body anterior and posterior scan is performed at 48 hours, plus high-count spot views of the neck and chest, and a pinhole collimator of the neck help to resolve the individual neck remnant foci (Figure 8.4a). If it is suspected that metastatic disease is present, imaging with single-photon emission computed tomography–computed tomography (SPECT-CT) can help in localization for future follow-up and for possible surgical or radiotherapy, as in Figure 8.4d. The uptake in the neck, and any other area of uptake, is calculated.

USE OF IODINE-123 FOR DIAGNOSTIC WHOLE BODY IMAGING

Iodine-123 for diagnostic whole body imaging is an alternative to I-131. A 5–10 mCi (185–370 MBq) dose of I-123 orally is followed by a whole body scan approximately 4 hours later, with additional neck and chest views, and pinhole or magnified views of the neck. The advantages include a lower dose of radiation absorbed by the patient, a lower likelihood of stunning, and improved image quality due to more counts and higher resolution. The disadvantage of I-123 is its higher cost, and the shorter time available for optimal target tissue uptake and blood pool clearance. Comparisons show good correlation between I-123 and I-131 for tumor detection [30], although some studies found slightly lower sensitivity of I-123 imaging [31], while others [32] found higher sensitivity for metastatic disease.

EMPIRICAL POSTTHYROIDECTOMY ABLATION WITHOUT IMAGING

An alternative approach in patients who have undergone a thorough thyroidectomy omits diagnostic pretherapy imaging altogether, administering an empirical ablative dose of 50–150 mCi (1850–5550 MBq) of I-131, depending on risk (see below), followed by a posttherapy scan 2–7 days after the therapy. The aim of therapy is to perform ablation plus treatment of local disease, if any, while the posttherapy scan is used for staging, with further treatment at 6–12 months, if necessary (see example in Figure 8.5).

DETECTION OF LOCAL AND DISTAL METASTASES

One should be aware of normal structures that take up radioiodine avidly, such as the salivary glands, stomach, and excreted activity in the colon and kidneys and urinary bladder. Activity is frequently seen in the esophagus as a result of swallowed saliva, which is cleared by drinking liquids and eating a piece of solid food. Aspirated saliva can

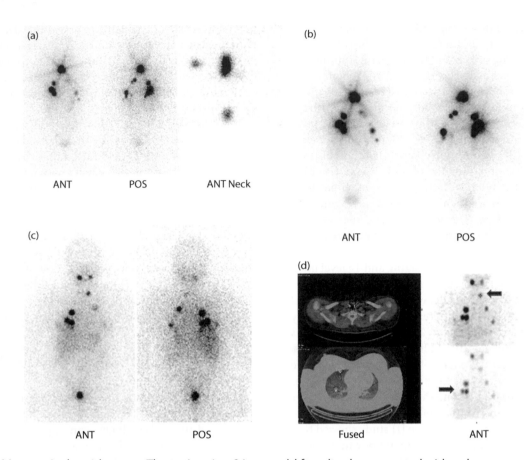

Figure 8.4 Metastatic thyroid cancer. The patient is a 36-year-old female who presented with pulmonary nodules detected incidentally on a CT scan of the abdomen obtained for obstetrical reasons. A lung biopsy revealed thyroid cancer, and a thyroid US revealed a 2.5 thyroid nodule, positive for follicular thyroid cancer on FNA. The patient underwent thyroidectomy. (a) An I-131 whole body diagnostic scan, which reveals a large thyroid remnant, with 9% uptake, plus multiple lung metastases, corresponding to lung nodules on CT. Because of the large remnant, the patient underwent a preliminary thyroid remnant ablation with 30 mCi of I-131. The immediate posttherapy scan (b) shows similar findings, although several additional lung metastases were detected. Six months later, the patient underwent a follow-up diagnostic scan (c), which showed ablation of the previously seen thyroid remnant, marked improvement on the scan, and a significant fall in the serum Tg level from 110 to 7.4. The fused SPECT-CT images (d) show localization of a residual metastatic lesion in the neck, and two of the lung metastases. The patient was treated with the maximal tolerated dose of 200 mCi of I-131 for the metastatic disease. POS, posterior.

occasionally be seen in the carina, verified by SPECT-CT imaging and resolution on repeat imaging on successive days. Sometimes, inflammatory lesions may take up RAI as an artifact [33]. Superficial contamination from saliva or urine may cause diagnostic confusion.

POSTABLATION THERAPY IMAGING

The large activity of I-131 used in therapy, 20–50 times the activity for diagnostic RAI imaging; significantly better image quality; and improved contrast all contribute to increased lesion detectability. This is illustrated in Figure 8.4. Scanning at 5 days allows SPECT-CT imaging with good quality. Additional metastatic foci have been detected in 10%–20% of patients imaged after high-dose radioiodine treatment compared with the pretherapy diagnostic scan [34]. New findings on the posttherapy scan have been shown to alter staging in approximately

10% of patients, affecting clinical management in 9%–15% of patients [35].

POSTABLATION FOLLOW-UP IMAGING

Patients are usually evaluated 6–12 months after ablation to assess the efficacy of ablation (Figures 8.4 and 8.5), and for the presence of metastatic disease, for possible additional treatment. If the patient has a low risk of tumor recurrence, and negative TSH-stimulated Tg levels and negative neck US, further follow-up diagnostic RAI scans are not considered necessary [15], unless clinical or Tg level measurements indicate otherwise. In patients with a higher risk of recurrence, annual scans and Tg measurements for 3–5 years, and then at longer intervals, are considered appropriate [15]. Patients with highly suspected or known metastases are often reexamined at 6 months after ablation [15]. Patients with known new or previously treated metastatic disease return for blood dosimetry measurement and imaging with a low diagnostic dose of I-131, and perform therapy with a high dose or maximal tolerated dose of I-131, followed by posttherapy imaging 5–7 days after therapy (Figures 8.4 and 8.5).

FOLLOW-UP MONITORING

Patients are frequently followed with Tg testing, at baseline and during rhTSH or withdrawal stimulation. Approximately 20% of patients who are clinically free of disease with a Tg level

of less than 1 ng/mL on suppression have a Tg level greater than 2 ng/mL after rhTSH stimulation or withdrawal. A RAI scan will be positive in about one-third of such patients [36]. The patient is then considered for further RAI treatment. If the RAI scan is negative but the Tg is positive, then one may consider F-18 fluorodeoxyglucose (FDG) PET imaging, as discussed below [15]. One can omit follow-up RAI scans once the initial therapy is performed if an undetectable serum Tg level on thyroxin therapy is found, although continued follow-up with Tg level measurements is recommended [15].

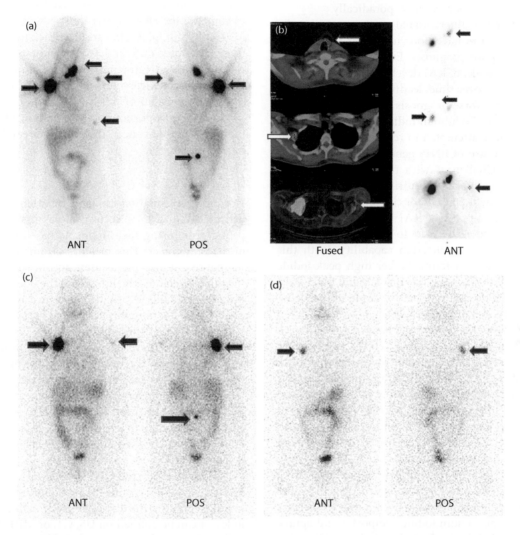

Figure 8.5 **(a and b)** The patient is a 55-year-old male, presenting with a neck mass, revealed to represent thyroid cancer. The patient underwent a total thyroidectomy for a 4.8 cm papillary thyroid carcinoma with only minimal capsular invasion, no lymphovascular invasion, and no regional lymph node involvement. Two months later, he underwent empirical radio-iodine ablation therapy with 50 mCi of I-131 for presumed thyroid remnants, with rhTSH stimulation. The postradiation whole body and SPECT-CT scan revealed two thyroid remnants in the neck, plus, surprisingly, a metastasis in the right second rib, associated with an expansile destructive lesion on CT, a metastasis in the left scapula, left fifth rib, and the spinous process of L4 **(a and b; see arrows)**. The Tg level was 134. **(c)** A follow-up whole body iodine scan 6 months later, on thyroid hormone withdrawal, shows resolution of the neck foci, with persistence of uptake in the right second rib, L4, and a faint focus in the left scapula, while a previous faint focus in the left fifth rib was no longer seen. Uptake in bilateral pulmonary metastases was seen, corresponding to small nodules on CT. The Tg level was 155. A second round of RAI therapy was administered with a maximal tolerated dose of 160 mCi, limited by blood dosimetry. **(d)** A follow-up diagnostic whole body RAI scan with I-131, 7 months later, shows resolution of all lesions except for the second rib lesion, which shows significantly reduced uptake, while the serum TG level had fallen to 14, with stable pulmonary nodules on CT.

SENSITIZATION METHODS FOR RAI IMAGING AND THERAPY

It was determined some time ago that lithium inhibits iodine release from thyroid tissues, without inhibiting the intake of iodine. The overall effect is greater RAI retention in normal thyroid tissue and thyroid tumors [37]. It has been estimated that the I-131 radiation dose in metastatic tumors is doubled, primarily in tumors with rapid clearance of iodine [38]. However, randomized data in support of lithium treatment as an adjuvant leading to a better outcome are lacking, and given its appreciable side effects, it is not recommended for routine use [15], and is used only sporadically.

Patients with poorly differentiated carcinoma and in the older age group tend to have poor uptake of I-131, which is associated with poor prognosis. Even patients with initially good tumor uptake of RAI develop loss of RAI uptake in metastatic disease over time, leading to poorer response to RAI therapy and worse prognosis. In these cases, there appears to be loss of the human iodide symporter (hNIS). Research efforts have attempted to restore the iodide symporter through the use of hNIS gene transfer into hNIS-defective tumors. Challenges with this approach include delivery of the gene, usually requiring direct local injection, and only transient efficacy for the carrier adenovirus. Moreover, increased uptake of RAI by the restored symporter does not necessarily lead to prolonged retention, if there is also poor organification capability. With this approach, Smit et al. [39] found higher high peak iodide accumulation, and the half-life was increased in hNIS-deficient mice. A lethal dose of radioiodine could not be delivered, however, although tumor development was delayed in thyroid-ablated, low-iodide-diet mice treated with radioiodine therapy. This has been tried as well in cancers other than thyroid cancer. Park et al. [40] investigated in mice the feasibility of combination gene therapy and noninvasive radionuclide imaging after expression of human hNIS and inhibition of multidrug resistance (MDR1) with the aid of a cytomegalovirus promoter, in order to effect enhanced response to both I-131 and doxorubicin, with encouraging results.

Along another line of research, in mouse models of thyroid cancer, selective mitogen-activated protein kinase (MAPK) pathway antagonists have been found to increase the expression of the sodium iodide symporter and uptake of iodine. Ho et al. [41] conducted a study to determine whether the MAPK kinase (MEK) 1 and MEK2 inhibitor selumetinib could reverse refractoriness to radioiodine in patients with metastatic thyroid cancer. Using stimulation with thyrotropin alfa, and metastatic tumor lesion dosimetry with quantitative iodine-124 PET imaging before and 4 weeks after treatment with selumetinib in 20 patients with thyroid cancer refractory to RAI treatment, it was found that selumetinib increased the uptake of iodine-124 in 12 of the 20 patients, such that 8 of these 12 patients reached the lesion dosimetry threshold to qualify for RAI therapy. Of the eight patients treated with radioiodine, five had confirmed partial responses and three had stable disease; all patients had decreases in serum Tg levels, with a mean reduction of 89%. No toxic effects of grade 3 or higher attributable by the investigators to selumetinib were observed. Selumetinib produces clinically meaningful increases in iodine uptake and retention in a subgroup of patients with thyroid cancer that are refractory to radioiodine; the effectiveness may be greater in patients with *RAS* mutant disease.

These encouraging preliminary results led to a multicenter clinical trial. The ASTRA study (Adjuvant Selumetinib for Differentiated Thyroid Cancer, Remission after RAI) is a randomized, double-blind, placebo-controlled study designed to compare the efficacy of a short course of selumetinib, a MEK inhibitor, plus adjuvant RAI therapy in patients with newly diagnosed differentiated thyroid cancer (DTC) at high risk of primary treatment failure. The study design aims to improve the complete remission rate and clinical outcome in a high-risk population [42].

Given the importance of restoration of sensitivity to iodine in thyroid cancer, this line of research is of obvious importance.

DOSIMETRY CALCULATION

Dosimetry calculation is the estimation of the expected delivered radiation dose to a target tissue from a therapeutic dose, using measurements based on a tracer dose of the radiotracer. This includes dosimetry to the thyroid remnant(s), tumor metastases, and other tissues, such as the salivary glands, the lungs, and the bone marrow. While dosimetry should ideally be performed in all instances of radionuclide therapy, it is performed in thyroid cancer therapy in selected settings only.

Maxon et al. have demonstrated the utility of dosimetry calculation to the thyroid remnants, by estimating the volume from Tc-99m pertechnetate images and estimating the residence time by serial I-131 uptake measurements, in deciding on the ablation therapy dose to achieve treatment efficacy, as opposed to an arbitrary dose [43]. This approach, however, is rarely used clinically, as it is time-consuming and costly.

Dosimetry estimation to RAI-avid metastatic lesions can be carried out in the same manner. It is difficult to carry out in practice, due to the difficulty in estimating lesion volume, unless it can be defined on US, CT, or MRI. The resolution with I-131 is too poor to accurately measure volume, and only slightly better with I-123. The use of I-124 with PET imaging allows uptake to be quantified, and volumes estimated with greater accuracy than with conventional imaging, thus offering a chance at real dosimetry and a rational approach to tumor therapy, but it is still used only investigationally [44].

With pulmonary metastases, as in the patient in Figure 8.4, the delivered dose to the lungs needs to be assessed to avoid the rare but possible pulmonary pneumonitis and eventual fibrosis due to a high dose of radiation from I-131 therapy [45]. If the RAI uptake is distributed uniformly, one can estimate the dosimetry to the lungs. The recognized upper limit of radiation tolerance to the lungs is 30 Gy [46]. If the lung uptake is nodular, the method would need to revert to one discussed above for discrete metastases. In practice, most centers use an empirical method. A limit of 40 mCi lung uptake or 80 mCi whole body retention at 48 hours should be observed in patients with diffuse pulmonary I-131 uptake [47].

The calculation of dosimetry to the bone marrow assumes all exposure derived from the blood activity bathing the bone marrow, and the gamma radiation from the rest of the body. The activity in the blood is sampled at the time of administration of the diagnostic tracer dose of I-131 at 24, 48, and 72 hours. By graphic or analytic methods, the area under the curve, the maximal uptake, and the administered activity yield the radiation dose to the blood, which is assumed to equal the dose to the bone marrow [41,45]. The result is then used to calculate the activity of I-131 required to deliver a 200 rad (cGy) dose. Below this limit, one can avoid radiation-induced bone marrow suppression. The actual radiation dose absorbed by the bone marrow from the blood is believed to range from 30% to 60% of the dose to the blood [41], thus providing a margin of extra safety.

F-18 FLUORODEOXYGLUCOSE PET IMAGING

Radioiodine imaging is only 60%–70% sensitive for thyroid cancer. Frequently, RAI-non-avid tumors, including poorly differentiated cancer, tall cell papillary cancer variants, and Hurthle cell carcinoma, and patients with well-differentiated thyroid cancer that start out I-131 avid may, over time and with multiple I-131 treatments, become I-131 negative. FDG PET imaging has become a modality of choice when thyroid cancer is I-131 nonavid [15]. The detection and localization of disease may prompt decision making regarding therapy, whether surgical reception, local external beam radiotherapy, or even a trial of I-131 after diligent patient preparation with a low-iodine diet and proper TSH stimulation.

FDG, an analog of glucose, is transported into living cells by facilitated diffusion and trapped in the cell after hexokinase-mediated phosphorylation, while not being able to enter into further metabolic pathways. FDG is not dephosphorylated back into FDG because of low levels of glucose-6-phosphatase in most tumors. For all practical purposes, FDG accumulation is an indication of glucose utilization.

The method of FDG PET imaging for thyroid cancer is the same standard method as for other malignancies. After fasting for 4–6 hours, the patient is injected with 10 mCi (370 MBq) of FDG and is instructed to rest for 45–60 minutes. The patient then undergoes imaging from the base of the brain down to the thighs. The use of CT along with PET as PET/CT imaging has significantly improved the value of FDG PET imaging in the localization of FDG uptake, improving specificity, and the guiding of surgical resection and external beam radiotherapy [48]. In some studies, stimulation with rhTSH [49] was found to enhance disease

detection sensitivity. Other studies showed that an increase in TSH levels did not increase the ability of FDG PET to detect lesions [50].

The use of FDG partly overlaps as well as complements the use of RAI in thyroid cancer. In some patients with thyroid cancer, there is uptake of both RAI and FDG, while in other patients, only RAI imaging is positive, and in yet others, only FDG scanning is positive. Together, however, the two agents achieve a high sensitivity of detection [51]. Wang et al. [52] noted that the degree of FDG uptake correlated with increased aggressiveness of thyroid cancer, and inversely correlated with RAI uptake. The FDG PET scans were positive in all patients with stage IV disease and increased Tg levels. At the same time, the methodology is not sensitive enough to detect minimal residual disease in the cervical nodes [53].

FDG PET imaging is currently indicated in patients with evidence of thyroid cancer, on the basis of clinical evidence or an elevated Tg level, where I-131 imaging is negative [15] (Figure 8.6). The ability to detect tumor metastases, in the presence of a negative RAI scan, helps direct therapy to either surgical resection, if feasible, or external beam radiotherapy, or in patients with progressing cancer, to chemotherapy with tyrosine kinase inhibitors.

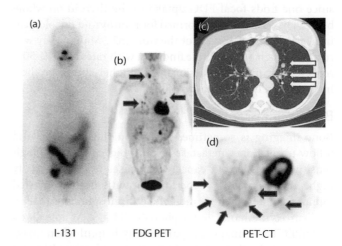

I-131   FDG PET   PET-CT

Figure 8.6 Metastatic RAI-non-avid thyroid cancer. The patient is a 60-year-old female who had undergone a total thyroidectomy for locally invasive papillary thyroid carcinoma. A preablation RAI scan showed tumor nodal involvement. She received high-dose RAI therapy with 200 mCi of I-131 with successful ablation of all tumor uptake. Three years later, she received another 260 mCi of RAI because of rising serum TG level. The anterior whole body posttherapy I-131 scan **(a)** was negative despite an abnormal CT scan of the chest **(c)**, which showed multiple new pulmonary nodules (arrows). A FDG PET whole body scan **(b)** showed hypermetabolic lymph nodes in the neck and hila with multiple foci in the lung fields (arrows), as well as mild diffuse FDG uptake in the basal lung parenchyma **(d, arrows)**, corresponding to multiple small lung nodules on the CT.

FDG PET imaging also provides prognostic information. Robbins et al. [54] found that the combination of FDG-negative and either RAI-positive or -negative results predicted a good prognosis, while PET-positive uptake with either radioiodine-negative or radioiodine-positive results predicted a much worse prognosis.

The challenge in poorly differentiated and anaplastic carcinoma of the thyroid is early diagnosis and complete surgical resection as the only chance for cure and early diagnosis of recurrence, with conventional methods having poor sensitivity, and these tumors are not radioiodine avid. FDG PET imaging can be helpful in evaluating disease extent, and evaluating therapeutic results [15,55].

INCIDENTAL FDG PET FINDINGS IN THE THYROID

Incidental findings in the thyroid gland on US or CT are common, ranging from 19% to 46%; 1.5% to 10% prove to represent thyroid carcinoma. Studies on the ability of FDG PET to evaluate thyroid nodules for malignancy vary, from 100% sensitivity and 63% specificity [53] to 60% sensitivity and 91% specificity [56]. These results underline the fact that many well-differentiated thyroid cancers do not avidly take up FDG, so that FDG PET should not be used routinely for the evaluation of thyroid nodules [15], and the diagnostic use of FDG PET for this situation is neither indicated nor reimbursed. This is of interest mainly for incidental findings, since one finds focal FDG uptake in the thyroid on whole body FDG PET scans performed for nonthyroid oncological indications about 1%–2% of the time [57]. Malignancy was relatively high among these findings, with rates of 25%–50% representing malignant lesions, with higher uptake predicting more likely malignancy [58].

Bone scintigraphy

Bone imaging is sometimes helpful in the detection and follow-up of bone metastases of thyroid cancer, although sensitivity for thyroid cancer metastases is not especially high. Bone imaging is performed with Tc-99m-labeled diphosphanates such as methylene diphosphonate (MDP) or hydroxymethane diphosphonate (HDP). Whole body and SPECT-CT imaging is particularly helpful when imaging suspected lesions of the skull, spine, and pelvis. Thyroid cancer metastases are typically osteolytic, that is, appear photopenic, with a small osteoblastic rim on the edges. Small lesions simply appear as foci of increased uptake. Multiple studies reveal bone imaging to have a sensitivity ranging from 45% to 100% for bone lesions [59].

RADIONUCLIDE THERAPY OF THYROID CANCER

Iodine-131 has been a mainstay of well-differentiated thyroid cancer management to this day, ever since the first application of I-131 to the treatment of thyroid cancer by Seidlin et al. in 1946 [60], and is closely integrated with diagnostic anatomical and scintigraphic RAI, as well as non-RAI scintigraphic imaging methods.

Thyroid cancer therapy begins with surgical removal of the thyroid gland and the primary tumor, along with identification and removal of involved lymph nodes, covered elsewhere in this volume. Patients with well-differentiated thyroid cancer who are not considered cured by surgery, or considered at moderate to high risk of cancer recurrence, frequently undergo radioiodine therapy [15]. In the appropriate setting, I-131 therapy reduces the rate of cancer recurrence, and extends the disease-free interval, or helps to control the tumor after recurrence that cannot be surgically managed. Most patients with metastatic disease can be managed for many years with I-131 therapy, and occasionally, some patients are cured with I-131 therapy.

Risk assessment

Various systems of clinical risk assessment for well-differentiated carcinoma exist. Because of its utility in predicting disease mortality, and its requirements for cancer registries, the American Joint Committee on Cancer/Union for International Cancer Control (AJCC/UICC) staging is currently recommended for all patients with DTC [15]. In the most benign setting, a young woman with a small, well-differentiated, well-encapsulated thyroid tumor, without lymphovascular invasion or abnormal lymph nodes, with no history of radiation exposure, carries a risk of death of less than 2% in the 20 years after initial treatment [15]. Increasing age, male gender, increasing size of the primary lesion, penetration of the thyroid capsule and invasion of surrounding tissues, invasion of blood vessels, the presence of metastases in local lymph nodes, and the presence of distant metastases progressively increase the likelihood of tumor recurrence and disease: 20-year mortality of 25%–40% [15]. Similar risk stratification holds for follicular carcinoma. Low-risk patients have about 5% risk of mortality in 10 years, and 10%–12% at 20 years. Patients at high risk have a 70% mortality at 10 years and about 90% at 20 years [61].

Mazzaferri and Young [62] and Mazzaferri and Jhiang [63] showed that I-131 therapy has a beneficial effect on survival, cutting the death rate down to no reported deaths out of 138 patients, and a rate of recurrence of about 7%–8% in 20–35 years in 802 patients. These results have served as a rationale for radioiodine therapy in stage II or stage III patients. In addition, RAI ablation therapy removes residual normal thyroid tissue, which is almost always seen even after "complete" thyroidectomy [64], that interferes with the interpretation of radioiodine scans on follow-up, and may result in slightly elevated serum Tg assays.

The goals of postoperative RAI ablation therapy are to destroy residual thyroid tissue in an effort to decrease the risk of recurrent locoregional disease and to facilitate long-term surveillance with whole body RAI imaging and Tg measurements [15]. The latter has been a rationale for ablation in patients with stage I disease. In larger remnants that secrete sufficient amounts of thyroid hormone to prevent therapy of known residual or new metastatic disease, ablation removes this possible cause of ineffective therapy.

In addition to complete surgical removal of the primary tumor and local extension or local lymph node metastases, radioiodine treatment is used, together with TSH suppression therapy and local external beam radiation therapy, to control disease [15]. A number of large, retrospective studies show a significant reduction in the rates of disease recurrence, as well as cause-specific mortality [15]. On the other hand, studies show that the majority of patients with papillary thyroid carcinoma, those at the lowest risk for mortality, did not find any clear benefit of radioiodine ablation therapy [15]. In those studies that show benefit, the advantage appeared to be restricted to patients with larger tumors (>4.0 cm), or with residual disease after surgery. Therefore, the current consensus recommendation is that radioiodine ablation is recommended for patients with stage III and IV disease, all patients with stage II disease younger than age 45, most patients with stage II disease 45 years or older, and selected patients with stage I disease, especially those with multifocal disease, nodal metastases, extrathyroidal or vascular invasion, or more aggressive histologies [15].

Patient preparation

The dietary iodine preparation and TSH stimulation are the same as for diagnostic imaging. While rhTSH stimulation was Food and Drug Administration (FDA) approved for a diagnostic stimulation for I-131 or I-123 imaging or a stimulated Tg measurement [15], remnant ablation has been shown to be equally successful with I-131 in patients after thyroid hormone withdrawal compared with rhTSH stimulation [15]. RhTSH results in enhanced iodine excretion compared with withdrawal, which shortened the length of stay in some patients hospitalized for therapy, thus helping to offset the cost of the rhTSH, as well as resulting in a lower absorbed dose to the blood; however, the effective half-time in the remnant thyroid tissue was significantly longer than that of hormone withdrawal [65,66].

RAI dosage regiments and effectiveness

Given the wide range of therapeutic options available, risk factors influencing the likelihood of tumor recurrence and progression and mortality generally guide therapy, with increasing aggressiveness of therapy matching the increasing clinical risk. Activities ranging from 30 to 100 mCi (1110–3700 MBq) of I-131 generally show similar rates of successful remnant ablation [15], as defined by the absence of visible radioiodine uptake on a subsequent diagnostic radioiodine scan, although there is a trend toward higher success rates with higher activity. While a dose of 30 mCi (1110 MBq) was found to be effective in most patients, it was not entirely reliable, with a range of success ranging from 20% to 83% [67,68]. Rosario et al. [69] found that after 100 mCi of I-131 ablation dose, uptake and ablation efficacy were inversely related, ranging from 46 of 48 patients who had uptake less than 1% to only 6 of 12 patients with uptake greater than 10%. The goal is to use the minimum activity

necessary to achieve successful thyroid remnant ablation, particularly for low-risk patients [15].

Treatment of residual or recurrent cancer

Although postoperative ablation of thyroid remnants undoubtedly destroys some micrometastases, the common site of recurrence is in the cervical lymph nodes. The presence of residual or recurrent thyroid cancer may be evident at the time of remnant ablation, or may become evident sometime after thyroid remnant ablation, as a result of detection of elevated Tg levels, detection of regional neck lymph node enlargement by CT, or uptake on a follow-up RAI scan (Figures 8.4 and 8.5). Generally, higher activities of 100–200 mCi are used for ablation of thyroid remnants when residual microscopic disease is suspected or documented, or if there is a more aggressive tumor histology [15]. Although metastases that appear on follow-up are difficult to eradicate completely with RAI therapy, and thus should also be considered for surgical resection, if accessible, or treated with radiotherapy in combination with RAI therapy, many patients may benefit with additional RAI treatment because of the reduction of tumor burden that may improve survival or provide palliative benefit [15].

The approach to treatment may use fixed empirical disease, or doses based on maximal tolerated dose. Dosimetry to the tumor has been used mainly for investigational purposes. These approaches presume that higher RAI activity absorbed by the tumor leads to better outcome, as suggested by some data [70], while not confirmed by other data [71].

Empirical fixed doses

This approach uses standard fixed doses from 100 to 200 mCi, based on the site of tumor location. The recommended treatment of recurrent tumor in the thyroid bed was 100–150 mCi, while treatment of neck lymph nodes called for 150–180 mCi. Treatment of tumor outside of the neck involved doses of 200 mCi [72]. The main argument for the use of simple empirical doses is that this approach is simple and the least expensive, and little evidence compels that more patient- or tumor-specific approaches are more effective [15].

Maximum safe dose method

Peripheral metastases often have weak uptake of radioiodine, and in the effort to deliver as much radiation as is feasible, one would like to give doses in excess of the 200 mCi dose recommended in the empirical approach, if it can be given safely, while avoiding a dose to the marrow in excess of the "safe" limit, even if the activity given is 200 mCi or less, especially in patients with a small body mass, and the elderly, with decreased renal clearance (see example in Figures 8.4 and 8.5). Generally, a rapid turnover in I-131 results in a higher tolerated dose, while slow turnover results in a low tolerated dose. As a result, 80% of patients can tolerate activities greater than 200 mCi of I-131, sometimes reaching up to 400–500 mCi, although there is no evidence that this results in better outcome than an empirical dose of 200 mCi [15]. In 20% of patients, this maximal activity is less than 200 mCi. The use of Thyrogen for TSH stimulation for therapy results in a more rapid turnover of I-131, with the results that the maximal tolerated dose is higher.

Individual lesion dosimetry

As discussed above, the use of dosimetry for individual lesions, including the use of iodine-124 PET imaging, which was detailed earlier, has not been routine. In addition, even if one sees a single or a few lesions on the diagnostic scan, one often sees additional lesions on the posttherapy scan. Thus, it is still most appropriate to try to deliver either a high empirical dose or the maximal tolerated dose for peripheral metastases.

Use of rhTSH for recurrent or metastatic disease

While no randomized studies exist that compare the use of rhTSH stimulation with thyroid hormone withdrawal for the treatment of metastatic disease, there have been a number of studies regarding its usefulness [73,74]. Early on, rhTSH stimulation was targeted in patients with brain or spinal cord metastases with the aim of avoiding prolonged tumor stimulation that could cause neurological signs or symptoms from tumor swelling. Nonetheless, the use of rhTSH does not eliminate the danger of possible swelling of the tumor causing neurological sequelae [75–77]. More recently, many centers have used rhTSH stimulation for the treatment of metastases in patients with other medical comorbidities where thyroid hormone withdrawal might cause a significant deterioration in health status, although rhTSH is not yet recommended for routine use with peripheral metastases [15].

Treatment of distant metastatic disease

Morbidity and mortality are increased in patients with distant metastases, although other factors, such as distribution (e.g., lung, brain, and bone), the number of metastatic lesions, and the amount of tumor burden and age, are important. Responsiveness to surgery or radioiodine is associated with improved survival [15]. Even if improved survival is not demonstrated, significant palliative objectives and decreased morbidities can be achieved with therapy [15]. If isolated, pulmonary and bone metastases can be treated surgically to decrease tumor bulk and, in the case of bone metastases, to provide stabilization. External beam radiotherapy is also used for this purpose to stabilize critical weight-bearing bones. This approach is often combined with radioiodine therapy, since other disseminated disease

is likely, even if not visible on the I-131 scan [15]. The ablation of tumor outside of local cervical lymph nodes may require larger absorbed radiation doses.

Treatment of pulmonary metastases

Pulmonary metastases can be detected by chest radiography and CT if macronodular disease, and by CT and radioiodine if micronodular metastatic disease. Pulmonary micrometastases are the most responsive to radioiodine treatment among peripheral metastases, and can be treated every 6–12 months as long as responsiveness is observed [15]. The amount of I-131 activity given is most frequently determined empirically, ranging from 100 to 300 mCi, subject to limitation by whole body retention of 80 mCi at 48 hours, and 200 Gy dosimetry to the bone marrow estimated by blood dosimetry measurements [15]. Macronodular pulmonary metastases can also be treated with radioiodine, as discussed previously, if they are radioiodine avid, and this is repeated if they show to be responsive (Figure 8.4).

Generally, survival is related to early detection of localized or low-volume residual or metastatic disease, and is related to a high uptake of I-131 in the tumor, as opposed to low uptake [15]. The percentage of patients surviving 5 years increased from 8% to 72% with I-131 in this category. At 8 years, 50% of patients with lung metastases treated with I-131 survived, while none survived without treatment [78]. Others [79] found good outcome in patients with a high RAI uptake and low disease volume, after I-131 therapy. The 10-year survival was 84%. Even in the presence of advanced disease, long-term survival was possible with continued I-131 treatments.

Macronodular pulmonary metastases that do not show radioiodine uptake on diagnostic radioiodine scans often demonstrate FDG uptake on PET imaging, have a relatively poor prognosis [80], and have been shown to be poorly responsive to radioiodine treatment. Chemotherapy agents, such as the tyrosine kinase inhibitors, are being investigated in this group of patients [81].

Treatment of bone metastases

Radioiodine therapy of iodine-avid bone metastases has been found to be associated with improved survival, with empirical doses ranging from 150 to 300 mCi, or doses determined by dosimetry [15] (see example in Figure 8.5). Usually, high-dose RAI treatment is given, since these lesions are relatively resistant to RAI therapy compared with micronodular pulmonary metastases. Bone lesions are frequently also treated with external beam radiation, especially when pathologic fracture threatens, and as palliative measures for painful bone metastases. Local sites of metastasis are frequently amenable to external beam radiotherapy with successful control [15], with improved relapse-free survival [82]. Since the presence of bone metastases generally predicts a lower response to I-131 therapy, a poorer prognosis than soft tissue metastases, surgical therapy or external beam radiotherapy is used for control of the tumor. Nonetheless, I-131 therapy is still often used because there is usually additional disseminated tumor, even if not seen on I-131 imaging. The response to treatment of bone metastases is still related to the degree of I-131 uptake. In general, an aggressive approach as possible is used [15].

Treatment for elevated thyroglubulin even though the RAI scan is negative

When a patient presents with an elevated Tg level or a positive FDG PET scan or other evidence of tumor with no RAI uptake on a RAI diagnostic scan, as illustrated Figure 8.6, there is low likelihood that one can deliver sufficient radiation dose with even high-dose RAI therapy to effect substantial benefit. It is then usually preferred to wait and follow the patient until more tumor appears that can be seen on a RAI scan and more activity can be delivered with I-131 therapy. A counterargument can be made that despite no visible tumor uptake on a diagnostic RAI scan, after a therapeutic RAI dose is given, one can see the tumor on the posttherapy scan about one-third of the time [83,84]. In 30%–50% of such patients, the Tg levels may decrease significantly after therapy [85–87].

Thus, empiric therapy with 100–200 mCi may be considered to aid in localization of the responsible tumor, possibly leading to partial reduction in tumor volume, or possible surgical resection. Such an approach has been reported to aid in the location of persistent disease in up to 50% of patients [88,89]. Nonetheless, there is no reported evidence of improved survival in the empiric treatment of elevated Tg levels in the setting of a negative RAI scan [90].

Use of external beam radiotherapy in combination with RAI therapy

Unresectable disease in regional lymph nodes or in bone (see example in Figure 8.5) is frequently unresponsive or only partially responsive to RAI therapy alone. Painful bone lesions that cannot be resected can be treated with combinations of external beam radiotherapy, radioiodine, and other palliative approaches, discussed above [15]. Likewise, brain metastases that occur in more advanced disease are treated with surgical resection and external beam radiotherapy, along with radioiodine treatment of other lesions [15].

SIDE EFFECTS AND COMPLICATIONS OF RAI THERAPY

Side effects

Patients who undergo treatment with radioiodine are expected to experience individual dose- and cumulative dose-related risks of nausea, salivary gland and nasolacrimal duct damage, and increased risk of new malignancies. Thus, it is important to ensure that the benefits of treatment outweigh the possible risks, and that counseling and efforts in prophylaxis are standard procedures [15].

Younger patients who are being prepared for treatment with 200 mCi of I-131 or more, older patients with intended doses greater than 180 mCi, or those with small body habitus or reduced renal function should undergo blood dosimetry calculation as discussed above (see cases in Figures 8.4 and 8.5). Patients with blood dosimetry at or below 200 cGy (200 rads) rarely show serious bone marrow toxicity, such as aplastic anemia or prolonged bone marrow suppression [15]. The precautions relating to prevention of pulmonary toxicity have already been discussed as part of dosimetric considerations.

Swallowed activity in saliva and activity excreted in the GI tract, namely, in the stomach, are not completely absorbed and partially excreted in the colon, as documented on diagnostic and posttherapy RAI scans. To avoid excessive exposure to the colon, avoidance of constipation through the use of a high-fiber diet and laxatives is recommended.

Carcinogenesis

Long-term studies demonstrate a small additional risk of secondary malignancies, such as bone and soft tissue malignancies, colorectal cancer, salivary tumors, and leukemia, in patients who have undergone radioiodine therapy, in proportion to the cumulative dose. A European study showed an increased risk of 14.4 additional solid tumors and 0.8 leukemia cases per gigabecquerel (27 mCi) of I-131 per 10^5 person-years, or 53 excess cases out of 576 of solid malignancies and 3 cases of leukemia per 10 years among 10,000 patients treated with 100 mCi (3700 MBq) of I-131 [91]. The mean time between radioiodine therapy and the secondary malignancy was 15 years. The relative risk ranged from 2.2 to 4.0. Another study suggested increased risk of breast cancer in patients with thyroid cancer; it is unclear if this was due to radioiodine therapy or a referral bias [92].

Effects on fertility in women

Although temporary amenorrhea or oligomenorrhea lasting 4–10 months has been reported in 17%–20% of menstruating women following I-131 therapy for thyroid cancer, long-term rates of fertility, miscarriage, and fetal malformation do not appear to be elevated in women after radioiodine therapy, as long as they avoided pregnancy for 6–12 months [93–95].

Effects on fertility in men

Dose-dependent oligospermia and elevated follicle-stimulating hormone (FSH) levels have been observed in men treated with I-131 [96–98]. Usually, the oligospermia is transient with low and moderate doses of I-131, but more prolonged with high doses. High cumulative doses (500–800 mCi) in men are associated with an increased risk of persistent elevation of serum FSH levels, but fertility and risks of miscarriage or congenital abnormalities in subsequent pregnancies are not changed with moderate single radioiodine doses of approximately 200 mCi [99]. There is a possibility of cumulative damage with multiple treatments, and sperm banking while the patient is euthyroid may be advised for cumulative doses greater than 400 mCi. Gonadal radiation exposure in both men and women is reduced with good hydration, frequent urinary voiding, and avoidance of constipation [100].

Therapy in postpartum women

Since uptake in the breasts is increased in lactating or postpartum women, radioiodine treatment should be avoided, until after breast feeding has been stopped for at least 6–8 weeks [15], to avoid both radiation breast exposure and adverse effects to the infant's thyroid gland.

Therapy in children

Although thyroid cancer tends to be more aggressive and have higher incidence of multifocal disease and nodal and pulmonary metastases in children, well-differentiated thyroid cancer usually carries a good prognosis in younger patients. Studies of 5–10 years of follow-up and longer generally show good quality of life. A partial response with reduction of metastatic disease was usually possible with RAI therapy, with no further progression, and a low mortality rate, with 97% survival at 11 years of follow-up in one study, and lack of pulmonary side effects despite therapy [101,102]. The high rate of extensive disease in children also argues for preablation therapy diagnostic imaging, ablation therapy, and close follow-up. The diagnostic dose is adjusted according to body weight or body surface area, and the therapy dose, as in adults, is adjusted depending on whether the dose of I-131 is used for mere ablation or treatment of locoregional disease or peripheral metastases.

Regulations regarding hospitalization of patients treated with RAI

As a result of recent revision of regulations by the U.S. Nuclear Regulatory Commission for release of patients receiving RAI doses, patients with doses larger than 30 mCi (1110 MBq) can be released if it can be demonstrated that family members and caregivers do not receive more than 5 mSv (500 mrem), and other members of the public do not receive more than 1 mSv (100 mrem), under Title 10 of the Code of Federal Regulations (CFR), Part 35.75. Recent studies confirmed that with proper counseling and observation of precautions under this rule, exposure of family members of patients treated with 75–150 mCi (2.8–5.6 GBq) is minimal [103].

In the absence of patient-specific calculations, one may use group-defined exposures for I-131 dose ranging from 30 to 200 mCi (1110–7400 MBq) for outpatient management and hospitalize patients with doses greater than 200 mCi

(7400 MBq). Others have developed models for estimating exposure to others [104], allowing outpatient treatment with activities even greater than 200 mCi (7400 MBq).

Proper counseling requires an evaluation of the patient's home and work conditions. The patient must receive clear and simple written instructions about appropriate behavior and precautions, which usually need a consultation in advance of the treatment, plus a review at the time of the treatment.

OUTSTANDING ISSUES ON RADIOIODINE USE IN DIAGNOSIS AND THERAPY

The first and foremost challenge in the management of thyroid cancer is the relative lack of randomized controlled multicenter clinical trials examining various aspects of diagnosis and treatment, due to the longevity of patients and low mortality. There is a need for improvements in understanding the long-term risks of radioiodine therapy, the limitation of side effects on the salivary glands, the long-term effects on reproductive organs, and the risk of second malignancies. There are also challenges in finding effective therapy for poorly differentiated thyroid cancer or differentiated cancer that loses avidity for iodine.

REFERENCES

1. Berson SA, Yalow RS, Sorrentino J et al. The determination of thyroidal and renal plasma I-131 clearance rates as a routine diagnostic test of thyroid dysfunction. J Clin Invest 1952;31:141.
2. Castro MR, Bergert ER, Goellner JR et al. Immunohistochemical analysis of sodium iodide symporter expression in metastatic differentiated thyroid cancer: Correlation with radioiodine uptake. J Clin Endocrinol Metab 2001;86:5627–32.
3. Honor AJ, Myant NB, Rowlands EN. Secretion of radioiodine in digestive juices and milk in man. Clin Sci 1952;11:447.
4. Chapman EM, Corner GW Jr, Robinson D et al. The collection of radioactive iodine by the human fetal thyroid. J Clin Endocrinol 1984;8:717.
5. Wolff J, Maurey JR. Thyroidal iodide transport IV. The role of ion size. Biochim Biophys Acta 1963;69:48.
6. Atkins HL, Richards P. Assessment of thyroid function and anatomy with technetium-99m as pertechnetate. J Nucl Med 1968;9:7.
7. Wegst A, Goin J, Robinson R. Cumulated activities determined from biodistribution data in pregnant rats ranging from 13 to 21 days gestation. I. Tc-99m pertechnetate. Med Phys 1983;10:841.
8. Hahn V, Brod K, Wolf R. The radiation dose to the fetus during isotope investigations of the mother. Fortschr Rontgenstr 1980;132:326.
9. Wyburn J. Human breast milk excretion of radionuclides following administration of radiopharmaceuticals. J Nucl Med 1973;14:115.

10. Romney BM, Nickoloff EL, Esser PD et al. Radionuclide administration to nursing mothers: Mathematically derived guidelines. *Radiology* 1986;160:549.

11. Gharib H, Zimmerman D, Goellner JR et al. Fine-needle aspiration biopsy: Use in diagnosis and management of pediatric thyroid diseases. *Endocr Pract* 1995;1:9–13.

12. Kocher DC. Radioactive decay data table. DOE/TIC 1981;11026:133.

13. Pentlow KS, Graham MC, Lambrecht RM et al. Quantitative imaging of iodine-124 with PET. *J Nucl Med* 1996;37:1557–62.

14. Ridgeway EC. Clinician evaluation of a solitary thyroid nodule. *J Clin Endocrinol Metab* 1992;8:215–24.

15. Cooper DS, Doherty GM, Haugen BR et al. Revised management guidelines for patients with thyroid nodules and differentiated thyroid cancer. *Thyroid* 2009;19:1167–214.

16. Sachmechi I, Miller E, Varatharajah R et al. Thyroid carcinoma in single cold nodules and in cold nodules of multinodular goiters. *Endocr Pract* 2000;6:5–7.

17. Rallison ML, Dobyns BM, Keating FR Jr et al. Thyroid nodularity in children. *JAMA* 1975;233:1069–72.

18. Corrias A, Einaudi S, Chiorboli E et al. Accuracy of fine needle aspiration biopsy of thyroid nodules in detecting malignancy in childhood: Comparison with conventional clinical, laboratory, and imaging approaches. *J Clin Endocrinol Metab* 2001;86:4644–48.

19. Kusic Z, Becker DV, Saenger EL et al. Comparison of technetium-99m and iodine-123 imaging of thyroid nodules: Correlation with pathologic findings. *J Nucl Med* 1990;31:393–9.

20. Pluijmen MJ, Eustatia-Rutten C, Goslings BM et al. Effects of low-iodide diet on postsurgical radioiodide ablation therapy in patients with differentiated thyroid carcinoma. *Clin Endocrinol (Oxf)* 2003;58:428–35.

21. Maxon HR, Thomas SR, Boehringer A et al. Low iodine diet in I-131 ablation of thyroid remnants. *Clin Nucl Med* 1983;8:123–26.

22. Hladik WB, Nigg KK, Rhodes BA. Drug-induced changes in the biologic distribution of radiopharmaceuticals. *Semin Nucl Med* 1982;12:184.

23. Edmonds CJ, Hayes S, Kermode JC et al. Measurement of serum TSH and thyroid hormones in the management of treatment of thyroid carcinoma with radioiodine. *Br J Radiol* 1977;50:799–807.

24. Thyrogen package insert. Cambridge, MA: Genzyme Corporation, November 1998.

25. Serhal DI, Nasrallah MP, Arafah BM. Rapid rise in serum thyrotropin concentrations after thyroidectomy or withdrawal of suppressive thyroxine therapy in preparation for radioactive iodine administration to patients with differentiated thyroid cancer. *J Clin Endocrinol Metab* 2004;89:3285–9.

26. Haugen RB, Pacini F, Reiners C et al. A comparison of recombinant human thyrotropin and thyroid hormone withdrawal for the detection of thyroid remnant or cancer. *J Clin Endocrinol Metab* 1999;84:3877–85.

27. Ladenson PW, Braverman LE, Mazzaferri EL et al. Comparison of administration of recombinant human thyrotropin with withdrawal of thyroid hormone for radioactive iodine scanning in patients with thyroid carcinoma. *N Engl J Med* 1997;337:888–96.

28. Carril JM, Quirce R, Serrano J et al. Total-body scintigraphy with thallium-201 and iodine-131 in the follow-up of differentiated thyroid cancer. *J Nucl Med* 1997;38:686–92.

29. Hilditch TE, Dempsey MF, Bolster AA et al. Self-stunning in thyroid ablation: Evidence from comparative studies of diagnostic I-131 and I-123. *Eur J Nucl Med Mol Imaging* 2002;29:783–8.

30. Anderson GS, Fish S, Nakhoda K et al. Comparison of I-123 and I-131 for whole-body imaging after stimulation by recombinant human thyrotropin: A preliminary report. *Clin Nucl Med* 2003;28:93–6.

31. Sarkar SD, Kalapparambath TP, Palestro CJ et al. Comparison of I-123 and I-131 for whole-body imaging in thyroid cancer. *J Nucl Med* 2002;43:632–4.

32. Thomas DL, Menda Y, Bushnell D et al. A comparison between diagnostic I-123 and post-therapy I-131 scans in the detection of remnant and locoregional thyroid disease. *Clin Nucl Med* 2009;34:745–8.

33. Regalbuto C, Buscema M, Arena S et al. False-positive findings on I-131 whole-body scans because of post-traumatic superficial scabs. *J Nucl Med* 2002;43:207–9.

34. Fatourechi V, Hay ID, Mullan BP et al. Are post-therapy radioiodine scans informative and do they influence subsequent therapy of patients with differentiated thyroid cancer? *Thyroid* 2000;10:573–7.

35. Souza Rosario PW, Barroso AL, Rezende LL et al. Post-131 therapy scanning in patients with thyroid carcinoma metastases: An unnecessary cost or a relevant contribution? *Clin Nucl Med* 2004;29:795–8.

36. David A, Blotta A, Bondanelli M et al. Serum thyroglobulin concentrations and I-131 whole body scan results in patients with differentiated thyroid carcinoma after administration of recombinant human thyroid stimulating hormone. *J Nucl Med* 2001;42:1470–5.

37. Pons F, Carrio I, Estorch M et al. Lithium as an adjuvant of iodine-131 uptake when treating patients with well-differentiated thyroid carcinoma. *Clin Nucl Med* 1987;12:644–7.

38. Koong SS, Reynolds JC, Movius EG et al. Lithium as a potential adjuvant to I-131 therapy of metastatic, well-differentiated thyroid carcinoma. *J Clin Endocrinol Metab* 1999;84:912–6.

39. Smit JWA, Schroder-van der Elst JP, Karperien M et al. Iodide kinetics and experimental I-131 therapy in a xenotransplanted human sodium-iodide symporter-transfected human follicular thyroid carcinoma cell line. *J Clin Endocrinol Metab* 2002;87:1247–53.

40. Park SY, Kwak W, Tapha N et al. Combination therapy and noninvasive imaging with a dual therapeutic vector expressing MDR1 short hairpin RNA and a sodium iodide symporter. *J Nucl Med* 2008;49:1480–8.

41. Ho AL, Grewal RK, Leboeuf R. Selumetinib-enhanced radioiodine uptake in advanced thyroid cancer. *N Engl J Med* 2013;368:623–32.

42. http://clinicaltrials.gov/ct2/show/NCT01843962?term=NCT01843062rank=1.

43. Maxon HR, Thomas SR, Hetzberg VS et al. Relation between effective radiation dose and outcome of radioiodine therapy for thyroid cancer. *N Engl J Med* 1983;309:937–41.

44. Kolbert KS, Pentlow KS, Pearson JR et al. Prediction of absorbed dose to normal organs in thyroid cancer patients treated with I-131 by use of I-124 PET and 3-dimensional internal dosimetry software. *J Nucl Med* 2007;48:143–9.

45. Beierwalters WH. The treatment of thyroid carcinoma with radioactive iodine. *Semin Nucl Med* 1978;8:79.

46. Stabin MG. MIRDOSE: Personal computer software for internal dose assessment in nuclear medicine. *J Nucl Med* 1996;37:538–46.

47. Benua RS, Cicale NR, Sonenberg M et al. The relation of radioiodine dosimetry to results and complications in the treatment of metastatic thyroid cancer. *AJR Am J Roentgenol* 1962;87:171.

48. Zimmer LA, McCook B, Meltzer C et al. Combined positron emission tomography/computed tomography imaging of recurrent thyroid cancer. *Otolaryngol Head Neck Surg* 2003;128:178–84.

49. Moog F, Linke R, Manthey N et al. Influence of thyroid-stimulating hormone levels on uptake of FDG in recurrent and metastatic differentiated thyroid carcinoma. *J Nucl Med* 2000;41:1989–95.

50. Bertagna F, Bosio G, Biasiotto G et al. F-18 FDG-PET/CT evaluation of patients with differentiated thyroid cancer with negative I-131 total body scan and high thyroglobulin level. *Clin Nucl Med* 2009;34:756–61.

51. Wang, W, Macapinlac H, Finn R et al. PET scanning with F-18-fluorodeoxyglucose can localize differentiated thyroid carcinoma in patients with negative I-131 whole body scans. *J Clin Endocrinol Metab* 1999;84:2291–302.

52. Wang W, Larson SM, Fazzari M et al. Prognostic value of [18F]fluorodeoxyglucose positron emission tomographic scanning in patients with thyroid cancer. *J Clin Endocrinol Metab* 2000;85:1107–13.

53. Kresnik E, Gallowitsch HJ, Mikosch P et al. Flurine-18-fluorodeoxyglucose positron emission tomography in the preoperative assessment of thyroid nodules in an endemic goiter area. *Surgery* 2003;133:294–9.

54. Robbins RJ, Wan W, Grewal RK et al. Real-time prognosis for metastatic thyroid carcinoma based on 2-[F-18] fluoro-2-deoxy-d-glucose-positron emission tomography scanning. *J Clin Endocrinol Metab* 2006;91:498–505.

55. Smallridge RC, Ain KB, Asa SL et al. American Thyroid Association guidelines for management of patients with anaplastic thyroid cancer. *Thyroid* 2012;22:1104–39.

56. Mitchell JC, Grant F, Evenson AR et al. Preoperative evaluation of thyroid nodules with F-18 FDG PET/CT. *Surgery* 2005;138:1166–75.

57. Van Den Bruel A, Maes A, De Potter T et al. Clinical relevance of thyroid fluorodeoxyglucose-whole body positron emission tomography incidentaloma. *J Clin Endocrinol Metab* 2002;87:1517–20.

58. Chu QD, Connor MS, Lilien DL et al. Positron emission tomography (PET) positive thyroid incidentaloma: The risk of malignancy observed in a tertiary referral center. *Am Surg* 2006;72:272–5.

59. Alam MS, Takeuchi L, Kasagi K et al. Value of combined technetium-99m hydroxymethylene diphosphanate and thallium-201 imaging in detecting bone metastases from thyroid carcinoma. *Thyroid* 1997;7:705–12.

60. Seidlin SM, Marinelli LD, Osher E et al. Radioactive iodine therapy. Effect on functioning metastases of adenocarcinoma of the thyroid. *JAMA* 1946;232:838–47.

61. Brennan MD, Bergstrahl EJ, VanHerrden JA et al. Follicular thyroid cancer treated at the Mayo Clinic, 1946 through 1970: Initial manifestations, pathologic findings, therapy, and outcome. *Mayo Clin Proc* 1991;66:11–22.

62. Mazzaferri EL, Young RL. Papillary thyroid carcinoma: A 10-year follow-up report of the impact of therapy in 576 patients. *Am J Med* 1981;70:511–8.

63. Mazzaferri EL, Jhiang SM. Long-term impact of initial surgical and medical therapy on papillary and follicular thyroid cancer. *Am J Med* 1994;97:418–28.

64. Mazzaferri EL. An overview of the management of papillary and follicular thyroid carcinoma. *Thyroid* 1999;9:421–7.

65. Borget I, Remy H, Chevalier J et al. Length and cost of hospital stay of radioiodine ablation in thyroid cancer patients: Comparison between preparation with thyroid hormone withdrawal and Thyrogen. *Eur J Nucl Med Mol Imaging* 2008;35:1457–63.

66. Hanscheid H, Lassmann M, Luster M et al. Iodine biokinetics and dosimetry in radioiodine therapy of thyroid cancer: Procedures and results of a prospective international controlled study of ablation after rhTSH or hormone withdrawal.

67. Sisson JC. Applying the radioactive eraser: I-131 to ablate normal thyroid tissue in patients from whom thyroid cancer has been resected. *J Nucl Med* 1983;24:743–5.

68. Goolden AW. The indications for ablating normal thyroid tissue with I-131 in differentiated thyroid cancer. *Clin Endocrinol* 1985;23:81–6.

69. Rosario PWS, Ribeiro Maia FF, Cardoso LD et al. Correlation between cervical uptake and results of post-surgical radioiodine ablation in patients with thyroid carcinoma. *Clin Nucl Med* 2004;29:358–61.

70. Liel Y. Preparation for radioactive iodine administration in differentiated thyroid cancer patients. *Clin Endocrinol (Oxf)* 2002;57:523–7.

71. Robbins RJ, Schlumberger MJ. The evolving role of I-131 for the treatment of differentiated thyroid carcinoma. *J Nucl Med* 2005;46:28S–37S.

72. Beierwaltes WH. The treatment of thyroid carcinoma with radioactive iodine. *Semin Nucl Med* 1978;8:79–94.

73. Pellegriti G, Scollo C, Giuffrida D et al. Usefulness of recombinant human thyrotropin in the radiometabolic treatment of selected patients with thyroid cancer. *Thyroid* 2001;11:1025–30.

74. Adler ML, Macapinlac HA, Robbins RJ. Radioiodine treatment of thyroid cancer with the aid of recombinant human thyrotropin. *Endocr Pract* 1998;4:282–6.

75. Vargas GE, Uy H, Bazan C et al. Hemipegia after thyrotropin alfa in a hypothyroid patient with thyroid carcinoma metastatic to the brain. *J Clin Endocrinol Metab* 84:3867–71.

76. Robbins RJ, Voelker E, Wang W et al. Compassionate use of recombinant human thyrotropin to facilitate radioiodine therapy: Case report and review of the literature. *Endocr Pract* 2000;6:460–4.

77. Braga M, Ringel MD, Cooper DS. Sudden enlargement of local recurrent thyroid tumor after recombinant human TSH administration. *J Clin Endocrinol Metab* 2001;86:5148–51.

78. Ilgan S, Karacalioglu AO, Pabuscu Y et al. Iodine-131 treatment and high-resolution CT: Results in patients with lung metastases form differentiated thyroid carcinoma. *Eur J Nucl Mol Imaging* 2004;3:825–30.

79. Hindie E, Melliere D, Lange F et al. Functioning pulmonary metastases of thyroid cancer: Does radioiodine influence the prognosis? *Eur J Nucl Med Mol Imaging* 2003;30:974–81.

80. Fatourechi V, Hay ID, Javedan H et al. Lack of impact of radioiodine therapy in thyroglobulin-positive, diagnostic whole-body scan-negative patient with follicular cell-derived thyroid cancer. *J Clin Endocrinol Metab* 2002;87:1521–6.

81. Sarlis NJ. Metastatic thyroid cancer unresponsive to conventional therapies: Novel management approaches through translational clinical research. *Curr Drug Targets Immune Endocr Metabol Disord* 2001;1:103–15.

82. Tsang RW, Brierley JD, Simpson WJ et al. The effects of surgery, radioiodine, and external radiation therapy on the clinical outcome of patients with differentiated thyroid carcinoma. *Cancer* 1998;82:375–88.

83. Pineda JD, Lee T, Ain K et al. Iodine-131 therapy for thyroid cancer patients with elevated thyroglobulin and negative diagnostic scans. *J Clin Endocrinol Metab* 1995;80:1488–92.

84. Pacini F, Lippi F, Formica N et al. Therapeutic doses of iodine-131 reveal undiagnosed metastases in thyroid cancer patients with detectable serum thyroglobulin levels. *J Nucl Med* 1987;28:1888–91.

85. Kabasakal L, Selcuk NA, Shafipour H et al. Treatment of iodine-negative thyroglobulin-positive thyroid cancer: Differences in outcome in patients with macrometastases. *Eur J Nucl Med Mol Imaging* 2004;31:1500–4.

86. Ma C, Xie J, Kunag A. Is empiric I-131 therapy justified for patients with positive thyroglobulin and negative I-131 whole-body scanning results? *J Nucl Med* 2005;46:1164–70.

87. Pacini F, Agate L, Elisei R et al. Outcome of differentiated thyroid cancer with detectable serum Tg and negative diagnostic I-131 whole body scan: Comparison of patients treated with high I-131 activities versus untreated patients. *J Clin Endocrinol Metab* 2001;86:4092–7.

88. Schlumberger M, Mancusi F, Baudin E et al. I-131 therapy for elevated thyroglobulin levels. *Thyroid* 1997;7:273–6.

89. Van Tol KM, Jager PL, de Vries EG et al. Outcome in patients with differentiated thyroid cancer with negative diagnostic whole-body scanning and detectable stimulated thyroglobulin. *Eur J Endocrinol* 2003;148:589–96.

90. Kabasakal L, Selcuk NA, Shafipour H et al. Treatment of iodine-negative thyroglobulin positive thyroid cancer: Differences in outcome in patients with macrometastases and patients with micrometastases. *Eur J Nucl Med Mol Imaging* 2004;31:1500–4.

91. Rubino C, de Vathaire F, Dottorini ME et al. Second primary malignancies in thyroid cancer patients. *Br J Cancer* 2003;89:1638–44.

92. Chen AY, Ley L, Goepfeert H et al. The development of breast carcinoma in women with thyroid carcinoma. *Cancer* 2001;92:225–31.

93. Vini L, Hyer S, Al-Saadi A et al. Prognosis for fertility and ovarian function after treatment with radioiodine for thyroid cancer. *Postgrad Med J* 2002;78:92–3.

94. Dottorini ME, Lomuscio G, Mazzucchelli L et al. Assessment of female fertility and carcinogenesis after I-131 therapy for differentiated thyroid carcinoma. *J Nucl Med* 1995;36:21–7.

95. Sarkar SD, Beierwaltes WH, Gill SP et al. Fertility and birth histories of patients treated with I-131 for thyroid cancer before 1969 at 20 years or less. *J Nucl Med* 1976;17:460.

96. Pacini F, Gasperi M, Fugazzola L et al. Testicular function in patients with thyroid carcinoma treated with radioiodine. *J Nucl Med* 1994;35:1418–22.

97. Wichers M, Benz E, Palmedo H et al. Testicular function after radioiodine therapy for thyroid carcinoma. *Eur J Nucl Med* 2000;27:503–7.

98. Hyer S, Vini L, O'Connell M et al. Testicular dose and fertility in men following I-131 therapy for thyroid cancer. *Clin Endocrinol (Oxf)* 2002;56:755–8.

99. Lushbaugh CC, Casarett GW. The effects of gonadal irradiation in clinical radiation therapy: A review. *Cancer* 1976;37:1111–25.

100. Mazzaferri E. Gonadal damage from I-131 therapy for thyroid cancer. *Clin Endocrinol* 2002;57:313–4.

101. Samuel AM, Rajashekharrao B, Shah DH. Pulmonary metastases in children and adolescents with well-differentiated thyroid cancer. *J Nucl Med* 1998;39:1531–6.

102. Hod N, Hagag P, Baumer M et al. Differentiated thyroid carcinoma in children and young adults: Evaluation of response to treatment. *Clin Nucl Med* 2005;30:387–90.

103. Grigsby PW, Siegel BA, Baker S et al. Radiation exposures from outpatient radioactive I-131 therapy for thyroid carcinoma. *JAMA* 2000;283:2272–4.

104. Coover LR, Silberstein EB, Kuhn PJ et al. Therapeutic I-131 in outpatients: A simplified method conforming to the Code of Federal Regulations, title 10, part 35.75. *J Nucl Med* 2000;41:1868–75.

9

Mediastinal goiters

YAMIL CASTILLO BEAUCHAMP AND ASHOK R. SHAHA

DEFINITION

There are several theories regarding substernal goiter, but the most popular is that the goiter represents an inferior growth from the cervical thyroid gland that is supplied by the vessels in the neck. The upright posture of human beings combined with normal swallowing and breathing mechanisms induces negative intrathoracic pressure. The weight of the enlarging mass allows the gland to grow and descend through the thoracic inlet into the substernal position. Inferiorly, there is no anatomic structure that can restrict the growth of the thyroid gland. This leads to the path of "least resistance"—toward the thoracic inlet.

Coming from the Latin word *gutteria*, the basic definition of *goiter* is swelling of the neck resulting from enlargement of the thyroid gland associated with a thyroid gland that is functioning properly or not. There have been several different definitions for intrathoracic goiter published since it was initially described by Haller in 1729. Albeit inconsistently, and with varying degrees of clinical significance, these definitions have attempted to describe the characteristics of the mediastinal goiter and predict the risks for complications. The clinical definition defines the mediastinal goiter as a thyroid that, on neck examination, has a portion that remains permanently retrosternal. *Hsu* defined it as a thyroid gland (clinically or radiologically) below the manubrium. *Kocher* proposed that it was a thyroid goiter in which some portion remained permanently retrosternal. *Torre* defined is as a thyroid gland with its lower position remaining below the sternal notch with the neck hyperextended. *Escharpase* classified it as a goiter that is totally or partially located in the mediastinum and, in the operating room, has its edge at least 3 cm below the sternal manubrium. *Lahey* stated that it was a goiter that needs excision to be performed from the upper mediastinum. *Linskog*'s definition stated that it was a thyroid growth up to the level of the fourth thoracic vertebrae on x-ray examination. *Crile*'s definition referred to it as a goiter with thyroid growth up to the aortiuc arch. *Katlic* defined it as a goiter that was at least 50% restrosternal. The subcarinal definition described by *Sancho* et al. stated that it was a goiter with thyroid growth that reached the tracheal carina [1,2].

The most common cause of goiter is iodine deficiency, usually seen in Third World countries; it is one of the most common problems in mountainous regions such as the Alps and the Himalayas [3,4]. Iodine deficiency, resulting in increased thyroid-stimulating hormone (TSH) output in an attempt to maintain the euthyroid state, is often associated with large multinodular goiters rather than a homogeneous expansion of all thyroid follicular cells. The incidence of goiter (colloid or endemic) is rare in the United States because of the compulsory use of iodized salt. However, goiters may also be associated with Graves' disease, Hashimoto's thyroiditis, and benign and malignant thyroid neoplasms.

Thyroid tumors, of course, develop in the neck but can extend downward into the mediastinal region as they grow. Most enlarge over a long period of time and occasionally remain asymptomatic. When symptoms are present, they are most commonly respiratory in nature with an accompanying neck mass. The tumor may be almost entirely substernal at times, with no significant mass appearing in the neck. As a result of the bony confines of the thoracic inlet, mediastinal goiters lead to compression symptoms—mainly related to the trachea and esophagus, but also at times producing venous obstruction [5,6].

Mediastinal goiters can be classified as primary or secondary. Primary mediastinal goiters arise from ectopic thyroid in the mediastinum. Although rare (fewer than 1% of cases), it is important to note that when it is present, it receives its vascular supply from intrathoracic vessels. The far more common secondary mediastinal goiter develops from the downward growth of cervical thyroid tissue. This growth occurs more frequently into the anterior mediastinum, anterior to the ipsilateral recurrent laryngeal nerve and anterolateral to the trachea. In approximately 10%–15% of cases, the cervical thyroid tissue may grow into the posterior mediastinum, and hence posterior to the ipsilateral recurrent laryngeal nerve and the carotid sheath. When this occurs, it is predominantly on the right side, due to the presence of the aortic arch. Regardless of whether it is anterior or posterior, secondary mediastinal goiters receive their vascular supply from the superior and inferior thyroid arteries.

The management of mediastinal goiters is engrossing because of the complexity of surgical procedures and associated risks. Most frequently, surgery is advised to avoid problems related to airway, venous obstruction, and malignancy [7–13].

Historical reports of goiters date back to 2700 BC, and management of can be traced to as far back as 1600 BC, when burnt sponges and seaweed were used in ancient China as medical treatment. Other historical accounts of treatment of goiters have referred to the use of toad's blood and to the stroking of the goiter with a cadaveric hand. Ali Ibn Abbas recorded in 952 AD the removal of a large goiter under opium sedation using simple ligatures and hot cautery irons as the patient sat with a bag around his neck to catch the blood. Eventually, surgical treatment evolved, although as late as 1866, Samuel Gross from the University of Pennsylvania remarked that thyroid surgery was "butchery" and that "no honest and sensible surgeon would ever engage in thyroid surgery." Clearly, this was an era before antisepsis, hemostats, and the use of iodine to control hyperthyroidism.

Klein, a German surgeon in 1820, first reported removal of a substernal goiter. The mortality from thyroid surgery before the Kocher era was almost 40%. Credit goes to Kocher, Halsted, and Lahey for perfecting the technique of thyroid surgery. Kocher, with his vast experience in thyroid surgery, studied the physiology, improved the techniques of thyroid surgery, and was the first surgeon to receive the Nobel Prize for his contributions in thyroid diseases [14].

CLINICAL PRESENTATION AND SYMPTOMS

Respiratory

Most intrathoracic goiters present in elderly females and appear more frequently in the fifth or sixth decade. Thirty to forty percent are asymptomatic, and in about 20% of patients there is no palpable neck mass. The diagnosis is sometimes made by a routine chest x-ray disclosing a mediastinal mass. Reeve et al. reviewed 967,759 screening radiographs in Sydney, Australia, and reported the incidence of substernal goiter to be 1 in 5040 [15]. Seventy to eighty percent of all patients, however, can be demonstrated to be symptomatic at the time of initial evaluation (Figure 9.1).

Respiratory symptoms are the most common presentation of intrathoracic goiters, and they can range from a mild cough to life-threatening asphyxia. Even though those affected may not be aware of a problem, dyspnea can often be provoked in approximately 85% of cases by raising both arms above the shoulders (Pemberton's sign). Hoarseness is a rare symptom. The recurrent nerve may be paralyzed due to the long-standing compression or stretching of a benign

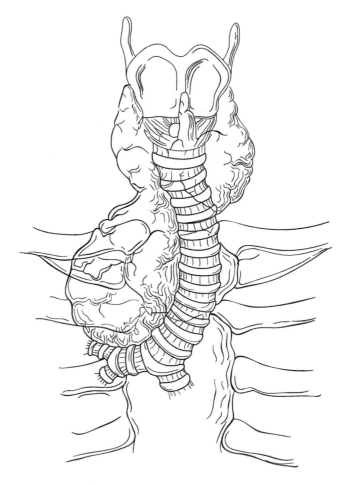

Figure 9.1 Schematic picture of mediastinal goiter with tracheal deviation. The bony confines of the thoracic inlet causing compression.

goiter, but the presence of hoarseness and a paretic recurrent nerve raises a suspicion of thyroid malignancy. Patients may be totally asymptomatic, but because of the bony confines of the thoracic inlet, the thyroid can act like an expanding mass within a rigid cage—leading to compression of vital structures. The most common symptom is related to compression of the upper airway. Ninety percent of symptomatic patients mainly have respiratory symptoms, including cough, hoarseness of voice, and shortness of breath. Although rare, occasional dyspnea, cough, cyanosis, choking accompanied by suffocation, and respiratory collapse requiring emergency treatment may be seen. Shaha et al. [35] reported 24 patients with life-threatening respiratory symptoms, with nine requiring immediate intubation [16]. Patients with acute airway obstruction require intervention on an urgent basis and should remain on a ventilator until surgery because acute asphyxia may result if it is discontinued [17–19].

Esophageal

Approximately one-third of the patients will experience some degree of dysphagia or difficulty in swallowing as a result of pressure on the esophagus as it is displaced posteriorly and laterally by the goiter. This can be confirmed by esophagram but is not usually a major problem.

Vascular obstruction

Obstruction of venous return occurs in less than 10% of cases. It may be minimal but can be demonstrated by elevating the patient's arms (Pemberton's sign) and observing the distention of neck veins. The symptoms and signs may become more severe as the intrathoracic mass becomes larger, progressing to a full-blown superior vena cava syndrome with dilatation of the veins of the neck, face, and descending collateral venous circulation, as well as cyanosis. Other rare symptoms may be related to compression of the mediastinal vessels, such as downward esophageal varices, Horner's syndrome, pleural effusion, and transient ischemic attacks secondary to the goiter stealing the blood from cerebral circulation [20–26]. Although rare, the appearance of symptoms of venous obstruction is an urgent indication for surgery. The obstruction may be due to the encroaching bulk of a benign nodular goiter or the result of malignant infiltration.

Hyperthyroidism

Multinodular goiters, whether they are in the neck or in the mediastinum, can develop autonomous hyperfunctioning nodules, particularly if the goiter is long standing. Hyperthyroidism, as well as the presence of mediastinal goiter, is more common in elderly patients. Cougard et al. [19] reported an incidence of hyperthyroidism in 35% of 218 intrathoracic goiters in patients over 70 years of age. The cardiac effects of hyperthyroidism can be serious, and often appear insidiously; arrhythmias, congestive failure, and ischemic heart disease carry a more serious implication in the elderly and may be life threatening.

Radioactive iodine has been used to control the hyperthyroidism of large multinodular goiters. It may significantly reduce the size of the mediastinal goiter in up to 30%–40%, especially if used in combination with recombinant TSH, as reported by Bonnema and Hegedus [27] in 2012. It often requires, however, repeated doses and a long time period to be effective. Due to concerns such as the risk of goiter recurrence, overlooking a malignancy, and the development of short-term side effects such as radiation thyroiditis following radioactive iodine, which may precipitate acute airway obstruction, and the long-term risk of developing a secondary malignancy, it remains an option that should only be offered to those patients with prohibitive surgical risks or who refuse surgery.

Malignancy

The incidence of overt cancer, as well as incidental papillary carcinoma, in mediastinal goiters has been estimated to be anywhere from 3% to 15% [17,18]. In his review of substernal goiters, White et al. [28] concluded that the incidence of malignancy in substernal goiters was no higher than that of cervical goiters. Risk factors such as family history of thyroid cancer, prior radiation to the neck area, recurrent thyroid mass, and the presence of cervical adenopathy had the same impact on risk of malignancy as cervical goiters. The distribution of the types of thyroid malignancies found was also no different when considering referral bias [28,29,40]. The preoperative presence of dysphonia should raise the suspicion of malignancy regardless of the anatomical location of the goiter. It may suggest the invasion of adjacent structures, which may pose a formidable surgical problem should the laryngeal nerves or great vessels be involved. Lymphomas and thymomas are the most common malignant tumors following intrinsic thyroid carcinoma.

Diagnostic procedures

Many unsuspected intrathoracic goiters are revealed by routine anteroposterior and lateral chest x-rays. This can indicate the extent of substernal mass and its location in the mediastinum. It may also disclose tracheal displacement and compression, calcifications, soft tissue masses, or displacement of the pleural reflection.

As noted previously, there may be no thyroid enlargement in the neck. But if a thyroid mass is present and the inferior margin cannot be defined, substernal extension is likely. Direct or fiber-optic laryngoscopy should be performed and may define laryngeal compression, distortion, or vocal cord paresis. A normal laryngoscopy exam does not rule out compression, as the airway compromise may be located well below the level of the larynx, requiring evaluation by imaging procedures.

Computerized tomography offers additional important information that is of great value in the management of the substernal goiter [30,31]. It outlines the continuity of the intrathoracic mass with the cervical thyroid. The addition of contrast material increases its value. The extent, location, and borders of the intrathoracic goiter can be precisely defined. The integrity of the airway, as well as the presence and sites of distortion or compression, can be accurately evaluated. Calcifications and the homogeneity of the tumor, which can be easily assessed, can raise the suspicion of cancer. By establishing the relationship of the goiter to the airway, esophagus, and great vessels, important information becomes available to the surgeon in determining the operative approach.

Magnetic resonance offers high-resolution imaging without the need for contrast agents. It offers a choice of tomographic cuts, and because of its greater accuracy in delineating soft tissue, it may more accurately delineate the goiter and adjacent structures, such as trachea and vascular involvement.

Ultrasound, although of great help in evaluation of cervical goiters, is not useful in substernal goiters because the bony thorax limits visibility. Barium swallow may evaluate and locate the position of the esophagus and determine if there is any major compression. Thyroid scanning is rarely helpful and may often be misleading due to the nonfunctional portion of the substernal goiter. Thyroid function tests are generally within normal limits, although, as mentioned before, hyperthyroidism may accompany toxic nodules.

Since most of the patients with substernal goiter are elderly, it is important not to assume that dyspnea is due solely to the goiter. Cardiac or pulmonary disease may account for part or even all of the symptoms. Pulmonary flow-loop studies can document the extent of pulmonary and extrapulmonary components of the dyspnea.

Pathology

The majority of substernal goiters are benign multinodular goiters or follicular adenomas. Perhaps 10%–15% are malignant; papillary or follicular cancers and thymomas predominate. Incidental papillary carcinomas are not unusual. Hyperplastic toxic nodules, lymphomas, and thyroiditis are also well recognized. Fifty percent of Hodgkin's and 20% of non-Hodgkin's lymphoma present as mediastinal masses. Due to the right-sided predominance of paratracheal nodes, superior vena cava syndrome is present in 20% of patients, particularly in those with non-Hodgkin's lymphoma. Occasionally, anaplastic thyroid cancer may present as a substernal goiter; this condition produces rapid progression of disease and severe symptoms, and carries a dismal prognosis.

Surgical approach

After careful history and physical examination, most patients are found to be symptomatic. In addition, the growth of the goiter can be unpredictable, especially if a malignancy is present. Although there is, at times, a role for radioactive iodine, there really is no satisfactory medical treatment for mediastinal goiter. The minimal regression seen with thyroid suppression offers no significant benefit, particularly if the mass is large. The majority of patients with substernal goiters should be considered for surgical intervention, unless there are prohibitive surgical risks or the patient refuses.

Kocher was the first surgeon to develop a technique of surgery for substernal goiter and invented tools to facilitate its removal. He also described the technique of morcellation (piecemeal removal of the substernal goiter) in difficult cases. Lahey reported that nearly all the cases of substernal goiters could be easily removed through the neck [32–35]. He stated, "It is a surprising fact that if the dissection is gentle and within the line of clearage, enormous masses may be removed into the neck with virtually no bleeding" [23]. Lahey also popularized the technique of morcellation for removal of large substernal goiters, as well as the use of modified sternal splitting or widening using wedges in difficult cases. Although there is still some debate regarding partial or complete sternal split, a lateral thoracotomy may occasionally be necessary.

The overwhelming number of substernal goiters, even though they may extend deep into the thorax, can be removed through a neck incision because of their cervical blood supply. Only 1%–3% require exploration through the chest wall. There have been several retrospective reviews evaluating the need for extracervical approaches and the associated predictive factors. White et al. [28] found that expert surgeons utilized extracervical approaches for the removal of substernal goiters only 2% of the time. This was more likely in the presence of primary mediastinal goiters or when the mediastinal mass was larger than the thoracic inlet opening. This may be influenced by surgeon experience, referral bias, case complexity, and differences in the definition of substernal goiter. Other authors have also considered other factors, such as malignancy, history of prior or revision surgery, extension into the posterior mediastinum, extension down to the level of the aortic arch, and lack of solid attachment between the cervical component and the substernal component, as factors predictive of the need for sternotomy [29,36].

SURGICAL TECHNIQUE

A variety of techniques and technical details are described in the literature [37–39]. The standard technique is as follows: a generous skin incision should be used. This is carried through the platysma and flaps are raised in the plane beneath this muscle. The dissection is continued in the midline. Generally, the strap muscles are divided to obtain better exposure. At the minimum, the strap muscles should be transected on the side of a large substernal goiter. The middle thyroid vein is divided and ligated, and the superior thyroid vessels are divided and ligated close to the thyroid parenchyma. The location of the laryngeal nerve is usually at its normal anatomical location; however, several studies have reported an increased incidence of recurrent laryngeal nerve injury in surgery for substernal goiter. The identification of the recurrent laryngeal nerve may be quite difficult due to the large size of the substernal goiter and the displacement of the nerve, especially when there is extension into the posterior mediastinum. As the strap muscles are divided, they should be retracted away from the thyroid. A careful attempt is made to stay on the thyroid capsule to perform a subcapsular dissection. It is important to be aware of the possibility that the recurrent nerve may be stretched over the thyroid mass in an unusual manner. Multiple inferior thyroid veins should be clamped and ligated carefully. Hemoclips or the use of modern ultrasonic or electrocoagulation devices may be helpful in this region. Special attention should be given to the identification and preservation of the superior parathyroid glands since the lower glands are more vulnerable to injury or devascularization as the goiter is delivered and removed from its substernal location. The increased incidence of hypoparathyroidism in the setting of surgery for substernal goiter has also been confirmed by several retrospective studies. Gentle blunt dissection is helpful in the substernal area under the strap muscles; it is best approached starting laterally from the under aspect of the sternomastoid muscle and extending medially (Figure 9.2). Occasionally, the medial head of the sternomastoid may require transection for better exposure. Injury to the inferior thyroid veins can produce serious bleeding; retraction of these veins into the mediastinum or the tearing of veins below the level of the sternum can become a critical problem, sometimes requiring a sternotomy for control of the bleeding.

As the finger dissection is continued from the lateral surface and after ligation of multiple small inferior veins, the thyroid is generally delivered into the neck. At the beginning of the operation, it is important to determine whether the goiter is in the posterior mediastinum, with displacement and stretching of the recurrent laryngeal nerve anteriorly over the mass. It is advisable, whether the goiter is in the anterior or posterior mediastinum, to trace the course of the nerve, if possible, before removal of the substernal mass, protecting it from injury. If there is difficulty in finding the recurrent nerve inferiorly, a good alternative is to identify the nerve as it enters the trachea under the cricothyroid muscle at the junction of its middle and anterior third and then follow it downward. At times, however, identification and tracing of the recurrent laryngeal nerve may be difficult or impossible without delivering the substernal thyroid mass from the mediastinum and then dissecting laterally to find the nerve and the parathyroids.

The surgical procedure is usually a total thyroid lobectomy with excision of the substernal goiter. As previously noted, this is possible since most intrathoracic goiters originate from one thyroid lobe or the other, although at times a total thyroidectomy may be required if there is significant enlargement of the opposite lobe. In this situation,

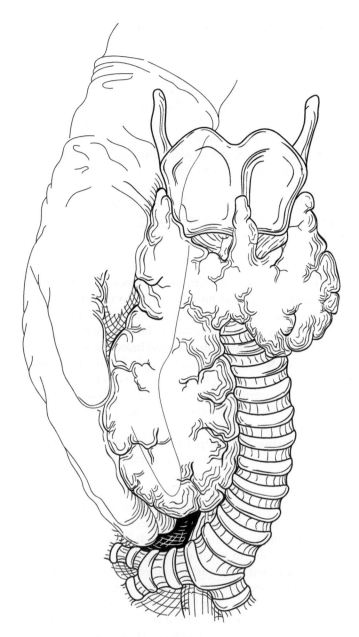

Figure 9.2 The technique of surgery for the mediastinal goiter. Careful ligation of the inferior thyroid veins is necessary to avoid unexpected bleeding.

a near-total thyroidectomy on the lesser side may occasionally be advisable, to avoid injury to the parathyroid glands, if there is doubt about their integrity on the primary side. If a parathyroid gland is injured, it should transplanted into the sternomastoid muscle. Although there is controversy about the use of drains in a routine thyroidectomy, the author prefers to use a suction drain such as a Hemovac or a Jackson–Pratt, because of the extensive dead space following substernal thyroid surgery [9].

THORACIC APPROACH

Most substernal goiters can be easily retrieved using the above technique. However, as stated previously, a sternal split may sometimes be necessary—as well as other adjunct techniques, such as the drawer maneuver, where the substernal thyroid is held by two hands from the neck and pulled like a drawer. Lahey popularized the morcellation and fragmentation of the mass, as well as suctioning colloid from within the mass to facilitate its removal through the neck. Many authors advise against this method because of the risk of serious bleeding and the possibility of spilling and disseminating malignant disease. Nevertheless, it is still occasionally used with success.

TRANSSTERNAL AND LATERAL THORACOTOMY APPROACH

Sternotomy

The main concept of performing a sternotomy is to enlarge the thoracic inlet and provide access to the great vessels, offering a much safer dissection and ease of removal of the goiter. It may help in identifying the recurrent nerve. The vessels to the thyroid are divided and ligated prior to the sternal incision, to reduce its blood supply, facilitating removal of the substernal mass. In the case of venous obstruction, however, the sternotomy might be best performed initially to decompress the distended veins and make the dissection easier and safer.

The anterior sternal-splitting incision has become the preferred choice because of the advantages it offers: it is easily combined with a neck incision and does not require repositioning of the patient. In patients with an aberrant mediastinal thyroid, or primary mediastinal goiter, which is separate from the thyroid and derives its blood supply from intrathoracic mediastinal vessels, the sternal approach makes it possible to avoid avulsion of thoracic vessels and the severe hemorrhage that would result; there is excellent access to the large vessels of the chest, and it is usually possible to dissect the goiter free from its attachments under direct vision. In contrast, lateral thoracotomy incisions are reported to have a higher incidence of recurrent nerve injuries because of the difficulty in visualizing them through this approach.

Anesthesia

Preoperative evaluation of the laryngeotracheal tree will help locate the position and opening of the laryngeal aditus [8]. Even though there may be considerable deviation of the trachea, the larynx will generally be in a normal position with a patent and open airway. Therefore, intubating these patients is usually not a difficult problem, especially if a small endotracheal tube is used. Although there appears to be considerable enthusiasm for intubating these patients while awake, it may be more dangerous due to trauma associated with endotracheal injury. Some anesthesiologists consider fiber-optic intubation, sometimes over a flexible bronchoscope, but any intubation in substernal goiter must be totally nontraumatic. The cuff of the endotracheal tube should also be well below the vocal cords and the patient extubated smoothly to avoid any intrathoracic rise of pressure—causing postoperative bleeding.

Complications

The main complications are related to recurrent laryngeal nerve injury, generally less than 1%, which is low, but may be higher than the incidence in nonsubsternal thyroidectomies. Important consideration should be given intraoperatively to localization of the parathyroid glands and careful preservation. As mentioned above, parathyroid autotransplantation may be necessary if the parathyroids are rendered avascular. Postoperative hematoma is a well-known complication and occurs in approximately 3% of the patients. Other complications, such as pneumothorax and pneumonia, are quite rare. Tracheomalacia may be the result of long-standing tracheal compression by the goiter; however, it appears to be an overstated condition. In his review of substernal goiters, White et al. [28] published an incidence ranging from 0% to 10%, depending on the varying definitions of tracheomalacia. True tracheomalacia with disintegration of the tracheal rings is quite rare [40,41]. A majority of the time—even with considerable deviation and compression of the trachea—the cartilage and rings of the trachea generally are intact, and in most cases, the trachea returns to an almost normal position within 24–48 hours of surgery. If the trachea appears to be weak, a trachelopexy may occasionally be performed by suturing the tracheal wall to the surrounding musculature or sternal periosteum. Techniques such as support with silastic rings or a Gortex graft are well described in the literature. However, the clinical experience is limited to only a few patients. Most of the time, the patients may be left intubated for 24–48 hours and extubated under close observation without any major problems related to tracheomalacia. Cattel and Hare [41] noted that compression of tracheal rings was rapidly reversed after removal of substernal goiters, but deviation of the trachea took months to return. Airway obstruction is more likely from kinking of an elongated trachea or injury on intubation. In rare instances (reported from 0%–4%), a patient may require temporary tracheostomy. A long-standing (>5 years) history of tracheal compression has been reported to predict the possible need for tracheostomy.

The results of the surgery for substernal goiters are excellent, with a rare operative mortality. However, the risks to the recurrent laryngeal nerve and permanent hypoparathyroidism are slightly higher than in routine thyroidectomy. The extent of thyroidectomy is generally dictated by the size of the thyroid gland and the histopathology. Total thyroidectomy may be required because of the multiglandular nature of the disease and the absence of essentially normal thyroid tissue. A contralateral subtotal thyroidectomy may be considered to avoid injury to the parathyroids or recurrent laryngeal nerve. The sternoclavicular disarticulation, although described in the literature, is technically quite a difficult procedure and is not generally helpful in surgery for substernal goiter. A median sternotomy is preferred, and the need for this may be predicted by the factors discussed above.

SUMMARY

Even though thyroid disease is very common, the incidence of substernal goiter is not high in the United States. However, it is a frequent condition noted in areas of endemic goiter. The main indication for surgery is tracheoesophageal compression and fear of malignancy. The preoperative workup includes careful laryngoscopic evaluation, chest x-ray, and computerized tomography scanning. The latter will give a better definition of the extent of the substernal goiter, along with the location of the trachea. Substernal goiter has been described by a large number of authors but can be commonly defined as the thyroid gland being more than 50% in the mediastinal location. The most common presenting and compelling symptom for treatment is airway compression. Surgical intervention is commonly indicated—with a majority of substernal goiters retrieved through the neck. In less than 2% of the patients, surgical intervention may include sternal split. The operative mortality is negligible, and the incidence of life-threatening complications is very rare. The risk of injury to the recurrent laryngeal nerve or permanent hypoparathyroidism needs to be kept in mind and appropriate techniques used to minimize these distressing complications. Overall, surgery should be undertaken with a diagnosis of substernal goiter to avoid future problems related to the airway.

REFERENCES

1. Rios A, Rodriguez JM, Balsalobre MD, Tebar FJ, Parrilla P. The value of various definitions of intrathoracic goiter for predicting intra-operative and postoperative complications. *Surgery* 2010;147:233–8.
2. Shaha A. Substernal goiter: What is in a definition? *Surgery* 2010;239–40.
3. Gaitan E, Nelson NC, Poole GV. Endemic goiter and endemic thyroid disorders. *World J Surg* 1991;15:205–15.
4. Kelly FC, Sneeden WW. Prevalence and geographical distribution of endemic goiter. In: World Health Organization, *Endemic Goiter*. Monograph Series 44. Geneva: World Health Organization, 1960:9–25.
5. Shaha AR, Burnett C, Alfonso AE, Jaffe BM. Goiters and airway problems. *Am J Surg* 1989;158:378–80.
6. Alfonso A et al. Tracheal or esophageal compression due to benign thyroid disease. *Am J Surg* 1981;142:350–3.
7. Shaha AR, Alfonso AE, Jaffe BM. Operative treatment of substernal goiter. *Head Neck* 1988;11:325–30.
8. Shaha AR. Surgery for benign thyroid disease causing tracheoesophageal compression. *Otolaryngol Clin N Am* 1990;23:391–401.
9. Blum M, Biller B, Bergman DA. The thyroid cork: Obstruction of the thoracic inlet due to retroclavicular goiter. *JAMA* 1974;227:189–91.
10. Kelley TS, Mayors DJ, Boutsicaris PS. "Downhill" varices: A cause of upper gastrointestinal hemorrhage. *Am Surg* 1982;48:35–8.
11. Parker DR, el-Shaboury AH. Fatal haematemesis due to benign retrosternal goitre. *Postgrad Med J* 1992;68:756–7.
12. Cohen P et al. Superior vena cava syndrome and right pleural effusion due to giant goiter. *NY State J Med* 1990;90:467–8.
13. Cengiz K, Aykin A, Demirci A, Diren B. Intrathoracic goiter with hyperthyroidism, tracheal compression, superior vena cava syndrome and Horner's syndrome. *Chest* 1990;97:1005–6.
14. Becker WF. Pioneers in thyroid surgery. *Ann Surg* 1977;185:493–504.
15. Reeve TS, Rubenstein C, Rundle FF. Intrathoracic goiter: Its prevalence in Sydney metropolitan mass x-ray surveys. *Med J Aust* 1957;2:149–52.
16. Shaha AR, Alfonso AE, Jaffe BM. Acute airway distress due to thyroid pathology. *Surgery* 1987;102(6):1068–74.
17. Newman E, Shaha AR. Substernal goiter. *J Surg Oncol* 1995;60(3):207–12.
18. Singh B, Lucente FE, Shaha AR. Substernal goiter—A clinical review. *Am J Otolaryngol* 1994;15:409–16.
19. Cougard P et al. Substernal goiters: 218 operated cases. *Ann Endocrinol (Paris)* 1992;53:230.
20. Katlic MR, Wang C, Grillo HC. Substernal goiter. *Ann Thor Surg* 1985;39:391–399.
21. Michel LA, Bradpiece HA. Surgical management of substernal goiter. *Br J Surg* 1988;75:565–9.
22. Milliere D et al. Goiter with severe respiratory compromise: Evaluation and treatment. *Surgery* 1988;103:367–73.
23. Sanders LE, Rossi RL, Shahian DM, Williamson WA. Mediastinal goiter: The need for an aggressive approach. *Arch Surg* 1992;127:609–13.
24. Cho HT, Cohen JP, Som ML. Management of substernal and intrathoracic goiters. *Otolaryngol Head Neck Surg* 1986;94:282–7.
25. Wax MK, Briant DR. Management of substernal goiter. *J Otolaryngol* 1992;21:165–70.
26. Manning PB, Thompson NW. Bilateral phrenic nerve palsy associated with benign thyroid goiter. *Acta Chir Scand* 1989;155:429–31.
27. Bonnema SJ, Hegedus L. Radioiodine therapy in benign thyroid diseases: Effects, side effects, and factors affecting therapeutic outcome. *Endocr Rev* 2012;33(6):920–80.

28. White M, Doherty G, Gauger P. Evidence-based surgical management of substernal goiter. *World J Surg* 2008;32:1285–300.
29. Hajhosseini B, Montazeri V, Hajhosseini L, Nezami N, Beygui RE. Mediastinal goiter: A comprehensive study of 60 consecutive cases with special emphasis on identifying predictors of malignancy and sternotomy. *Am J Surg* 2012;203:442–7.
30. Bashist B, Ellis K, Gold RP. Computerized tomography of intrathoracic goiters. *Am J Radiol* 1983;140:455–60.
31. Miller RD, Hyatt RE. Obstructive lesions of the larynx and trachea: Clinical and physiologic characteristics. *Mayo Clin Proc* 1969;44:145–61.
32. Lahey FH, Swinton NW. Intrathoracic goiter. *Surg Gynecol Obstet* 1934;59:627–37.
33. Crile G. Intrathoracic goiter. *Cleve Clin Q* 1939;6:313–22.
34. Lahey FH. Diagnosis and management of intrathoracic goiter. *JAMA* 1920;75:163–6.
35. Lahey FH. Intrathoracic goiters. *Surg Clin N Am* 1945;25:609–18.
36. Casella C et al. Preoperative predictors of sternotomy need in mediastinal goiter management. *Head Neck* 2010;32:1131–5.
37. Allo MD, Thompson NW. Rationale for the operative management of substernal goiter. *Surgery* 1983;94:969–77.
38. Sand ME, Laws HL, McElevin RB. Substernal and intrathoracic goiter. Reconsideration of surgical approach. *Am Surg* 1983;49:196–202.
39. DeSouza FM, Smith PE. Retrosternal goiter. *J Otolaryngol* 1983;12:393–6.
40. Geelhoed GW. Tracheomalacia from compressing goiter: Management after thyroidectomy. *Surgery* 1988;104:1100–8.
41. Cattel RB, Hare HF. The position of the trachea before and after removal of substernal goiter. *Surg Clin N Am* 1948;28:781–92.

10

Hyperthyroidism

ALEXANDRIA ATUAHENE AND TERRY F. DAVIES

INTRODUCTION

Hyperthyroidism and thyrotoxicosis are terms that are used interchangeably by most clinicians, yet they can mean different things. *Hyperthyroidism* is defined as a process causing excess production and secretion of thyroid hormones by the thyroid gland, while *thyrotoxicosis* often refers to the clinical signs of a hypermetabolic state. An increase in sympathetic nervous system symptoms usually characterizes this hypermetabolic state. It should be noted that clinical manifestations of thyrotoxicosis can differ based on age, and that the degree of biochemical abnormality does not always correlate with symptom presentation. The major causes of hyperthyroidism are summarized in Table 10.1, with the vast majority of cases being secondary to Graves' disease, toxic multinodular goiter (TMG), and toxic adenoma.

GRAVES' DISEASE

Presentation

Graves' disease is the most common cause of hyperthyroidism. It is an autoimmune process, caused by circulating autoantibodies that bind to thyrotropin receptors (thyroid-stimulating hormone receptors [TSHRs]) and act as TSHR agonists. This results in thyroid gland growth and subsequent increased synthesis of thyroid hormones. Patients usually present with signs and symptoms suggestive of thyrotoxicosis (Table 10.2), a diffuse goiter, and sometimes a unique ophthalmopathy, referred to as Graves' eye disease or Graves' orbitopathy, and a dermopathy, referred to as pretibial myxedema (Figure 10.1).

Typically a disease of young women, Graves' disease can occur in persons of any age, although it is rarely seen before

Table 10.1 Causes of thyrotoxicosis

Graves' disease
Toxic adenoma or TMG
Excess thyroid-stimulating hormone
   TSH-producing pituitary adenoma
   Trophoblastic disease
Ectopic thyroid-producing tissue
   Extensive metastases from follicular carcinoma
   Struma ovarii
Factitious ingestion of thyroid hormone
Painless (silent) thyroiditis
Amiodarone-induced thyroiditis
Subacute (granulomatous, de Quervain's) thyroiditis
Iatrogenic thyrotoxicosis
Acute thyroiditis
Resistance to thyroid hormone (T3 receptor mutation)

Table 10.2 Major signs of thyrotoxicosis

Specific for Graves' Disease

Eyes—proptosis, periorbital edema, muscle dysfunction
Diffuse, vascular goiter
Localized pretibial myxedema
Acropatchy
Splenomegaly and lymphadenopathy

Nonspecific

Eyes—stare, lid lag, tearing
Tachycardia and atrial fibrillation
Systolic hypertension
Apical systolic flow murmur
Weight loss
Proximal muscle weakness
Moist skin
Tremor
Brisk tendon reflexes
Hair loss

the age of 10. The incidence increases until roughly 30 years of age, when it stabilizes. Like other thyroid diseases, it is more common in women, with an overall prevalence of 1%–2%, and a female-to-male ratio of approximately 7–8:1. The incidence in women has been estimated to be 1 case per 1000 per year over a 20-year follow-up [1].

Evidence for an autoimmune etiology

Environmental and genetic factors play a role in the autoimmune process seen in Graves' disease. To date, a number of susceptibility genes have been identified [2]. Most patients with Graves' disease display serum autoantibodies against thyroid peroxidase (TPO) (the "microsomal" antigen), thyroglobulin (Tg), and the TSHR. T cell–mediated autoimmunity can also be demonstrated against these three thyroid antigens. In addition, patients and their relatives may show

an increased frequency of other autoimmune disorders, e.g., type I diabetes mellitus, myasthenia gravis, or rheumatoid arthritis [3]. The autoantibodies specific to hyperthyroid Graves' disease are those detected against the TSHR (TSHR-Ab), which behave as TSH agonists and are referred to as thyroid-stimulating antibodies [4]. These antibodies compete for the binding of TSH to the TSHR on the surface of the thyroid epithelial cells. Their direct stimulation of the gland removes the thyroid from pituitary TSH control (Figure 10.2). Evidence suggests that the thyroid gland is itself the major site of thyroid autoantibody secretion in Graves' disease, and many of the responsible B cells can be found among the intrathyroidal lymphocytic infiltrate.

Pathology

The thyroid in Graves' disease typically shows a nonhomogeneous lymphocytic infiltration by T cells and B cells, with an absence of the gross follicular destruction seen in patients with Hashimoto's thyroiditis (Figure 10.3). Presurgical antithyroid drug treatment may reduce the relative degree of infiltration, resulting in many pathological reports of sparse or absent infiltrate [5]. Follicular epithelial cell size has been found to correlate with the intensity of the local infiltrate, and this could be explained by local production of thyroid-stimulating antibodies.

It is important to note that as a result of the lymphocytic infiltration, the disease may eventually change to thyroid failure because of the development of clinical autoimmune (Hashimoto's) thyroiditis. Furthermore, both these diseases may occur within the same family, indicating their close relationship.

Pathogenesis of Graves' orbitopathy and dermopathy

Nearly half of patients with Graves' disease report symptoms of Graves' ophthalmopathy, including excessive tearing, a gritty sensation, photophobia, and increased pressure sensation behind the eyes. In contrast, the dermopathy is rare and seen only in patients with the most severe disease. With such a close clinical and temporal relationship among Graves' orbitopathy, hyperthyroidism, and thyroid dermopathy, it is thought that these conditions arise from a single systemic process associated with the TSHR, as the major antigen and their pathogenesis is beginning to be better understood [6].

Histologically, the extraocular muscles and adipose tissue are swollen by the accumulation in the extracellular matrix of glycosaminoglycans. These are elaborated by fibroblasts under the influence of cytokines secreted by lymphocytes as part of the associated lymphocytic infiltration. This accumulation causes osmotic changes; the resulting swelling disrupts and impairs the function of the extraocular muscles, which eventually become fibrosed. A similar phenomenon has been proposed to explain pretibial myxedema. The antigen to which the infiltrating T cells react appears to be the

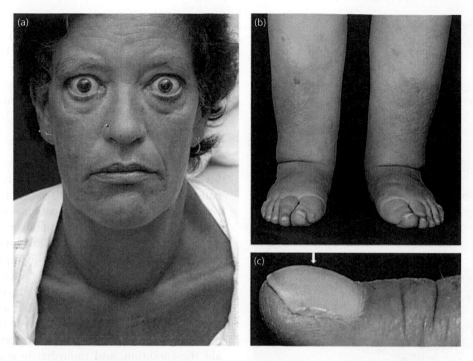

Figure 10.1 (a) Graves' patient with ophthalmopathy symmetrical goiter. (b) Pretibial myxedema and (c) clubbing and swelling of the fingers, now rare, called thyroid acropatchy and thought to be secondary to increased blood flow. (Adapted from Vaidya B, Pearce SH. *BMJ* 2014;349:g5128.)

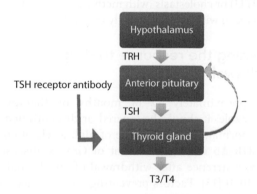

Figure 10.2 Loss of pituitary control of TSH function in Graves' disease. TSHR antibodies (thyroid-stimulating immunoglobulins) increase thyroid hormone synthesis and release, which suppresses the action of endogenous TRH on TSH and suppresses TSH directly. Hence, TSH levels are low but radioiodine uptake is high because it is under the control of the stimulating antibody rather than TSH.

TSHR itself. Evidence in support of this hypothesis includes the observation that TSHR mRNA and protein have been shown to be overexpressed in retro-orbital fibroblasts and adipocytes when compared with many different cells where they are found [6,7].

TREATMENT OF GRAVES' DISEASE HYPERTHYROIDISM

Unfortunately, it is not yet possible to target the basic immunopathogenic factors in Graves' disease. Available for use are three effective and relatively safe long-used options: antithyroid medications, radioactive iodine, and surgery. Once the diagnosis of hyperthyroidism secondary to Graves' disease has been established, the physician and patient should discuss which treatment modality will be implemented. There is no consensus on which treatment modality is best because none is ideal, which further highlights the need to take an individualized patient-specific approach.

Antithyroid medications

The major agents for treating thyrotoxicosis are drugs of the thionamide class, most commonly methimazole (Tapazole) and less commonly propylthiouracil (PTU). These agents inhibit the oxidation and organic binding of thyroid iodide. In addition, large doses of PTU (400 mg) impair the conversion of T4 to T3 by deiodinase type I in the thyroid and peripheral tissues [8]. The half-life of methimazole is about 6 hours, whereas that of PTU is about 1½ hours. Hence, a single daily dose of methimazole may be sufficient. Thionamide drugs may also directly influence the immune response within the thyroid gland of patients with Graves' disease, where the drugs are concentrated [9]. The clinical importance of this immunosuppression and coincidental induction of apoptosis is unclear.

Use of thionamides

Although PTU is considered less teratogenic than methimazole because of its hepatic toxicity, the drug of first choice is methimazole at a dose of 10–20 mg daily.

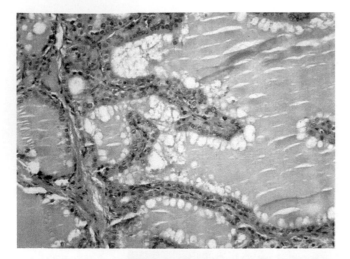

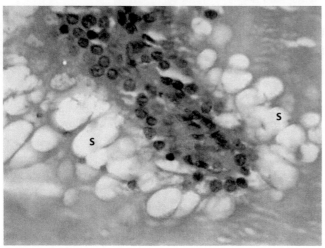

Figure 10.3 Histology of Graves' disease. Top: Graves' hyperthyroidism is characterized by thyrocytic hyperplasia forming pseudopapillae that can mimic papillary thyroid carcinoma. Bottom: The scalloped colloid (S) and thyrocyte distinguish Graves' disease from papillary thyroid carcinoma (hematoxylin and eosin).

When methimazole is contraindicated because of allergy or pending pregnancy, the initial dose of PTU most commonly employed is 50–150 mg given orally every 8 hours. Higher doses of these drugs may be required in patients with severe thyrotoxicosis and large thyroid glands. The therapeutic response appears after a latent period because both of these agents inhibit the synthesis but not the release of preformed thyroid hormone. There appears to be little difference in the duration of the latent period when either of these agents is employed alone in the usual dosage. In a thyroid gland rich in iodine, as when the patient has received medications containing iodine, the clinical response to antithyroid agents may be delayed for months. However, under normal circumstances, a return to euthyroidism is obtained within about 6 weeks. During antithyroid drug treatment, the size of the thyroid decreases in many patients; indeed, a failure for this to be achieved may signal an intensification and prolongation of the disease process. Since the serum TSH

concentration may remain subnormal for many months, presumably secondary to accelerated conversion of T4 to T3 within the pituitary gland, it is best to monitor the response to drug treatment using free T4 levels. It should also be noted that an enlarging thyroid gland in a treated patient with Graves' disease might signal the onset of tumor growth, requiring prompt sonographic investigation.

Adverse reactions

Serious adverse reactions develop in only a small number of patients taking thionamide drugs. Agranulocytosis, occurring in less than 0.5% of the patients, is of most concern. Because of the frequency of lymphopenia in hyperthyroidism, a complete blood count and differential is recommended before starting antithyroid drug therapy. Serial leukocyte counts are prudent; if they display a downward trend, the antithyroid drugs should be discontinued. Agranulocytosis, however, can appear suddenly without a gradual decline in the leukocyte count [10,11]. The patient must be made alert to the appearance of a sore throat and fever, which can herald the condition, and immediately seek medical advice. A thionamide rash that can take many forms, including hives, occurs in less than 10% of patients. Less frequent reactions include arthralgias, myalgias, neuritis, hepatitis (with PTU) or cholestasis (with methimazole), and rare liver necrosis seen with PTU, especially in children [12].

Predicting the response to drug withdrawal

After approximately 12–18 months of therapy with methimazole, it should be tapered or discontinued if the TSH is normal. The persistence of high levels of circulating TSHR-Ab during treatment of Graves' disease portends a recurrence after withdrawal of antithyroid drugs (Table 10.3) [13]. Factors preventing a recurrence include a change from TSHR-stimulating antibody to blocking antibody (a rare occurrence), or the progression of concomitant thyroiditis and the onset of thyroid failure with inability to respond to the thyroid-stimulating antibodies.

Table 10.3 Factors predicting recurrence of Graves' disease

High titer of TSHR antibody
Continuing suppressed TSH levels
Failure to suppress radioiodine uptake or serum Tg or T3 (indirect measure of TSHR-Ab)
High T3 levels at diagnosis
Large thyroid size
Male sex
Smoking
Previous recurrence
Postpartum period
Large iodine load
Major trauma—physical or mental

Furthermore, iodine deficiency itself may prevent the recurrence of Graves' disease.

Additional features associated with the likelihood of long-term remission after withdrawal of therapy include the initial presence of T3 toxicosis, a small thyroid or a decrease in size of the gland, and, in particular, return of the serum TSH concentration to normal during treatment. Conversely, smokers and patients with large goiters (>80 g) have lower remission rates. In practice, treatment should generally be continued for about 12–18 months and then withdrawn if the serum is TSHR-Ab negative [14,15]. About three-quarters of relapses occur in the first 3 months after withdrawal of therapy, and most of the remainder occur during the subsequent year. The frequency of long-term remission, after withdrawal of antithyroid therapy, has decreased over the past 30 years, perhaps because of the increase in dietary iodine intake. At present, only about one-third of patients experience a lasting remission.

Iodine

Iodine is rarely used as sole therapy. Large doses of iodine inhibit hormone release rather than formation [16]. Hence, the beneficial effect of iodine is evident more quickly than the effects of even large doses of agents that inhibit hormone synthesis. However, the addition to glandular organic iodine stores may retard the clinical response to subsequently administered thionamide drugs.

The decrease in radioiodine uptake produced by iodine also prevents the use of radioiodine as treatment for many weeks. Therefore, aside from its use in preparation for surgery (see below), iodine is useful mainly in patients with highly accelerated thyrotoxicosis ("thyroid storm") or severe thyrocardiac disease. Six milligrams of iodine daily is sufficient to control thyrotoxicosis. This is the amount present in one-eighth of a drop of saturated solution of potassium iodide (SSKI) or eight-tenths of a drop of Lugol's solution. Large doses are more likely to produce adverse reactions. In practice, two or three drops of SSKI two times daily is recommended, and it should be administered with doses of a thionamide drug [17–19]. Adverse reactions to iodine are unusual and are generally not serious. They include a rash that may be acneiform, drug fever, sialadenitis, conjunctivitis, and rhinitis.

Radioiodine

Radioiodine therapy has been used to treat hyperthyroidism for more than 60 years. The advantage is that it produces thyroid ablation without the potential complications of surgery. This can be accomplished by delivering a fixed dose or a calculated dose of radioactivity to achieve hypothyroidism [20]. Doses of 10 and 15 mCi are associated with 69% cure at 1 year and 75% cure at 6 months, respectively [21], while 20 mCi will produce almost a 100% cure.

Calculating the delivered radioactivity requires determining three unknowns: the uptake of radioactive iodine,

the size of the thyroid (by palpation or ultrasound), and the quantity of radiation to be deposited per gram of thyroid. Although attempts have been made to standardize the dose of radiation delivered to the thyroid gland, these calculations have not provided uniform results, and no data currently report an advantage with calculated- versus fixed-dose radiation. In addition to radioiodine therapy, pretreatment with methimazole is normally provided to reduce the increased risk of complications from worsening hyperthyroidism, which may occur postradioiodine due to radiation-induced thyroiditis [22,23].

Complications of radioiodine

In theory, radioiodine may affect extrathyroidal tissues that concentrate iodide, e.g., the salivary and gastric glands and the breasts. As mentioned above, radiation thyroiditis itself may lead to an exacerbation of thyrotoxicosis 10–14 days after the radioiodine is administered and has occasionally had serious consequences, including the precipitation of arrhythmias or a thyrotoxic crisis. Radioiodine may also worsen Graves' ophthalmopathy, if only transiently [24]. This treatment is also accompanied by a high frequency of late hypothyroidism. Many reports have documented that the incidence of hypothyroidism after calculated doses or standardized doses of radioiodine is high during the first year or two after radioiodine treatment and continues to increase at a rate of approximately 5% per year thereafter. The incidence of postradioiodine hypothyroidism at 5 years has been reported up to 70% with calculated dosing. For this reason, many physicians advocate an ablative approach to treatment. There is no evidence of a major increase in thyroid carcinoma, leukemia, or mutation rates in patients followed many years after treatment for Graves' disease [25]. The conventional dose of radioiodine employed in the treatment of thyrotoxicosis delivers a radiation dose to the gonads that is roughly equivalent to that delivered by a barium enema examination or intravenous urogram. However, experience from the Chernobyl nuclear accident, which caused a large increase in the number of childhood thyroid cancers [26,27], has caused many physicians to think that the use of any radioactivity in children should be avoided, despite some studies that have shown no increase in the incidence of thyroid carcinoma in adolescents and children treated with radioactive iodine [28]. The available evidence supports the concept that, in children, low doses of radiation from fallout (6.5–1500 cGY) stimulate the development of thyroid nodules and cancer, while higher doses (10,000 cGY), as in radioiodine therapy, which ablate thyroid tissue, are not associated with an increase in thyroid neoplasia.

Orbitopathy and radioiodine

As discussed earlier, Graves' ophthalmopathy is most likely the result of crossover specificity between retro-orbital and thyroid antigens, perhaps to the TSHR itself. Following radioiodine therapy, the levels of circulating TSHR-Ab increase secondary to impairment of immune restraint caused by intrathyroidal irradiation because regulatory T cells are especially sensitive to irradiation. Carefully conducted studies indicate that eye disease worsens in patients with Graves' ophthalmopathy who are treated with radioiodine, and some physicians advocate the use of glucocorticoids at the time of radioiodine treatment to prevent such effects [29,30]. As discussed later, some authors prefer surgical thyroidectomy for the management of Graves' disease with ophthalmopathy.

SURGERY FOR GRAVES' DISEASE

Thyroidectomy, for the appropriate patient with Graves' disease, offers swift and certain treatment, with a high degree of safety. It can be a same-day or overnight procedure and was the original treatment of choice prior to radioiodine and antithyroid drugs. In skilled hands, the risk of recurrent nerve injury is less than 1%, and the incidence of permanent hypocalcemia is less than 1%–1.5%. Because of the occasional recurrence of hyperthyroidism associated with subtotal thyroidectomy, near-total thyroidectomy has become the preferred surgical procedure [31].

History

Theodor Kocher, who in 1909 was awarded the Nobel Prize for Medicine or Physiology for his work on the thyroid gland, pioneered the development of thyroidectomy [32,33]. However, the disastrous results of myxedema and tetany following total thyroid resection moved him to eventually condemn the procedure. He noted, however, that patients fared better if only one lobe was removed or if the posterior capsule with a portion of the parenchyma of the thyroid lobe was left in place—a subtotal thyroidectomy. The reasons were not understood at the time, but he had performed 2000 such thyroid resections by 1912, reducing the mortality of the operation from 18% to 0.5%.

Plummer's observation in 1923 that iodine blocked the release of thyroid hormone was a watershed event. The use of Lugol's solution for the preparation of hyperthyroid patients before surgery introduced a new era of reduced mortality and reduced postoperative complications. Subtotal thyroidectomy was transformed from a hazardous endeavor to a safe and reliable procedure. In 1943, the advent of the antithyroid drugs also made it possible to render patients euthyroid before surgery. This was supplemented by iodine for 2–3 weeks before surgery because of its antithyroid activity and its additional value in decreasing the vascularity of the gland [17–19]. The preparation of the patient in this fashion, as well as refinements in surgical technique, ushered in a new epoch of consistency and reliability in the treatment of hyperthyroidism. The use of beta-adrenergic blocking agents such as propranolol and atenolol added to the safety of the operation. With modern preoperative preparation, the patient arrives in the operating room in a euthyroid state.

Indications for surgery

Surgery is not a common choice of treatment for Graves' disease. Past surveys in the United States suggest that >50% of clinicians still prefer to first offer radioactive iodine ablation compared with >80% of European physicians offering antithyroid drugs as first-line treatment [34]. Nevertheless, surgery retains a place in the therapeutic options for treatment of the condition. The indications are not precise, rigid, or absolute. Patient preference and especially the availability of surgical expertise are important factors in making a choice. Surgery achieves euthyroidism more rapidly than radioiodine, which requires 6 weeks or more to reach this status. In a situation when antithyroid drugs do not control hyperthyroidism or the patient becomes allergic to them, surgery can render the patient euthyroid in days [35].

Currently, surgery is recommended for

1. Patients with markedly enlarged glands that may encroach on the upper airway and digestive tract. In this situation, there is often an accompanying cosmetic deformity that is simultaneously corrected.
2. Patients with accompanying thyroid nodules not designated benign on biopsy. Up to 20% of nodules in patients with Graves' disease may be suspicious.
3. Patients who wish to become pregnant within 4–6 months of treatment. They may be treated surgically to avoid any concern about the effect of radioiodine on the ovaries.
4. Already pregnant patients who cannot be adequately controlled by antithyroid drugs or who develop drug reactions. They may be considered for surgery. The optimum time is the second trimester.
5. Patients who are noncompliant in the use of antithyroid drugs and refuse radioactive iodine ablation.
6. Patients, especially children, who have a fear of radioactivity—although there is no definitive evidence to support an adverse effect [31,36].

Note: In recurrent or persistent hyperthyroidism, radioactive iodine is the universal choice because of the vulnerability of the parathyroid glands and recurrent nerves in reoperation.

Surgery in special situations

CHILDHOOD

Many authors advise surgery for Graves' disease in children if definitive treatment is required. Antithyroid drugs have a failure rate of 60% or higher after withdrawal and are therefore best continued through puberty. But if there are problems with side effects, allergies, and compliance, a different approach may be needed [36,37]. If antithyroid drugs cannot be continued or radioactive iodine is declined, total thyroidectomy with subsequent thyroid hormone replacement offers effective and rapid management with few complications when experienced surgical expertise is available.

OPHTHALMOPATHY

Although the issue is not settled, some authors believe that surgical thyroidectomy, rather than radioactive iodine and high-dose steroids, is the preferred management of hyperthyroid Graves' disease in the presence of ophthalmopathy [38,39]. In a prospective randomized trial of total versus subtotal thyroidectomy on 150 patients for the control of Graves' orbitopathy, 70%–74% improved after a period of 6–36 months regardless of whether total or subtotal thyroidectomy was performed [40]. Furthermore, the addition of radioiodine ablation after total thyroidectomy to obtain a "complete" thyroidectomy has also been advocated [41].

Preparation for surgery

The usual preparation of hyperthyroid patients for surgery involves utilizing methimazole to achieve a euthyroid state by blocking iodination, and an iodine-containing product (potassium iodide, SSKI, or inorganic iodide, two or three drops twice daily 7–10 days before surgery), which decreases thyroid blood flow and vascularity, resulting in decreased intraoperative blood loss [18,19,42]. Beta blockade can be used as adjunctive therapy or alone to control signs and symptoms of thyrotoxicosis. Propranolol 10–20 mg up to four times a day can rapidly control overt thyrotoxic symptoms by blocking the catecholamine response in hyperthyroidism. In patients who cannot be given thionamides, iodine and beta blockers alone can be used for rapid preoperative preparation, with the caution that providing iodine in the absence of antithyroid drugs may worsen the hyperthyroidism in the longer term, since thyroid hormone synthesis has not been blocked. This regimen is not as reliable as the use of all three drugs, but is usually effective in bringing thyroid function to normal within 10 days. No date for surgery should be set until a normal metabolic state has been restored. Much too often, the operation is planned well in advance and the patient is given a standardized regimen independent of the clinical progress. In addition, iodine should not be relied on to complete an as yet incomplete response to antithyroid therapy because iodine will enrich glandular hormone stores if the antithyroid drug is not entirely effective.

Choice of operative procedure in Graves' disease

Most physicians and surgeons now recommend total thyroidectomy, claiming that the operation is equal in safety to subtotal thyroidectomy and can be completely relied upon to control hyperthyroidism with no risk of recurrence, assuming it is performed by a high-volume surgeon [43–45].

The technique of total thyroid lobectomy and contralateral, near-total thyroidectomy for the opposite side (Hartley–Dunhill operation) is also still being used and

has valid reason to be considered. Lobectomy is undertaken on the side that is problematic, i.e., the one containing nodules or the one that is larger. The entire course of the recurrent nerve and superior parathyroid gland on the side of lobectomy are carefully dissected and preserved, but on the opposite side, the upper portion of the nerve and the upper parathyroid are left in place, undisturbed, protected by the posterior capsule, and with less exposure to injury. The size of the remnant remaining on the near-total side can be accurately controlled; approximately 4–5 g is recommended. Most studies show no higher rate of nerve injury or hypocalcemia than earlier subtotal resections, but a 5%–8% recurrence rate occurs [44].

Recurrence

If recurrence of Graves' disease develops, surgery cannot be safely repeated because of the scarring and distortion in the positions of the parathyroid glands and recurrent nerve, which make reoperation hazardous. The patient would be left with the choice of radioiodine, which may have been declined in the first place, or the use of antithyroid drugs. Subsequent hypothyroidism can be completely controlled and is easily managed by oral administration of thyroxine, which replaces all thyroid functions and is readily monitored by thyroid function studies [35].

Results of surgery for Graves' disease

The rate of recurrent or persistent hyperthyroidism after subtotal (near-total) thyroidectomy has been an unacceptable 8%. It is, of course, not just a function of the amount of tissue left in place, but also the varying influence of TSHR antibodies and ongoing thyroiditis. The rate of hypothyroidism in subtotal thyroidectomy has ranged around 30%, but again, it is a reflection of the remnant size and other variables. Furthermore, the incidence of hypothyroidism increases over the years, since the remnant frequently becomes impaired by thyroiditis. In contrast, there is 0% recurrence of hyperthyroidism for total thyroidectomy, but all patients become hypothyroid [35]. Hypothyroidism is easily controlled, but recurrent or persistent hyperthyroidism is bad news.

Complications of surgery

The complications of surgery for hyperthyroidism are the same as for other thyroid surgery. Postoperative bleeding may require reopening the neck. The incidence is low, <1%, and usually easily controlled. Postoperatively bleeding into the neck creates pressure in a closed space that can threaten the airway and the life of the patient. In a hospital setting with close monitoring, experienced personnel can open the wound and preserve the airway [46]. If bleeding occurs where trained help is not available, the result can be catastrophic. Recurrent nerve injury in thyroid surgery in experienced hands occurs in <1% of cases. The principle of exposure and dissection of the nerve, as well as nerve monitoring, has substantially reduced the incidence of palsy.

Hypoparathyroidism

Hypocalcemia is more frequent and severe after thyroidectomy for Graves' disease rather than other conditions. This is attributed to "hungry bones," as well as the effect of manipulation of the parathyroid glands and interference with their blood supply [47]. This problem is usually transient, but there is a wide variation in the frequency of permanent hypoparathyroidism after thyroid surgery for Graves' disease. In experienced hands, it is approximately <1% of patients, and there are some series reporting close to 0%. Transient hypocalcemia is more common; it occurred in 14.6% of a series of 150 Graves' patients [40].

Permanent hypoparathyroidism is a distressing problem and may produce serious metabolic problems that require lifelong surveillance. Despite conventional replacement treatment with calcium and vitamin D, surgical hypoparathyroidism can result in cataracts occurring in up to 70% of patients, fatigue, paresthesias, and muscular irritability [48]. The measurement of intraoperative PTH levels during total thyroidectomy has been advocated to help avoid this [49]. In addition, the recent availability of recombinant parathyroid hormone for the treatment of hypoparathyroidism may abrogate many of the long-term side effects of the condition [50].

TOXIC MULTINODULAR GOITER AND TOXIC SINGLE NODULES

TMG is a disorder in which thyroid overactivity is secondary to thyroid nodules that secrete thyroid hormone autonomously, resulting in hyperthyroidism. On radioiodine scanning, these patients present as a mixture of "hot" and "cold" nodules. A single hot toxic adenoma is a less common form of hyperthyroidism. Patients with either TMG or a single toxic adenoma are often referred to as having Plummer's disease [51].

Pathogenesis

TMG arises in patients with multinodular goiters of long duration. Thyroid hormone secretion is secondary to somatic mutations that result in constitutive activation of the TSHR or TSHR signal transduction pathways. The precise mutations in the TSHR itself may differ from nodule to nodule [52,53]. A small number of autonomous adenomas have mutations in the G protein genes that lead to a similar state of constitutive activation [53]. The constitutive activation of the TSHR results initially in functional autonomy of the nodules, as shown by the lack of pituitary TSH control. Hyperthyroidism may develop quite suddenly after exposure to excess dietary iodine or iodine-containing contrast medium, which permits autonomous thyroid cells to increase hormone secretion to excessive levels. In addition,

toxicity in patients with multinodular goiter may be the result of Graves' disease, which can develop within a multinodular gland or be the primary cause of the nodule formation [54]. In the absence of Graves' disease, the remaining normal tissue between the nodules appears inactive as a result of the suppression of pituitary TSH by the excess thyroid hormones secreted by the active nodules. Hence, radioiodine scanning may distinguish between these conditions.

Clinical presentation

TMG usually occurs after the age of 50 in patients who have had nontoxic multinodular goiter for many years; it is more frequent in women than in men. However, thyroid hormone excess in patients with multinodular goiters is usually less than that seen in Graves' disease. Since the hyperthyroidism is due to autonomously functioning adenomas, rather than autoimmune disease, there are no spontaneous remissions; a continued growth of the adenomas and a progression of hyperthyroidism may continue. Eye and skin disease, a reflection of the autoimmune process seen in Graves' disease, is absent in TMG (Table 10.2). Serum T4 and T3 concentrations may be only slightly above normal, and a suppressed TSH may be the only finding. Cardiovascular manifestations, including tachycardia and atrial fibrillation, are more common than seen in Graves' disease because of the age of the patients with multinodular goiter. Obstructive symptoms are not unusual because the enlarged thyroid gland may be retrosternal in the older population. On palpation, the goiter is identical to a nontoxic multinodular goiter.

Single toxic adenomas occur in a younger age group than TMG, frequently in patients in their third or fourth decade. Often, there is a history of a long-standing, slowly growing lump in the anterior neck. It is unusual for adenomas to produce thyrotoxicosis until they have achieved a diameter of 2.5–3 cm. There may be progressive growth and increasing function over many years. At first, the adenoma may present as a small nodule or may be nonpalpable, but it can be detected by sonography or radioiodine scanning as a localized area of increased isotope accumulation. Ultimately, the normal thyroid tissue is completely suppressed and atrophic, with a radioiodine scan revealing function limited to the adenoma ("hot nodule"). The mass is usually smooth, well defined, round, or ovoid. It is firm and moves with swallowing. Often, the remainder of the gland is not palpable. In contrast to Graves' disease, a bruit is never present.

Investigation

Serum thyroid function testing reveals a suppressed TSH and often an increased free T4 and free T3. However, a suppressed TSH may be the only abnormality. In addition to hyperthyroidism, other reasons for treatment may be present, e.g., an accelerating loss of bone density or cardiac arrhythmias. Ultrasonography offers accurate sizing of the major nodules present: radioiodine scanning will reveal which of the nodules are toxic. Rarely, thyroid carcinoma may be present in a gland with a hyperfunctioning adenoma, but autonomous malignant nodules resulting in hyperthyroidism are extremely rare. A rapidly enlarging nodule may suggest the need for an aspiration biopsy, but cytology of active nodules can be difficult to interpret because they may simulate papillary carcinoma. An MRI or computed tomography scan may be required to assess retrosternal extension and tracheal compression. Pulmonary flow studies can indicate the severity of tracheal obstruction.

TREATMENT OF TOXIC NODULES

Treatment of asymptomatic patients with functional nodules is best decided on an individual basis. Rather than thyroid hormone measurements, the degree of TSH suppression is an index of the progression of thyroid hormone production by the autonomous cells. Suppression of TSH below the lower limits of normal indicates that hyperthyroidism is present and that therapy should be considered.

The same three therapies are most appropriate: antithyroid drugs, radioiodine, and surgery. Large nodules with concomitant physical symptoms are most readily treated with surgical excision. Surgical excision is also employed in patients younger than age 20, in whom radiation from radioiodine to the perinodular normal thyroid tissue could theoretically predispose to the development of radiation-related thyroid neoplasia, although there is no direct evidence for this caution. In addition, determining the dosage of radioactive iodine may be difficult, sometimes requiring repeat treatments.

Radioiodine

In terms of the specificity of treatment, multiple functioning thyroid nodules are ideal candidates for radioiodine therapy [31,55]. The radiation is directed almost exclusively to the diseased tissue. Since TSH is suppressed, the normal thyroid tissue surrounding the nodule should not take up radioiodine, although in practice many patients develop thyroid failure. For the patient older than age 18 with a single autonomous nodule 5 cm in diameter or smaller, ^{131}I is an appropriate treatment if the risk of eventual hypothyroidism is acceptable [56]. A dose of 8–10 mCi deposited at 24 hours is used. Because of the potential for hypothyroidism, prolonged follow-up is mandatory [57].

Surgery

When a toxic nodular goiter is sizable and enlarging, surgery can rapidly return the patient to a euthyroid state and simultaneously remove any suspicious cold nodules. In such patients, a bilateral subtotal thyroidectomy (near-total thyroidectomy) or total thyroidectomy may be preferred [58,59]. Surgery for a single autonomous adenoma has the advantage of avoiding the problem of hypothyroidism that may occur after radioiodine ablation. In this situation, an ipsilateral thyroid lobectomy is curative [60].

THYROTOXICOSIS IN SPECIAL CIRCUMSTANCES

Accelerated hyperthyroidism

Thyroid storm, a severe and accelerated form of hyperthyroidism, may be seen in postoperative thyrotoxic patients who were not adequately prepared for surgery. This condition has become a rarity because virtually every patient now arrives at the operating table in either a euthyroid state or with only mild persisting hyperthyroidism. Storm is usually abrupt in onset and characterized by symptoms of severe thyrotoxicosis and a change in mental status. Extreme hypermetabolism with body temperatures rising to 40°C or more is a distinguishing feature of the condition, which is most commonly precipitated by a medical complication, such as infection, rather than surgery. If not treated, the outcome can be lethal within 24–48 hours. Management is directed to stopping the synthesis and secretion of thyroid hormones and blocking their effects on peripheral tissues by inhibiting peripheral deiodination and adrenergic overactivity. Corticosteroids (dexamethasone 1–2 mg twice daily), beta-adrenergic blocking agents, thionamides, and Lugol's solution are used. A controlled cooling blanket is valuable in the attempt to decrease body temperature [61,62].

Amiodarone-induced thyrotoxicosis

This antiarrhythmic drug has complex effects on the thyroid, although the majority (~80%) of patients remain euthyroid [63]. The drug resembles T4 and contains 37% iodine and has a half-life of 50–60 days, and therefore remains available for a long period even after drug withdrawal. Amiodarone also has a direct cytotoxic effect on thyroid cells, which may cause thyroid failure. However, the iodine load or the cell damage may also precipitate Graves' disease in susceptible individuals, particularly in areas of iodine deficiency. Amiodarone-induced hyperthyroidism may develop either rapidly in a patient or after a few years of treatment. Antithyroid drugs and radioiodine may be ineffective because of the large intrathyroidal iodine load. Thyroidectomy is therefore often the treatment of choice, and allows the continuation of the drug [64].

REFERENCES

1. Vanderpump MP et al. The incidence of thyroid disorders in the community: A twenty-year follow-up of the Whickham Survey. *Clin Endocrinol (Oxf)* 1995;43(1):55–68.
2. Jacobson EM, Tomer Y. The CD40, CTLA-4, thyroglobulin, TSH receptor, and PTPN22 gene quintet and its contribution to thyroid autoimmunity: Back to the future. *J Autoimmun* 2007;28(2–3):85–98.
3. Weetman AP. Diseases associated with thyroid autoimmunity: Explanations for the expanding spectrum. *Clin Endocrinol* 2011;74(4):411–8.

4. Rees Smith B et al. TSH receptor—Autoantibody interactions. *Horm Metab Res* 2009;41(6):448–55.

5. McGregor AM et al. Carbimazole and the autoimmune response in Graves' disease. *N Engl J Med* 1980;303(6):302–7.

6. Bahn RS. Graves' ophthalmopathy. *N Engl J Med* 2010;362(8):726–38.

7. Wang Y, Smith TJ. Current concepts in the molecular pathogenesis of thyroid-associated ophthalmopathy. *Invest Ophthalmol Vis Sci* 2014;55(3):1735–48.

8. Abuid J, Larsen PR. Triiodothyronine and thyroxine in hyperthyroidism. Comparison of the acute changes during therapy with antithyroid agents. *J Clin Invest* 1974;54(1):201–8.

9. Davies TF. A new role for methimazole in autoimmune thyroid disease: Inducing T cell apoptosis. *Thyroid* 2000;10(7):525–6.

10. Tajiri J et al. Antithyroid drug-induced agranulocytosis. The usefulness of routine white blood cell count monitoring. *Arch Intern Med* 1990;150(3):621–4.

11. Kobayashi S et al. Characteristics of agranulocytosis as an adverse effect of antithyroid drugs in the second or later course of treatment. *Thyroid* 2014;24(5):796–801.

12. Rivkees SA. 63 years and 715 days to the "boxed warning": Unmasking of the propylthiouracil problem. *Int J Pediatr Endocrinol* 2010;2010:658267.

13. Davies TF et al. Thyroid controversy—Stimulating antibodies. *J Clin Endocrinol Metab* 1998;83(11):3777–85.

14. Nedrebo BG et al. Predictors of outcome and comparison of different drug regimens for the prevention of relapse in patients with Graves' disease. *Eur J Endocrinol* 2002;147(5):583–9.

15. Orgiazzi J, Madec AM. Reduction of the risk of relapse after withdrawal of medical therapy for Graves' disease. *Thyroid* 2002;12(10):849–53.

16. Emerson CH et al. Serum thyroxine and triiodothyronine concentrations during iodide treatment of hyperthyroidism. *J Clin Endocrinol Metab* 1975;40(1):33–6.

17. Marigold JH et al. Lugol's iodine: Its effect on thyroid blood flow in patients with thyrotoxicosis. *Br J Surg* 1985;72(1):45–7.

18. Chang DC et al. The effect of preoperative Lugol's iodine on thyroid blood flow in patients with Graves' hyperthyroidism. *Surgery* 1987;102(6):1055–61.

19. Erbil Y et al. Effect of Lugol solution on thyroid gland blood flow and microvessel density in the patients with Graves' disease. *J Clin Endocrinol Metab* 2007;92(6):2182–9.

20. Vaidya B, Pearce SH. Diagnosis and management of thyrotoxicosis. *BMJ* 2014;349:g5128.

21. Peters H et al. Radioiodine therapy of Graves' hyperthyroidism: Standard vs. calculated 131 iodine activity. Results from a prospective, randomized, multicentre study. *Eur J Clin Invest* 1995;25(3):186–93.

22. Burch HB et al. The effect of antithyroid drug pretreatment on acute changes in thyroid hormone levels after (131)I ablation for Graves' disease. *J Clin Endocrinol Metab* 2001;86(7):3016–21.

23. Andrade VA, Gross JL, Maia AL. Effect of methimazole pretreatment on serum thyroid hormone levels after radioactive treatment in Graves' hyperthyroidism. *J Clin Endocrinol Metab* 1999;84(11):4012–6.

24. Bartalena L et al. Relation between therapy for hyperthyroidism and the course of Graves' ophthalmopathy. *N Engl J Med* 1998;338(2):73–8.

25. Franklyn JA et al. Cancer incidence and mortality after radioiodine treatment for hyperthyroidism: A population-based cohort study. *Lancet* 1999;353(9170):2111–5.

26. Nikiforov Y, Gnepp DR. Pediatric thyroid cancer after the Chernobyl disaster. Pathomorphologic study of 84 cases (1991–1992) from the Republic of Belarus. *Cancer* 1994;74(2):748–66.

27. Pacini F et al. Thyroid consequences of the Chernobyl nuclear accident. *Acta Paediatr Suppl* 1999;88(433):23–7.

28. Hamburger JI. Management of hyperthyroidism in children and adolescents. *J Clin Endocrinol Metab* 1985;60(5):1019–24.

29. Bartalena L, Pinchera A, Marcocci C. Management of Graves' ophthalmopathy: Reality and perspectives. *Endocr Rev* 2000;21(2):168–99.

30. Bartalena L. Prevention of Graves' ophthalmopathy. *Best Pract Res Clin Endocrinol Metab* 2012;26(3):371–9.

31. Bahn Chair RS et al. Hyperthyroidism and other causes of thyrotoxicosis: Management guidelines of the American Thyroid Association and American Association of Clinical Endocrinologists. *Thyroid* 2011;21(6):593–646.

32. Schussler-Fiorenza CM, Bruns CM, Chen H. The surgical management of Graves' disease. *J Surg Res* 2006;133(2):207–14.

33. Alsanea O, Clark OH. Treatment of Graves' disease: The advantages of surgery. *Endocrinol Metab Clin North Am* 2000;29(2):321–37.

34. Bartalena L, Burch HB, Burman KD, Kahaly GF. A 2013 European survey of clinical practice patterns in the management of Graves' disease. *Clin Endocrinol* 2016;84:115–20.

35. Palit TK, Miller CC 3rd, Miltenburg DM. The efficacy of thyroidectomy for Graves' disease: A meta-analysis. *J Surg Res* 2000;90(2):161–5.

36. Sinha CK et al. Thyroid surgery in children: Clinical outcomes. *Eur J Pediatr Surg* 2015;25:425–9.

37. Witte J, Goretzki PE, Roher HD. Surgery for Graves disease in childhood and adolescence. *Exp Clin Endocrinol Diabetes* 1997;105(Suppl 4):58–60.

38. Torring O et al. Graves' hyperthyroidism: Treatment with antithyroid drugs, surgery, or

radioiodine—A prospective, randomized study. Thyroid Study Group. *J Clin Endocrinol Metab* 1996;81(8):2986–93.

39. Sridama V, DeGroot LJ. Treatment of Graves' disease and the course of ophthalmopathy. *Am J Med* 1989;87(1):70–3.

40. Witte J et al. Surgery for Graves' disease: Total versus subtotal thyroidectomy—Results of a prospective randomized trial. *World J Surg* 2000;24(11):1303–11.

41. Menconi F, Leo M, Vitti P, Marcocci C, Marino M. Total thyroid ablation in Graves' orbitopathy. *J Endocrinol Invest* 2015;38:809–15.

42. Ansaldo GL et al. Doppler evaluation of intrathyroid arterial resistances during preoperative treatment with Lugol's iodide solution in patients with diffuse toxic goiter. *J Am Coll Surg* 2000;191(6):607–12.

43. Snyder S et al. Total thyroidectomy as primary definitive treatment for Graves' hyperthyroidism. *Am Surg* 2013;79(12):1283–8.

44. Yamanouchi K et al. Evaluation of the operative methods for Graves' disease. *Minerva Chir* 2015;70:77–81.

45. Bojic T et al. Total thyroidectomy as a method of choice in the treatment of Graves' disease—Analysis of 1432 patients. *BMC Surg* 2015;15:39.

46. Schwartz AE et al. Therapeutic controversy: Thyroid surgery—The choice. *J Clin Endocrinol Metab* 1998;83(4):1097–105.

47. Yamashita H et al. Postoperative tetany in patients with Graves' disease: A risk factor analysis. *Clin Endocrinol (Oxf)* 1997;47(1):71–7.

48. Ireland AW et al. The crystalline lens in chronic surgical hypoparathyroidism. *Arch Intern Med* 1968;122(5):408–11.

49. Kai M et al. Intraoperative parathyroid hormone levels measured by intact and whole parathyroid hormone assays in patients with Graves' disease. *Surg Today* 2008;38(3):214–21.

50. Cusano NE, Rubin MR, Bilezikian JP. PTH(1-84) replacement therapy for the treatment of hypoparathyroidism. *Expert Rev Endocrinol Metab* 2015;10(1):5–13.

51. Porterfield JR Jr et al. Evidence-based management of toxic multinodular goiter (Plummer's disease). *World J Surg* 2008;32(7):1278–84.

52. Van Sande J et al. Somatic and germline mutations of the TSH receptor gene in thyroid diseases. *J Clin Endocrinol Metab* 1995;80(9):2577–85.

53. Tonacchera M et al. Hyperfunctioning thyroid nodules in toxic multinodular goiter share activating thyrotropin receptor mutations with solitary toxic adenoma. *J Clin Endocrinol Metab* 1998;83(2):492–8.

54. Kraiem Z et al. Toxic multinodular goiter: A variant of autoimmune hyperthyroidism. *J Clin Endocrinol Metab* 1987;65(4):659–64.

55. Nygaard B et al. Radioiodine treatment of multinodular non-toxic goitre. *BMJ* 1993;307(6908):828–32.

56. Hegedus L, Bonnema SJ, Bennedbaek FN. Management of simple nodular goiter: Current status and future perspectives. *Endocr Rev* 2003;24(1):102–32.

57. Kang AS et al. Current treatment of nodular goiter with hyperthyroidism (Plummer's disease): Surgery versus radioiodine. *Surgery* 2002;132(6):916–23; discussion 923.

58. Hisham AN et al. Total thyroidectomy: The procedure of choice for multinodular goitre. *Eur J Surg* 2001;167(6):403–5.

59. Reeve TS et al. Total thyroidectomy. The preferred option for multinodular goiter. *Ann Surg* 1987;206(6):782–6.

60. Vidal-Trecan GM, Stahl JE, Eckman MH. Radioiodine or surgery for toxic thyroid adenoma: Dissecting an important decision. A cost-effectiveness analysis. *Thyroid* 2004;14(11):933–45.

61. Angell TE et al. Clinical features and hospital outcomes in thyroid storm: A retrospective cohort study. *J Clin Endocrinol Metab* 2015;100(2):451–9.

62. Chiha M, Samarasinghe S, Kabaker AS. Thyroid storm: An updated review. *J Intensive Care Med* 2015;30(3):131–40.

63. Bogazzi F et al. Amiodarone and the thyroid: A 2012 update. *J Endocrinol Invest* 2012;35(3):340–8.

64. Pierret C et al. Total thyroidectomy for amiodarone-associated thyrotoxicosis: Should surgery always be delayed for pre-operative medical preparation? *J Laryngol Otol* 2012;126(7):701–5.

11

Thyroid nodules

SALEM I. NOURELDINE AND RALPH P. TUFANO

INTRODUCTION

Thyroid nodules are quite prevalent in the United States, and are often discovered as incidental findings on a physical exam, or through radiographic studies. The clinical importance of thyroid nodules rests with the need to exclude ones that may harbor malignancy, or in a patient with hyperthyroidism, to identify if the nodule is the autonomous source of excessive thyroid hormone production. This is usually accomplished by obtaining a detailed history, physical exam, and thyroid function tests, in addition to a thyroid and neck ultrasound. The information obtained will then direct subsequent evaluation, including the need for fine-needle aspiration (FNA) biopsy assessment. The management of the nodule is dictated by these findings and subsequent behavior. This chapter encompasses the clinical description of thyroid nodules, in addition to diagnosis and management.

EPIDEMIOLOGY OF THYROID NODULES

The prevalence of thyroid nodules increases with age, and population surveys suggest nearly 5%–15% of the adult population may harbor a clinically significant nodule requiring evaluation [1]. Palpable thyroid nodules are found in approximately 5% of women and 1% of men living in iodine-sufficient parts of the world. High-resolution ultrasound can detect thyroid nodules in 19%–67% of randomly selected individuals, with higher frequencies in women and the elderly [2]. In contrast, the prevalence of thyroid nodular lesions from autopsy studies in clinically normal thyroid glands is approximately 50%–60%.

The differences between the prevalence of thyroid nodules found on clinical examination and those found on ultrasound or at autopsy relate to the skill of the individual performing the examination, the size of the nodule, and the location of the nodule, as small posterior nodules are more difficult to identify than the same nodules located anteriorly. Usually, nodules less than 5 mm are not palpable, about 35% of 1 cm nodules are palpated, 80% of 1.5 cm nodules are palpated, and almost all 2 cm nodules can be appreciated [3].

MALIGNANCY RATE OF THYROID NODULES

Numerous studies have documented that the risk of malignancy in patients with thyroid nodules is 5%–17%, whether detected by palpation or ultrasonography. Usually, the size of the thyroid nodule does not predict the likelihood of thyroid cancer. Only 8% of incidentally found thyroid nodules measuring <5 mm, 15% of nodules measuring 5–10 mm, and 13% of nodules measuring 10–15 mm are found to be malignant [4]. In addition, the cancer rates for patients with solitary nodules versus those with multiple nodules are virtually identical.

Autopsy series have found that 0.5%–35.6% of populations from North America, Europe, and Japan have at least microscopic thyroid cancer. The median prevalence from these studies is 6.5% [5]. The majority of the tumors found at autopsy are microcarcinomas, measuring less than a centimeter [6].

EVALUATION OF A PATIENT WITH THYROID NODULES

The majority of thyroid nodules are benign and represent hyperplastic multinodular goiter, colloid nodules, Hashimoto's thyroiditis, simple or hemorrhagic cysts, or follicular adenomas, all of which need to be differentiated from thyroid cancer. Malignancies of the thyroid gland include papillary, follicular, Hurthle cell, medullary, and anaplastic carcinomas, as well as primary thyroid lymphomas and extrathyroid metastases to the thyroid gland. In most instances, the patient's history, physical examination, laboratory testing, ultrasonography, and FNA biopsy will allow a diagnosis to be made.

History and physical examination

Several clinical features must be considered during thyroid nodule evaluation, including age, sex, status of thyroid function, history of radiation exposure, family history, and pre-existing thyroid disorders.

First-, second-, and third-degree relatives of papillary thyroid cancer (PTC) patients have a significant increased risk of developing the same cancer. First-degree relatives have a fivefold increased risk of being diagnosed as having this cancer themselves. Second- and third-degree relatives have a twofold increased risk. Siblings are at highest risk and have a sevenfold increased risk [7]. There is also an increased risk of developing a thyroid cancer with several complex familial syndromes, if first-degree relatives are involved [8]. These include familial adenomatous polyposis (colonic polyps, epidermoid cysts, and desmoid tumors of the abdominal wall), Gardner's syndrome (familial polyposis coli and bone osteomas), Cowden disease (phosphatase and tensin homolog [PTEN] hamartomas tumor syndrome), and Carney complex (skin and mucosal lentigines and cardiac myxomas, in addition to adrenal, pituitary, and testicular neoplasms). A familial history of isolated medullary thyroid cancer (MTC) or multiple endocrine neoplasia (MEN) type 2 also raises the risk of thyroid cancer, especially if the nodule is discovered in a young individual.

External beam radiation had been used in the past to shrink the thymus glands in infants with respiratory symptoms; to treat birthmarks, ringworm, and scrofula in children; and to treat acne in adolescents. Radium implants were used to shrink tonsils and adenoids in childhood. This radiation to the head and neck region has led to the development of benign and malignant thyroid nodules and hyperparathyroidism, including other neoplasms depending on the site of treatment. The risk of a malignancy in thyroids exposed to such irradiation is 33% [9].

Patients under the age of 20 or over 70 years with thyroid nodules have an increased risk of malignancy, as do men. A history of persistent hoarseness, dysphagia, or dyspnea also increases the risk, although these symptoms may also occur with benign nodules. A rapid painless growth of a solid nodule is concerning and also raises the suspicion for thyroid cancer. A thyroid nodule that is metabolically active on ^{18}F-fluorodeoxyglucose positron emission tomography (FDG-PET) scan performed for non-thyroid-related reasons has an approximately 30% chance of being malignant [10].

Symptoms of hyperthyroidism, such as weight loss, tremor, palpitations, increased sweating, heat intolerance, and insomnia, should be sought, as their presence suggests that the nodule may be autonomously functioning and causing the hyperthyroidism state. Nodules can be present in patients with a diffuse toxic goiter from Graves' disease, and about 9% of such nodules are malignant. Therefore, additional studies, such as a thyroid scan and possibly a FNA biopsy, should be performed.

On physical examination, thyroid nodules may be smooth or nodular, diffuse or localized, soft or hard, mobile or fixed, and painful or nontender. While palpation is the clinically relevant method of examining the thyroid gland, it can be insensitive and inaccurate, depending on the skill of the examiner. Nonetheless, a nodule that is firm, fixed to the adjacent structures in the neck, and associated with cervical lymphadenopathy or paralysis of the vocal folds should be considered highly suspicious for thyroid cancer.

Laboratory testing

As a basic diagnostic step, all patients with thyroid nodules should have their thyroid function assessed. The blood levels of thyroid-stimulating hormone (TSH) can provide valuable information about how well the thyroid gland is functioning. A low-serum TSH concentration indicates overt or subclinical hyperthyroidism, increasing the possibility that the nodule is hot, and thus a radioisotope thyroid scan should be obtained to document whether the nodule is hyperfunctioning, isofunctioning, or nonfunctioning. Conversely, an elevated TSH level indicates hypothyroidism, and a serum antithyroid peroxidase antibody should be measured to determine if the patient has Hashimoto's thyroiditis. Most patients with thyroid cancer have TSH levels within the normal range. However, higher-serum TSH, even within the upper part of the reference range, is associated with increased risk of malignancy in a thyroid nodule.

Serum thyroglobulin (Tg) measurement for initial evaluation of thyroid nodules has no predictive value for thyroid malignancy. Serum Tg levels can be elevated in most thyroid diseases and are an insensitive and nonspecific test for thyroid cancer. An unstimulated serum calcitonin greater than 100 pg/mL is likely to be associated with MTC. The data suggest that serum calcitonin should be measured routinely in patients with nodular thyroid disease in order to detect C-cell hyperplasia and MTC at an earlier stage, and that this may improve overall survival. In addition, a recent cost-effectiveness analysis suggested that calcitonin screening would be cost-effective in the United States [11]. However, the most recent American Thyroid Association (ATA) guidelines do not recommend for or against the routine measurement of serum calcitonin [12]. DNA analysis for specific mutations in the *RET* proto-oncogene allows screening for MEN type 2.

Ultrasound assessment

Imaging studies characterize the thyroid nodule and help determine the extent of disease, providing an anatomical road map for surgical planning. Ultrasound is often the first imaging modality employed to evaluate a patient with a thyroid nodule since it is readily accessible, inexpensive, and noninvasive. Ultrasound is effective at delineating intrathyroidal architecture, distinguishing cystic from solid lesions, determining if a nodule is solitary or part of a multinodular gland, and accurately locating and measuring a nodule. In addition, ultrasound is extremely useful in patients who are managed conservatively for follow-up of possible increased volume of a suspicious lesion.

Ultrasound has been proven highly effective in determining the location and characteristics of nodules; however, by itself, it cannot reliably be used to distinguish a benign nodule from a malignant one. Combining high-resolution ultrasonography with Doppler and spectral analysis of the vascular characteristics of a thyroid nodule holds promise as a useful tool for diagnosing benign lesions and in screening thyroid nodules for malignancy. Studies have shown that the risk of malignancy is lower in nodules with a predominantly perinodular vascular pattern than in nodules with an exclusively central vascular pattern. Furthermore, if the vascular characteristics of thyroid nodules are combined with their ultrasonographic parameters, including microcalcifications, cross-sectional diameter, and echogenicity, the predictive value of this imaging approach may increase (Table 11.1).

Ultrasound has the added advantages of demonstrating any associated lymphadenopathy. Sonographic appearances

Table 11.1 Features of thyroid lesions on ultrasonography

Malignant	Benign
• Hypoechogenicity	• Hyperechogenicity
• Increased intranodular vascularity	• A pure cystic nodule
• Irregular infiltrative margins	• Spongiform appearance (multiple microcysts in >50% of nodule)
• Presence of microcalcifications	
• Absent halo	• Present halo
• Shape taller than wide measured in the transverse dimension	• Round shaped

of normal nodes differ from those of abnormal nodes. Abnormal lymph nodes have sonographic features that include round shape, absent hilus, calcification, intranodal necrosis, reticulation, matting, soft tissue edema, and peripheral vascularity. However, many nodal metastases demonstrate a wide variety of nondiagnostic features. Children and adolescents command an important degree of attention to cystic lesions. Approximately 8% of cystic lesions represent malignancy in this population.

Thyroid ultrasonography should be used routinely to guide FNA Biopsy. Data have suggested that ultrasound-guided FNA biopsy is preferable to palpation-guided FNA biopsy, especially in the assessment of nonpalpable or small nodules, nodules with cystic components or nodules that are located posteriorly in the thyroid gland. Table 11.2 summarizes the consensus recommendations of the ATA concerning the criteria for which nodules should undergo FNA biopsy [12].

Radioisotope thyroid scan

Radioiodine scans, using ^{123}I, are useful for determining whether a thyroid nodule is autonomous in a patient with a suppressed serum TSH level. The term *hot nodule* is used when the nodule is suppressing the surrounding normal thyroid tissue, and *warm nodule* when it is functioning but does not suppress the surrounding thyroid tissue. A *cold nodule* is a nodule that is hypofunctioning in comparison with the surrounding thyroid tissue. Approximately 95% of nodules are cold on radioisotope scanning. The frequency of malignancy in cold nodules is 10%–15%, and 4% in hot nodules [13]. Thus, both hot and cold nodules are likely to be benign, and malignancy is only slightly more likely in cold nodules.

Radioisotope scanning can also help differentiate between a toxic nodule greater than 1 cm and the diffuse pattern in Graves' disease; the resolution of scans is inferior to that of ultrasound, as they generally are unable to detect lesions of <1 cm. Isotope scanning can also detect metastatic disease, when the cancer is iodine avid. The recent ATA guidelines recommend that radioisotope scanning should also be considered in patients with multiple thyroid nodules, if the serum TSH is in the low or low–normal range, with FNA being reserved for those that are shown to be hypofunctioning [12].

Other imaging modalities

Computed tomography (CT) scanning, magnetic resonance imaging (MRI), and PET scanning are generally not recommended as the initial evaluation of solitary thyroid nodules. In addition, the sensitivities of CT, MRI, and PET for the detection of cervical lymph node metastases are relatively low (30%–40%). Such studies may be useful in the assessment of thyroid masses that are largely substernal and rapidly growing, or for invasive tumors, to assess the involvement of extrathyroidal tissues. A CT with iodinated

Table 11.2 ATA recommendations for FNA biopsy based on ultrasound and clinical features of thyroid nodules

Nodule features	Recommended nodule	Strength of recommendation
High-risk history[a]		
Suspicious ultrasound features[b]	>5 mm	Strong—based on good evidence
No suspicious ultrasound features	>5 mm	Recommends neither for or against
Abnormal cervical lymph nodes	All	Strong—based on good evidence
Microcalcifications present	≥1 cm	Recommends—based on fair evidence
Solid nodule		
Hypoechoic	>1 cm	Recommends—based on fair evidence
Isoechoic or hyperechoic	≥1–1.5 cm	Recommends—based on expert opinion
Mixed nodule		
With any suspicious ultrasound features	≥1–2 cm	Recommends—based on fair evidence
Without suspicious ultrasound features	≥2 cm	Recommends—based on expert opinion
Spongiform nodule	≥2 cm	Recommends—based on expert opinion
Purely cystic nodule	—	Recommends against—based on fair evidence

[a] History of thyroid cancer in one or more first-degree relatives, history of irradiation, prior lobectomy with discovery of thyroid cancer, ^{18}FDG avidity on PET scanning, MEN2/FMTC-associated RET proto-oncogene mutation, >100 pg/mL calcitonin.

[b] Microcalcifications, hypoechoic, increased nodular vascularity, infiltrative margins, taller than wide on transverse view.

contrast is considered extremely helpful to evaluate the extent of retroesophageal, parapharyngeal, and mediastinal lymphadenopathy, as it helps define the extent of surgery necessary to plan clearance of all gross disease in the neck [14].

Recently, FDG-PET scanning has been utilized in an effort to distinguish indeterminate nodules that are benign from those that are malignant. FDG-PET scans appear to have relatively high sensitivity for malignancy but low specificity. Approximately 1%–2% of people undergoing FDG-PET imaging for other reasons have thyroid nodules discovered incidentally; such lesions require prompt evaluation due to the 33% risk of malignancy in FDG-avid nodules [15]. Diffuse FDG-PET uptake is seen with autoimmune thyroiditis.

Fine-needle aspiration biopsy

FNA biopsy has resulted in substantial improvements in diagnostic accuracy and a higher malignancy yield at time of surgery. FNA biopsy is the most cost-effective and reliable technique available to differentiate between benign and malignant diseases of the thyroid. It is estimated that its use reduces the need for diagnostic thyroidectomy by half and the overall cost of thyroid nodule medical care by one-quarter, while doubling the surgical confirmation of carcinoma. Cytopathologic evaluation has improved significantly over the past two decades, but good aspiration technique and an experienced cytopathologist are necessary to reach the modern high standards. Ultrasound-guided FNA biopsy, combined with on-site cytology verification of the adequacy of the specimen by a cytotechnologist or pathologist, may likely provide the highest sensitivity and specificity. Current sensitivity and specificity generally exceed 90% and 70%, respectively. However, negative cytology

results should never override strong clinical suspicion of malignancy. After an initial nondiagnostic cytology result, repeat FNA with ultrasound guidance will yield a diagnostic cytology specimen in 75% of solid nodules and 50% of cystic nodules [16]. For patients who proceed to an operation, prior use of FNA biopsy reduces the need for frozen section analysis for diagnosis, reducing operative time and pathology fees.

FNA biopsy of thyroid nodules can be used to categorize tissue into the following diagnostic categories: nondiagnostic, benign, follicular lesion of undetermined significance (atypia of undetermined significance), follicular or Hurthle cell neoplasm (or suspicious for follicular or Hurthle cell neoplasm), suspicious for malignancy, and malignant. The diagnostic category should be clearly elucidated by labeling it with the terminology from The Bethesda System for Reporting Thyroid Cytopathology [17] (Table 11.3). In the malignant category, FNA biopsy can be used to distinguish papillary carcinoma, medullary carcinoma, anaplastic

Table 11.3 The Bethesda System for Reporting Thyroid Cytopathology: Risk of malignancy

Cytology diagnostic category	Malignancy rate (%)
Nondiagnostic or unsatisfactory	1–4
Benign	0–3
AUS/FLUS	5–15
FN/SFN or SHCN	15–30
Suspicious for malignancy	60–75
Malignant	97–99

Note: AUS, atypia of undetermined significance; FLUS, follicular lesion of undetermined significance; FN, follicular neoplasm; SFN, suspicious for follicular neoplasm; SHCN, suspicious for Hurthle cell neoplasm.

carcinoma, and carcinoma metastatic to the thyroid gland, and it can be used to distinguish malignant lymphoma from other disease [12].

Genetic testing

The recent development of diagnostic molecular methods, including BRAF, RAS, RET/PTC, and PAX8/PPARγ, applied to FNA specimens offers improved diagnostic accuracy, and may become a more commonly available component of needle aspirate evaluation in the future. Recent large prospective studies have confirmed the ability of genetic markers (BRAF, RAS, RET/PTC, and PAX8/PPARγ), a gene expression classifier, and protein markers (galectin-3) to improve the preoperative diagnostic accuracy for patients with indeterminate thyroid nodules [18,19]. In addition, reverse transcription–polymerase chain reaction to detect Tg mRNA and thyrotropin receptor mRNA from a lymph node is accurate for diagnosing metastatic thyroid cancer. The use of molecular markers is now formally recommended in the current ATA management guidelines for specific patients with thyroid nodules and differentiated thyroid cancer [12].

The presence of a BRAF V600E mutation has been associated in many studies with the aggressiveness of PTC (extrathyroidal invasion, lymph node metastasis, and advanced stage) and also with disease-specific mortality when associated with other aggressive features, such as extrathyroidal extension. However, BRAF V600E mutation analysis offers a limited positive predictive value (28%) for disease recurrence [20]. RAS mutations are associated with a follicular pattern of thyroid neoplasms, and have also been reported in poorly differentiated thyroid cancer. The clinical significance of RAS mutations in thyroid cancer is controversial; some reports show that RAS mutations are associated with tumor-aggressive phenotypes and poor prognosis, while others could not confirm this association. Similarly, RET/PTC rearrangements are associated in some reports with lymph node metastasis and extrathyroidal extension, and with a better prognosis in other studies. PAX8/PPARγ rearrangements have been associated with multifocality of the tumors and vascular invasion, conferring an invasive potential. Despite this, the consistent detection of PAX8/PPARγ rearrangements in benign tumors hinders its value as a diagnostic molecular marker. To date, none of these markers have been demonstrated to be clear, independent prognostic indicators, thus preventing their widespread acceptance and utilization in clinical practice.

MANAGEMENT OF PATIENTS WITH THYROID NODULES

Observation

Nonfunctioning thyroid nodules diagnosed as benign require follow-up for a change in size and a low, but not

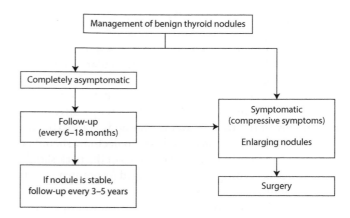

Figure 11.1 Management of benign, nonautonomous functioning thyroid nodules.

negligible, false-negative rate of up to 5% with FNA, which may be even higher with nodules of >4 cm. It is recommended that all benign thyroid nodules be followed with serial ultrasound examinations 6–18 months after FNA biopsy. If the nodule size is stable (no more than 50% change in volume or <20% increase in at least two nodule dimensions in solid nodules or in the solid portion of mixed cystic–solid nodules), the interval before the next follow-up clinical examination or ultrasound may be longer [12]. Possible exceptions include large intrathoracic goiters, nodules that are exerting pressure on surrounding structures, and those that are cosmetically unacceptable. Cystic nodules may be drained at the time of initial biopsy, but there is a high rate of fluid reaccumulation, often from recurrent hemorrhage into the lesion. With such lesions, it is important to monitor the size of the solid portion of the lesion for growth, which should prompt an ultrasound-guided FNA biopsy.

Patients with growing nodules that are benign after repeat FNA biopsy should be considered for continued monitoring or intervention, with surgery based on symptoms and clinical concern. The management of benign thyroid nodules is summarized in Figure 11.1.

Levothyroxine suppressive therapy

Evidence from multiple prospective randomized trials and meta-analyses suggests that thyroid hormone supplementation in doses that suppress the serum TSH to subnormal levels may result in a decrease in nodule size and may prevent the appearance of new nodules. However, the effect is modest, with most studies suggesting an average 5%–15% reduction in nodule volume when treated with suppressive levothyroxine therapy for 6–18 months [21]. Hyperthyroidism to this degree has been significantly associated with an increased risk of cardiac arrhythmias and osteoporosis, as well as adverse symptomology. Therefore, neither the ATA nor the American Association of Clinical Endocrinologists recommends routine suppression therapy in patients with growing nodules that are benign after FNA [12,22].

Surgery

Surgery is indicated for nodules that are malignant or suspicious for malignancy, in addition to follicular lesions that are cold, especially if the nodule is >4 cm with atypical features in an older male patient. For patients with lesions compatible with or suspicious for PTC, preoperative ultrasonography of the thyroid and lymph node compartments of the neck should be considered. Thyroidectomy should be performed and the nodal compartments of the neck should be managed according to evidence-based recommendations and the multidisciplinary management team consensus, which includes the patient. Patients with unifocal tumors of <1 cm, which are confined to the thyroid gland and without a history of head and neck irradiation, may only require a hemithyroidectomy. Patients with small follicular neoplasms or with a follicular lesion of undetermined significance may undergo a diagnostic hemithyroidectomy, with the understanding that a completion thyroidectomy may be necessary should the surgical pathology and multidisciplinary management team dictate [12].

Surgery should also be considered for patients with large nodules or a multinodular goiter that causes symptoms such as dysphagia, choking, dysphonia, shortness of breath, dyspnea on exertion, and neck pressure or neck pain. Continued growth of a thyroid nodule is another indication to consider surgery [5].

Radioactive iodine

^{131}I therapy can be used to treat toxic nodules or Graves' disease. The therapy is successful in controlling hyperthyroidism in more than 75% of patients at 2 years [23]. The major side effect is hypothyroidism that occurs in about 10% of patients by 5 years. Nonetheless, there has been a noticeable shift toward the use of total thyroidectomy in lieu of radioactive iodine ablation for the surgical management of Graves' disease [24].

FUTURE DEVELOPMENTS

Significant progress has been made over the last several years in understanding the genetic mechanisms of thyroid cancer and creating molecular tests for cancer diagnosis in thyroid nodules. This process is currently going through the accelerated phase, which is expected to continue in the future and result in a significantly improved accuracy of cancer detection in thyroid nodules compared with the currently available clinical tests.

Ultrasound elastography is a new technique that measures the change of the ultrasound beam that occurs when pressure is applied to a thyroid nodule [25]. Thyroid cancers tend to be firmer than benign lesions; therefore, the external pressure will distort cancers less than it would for benign nodules. This technique has been shown to have sensitivity up to 97% and specificity of 77%–100% for predicting malignancy [25].

Percutaneous ethanol injection therapy, radiofrequency ablation, and laser ablation have each been reported as effective for treating benign and malignant thyroid nodules, as well as for locoregional control of cancer or for improving tumor-related symptoms in selected patients. Nonsurgical ablation seems likely to have a future role in managing benign and malignant thyroid nodules [26]. Its specific indications, however, remain to be determined. At present, due to small series reports from single centers, the use of these techniques should be relegated to an alternative therapy category rendered at large medical centers with the most significant experience with these techniques [27].

REFERENCES

1. Tomimori E, Pedrinola F, Cavaliere H, Knobel M, Medeiros-Neto G. Prevalence of incidental thyroid disease in a relatively low iodine intake area. *Thyroid* 1995;5(4):273–6.
2. Tan GH, Gharib H. Thyroid incidentalomas: Management approaches to nonpalpable nodules discovered incidentally on thyroid imaging. *Ann Intern Med* 1997;126(3):226–31.
3. Takahashi T, Trott KR, Fujimori K et al. An investigation into the prevalence of thyroid disease on Kwajalein Atoll, Marshall Islands. *Health Phys* 1997;73(1):199–213.
4. Nam-Goong IS, Kim HY, Gong G et al. Ultrasonography-guided fine-needle aspiration of thyroid incidentaloma: Correlation with pathological findings. *Clin Endocrinol (Oxf)* 2004;60(1):21–8.
5. Braunstein GD, Sacks W. Thyroid nodules. In: Braunstein GD, ed., *Thyroid Cancer*. New York: Springer US, 2012:45–61.
6. Harach HR, Franssila KO, Wasenius VM. Occult papillary carcinoma of the thyroid. A "normal" finding in Finland. A systematic autopsy study. *Cancer* 1985;56(3):531–8.
7. Oakley GM, Curtin K, Pimentel R, Buchmann L, Hunt J. Establishing a familial basis for papillary thyroid carcinoma using the Utah Population Database. *JAMA Otolaryngol Head Neck Surg* 2013;139(11):1171–4.
8. Loh KC. Familial nonmedullary thyroid carcinoma: A meta-review of case series. *Thyroid* 1997;7(1):107–13.
9. Mihailescu DV, Schneider AB. Size, number, and distribution of thyroid nodules and the risk of malignancy in radiation-exposed patients who underwent surgery. *J Clin Endocrinol Metab* 2008;93(6):2188–93.
10. Boelaert K, Horacek J, Holder RL, Watkinson JC, Sheppard MC, Franklyn JA. Serum thyrotropin concentration as a novel predictor of malignancy in thyroid nodules investigated by fine-needle aspiration. *J Clin Endocrinol Metab* 2006;91:4295–301.
11. Cheung K, Roman SA, Wang TS, Walker HD, Sosa JA. Calcitonin measurement in the evaluation of thyroid nodules in the United States: A cost-effectiveness and decision analysis. *J Clin Endocrinol Metab* 2008:93;2173–80.

12. Cooper DS, Doherty GM, Haugen BR et al. Revised American Thyroid Association management guidelines for patients with thyroid nodules and differentiated thyroid cancer. *Thyroid* 2009;19(11):1167–214.

13. Ashcraft MW, Van Herle AJ. Management of thyroid nodules. I. History and physical examination, blood tests, x-ray tests, and ultrasonography. *Head Neck Surg* 1981;3(3):216–30.

14. Yeh MW, Bauer AJ, Bernet V et al. American Thyroid Association statement on preoperative imaging for thyroid cancer surgery. *Thyroid* 2015;25:3–14.

15. Kim TY, Kim WB, Ryu JS, Gong G, Hong SJ, Shong YK. 18F-fluorodeoxyglucose uptake in thyroid from positron emission tomogram (PET) for evaluation in cancer patients: High prevalence of malignancy in thyroid PET incidentaloma. *Laryngoscope* 2005;115(6):1074–8.

16. Alexander EK, Heering JP, Benson CB et al. Assessment of nondiagnostic ultrasound-guided fine needle aspirations of thyroid nodules. *J Clin Endocrinol Metab* 2002;87(11):4924–7.

17. Baloch ZW, LiVolsi VA, Asa SL et al. Diagnostic terminology and morphologic criteria for cytologic diagnosis of thyroid lesions: A synopsis of the National Cancer Institute Thyroid Fine-Needle Aspiration State of the Science Conference. *Diagn Cytopathol* 2008;36(6):425–37.

18. Nikiforov YE, Ohori NP, Hodak SP et al. Impact of mutational testing on the diagnosis and management of patients with cytologically indeterminate thyroid nodules: A prospective analysis of 1056 FNA samples. *J Clin Endocrinol Metab* 2011;96(11):3390–7.

19. Alexander EK, Kennedy GC, Baloch ZW et al. Preoperative diagnosis of benign thyroid nodules with indeterminate cytology. *N Engl J Med* 2012;367(8):705–15.

20. Xing M. Prognostic utility of BRAF mutation in papillary thyroid cancer. *Mol Cell Endocrinol* 2010;321(1):86–93.

21. Papini E, Petrucci L, Guglielmi R et al. Long-term changes in nodular goiter: A 5-year prospective randomized trial of levothyroxine suppressive therapy for benign cold thyroid nodules. *J Clin Endocrinol Metab* 1998;83(3):780–3.

22. Gharib H, Papini E, Valcavi R et al. American Association of Clinical Endocrinologists and Associazione Medici Endocrinologi medical guidelines for clinical practice for the diagnosis and management of thyroid nodules. *Endocr Pract* 2006;12(1):63–102.

23. Sywak M, Cornford L, Roach P, Stalberg P, Sidhu S, Delbridge L. Routine ipsilateral level VI lymphadenectomy reduces postoperative thyroglobulin. *Surgery* 2006;140(6):1000–5; discussion 1005–7.

24. Genovese BM, Noureldine SI, Gleeson EM, Tufano RP, Kandil E. What is the best definitive treatment for Graves' disease? A systematic review of the existing literature. *Ann Surg Oncol* 2013;20(2):660–7.

25. Hong Y, Liu X, Li Z, Zhang X, Chen M, Luo Z. Real-time ultrasound elastography in the differential diagnosis of benign and malignant thyroid nodules. *J Ultrasound Med* 2009;28(7):861–7.

26. Hay ID, Lee RA, Davidge-Pitts C, Reading CC, Charboneau JW. Long-term outcome of ultrasound-guided percutaneous ethanol ablation of selected "recurrent" neck nodal metastases in 25 patients with TNM stages III or IVA papillary thyroid carcinoma previously treated by surgery and 131I therapy. *Surgery* 2013;154(6):1448–54; discussion 1454–5.

27. Na DG, Lee JH, Jung SL et al. Radiofrequency ablation of benign thyroid nodules and recurrent thyroid cancers: Consensus statement and recommendations. *Korean J Radiol* 2012;13(2):117–25.

12

Molecular testing of thyroid nodules

LINWAH YIP

INTRODUCTION

Thyroid cancer is one of the few malignancies that are increasing in incidence. Although early detection may be one reason for the rise, other variables may also be contributing to the observed increase, as the trend has been observed in both genders, and in patients of all ages and racial and ethnic groups [1–3]. Thyroid cancer is commonly diagnosed during the evaluation of a thyroid nodule that is detected either on physical examination or as an incidental finding on imaging, such as carotid ultrasound (US) or computed tomography (CT) scans of the neck or chest. With today's sensitive CT and US technology, clinically occult nodules are being diagnosed with rising frequency. In a recent study of 635 German patients who were screened with neck US, thyroid nodules were detected in up to 68% of adults and the incidence was age dependent, with nodules diagnosed in nearly 80% of those who were >61 years old [4]. Thus, as the population ages and receives more diagnostic testing, thyroid nodules will become a commonplace finding. In the routine evaluation of thyroid nodules, the goal should be to exclude malignancy [5].

US and US-guided fine-needle aspiration biopsy (FNAB) are the diagnostic modalities typically used to risk-stratify thyroid nodules [5]. US-guided FNAB is reliable, and cytology results are classified into one of the six Bethesda System for Reporting Thyroid Cytopathology categories (Table 12.1) [6]. Benign results are highly accurate and have a low false-negative rate that ranges from 1% to 3% [7,8]. However, up to 20%–30% of biopsy results are classified into one of the three indeterminate categories: atypia or follicular lesion of undetermined significance (AUS/FLUS), follicular neoplasm or

suspicious for follicular neoplasm (FN), and suspicious for malignancy [5,6]. In a meta-analysis inclusive of 4212 nodules with cytohistologic correlation, the risk of malignancy in the AUS/FLUS, FN, and suspicious categories was 16%, 26%, and 75%, respectively (Table 12.1) [7]. Because nodules with AUS/FLUS biopsy results have a lower risk of malignancy, repeat biopsy can be helpful. However, for definitive diagnosis, surgery is still often necessary for the majority of nodules with indeterminate cytology, despite the fact that many will be histologically benign.

Recent advancements in molecular testing technology have led to an improved understanding of the molecular mechanisms that contribute to thyroid carcinogenesis, and have allowed significant progress in expanding diagnostic options for patients with thyroid nodules [9–11]. Preoperative testing would ideally guide the initial operative procedure, allowing oncologic concerns to be balanced with quality of life considerations while potentially also leading to algorithms that could appropriately guide consideration for nonoperative management in patients with low-risk cancers [12]. Improving risk stratification of thyroid nodules and avoiding unnecessary surgery will also have population-level policy implications, as recent evaluation of healthcare utilization data has shown a 12% annual percentage change increase in the number of thyroid operations in the United States from 2008 to 2011 [13]. Using molecular-based tests as a diagnostic adjunct will likely significantly augment the accuracy of current nodule management algorithms. Molecular tests that have been studied for thyroid nodule evaluation include circulating markers of malignancy that can be detected by sampling of peripheral blood, and specific testing of FNAB cytology

Table 12.1 The Bethesda System for Reporting Cytopathology classification system: Frequency of category use and cancer risk

	Cytology diagnosis	Theorized risk of cancer [6]	Frequency of diagnosis, % (range) [7]	Actual risk of cancer [7]
I	Nondiagnostic	1%–4%	13 [2–24]	17%
II	Benign	0%–3%	59 [39–74]	4%
III	AUS/FLUS	5%–15%	10 [1–27]	16%
IV	FN	15%–30%	10 [1–25]	26%
V	Suspicious for malignancy	60%–75%	3 [1–6]	75%
VI	Malignant	97%–99%	5 [2–16]	99%

Source: Adapted from Baloch ZW et al. Diagn Cytopathol 2008;36(6):425–37; Bongiovanni M et al. Acta Cytol 2012;56(4):333–9.

Table 12.2 Types of molecular testing used in thyroid cancer diagnosis

Circulating molecular markers
  TSHR mRNA
  Cell-free BRAF V600E
ICC analysis
MiRNA expression
Multigene expression panels
  GEC
Genetic mutation and rearrangements
  BRAF V600E
  7-Gene MT
  NGS-based thyroid-specific panel

for protein-based markers by immunocytochemical (ICC) methods, differential microRNA (miRNA) expression patterns, differential expression patterns using multigene expression panels, or detection of somatic DNA mutations and rearrangements (Table 12.2).

CIRCULATING MOLECULAR MARKERS

Circulating molecular markers have been an appealing area of study due to ease of patient sampling. The presence of circulating TSHR mRNA may be a marker of thyroid malignancy and can be detected using quantitative reverse transcription–polymerase chain reaction (RT-PCR) when present in >10 cancer cells per milliliter of peripheral blood. In a study of 54 patients with FNAB cytology classified as FN, an elevated TSHR mRNA level of >1 ng/µg was associated with 85% diagnostic accuracy [14]. In order to optimize the diagnostic discriminancy, an algorithm was developed that incorporated nodule size (<3.5 cm or ≥3.5 cm), TSHR mRNA detection, and number of suspicious US characteristics (hypervascularity, microcalcifications, irregular shape, and indistinct margins). The algorithm was able to preoperatively predict thyroid cancer with 91% accuracy, 97% sensitivity, 95% negative predictive value (NPV), 84% specificity, and 88% positive predictive value (PPV) [14]. TSHR mRNA levels usually normalized within 1 day of thyroid surgery, and this correlated to being disease-free at follow-up. However, a persistent postoperative elevation in TSHR

mRNA was predictive of recurrent disease or distant metastasis, and provides some prognostic utility [15].

Detection of circulating cell-free BRAF V600E using allele specific-quantitative PCR has also been investigated as another diagnostic tool. BRAF V600E is the most common gene alteration in thyroid cancer, and is associated with up to 40%–50% of conventional papillary thyroid cancer (PTC). Pupilli et al. were able to detect a higher percentage of mutated circulating BRAF V600E in patients with histologic PTC compared with patients with benign nodular disease [16]. After calculating a cutoff value that could be used preoperatively to predict the presence of thyroid cancer, the percentage of circulating BRAF V600E correlated to histologic malignancy in a cohort of patients with cytology classified as FN with a PPV of 33% and an NPV of 80%. In their pilot study, the proportion of circulating BRAF V600E also decreased after surgery [16]. To date, preliminary data from these studies suggest that circulating markers may be a useful diagnostic adjunct. However, detection of circulating markers will likely be more useful in the surveillance of thyroid cancer patients who have already completed initial treatment.

PROTEIN-BASED MARKERS

ICC analysis of markers expressed in PTC can be helpful for further characterization of indeterminate FNAB results, may be less costly than other forms of molecular testing, and uses resources that are likely readily available in any pathology laboratory. The three most commonly used markers are cytokeratin-19 (CK-19), galectin-3 (Gal-3), and Hector Battifora mesothelial-1 (HBME-1), all of which have higher expression in differentiated thyroid cancers compared with benign lesions. In a recent meta-analysis, HBME-1 has been the most studied ICC marker, although Gal-3 had the highest sensitivity (85%) and specificity (90%) for malignancy [17]. Gal-3 as an adjunct to FNAB cytology was evaluated in a multi-institutional study inclusive of 465 FNAB samples that were classified as follicular neoplasm or suspected follicular neoplasm and had an overall malignancy rate of 28% [18]. False-negative staining occurred in 9%, and included histologic follicular-variant PTC (FVPTC), follicular thyroid cancer (FTC), oncocytic-variant FTC, and poorly differentiated thyroid cancers. False-positive staining occurred in 25% with an overall accuracy of 88% [18]. Thus, using Gal-3 ICC analysis alone is insufficient to exclude cancer or to guide surgery.

Using panels with more than one marker may increase the accuracy of ICC. In a small series of 115 indeterminate FNAB specimens evaluated by HBME-1 and CK-19, there were no false-negative ICC results. However, four false-positive cases occurred and specificity was 85%. Moreover, inconclusive ICC results were obtained in 38% of FNAB specimens, further limiting the described technique [19]. In another study of 50 indeterminate FNAB specimens evaluated by HBME-1, Gal-3, and p27 ICC, sensitivity was high (100%); however, specificity was again limited (86%). Colocalization of both Gal-3 and HBME-1 in the same cell was seen in 86% of the histologic malignancies and, when present, was 100% predictive of thyroid cancer [20]. Limitations of ICC include the higher cost incurred with the use of additional markers and variability in interpretation of immunostaining results. In addition, accurate results are reliant on obtaining enough cells by FNA alone, and some of the tests have been optimized on formalin-fixed, paraffin-embedded preparations that are not the current standard method for cytology smears used for routine diagnosis.

MICRORNA EXPRESSION ANALYSIS

MiRNAs are small, noncoding, single-strand RNAs that can regulate gene expression. Dysregulation of miRNA has been associated with a number of human malignancies, such as breast cancer and melanoma [21]. Differential miRNA expression can be seen in thyroid malignancies, is predictive of specific histologic subtypes, may vary by tumor aggressiveness, and can usually be detected in FNAB specimens. miRNA analysis of thyroid lesions was evaluated by Nikiforova et al. by initial screening of 62 benign and malignant thyroid lesions with an assay of 158 human miRNAs, and differential expression patterns were observed according to histology [22]. Furthermore, different patterns were present among histologic subtypes and in tumors with different oncogenic mutations. When 13 FNAB specimens were evaluated using a panel of seven selected miR-NAs (miR-187, -221, -222, -146b, -155, -224, and -197) and expression patterns correlated to histology, upregulation of three or more miRNAs was predictive of malignancy with 100% specificity, 88% sensitivity, and 98% accuracy [22]. MiRNA expression that could further augment diagnostic FNAB analysis has been further explored in three studies, and the accuracy ranges from 85% to 90%. Each of the studies (including the initial study by Nikiforova et al.) used a different miRNA panel, although miR-146b, -221, and -222 were evaluated in two of the three studies [23–25].

Identification of the specific miRNA expression patterns has been evaluated recently in FVPTC and FTC, the two histologies most often associated with indeterminate FNAB results. Dysregulation of miR-885-5p, -221, and -574-3p was identified in conventional and oncocytic FTC compared with normal thyroid tissue, and in a preliminary series of 19 FNAB specimens, analysis of these miRNAs was able to diagnose FTC with 100% accuracy [26]. In another study of miRNA expression patterns using microarray analysis, FVPTC compared with classic PTC was characterized by dysregulation of miR-125a, -3p, -1271, and -153 [27].

Thus far, miRNA analysis shows some promise in improving preoperative diagnostic discrimination, but whether these markers will readily translate into cost-effective and routine use still remains to be seen in larger multi-institutional and prospective studies.

MULTIGENE EXPRESSION PANELS

Identifying characteristic gene expression patterns has been another molecular testing modality used to differentiate malignant from benign nodules. In one approach that focused predominantly on the use of gene expression patterns as a diagnostic adjunct, >240,000 gene and exon transcripts were screened in 178 thyroid samples. The variable expression of 167 genes was then identified as most likely to be associated with histologically benign nodules. Only 24 indeterminate FNAB samples were included in the initial validation cohort, and an observed sensitivity of 100% and specificity of 73% were reported [28]. The performance of the commercially available gene expression classifier (GEC) was further analyzed in a study of 265 nodules with indeterminate FNAB cytology results and histology [29]. The overall rate of histologic malignancy was 32%, and the panel had a specificity of 52%, PPV 47%, sensitivity 92%, and NPV 93%. In nodules with AUS/FLUS and FN cytology results, the NPVs were 95% and 94%, respectively. Thus, negative GEC panel results decreased but did not completely eliminate the cancer risk. Furthermore, the malignancy risk with GEC-benign results was not equivalent to an FNAB with benign cytology, which was 3.7% in the previously discussed meta-analysis [7].

The GEC panel had false-negative results for 7/85 (8%) malignancies; four were papillary (size range 0.6–1.2 cm), two were FVPTC (size range 1–3 cm), and most concerning, one was a 3.5 cm oncocytic carcinoma [29]. For nodules with suspicious cytology, the GEC was not reliable, as the NPV of 85% was not high enough to exclude the possibility of cancer. Another limitation of GEC testing is that the overall high false-positive rate of 53% prevented use of GEC results to indicate the possible need for initial total thyroidectomy [29]. Furthermore, lesions with oncocytic features have been a source of both false-positive and false-negative GEC testing. In a study of 132 FNABs with indeterminate cytology and GEC testing, the PPV for cytology that was classified as FN with oncocytic features was only 15%, and significantly lower than the 53% PPV for cytology classified as FN [30].

The cytology specimen for the GEC test is typically collected by the ordering clinician and classified into one of the Bethesda categories by a selected commercial cytopathology group. The quality data, including cancer prevalence in each Bethesda category for this cytopathology group, are not known [31], and only a limited number of academic

Table 12.3 Performance of common molecular tests of indeterminate FNAB results

Reference	Test	Specimens with histology evaluated, n	Sensitivity	Specificity	NPV	PPV	Malignancy rate	Missed cancers
29	GEC	265	92	52	93	47	32	HCC, FVPTC, PTC
32	GEC	36	83	10	75	16	17	FTC
33	GEC	35	94	24	80	57	51	PTC
39	7GMT	513	61	98	89	89	24	FVPTC, PTC, FTC
63	7GMT	53	44	89	64	79	47	FVPTC, PTC
68	NGS[a]	143	90	93	96	83	27	FVTPC, PTC, FTC

Note: 7GMT, seven-gene mutation testing; HCC, Hurthle cell carcinoma.
[a] Included results in the FN category only.

centers are allowed to use in-house cytopathologists that are not part of the selected commercial group. The GEC assay is then performed only on cytology results that are either AUS/FLUS or FN, and reported as either GEC benign or GEC suspicious.

Two recent reports that independently evaluated GEC use in single-center studies highlighted the importance of cancer prevalence on derivation of NPV and PPV [32,33]. Harrell et al. evaluated 35 patients with indeterminate cytology, histology, and GEC results, and observed a high cancer rate of 51%. Although the calculated sensitivity was 94% and similar to the previously published sensitivity rate, the high malignancy rate in their series resulted in a lower than expected NPV of 80% [33]. Utilizing in-house cytology and pathology for interpretation of their specimens, McIver et al. analyzed 36 FNAB specimens with indeterminate cytology, histology, and GEC results. In contrast to the previous study, the cancer incidence was quite low at 17%, and test sensitivity and specificity were 83% and 10%, respectively. Because of the lower pretest probability of malignancy and diminished sensitivities and specificities, significant decreases in NPV (75%) and PPV (16%) were observed [32]. Thus, the interpretation of GEC results should ideally take into account institutional and geographical cancer prevalence for each cytology category, and the clinical application should be modified accordingly (Table 12.3).

GENETIC MUTATIONS AND REARRANGEMENTS

Gene mutations and rearrangements commonly associated with thyroid cancer can be detected in both FNAB and histology specimens. The most frequent gene alterations affect the MAPK and PI3K-AKT pathways, which have both been implicated in thyroid carcinogenesis. Activating mutations in both of these pathways have been shown to lead to upregulation of genes that regulate cellular proliferation, differentiation, and survival [10]. Mutations may often also correspond to histologic subtype, providing additional preoperative risk stratification (Table 12.4) [9–11,34]. For example, FTCs are more likely to have mutations in the RAS and PTEN genes, while conventional PTCs are more likely

Table 12.4 Gene alterations associated with thyroid cancer

Histology	Mutations
Papillary thyroid cancer	
Conventional	BRAF V600E
	H-, K-, or N-RAS (occasional)
	PTEN mutation
	RET fusions (including RET/PTC)
	BRAF fusions
Follicular variant	H-, K-, or N-RAS
	BRAF K601E
	TSHR
	EIF1AX
	PAX8/PPARγ
	RET/PTC (rare)
Tall cell variant	BRAF V6000E
Follicular thyroid cancer	RAS
	PTEN deletion or mutation
	PIK3-CA
	TSHR
	PAX8/PPARγ
Poorly differentiated thyroid cancer	BRAF V600E
	p53
	RAS
	CTNNB1
	PIK3CA
Anaplastic thyroid cancer	p53
	CTNNB1
	AKT1
	PIK3CA
	RAS
	BRAF V600E
	PTEN mutation
	ALK rearrangements
Medullary thyroid cancer, sporadic	H- or K-RAS
	RET mutations (M918T)

to have the *BRAF* V600E mutation or *RET/PTC* rearrangements. Interestingly, FVPTC has morphologic features that are usually consistent with PTC, but has biologic behavior that may be more similar to FTC, and shares gene alterations with both histologic types.

As mentioned previously, *BRAF* V600E is the most common gene alteration in thyroid cancer. When identified in preoperative biopsy specimens, *BRAF* V600E has greater than 99% PPV for PTC. The presence of *BRAF* V600E has also been associated with aggressive histologic PTC features, including tall cell variant subtype, extrathyroidal extension, lymph node metastasis, recurrence, and disease-specific mortality [11,35]. The additional prognostic information gained from preoperative *BRAF* V600E testing may help direct surgical management, such as whether to perform prophylactic central compartment lymph node dissection, but this is controversial [36]. The second most common *BRAF* mutation detected in thyroid cancer, *BRAF* K601E, is associated with PTCs that typically have more indolent features despite the fact that the mutation involves the same exon. In a study evaluating characteristics of 120 *BRAF*-positive indeterminate FNAB results, *BRAF* K601E was detected in ~50% of the results categorized as either AUS/FLUS or FN, and the majority were histologic FVPTC [37].

RAS has a key role in signal transduction, from tyrosine kinase and G protein-coupled receptors to effectors of both the MAPK and PI3K-AKT pathways. Point mutations cause increased affinity of *RAS* to guanosine triphosphate (GTP) or inhibit the autocatalytic GTP-ase function, and both cause constitutive activation of downstream pathways [38]. In indeterminate FNAB specimens, *RAS* mutations are the most common gene alterations identified and can include point mutations in the *N-*, *K-*, and *H-RAS* hotspots in codons 12/13 and 61 [39]. All three mutant isoforms have been identified in up to 48% of benign follicular adenomas, 50%–60% of FTCs, and 20% in PTCs [38]. In one recent study that included 63 FNAB specimens, the preoperative detection of *RAS* in FNAB cytology had an 80%–85% risk of malignancy and was most frequently associated with histologic FVPTC (90%) [40]. Bilateral multifocal disease was diagnosed in 50%, and lymph node metastasis was rare. The majority of *RAS*-associated thyroid cancers are indolent; however, *RAS* mutations have also been identified in medullary thyroid, poorly differentiated, and anaplastic thyroid cancers. Although 15%–20% of *RAS*-positive biopsies are histologically benign follicular adenoma (FA), these are still likely to be lesions with malignant potential [11,41].

RET rearrangements in PTC have been well documented, and more than 10 different types of translocations have been described that are identified in 10%–20% of PTC [42,43]. A ligand-independent dimerization and constitutive activation of effector genes in both the MAPK and PI3-AKT pathways results when the 3′ tyrosine kinase portion of the *RET* gene fuses with the 5′ portion of a different gene. The two most common fusion rearrangements are *RET/PTC1* and *RET/PTC3*, which are paracentric versions

with the 5′ domain of two genes on chromosome 10: *CCDC6* and *NCOA4*, respectively [42]. A higher incidence of *RET/PTC* rearrangements is seen in PTC patients with a previous history of radiation exposure (50%–80%) and in younger patients (40%–70%) [44–46]. *RET/PTC1*-positive tumors demonstrate either classic papillary architecture or diffuse sclerosing features, and *RET/PTC3* is associated with solid-variant PTC. All of the *RET/PTC* tumor subtypes have a higher rate of lymph node metastases [47]. In an evaluation of temporal changes in molecular profiles of thyroid cancers, the proportion of *RET/PTC*-positive PTC has diminished over time, suggesting that exposure to ionizing radiation has a decreasing contribution to thyroid carcinogenesis [48].

A gene rearrangement leading to the fusion of the thyroid-specific paired domain transcription factor, *PAX8*, and the peroxisome proliferator-activated receptor gene, *PPARγ*, which plays an important role in lipid metabolism, was discovered in FTC in 2000 [49]. The *PAX8/PPARγ* rearrangement results in overexpression of the fusion protein, but the carcinogenic mechanism of action is still unclear. *PAX8* plays an essential role in thyrocyte development, as well as in the differential gene expression of the sodium iodide symporter, thyroglobulin, and the TSH receptor [50]. The fusion protein antagonizes the action of *PPARγ* via a dominant-negative inhibition that has been shown to be a potential causative agent in FTC tumorigenesis [51]. *PAX8/PPARγ* translocation is found in 30%–40% of classic FTCs, 2%–10% of FAs, and in FVPTC [52,53]. Similar to *RAS*-positive FAs, *PAX8/PPARγ*-positive FA may actually represent carcinomas *in situ*. *PAX8/PPARγ*-positive FTCs tend to occur in younger patients with tumor characteristics that have solid patterns and vascular invasion [52].

Diagnostic utility of single-gene testing

Studies that have evaluated preoperative FNAB testing for *BRAF* V600E only have produced variable results. In a study of 814 patients with 966 FNABs who all had *BRAF* V600E mutation analysis, 17 (1.8%) of the FNABs were positive for *BRAF* V600E [54]. All 17 had PTC in the biopsied nodule, even though five FNABs had cytology that was classified as benign and five classified as FN. Overall, *BRAF* V600E detection increased the sensitivity of preoperative testing for thyroid cancer from 50% to 67% [54]. The improvement in diagnostic sensitivity with *BRAF* V600E cytology testing has also been reported by others [55,56], but it has been refuted in other studies. For example, in a study of 960 patients with indeterminate FNAB cytology, only 13 (1.4%) were *BRAF* V600E positive [57]. Furthermore, 11 of the *BRAF* V600E-positive FNABs had cytology that was also suspicious for malignancy and total thyroidectomy was already indicated. Therefore, the authors concluded that preoperative *BRAF* V600E testing did not provide additional diagnostic information to justify its routine use in cytologically indeterminate nodules [57]. The added utility of *BRAF* V600E testing likely depends on regional incidence and histologic subtype of malignancies that are characteristically missed when cytology is interpreted as inadequate or benign.

Mutation testing for one of the three *RAS* isoforms has not typically been used in single-gene diagnostic tests; however, *RAS* is the most frequently detected mutation when cytology is AUS/FLUS or FN [39]. *NRAS* 61 is the most common *RAS* point mutation detected and is associated with a 75%–88% risk of histologic malignancy. The most common subtype is FVPTC, although PTC, FTC, and poorly differentiated thyroid cancer can also be *NRAS* 61 positive. *HRAS* 61 and *KRAS* 12/13 are associated with variable risks of malignancy that range from 56% to 96% and 40% to 100%, respectively [58,59]. The reported differences likely are due to interobserver variability in diagnosing follicular-patterned neoplasms, as well as regional variances in the contribution of *RAS* positivity on thyroid malignancy [60]. Medullary thyroid cancer can be *HRAS* 61 or *KRAS* 12/13 positive and should be considered in the differential when one of these mutations is detected.

Diagnostic utility of 7-gene MT

Because of the number of gene alterations involved in thyroid carcinogenesis, testing for a panel of mutations instead of for a single gene improves the sensitivity for thyroid cancer detection. In the first two studies that evaluated gene testing of indeterminate cytology specimens by Cantara et al. and Nikiforov et al., a mutation was identified in 45% and 29%, respectively. These studies included biopsies classified in the suspicious category, and molecular testing added diagnostic sensitivity and accuracy [61,62]. Nikiforov et al. reported results from an independent and consecutive cohort of 513 indeterminate FNAB specimens that had prospective mutation testing for *BRAF*, *RAS* mutations, and *PAX8/PPARγ* and *RET/PTC1* and *3* rearrangements (seven-gene mutation testing [7-gene MT]) with cytologic and histologic correlation. The cancer rate was 24%, and false-positive mutation testing results occurred in 11% [39]. *RAS* positivity was the primary source of false-positive testing results. When *BRAF*, *RET/PTC1* or *3*, or *PAX8/PPARγ* was detected preoperatively, the risk of malignancy was 100% regardless of cytology category. For all indeterminate FNAB results, 7-gene MT had specificity 98%, PPV 89%, sensitivity 61%, and NPV 89% (Table 12.3) [39]. The high PPV and specificity allowed appropriate stratification into those FNAB results that carry a high risk of cancer, and can be used to direct the appropriate extent of initial thyroidectomy or lymphadenectomy.

The high diagnostic specificity of 7-gene MT was recently verified in an industry-sponsored multi-institutional non-interventional study using in-house pathologists who were blinded to 7-gene MT results [63]. A total of 53 patients had indeterminate FNAB results, 7-gene MT, and histology. The malignancy rate was 47%, and the test sensitivity and specificity were 44% and 89%, respectively. The most commonly missed malignancy was FVPTC (Table 12.3).

The cost outcomes of adding prospective 7-gene MT have been modeled in hypothetical decision tree analysis, which showed that added costs of preoperative mutation testing were offset by reductions in the number of necessary two-stage thyroidectomies [64]. Furthermore, in a study of patient outcomes after incorporation of an institutional algorithm for prospective 7-gene MT, when preoperative mutation testing was routinely performed for FNAB results classified as AUS/FLUS or FN, a 2.5-fold reduction in two-stage thyroidectomy for clinically significant thyroid cancer ($p < 0.001$) was observed [65].

Although the risk of malignancy is lower when 7-gene MT results are negative, the risk is not low enough to reliably exclude the possibility of malignancy. Indeterminate cytology biopsy results with negative 7-gene MT results are still associated with an overall 11% risk of cancer, but this varies by cytology category. 7-Gene MT negative cytology results should therefore be conventionally managed with either repeat FNAB or surgery, as indicated (Figure 12.1).

Diagnostic utility of high-throughput sequencing techniques

New techniques, such as next-generation sequencing (NGS) technology, will likely allow for cost-effective and sensitive screening of multiple gene alterations, and have already

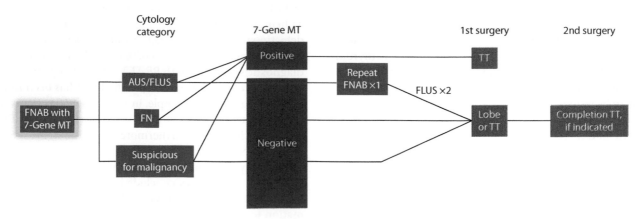

Figure 12.1 Proposed algorithm for the management of indeterminate cytology results when 7-Gene MT is used. TT, total thyroidectomy; Lobe, lobectomy.

been investigated for mutations that are thyroid specific. Accurate testing is observed using either paraffin-embedded or FNAB samples with acceptable concordance to conventional Sanger sequencing methods [66]. Using the Ion Torrent platform and an expanded 12-gene panel that is inclusive of 284 mutational hotspots, Nikiforova et al. were able to detect mutations in genes such as *TSHR*, *PIK3CA*, and *p53* [67]. Two of 27 conventional PTCs had coexistent *BRAF* V600E with *p53* or *PIK3CA* mutations, which are typically more characteristic of aggressive thyroid cancers. The identification of more than one driver mutation may provide preoperative prognostic information that may beneficially guide surgical management [11,67].

The utility of NGS testing on a series of FNAB classified as FN and inclusive of 91 patients studied retrospectively and 52 patients studied prospectively was reported by Nikiforov et al. [68]. The testing incorporated the previously described 12-gene panel and added evaluation for *TERT* hotspots (C228T and C250T), and an RNA panel that tested for 38 types of *RET* fusion genes in addition to eight genes used to characterize the types of cells in the biopsy specimen (e.g., thyroid follicular, C-, nonthyroidal epithelial, and parathyroid cells). All patients had surgical histology, and the overall malignancy rate was 27%. The performance parameters of NGS testing using this thyroid-specific marker panel were 90% sensitivity, 93% specificity, 83% PPV, and 96% NPV (Table 12.3) [68]. If these performance parameters are validated in ongoing multi-institutional studies, then this testing methodology appears to provide both the high sensitivity and specificity needed to optimally risk-stratify nodules with indeterminate FNAB results into observation versus surgical treatment.

Molecular testing in pediatric patients

The incidence of thyroid nodules in pediatric patients (age < 21 years) is 0.5%–2%, and the likelihood of malignancy is higher [69]. *RET/PTC* rearrangements have been reported to be more prevalent in the pediatric population, while *BRAF* V600E has a lower prevalence. In a series of 66 FNAB results in pediatric patients that also had 7-gene MT, *RAS* and *RET/PTC1* were the most common molecular alterations identified. Overall, the rate of thyroid cancer in the study cohort was 35% and the majority of malignancies (95%) were PTC [70]. All nodules that were mutation positive were histologic malignancies. However, in a subset of nodules that had both negative mutation testing and histology, 49% were malignant and there was a false-negative rate that was much higher than reported in the adult population. The molecular mechanisms leading to pediatric thyroid cancer are likely distinct from the mechanisms that lead to adult-onset thyroid cancer, and thus 7-gene MT testing may have decreased utility in the pediatric population. The expanded molecular panel via NGS testing includes a wider range of genetic rearrangements, which may help improve the diagnostic accuracy in pediatric thyroid nodules.

SUMMARY

Molecular testing of thyroid nodules can be used successfully as a diagnostic adjunct, particularly in nodules with indeterminate FNAB cytology results. Tests with high specificity are already available that can help direct the initial extent of surgery, and NGS-based testing may eventually provide high sensitivity to allow reliable nonoperative management options. The correlation of somatic genetic alteration to type of thyroid cancer provides added prognostic significance that may allow further optimization of preoperative clinical decision making.

REFERENCES

1. Davies L, Welch HG. Increasing incidence of thyroid cancer in the United States, 1973–2002. *JAMA* 2006;295(18):2164–7.
2. Chen AY, Jemal A, Ward EM. Increasing incidence of differentiated thyroid cancer in the United States, 1988–2005. *Cancer* 2009;115(16):3801–7.
3. Aschebrook-Kilfoy B, Kaplan EL, Chiu BC, Angelos P, Grogan RH. The acceleration in papillary thyroid cancer incidence rates is similar among racial and ethnic groups in the United States. *Ann Surg Oncol* 2013;20(8):2746–53.
4. Guth S, Theune U, Aberle J, Galach A, Bamberger CM. Very high prevalence of thyroid nodules detected by high frequency (13 MHz) ultrasound examination. *Eur J Clin* 2009;39(8):699–706.
5. American Thyroid Association Guidelines Taskforce on Thyroid N, Differentiated Thyroid C, Cooper DS, Doherty GM et al. Revised American Thyroid Association management guidelines for patients with thyroid nodules and differentiated thyroid cancer. *Thyroid* 2009;19(11):1167–214.
6. Baloch ZW, LiVolsi VA, Asa SL et al. Diagnostic terminology and morphologic criteria for cytologic diagnosis of thyroid lesions: A synopsis of the National Cancer Institute Thyroid Fine-Needle Aspiration State of the Science Conference. *Diagn Cytopathol* 2008;36(6):425–37.
7. Bongiovanni M, Spitale A, Faquin WC, Mazzucchelli L, Baloch ZW. The Bethesda System for Reporting Thyroid Cytopathology: A meta-analysis. *Acta Cytol* 2012;56(4):333–9.
8. Cap J, Ryska A, Rehorkova P, Hovorkova E, Kerekes Z, Pohnetalova D. Sensitivity and specificity of the fine needle aspiration biopsy of the thyroid: Clinical point of view. *Clin Endocrinol* 1999;51(4):509–15.
9. Cancer Genome Atlas Research N. Integrated genomic characterization of papillary thyroid carcinoma. *Cell* 2014;159(3):676–90.
10. Xing M. Molecular pathogenesis and mechanisms of thyroid cancer. *Nat Rev Cancer* 2013;13(3):184–99.

11. Nikiforov YE, Nikiforova MN. Molecular genetics and diagnosis of thyroid cancer. *Nat Rev Endocrinol* 2011;7(10):569–80.

12. Ito Y, Miyauchi A, Inoue H et al. An observational trial for papillary thyroid microcarcinoma in Japanese patients. *World J Surg* 2010;34(1):28–35.

13. Sosa JA, Hanna JW, Robinson KA, Lanman RB. Increases in thyroid nodule fine-needle aspirations, operations, and diagnoses of thyroid cancer in the United States. *Surgery* 2013;154(6):1420–6; discussion 1426–7.

14. Milas M, Shin J, Gupta M et al. Circulating thyrotro-pin receptor mRNA as a novel marker of thyroid cancer: Clinical applications learned from 1758 samples. *Ann Surg* 2010;252(4):643–51.

15. Chia SY, Milas M, Reddy SK et al. Thyroid-stimulating hormone receptor messenger ribonucleic acid measurement in blood as a marker for circulating thyroid cancer cells and its role in the preoperative diagnosis of thyroid cancer. *J Clin Endocrinol Metab* 2007;92(2):468–75.

16. Pupilli C, Pinzani P, Salvianti F et al. Circulating BRAFV600E in the diagnosis and follow-up of differentiated papillary thyroid carcinoma. *J Clin Endocrinol Metab* 2013;98(8):3359–65.

17. de Matos LL, Del Giglio AB, Matsubayashi CO, de Lima Farah M, Del Giglio A, da Silva Pinhal MA. Expression of CK-19, galectin-3 and HBME-1 in the differentiation of thyroid lesions: Systematic review and diagnostic meta-analysis. *Diagn Pathol* 2012;7:97.

18. Bartolazzi A, Orlandi F, Saggiorato E et al. Galectin-3-expression analysis in the surgical selection of follicular thyroid nodules with indeterminate fine-needle aspiration cytology: A prospective multicentre study. *Lancet Oncol* 2008;9(6):543–9.

19. Cochand-Priollet B, Dahan H, Laloi-Michelin M et al. Immunocytochemistry with cytokeratin 19 and anti-human mesothelial cell antibody (HBME1) increases the diagnostic accuracy of thyroid fine-needle aspirations: Preliminary report of 150 liquid-based fine-needle aspirations with histological control. *Thyroid* 2011;21(10):1067–73.

20. Zhang L, Krausz T, DeMay RM. A pilot study of galectin-3, HBME-1, and p27 triple immunostaining pattern for diagnosis of indeterminate thyroid nodules in cytology with correlation to histology. *Appl Immunohistochem Mol Morphol* 2015;23:481–90.

21. Mazeh H. MicroRNA as a diagnostic tool in fine-needle aspiration biopsy of thyroid nodules. *Oncologist* 2012;17(8):1032–8.

22. Nikiforova MN, Tseng GC, Steward D, Diorio D, Nikiforov YE. MicroRNA expression profiling of thyroid tumors: Biological significance and diagnostic utility. *J Clin Endocrinol Metab* 2008;93(5):1600–8.

23. Shen R, Liyanarachchi S, Li W et al. MicroRNA signature in thyroid fine needle aspiration cytology applied to "atypia of undetermined significance" cases. *Thyroid* 2012;22(1):9–16.

24. Keutgen XM, Filicori F, Crowley MJ et al. A panel of four miRNAs accurately differentiates malignant from benign indeterminate thyroid lesions on fine needle aspiration. *Clin Cancer Res* 2012;18(7):2032–8.

25. Mazeh H, Levy Y, Mizrahi I et al. Differentiating benign from malignant thyroid nodules using micro ribonucleic acid amplification in residual cells obtained by fine needle aspiration biopsy. *J Surg Res* 2013;180(2):216–21.

26. Dettmer M, Vogetseder A, Durso MB et al. MicroRNA expression array identifies novel diagnostic markers for conventional and oncocytic follicular thyroid carcinomas. *J Clin Endocrinol Metab* 2013;98(1):E1–7.

27. Dettmer MS, Perren A, Moch H, Komminoth P, Nikiforov YE, Nikiforova MN. Comprehensive microRNA expression profiling identifies novel markers in follicular variant of papillary thyroid carcinoma. *Thyroid* 2013;23:1383–9.

28. Chudova D, Wilde JI, Wang ET et al. Molecular classification of thyroid nodules using high-dimensionality genomic data. *J Clin Endocrinol Metab* 2010;95(12):5296–304.

29. Alexander EK, Kennedy GC, Baloch ZW et al. Preoperative diagnosis of benign thyroid nodules with indeterminate cytology. *N Engl J Med* 2012;367(8):705–15.

30. Lastra RR, Pramick MR, Crammer CJ, LiVolsi VA, Baloch ZW. Implications of a suspicious Afirma test result in thyroid fine-needle aspiration cytology: An institutional experience. *Cancer Cytopathol* 2014;122(10):737–44.

31. Krane JF. Lessons from early clinical experience with the Afirma gene expression classifier. *Cancer Cytopathol* 2014;122(10):715–9.

32. McIver B, Castro MR, Morris JC et al. An independent study of a gene expression classifier (Afirma) in the evaluation of cytologically indeterminate thyroid nodules. *J Clin Endocrinol Metab* 2014;99:4069–77.

33. Harrell RM, Bimston DN. Surgical utility of Afirma: Effects of high cancer prevalence and oncocytic cell types in patients with indeterminate thyroid cytology. *Endocr Practice:* 2014;20(4):364–9.

34. Romei C, Elisei R. RET/PTC translocations and clinico-pathological features in human papillary thyroid carcinoma. *Front Endocrinol* 2012;3:54.

35. Xing M, Alzahrani AS, Carson KA et al. Association between BRAF V600E mutation and mortality in patients with papillary thyroid cancer. *JAMA* 2013;309(14):1493–501.

36. Howell GM, Nikiforova MN, Carty SE et al. BRAF V600E mutation independently predicts central compartment lymph node metastasis in patients with papillary thyroid cancer. *Ann Surg Oncol* 2013;20(1):47–52.

37. Ohori NP, Singhal R, Nikiforova MN et al. BRAF mutation detection in indeterminate thyroid cytology specimens: Underlying cytologic, molecular, and pathologic characteristics of papillary thyroid carcinoma. *Cancer Cytopathol* 2013;121(4):197–205.

38. Howell GM, Hodak SP, Yip L. RAS mutations in thyroid cancer. *Oncologist* 2013;18(8):926–32.

39. Nikiforov YE, Ohori NP, Hodak SP et al. Impact of mutational testing on the diagnosis and management of patients with cytologically indeterminate thyroid nodules: A prospective analysis of 1056 FNA samples. *J Clin Endocrinol Metab* 2011;96(11):3390–7.

40. Gupta N, Dasyam AK, Carty SE et al. RAS mutations in thyroid FNA specimens are highly predictive of predominantly low-risk follicular-pattern cancers. *J Clin Endocrinol Metab* 2013;98:E914–22.

41. Fukahori M, Yoshida A, Hayashi H et al. The associations between RAS mutations and clinical characteristics in follicular thyroid tumors: New insights from a single center and a large patient cohort. *Thyroid* 2012;22(7):683–9.

42. Tallini G, Asa SL. RET oncogene activation in papillary thyroid carcinoma. *Adv Anat Pathol* 2001;8(6):345–54.

43. Nikiforov YE. RET/PTC rearrangement in thyroid tumors. *Endocr Pathol* 2002;13:3–16.

44. Nikiforov YE, Rowland JM, Bove KE, Monforte-Munoz H, Fagin JA. Distinct pattern of ret oncogene rearrangements in morphological variants of radiation-induced and sporadic thyroid papillary carcinomas in children. *Cancer Res* 1997;57(9):1690–4.

45. Rabes HM, Demidchik EP, Sidorow JD et al. Pattern of radiation-induced RET and NTRK1 rearrangements in 191 post-Chernobyl papillary thyroid carcinomas: Biological, phenotypic, and clinical implications. *Clin Cancer Res* 2000;6(3):1093–103.

46. Fenton CL, Lukes Y, Nicholson D, Dinauer CA, Francis GL, Tuttle RM. The ret/PTC mutations are common in sporadic papillary thyroid carcinoma of children and young adults. *J Clin Endocrinol Metab* 2000;85(3):1170–5.

47. Adeniran AJ, Zhu Z, Gandhi M et al. Correlation between genetic alterations and microscopic features, clinical manifestations, and prognostic characteristics of thyroid papillary carcinomas. *Am J Surg Pathol* 2006;30(2):216–22.

48. Jung CK, Little MP, Lubin JH et al. The increase in thyroid cancer incidence during the last four decades is accompanied by a high frequency of BRAF mutations and a sharp increase in RAS mutations. *J Clin Endocrinol Metab* 2014;99(2):E276–85.

49. Kroll TG, Sarraf P, Pecciarini L et al. PAX8-PPARgamma1 fusion oncogene in human thyroid carcinoma [corrected]. *Science* 2000;289(5483):1357–60.

50. Eberhardt NL, Grebe SK, McIver B, Reddi HV. The role of the PAX8/PPARgamma fusion oncogene in the pathogenesis of follicular thyroid cancer. *Mol Cell Endocrinol* 2010;321(1):50–6.

51. McIver B, Grebe SK, Eberhardt NL. The PAX8/PPAR gamma fusion oncogene as a potential therapeutic target in follicular thyroid carcinoma. *Curr Drug Targets Immune Endocr Metab Disord* 2004;4(3):221–34.

52. Nikiforova MN, Lynch RA, Biddinger PW et al. RAS point mutations and PAX8-PPAR gamma rearrangement in thyroid tumors: evidence for distinct molecular pathways in thyroid follicular carcinoma. *J Clin Endocrinol Metab* 2003;88(5):2318–26.

53. Armstrong MJ, Huaitao Y, Yip L et al. PAX8/PPARgamma rearrangement in thyroid nodules predicts follicular-pattern carcinomas, in particular the encapsulated follicular variant of papillary carcinoma. *Thyroid* 2014;24:1369–74.

54. Canadas-Garre M, Becerra-Massare P, Lopez de la Torre-Casares M et al. Reduction of false-negative papillary thyroid carcinomas by the routine analysis of BRAF(T1799A) mutation on fine-needle aspiration biopsy specimens: A prospective study of 814 thyroid FNAB patients. *Ann Surg* 2012;255(5):986–92.

55. Johnson SJ, Hardy SA, Roberts C, Bourn D, Mallick U, Perros P. Pilot of BRAF mutation analysis in indeterminate, suspicious and malignant thyroid FNA cytology. *Cytopathology* 2014;25(3):146–54.

56. Kim SW, Lee JI, Kim JW et al. BRAFV600E mutation analysis in fine-needle aspiration cytology specimens for evaluation of thyroid nodule: A large series in a BRAFV600E-prevalent population. *J Clin Endocrinol Metab* 2010;95(8):3693–700.

57. Kleiman DA, Sporn MJ, Beninato T et al. Preoperative BRAF(V600E) mutation screening is unlikely to alter initial surgical treatment of patients with indeterminate thyroid nodules: A prospective case series of 960 patients. *Cancer* 2013;119(8):1495–502.

58. Radkay LA, Chiosea SI, Seethala RR et al. Thyroid nodules with KRAS mutations are different from nodules with NRAS and HRAS mutations with regard to cytopathologic and histopathologic outcome characteristics. *Cancer Cytopathol* 2014;122(12):873–82.

59. Vasko V, Ferrand M, Di Cristofaro J, Carayon P, Henry JF, de Micco C. Specific pattern of RAS oncogene mutations in follicular thyroid tumors. *J Clin Endocrinol Metab* 2003;88(6):2745–52.

60. Elsheikh TM, Asa SL, Chan JK et al. Interobserver and intraobserver variation among experts in the diagnosis of thyroid follicular lesions with borderline nuclear features of papillary carcinoma. *Am J Clin Pathol* 2008;130(5):736–44.

61. Cantara S, Capezzone M, Marchisotta S et al. Impact of proto-oncogene mutation detection in cytological specimens from thyroid nodules improves the diagnostic accuracy of cytology. *J Clin Endocrinol Metab* 2010;95(3):1365–9.

62. Nikiforov YE, Steward DL, Robinson-Smith TM et al. Molecular testing for mutations in improving the fine-needle aspiration diagnosis of thyroid nodules. *J Clin Endocrinol Metab* 2009;94(6):2092–8.

63. Beaudenon-Huibregtse S, Alexander EK, Guttler RB et al. Centralized molecular testing for oncogenic gene mutations complements the local cytopathological diagnosis of thyroid nodules. *Thyroid* 2014;24:1479–87.

64. Yip L, Farris C, Kabaker AS et al. Cost impact of molecular testing for indeterminate thyroid nodule fine-needle aspiration biopsies. *J Clin Endocrinol Metab* 2012;97(6):1905–12.

65. Yip L, Wharry L, Armstrong MJ et al. A clinical algorithm for fine-needle aspiration molecular testing effectively guides the appropriate extent of initial thyroidectomy. *Ann Surg* 2014;260:163–8.

66. Hadd AG, Houghton J, Choudhary A et al. Targeted, high-depth, next-generation sequencing of cancer genes in formalin-fixed, paraffin-embedded and fine-needle aspiration tumor specimens. *J Mol Diagn* 2013;15(2):234–47.

67. Nikiforova MN, Wald AI, Roy S, Durso MB, Nikiforov YE. Targeted next-generation sequencing panel (ThyroSeq) for detection of mutations in thyroid cancer. *J Clin Endocrinol Metab* 2013;98(11):E1852–60.

68. Nikiforov YE, Carty SE, Chiosea SI et al. Highly accurate diagnosis of cancer in thyroid nodules with follicular neoplasm/suspicious for a follicular neoplasm cytology by ThyroSeq v2 next-generation sequencing assay. *Cancer* 2014;120(23):3627–34.

69. Niedziela M. Pathogenesis, diagnosis and management of thyroid nodules in children. *Endocr Relat Cancer* 2006;13(2):427–53.

70. Buryk MA, Monaco SE, Witchel SF et al. Preoperative cytology with molecular analysis to help guide surgery for pediatric thyroid nodules. *Int J Pediatr Otorhinolaryngol* 2013;77(10):1697–700.

13

Surgery for well-differentiated thyroid cancer

KELLY L. MCCOY AND SALLY E. CARTY

SURGICAL ANATOMY AND PHYSIOLOGY

The thyroid gland lies in the central neck draped over the anterior trachea, with the isthmus sitting below the cricoid cartilage at the level of the second to fourth tracheal rings. The gland is covered by pretracheal fascia, and moves upward with deglutition. The tubercle of Zuckerkandl is a bilateral posterior tissue projection that lies over the laryngeal insertion of the recurrent laryngeal nerve (RLN) and can aid in identification of the RLN during surgery [1]. Behind the tubercle, a thick fibrous band, termed the ligament of Berry, attaches the medial lobe to the trachea. The thyroid gland typically weighs 20–25 g, but its shape and weight vary widely in adults. The anatomy of the thyroid, parathyroid glands, and RLN is depicted in Figure 13.1.

Primary arterial flow to the thyroid is via paired superior and inferior thyroid arteries. On the right and left, the superior thyroid artery descends as the first branch of the external carotid artery to the superior pole of each thyroid lobe, following the path of the external branch of the superior laryngeal nerve (SLN). The posterior branches of the superior thyroid artery may supply the superior parathyroid glands (15%) and are therefore important to preserve. The inferior thyroid arteries come off of the thyrocervical trunk to supply the lower thyroid poles and the inferior parathyroid glands, as well as the superior parathyroid glands in 85% of patients. The thyroid gland is also supplied uncommonly (3%) by a midline thyroidea ima artery that arises from the aortic arch or innominate artery. Anatomic variation of the three paired major thyroid veins is common. The superior and middle veins drain into the internal jugular veins, and the inferior veins into the innominate vein. The vasculature of the thyroid gland can be hypertrophied in disease states such as hyperthyroidism or goiter.

The superior and recurrent laryngeal nerves arise bilaterally from the vagi as they descend caudally [2]. The SLN divides into an internal branch that enters the thyrohyoid membrane, providing sensation to the larynx, and an external motor branch that innervates the cricothyroid muscles to affect vocal cord tension. The SLN motor branch is often referred to as the "opera singer's nerve" because division can permanently alter voice pitch [3]; to avoid this injury, careful ligation of each superior thyroid artery branch on the anterior surface of the superior thyroid capsule is recommended. Vocal cord motor function is controlled by the RLN, which innervates all laryngeal muscles except for the cricothyroid muscle and also provides sensation to the subglottic area. Coursing posterior to the subclavian artery on the right, and posterior to the aortic arch on the left, each RLN "recurs" to course cranially and then insert at the inferior edge of the thyroid cartilage. RLN anatomic variants are common (up to 25%). When the RLN branches before insertion, motor function is provided by the anterior branch [4]. A right nonrecurrent RLN occurs in <1%, extending straight to the larynx from the cervical vagus in association with a vascular malformation in which the right common carotid artery comes directly off the aortic arch and a right retroesophageal subclavian artery arises as a fourth branch of the arch with an absent innominate artery. A left nonrecurrent laryngeal nerve occurs only in the setting of situs

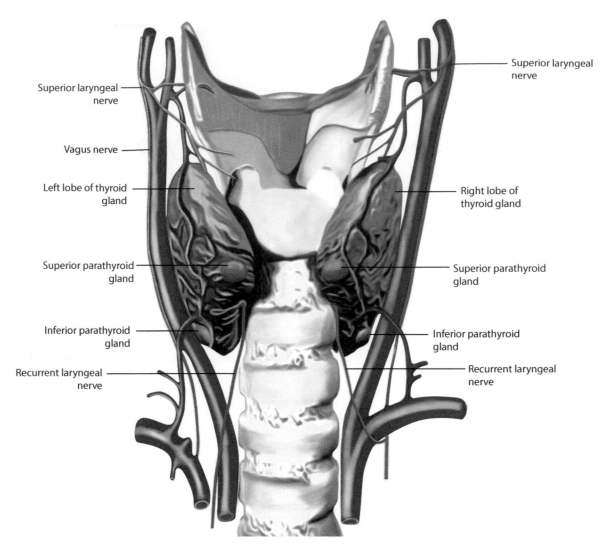

Figure 13.1 Thyroid, parathyroid, and recurrent laryngeal nerve anatomy.

inversus, with a left retroesophageal subclavian artery from a right-sided aortic arch, and is thus exceedingly rare [5].

The thyroid secretes hormones that play a critical role in metabolism, growth, and temperature regulation. Dietary iodide is taken up from the blood into thyroid follicular cells via the sodium iodine transporter and then oxidized to tyrosyl residues and incorporated into thyroxine (T4), which is bound to thyroglobulin and stored as colloid in thyroid follicles. T4 is secreted into the blood in response to thyroid-stimulating hormone (TSH) secretion by the anterior pituitary gland, which in turn is stimulated by hypothalamic thyroid-releasing hormone (TRH). T4 is converted peripherally to triiodothyronine (T3) primarily in the liver and kidney. More than 99% of peripheral T3 and T4 is bound to serum binding proteins [6].

WELL-DIFFERENTIATED THYROID CARCINOMA

Differentiated thyroid carcinoma (DTC) accounts for about 85% of thyroid cancers and carries an overall excellent prognosis. DTC is comprised of both papillary and follicular types. The incidence is steeply rising in the United States, a phenomenon that is not thought to be due solely to improved screening, and the mortality rate remains stable, while the rates for other adult tumors have decreased [7,8]. DTC is three to four times more common in women [9]. Consonant with its generally excellent outcomes, traditional staging is not useful, but certain clinical and pathologic factors do portend a higher risk of recurrence and mortality, including age of >45 years, large tumor size, extrathyroidal extension, and the presence of distant metastases. These factors are utilized in the commonly employed staging systems for DTC, which are TNM, MACIS, and the National Thyroid Cancer Treatment Cooperative Study (NTCTCS). TNM staging includes patient age, tumor size, extension beyond the thyroid capsule, lymph node status, and presence of distant metastases (Table 13.1). The MACIS score is based on metastases, patient age, completeness of resection, invasion, and tumor size [10]. NTCTCS staging includes tumor size, tumor characteristics, and the presence of metastases, as well as specific histology [11].

Table 13.1   TNM staging system for thyroid cancer

Primary tumor (T)[a]

TX	Primary tumor cannot be assessed
T0	No evidence of primary tumor
T1	Tumor 2 cm or less in greatest dimension, limited to the thyroid
T1a	Tumor 1 cm or less, limited to the thyroid
T1b	Tumor more than 1 cm but not more than 2 cm in greatest dimension, limited to the thyroid
T2	Tumor more than 2 cm but not more than 4 cm in greatest dimension, limited to the thyroid
T3	Tumor more than 4 cm in greatest dimension, limited to the thyroid, or any tumor with minimal extrathyroid extension (e.g., extension to sternothyroid muscle or perithyroid soft tissues)
T4a	Moderately advanced disease
	Tumor of any size extending beyond the thyroid capsule to invade subcutaneous soft tissues, larynx, trachea, esophagus, or RLN
T4b	Very advanced disease
	Tumor invades prevertebral fascia or encases carotid artery or mediastinal vessels

All anaplastic carcinomas are considered T4 tumors

T4a	Intrathyroidal anaplastic carcinoma
T4b	Anaplastic carcinoma with gross extrathyroid extension

Regional lymph nodes (N)[b]

NX	Regional lymph nodes cannot be assessed
N0	No regional lymph node metastasis
N1	Regional lymph node metastasis
N1a	Metastasis to level VI (pretracheal, paratracheal, and prelaryngeal/Delphian lymph nodes)
N1b	Metastasis to unilateral, bilateral, or contralateral cervical (level I, II, III, IV, or V) or retropharyngeal or superior mediastinal lymph nodes (level VII)

Distant metastasis (M)

M0	No distant metastasis
M1	Distant metastasis

Anatomic stage/prognostic groups[c]

Papillary or follicular (differentiated)

Under 45 years

Stage I	Any T	Any N	M0
Stage II	Any T	Any N	M1

45 years and older

Stage I	T1	N0	M0
Stage II	T2	N0	M0
Stage III	T3	N0	M0
	T1	N1a	M0
	T2	N1a	M0
	T3	N1a	M0
Stage IVA	T4a	N0	M0
	T4a	N1a	M0
	T1	N1b	M0
	T2	N1b	M0
	T3	N1b	M0
	T4a	N1b	M0
Stage IVB	T4b	Any N	M0
Stage IVC	Any T	Any N	M1

Source: Reproduced with permission from the American Joint Committee on Cancer (AJCC), Chicago, Illinois. The original source for this material is the *AJCC Cancer Staging Manual*, 7th ed., Springer, New York, 2010.

Note: cTNM is the clinical classification, pTNM is the pathologic classification.

[a]   All categories may be subdivided: (s) solitary tumor and (m) multifocal tumor (the largest determines the classification).

[b]   Regional lymph nodes are the central compartment, lateral cervical, and upper mediastinal lymph nodes.

[c]   Separate stage groupings are recommended for papillary or follicular (differentiated), medullary, and anaplastic (undifferentiated) carcinoma.

Papillary thyroid cancer (PTC) is the most common type of thyroid cancer overall (85%). It has an excellent prognosis with a 5-year survival of 95%–97% combining all stages [12], and a 20-year survival of 95%. Most patients present with an incidentally discovered thyroid nodule on examination or imaging obtained for another reason; because PTC is typically indolent, symptoms due to invasion or compression are rare. Known risk factors include prior radiation exposure to the head, upper chest, or neck, and one or more first-degree relatives with PTC. The diagnosis is often made preoperatively by fine-needle aspiration biopsy (FNAB), but PTC is also often diagnosed only on histology after thyroidectomy is performed for another reason. Several distinct histologic subtypes have varying profiles of aggressiveness, including follicular-variant PTC (generally indolent), as well as the more aggressive tall cell, insular, cribriform-morular, and diffuse sclerosing types. PTC is frequently multifocal within the thyroid gland. Although PTC rarely spreads to distant sites, cervical lymph node involvement is common, seen microscopically in as many as 78% of patients undergoing neck dissection [13]. Lymph node involvement does not affect survival, but it does predict local recurrence, which in the past occurred in the central neck in up to 30% of patients [14].

Follicular thyroid cancer (FTC) is the second most commonly diagnosed type overall (12%), with a 20-year survival rate of 81% [15]. Most FTC patients present with FNAB cytology results in the Bethesda III category of follicular neoplasm or follicular lesion of undetermined significance [16]. FTC is diagnosed when a follicular lesion is histologically identified to have tumor capsular invasion or vascular invasion—thus, FNAB is unable to differentiate benign from malignant follicular neoplasms. Molecular testing, however, can improve this preoperative diagnostic dilemma (below). Histologically, FTC lacks the typical nuclear changes seen in PTC. Unlike PTC, FTC spreads hematogenously, rarely involving regional lymph nodes.

Hurthle cell (oncocytic) carcinoma (HCC) is considered a subtype of follicular tumors. It is characterized by an abundant cytoplasmic accumulation of abnormal mitochondria [17]. The determination of malignancy in Hurthle cell neoplasms requires the identification of tumor capsule or vascular invasion and is managed similarly to FTC, but it has a worse prognosis, potentially due to the tumors' decreased avidity for radioactive iodine [18].

EVALUATION OF THYROID NODULES

Once a dominant thyroid nodule is detected on self-exam or incidentally on imaging, the next step is thorough physical exam and TSH measurement. All patients with nodular thyroid disease should also be assessed for key risk factors and signs of thyroid cancer, such as a rapidly growing mass, hoarseness, dysphagia to solids, positional dyspnea, local pain, radiation history, or pertinent family history. In hypothyroid patients, T4 is adequately replaced and nodule size is monitored briefly for stability. Hyperthyroidism is uncommon in thyroid nodule patients, and their evaluation follows a different diagnostic algorithm that includes nuclear imaging, as well as ultrasound (US). Of nodules detected on ^{18}F-fluorodeoxyglucose positron emission tomography (FDG-PET) scan, about 30% are found to be DTC, and further workup with US-directed FNAB is recommended [19].

In euthyroid patients, the next step in thyroid nodule evaluation is cervical US, including systematic survey of the central and lateral lymph nodes. US identifies concerning nodule characteristics, other thyroid nodules, and cervical lymphadenopathy. The six thyroid nodule US features that predict malignancy are hypoechogenicity, intranodular hypervascularity, calcifications, taller than wide shape, irregular margins, and solid composition [20]. Computed tomography (CT) is additionally useful to characterize deep or bulky adenopathy, or to assess for local invasion in the setting of fixed adenopathy.

FNAB is the standard of care for evaluation of thyroid nodules of >1 cm or subcentimeter nodules with concerning US characteristics [21]. It is best performed under US guidance, and when available, on-site cytopathology allows immediate assessment of adequacy [22,23]. The Bethesda classification has standardized the coding of thyroid cytology results and includes six categories; the categories and their corresponding risk of thyroid cancer are shown in Table 13.2 [24,25]. About 65%–70% of FNAB results are benign. Benign nodules may be followed with neck US to document stability, with repeat FNAB or resection performed for significant growth or new concerning imaging findings. Significant growth has been defined as a 20% increase in nodule diameter, with an increase in two or more dimensions of more than 2 mm or a 50% increase in nodule volume [21]. About 5%–7% of thyroid nodules

Table 13.2 The Bethesda System for Reporting Thyroid Cytopathology and corresponding malignancy risk

Diagnostic category	Risk of malignancy	Risk of malignancy in practice (Nikiforov et al. [24])
Benign	0%–3%	
Atypia of undetermined significance (AUS) or follicular lesion of undetermined significance (FLUS)	5%–19%	14%
Follicular neoplasm or suspicious for follicular neoplasm	20%–30%	27%
Suspicious	50%–75%	54%
Malignant	97%–99%	

are malignant on cytology. The cancer risk for the malignant cytology category is >99%, and thyroidectomy is indicated [21]. One-fourth of FNAB cytology results are classed as "indeterminate," and the three indeterminate categories, in order of rising cancer risk, are comprised of atypia/follicular lesion of undetermined significance (AUS/FLUS), follicular neoplasm (FN), and suspicious for papillary thyroid cancer (SUSP) [21]. The risk of cancer ranges widely across the indeterminate categories from 6% to 87%, but molecular testing has helped to further define specific nodule risk.

MOLECULAR TESTING

Molecular testing of thyroid cytology (MT) specimens is an adjunct to help decrease the number of diagnostic thyroidectomies performed for benign disease and to guide the initial extent of surgery for cytology results in the three indeterminate categories [24,26]; MT may also be used in selected patients with inadequate, benign, or malignant FNAB results if prognostic information is desired [27]. The seven-gene MT panel is based on genetic alterations in the MAPK and PI3K-AKT pathways, including *BRAF* V600E and *RAS* point mutations, as well as *RET/PTC* and *PAX8/ PPAR*γ rearrangements, which together account for more than 70% of known DTC mutations. In 2011, a large prospective study with cytologic, molecular, and histologic correlation showed an 88%–99% cancer risk in those with indeterminate cytology and positive mutational testing [24]. A clinical algorithm using the seven-gene MT panel to guide the optimal extent of initial thyroidectomy has been shown to increase rates of appropriate initial total thyroidectomy for DTC, as well as to increase appropriate lobectomy for papillary microcarcinoma [28].

An alternative method for risk-stratifying nodules with indeterminate FNAB cytology uses a gene expression classifier (GEC) panel that measures the expression of 167 gene transcripts and is marketed as a "rule-out" test for thyroid cancer [29]. This test is commercially available but mandates cytology review by commercial pathologists with few exceptions. The GEC classifies results as benign or suspicious. Its efficacy in reducing the rate of thyroidectomy for benign disease has not yet been proven; moreover, a positive or "suspicious" result correlates with only a 40% risk of cancer, so the GEC does not help to guide the extent of thyroid surgery.

Very recently developed, the next-generation sequencing panel (ThyroSeq v2) tests for point mutations in 13 genes and 42 gene fusions accounting for more than 90% of thyroid cancers. The test provides improved sensitivity over the seven-gene MT panel. For example, thyroid nodules in the cytology category of FN have historically required diagnostic lobectomy because of a 14%–34% cancer risk, together with an inability to differentiate benign and malignant tumors based on cytology alone. However, an FN lesion with negative results by ThyroSeq v2 has a cancer risk of only 4%, allowing for the first time the active surveillance of FN lesions [30]. The high specificity (93%) and sensitivity (90%) of the Thyroseq v2 panel may sufficiently merge the capabilities of the early high PPV/ NPV tests (seven-gene MT and GEC, respectively) for both "rule-in" and "rule-out" proficiency. The ThyroSeqv2 panel also provides genotype–phenotype prognostic information [31].

INDICATIONS

Today thyroid lobectomy is considered to be the minimal acceptable operation in management of thyroid nodular disease, largely because it removes any need for future reoperation on that side, which also could endanger the RLN or parathyroid glands embedded in scar tissue. For the same reasons, subtotal thyroidectomy is no longer performed, although occasionally a very small amount of thyroid tissue (<50 mg, <3 mm) must be left behind to protect the RLN at the ligament of Berry. Although intraoperative frozen section was once used to help determine the initial extent of thyroidectomy, it has a low predictive value for DTC and has largely been abandoned [32,33].

The standard treatment of differentiated thyroid cancer of >1 cm based on prior and current American Thyroid Association (ATA) guidelines is total thyroidectomy; however, the upcoming revised ATA guidelines are expected to acknowledge that a more conservative approach is feasible for low-risk, small tumors [21]. The standard treatment of preoperatively diagnosed papillary thyroid microcarcinoma may be limited to lobectomy and isthmusectomy given the excellent prognosis of such lesions [21]. Besides DTC, thyroidectomy is also indicated by conditions that include positive MT results, twice-inadequate FNAB results, concerning US features, toxic nodular goiter, mass size of >4 cm, a substernal (i.e., unbiopsiable) nodule, tracheal compression by substernal goiter, a hot nodule of >2.5 cm, a recurrent cyst, Graves' disease with ophthalmopathy or failed ablation, positional dyspnea, dysphagia to solids, and clinical judgment [21,34,35]. The initial extent of thyroidectomy is influenced by MT and FNAB results; a contralateral dominant thyroid nodule; a history of head, neck, or chest irradiation, especially in childhood; a familial DTC setting; medical comorbidities; and other conditions of the contralateral lobe [21], as well as by chronic hypothyroidism requiring T4 replacement (if total thyroidectomy can be done safely). Completion (reoperative) total thyroidectomy is indicated when initial lobectomy removes a clinically significant thyroid carcinoma and adjuvant radioactive iodine ablation is planned, and also facilitates use of serum thyroglobulin levels as a marker for future recurrence.

Patients with preoperatively diagnosed PTC should have thorough US lymph node mapping to identify central and lateral involvement. A suspicious enlarged lateral lymph node undergoes FNAB, preferably with thyroglobulin assay on the aspirate to confirm tissue identity. Positive nodes are treated by compartment-oriented lymph node dissection of involved

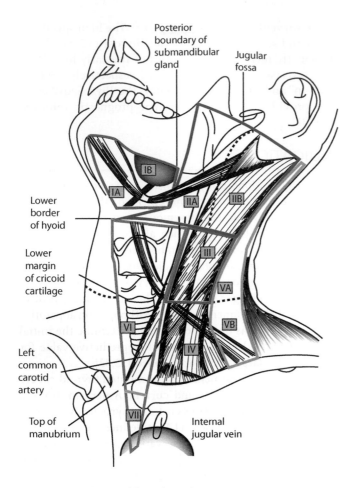

Figure 13.2 Cervical lymph node compartments.

and adjacent lymph node groups (Figure 13.2). Prior to thyroidectomy, the serum calcium level is checked to screen for concomitant primary hyperparathyroidism (pHPT), which is not at all uncommon and is best managed concurrently [36]. Preoperative vocal cord examination (by US, mirror, or laryngoscope) is recommended for any patient undergoing initial thyroidectomy who has clinical hoarseness or apparent extensive DTC, as well as for all patients with a history of prior anterior cervical or thoracic surgery. The cost-effectiveness of routine preoperative laryngoscopy has yet to be examined.

THYROIDECTOMY FOR DTC

Lobectomy and isthmusectomy

Thyroidectomy can be performed safely under regional anesthesia in selected patients but is most commonly performed with general endotracheal anesthesia. Patients with large goiters, severe tracheal compression, or a difficult airway may require awake, fiber-optic intubation. After intubation, the patient is placed in a modified beach chair position that facilitates safe access and a short incision length (Figure 13.3). A roll is placed under the shoulder blades to improve exposure, the arms are tucked bilaterally with shoulders dropped, and any pressure points (elbows and heels) are padded. Appropriate DVT prophylaxis is employed and procedure-specific antibiotics are administered.

The incision is sited midneck, well below the level of the cricothyroid membrane and ideally in a natural skin crease,

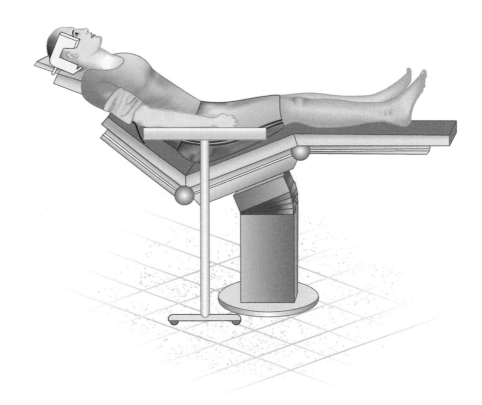

Figure 13.3 Beachchair position.

with incision length varying based on patient habitus and gland size [37]. Long-acting local anesthetic (bupivacaine 0.5%) is injected along the planned incision for preemptive analgesia. Once the incision is made, dissection is carried through the platysmal fibers with cautery and subplatysmal flaps are raised. To allow adequate exposure, the median raphe is divided entirely (from the thyroid cartilage cranially down to the sternal notch caudally) and the strap muscles are then bluntly mobilized and retracted laterally, away from the underlying thyroid lobe. The strap muscles rarely require division. Dissection is performed meticulously in a near-bloodless field. Care should be taken during thyroid cancer resection to avoid capsular rupture and to resect *en bloc* any adherent lymphatic or areolar tissue.

Typically, the upper thyroid pole is mobilized first, but not uncommonly, there are variations in anatomy that make the inferior vascular pedicle a better first target. The upper pole is retracted and rotated medially to expose the upper pole vessels and their branches, which usually course on the anterior surface of the superior pole. With care taken to identify and preserve the SLN and the superior parathyroid gland, the superior vascular branches are ligated on the anterior superior capsule using ties or a vessel sealing device [38]. The lower-pole vascular branches are then divided directly on the thyroid capsule, along with gentle dissection to preserve the RLN and the inferior parathyroid gland on its vascular pedicle.

As the thyroid lobe is rotated medially and circumferentially devascularized, multiple small unnamed vessels may also require division. The tubercle of Zuckerkandl is then gently freed from the underlying RLN or its anterior branch, taking note of the commonly present RLN anatomic variations to avoid injury; as described earlier, although the RLN typically courses in the tracheoesophageal groove, it can also reside in a more anterior plane, intertwine with the inferior thyroid artery, be nonrecurrent, or run up on the anterior trachea, tethered by tumor or prior scar.

Delicately preserving the RLN throughout its length, dissection continues behind the gently rotated thyroid lobe until the ligament of Berry is divided and any remaining attachments between the anterior trachea and the isthmus are freed. If a pyramidal lobe is present (and these can be bifid), it is dissected to its full extent and resected. When lobectomy and isthmusectomy is the planned operation, the isthmus is then divided at its junction with the contralateral thyroid lobe using a vessel sealing device or scalpel; if sharply divided, the isthmus is oversewn with nonabsorbable suture. Prior to being sent to pathology, the resected thyroid specimen is oriented and its posterior capsule is inspected for the occasional adherent parathyroid gland. If a normal parathyroid is accidentally removed or devascularized, it should be retrieved, kept sterile on ice, confirmed as parathyroid tissue on frozen section, and immediately autotransplanted as minced 1 mm fragments into an ipsilateral strap muscle pocket that is marked with a nonabsorbable suture. Meticulous hemostasis is ensured prior to closure (discussed below).

Total thyroidectomy

If total thyroidectomy is planned, or is (rarely) required by intraoperative findings in a consenting patient, the contralateral thyroid lobe is similarly mobilized, taking care to identify and preserve the contralateral RLN, SLN, and parathyroid glands. The entire thyroid gland is removed and oriented for pathology. Prior to proceeding with contralateral thyroidectomy, if there is significant concern about the integrity of the initially dissected RLN, the alternative of completion thyroidectomy at a later date may be considered. Compared with RLN monitoring, this occasional strategy allows for accurate functional assessment and also helps to avoid the rare but dreaded complication of bilateral RLN injury.

CENTRAL COMPARTMENT LYMPH NODE DISSECTION

There is little or no controversy regarding therapeutic level VI central compartment lymph node dissection (CND) for PTC [21,39]. Abnormal LN may be suspected preoperatively on exam or imaging, and may also be identified during thyroidectomy for DTC. US characteristics that increase suspicion for malignancy in a cervical lymph node include microcalcifications or cystic spaces, rounded shape, lack of a defined fatty hilum, and increased vascularity [40]. Grossly, malignant lymph nodes may appear rounded or cystic or have a characteristic blue color.

In the setting of malignant FNAB results, prophylactic CND is controversial because it has not been shown to improve survival and is also suspected to have higher complication rates, including permanent hypoparathyroidism and RLN injury [21,41,42]. Prophylactic CND in the management of PTC is intended to decrease the risk of local recurrence and allow more selective use of radioiodine ablation when disease is upstaged by the presence of positive lymph nodes. The feasibility of achieving reasonable statistical power to determine differences in the survival benefit of prophylactic CND is thought to be precluded by the high survival rate and low morbidity [43]. However, a recent small ($n = 181$) prospective randomized trial showed no difference in disease outcome, but did find that those treated with total thyroidectomy alone required more frequent retreatment with radioactive iodine, and those treated with prophylactic CND had a higher rate of permanent hypoparathyroidism [44]. In a review of existing studies evaluating the role of CND in clinically node-negative disease, McHenry and Stulberg concluded that the risk of prophylactic CND does not outweigh the apparent limited benefit [45].

During CND on the side ipsilateral to the diagnosed cancer, all fibroadipose and lymphatic tissue is removed *en bloc*, with dissection extending from the hyoid bone/thyroid cartilage cranially down to the innominate artery, and from the midline anterior trachea over to the carotid sheath laterally to include removal of the prelaryngeal, pretracheal, and one paratracheal nodal basins [39]. *En bloc* with the thyroid gland, some level VI central lymph nodes are often removed as well, of course. Although during CND the inferior parathyroid gland should be carefully preserved on its vascular pedicle, this is not always possible anatomically; moreover, the ipsilateral thymus is routinely removed, particularly when enlarged lymph nodes are palpated or imaged within it. During prophylactic CND, the deep aspect of dissection is the RLN, which is exposed and carefully preserved. During therapeutic CND, abnormal lymph nodes imaged or palpated deep to the RLN indicate the removal of all ipsilateral deep lymphatic tissue as well [38]. Because the benefit of CND is still unclear, in the setting of limited exposure or concern for RLN integrity, prophylactic CND may not be prudent. In addition, to reap any potential benefit, CND should be performed only by surgeons with low surgical morbidity rates.

LATERAL COMPARTMENT LYMPH NODE DISSECTION

In DTC, lateral compartments III and IV are the most common sites of metastatic spread, but levels II, V, and VII (upper mediastinal lymph nodes) may also be involved (Table 13.2). Compartment-oriented or selective lateral neck dissection (SLND) is performed for clinical (on imaging or exam) and biopsy-proven metastatic disease [46]. "Berry picking" is not indicated.

When LND is planned concurrently with thyroidectomy, the regular transverse cervical incision is extended to the anterior border of the ipsilateral sternocleidomastoid muscle (SCM). This allows adequate exposure in most patients with excellent cosmetic results. In a patient with a long neck and level II disease, a higher counterincision may be necessary, but this is infrequent. A standard "hockey stick" incision along the anterior border of the SCM can maximize exposure when lateral neck involvement is extensive, but today this is rarely required.

Selective LND involves removal of only involved compartments and less than the five standard cervical levels of classic lymph node dissection (modified radical neck dissection [MRND]) [46]. The SCM is freed anteriorly from the lateral border of the strap muscles and is retracted laterally. The internal jugular vein is carefully exposed, encircled with a vessel loop, and retracted medially. Dissection begins low, at the internal jugular vein and the subclavian vein confluence. On the left, it is important to locate and preserve the thoracic duct, which resides low in level IV. Injury to the thoracic duct is a major problem that can lead to persistent lymphatic leak, infection, and malnutrition, often requiring re-exploration. The nodal tissue is dissected in an *en bloc* packet that is sequentially retracted cranially, exposing and preserving the phrenic nerve as it courses atop the anterior scalene muscle. All lymphatic tissue is systematically freed from the internal jugular vein medially and from the level V area at the lateral border of the SCM up to the level of the hyoid bone

for a level III/IV dissection. Because there is no clear anatomic division between levels III and IV, both compartments are resected in continuity when either is involved. Careful identification and preservation of the phrenic nerve, spinal accessory nerve, and cervical sensory nerve branches is essential.

An MRND includes removal of all lymph nodes from levels I to V while sparing the spinal accessory nerve, internal jugular vein, and SCM [46]. For a classic radical neck dissection, on the other hand, lymph nodes from all five lateral cervical compartments are removed and the jugular vein, SCM, and spinal accessory nerve sacrificed [46]. Modified and radical neck dissections are rarely required for DTC. After completion of a compartment III/IV dissection, we routinely perform intraoperative US to identify suspicious adenopathy missed on preoperative imaging. Although most involved lymph nodes are identified on preoperative imaging, habitus and extent of disease may hinder visualization.

CLOSURE

Once adequate hemostasis in confirmed, the use of hemostatic agents is uncommonly required and is based on risk factors. Drains do not prevent hematoma after thyroidectomy, but can facilitate the detection of bleeding, whereas after LND, they can help to identify lymphatic leak. We reserve drain use for LND and for the uncommon thyroidectomy patient with difficult habitus, massive goiter resection, or known coagulopathy. The strap and platysma muscles are closed with absorbable suture. The skin is cosmetically closed with running subcuticular absorbable suture. Steri strips or medical glue is applied as a dressing. Figure 13.4a and b shows the typical immediate postoperative and initial follow-up incision appearance. It is important to communicate in the dictated operative report all essential intraoperative findings [47].

SPECIAL CONSIDERATIONS

Locally advanced thyroid cancer

With a history of rapid nodule growth or new-onset hoarseness, or with findings of a firm nonmobile mass, or suspicious imaging characteristics, a locally advanced thyroid cancer should be suspected, potentially altering the operative plan. In this setting, preoperative laryngoscopy should be done to assess involvement of the RLN. If RLN dysfunction is present, intraoperative neuromonitoring may be indicated to help identify the nerve during dissection. Preoperative esophagoscopy and bronchoscopy are indicated when aerodigestive tract invasion is suspected. Medullary thyroid cancer and rare thyroid tumor types like paraganglioma can occasionally be misdiagnosed as DTC, are often locally aggressive, and should be considered in the setting of apparent locally advanced disease [48].

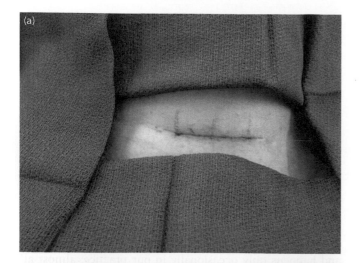

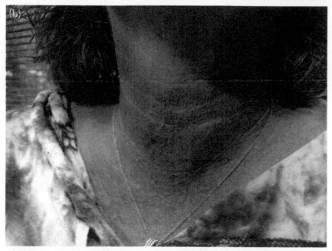

Figure 13.4 (a) Closed incision immediately postop. **(b)** Incision at initial postoperative follow-up.

When the RLN is involved by known DTC, unless the involvement is circumferential, the cancer can usually be shaved off carefully with a scalpel. All efforts should be made to preserve the RLN in DTC, including, if necessary, a microscopically incomplete resection—because radioactive iodine ablation is available postoperatively. However, if poorly differentiated or anaplastic carcinoma is suspected, sacrifice of an invaded nerve segment with reapproximation or grafting may be necessary to achieve best outcomes. The possibility of primary thyroid lymphoma or anaplastic thyroid carcinoma should always be considered when a patient presents with a rapidly enlarging neck mass, but specific management is outside of the scope of this chapter. During resection of presumed DTC, if a large fixed mass is encountered, incisional biopsy for definitive diagnosis and delayed treatment planning is prudent. Comprehensive resection of adjacent involved structures, such as the esophagus, larynx, carotid artery, or trachea, is rarely indicated for poorly differentiated or anaplastic cancers, but when deemed appropriate, it includes a multidisciplinary approach potentially involving otolaryngology, thoracic surgery, and vascular surgery.

Reoperation

Due to the limitations of existing scar tissue, thyroid reoperation for DTC has a different strategy and risks than does initial surgery, as described above. Prior anterior cervical surgery includes thyroidectomy, parathyroidectomy, tracheostomy, carotid endarterectomy, cervical discectomy, and several thoracic operations, such as mediastinoscopy, which can injure the RLN. A history of such prior surgery warrants additional evaluation, including preoperative laryngoscopy and, in certain cases, additional imaging. Even in expert hands, in reoperative thyroidectomy the risk of injury to the ipsilateral RLN and parathyroid glands is two to five times higher than in initial surgery [49]. Reoperation for recurrent or persistent DTC also requires current imaging with US or CT to identify extent and resectability of disease, as well as potential involvement of adjacent structures. With documented RLN injury from any cause, a staged approach should be considered to allow interim assessment of vocal cord movement and further discussion with the patient regarding optimal subsequent management. In reoperation, RLN monitoring may facilitate nerve identification and thus be helpful [50].

COMPLICATIONS, POSTOPERATIVE MANAGEMENT, AND OUTCOMES

Cervical hematoma is a rare but potentially lethal complication of thyroid surgery. The incidence is low (0.05%–1.2%) but is increased by technical, patient-specific, and thyroid-specific factors [51]. Hematoma occurs most commonly in the initial 8 hours after surgery, and early diagnosis of this emergency is facilitated by a high level of suspicion and careful postoperative examination. The treatment is emergency operative evacuation; there is no safe observation of post-thyroidectomy hematoma. Reintubation requires close communication with anesthesia colleagues to avoid airway compromise, and if the patient is in severe respiratory distress, bedside evacuation may be required as a life-saving maneuver. Unilateral permanent RLN injury rates vary with high-volume expertise. Permanent RLN paralysis occurs in less than 1% of initial cases for high-volume surgeons, and more often otherwise [52,53]. Patients should be informed preoperatively about the national risks and about the surgeon's own risks for this complication. Infrequently, intubation can also lead to vocal fold dysfunction by arytenoid dislocation. Permanent RLN paralysis is not diagnosed until >6 months postoperatively and before that time is termed paresis. Dysfunction can be asymptomatic or can result in a hoarse, weak, or characteristically high-pitched voice. If transection of the RLN is noted intraoperatively, direct tension-free repair with fine suture is recommended; although function will not be restored, RLN anastomosis can improve voice outcomes by increasing tone of the vocal fold [54]. Over time, voice quality generally improves, but some patients may develop dyspnea on exertion as the paralyzed RLN medializes. Laryngeal electromyography may help to determine prognosis for recovery, and temporary measures, including vocal cord injection, may improve voice and decrease aspiration risk. Laryngoplasty may be necessary once paralysis is determined to be permanent. Off-label use of nimodipine has shown decreased time to recovery and an improved recovery rate in RLN paralysis [55].

Bilateral RLN paresis after total thyroidectomy is an exceedingly rare complication occurring in 0.1%–0.4% of patients. Early bilateral RLN injury can result in dyspnea with a breathy, whispery voice, aspiration, or severe stridor requiring urgent tracheostomy. Permanent tracheostomy or vocal fold surgery may ultimately be required months later as the paralyzed cords medialize. Immediately after thyroidectomy, because stridor can indicate hematoma or airway obstruction, the situation requires immediate examination, but fortunately, the vast majority of cases are due to bronchospasm, which quickly responds to racemic epinephrine.

SLN injury after thyroidectomy may affect up to 5% of patients, but the actual rate remains unknown due to difficulties in accurate diagnosis. SLN paralysis can result in impaired voice projection, loudness, or pitch, and patients should be informed preoperatively about this risk [3].

Permanent hypoparathyroidism is not anatomically possible after initial thyroid lobectomy. However, after total or reoperative thyroidectomy, routine calcium measurement should be performed to preemptively identify and manage symptoms of hypocalcemia. In addition, after total or reoperative thyroidectomy, many high-volume surgeons prescribe routine postoperative oral calcium supplementation, which is dose adjusted according to any symptoms and to the calcium level the morning after surgery. We find that with such routine supplementation, circumoral or digital paresthesias are typically specific, transient, and mild, occurring in about 15% of cases and easily managed on an outpatient basis. Almost all patients are able to stop calcium supplementation at the first visit 1–2 weeks postoperatively. The uncommon patient with persistent symptoms or hypocalcemia requires laboratory evaluation with serum calcium, phosphorus, albumin, and magnesium levels. Significant hypocalcemia requires at least temporary administration of oral calcitriol; in weaning calcitriol off subsequently, it is important to keep in mind that on this medication, parathyroid hormone levels are often nonevaluable due to reflex suppression.

Permanent hypoparathyroidism typically requires an ongoing requirement for full oral calcitriol dosing for >6 months after surgery, results from removal or devitalization of all parathyroid glands, and in the literature, should occur in no more than 2% of patients after total thyroidectomy (over two decades, our rate is about 0.3%). The condition requires lifelong calcium and calcitriol medication and, when necessary, magnesium supplementation, and can also lead to bone, skin, and eye disorders, including cataracts [56].

Chronic hypothyroidism occurs in 22%–33% of patients after lobectomy. After lobectomy, all patients should be screened for elevated TSH at 6–8 weeks. Immediately after total thyroidectomy, patients begin a weight-based daily thyroxine dose (1.5 µg/kg). Thyroid function is checked at 6–8 weeks postoperatively, and the dose is adjusted as required.

Complications of LND can include thoracic duct injury with chyle leak, infection, and injury to the internal jugular vein and carotid artery, as well as injury to the phrenic nerve, the spinal accessory nerve, or the cervical sensory nerves. The brachial plexus branches are deep and very rarely injured [46].

After uneventful thyroid lobectomy, patients may be safely discharged the day of surgery following 4–6 hours of observation. Same-day discharge of total thyroidectomy patients [57,58] has been proposed on a very selective basis and happens only occasionally in our practice; almost all such patients are discharged the morning after surgery. Patients are seen surgically 7–14 days postoperatively and again at 3–6 months. If completion thyroidectomy is required, it is performed either within 1–2 weeks of initial operation or >6 weeks later to give scarring the opportunity to diminish.

SURVEILLANCE

Surveillance of DTC is typically managed by or in conjunction with the patient's endocrinologist, and can include radioactive iodine ablation, thyroid suppression, serial imaging with US or radioactive whole body scan, and thyroglobulin assessment. Remnant ablation may be recommended to facilitate surveillance with thyroglobulin, although the recommendation for ablation is currently widely variable and based on increasingly subtle histologic details [21,59]. A properly performed total thyroidectomy routinely produces less than 1% uptake on the initial postoperative whole body scan [52]. Referral to medical oncology and radiation oncology is uncommonly necessary for patients with DTC, the exceptions being cases of widely metastatic, unresectable, locally recurrent, radioiodine refractory, or differentiated thyroid carcinomas with a molecular profile indicative of aggressive phenotype [60].

REFERENCES

1. Pelizzo MR, Toniato A, Gemo G. Zuckerkandl's tuberculum: An arrow pointing to the recurrent laryngeal nerve (constant anatomical landmark). *J Am Coll Surg* 1998;187:333–6.
2. Droulias C, Tzinas S, Harlaftis N et al. The superior laryngeal nerve. *Am Surg* 1976;42:635.
3. Crookes PF, Recabaren, JA. Injury to the superior laryngeal branch of the vagus during thyroidectomy: Lesson or myth? *Ann Surg* 2001;233:588.
4. Serpell JW, Yeung MJ, Grodski S. The motor fibers of the recurrent laryngeal nerve are located in the anterior extralaryngeal branch. *Ann Surg* 2009;249:648.

5. Henry JF, Audiffret J, Denizot A, Plan M. The nonrecurrent inferior laryngeal nerve: Review of 33 cases, including two on the left side. *Surgery* 1988;104:977.

6. Kopp P. Thyroid hormone synthesis. In: Braverman LE, Utiger RD, eds., *The Thyroid: Fundamental and Clinical Text*. 9th ed. Philadelphia: Lippincott Williams & Wilkins, 2005:52.

7. American Cancer Society, Facts and Figures, 2013. http://www.cancer.org/acs/groups/content/@epidemiologysurveilance/documents/document/acspc-036845.pdf

8. Ries LAG, Melbert D, Krapcho M et al. SEER cancer statistics review 1975–2004. Bethesda, MD: National Cancer Institute. http://seer.cancer.gov/csr/1975_2004.

9. National Cancer Institute, Surveillance, Epidemiology, and End Results. SEER stat fact sheets: Thyroid cancer. http://seer.cancer.gov/statfacts/html/thyro.html.

10. Hay ID, Bergstralh EJ, Goellner JR et al. Predicting outcome in papillary thyroid carcinoma: Development of a reliable prognostic scoring system in a cohort of 1779 patients surgically treated at one institution during 1940 through 1989. *Surgery* 1993;114:1050.

11. Sherman SI, Brierley JD, Sperling M et al. Prospective multicenter study of thyroid carcinoma treatment: Initial analysis of staging and outcome. National Thyroid Cancer Treatment Cooperative Study Registry Group. *Cancer* 1998;83:1012.

12. Howlader N, Noone AM, Krapcho M et al. SEER cancer statistics review, 1975–2009 (vintage 2009 populations). Bethesda, MD: National Cancer Institute, April 2012.

13. Wada N, Suganuma N, Nakayama H et al. Microscopic regional lymph node status in papillary thyroid carcinoma with and without lymphadenopathy and its relation to outcomes. *Langenbecks Arch Surg* 2007;392:417.

14. Mazzaferri EL, Jhiang SM. Long-term impact of initial surgical and medical therapy on papillary and follicular thyroid cancer. *Am J Med* 1994;97:418.

15. Kosary C. Cancer of the thyroid. In: Ries LAG, Young JL, Keel GE, Eisner MP, Lin YD, Horner M-J, eds., *SEER Survival Monograph: Cancer Survival among Adults: US SEER Program, 1988–2001, Patient and Tumor Characteristics*. Bethesda, MD: National Cancer Institute, SEER Program, 2007:217.

16. Baloch ZW, Livolsi VA. Follicular-patterned afflictions of the thyroid gland: Reappraisal of the most discussed entity in endocrine pathology. *Endocr Pathol* 2014;25:12–20.

17. Maximo V, Lima J, Prazeres H et al. The biology and genetics of Hurthle cell tumors of the thyroid. *Endocr Relat Cancer* 2012;19:131–47.

18. Kushchayeva Y, Duh QY, Kebebew E et al. Comparison of clinical characteristics at diagnosis and during follow up in 118 patients with Hurthle cell or follicular thyroid cancer. *Am J Surg* 2008;195:457.

19. Kang KW, Kim SK, Kang HS et al. Prevalence and risk of cancer of focal thyroid incidentaloma identified by 18F-fluorodeoxyglucose positron emission tomography for metastasis evaluation and cancer screening in healthy subjects. *J Clin Endocrinol Metab* 2003;88:4100.

20. Yoon JH, Kwak JY, Moon HJ et al. The diagnostic accuracy of ultrasound-guided fine-needle aspiration biopsy and the sonographic differences between benign and malignant thyroid nodules 3 cm or larger. *Thyroid* 2011;21:993.

21. Cooper DS, Doherty GM, Haugen BR et al. Revised American Thyroid Association Management guidelines for patients with thyroid nodules and differentiated thyroid cancer. *Thyroid* 2009;19:1167.

22. Danese D, Sciacchitano S, Farsetti A et al. Diagnostic accuracy of conventional versus sonography-guided fine-needle aspiration biopsy of thyroid nodules. *Thyroid* 1998;8:15.

23. Layfield LJ, Cibas ES, Baloch Z. Thyroid fine-needle aspiration cytology: A review of the National Cancer Institute state of the science symposium. *Cytopathology* 2010;21:75.

24. Nikiforov YE, Ohori NP, Hodak SP et al. Impact of mutational testing on the diagnosis and management of patients with cytologically indeterminate thyroid nodules: A prospective analysis of 1056 FNA samples. *J Clin Endocrinol Metab* 2011;96:3390.

25. Yip L, Farris C, Kabaker AS et al. Cost impact of molecular testing for indeterminate thyroid nodule fine-needle aspiration biopsies. *J Clin Endocrinol Metab* 2012;97:1905.

26. Ferris RL, Baloch Z, Bernet V et al. American Thyroid Association statement on surgical application of molecular profiling for thyroid nodules: Current impact on perioperative decision making. *Thyroid* 2015;25:760–8.

27. Yip L, Nikiforova MN, Carty SE et al. Optimizing surgical treatment of papillary thyroid carcinoma associated with BRAF mutation. *Surgery* 2009;146:1215–23.

28. Yip L, Wharry LI, Armstrong MJ et al. A clinical algorithm for fine-needle aspiration molecular testing effectively guides the appropriate extent of initial thyroidectomy. *Ann Surg* 2014;260:163–8.

29. Alexander EK, Kennedy GC, Baloch ZW et al. Preoperative diagnosis of benign thyroid nodules with indeterminate cytology. *N Engl J Med* 2012;367:705.

30. Nikiforov YE, Carty SE, Chiosea SI et al. Highly accurate diagnosis of cancer in thyroid nodules with follicular neoplasm/suspicious for a follicular neoplasm cytology by ThyroSeq v2 next-generation sequencing assay. *Cancer* 2014;120:3627–34.

31. Yip L, Nikiforova MN, Yoo JY et al. Tumor genotype determines phenotype and disease-related

outcomes in thyroid cancer: A study of 1510 patients. *Ann Surg* 2015;262:519–25.

32. Chen H, Nicol TL, Udelsman R. Follicular lesions of the thyroid. Does frozen section evaluation alter operative management? *Ann Surg* 1995;222:101.

33. McCoy KL, Carty SE, Armstrong MJ et al. Intraoperative pathologic examination in the era of molecular testing for differentiated thyroid cancer. *J Am Coll Surg* 2012;215:546.

34. McCoy KL, Jabbour N, Ogilvie JB et al. The incidence of cancer and rate of false negative cytology in thyroid nodules greater than or equal to 4 cm in size. *Surgery* 2007;142:837.

35. Stang MT, Armstrong MJ, Ogilvie JB et al. Positional dyspnea and tracheal compression as indications for goiter resection. *Arch Surg* 2012;147:621–6.

36. Morita SY, Somervell H, Umbricht CB et al. Evaluation for concomitant thyroid nodules and primary hyperparathyroidism in patients undergoing parathyroidectomy or thyroidectomy. *Surgery* 2008;144:862.

37. Brunaud L, Zarnegar R, Wada N et al. Incision length for standard thyroidectomy and parathyroidectomy. *Arch Surg* 2003;138:1140.

38. Ecker T, Carvalho AL, Choe JH et al. Hemostasis in thyroid surgery: Harmonic scalpel versus other techniques—A meta-analysis. *Otolaryngol Head Neck Surg* 2010;143:17.

39. Carty SE, Cooper DS, Doherty GM et al. Consensus statement on the terminology and classification of central neck dissection for thyroid cancer. *Thyroid* 2009;19:1153.

40. Leboulleux S, Girard E, Rose M et al. Ultrasound criteria of malignancy for cervical lymph nodes in patients followed up for differentiated thyroid cancer. *J Clin Endocrinol Metab* 2007;92:3590.

41. White ML, Gauger PG, Doherty GM. Central lymph node dissection in differentiated thyroid cancer. *World J Surg* 2007;31:895–904.

42. Carling T, Long WD 3rd, Udelsman R. Controversy surrounding the role for routine central lymph node dissection for differentiated thyroid cancer. *Curr Opin Oncol* 2010;22(1):30–4.

43. Carling T, Carty SE, Ciarleglio MM et al. American Thyroid Association design and feasibility of a prospective randomized controlled trial of prophylactic central lymph node dissection for papillary thyroid carcinoma. *Thyroid* 2012;22:237–44.

44. Viola D, Materazzi G, Valerio L et al. Prophylactic central compartment lymph node dissection in papillary thyroid carcinoma: Clinical implications derived from the first prospective randomized controlled single institution study. *J Clin Endocrinol Metab* 2015;100:1316–24.

45. McHenry CR, Stulberg JJ. Prophylactic central compartment neck dissection for papillary thyroid cancer. *Surg Clin North Am* 2014;94:529–40.

46. Stack BC, Ferris RL, Goldenberg D et al. American Thyroid Association consensus review and statement regarding the anatomy, terminology, and rationale for lateral neck dissection in differentiated thyroid cancer. *Thyroid* 2012;22:501.

47. Carty SE, Doherty GM, Inabnet WB III et al. American Thyroid Association statement on the essential elements of interdisciplinary communication of perioperative information for patients undergoing thyroid cancer surgery. *Thyroid* 2012;22:395.

48. Armstrong MJ, Chiosea SI, Carty SE et al. Thyroid paragangliomas are locally aggressive. *Thyroid* 2012;22:88–93.

49. Mitchell J, Milas M, Barbosa G et al. Avoidable reoperations for thyroid and parathyroid surgery: Effect of hospital volume. *Surgery* 2008;144:899–906; discussion 906–7.

50. Dralle H, Sekulla C, Haerting J et al. Risk factors of paralysis and functional outcome after recurrent laryngeal nerve monitoring in thyroid surgery. *Surgery* 2004;136:1310.

51. Campbell MJ, McCoy KL, Shen WT et al. A multi-institutional international study of risk factors for hematoma after thyroidectomy. *Surgery* 2013;154:1283.

52. Adkisson CD, Howell GM, McCoy KL et al. Surgeon volume and adequacy of thyroidectomy for differentiated thyroid cancer. *Surgery* 2014;156:1453–59.

53. Sosa JA, Bowman HM, Tielsch JM et al. The importance of surgeon experience for clinical and economic outcomes from thyroidectomy. *Ann Surg* 1998;228(3):320–30.

54. Miyauchi A, Inoue H, Tomoda C et al. Improvement in phonation after reconstruction of the recurrent laryngeal nerve in patients with thyroid cancer invading the nerve. *Surgery* 2009;146:1056.

55. Hydman J, Remahl S, Bjorck G et al. Nimodipine improves reinnervation and neuromuscular function after injury to the recurrent laryngeal nerve in the rat. *Ann Otol Rhinol* 2007;116:623.

56. Stein R, Godel V. Hypocalcemic cataract. *J Pediatr Ophthalmol Strabismus* 1980;17:159.

57. Inabnet WB, Shifrin A, Ahmed L et al. Safety of same day discharge in patients undergoing sutureless thyroidectomy: A comparison of local and general anesthesia. *Thyroid* 2008;18:57.

58. Vrabec S, Oltmann SC, Clark N et al. A short-stay unit for thyroidectomy patients increases discharge efficiency. *J Surg Res* 2013;184:204.

59. Haugen BR, Alexander EK, Bible KC et al. 2015 American Thyroid Association Guidelines for adult patients with thyroid nodules and differentiated thyroid cancer: The American Thyroid Association Guidelines Task force on thyroid nodules and differentiated thyroid cancer. *Thyroid* 2016;26:1–133.

60. Xing M, Liu R, Liu X et al. BRAF V600E and TERT promoter mutations cooperatively identify the most aggressive papillary thyroid cancer with highest recurrence. *J Clin Oncol* 2014;32:2718–26.

14

Medullary thyroid cancer

DANIEL RUAN AND SUSAN C. PITT

In 2014, nearly 63,000 new cases of thyroid cancer were diagnosed in the United States [1]. Medullary thyroid cancer (MTC) represents only 4%–5% of these thyroid cancers, or approximately 2800 newly diagnosed patients each year [2]. Unlike differentiated thyroid cancers that arise from follicular cells, such as papillary (PTC) or follicular (FTC) types, MTCs arise from neural crest-derived, parafollicular C-cells that possess the ability to secrete bioactive peptides and hormones, particularly calcitonin. On gross pathology, MTCs have a distinct whitish-grey, firm appearance. Histologically, they appear as uniform spindle- or polygonal-shaped cells with a fine granular eosinophylic cytoplasm and stromal amyloid (Figure 14.1) [3,4]. These tumors exhibit a wide variety of behaviors from indolent to aggressive and are hereditary in 25% of cases. As such, the treatment, prognosis, and outcomes may also vary.

CLINICAL PRESENTATION

MTC manifests itself with a wide spectrum of clinical disease that depends on whether the cancer is sporadic or familial, and further, which codon in the RET (rearranged during transfection) proto-oncogene is mutated. At one end of the spectrum, in approximately 10% of all MTC cases, the disease is found incidentally when thyroidectomy is performed for another reason [5]. However, most patients are diagnosed before surgery via fine-needle aspiration (FNA) of a palpable neck mass, either a solitary thyroid nodule or clinically apparent cervical lymphadenopathy [6]. The majority of MTC patients (75%) have sporadic disease, although a quarter of the sporadic MTCs still harbor a RET mutation. The remaining 25% of all MTC patients have hereditary disease, in the form of either multiple endocrine neoplasia syndrome type 2A or 2B (MEN2A or MEN2B) or familial MTC (FMTC). In contrast to sporadic disease, greater than 95% of patients with hereditary MTC have an identifiable RET mutation [4]. The continuum of disease aggressiveness in MTC ranges from sporadic, which is the most benign, to MEN2B, which is the most aggressive.

Patients with sporadic MTC typically present in their 50s or 60s, most often with a solitary palpable nodule. On the contrary, those with MEN2A and FMTC present in their 30s or 40s, while patients with MEN2B are even younger at diagnosis, ranging from infancy in patients with known germline mutations to the teens or 20s when no genetic syndrome has been identified [7]. Patients with these hereditary forms of MTC are more likely to have multifocal or bilateral disease at the time of diagnosis, and greater than 50% will also have lymph node metastases [8]. This nodal spread is most commonly in the central neck (level VI), followed by the ipsilateral lateral neck (levels II–V), the contralateral neck, and last, the anterior mediastinum (level VII). While a palpable neck mass is the most common presentation, symptoms of compression, such as dysphagia, hoarseness, and respiratory difficulty, are seen in approximately 15% of patients, often due to the posterior locations of these tumors [9]. Diarrhea, flushing, and weight loss are other symptoms that may be seen and are secondary to elevated calcitonin levels [3,9]. Very rarely, Cushing's syndrome is present due to ectopic production of corticotropin by the tumor [10,11]. Distant metastases are observed in approximately 10%–15% of patients at the time of presentation, and the most common sites include the lungs, liver, bone, and brain.

In patients with hereditary MTC, the presentation may vary because some patients may have no disease at all if they have a known family history or have had prior genetic

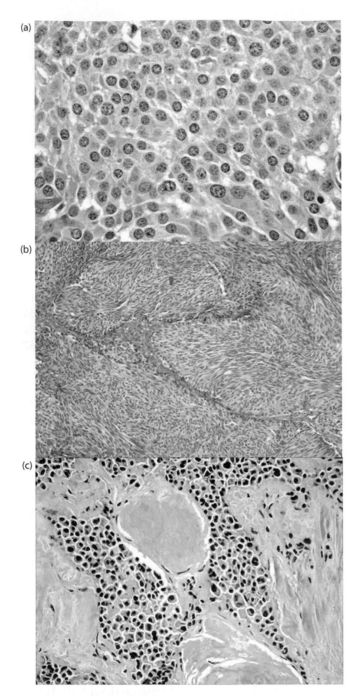

Figure 14.1 Histology of MTC demonstrates (a) epithelioid morphology with "salt and pepper" chromatin and fine, granular eosinophylic cytoplasm, as well as (b) spindle-cell morphology. (c) Cells can also have a plasmacytoid morphology with amyloid present in the stroma.

testing. In addition, patients may be diagnosed in the setting of other diseases within a specific syndrome. At present, a large proportion of patients with either FMTC or an MEN2 disorder are recognized after the diagnosis of a family member with a germline RET mutation located on chromosome 10q11 [7]. Genetic counseling in these patients and families is critical when performing mutational analysis of the RET

proto-oncogene. Transmission of a RET mutation is autosomal dominant, meaning that offspring have a 50% chance of inheriting the given disorder. Once inherited, penetrance of MTC is 100% [12,13].

The variable presentation of patients with hereditary MTC that is not diagnosed prior to disease development (due to genetic testing) is directly related to the other diseases within each disorder. These associated diseases are summarized in Table 14.1. MEN2A, or Sipple's syndrome, is the most common form of hereditary MTC, accounting for 75%–80% of patients in this class. The diseases associated with MEN2A other than MTC include pheochromocytoma and hyperparathyroidism, which are seen in 40%–50% and 20%–35% of these patients, respectively [7,10,11]. Cutaneous lichen amyloidosis (CLA) and Hirschsprung's disease can also be seen in MEN2A patients, but much less commonly [4], MEN2B accounts for 5%–15% of hereditary MTC, also has 100% penetrance of MTC, and is associated with pheochromocytoma in 40%–50% of cases [12,14]. Additional features of MEN2B include mucosal neuromas (of the lips, tongue, and eyelids), gastrointestinal ganglioneuromatosis, marfanoid body habitus, and chronic constipation with megacolon [12,14]. The marfanoid habitus and physical attributes can include a decreased ratio of the upper to lower body, joint laxity, low body fat, lack of aortic abnormalities or ectopia lentis typically associated with Marfan's syndrome, increased myelination of the corneal nerves, and everted eyelids [7,12,14]. Either MEN2A or MEN2B can present with a pheochromocytoma, although MTCs usually manifest first. In MEN2B, the median age at presentation is in the mid-20s [15]. Therefore, when evaluating a patient with a pheochromocytoma, a detailed family history should be obtained and further workup performed as indicated [9]. Patients with FMTC represent 5%–15% of hereditary MTC patients and typically present in a manner similar to that of MEN2A, but without the risk of other associated diseases [14].

GENOTYPE–PHENOTYPE OF MTC

The RET gene, which is mutated in approximately 25% of sporadic and 95% of hereditary MTCs, codes for a transmembrane tyrosine kinase receptor that is involved in renal and enteric nervous system development [4,16]. Mutations of the RET gene lead to gain-of-function or dominant-activating alterations, causing continuous phosphorylation of tyrosine residues and activation of intracellular signal transduction [17,18]. Only a single point missense mutation is necessary to cause malignant transformation and perpetually activate signaling pathways such as RAS/MAPK, JUN kinase, and PI3 K/AKT. A unique aspect of the association between mutations in the RET gene and the development of MTC is that various mutations in the RET domains are correlated with specific phenotypes expressed in patients. Table 14.2 summarizes the genotype–phenotype relationship in terms of MTC aggressiveness that is observed in MEN2 and FMTC patients.

Table 14.1 Hereditary MTC syndromes: Clinical features

Hereditary MTC type	Common clinical features (% penetrance)	Other features
MEN2A (75%–80%) (Sippel's syndrome)	MTC (100%) Pheochromocytoma (40%–50%) Primary hyperparathyroidism (20%–35%)	CLA (rare) Hirschsprung's disease (rare)
MEN2B (5%–15%)	MTC (100%) Pheochromocytoma (40%–50%) Variable (see right)	Mucosal neuromas, marfanoid body habitus, ganglioneuromatosis of gastrointestinal tract
FMTC (5%–10%)	MTC only (requires no diagnosis of either pheochromocytoma or hyperparathyroidism, ≥10 RET mutation carriers, and diagnosis after age 50 in multiple family members)	

Table 14.2 Genotype–phenotype relationships of hereditary MTC syndromes and therapeutic recommendations

Hereditary MTC syndrome	ATA risk level[a]	RET mutation[b]	Prophylactic thyroidectomy recommendations	Age recommendations to start PHEO and HPT screening
MEN2A	A (low)	609, 790, 791, 804, 891	Before age 5; may delay[c]	Age 20
	B	611, 618, 620, 630, 633, 634, V804M + V778I	Before age 5; may delay[c]	Age 20, except for 630 mutation, which is age 8
	C	C634R	Before age 5	Age 8
	D (high)	—		
MEN2B	A	—		
	B	—		
	C	—		
	D	883, 918, V804M + E805K or Y806 or S904C, 922	As soon as possible in first year of life	Age 8 for PHEO
FMTC	A	532, 609, 768, 790, 791, 804, 891, 912	Before age 5; may delay[c]	No screening guidelines[d]
	B	633, 634	Before age 5; may delay[c]	
	C	C634R	Before age 5	
	D	—		

Note: PHEO, pheochromocytoma; HPT, hyperparathyroidism. Other known mutations in hereditary MTC include codons 292, 533, 649, 666, and 891 in MEN2A, and codons 321, 510, 511, 515, 531, 600, 603, 606, 611, 620, 630, 632, 666, 770, 777, 778, 781, 819, 833, 844, 848, 904, 881, and 886 in FMTC.

[a] Level A mutations have the least risk of MTC and aggressiveness. Risk of MTC is the highest and most aggressive with level D mutations.
[b] Bolded mutations are the most commonly seen in each hereditary syndrome.
[c] For level A and B mutations, thyroidectomy may be delayed if the patient is screened with US and serum calcitonin levels remain normal, the family history phenotype is a poorly aggressive MTC form, or this is the patient's or family's preference.
[d] Screening guidelines do not exist for patients with FMTC, but the possibility of a PHEO remains with diagnostic error. One should have a low threshold for workup if the patient develops symptoms. The chance of missing a PHEO increases once a family is labeled with FMTC [7].

More than 50 mutations in the RET gene have been identified and are associated with one or more of the hereditary forms of MTC [19]. Furthermore, each mutation has been classified into levels of aggressiveness in terms of the risk of MTC development, associated outcomes, and recommendations for treatment (Table 14.2) [12]. The most common mutation in hereditary MTC is seen in MEN2A and FMTC and is in codon 634 in exon 11 of RET. A single point mutation at this cysteine codon results in an American Thyroid Association (ATA) level B risk mutation. MEN2A has a C634R mutation most commonly, whereas FMTC has a C634Y mutation the majority of the time. This RET 634 mutation is associated with CLA. Table 14.2 lists many of the mutations observed in the three hereditary MTC syndromes in terms of their ATA risk level. The lowest level of risk in the ATA system is level A, while the highest level of risk is level D [15]. In MEN2A, codons 609, 611, 618, and 620 in exon 11 also are observed with some frequency. These same mutations are linked to FMTC, as well as to mutations in codon 768 of exon 13 and codon 804 in exon 14. As opposed to the mutations in MEN2A and FMTC, those causative in MEN2B are rare, aggressive, and more often de novo germline RET mutations. The phenotype of MEN2B mutations, most commonly codon 918 in exon 16 and less commonly codon 883 in exon 15, leads to a younger age at diagnosis, a more advanced stage at presentation, and a higher mortality. The specific RET mutations can be used clinically to predict the phenotype of a particular patient in terms of both clinical course and likelihood of associated disease development, which may aid in surveillance, diagnosis, treatment decisions, and screening of additional family members.

DIAGNOSIS

The diagnosis of MTC is akin to that of other thyroid tumors when clinical manifestations of the disease are present. However, germline *RET* mutation testing and screening of individuals at risk for disease development provides an opportunity for performing a detailed history. Questioning about symptoms, such as voice changes, dysphagia, flushing, diarrhea, and bone pain, should be included. Eliciting a family history of thyroid cancer, primary hyperparathyroidism, pheochromocytoma, or other MEN2 diseases is important in discovering a yet undiagnosed hereditary MTC syndrome. Furthermore, attention should be paid to any history of hypertensive crises, headaches, palpitations, or hypercalcemia-associated symptoms (i.e., nephrolithiasis or osteoporosis).

On physical exam, one should note the size, mobility, and firmness of any neck mass, as well as any accompanying cervical lymphadenopathy. Because of the aggressiveness of MTC, signs or symptoms of tracheal or recurrent laryngeal nerve (RLN) involvement should also be noted. Manifestations of hereditary disease, such as the presence of any skin changes on the upper back, mucosal lesions, or marfanoid body habitus, should be included in the physical exam.

Since the most common presentation of MTC is a palpable neck mass, ultrasound (US) and FNA are typically the next diagnostic steps. US allows for characterization of the mass, thyroid, anatomy, and cervical lymph nodes (Figure 14.2). The US should be performed by a skilled ultrasonographer and include a scan of the ipsilateral and contralateral neck, as well as the superior mediastinum [15]. In addition, US can guide FNA attainment. Interpretation of the cytology specimen can be difficult with traditional staining based on the

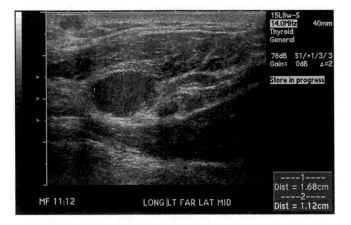

Figure 14.2 US imaging of a lateral cervical lymph node in a patient with MTC identifies a metastatic abnormal (enlarged, round) node.

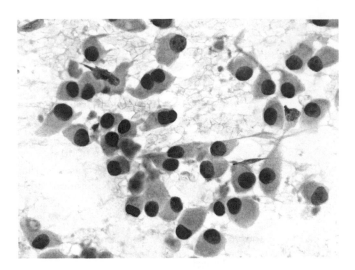

Figure 14.3 Medullary thyroid carcinoma, FNA. Cytologic preparations are usually highly cellular. The neoplastic cells can be epithelioid (as seen here), spindle shaped, or both. Amyloid is present. This patient presented with a cervical lymph node metastasis (Papanicolaou-stained smear).

cellular appearance alone—amyloid in the stroma and a paucity of thyroid follicles. Immunohistochemical (IHC) staining for calcitonin aids in the diagnosis, although the diagnostic accuracy of FNA remains limited [20,21] (Figure 14.3).

In addition to US and FNA, laboratory studies are also implemented in the diagnosis of MTC. Serum calcitonin testing is often confirmatory for MTC since a level greater than 100 pg/mL has a positive predictive value of 100% [22]. The serum calcitonin level can be implemented as a tumor marker to predict clinical behavior, as well as in following patients for disease recurrence postoperatively or screening those with potential hereditary MTC. A calcitonin level of 10–40 pg/mL suggests localized disease, whereas a level greater than 150 pg/mL is indicative of distant metastases [7]. When utilized as a screening test, a calcitonin level of more than 100 pg/mL raises suspicion for the presence of MTC. The 2010 National Comprehensive Cancer Network (NCCN) guidelines recommend a serum carcinoembryonic antigen (CEA) level as well, which is elevated in more than 50% of patients and correlates with disease prognosis. A CEA level of more than 30 mg/mL indicates that a poor prognosis is likely, while a level above 100 ng/mL is associated with extensive disease spread to the lymph nodes and distant sites [23]. Additional laboratory tests that are indicated in the diagnosis and workup of patients with MTC are plasma or urine metanephrines and catecholamines, looking for a pheochromocytoma and a serum calcium level that screens for hyperparathyroidism. Some also recommend chromogranin A. If the calcium is elevated, a serum parathyroid hormone (PTH) level should be obtained as well.

Various adjuncts and imaging studies in addition to US are frequently indicated to completely evaluate patients with MTC. Direct or indirect laryngoscopy is recommended in all patients to examine vocal cord function that may impact the operative planning [24]. In the presence of palpable nodal disease or a serum calcitonin level greater than 400 pg/mL, cross-sectional imaging of the chest and neck with a computed tomography (CT) and the abdomen with a CT or magnetic resonance imaging (MRI) is prudent (Figure 14.4a) [24]. The appearance of MTC on CT scan classically depicts calcifications within the metastases. ^{18}F-fluorodeoxyglucose positron emission tomography (FDG-PET) imaging plays a limited role in MTC diagnosis due to the decreased sensitivity of this modality. Nonetheless, in patients with occult metastatic disease undetectable on more conventional imaging methods, FDG-PET may be revealing, particularly if calcitonin levels exceed 1000 mg/mL (Figure 14.4). For persistently undetectable disease, laparoscopic evaluation of the liver may be necessary to identify metastases since the pattern of hepatic spread is miliary and results in multiple subcentimeter lesions. Abdominal imaging with an adrenal protocol CT or MRI is also indicated in patients with positive laboratory studies suggestive of pheochromocytoma. These preoperative studies allow for staging of patients who present with disease. While several staging systems have been proposed for MTC, the 2010 American Joint Committee on Cancer (AJCC) system is the most commonly employed (Table 14.3).

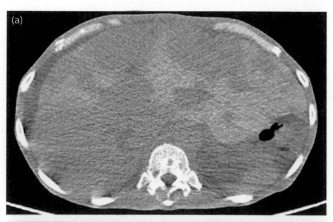

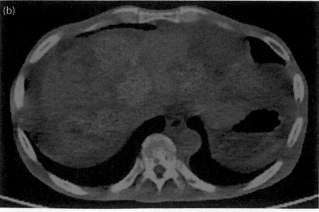

Figure 14.4 CT **(a)** and FDG-PET **(b)** demonstrate MTC hepatic metastases, a common location for MTC metastasis.

Genetic counseling and mutational *RET* testing is another useful tool in the diagnostic algorithm of MTC patients and their kindred. Current ATA guidelines recommend that all patients with a diagnosis of MTC or C-cell hyperplasia be offered *RET* testing for identification of possible germline mutations. C-cell hyperplasia is a precursor of MTC and is defined as greater than six C-cells/follicle or greater than 50 C-cells/low-power field (lpf). Working in conjunction with a genetic counselor to discuss issues related to the risks and benefits of the analysis is crucial for patients and families to make informed decisions. Those impacted by the results absolutely need to comprehend the interpretation and implications of a positive finding.

TREATMENT

Once the diagnostic evaluation and staging of MTC patients is complete, the appropriate therapy can be implemented. Surgery is the mainstay of treatment for MTC and the only curative treatment option. The type of surgical resection depends on whether the cancer is sporadic or hereditary, and also on the extent of disease at presentation. In patients with a hereditary *RET* mutation, disease may be absent, and thus treatment prophylactic. The recommendations for the operative management of hereditary MTC are included in Table 14.2, along with the appropriate timing for prophylactic surgery.

Surgical

In all patients with clinically apparent MTC, a total extracapsular thyroidectomy and bilateral central neck dissection (level VI) is the procedure of choice. At the time of surgery, disease is present in the central neck in the majority of these patients. Consequently, a central neck dissection is more likely to be curative than a total thyroidectomy alone. Whether a routine lateral neck dissection (levels IIA–V) is indicated remains under debate and is often guided by tumor size, calcitonin level, and preoperative US findings. Tumor size greater than 1 cm, a calcitonin level of more than 40 pg/mL, and suspicious lateral lymphadenopathy are all indications for a lateral neck dissection. In patients with sporadic MTC, an ipsilateral lateral neck dissection should generally only be performed when high-quality imaging detects nodal disease, although much controversy surrounds this issue. Overall, the treatment and extent of surgical resection for MTC patients is much debated since the literature in this area is conflicting. Because biochemical cure is often not attainable in patients with MTC, the risks associated with a lateral neck dissection, particularly in patients with sporadic disease, need to be weighed against the morbidity of the procedure. When evidence of nodal disease is present preoperatively in any patient with MTC, a bilateral neck dissection is recommended by many, in addition to a central neck dissection, because of the high likelihood of concurrent disease

Table 14.3 MTC staging (AJCC 2012, 7th edition) and corresponding survival

TNM Classification

Primary Tumor (T)

TX	Primary tumor cannot be assessed
T0	No evidence of primary tumor
T1	Tumor ≤2 cm in greatest dimension, limited to the thyroid
T1a	Tumor ≤1 cm
T1b	Tumor >1 cm but ≤2 cm in greatest dimension
T2	Tumor >2 cm but ≤4 cm in greatest dimension, limited to the thyroid
T3	Tumor >4 cm in greatest dimension, limited to the thyroid, or T1–T3 with minimal extrathyroid extension (within the sternothyroid muscle or perithyroid soft tissues)
T4a	Any T extending beyond the thyroid capsule and invading into the subcutaneous soft tissues, larynx, trachea, esophagus, or recurrent laryngeal nerve
T4b	Any T invading the prevertebral fascia and/or encasing the carotid artery or mediastinal vessels

Regional Lymph Nodes (N)

NX	Regional lymph nodes cannot be assessed
N0	No regional lymph node metastasis
N1	Regional lymph node metastasis (includes central compartment, lateral cervical, and upper mediastinal nodal basins)
N1a	Level VI lymph node metastasis (pretracheal, paratracheal, and/or prelaryngeal/Delphian lymph nodes)
N1b	Unilateral, bilateral, or contralateral cervical (levels I–V), retropharyngeal, or superior mediastinal (level VII) lymph node metastasis

Distant Metastases (M)

MX	Distant metastasis cannot be assessed
M0	No distant metastasis
M1	Distant metastasis

MTC Stage and Corresponding Survival

Stage	TNM category			Survival (%) [25–27]
I	T1a–T1b	N0	M0	98–100
II	T2	N0	M0	98–99
	T3	N0	M0	
III	T1–T3	N1a	M0	73–96
	T3	N0	M0	
IVA	T1–T3	N1a	M0	Stage IVA–C
	T4a	N0–N1a	M0	40–82
	T1–T4a	N1b	M0	
IVB	T4b	Any N	M0	
IVC	Any T	Any N	M1	

Source: Edge S. et al. eds., *AJCC Cancer Staging Manual*, 7th ed., Springer, New York, 2012.
Note: TNM, tumor, node, metastasis.

in other nodal basins [14]. However, some surgeons in this situation would not perform a contralateral neck dissection because of the increased risks and lack of clear evidence of a survival benefit.

When germline *RET* mutations are known, prophylactic thyroidectomy is indicated [28]. The ATA recommendations for timing of prophylactic surgery are listed in Table 14.2. Additional groups, including the International Workshop on Multiple Endocrine Neoplasia, the North American Neuroendocrine Tumor Society (NANETs), and the NCCN, have published their own set of guidelines. These other guidelines all utilize a three-level system (1, 2, 3 or low, medium, high) for stratifying risk instead of the four levels (A, B, C, D) used by the ATA. In addition, each group considered ATA levels C and D, the highest level, as one category. The main differences of these other guidelines are related to the timing of thyroidectomy in the lowest-risk (ATA level A) group.

According to ATA guidelines, in MEN2A and FMTC, prophylactic thyroidectomy should be performed by age 5 (or at the time of diagnosis if later) for levels A, B, and C. However, level A and B patients can delay prophylactic thyroidectomy and be followed with annual serum calcitonin and US screening as long as these studies remain normal and there is no family history of aggressive MTC. The other sets of guidelines recommend prophylactic thyroidectomy for equivalent group A patients between the ages of 5 and 10 years. For these low-risk patients, when the serum calcium and US are normal, no concomitant lymphadenectomy is necessary. However, if the serum calcitonin is more than 40 pg/mL or US is suspicious for disease, a bilateral central neck dissection is recommended. In the more aggressive MEN2B, a prophylactic total thyroidectomy and bilateral central neck dissection before the age of 1 is the optimal surgical management. An ipsilateral lateral neck dissection should be considered if a tumor greater than 0.5 cm is present. In addition, due to the technical difficulty of the procedure in infancy, an experienced surgeon should perform surgery in order to avoid complications.

During surgical intervention in all patients with MTC, the parathyroids are at risk for devascularization because a total extracapsular thyroidectomy is central to operative management. When the parathyroids have lost their blood supply in patients with sporadic MTC, FMTC, or MEN2B, standard autograft into the sternocleidomastoid muscle is appropriate. However, patients with MEN2A are at risk for developing hyperparathyroidism; therefore, autotransplantation into the forearm and cryopreservation of tissue should be strongly considered to aid future management. If hyperparathyroidism is already present in a patient with MEN2A and hyperplasia is the underlying cause, then a total parathyroidectomy with forearm transplantation is indicated. If an adenoma is the underlying mechanism, then the usual management should be performed. A prophylactic parathyroidectomy at the time of thyroidectomy is not prudent. If preoperative workup detects a pheochromocytoma in a patient with MEN2A or 2B, the pheochromocytoma should be treated first.

Locoregional therapies

Alternative invasive and noninvasive medical therapies may be indicated in patients with unresectable MTC. Unlike patients with PTC or FTC, those with MTC do not respond to radioactive iodine (RAI) or thyroid suppression with thyroxine. Radiofrequency ablation (RFA) or chemoembolization can be employed in patients with nonmiliary hepatic metastases. Patients with MTC that is not amenable to such treatment can also be treated medically. Symptomatic treatment may include narcotics for pain or somatostatin analogs for diarrhea or flushing. Bisphosphonates and radiotherapy can be useful in treating bony metastases. External beam radiation therapy (XRT) also has commonly been used for cervical and mediastinal disease and has a potential role in MTC therapy [29]. In patients at high risk for local recurrence due to features of their primary tumor, such as local invasion, positive margin status, significant nodal burden, and extranodal extension, XRT has been shown to decrease the 10-year local recurrence rate [30]. Traditional chemotherapy, however, is not terribly effective for MTC. Less than 30% of patients respond to single agents, such as doxorubicin, capecitabine, or 5-fluorouracil [31].

Targeted therapies

More recently, small-molecule inhibitors targeted at RET have been employed. These receptor tyrosine kinases act by binding to the adenosine triphosphate (ATP) site of the RET catalytic domain and inhibiting downstream signaling by interfering with autophosphorylation. Imatinib, sorafenib, sunitinib, motesanib, axitinib, vandetamib, and cabozantinib have all been investigated and demonstrated variable response rates, although all are not approved Food and Drug Administration (FDA) therapies. The efficacy of these agents has ranged from stable disease to partial response. Additional therapies aimed at intracellular signaling pathways are being investigated *in vitro* and may eventually play a role in MTC treatment [18,32–38].

SURVEILLANCE

Postoperatively, MTC patients should undergo surveillance to detect disease recurrence early. A baseline serum calcitonin and CEA levels should be checked in the postoperative period approximately 72 hours after surgery to allow for a new steady state to be reached [3]. If the calcitonin level is undetectable and the CEA level normal, then levels should be checked annually with a US of the neck. Some surgeons also check levels 3–6 months after surgery when the calcitonin nadir is sometimes reached [14]. In patients with MEN syndromes, surveillance at the same time intervals should include screening laboratories for pheochromocytoma in both MEN2A and MEN2B, and hyperparathyroidism in MEN2A.

As a tumor marker, calcitonin is very sensitive for the detection of microscopic persistent or recurrent disease, and is elevated in more than 50% of MTC patients at some point in the postoperative period. However, an elevated calcitonin level is often observed in the setting of occult disease on conventional imaging, and the management of such patients can be difficult and controversial. In asymptomatic patients with elevated calcitonin or CEA levels and no evidence of disease on imaging, including US of the neck; CT of the neck, chest, and abdomen; or MRI of the liver and axial skeleton, surveillance should continue with tumor marker levels and cervical US every 6 months. If a further rise in calcitonin or CEA is observed, or if the calcitonin level is greater than 150 pg/mL, then a metastatic workup should be performed or repeated. Observation in the setting of elevated tumor markers can be unsettling, especially if inadequate lymphadenectomy was performed at the initial operation. Nevertheless, reoperation is not recommended unless disease is clinically evident on exam or imaging. Once postoperative surveillance has identified persistent or recurrent MTC, management is operative when possible and may result in biochemical normalization in more than 25% of patients [39,40]. For patients with hereditary MTC who undergo prophylactic thyroidectomy with no evidence of MTC on final pathology, the role of surveillance is less well defined.

PROGNOSIS

The survival for patients with MTC has improved over the last few decades, but remains worse than that of differentiated thyroid cancers, like PTC and FTC. The mean survival of MTC from the time of diagnosis is approximately 8.5 years [25]. Overall, the survival rates for all patients with MTC are reported to be 80%–97% at 5 years and 75%–88% at 10 years [26,41]. When examined by AJCC stage, the 5-year overall survival rates for stages I–IV, respectively, are 100%, 99%, 96%, and 82% [42]. The greatest improvement in survival has been in patients with stages III and IV disease, whose 5-year overall survival has improved from 73% to 96% in stage III patients and from 40% to 82% in stage IV patients over the last 30 years [26,42]. The development of novel therapies and improved imaging techniques will likely continue to improve the outcomes of patients with MTC.

Several factors have been shown to be associated with the prognosis of patients with MTC, including disease stage, age at presentation, and extent of surgery [25,27]. Patients with distant metastases have been shown to have a 4.5-fold increased risk of death when compared with patients with localized disease [25]. In addition, patients over the age of 65 are also at increased risk of death. Male gender has also been associated with a worse prognosis. Not surprisingly, pathology-related factors likened to improved outcomes include small tumor size, well-differentiated status, lack of extracapsular extension, and absence of lymphatic involvement [9,25,27,41]. A postsurgical undetectable calcitonin level is also associated with a better prognosis.

CONCLUSION

MTC is an aggressive form of thyroid cancer that is distinct from differentiated thyroid cancers, like PTC and FTC, and requires a different diagnostic, surgical, and adjuvant treatment algorithm. Notably, 25% of MTC is associated with three hereditary syndromes, MEN2A, MEN2B, and FMTC, which have germline mutations in the *RET* gene. Therefore, genetic screening is indicated in all patients with MTC, and prophylactic thyroidectomy is often appropriate if a mutation is discovered. The various *RET* mutations have a genotype–phenotype correlation that should direct therapeutic decisions like the timing and extent of resection. When evaluating a patient with MTC, screening for pheochromocytoma and hyperparathyroidism should be performed, and if found, a pheochromocytoma should be treated first. Calcitonin and CEA measurement are important in the diagnosis and surveillance of this disease, as well as in screening patients with hereditary MTC. The extent of

surgical resection is also different in patients with clinically proven MTC and should include a bilateral central neck dissection. Adjuvant treatment is dissimilar as well since MTC does not respond to RAI. MTC also differs from PTC or FTC in that it has a worse prognosis, although outcomes for MTC patients have appreciably improved in the last 20–30 years.

REFERENCES

1. American Cancer Society. Cancer facts & figures ACS. http://www.cancer.org/acs/groups/content/@research/documents/webcontent/acspc-042151.pdf (accessed August 18, 2014).
2. Panigrahi B, Roman S, Sosa J. Medullary thyroid cancer: Are practice patterns in the United States discordant from American thyroid association guidelines? *Ann Surg Oncol* 2010;17:1490–8.
3. Fialkowski E, Moley J. Current approaches to medullary thyroid carcinoma, sporadic and familial. *J Surg Oncol* 2006;94(8):737–47.
4. Pitt SC, Moley JF. Medullary, anaplastic, and metastatic cancers of the thyroid. *Semin Oncol* 2010;37(6):567–79.
5. Ahmed RA, Ball DW. Incidentally discovered medullary thyroid cancer: Diagnostic strategies and treatment. *J Clin Endocrinol Metab* 2011;96(5):1237–45.
6. Saad MF, Ordonez NG, Rashid RK et al. Medullary carcinoma of the thyroid. A study of the clinical features and prognostic factors in 161 patients. *Medicine* 1984;63(6):319–42.
7. Roy M, Chen H, Sippel RS. Current understanding and management of medullary thyroid cancer. *Oncologist* 2013;18(10):1093–100.
8. Moley JF, DeBenedetti MK. Patterns of nodal metastases in palpable medullary thyroid carcinoma: Recommendations for extent of node dissection. *Ann Surg* 1999;229(6):880–7; discussion 887–8.
9. Kebebew E, Ituarte PH, Siperstein AE, Duh QY, Clark OH. Medullary thyroid carcinoma: Clinical characteristics, treatment, prognostic factors, and a comparison of staging systems. *Cancer* 2000;88(5):1139–48.
10. Mure A, Gicquel C, Abdelmoumene N et al. Cushing's syndrome in medullary thyroid carcinoma. *J Endocrinol Invest* 1995;18(3):180–5.
11. Smallridge RC, Bourne K, Pearson BW, Van Heerden JA, Carpenter PC, Young WF. Cushing's syndrome due to medullary thyroid carcinoma: Diagnosis by proopiomelanocortin messenger ribonucleic acid *in situ* hybridization. *J Clin Endocrinol Metab* 2003;88(10):4565–8.
12. Brandi ML, Gagel RF, Angeli A et al. Guidelines for diagnosis and therapy of MEN type 1 and type 2. *J Clin Endocrinol Metab* 2001;86(12):5658–71.
13. Howe JR, Norton JA, Wells SA Jr. Prevalence of pheochromocytoma and hyperparathyroidism in multiple endocrine neoplasia type 2A: Results of long-term follow-up. *Surgery* 1993;114(6):1070–7.

14. Callender GC, Hu MI, Evans DB, Perrier, ND. Medullary thyroid cancer. In: Morita SY, Dackiw APB, Zeiger MA, eds., *McGraw-Hill Manual Endocrine Surgery.* New York: McGraw-Hill, 2009: chapter 6.

15. American Thyroid Association Guidelines Task F, Kloos RT, Eng C et al. Medullary thyroid cancer: Management guidelines of the American Thyroid Association. *Thyroid* 2009;19(6):565–612.

16. Liu Z, Falola J, Zhu X et al. Antiproliferative effects of Src inhibition on medullary thyroid cancer. *J Clin Endocrinol Metab* 2004;89(7):3503–9.

17. Wells SA Jr, Pacini F, Robinson BG, Santoro M. Multiple endocrine neoplasia type 2 and familial medullary thyroid carcinoma: An update. *J Clin Endocrinol Metab* 2013;98(8):3149–4.

18. Pitt SC, Chen H. The phosphatidylinositol 3-kinase/akt signaling pathway in medullary thyroid cancer. *Surgery* 2008;144(5):721–4.

19. Krampitz GW, Norton JA. RET gene mutations (genotype and phenotype) of multiple endocrine neoplasia type 2 and familial medullary thyroid carcinoma. *Cancer* 2014;120(13):1920–31.

20. Chang TC, Wu SL, Hsiao YL. Medullary thyroid carcinoma: Pitfalls in diagnosis by fine needle aspiration cytology and relationship of cytomorphology to RET proto-oncogene mutations. *Acta Cytologica* 2005;49(5):477–82.

21. Papaparaskeva K, Nagel H, Droese M. Cytologic diagnosis of medullary carcinoma of the thyroid gland. *Diagnostic Cytopathology* 2000;22(6):351–8.

22. Costante G, Filetti S. Early diagnosis of medullary thyroid carcinoma: Is systematic calcitonin screening appropriate in patients with nodular thyroid disease? *Oncologist* 2011;16(1):49–52.

23. Machens A, Dralle H. Pretargeted anti-carcinoembryonic-antigen radioimmunotherapy for medullary thyroid carcinoma. *J Clin Oncol* 2006;24(20):e37; author reply e38.

24. Tuttle RM, Ball DW, Byrd D et al. Medullary carcinoma. *J Natl Compr Canc Netw* 2010;8(5):512–30.

25. Roman S, Lin R, Sosa JA. Prognosis of medullary thyroid carcinoma: Demographic, clinical, and pathologic predictors of survival in 1252 cases. *Cancer* 2006;107(9):2134–42.

26. Hundahl SA, Fleming ID, Fremgen AM, Menck HR. A National Cancer Data Base report on 53,856 cases of thyroid carcinoma treated in the U.S., 1985–1995 [see comments]. *Cancer* 1998;83(12):2638–48.

27. Gilliland FD, Hunt WC, Morris DM, Key CR. Prognostic factors for thyroid carcinoma. A population-based study of 15,698 cases from the Surveillance, Epidemiology and End Results (SEER) program 1973–91. *Cancer* 1997;79(3):564–73.

28. Chen H, Sippel RS, O'Dorisio MS et al. The North American Neuroendocrine Tumor Society consensus guideline for the diagnosis and management of neuroendocrine tumors: Pheochromocytoma, paraganglioma, and medullary thyroid cancer. *Pancreas* 2010;39(6):775–83.

29. Schwartz DL, Rana V, Shaw S et al. Postoperative radiotherapy for advanced medullary thyroid cancer—Local disease control in the modern era. *Head Neck* 2008;30(7):883–8.

30. Brierley J, Tsang R, Simpson WJ, Gospodarowicz M, Sutcliffe S, Panzarella T. Medullary thyroid cancer: Analyses of survival and prognostic factors and the role of radiation therapy in local control. *Thyroid* 1996;6(4):305–10.

31. Sippel RS, Kunnimalaiyaan M, Chen H. Current management of medullary thyroid cancer. *Oncologist* 2008;13(5):539–47.

32. Chen H, Carson-Walter EB, Baylin SB, Nelkin BD, Ball DW. Differentiation of medullary thyroid cancer by C-Raf-1 silences expression of the neural transcription factor human achaete-scute homolog-1. *Surgery* 1996;120(2):168–72; discussion 173.

33. Chen H, Kunnimalaiyaan M, Van Gompel JJ. Medullary thyroid cancer: The functions of raf-1 and human achaete-scute homologue-1. *Thyroid* 2005;15:511–21.

34. Cook M, Yu XM, Chen H. Notch in the development of thyroid C-cells and the treatment of medullary thyroid cancer. *Am J Transl Res* 2010;2(1):119–25.

35. Cook MR, Luo J, Ndiaye M, Chen H, Kunnimalaiyaan M. Xanthohumol inhibits the neuroendocrine transcription factor achaete-scute complex-like 1, suppresses proliferation, and induces phosphorylated ERK1/2 in medullary thyroid cancer. *Am J Surg* 2010;199(3):315–8; discussion 318.

36. Greenblatt DY, Cayo MA, Adler JT et al. Valproic acid activates Notch1 signaling and induces apoptosis in medullary thyroid cancer cells. *Ann Surg* 2008;247(6):1036–40.

37. Adler JT, Cook M, Luo Y et al. Tautomycetin and tautomycin suppress the growth of medullary thyroid cancer cells via inhibition of glycogen synthase kinase-3beta. *Mol Cancer Ther* 2009;8(4):914–20.

38. Alhefdhi A, Burke JF, Redlich A, Kunnimalaiyaan M, Chen H. Leflunomide suppresses growth in human medullary thyroid cancer cells. *J Surg Res* 2013;185(1):212–6.

39. Moley JF, Dilley WG, DeBenedetti MK. Improved results of cervical reoperation for medullary thyroid carcinoma. *Ann Surg* 1997;225(6):734–40; discussion 740–33.

40. Kebebew E, Kikuchi S, Duh QY, Clark OH. Long-term results of reoperation and localizing studies in patients with persistent or recurrent medullary thyroid cancer. *Arch Surg* 2000;135(8):895–901.

41. Clark JR, Fridman TR, Odell MJ, Brierley J, Walfish PG, Freeman JL. Prognostic variables and calcitonin in medullary thyroid cancer. *Laryngoscope* 2005;115(8):1445–50.

42. Boostrom SY, Grant CS, Thompson GB et al. Need for a revised staging consensus in medullary thyroid carcinoma. *Arch Surg* 2009;144(7):663–9.

15

Anaplastic thyroid carcinoma

ELIZABETH G. DEMICCO

INTRODUCTION

Anaplastic (undifferentiated) thyroid carcinoma is the least common form of primary thyroid carcinoma, with an incidence rate of 0.21 per 100,000 person years in the United States [1], and accounting for approximately 2% of all thyroid malignancy [2]. Worldwide, the incidence of anaplastic carcinoma varies regionally from 1% to as high as 26% of thyroid carcinoma [3]. Geographic variations in incidence are thought to be related to dietary iodine intake, as well as detection and management of precursor lesions (differentiated thyroid carcinomas) [2,4]. Although uncommon, anaplastic thyroid carcinoma is disproportionately fatal compared with differentiated forms of thyroid carcinoma and causes more than 50% of thyroid carcinoma-related deaths [4]. This chapter reviews the clinicopathologic features of anaplastic thyroid carcinoma, as well as the current state of knowledge as to the molecular underpinning of disease, and discusses current and emerging therapeutic options.

CLINICAL FEATURES

Anaplastic thyroid carcinoma is a disease of older patients, with a mean age of ~60 years at the time of diagnosis, and peak incidence occurring in the sixth or seventh decade of life [1]. Women are 1.5–3 times more likely to develop anaplastic thyroid carcinoma than men [1,5]. Risk factors for the development of anaplastic carcinoma include low socioeconomic status, lack of access to medical care, and endemic goiter [3].

The incidence of anaplastic thyroid carcinoma has shown dramatic declines over the past 40 years. These declines are variously attributed to improved medical screening and increased access to medical care [3], with subsequent increased resection rates of follicular-derived differentiated thyroid carcinoma (papillary and follicular carcinoma) [4]. Increased iodine prophylaxis may also contribute to the decline in anaplastic carcinoma [4], although concurrent gains in access to medical care in affected regions are a confounding factor in these analyses [3].

Patients present with a rapidly growing neck mass over a course of weeks to months [6]. Symptoms of airway compromise (dyspnea, cough) due to compression by tumor are frequently present. Other symptoms include vocal cord paralysis (seen in approximately 30% of patients), hoarseness, pain, and dysphagia. There is often a preexisting history of long-standing goiter or thyroid mass with a recent sudden and dramatic increase in size [5]. At the time of diagnosis, fewer than 10% of cases are confined to the thyroid, with the majority demonstrating extensive invasion of the soft tissues of the neck, or locoregional lymph node metastases [1]. Approximately 34% of cases have been reported to have distant metastases at diagnosis [1,7,8], with another 32% subsequently progressing to distant metastatic disease. Metastatic spread is typically hematogenous and most commonly involves the lungs, with the bones and brain being slightly less frequently involved [7,8].

STAGING

Because of its aggressive behavior and poor prognosis, anaplastic thyroid carcinoma is classified by the American Joint Committee on Cancer (AJCC) as a T4, stage 4 malignancy [9]. Tumors confined to the thyroid (stage 4a) account for <20% of cases, while those with locoregional spread (stage 4b) or distant metastasis (stage 4c) account for the majority of cases.

HISTOPATHOLOGY

Grossly, anaplastic thyroid carcinoma is a large, tan, soft fleshy tumor (Figure 15.1), which may be difficult to separate from adjacent structures due to extensive invasion. Foci of hemorrhage or necrosis are common. The mean size is 8 cm, and tumors can be as large as 20 cm [4].

As the name implies, anaplastic thyroid carcinomas lose morphologic and antigenic evidence of thyroid differentiation at both the microscopic and biochemical levels. Tumors are characterized by a diffusely infiltrative growth pattern and are only rarely confined to the thyroid at the time of diagnosis. Malignant cells may grow in small nests or cords, but are more commonly arranged in disorganized sheets or fascicles. Necrosis is nearly always present, as the tumor rapidly outgrows its vascular supply. A marked

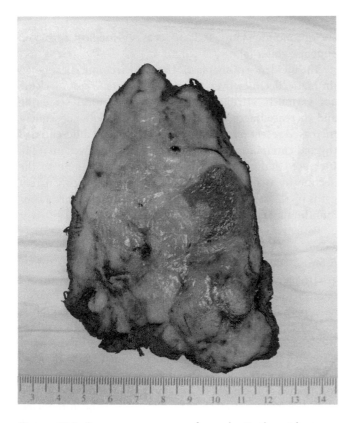

Figure 15.1 Gross appearance of anaplastic carcinoma. The tumor is a large, pink–white fleshy mass. At right, the darker tan, slightly gelatinous area represents residual thyroid parenchyma, partially invaded by the extensive carcinoma.

intratumoral inflammatory response with prominent neutrophils is a common finding, and may be associated with necrosis. A desmoplastic stromal reaction is also common. Mitoses are frequent, and may include atypical forms (e.g., tripolar mitotic spindles). Nuclear features vary, but nuclear enlargement, hyperchromasia, and marked nuclear membrane irregularities are typical findings.

Variants

Several morphologic variants of anaplastic thyroid carcinoma are recognized, including squamoid, spindle cell, pleomorphic (giant cell), giant cell rich, and paucicellular (Table 15.1). In general, the morphologic distinction between the variants is not thought to have prognostic significance, but is important for formulating a differential diagnosis and identifying potential mimics that must be excluded in order to confirm the diagnosis of anaplastic carcinoma.

The squamoid variant of anaplastic carcinoma usually arises from papillary thyroid carcinoma. Malignant cells are arranged in cohesive sheets, and have abundant eosinophilic cytoplasm and distinct cell borders (Figure 15.2a). Very rarely, true intracytoplasmic bridges or keratin pearls may be seen. The challenge in diagnosing the squamoid variant of anaplastic thyroid carcinoma lies in excluding a true squamous cell carcinoma. Squamous cell carcinomas of the skin or upper aerodigestive tract and larynx may involve the thyroid by direct extension or via spread from a locoregional neck metastasis. Pathologic distinction is easily made in well-differentiated tumors, or when the epicenter of the tumor is clearly arising outside of the thyroid. However, poorly differentiated carcinomas with extensive involvement of multiple structures in the neck are more difficult to characterize, particularly as squamoid anaplastic carcinoma expresses immunohistochemical markers of squamous differentiation (Figure 15.2b). In such cases, correct diagnosis relies upon the identification of a thyroid precursor differentiated carcinoma, or retention of markers of thyroid differentiation in malignant cells. Primary squamous cell carcinoma of the thyroid, a controversial entity, is also a consideration in the differential diagnosis. However, the prognosis is identical to squamoid anaplastic carcinoma, and it may not, in fact, represent a separate entity.

Spindle cell and pleomorphic (giant cell) variants of anaplastic thyroid carcinoma constitute a spectrum of sarcomatoid carcinoma. Spindle cell anaplastic thyroid carcinoma

Table 15.1 Morphologic variants of anaplastic thyroid carcinoma

Common
    Spindle cell
    Pleomorphic (Giant cell)
    Squamoid
Uncommon
    Giant cell rich
    Paucicellular

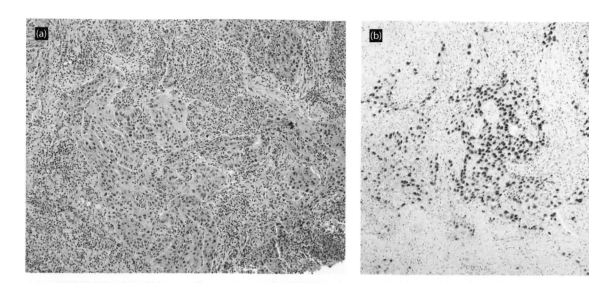

Figure 15.2 Squamoid variant of anaplastic thyroid carcinoma. **(a)** Malignant cells are arranged in anastomosing nests and cords within a desmoplastic fibrous stroma with a prominent inflammatory response. Cells are tightly cohesive and have abundant eosinophilic cytoplasm. H&E, hematoxylin and eosin stain. **(b)** Immunohistochemical study demonstrates antigenic evidence of aberrant squamous differentiation in the form of nuclear expression of p63 in malignant cells.

is composed of fascicles and sheets of atypical spindle cells (Figure 15.3a and b), while the pleomorphic variant is composed of wildly variable giant tumor cells with abundant cytoplasm and enlarged, bizarre, frequently multilobated nuclei with nuclear hyperchromasia or macronucleoli (Figure 15.3c and d). Spindle cell and pleomorphic anaplastic thyroid carcinoma is often a morphologic and immunohistochemical diagnosis of exclusion, as tumors may overgrow preexisting differentiated carcinoma and lose expression of both thyroid and epithelial markers. Foci of heterologous mesenchymal differentiation, including malignant osteoid, cartilage, or angiosarcoma, have been reported. Because the histologic appearance may be so variable from one patient to the next, spindle cell and pleomorphic anaplastic thyroid carcinomas have a broad differential diagnosis, including true sarcomas, anaplastic large cell lymphoma, medullary carcinomas, and metastatic sarcomatoid carcinomas of other sites. One important consideration in the differential diagnosis is a metastatic sarcomatoid renal cell carcinoma, which may be difficult to exclude on the basis of immunohistochemistry alone, and requires clinical correlation.

Giant cell-rich anaplastic thyroid carcinoma is also known as anaplastic thyroid carcinoma with osteoclast-like giant cells. The giant cells are not, themselves, the malignant cells but are secondarily recruited, nonneoplastic, tumor-infiltrating cells. These cells are large, and histologically resemble osteoclasts with multiple small, bland, oval nuclei with pale chromatin and small nucleoli. Osteoclast-like giant cells are more likely to be seen in anaplastic carcinomas with foci of hemorrhage, calcification, or ossification, and are thought to be reactive. It is important to note that the nomenclature in the literature may present some confusion as to the distinction between giant cell-rich and giant cell anaplastic carcinoma. In giant cell (pleomorphic) anaplastic carcinoma, the term *giant cell* is used to refer to

the massively enlarged malignant tumor cells, which may or may not possess multilobated bizarre nuclei, while in giant cell-rich anaplastic carcinoma, the giant cells are benign cells derived from monocytes, with true multinucleation.

The paucicellular variant of anaplastic thyroid carcinoma is uncommon, and rather than being a distinct histopathologic variant, it probably results from secondary changes affecting the tumor. Paucicellular anaplastic thyroid carcinomas are characterized by dense fibrosis and low cellularity, thought to be due to ischemic changes and tumor infarction. This variant must be distinguished from fibrosing processes such as immunoglobulin (Ig) G4-related sclerosing thyroiditis or Reidel's thyroiditis. Some studies have reported a possible association between paucicellular anaplastic carcinoma and younger patients, with improved survival compared with other variants [8].

Tumors previously reported as the small cell variant of anaplastic thyroid carcinoma are now considered to have been misclassified lymphomas, medullary carcinoma, or poorly differentiated carcinoma. Thus, with expansion of the diagnostic immunohistochemical arsenal, this histologic variant is no longer thought to exist.

Immunohistochemistry

Confirmatory immunohistochemical studies are of limited use in anaplastic carcinoma (Table 15.2). Conventional markers of thyroid follicular differentiation include thyroglobulin, TTF-1, and PAX8. Anaplastic carcinomas typically lose expression of these markers, or may only have patchy foci of positivity at best. PAX8 has been reported to be retained after loss of TTF-1 and thyroglobulin, particularly in squamoid anaplastic carcinoma, but is not entirely specific for thyroid origin, and also stains tumors of thymic origin or metastatic renal cell carcinomas, among others.

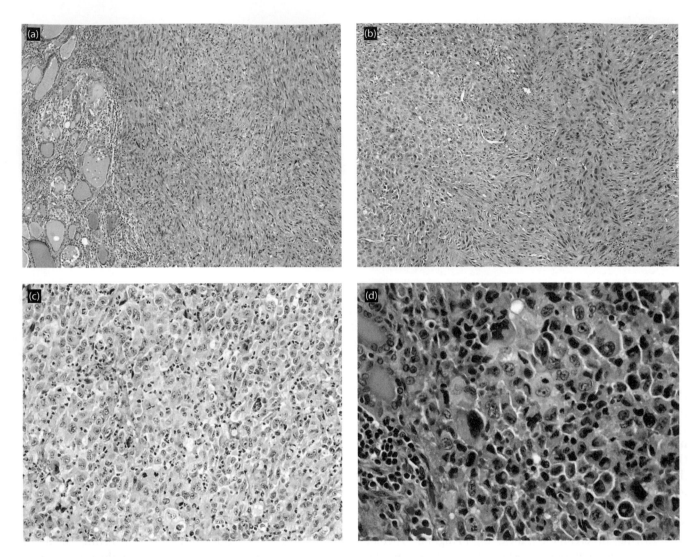

Figure 15.3 Spindle cell and pleomorphic variants of anaplastic thyroid carcinoma. **(a and b)** Spindle cell variant. **(a)** The undifferentiated spindle cell proliferation is juxtaposed to adjacent nonneoplastic thyroid at left. **(b)** Multiple morphologies may be seen within one tumor. Here, a more epithelioid population of tumor cells is seen at left, arranged in small nests. At right, the tumor transitions into a purely spindle cell morphology with fascicular growth pattern. **(c and d)** Pleomorphic variant. **(c)** Malignant cells are arranged in discohesive sheets. Cells have abundant cytoplasm and demonstrate marked variation in nuclear size and shape, with characteristic nuclear membrane irregularities. Numerous mitoses are present, including atypical forms. A neutrophilic infiltrate is present. **(d)** At high power, the marked pleomorphism of malignant cells is readily apparent. At upper left, two nonneoplastic thyroid follicles are present; anaplastic cells are markedly enlarged relative to these. H&E stain, all images.

Epithelial markers, including pancytokeratins and low-molecular-weight keratins (CK8/18), may be retained after loss of thyroid markers, but are often completely absent, and negative staining does not exclude the diagnosis. Anaplastic carcinomas may also gain aberrant expression of mesenchymal markers such as vimentin, or markers of squamous differentiation (p63, p40, CK5/6), as in the case of squamoid anaplastic carcinoma.

Immunohistochemistry is of more use in excluding potential morphologic mimics of anaplastic carcinoma, including medullary carcinoma (positive for neuroendocrine markers and calcitonin), metastatic melanoma (S100 protein, HMB-45, etc.), anaplastic large cell lymphoma (CD30 and ALK-1), and diffuse large B-cell lymphoma (CD45, CD20, and PAX5). Sarcomas of the neck, including undifferentiated pleomorphic sarcoma, postradiation sarcoma, and malignant peripheral nerve sheath tumor, among others, are also in the differential for anaplastic carcinoma, and may be difficult to exclude on the basis of immunohistochemistry. Fortunately, these only very rarely arise in the thyroid as a primary site.

Precursor lesions

Anaplastic carcinomas do not arise *de novo*. Rather, they are a consequence of long-standing, pre-existing thyroid disease, with goiter reported in more than 80% of cases. Thorough histologic exam of the thyroid gland typically

Table 15.2 Immunohistochemistry in the diagnosis of anaplastic thyroid carcinoma

Study	Anaplastic carcinoma		Medullary carcinoma	Squamous cell carcinoma	Anaplastic/large cell lymphoma	Spindle cell/pleomorphic sarcoma[a]
	Squamoid variant	Spindle cell/pleomorphic variant				
Pancytokeratin (AE1/AE3)	+	+/–	+	+	–[b]	–[b]
TTF-1	–/+	–/+	+/–	–	–	–
Thyroglobulin	–/+	–/+	–	–	–	–
PAX8	+	–/+	+/–	–	–	–
CK5/6	+/–	–	–	+	–	–
P63	+/–	–	–	+	–	–
Synaptophysin	–	–	+	–	–	–
Chromogranin	–	–	+	–	–	–
Calcitonin	–	–	+	–	–	–
TP53	+	+	–	+/–	+/–	+/–
Vimentin	–	+/–	–	–	–	+
CD45	–	–	–	–	–	–
E-cadherin	+/–	–	–	+	–	–

[a] There is a diverse array of spindle cell and pleomorphic sarcomas that may arise in the neck or mediastinum, and may require additional confirmatory or exclusionary studies to distinguish from anaplastic carcinoma, depending on tumor morphology.

[b] Some tumors may express weak or patchy aberrant keratin expression.

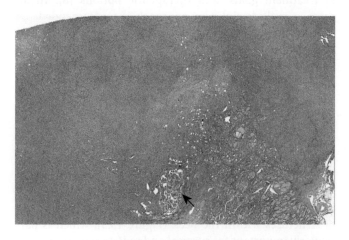

Figure 15.4 Anaplastic carcinoma arising in association with papillary thyroid carcinoma. Low-power view shows a spindle cell anaplastic thyroid carcinoma arising from the thyroid gland. At the lower left (arrow), a microscopic focus of residual papillary thyroid carcinoma can be seen adjacent to, and partially involved by, the anaplastic carcinoma. (H&E-stained image courtesy of Dr. W.C. Foo.)

yields microscopic evidence of a preexisting differentiated papillary or follicular carcinoma (Figure 15.4), although overgrowth of the anaplastic component can obliterate the originating tumor focus [4,5,10]. In large tumors or those which are diagnosed on biopsy without resection, lack of extensive sampling may also result in nondetection of precursor lesions. Follicular thyroid carcinoma is the most common precursor carcinoma to anaplastic carcinoma in regions with endemic goiter [3]. In other areas, papillary thyroid carcinoma, particularly the tall cell variant, is more frequently detected [8].

Poorly differentiated thyroid carcinoma is an intermediate stage in the morphologic continuum from differentiated carcinoma to anaplastic carcinoma. Poorly differentiated thyroid carcinomas retain morphologic similarity to follicular or papillary precursors, but typically show areas of increased proliferative activity (defined as three or more mitoses per 10 high-power fields), solid or trabecular growth, or foci of tumor necrosis [11]. Nuclear changes may also be seen, including convoluted nuclear membranes [11], sometimes with hyperchromasia and coarsening of chromatin. Generally, poorly differentiated carcinomas show monotonous nuclear features, without the pleomorphism typical of anaplastic carcinoma. In some cases of anaplastic carcinoma, residual foci of both well- and poorly-differentiated carcinomas are present, confirming the spectrum of disease progression.

Morphologic evidence of anaplastic carcinoma progression from differentiated carcinoma is echoed by the identification of sequential molecular alterations from well- to poorly-differentiated to anaplastic carcinoma.

MOLECULAR BIOLOGY

Anaplastic carcinomas are characterized by complex molecular alterations and increased genomic instability compared with differentiated thyroid carcinomas. Genomic studies have found frequent chromosomal gains and losses in anaplastic carcinoma, although there is little consensus as to which are most common or important in disease progression [12]. The finding of frequent aneuploidy with no recurrent pattern is typically a result of tumoral genomic instability combined with failures of cell cycle checkpoint regulation.

While conventional papillary carcinoma is frequently characterized by *BRAF* mutations, and both follicular carcinoma and the follicular variant of papillary carcinoma by *RAS* family mutations, anaplastic carcinoma may show either *RAS* or *BRAF* alterations, compatible with derivation from either follicular or papillary precursor lesions. Notably, neither *RET/PTC1* rearrangements nor *PAX8/PPAR*-gamma rearrangements, present in a subset of papillary and follicular carcinomas, respectively, have been identified in anaplastic carcinoma, suggesting that not all carcinomas are equally susceptible to dedifferentiation [12].

As differentiated carcinoma progresses to poorly differentiated to anaplastic carcinoma, a variety of additional mutations are acquired, commonly including inactivation of *TP53* and *PTEN*, and activating mutations in *PIK3CA* and *CTNNB1* (Table 15.3) [12–17]. Oncogenic signaling pathways involved in anaplastic thyroid tumorigenesis therefore include the MAPK pathway (activated in 65% of anaplastic carcinomas), the AKT/mTOR pathway (activated in ~90% of cases), and the Wnt pathway.

TERT promoter mutations have been identified in 45% of anaplastic thyroid carcinomas, compared with <20% of differentiated thyroid carcinoma [18–21]. hTERT contributes to telomere maintenance, and *TERT* promoter mutations reactivate telomerase activity, contributing to immortalization of malignant cells.

Consistent with the above genetic and genomic profiles, gene expression studies in anaplastic thyroid carcinoma demonstrate alterations in the regulation of focal adhesion and cell migration, cell growth and proliferation, and the regulation of chromosomal stability and cell cycle arrest. Compared with normal thyroid tissue, anaplastic thyroid carcinomas have shown altered expression of more than 900 genes, of which, by comparison, only 114 were altered in papillary carcinoma [22]. Many of the cell cycle regulatory alterations are favored to be a result of p53 loss or dysregulation. Cancer stem cell markers are also more frequently expressed in anaplastic carcinoma, and high expression may be associated with aggressive behavior [23].

Epigenetic alterations are another common feature of anaplastic carcinoma. Promoter hypermethylation, resulting in gene inactivation, is frequent and, as with other carcinomas, correlates with the presence of BRAF V600E mutation. In particular, PTEN, a negative regulator of AKT signaling, is highly susceptible to inactivation via promoter hypermethylation in anaplastic carcinoma [24,25].

The role of microRNA (miRNA) in anaplastic thyroid carcinoma is not well understood. However, evidence of alterations in miRNAs targeting E2F correlates well with the altered gene expression signature of anaplastic thyroid carcinomas [22]. Dysregulation of miRNAs involved in the regulation of hTERT, HMGA1, Rb, and PTEN has also been reported [26], emphasizing the importance of PTEN loss and hTERT expression in the pathogenesis of anaplastic thyroid carcinoma.

MANAGEMENT

Due to the rapid progression and high lethality of anaplastic thyroid carcinoma, it is necessary to efficiently evaluate disease and triage patients for appropriate management. The American Thyroid Association has published guidelines on the management of anaplastic thyroid carcinoma, including approach to diagnostic workup, establishment of treatment goals, and therapeutic options [8]. In all cases, a multidisciplinary approach is recommended. Of note, at the present time, quality of evidence for recommended treatment options is limited, as no randomized clinical trial data have been reported for anaplastic thyroid carcinoma [8], and only approximately 200 patients have been reported in nonrandom clinical trials over the past 20 years [27].

Prior to determining a course of treatment, it is necessary to define the extent of disease and confirm the diagnosis. Ultrasound may be used to rapidly assess the tumor and identify lymph node metastasis, while computed tomography (CT) and magnetic resonance imaging (MRI) are used to define extent of tumor spread and evaluate involvement of structures within the neck (Figure 15.5), which is particularly important for surgical and radiation planning.

The lung should be evaluated for metastatic spread, and positron emission tomography (PET)-CT should be

Table 15.3 Genetic and epigenetic alterations in anaplastic thyroid carcinoma

Pathway	Affected gene	Mutation frequency (%)	Effect
RAS/AKT	*RAS*	23	Activation
RAS	*BRAF*	24	Activation
AKT	*PIK3CA*	15	Activation
	PTEN mutation	10	Inactivation
	PTEN promoter hypermethylation	69	Inactivation
Wnt	*CTNNB1*	20	Activation
	Axin	49	Inactivation
	APC	7	Inactivation
Apoptosis, cell cycle progression	*TP53*	41	Inactivation
Telomere maintenance	*TERT* promoter mutation	45	Activation

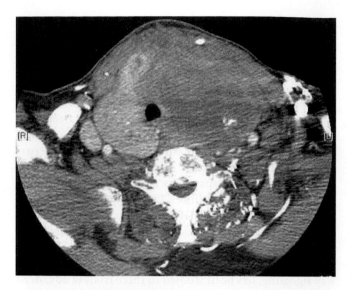

Figure 15.5 Radiographic features of anaplastic carcinoma on CT imaging. Anaplastic carcinoma (here, arising in the left thyroid lobe) frequently occurs in long-standing goiter (at right). Carcinoma has resulted in tracheal deviation to the right. Obliteration of normal tissue planes confirms extensive tumor involvement of the soft tissues of the neck.

considered to evaluate for sites of distant spread. Laboratory workup, including complete blood count and differential, as well as blood chemistries to assess for hematologic abnormalities and thyroid and parathyroid function, is recommended [8].

Establishing a tissue diagnosis is key to determining management options. As discussed earlier, the differential diagnosis for anaplastic thyroid carcinoma includes less lethal entities, such as lymphomas, for which appropriate systemic therapy may produce significant improvement in survival outcomes. Therefore, tissue biopsy is required prior to surgical resection. Biopsy options include fine-needle aspiration (FNA), core needle biopsy, and incisional biopsy.

Fine-needle aspiration

FNA is considered a reliable diagnostic modality for anaplastic thyroid carcinoma. Using the American Society for Clinical Pathology FNA performance assessment program test set of fine-needle aspirates with known diagnoses, 86.5% of 163 responding cytologists correctly classified the anaplastic thyroid carcinoma, with an additional 11% reporting anaplastic carcinoma as some other form of thyroid neoplasm (follicular or oncocytic neoplasm), and 2.5% correctly identifying malignancy, but misinterpreting the type of malignancy. None of the reporting cytopathologists misinterpreted anaplastic carcinoma as a benign lesion [28]. Adequate aspirate material should be taken for the creation of a cell block, on which to perform immunohistochemistry, as well as for flow cytometry, if lymphoma is considered in the differential diagnosis.

Core needle biopsy, open biopsy, and frozen section

FNA does not always yield diagnostic material, due to insufficiently cellular aspirate, largely necrotic tumor, or insufficient cell block material for definitive immunohistochemical studies. In such instances, core needle biopsy or open biopsy is required to establish tissue diagnosis. Intraoperative frozen section consultation on biopsy or resection tissue is not usually recommended in the workup for anaplastic thyroid carcinoma [8], but may be helpful in biopsy cases where tissue is extensively necrotic or fibrotic to confirm the presence of viable diagnostic lesional material for further workup, and to triage tissue for flow cytometry or molecular workup, as required. If tissue is sent for frozen section, it is useful to the pathologist to send a separate portion of tissue for permanent section, as previously frozen tissue may have a freezing artifact that can render morphologic interpretation difficult and may also render tissue less antigenic when immunohistochemistry is performed.

Surgical resection

The primary treatment modality for anaplastic carcinoma is surgery, which may be performed with curative intent, or palliatively to control airway symptoms. Because of the speed at which anaplastic carcinoma progresses, prompt surgical management is critical, and attempted neoadjuvant therapy is only rarely warranted.

Palliative surgical procedures in the management of anaplastic carcinoma include tracheostomy and tumor debulking in order to protect the airway from impending collapse. Although debulking of nonresectable disease and tracheostomy prevent acute asphyxiation and improve airway symptoms, these procedures do not significantly improve survival.

Surgical procedures performed with curative intent often require an aggressive approach, and include thyroidectomy with neck dissection, partial laryngectomy, and tracheal resection. Nevertheless, a true oncologic procedure with negative (R0) margins is difficult to achieve in anaplastic thyroid carcinoma due to extensive extrathyroidal disease at presentation [29]. Therefore, surgery alone is rarely enough to improve survival outcomes, and current guidelines do not recommend resection of major structures (e.g., total laryngectomy or esophagectomy), as the potential for disease clearance and survival benefit is low and outweighed by high morbidity and decreased quality of life [8]. As always, the prospective ability to achieve gross total tumor resection must be balanced with other patient factors when determining how aggressive a surgical approach to take. Some studies have shown a potential for complete resection to prolong patient survival, although selection bias, with most studies triaging the younger, most resectable patients for surgery, undoubtedly played a role in these results [8].

Adjuvant protocols in anaplastic carcinoma include both radiation and chemotherapy, although there is no standard protocol for the use of either. Moreover, results have been mixed with radiotherapy and chemotherapy, and the effectiveness of either in improving survival is uncertain, with no overall improvements seen in the outcome of anaplastic carcinoma over the past two decades [27].

Radiation therapy

External beam radiotherapy, with doses up to 65 Gray, may be used for locoregional control of anaplastic carcinoma. This may slow the spread of disease, but is not considered curative [30]. Thus, radiation therapy is more useful as a postoperative adjuvant therapy to improve margin control in R0–R1 disease, rather than as a single-modality treatment. As a combined modality with surgery, radiotherapy has been shown to offer some slight survival benefit [31].

High-dose accelerated radiation therapy and hyperfractionated radiotherapy have been described in the treatment of anaplastic carcinoma. Both pre- and postoperative regimens with or without concurrent chemotherapy have been utilized, with conflicting results as to the clinical benefit [8]. It is worth noting that survival benefits of radiotherapy in both resectable and nonresectable disease, when reported in the literature, are generally only on the order of 1–4 months, with median survivals remaining under 12 months [8].

Chemotherapy

Cytotoxic agents commonly used in the treatment of anaplastic thyroid carcinoma include doxorubicin, paclitaxel, docetaxel, cisplatin, carboplatinum, etoposide, cyclophosphamide, melphalan, and bleomycin. Due to disease rarity, randomized controlled trials and statistically significant data are lacking as to the benefits of different combinations and dosages in improving survival. However, the American Thyroid Association currently recommends a combination of taxane, anthracycline, and platin-based therapy in conjunction with radiotherapy in patients eligible for aggressive treatment [8]. Systemic chemotherapy may also be used for patients with bulky metastatic disease as a palliative modality, but has not been shown to improve survival or quality of life.

Multimodality therapy

Radiation may be used as an adjunct to surgery to improve local control. Concurrent chemoradiotherapy is suggested to be more efficacious than chemotherapy or radiotherapy alone, due to chemosensitization of tumor to the effects of radiation. However, the toxicity of combination regimens can be considerable. Nevertheless, a multimodality approach to the management of anaplastic thyroid carcinoma is commonly utilized.

Targeted therapy

Trials of targeted therapy in anaplastic thyroid carcinoma are currently very limited. Tyrosine kinase inhibitors (TKIs) are an active area of study for advance thyroid disease, and several phase II clinical trials have included patients with anaplastic thyroid carcinoma. Imatinib, targeting c-kit, as well as other receptor tyrosine kinases, has been studied in 11 anaplastic carcinomas with two of eight patients showing a partial response, and four with stable disease. In this study, 6-month progression-free survival was 36%, and 6-month overall survival was 45% [32]. Axitinib, another TKI, was tested in two anaplastic carcinomas, with one partial response [33]. In contrast, neither pazopanib, a multitarget TKI with primary specificity against angiogenic growth factor receptors, nor gefitinib, a TKI targeting the epidermal growth factor receptor (EGFR), demonstrated measurable benefit when respectively tested in 15 and five patients with anaplastic carcinoma.

Sorafenib, a combined inhibitor of RAS and AKT pathway signaling, has been studied in three trials of advanced thyroid carcinoma, including 24 patients with anaplastic thyroid carcinoma. In total, three partial responses and five stable disease responses were reported; however, median progression-free survival was 1.9 months, and 1-year survivals remained at <20% [34–36]. Everolimus, a specific inhibitor of the AKT signaling mediator mTOR, resulted in stable disease as the best response in three of six patient studied, with median progression-free survival of 10 weeks [37].

Although preliminary, these results suggest that some patients may show temporary benefit from targeted therapy. Clearly, more study is needed to identify agents with more dramatic and sustained efficacy against these lethal tumors, or to determine combinations of agents that may synergize more effectively.

OUTCOME

Anaplastic thyroid carcinoma represents the most aggressive form of thyroid carcinoma. Locoregional failure is common, even in patients with gross total tumor resection, and anaplastic carcinoma recurs in up to 92% of patients by 8 months' follow-up [8]. Distant metastases develop in more than 60% patients over the course of disease and are associated with a uniformly fatal, short disease course.

Reported median survivals for anaplastic thyroid carcinoma range between 4 and 5 months. One-year survival is <20% [2,26,27,31], with death ultimately resulting from overwhelming disease burden or airway collapse. Long-term survival is exceedingly rare, with an aggregate greater-than-2-year survival of 7% in series published between 1975 and 2002 [4]. Indeed, long-term survival is so infrequent that many authors question the diagnosis of anaplastic carcinoma in patients surviving for five or more years [4].

Prognostic indicators include age, sex, and tumor size [4]. Younger patients (<60 years) are reported to have less aggressive disease and prolonged survival. Likewise, patients with smaller tumors or those which are entirely confined to the thyroid (stage 4a) are predicted to do better. Some series have found that younger women treated with surgery or radiotherapy have improved outcomes, but these results are not consistently identified [8].

CONCLUSIONS

Although rare, anaplastic thyroid carcinoma is highly lethal. Improved access to medical care and management of precursor lesions has reduced the incidence of disease. However, options for patients diagnosed with anaplastic thyroid carcinoma remain limited, and outcomes have not improved in the past 20 years. In the last decade, understanding of the underlying genetic and epigenetic landscape responsible for the aggressive disease has expanded dramatically. It is hoped that this understanding will pave the way for future advances in targeted therapy, with resulting improvements in disease management and patient outcomes.

REFERENCES

1. Aschebrook-Kilfoy B, Ward MH, Sabra MM, Devesa SS. Thyroid cancer incidence patterns in the United States by histologic type, 1992–2006. *Thyroid* 2011;21:125–34.
2. O'Neill JP, Shaha AR. Anaplastic thyroid cancer. *Oral Oncol* 2013;49:702–6.
3. Harach HR, Galindez M, Campero M, Ceballos GA. Undifferentiated (anaplastic) thyroid carcinoma and iodine intake in Salta, Argentina. *Endocr Pathol* 2013;24:125–31.
4. Are C, Shaha AR. Anaplastic thyroid carcinoma: Biology, pathogenesis, prognostic factors, and treatment approaches. *Ann Surg Oncol* 2006;13:453–64.
5. Nishiyama RH, Dunn EL, Thompson NW. Anaplastic spindle-cell and giant-cell tumors of the thyroid gland. *Cancer* 1972;30:113–27.
6. McIver B, Hay ID, Giuffrida DF et al. Anaplastic thyroid carcinoma: A 50-year experience at a single institution. *Surgery* 2001;130:1028–34.
7. Kyriakides G, Sosin H. Anaplastic carcinoma of the thyroid. *Ann Surg* 1974;179:295–9.
8. Smallridge RC, Ain KB, Asa SL et al. American Thyroid Association guidelines for management of patients with anaplastic thyroid cancer. *Thyroid* 2012;22:1104–39.
9. Edge SB, Byrd DR, Compton CC, Fritz AG, Greene FL, Trotti A, eds. *AJCC Cancer Staging Manual.* 7th ed. New York: Springer, 2010.
10. Demeter JG, De Jong SA, Lawrence AM, Paloyan E. Anaplastic thyroid carcinoma: Risk factors and outcome. *Surgery* 1991;110:956–61; discussion 961–53.
11. Volante M, Collini P, Nikiforov YE et al. Poorly differentiated thyroid carcinoma: The Turin proposal for the use of uniform diagnostic criteria and an algorithmic diagnostic approach. *Am J Surg Pathol* 2007;31:1256–64.
12. Smallridge RC, Marlow LA, Copland JA. Anaplastic thyroid cancer: Molecular pathogenesis and emerging therapies. *Endocr Relat Cancer* 2009;16:17–44.
13. Pita JM, Figueiredo IF, Moura MM, Leite V, Cavaco BM. Cell cycle deregulation and TP53 and RAS mutations are major events in poorly differentiated and undifferentiated thyroid carcinomas. *J Clin Endocrinol Metab* 2014;99:E497–507.
14. Gauchotte G, Philippe C, Lacomme S et al. BRAF, p53 and SOX2 in anaplastic thyroid carcinoma: Evidence for multistep carcinogenesis. *Pathology* 2011;43:447–52.
15. Fugazzola L, Mannavola D, Cirello V et al. BRAF mutations in an Italian cohort of thyroid cancers. *Clin Endocrinol (Oxf)* 2004;61:239–43.
16. Puxeddu E, Moretti S, Elisei R et al. BRAF(V599E) mutation is the leading genetic event in adult sporadic papillary thyroid carcinomas. *J Clin Endocrinol Metab* 2004;89:2414–20.
17. Nikiforova MN, Wald AI, Roy S, Durso MB, Nikiforov YE. Targeted next-generation sequencing panel (ThyroSeq) for detection of mutations in thyroid cancer. *J Clin Endocrinol Metab* 2013;98:E1852–60.
18. Melo M, da Rocha AG, Vinagre J et al. TERT promoter mutations are a major indicator of poor outcome in differentiated thyroid carcinomas. *J Clin Endocrinol Metab* 2014;99:E754–65.
19. Liu T, Wang N, Cao J et al. The age- and shorter telomere-dependent TERT promoter mutation in follicular thyroid cell-derived carcinomas. *Oncogene* 2014;33:4978–84.
20. Landa I, Ganly I, Chan TA et al. Frequent somatic TERT promoter mutations in thyroid cancer: Higher prevalence in advanced forms of the disease. *J Clin Endocrinol Metab* 2013;98:E1562–6.
21. Liu X, Bishop J, Shan Y et al. Highly prevalent TERT promoter mutations in aggressive thyroid cancers. *Endocr Relat Cancer* 2013;20:603–10.
22. Salvatore G, Nappi TC, Salerno P et al. A cell proliferation and chromosomal instability signature in anaplastic thyroid carcinoma. *Cancer Res* 2007;67:10148–58.
23. Yun JY, Kim YA, Choe JY et al. Expression of cancer stem cell markers is more frequent in anaplastic thyroid carcinoma compared to papillary thyroid carcinoma and is related to adverse clinical outcome. *J Clin Pathol* 2014;67:125–33.
24. Hou P, Ji M, Xing M. Association of PTEN gene methylation with genetic alterations in the phosphatidylinositol 3-kinase/AKT signaling pathway in thyroid tumors. *Cancer* 2008;113:2440–7.
25. Frisk T, Foukakis T, Dwight T et al. Silencing of the PTEN tumor-suppressor gene in anaplastic thyroid cancer. *Genes Chromosomes Cancer* 2002;35:74–80.
26. Smallridge RC, Copland JA. Anaplastic thyroid carcinoma: Pathogenesis and emerging therapies. *Clin Oncol (R Coll Radiol)* 2010;22:486–97.

27. Bisof V, Rakusic Z, Despot M. Treatment of patients with anaplastic thyroid cancer during the last 20 years: Whether any progress has been made? *Eur Arch Otorhinolaryngol* 2015;272:1553–67.

28. Eilers SG, LaPolice P, Mukunyadzi P et al. Thyroid fine-needle aspiration cytology: Performance data of neoplastic and malignant cases as identified from 1558 responses in the ASCP Non-GYN Assessment program thyroid fine-needle performance data. *Cancer Cytopathol* 2014;122:745–50.

29. Cornett WR, Sharma AK, Day TA et al. Anaplastic thyroid carcinoma: An overview. *Curr Oncol Rep* 2007;9:152–8.

30. Wang Y, Tsang R, Asa S, Dickson B, Arenovich T, Brierley J. Clinical outcome of anaplastic thyroid carcinoma treated with radiotherapy of once- and twice-daily fractionation regimens. *Cancer* 2006;107:1786–92.

31. Kebebew E, Greenspan FS, Clark OH, Woeber KA, McMillan A. Anaplastic thyroid carcinoma. Treatment outcome and prognostic factors. *Cancer* 2005;103:1330–5.

32. Ha HT, Lee JS, Urba S et al. A phase II study of imatinib in patients with advanced anaplastic thyroid cancer. *Thyroid* 2010;20:975–80.

33. Cohen EE, Rosen LS, Vokes EE et al. Axitinib is an active treatment for all histologic subtypes of advanced thyroid cancer: results from a phase II study. *J Clin Oncol* 2008;26:4708–13.

34. Gupta-Abramson V, Troxel AB, Nellore A et al. Phase II trial of sorafenib in advanced thyroid cancer. *J Clin Oncol* 2008;26:4714–9.

35. Savvides P, Nagaiah G, Lavertu P et al. Phase II trial of sorafenib in patients with advanced anaplastic carcinoma of the thyroid. *Thyroid* 2013;23:600–4.

36. Capdevila J, Iglesias L, Halperin I et al. Sorafenib in metastatic thyroid cancer. *Endocr Relat Cancer* 2012;19:209–16.

37. Lim SM, Chang H, Yoon MJ et al. A multicenter, phase II trial of everolimus in locally advanced or metastatic thyroid cancer of all histologic subtypes. *Ann Oncol* 2013;24:3089–94.

16

Endoscopic and robotic thyroidectomy

CHO ROK LEE AND KEE-HYUN NAM

ENDOSCOPIC THYROIDECTOMY

Introduction

Beginning with the awarding of the 1909 Nobel Prize for Medicine to Theodor Kocher for thyroid surgery, the legacy of innovation and progress in conventional open thyroidectomy has continued through the modern era [1]. However, conventional open thyroidectomy is performed through a cervical incision (6–8 cm) on the anterior neck. This procedure is always open and occasionally leaves a prominent scar on the anterior neck. Since thyroid disease usually occurs in women, and the incidence rate is increasing in young women, there is now greater consideration of the cosmetic aspect of thyroid surgery. This consideration, along with associated sequelae that affect patients postoperatively, including paresthesias, hypesthesias, voice changes, and dysphagia without discrete clinical findings, has become a problem to both patients and doctors and needs to be addressed [2].

Recent technological and instrumental advances, such as the introduction of the endoscope and the surgical robotic system, have brought great changes to surgical methods, including remote-site removal of the thyroid gland, which leaves no neck scars [3]. Minimally invasive surgeries, including endoscopic operations, have also been developed to overcome these drawbacks.

Gagner first described endoscopic parathyroid surgery in 1996, and Huscher and colleagues completed a video-assisted thyroidectomy in 1997. Since then, the endoscopic approach to thyroidectomy has undergone many transitions and has been widely applied to minimize scarring [4–6]. Endoscopic thyroidectomy was developed as a scarless operation by Ikeda et al. and Ohgami et al. by using alternative techniques. Further, Miccoli et al. performed invasive video-assisted thyroidectomy in 2001. Various methods for scarless endoscopic thyroidectomy procedures have been subsequently performed in the decades that followed.

Based on the positions of the skin incisions, endoscopic procedures can be classified as cervical incisions (anterior and lateral) or remote incisions (anterior, axillary, breast, bilateral axillobreast, gasless, and transaxillary). In addition, according to the method used to create the working space, endoscopic procedures can also be classified as either "pure," in which steady gas flow through trocars is used, or "gasless," in which external retraction is used instead of gas insufflation [7,8].

In this chapter, a brief summary for each surgical technique of the endoscopic thyroidectomy methods is described.

Indications and contraindications of endoscopic thyroidectomy

INDICATIONS

In the early age of endoscopic thyroidectomy, the procedure was only used for benign tumors of the thyroid gland, while malignant tumors were considered one of the contraindications. With the continued development of operation instruments and progression of personal skills, indications for endoscopic thyroidectomy were expanded. The indications for endoscopic thyroidectomy in papillary carcinoma can be summarized as [1] papillary thyroid carcinoma size of less than 2 cm, [2] no local invasion, [3] no diffuse enlarged lymph node and no adhesion or fixation of enlarged lymph nodes, [4] no enlarged lymph node on the opposite side or in the superior mediastinum, and [5] patients who strongly request minimally invasive operations [9]. The indication for a follicular neoplasm is size less than 5 cm [10].

CONTRAINDICATIONS

Miccoli et al. have reported a list of contraindications of endoscopic thyroidectomy. A relative contraindication is having a clinical history of radiotherapy or surgery on the neck. Absolute contraindications are [1] the largest diameter of the tumor is more than 3.5 cm and [2] evidence of local or remote metastasis. Endoscopic thyroidectomy is also not a proper method for multiple infiltrates to the thyroid capsule or strap muscles or a lymph node metastasis [11,12].

Surgical technique of endoscopic thyroidectomy

CERVICAL INCISION APPROACH

Anterior cervical approach

The anterior cervical approach was first described by Gagner and Inabnet in 2003. They presented the results of 18 endoscopic thyroidectomies by anterior cervical approach for solitary nodules compared with 18 classical open thyroidectomies. Feasibility and safety of the anterior cervical approach were confirmed. Cosmetic results of the anterior cervical approach were superior, and the recovery period was reduced compared with the classical method. The anterior cervical approach incision uses a midline access and permits bilateral dissection of the thyroid. A 5 mm optical trocar is inserted just above the suprasternal notch. Carbon dioxide (CO_2) is insufflated with a pressure of 10 mmHg. Three additional trocars are used: one 5 mm trocar at the superior medial border of the sternocleidomastoid muscle and two 2 mm trocars. Using ultracision (Ethicon Endosurgery, Cincinnati, Ohio), all vital structures are identified and dissected as in a conventional procedure. The thyroid is extracted in a plastic bag through the superolateral trocar [13].

An alternative way has been proposed by Cougard et al. that starts with a 15 mm middle incision above the suprasternal notch, one 3 mm trocar on the side of the operator or lesion, and one 5 mm trocar at the other end with 8 mmHg CO_2 insufflation. A Veress needle is added in the upper midline to improve the working space whenever it is necessary for such improvement. The thyroid is extracted through the 15 mm median incision [14].

Lateral cervical approach

Henry et al. developed the lateral cervical approach. They described the technique developed for parathyroidectomy and performed in 38 patients. If the patient underwent a completion thyroidectomy, it was performed via a conventional cervicotomy. They used the plane between the carotid sheath laterally and the strap muscle medially based on the same approach and principles of the endoscopic parathyroidectomy performed in their institution. This "backdoor" approach can only be used for unilateral lesions and uses three trocars (a 10 mm optic port and two 3 mm ports placed on the anterior border of the sternocleidomastoid muscle on the lesion side). This approach can directly access the posterior aspect of the thyroid lobe without the need for a strap muscle dissection. Low-pressure (8 mmHg) CO_2 insufflation maintains the space. The freed gland is extracted through the 12–15 mm incision for division of the isthmus [15,16].

Another lateral approach has been described by Inabnet et al. After the initial 10–15 mm incision, a working space is created by CO_2 insufflation. Later, at the superior lateral area of the neck, three additional trocars (two 3 mm and one 5 mm) are inserted under direct vision. The specimen is extracted in a plastic bag through a 1 cm superolateral incision. In their publication, Inabnet et al. reported three conversions due to insufficient working space in a series of 38 patients [17].

REMOTE ACCESS APPROACH

Anterior approach

The anterior approach has been advocated mainly by Japanese and Korean groups. Successful surgery results in the total absence of a neck incision have been reported for bilateral thyroid dissection. The incisions are transposed to the anterior chest, subclavian areas, and circumareolar regions, so that the incision scar can be covered by an undergarment or dress.

Ikeda et al. performed one study that compared conventional, anterior chest, and axillary approaches. Three months after the operation, the swallowing discomfort incidence was higher in the open surgery group [18]. This approach has been favored for bilateral thyroid dissections. The working space is maintained by CO_2 insufflation. A 30 mm skin incision is made below the inferior border of the clavicle, while retracting the upper border of the pectoralis major muscle manually. Alternatively, cutaneous lifting devices are available. An additional two 5 mm trocars are inserted, one caudal to the sternal notch and the other caudal to the ipsilateral clavicle. The working space is dissected underneath the platysma muscle, advancing from the incision to the thyroid area and across the medial border of the sternocleidomastoid muscle. Dissection of the gland is performed with ultracision [19–21].

Axillary approach

This approach can be used for large tumors that do not extend contralaterally. Ikeda et al. reported a comparative study of axillary, anterior chest wall, and conventional approaches. Here, excellent cosmetic results were achieved in the axillary approach surgery group. This approach took the longest operation time. Swallowing discomfort was higher in the axillary approach than in open surgery [18]. In another study by Ikeda et al., the operative time was longer in the axillary approach and postoperative pain was similar in both the axillary approach and open surgery [22].

For this approach, the patient position must be supine, and the ipsilateral arm on the lesion side must be placed at a 90° angle to the axis of the body, thus exposing the operative axilla. Three 5 mm incisions are placed below the anterior axillary line equidistant apart, or one 30 mm incision and two 5 mm trocar incisions are made. CO_2 insufflation is kept up to 4–9 mmHg. A 0° optical scope or flexible laparoscope with CO_2 insufflation at 4–9 mmHg is inserted via a blunt and sharp dissection. With direct vision, the lower layer of the platysma is exposed through the upper surface of the pectoralis major muscle. All incisions are hidden in the axillary fossa [22,23].

Breast approach

This approach allows a bilateral dissection. Park et al. reported the endoscopic thyroidectomy by breast approach in 100 patients. The feasibility and safety for this type of thyroidectomy were confirmed [24]. The main goal is to avoid a scar in the neck. Through two incisions on both upper circumareolar areas, blunt subcutaneous tunnel dissections create a working space with the use of a Rochester clamp and a vascular tunneler with the use of a Dingmann dissector. CO_2 insufflation is used to create a working space. The third port (5 mm) can be inserted 3 cm below the clavicle on the lesion side or parasternal at the level of the nipple or in the axilla. Ipsilateral strap muscles are split longitudinally to achieve good exposure of the thyroid gland. The thyroid is then retrieved through the breast ports. Scars are present on parasternal, perimammillary, and axillary regions depending on the port placement [24–26].

Axillo-bilateral-breast approach

Shimazu et al. developed the axillo-bilateral-breast approach (ABBA) by modifying the breast approach method. They reported that the ABBA method improved endoscopic views of the structures and had feasibility for removing large goiters sized 5–6 cm. Furthermore, due to the multiangular nature of this approach, the ABBA procedure seemed easy to handle with surgical instruments, and led to avoiding collisions with major thyroid vessels and nerves. However, this method is limited by difficulty visualizing both lobes of the thyroid [26].

Bilateral axillo-breast approach

Youn et al. modified the ABBA method and developed a new endoscopic procedure by using the bilateral axillo-breast approach (BABA) [27]. A BABA has been developed to maintain optimal visualization of both thyroid lobes. The view with this approach resembles the conventional open thyroidectomy view. The BABA has several advantages: it provides symmetrical and familiar views of each thyroid lobe and good visualization of major structures. The surgeon can operate on both thyroid lobes using the same maneuvers. Choi et al. presented the results of this approach in 512 patients. In surgical completeness, postoperative complication, recurrence rate, and cosmetic results, the BABA endoscopic approach was superior to open thyroidectomy [28].

Under general anesthesia, patients are placed in the supine position with neck extension using a shoulder pillow. Both arms are mildly abducted to provide for insertion of 5 mm ports. Diluted (1:200,000) epinephrine solution is injected into the subcutaneous space in both breasts and the subplatysmal space in the neck to reduce bleeding during the dissection. Two 12 mm trocars are inserted via both upper circumareolar areas and two 5 mm trocars via the bilateral axillary incisions. With a blunt dissection using a Rochester clamp and vascular tunneler, the working space is produced. This space is extended to the level of thyroid cartilage superiorly and to the medial border of each sternocleidomastoid muscle laterally. The working space is established with CO_2 insufflation at a pressure up to 5–6 mmHg. The first step of the operation is making a midline incision and identification of the isthmus and trachea. The method then continues with the thyroidectomy. The view with this approach resembles the conventional open thyroidectomy view. The BABA has several advantages: it provides symmetrical and familiar views of each thyroid lobe and good visualization of major structures (such as parathyroid glands, recurrent laryngeal nerve (RLN), and superior and inferior thyroid vessels). The surgeon can operate on both thyroid lobes using the same maneuvers. This BABA has been performed using the da Vinci Surgical System (Intuitive Surgical, Inc., Sunnyvale, California) [27].

Gasless transaxillary approach

To maintain the working space constantly during the operation time, a gasless transaxillary approach (TAA) was developed by Chung et al. in Korea, and they developed a unique external retractor that can be connected with a continuous suction line by a canal in the midline of the retractor blade [7]. This approach allows for more superior cosmetic results than other remote approaches since there are no scars on the neck or anterior chest wall. The scar is completely covered by the arm in its natural position. During this procedure, the thyroid gland is visualized laterally and the RLN and the parathyroid glands are easily identified. This remote approach offers numerous advantages, including decreased CO_2-related complications, the use of conventional instruments, avoiding the dissection of strap muscle, and a wider and clearer surgical field of view by avoiding disturbance from smoke and fumes. The surgeon can preserve the sensory nerve around the anterior neck area, and postoperative hypesthesia in this region can be avoided. The most remarkable advantage of this method is that it can be focused for performance of central compartment node dissection (CCND) in malignant tumor patients. However, the contralateral region approach exhibits some difficulty and involves a widely invasive working space, which is a disadvantage. However, Chung et al. solved this problem by performing a subcapsular dissection of the anterior thyroid surface to create a working space until the contralateral lobe is exposed. Kang et al. reported the feasibility and safety of this method in 581 patients with benign nodules and thyroid cancer [10]. Hakim et al. reported long-term follow-up results of the transaxillary approach in 1085 patients, concluding that transaxillary endoscopic thyroidectomy is comparable to open thyroidectomy in terms of early surgical outcomes and complications, and it bridges the gap between conventional open surgery and robotic transaxillary thyroidectomy [29].

During the operation, the lesion-side arm is raised and fixed to shorten the distance from the axilla to the anterior neck. A vertical line is marked from the sternal notch to the hyoid in the midline (Figure 16.1). A 5–7 cm vertical skin incision is made along the line marked in the axilla at the posterior aspect of the pectoralis, and a tunnel is made from the axilla to the thyroid gland. A working space is created anterior to the surface of the pectoralis major muscle until the anterior border of the sternocleidomastoid muscle is exposed. The dissection continues through the space between the sternal and clavicular heads of the sternocleidomastoid muscle (SCM) and beneath the strap muscle until the contralateral lobe of the thyroid is exposed (Figure 16.2). After making a working space, an external retractor is inserted through the skin incision and is raised using a homemade lifting device to keep the working space open. A 0.5 cm second skin incision is made on the anterolateral chest wall for insertion of endoscopic instruments (Figure 16.3) [7]. For endoscopic thyroidectomy, under the endoscopic guidance of an assistant, dissection and resection are performed using a endoscopic dissector and Harmonic

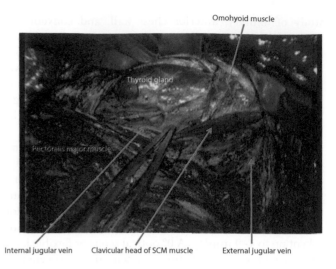

Figure 16.2 Approaching an adequate working space for the gasless transaxillary endoscopic thyroidectomy.

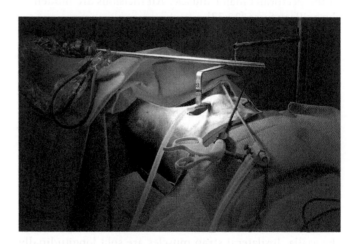

Figure 16.3 External view after positioning the retractor and inserting trocars in the gasless transaxillary endoscopic thyroidectomy. A second 0.5 cm skin incision was made on the anterolateral chest wall on an imaginary horizontal line starting from the lower end of the axillary incision and extending to 5–7 cm for the insertion of endoscopic instruments. (Adapted from Kang SW et al. *Endocr J* 2009;56:361–9.)

Scalpel (Johnson & Johnson, Cincinnati, Ohio). The operation proceeded in the same manner as conventional open thyroidectomy. This TAA has been performed using the da Vinci Surgical System [30].

Advantages and disadvantages of endoscopic thyroidectomy

ADVANTAGES

Compared with conventional open thyroidectomy, endoscopic thyroidectomy has a superior cosmetic result. It also has the additional benefits of significantly reducing the incidence of hypoesthesia, paresthesia of the anterior neck, and discomfort during swallowing by avoiding a transverse

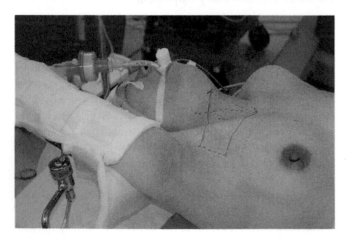

Figure 16.1 Patient position and skin markings for the gasless transaxillary endoscopic thyroidectomy. The primary incision is made along the axillary skin crease on the lateral border of the pectoralis major muscle within the anterior axillary fold, and the second incision on the anterior chest wall. (Adapted from Ryu HR et al. *J Am Coll Surg* 2010;211:e13–9.)

cervical incision [2,22,31]. Further, less pain is reported after this procedure compared with the traditional thyroidectomy [32].

DISADVANTAGES

The operation time of endoscopic thyroid surgery is longer than that of open thyroidectomy, especially for inexperienced surgeons [22,33]. This extended operation time is associated with making the working space and manipulating endoscopic instruments in a restricted area. In remote incision approaches, another drawback is the wider dissection needed to create a proper working space [7,34]. Another disadvantage is the higher cost compared with conventional open thyroidectomy due to the use of disposable instruments for cutting and sealing vessels.

Almost 15 years has passed since the idea of endoscopic neck surgery was turned into reality by Gagner. During this time, various approaches and techniques have been proposed and refined. Currently, it is not possible to recommend the use of endoscopic thyroidectomy based on evidence; however, there exists a general agreement that endoscopic thyroidectomy is a valid and feasible option for carefully selected patients.

Complications specific to conventional thyroidectomy can also occur after an endoscopic procedure. The major complication of endoscopic thyroidectomy is injury to the RLN and parathyroid gland. The incidence of transient or permanent RLN injury varies from 0% to 10%. Because of the similarity between the surgical equipment used by endoscopic and conventional operations, both procedures are associated with similar complications [9]. Dissection under a magnified endoscopic view demonstrating precise anatomic detail may likely enhance a patient's safety and contribute to a reduction of the 1%–3% incidence of RLN injury [35]. However, in endoscopic thyroidectomy, disposable instruments are usually used for sealing and cutting vessels. Although these instruments have advantages (less operation time and less bleeding), several studies have warned against the increased risk of thermal injury to adjacent tissues (mainly to the RLN and parathyroids, as well as to the trachea and esophagus) [36,37]. To prevent and reduce these complications, it is necessary to be cautious when using such devices.

Another complication in endoscopic thyroidectomy is caused by CO_2 insufflation. With a relatively high pressure of CO_2 (15–20 mmHg), patients may experience hypercapnea, pneumohypoderma, and mediastinal emphysema [9]. Therefore, it is prevailing current opinion that CO_2 insufflation is safe if insufflation is maintained at low pressures.

In remote incision access approaches, patients suffer from moderate to severe pain, which gradually subsides within 1 week. Postoperative paresthesias or numbness generally subside within 6 months [13].

Endoscopic thyroidectomy plays an important role in the surgical treatment of thyroid disease. It is a viable and safe procedure when based on good surgical principles and produces good outcomes both oncologically and cosmetically.

Trained surgeons can easily perform an endoscopic thyroidectomy with minimal equipment over and above the conventional laparoscopic equipment widely available in most institutions. The advantages of endoscopic thyroidectomy techniques and the need for better cosmetic outcomes both enhance further development of endoscopic thyroidectomy in the expert hands of endocrine surgeons.

ROBOTIC THYROIDECTOMY

In the beginning of this chapter, we investigated the suitability of endoscopic thyroidectomy for thyroid surgery. The advantages of endoscopic surgery over open surgery for thyroid diseases include reduced rates of hyperesthesia and paresthesia of the neck and highly improved cosmetic outcomes. However, despite the technical advances and proven benefits of endoscopic thyroidectomy for thyroid tumors, complex procedures, such as advanced thyroid cancer operations and radical neck dissections (RNDs), are typically still managed by conventional open approaches. Endoscopic instruments also have some limitations, including reduced range of motion, two-dimensional visualization, counterintuitive hand movement, difficulties in narrow and deep operative fields, ergonomic difficulties, and tremor amplification [38,39]. The da Vinci surgical robot was developed to address these limitations of conventional endoscopic surgery. The emergence of the da Vinci robot system has further progressed the surgical management of thyroid disease within the endoscopic environment. In 2007, Chung's group in South Korea successfully performed the first robotic thyroidectomy using a TAA [30]. The movement toward robotic thyroid surgery has reshaped the surgical approach for thyroid tumors in Asia and many parts of Western countries. Particularly in Asian countries, the impact has been remarkable and spread rapidly [39–41].

Since 2009, a large number of clinical trials have been published on robotic thyroid surgery. The safety and oncologic efficacy of robotic surgery for thyroid disease have been established. Several innovations at large-volume centers have enhanced quality of life outcomes in patients who have undergone robotic compared with conventional open thyroidectomy. The benefits of robotic surgery are excellent cosmetic results, reduction of sensory changes in the neck, and less swallowing discomfort after surgery [41–49]. From the surgeon perspective, robotic surgery has improved ergonomics that can shorten the learning curve compared with open or endoscopic surgery [50].

In this section, we define the indications and contraindications for robotic thyroid surgery and describe surgical tips for robotic thyroidectomy by the TAA and BABA.

Indications and contraindications of robotic thyroidectomy

Recently, robotic surgery for thyroid disease has been successfully extended to complete total thyroidectomy with RND for patients with thyroid cancer [44]. Patients selected for robotic thyroidectomy include those with [1] follicular proliferation without a substernal extension and tumor size of ≤5 cm and [2] differentiated thyroid cancer without contraindications to robotic surgery. Exclusion criteria include [1] a history of previous head-and-neck surgery or irradiation; [2] uncontrolled thyrotoxicosis; [3] unrelated pathologic conditions of the neck or shoulder; [4] lesions located in the dorsal thyroid area, especially in the region adjacent to the tracheoesophageal groove (because of possible injury during surgery to the trachea, esophagus, or RLN); [5] suspicious perinodal infiltration to adjacent structures, such as the internal jugular vein (IJV) or major nerves at the lateral metastatic lymph nodes; and [6] distant metastasis [39]. The extent of thyroidectomy and RND is determined based on American Thyroid Association (ATA) guidelines [51].

GASLESS TRANSAXILLARY ROBOTIC THYROIDECTOMY

The surgical procedure (patient positioning, working space making, and robotic console stage) of gasless transaxillary robotic thyroidectomy is the same as for gasless transaxillary endoscopic thyroidectomy. Under general anesthesia, the patient is placed in a supine position with the neck slightly extended. The arm is extended and a 5–6 cm vertical incision is marked in the anterior aspect of the ipsilateral axilla. The lesion-side arm is raised naturally, within the range of shoulder motion, to avoid brachial plexus paralysis. The arm is fixed to make the distance between the axilla and the anterior neck as short as possible. Modified patient positioning has been developed in the United States, especially for patients with obstacles due to a large body habitus [52,53]. In this alternative positioning, the lesion-side arm is extended to expose the patient's axillary area at the shoulder, followed by flexing the elbow to an angle of approximately 90°, such that the wrist is above the forehead of the patient with the palm facing the ceiling.

The subplatysmal skin flap from the axilla to the anterior neck area is dissected over the anterior surface of the pectoralis major muscle and clavicle using electrical cautery under direct vision. After the medial border of the SCM is exposed, the dissection is approached through the avascular space of the SCM branches (between the sternal and clavicular heads) and beneath the strap muscle until the contralateral lobe of the thyroid is exposed. Next, to maintain an adequate working space, an external retractor (Chung's retractor) is inserted through the skin incision in the axilla and raised using a lifting device (Figure 16.4).

In a two-incision robotic thyroidectomy, a second skin incision (0.8 cm in length) is made on the medial side of the anterior chest wall for insertion of the fourth robotic arm (2 cm superiorly and 6–8 cm medially from the nipple). Four robotic arms are used during the operation. Three arms are inserted through the axillary incision. The dual-channel endoscope is placed on the central arm, and Harmonic curved shears, together with a Maryland dissector, are placed on both lateral sides of the scope.

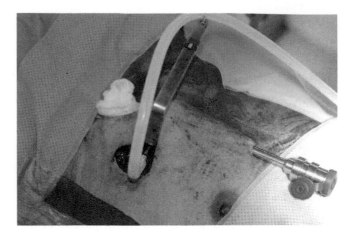

Figure 16.4 External view after positioning the retractor and anterior chest wall trocar in the gasless transaxillary robotic thyroidectomy (left-side approach, two incision). (Adapted from Kang SW et al. *Surgery* 2009;146:1048–55.)

ProGrasp forceps are inserted through the anterior chest arm (Figure 16.5a).

In a single-incision robotic thyroidectomy, the additional incision in the anterior chest is not made. All robotic arms are inserted through the single axillary incision. ProGrasp forceps are positioned beneath the anterior part of the skin incision parallel to the retractor blade (Figure 16.5b).

In the thyroidectomy procedure, all of the dissections and ligations of vessels are performed using Harmonic curved shears. The upper pole of the thyroid is drawn downward and medially by the ProGrasp forceps, and the superior thyroid vessels are identified and divided individually. The lower pole is dissected from the adipose and cervical thymic tissue. The inferior thyroid artery is then divided close to the thyroid gland. After the thyroid gland is retracted medially, the perithyroidal fascia is divided and sharply dissected. The inferior thyroid artery is divided, the entire cervical course of the RLN is exposed, and the thyroid gland is dissected from the trachea. The contralateral thyroidectomy is performed using the same method applied for medial traction of the thyroid. The specimen is extracted through the axillary skin incision [30].

GASLESS TRANSAXILLARY ROBOTIC MODIFIED RADICAL NECK DISSECTION

Under general anesthesia, the patient is placed in the supine position on a surgical table with a soft pillow under the shoulders. The neck is extended slightly and the face is turned away from the lesion. The lesion-side arm is then abducted 80° from the body to expose the axilla and lateral neck, and the head is tilted and rotated to face the nonlesion side (Figure 16.6).

A 7–8 cm vertical skin incision is made in the axilla along the anterior axillary fold and the lateral border of the pectoralis major muscle. The flap is dissected medially over the SCM toward the midline of the anterior neck. Laterally, the

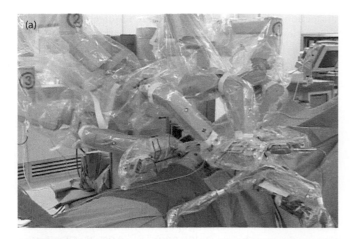

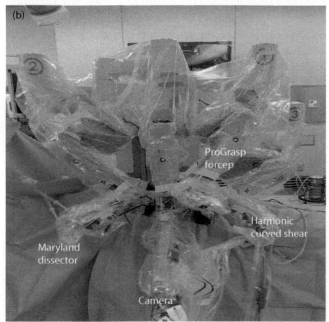

Figure 16.5 External view after port placement and instrument insertion of gasless transaxillary robotic thyroidectomy. **(a)** Two-incision robotic thyroidectomy (left-side approach): a second skin incision was created on the tumor side of the anterior chest wall to allow insertion of the fourth robotic arm (with ProGrasp forceps). **(b)** Single-incision robotic thyroidectomy (right-side approach): all four robotic instruments and the camera were inserted through the axillary incision.

trapezius muscle is identified and dissected upward along its anterior border. During flap dissection in the posterior neck area, the spinal accessory nerve is identified and preserved by skeletonization of the trapezius musle and is traced along its course until it passes on the undersurface of the SCM. After subplatysmal flap dissection, the clavicular head of SCM is transected at the level of the clavicle-attached point (to make full exposure of the junction area between the IJV and the subclavian vein). Soft tissue and lymph nodes are detached from the posterior surface of the SCM until the IJV and common carotid artery are exposed. To expose the level II area, the dissection proceeds upward along the

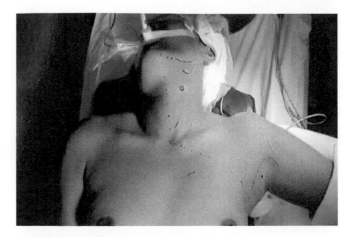

Figure 16.6 Patient position of gasless transaxillary robotic mRND. The neck was extended slightly and the face was turned away from the lesion. The lesion-side arm was abducted 80° from the body to expose the axilla and lateral neck, and the head was tilted and rotated to face the nonlesion side.

posterior surface of the SCM to expose the submandibular gland and the posterior belly of the digastric muscle. After flap dissection, the patient's head is returned to the natural position. A long, wide Chung's retractor blade (designed for robotic modified radical neck dissection [mRND]) is then inserted through the axillary incision to elevate the two heads of the SCM and strap muscles (Figure 16.7).

In a two-incision robotic mRND, a second skin incision (0.8 cm long) is then made on the medial side of the anterior chest wall to allow the fourth robotic arm to be inserted (2 cm superiorly and 6–8 cm medially from the nipple). The docking procedure for the robotic mRND is similar to that of the robotic thyroidectomy. Four robotic arms are used during the operation. Three arms are inserted through the axillary incision. The dual-channel endoscope is placed on the central arm, and Harmonic curved shears together with a Maryland dissector are placed on both lateral sides of

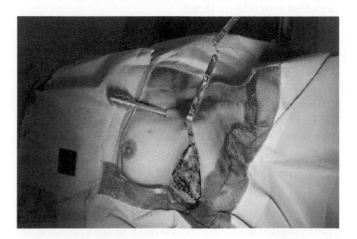

Figure 16.7 Initial position of the external retractor during gasless transaxillary robotic mRND of levels III, IV, and V (two-incision, left-side approach).

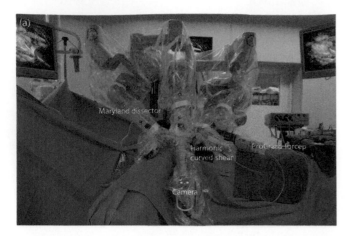

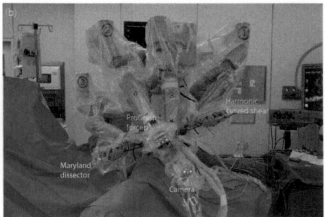

Figure 16.8 External view after port placement and instrument insertion of gasless transaxillary robotic mRND. **(a)** Two-incision robotic mRND (right-side approach): a second skin incision was created on the tumor side of the anterior chest wall to allow insertion of the fourth robotic arm (with ProGrasp forceps). **(b)** Single-incision robotic mRND (right-side approach): all four robotic instruments and the camera were inserted through the axillary incision.

the scope. ProGrasp forceps are inserted through the anterior chest arm (Figure 16.8a).

In a single-incision robotic mRND, the additional incision in the anterior chest is not made. All robotic arms are inserted through the single axillary incision. ProGrasp forceps are positioned beneath the anterior part of the skin incision parallel to the retractor blade (Figure 16.8b).

The total thyroidectomy with CCND is performed in the same manner as a double-incision thyroidectomy. The robotic mRND procedure is similar to the open mRND. After total thyroidectomy with central compartment neck dissection, lateral neck dissection is started at the level III/IV area. The IJV is pulled medially using the ProGrasp forceps, and the soft tissue and lymph nodes are detached from the IJV and common carotid artery. The dissection of the IJV is progressed upward from level IV to the upper level III area. Level VB dissection proceeds along the spinal accessory nerve in the superomedial direction, and is followed by level IV dissection. After the level III, IV, and VB node

dissections are finished, redocking is required to provide a better view for level II lymph node dissection. The external retractor is then reinserted through the axillary incision and directed toward the submandibular gland. After level II lymph node dissection, the specimen is extracted through the axillary skin incision [54].

Bilateral axillo-breast approach robotic thyroidectomy

The patient is under general anesthesia and placed in the supine position, with the neck extended. Then, the trajectory lines and working space are drawn on the chest and neck. Creation of a working space is started by hydrodissection, and epinephrine (1:200,000) in a 0.9% NaCl solution is injected subcutaneously in the working space under the platysma muscle in the neck. A bilateral incision is made at the superomedial edge of the breast areolas and at the axillary folds. After the working space is created, bilateral axillary and circumareolar 8–12 mm ports are inserted by using a vascular tunneler through the port incision. The flap is extended from the thyroid cartilage superiorly to 2 cm below the clavicle inferiorly and laterally from just beyond the medial border of the SCM. With CO_2 gas insufflations by low pressure (5–6 mmHg), the working space is created and maintained. The robot is docked, and a camera is inserted through the right breast. Monopolar electrocautery or ultrasonic shears are inserted through the left breast. Graspers are inserted through the right and left axillary ports.

The thyroidectomy procedure is begun with identification and separation of the midline of the strap muscle. After visualizing the cricothyroid membrane, isthmus, and trachea, the isthmus is divided with ultrasonic shears, which facilitate dissection of the gland laterally and posteriorly and allow for optimal visualization of the superior thyroid pedicle. The thyroidectomy is performed while identifying and preserving the parathyroid glands and RLN. The dissected thyroid lobe is extracted with an endoplastic bag. The contralateral lobe is dissected in the same manner [55].

Application of robotic technology to thyroid surgery has several advantages over conventional open or endoscopic thyroid surgery. Since our group published the feasibility of robotic thyroidectomy in 2009, many other centers have taken on robotic thyroidectomies for thyroid disease, and the number of publications describing robotic thyroidectomy has markedly increased [30]. In a recent study, a systematic review has analyzed each of these surgical outcomes [56].

Comparative studies of robotic and conventional open thyroidectomies have reported that robotic thyroidectomy is oncologically safe and feasible; however, it is associated with longer operation times and higher costs than conventional open surgery. The measured serum thyroglobulin concentration via radioactive iodine-131 (^{131}RI) scanning, the number of retrieved neck lymph nodes, and the overall morbidity rate are similar for robotic and conventional open surgery [39,43,50,57,58]. In studies comparing endoscopic with robotic thyroidectomy, postoperative complication rates and mean length of hospital stay have been shown to be similar, but the number of retrieved neck lymph nodes is higher in robotic surgery than in endoscopic surgery [59,60]. These findings suggest that robotic thyroidectomy is feasible and safe, and can overcome some of the technical limitations associated with conventional endoscopic procedures. However, due to short follow-up results, long-term outcomes cannot be compared currently among these operation methods. Therefore, prospective randomized clinical trials with long-term follow-up are necessary to compare the surgical outcomes of robotic with open and endoscopic methods.

Developments of new surgical techniques should be made toward improving the quality of life for patients. Several studies about quality of life after robotic thyroidectomy have been published. Patients undergoing robotic thyroidectomy have experienced higher satisfaction in terms of postoperative scarring than patients undergoing open thyroidectomy. In terms of functional measurements, including pain, neck discomfort, sensory changes in the neck, and voice and swallowing discomfort, improved results have been cited for robotic surgery. Therefore, robotic surgery results in increased cosmetic satisfaction and decreased discomforts following surgery [41,45,46,48].

Many studies have compared the operation times for robotic versus endoscopic or open surgery. The total operation time for robotic surgery was significantly longer than that for open surgery, but was similar or somewhat lower than that for endoscopic surgery. Because of the three stages associated with robotic surgery (working space creation stage, docking stage, and console stage), this approach usually consumes more time than open surgery. However, if a surgeon becomes familiar with the robotic method, the operation time decreases [47,59,60].

The main disadvantages of robotic thyroidectomy are longer operation time and higher costs than endoscopic or conventional open thyroid surgery. This method is more invasive due to the wide dissection from the axilla to the anterior neck area and a possibility of anterior chest numbness or CO_2 toxicity (BABA method). Further, the approach to the contralateral superior pole of the thyroid using this method (TAA method) is difficult because of the use of nonarticulating Harmonic curved shears in the deep and narrow area. Although the use of Harmonic curved shears results in minimal thermal spread compared with the various other energy sources, some limitations exist in applying the shears to taxing cases (such as RLN nerve invasion or trachea invasion). To overcome this limitation, many instrumental developments have been attempted.

Many studies have reported the advantages and disadvantages of robotic thyroidectomy; however, a consensus has not been reached. Clinicians should consider ideal patient selection (in terms of disease characteristics, patient characteristics, economic status, previous surgical history, and the patient's general medical condition) when deciding on the suitability of a patient for robotic surgery.

In the decision process, thoughtful discussions should be held with patients regarding postoperative results, based on patient-specific parameters and intraoperative challenges.

Robotic thyroidectomy is a safe, oncologically effective, and functionally superior surgery compared with conventional open or endoscopic surgery. Despite these advantages, its impact remains uncertain. Additional studies, including cost–benefit analyses and larger controlled trials, are needed to further assess cost-effectiveness, clinical outcomes, and patient satisfaction.

REFERENCES

1. Sakorafas GH. Historical evolution of thyroid surgery: From the ancient times to the dawn of the 21st century. *World J Surg* 2010;34:1793–804.
2. Lombardi CP, Raffaelli M, Princi P, De Crea C, Bellantone R. Video-assisted thyroidectomy: Report on the experience of a single center in more than four hundred cases. *World J Surg* 2006;30:794–800.
3. Tan CT, Cheah WK, Delbridge L. "Scarless" (in the neck) endoscopic thyroidectomy (SET): An evidence-based review of published techniques. *World J Surg* 2008;32:1349–57.
4. Gagner M. Endoscopic subtotal parathyroidectomy in patients with primary hyperparathyroidism. *Br J Surg* 1996;83:875–5.
5. Hüscher CS, Chiodini S, Napolitano C, Recher A. Endoscopic right thyroid lobectomy. *Surg Endosc* 1997;11:877.
6. Yeung HC, Ng WT, Kong CK. Endoscopic thyroid and parathyroid surgery. *Surg Endosc* 1997;11:1135.
7. Yoon JH, Park CH, Chung WY. Gasless endoscopic thyroidectomy via an axillary approach: Experience of 30 cases. *Surg Laparosc Endosc Percutan Tech* 2006;16:226–31.
8. Linos D. Minimally invasive thyroidectomy: A comprehensive appraisal of existing techniques. *Surgery* 2011;150:17–24.
9. Yang Y, Gu X, Wang X, Xiang J, Chen Z. Endoscopic thyroidectomy for differentiated thyroid cancer. *Sci World J* 2012;2012:456807.
10. Kang SW, Jeong JJ, Yun JS et al. Gasless endoscopic thyroidectomy using trans-axillary approach; surgical outcome of 581 patients. *Endocr J* 2009;56:361–9.
11. Miccoli P, Elisei R, Materazzi G et al. Minimally invasive video-assisted thyroidectomy for papillary carcinoma: A prospective study of its completeness. *Surgery* 2002;132:1070–3; discussion 1073–4.
12. Miccoli P, Materazzi G, Berti P. Minimally invasive thyroidectomy in the treatment of well differentiated thyroid cancers: Indications and limits. *Curr Opin Otolaryngol Head Neck Surg* 2010;18:114–8.
13. Gagner M, Inabnet BW, Biertho L. Endoscopic thyroidectomy for solitary nodules. *Ann Chir* 2003;128:696–701.

14. Cougard P, Osmak L, Esquis P, Ognois P. Endoscopic thyroidectomy. A preliminary report including 40 patients. *Ann Chir* 2005;130:81–5.

15. Henry JF, Sebag F. Lateral endoscopic approach for thyroid and parathyroid surgery. *Ann Chir* 2006;131:51–6.

16. Palazzo FF, Sebag F, Henry JF. Endocrine surgical technique: Endoscopic thyroidectomy via the lateral approach. *Surg Endosc* 2006;20:339–42.

17. Inabnet WB, Jacob BP, Gagner M. Minimally invasive endoscopic thyroidectomy by a cervical approach. *Surg Endosc* 2003;17:1808–11.

18. Ikeda Y, Takami H, Sasaki Y et al. Comparative study of thyroidectomies. Endoscopic surgery versus conventional open surgery. *Surg Endosc* 2002;16:1741–5.

19. Kim JS, Kim KH, Ahn CH et al. A clinical analysis of gasless endoscopic thyroidectomy. *Surg Laparosc Endosc Percutan Tech* 2001;11:268–72.

20. Shimizu K, Tanaka S. Asian perspective on endoscopic thyroidectomy—A review of 193 cases. *Asian J Surg* 2003;26:92–100.

21. Kitano H, Fujimura M, Hirano M et al. Endoscopic surgery for a parathyroid functioning adenoma resection with the neck region-lifting method. *Otolaryngol Head Neck Surg* 2000;123:465–6.

22. Ikeda Y, Takami H, Sasaki Y et al. Clinical benefits in endoscopic thyroidectomy by the axillary approach. *J Am Coll Surg* 2003;196:189–95.

23. Ikeda Y, Takami H, Tajima G et al. Total endoscopic thyroidectomy: Axillary or anterior chest approach. *Biomed Pharmacother* 2002;56(Suppl 1):72s–8s.

24. Park YL, Han WK, Bae WG. 100 cases of endoscopic thyroidectomy: Breast approach. *Surg Laparosc Endosc Percutan Tech* 2003;13:20–5.

25. Ohgami M, Ishii S, Arisawa Y et al. Scarless endoscopic thyroidectomy: Breast approach for better cosmesis. *Surg Laparosc Endosc Percutan Tech* 2000;10:1–4.

26. Shimazu K, Shiba E, Tamaki Y et al. Endoscopic thyroid surgery through the axillo-bilateral-breast approach. *Surg Laparosc Endosc Percutan Tech* 2003;13:196–201.

27. Choe J, Kim SW, Chung K et al. Endoscopic thyroidectomy using a new bilateral axillo-breast approach. *World J Surg* 2007;31:601–6.

28. Choi JY, Lee KE, Chung KW et al. Endoscopic thyroidectomy via bilateral axillo-breast approach (BABA): Review of 512 cases in a single institute. *Surg Endosc* 2012;26:948–55.

29. Hakim Darail NA, Lee SH, Kang SW et al. Gasless transaxillary endoscopic thyroidectomy: A decade on. *Surg Laparosc Endosc Percutan Tech* 2014;24:e211–5.

30. Kang S, Jeong JJ, Yun J et al. Robot-assisted endoscopic surgery for thyroid cancer: Experience with the first 100 patients. *Surg Endosc* 2009;23:2399–406.

31. Inukai M, Usui Y. Clinical evaluation of gasless endoscopic thyroid surgery. *Surg Today* 2005;35:199–204.

32. Alesina PF, Rolfs T, Ruhland K et al. Evaluation of postoperative pain after minimally invasive video-assisted and conventional thyroidectomy: Results of a prospective study. ESES Vienna presentation. *Langenbecks Arch Surg* 2010;395:845–9.

33. Inukai M, Usui Y. Clinical evaluation of gasless endoscopic thyroid surgery. *Surg Today* 2005;35:199–204.

34. Ikeda Y, Takami H, Sasaki Y, Kan S, Niimi M. Endoscopic neck surgery by the axillary approach. *J Am Coll Surg* 2000;191:336–40.

35. Naitoh T, Gagner M, Garcia-Ruiz A, Heniford BT. Endoscopic endocrine surgery in the neck. An initial report of endoscopic subtotal parathyroidectomy. *Surg Endosc* 1998;12:202–5; discussion 206.

36. Dionigi G. Energy based devices and recurrent laryngeal nerve injury: The need for safer instruments. *Langenbecks Arch Surg* 2009;394:579–80; author reply 581–6.

37. Agarwal BB, Agarwal S. Recurrent laryngeal nerve, phonation and voice preservation—Energy devices in thyroid surgery—A note of caution. *Langenbecks Arch Surg* 2009;394:911–2; author reply 913–4.

38. Gutt CN, Oniu T, Mehrabi A et al. Robot-assisted abdominal surgery. *Br J Surg* 2004;91:1390–7.

39. Lee J, Chung WY. Robotic surgery for thyroid disease. *Eur Thyroid J* 2013;2:93–101.

40. Bae DS, Koo DH, Choi JY et al. Current status of robotic thyroid surgery in South Korea: A web-based survey. *World J Surg* 2014;38:2632–9.

41. Lee KE, Kim E, Koo DH et al. Robotic thyroidectomy by bilateral axillo-breast approach: Review of 1,026 cases and surgical completeness. *Surg Endosc* 2013;27:2955–62.

42. Lee J, Yun JH, Nam KH et al. Perioperative clinical outcomes after robotic thyroidectomy for thyroid carcinoma: A multicenter study. *Surg Endosc* 2011;25:906–12.

43. Lee CR, Lee SC, Park S et al. Surgical completeness of robotic thyroidectomy: A prospective comparison with conventional open thyroidectomy in papillary thyroid carcinoma patients. *Surg Endosc* 2014;28:1068–75.

44. Kang S, Lee SH, Park JH et al. A comparative study of the surgical outcomes of robotic and conventional open modified radical neck dissection for papillary thyroid carcinoma with lateral neck node metastasis. *Surg Endosc* 2012;26:3251–7.

45. Lee J, Na KY, Kim RM et al. Postoperative functional voice changes after conventional open or robotic thyroidectomy: A prospective trial. *Ann Surg Oncol* 2012;19:2963–70.

46. Lee J, Nah KY, Kim RM et al. Differences in post-operative outcomes, function, and cosmesis: Open versus robotic thyroidectomy. *Surg Endosc* 2010;24:3186–94.

47. Tae K, Ji YB, Cho SH et al. Early surgical outcomes of robotic thyroidectomy by a gasless unilateral axillo-breast or axillary approach for papillary thyroid carcinoma: 2 years' experience. *Head Neck* 2012;34:617–25.

48. Tae K, Kim KY, Yun BR et al. Functional voice and swallowing outcomes after robotic thyroidectomy by a gasless unilateral axillo-breast approach: Comparison with open thyroidectomy. *Surg Endosc* 2012;26:1871–7.

49. Tae K, Song CM, Ji YB et al. Comparison of surgical completeness between robotic total thyroidectomy versus open thyroidectomy. *Laryngoscope* 2014;124:1042–7.

50. Lee J, Kang SW, Jung JJ et al. Multicenter study of robotic thyroidectomy: Short-term postoperative outcomes and surgeon ergonomic considerations. *Ann Surg Oncol* 2011;18:2538–47.

51. Cooper DS, Doherty GM, Haugen BR et al. Revised American Thyroid Association management guidelines for patients with thyroid nodules and differentiated thyroid cancer. *Thyroid* 2009;19:1167–214.

52. Perrier ND, Randolph GW, Inabnet WB et al. Robotic thyroidectomy: A framework for new technology assessment and safe implementation. *Thyroid* 2010;20:1327–32.

53. Kuppersmith RB, Holsinger FC. Robotic thyroid surgery: An initial experience with North American patients. *Laryngoscope* 2011;121:521–6.

54. Kang SW, Lee SH, Ryu HR et al. Initial experience with robot-assisted modified radical neck dissection for the management of thyroid carcinoma with lateral neck node metastasis. *Surgery* 2010;148:1214–21.

55. Lee KE, Choi JY, Youn Y. Bilateral axillo-breast approach robotic thyroidectomy. *Surg Laparosc Endosc Percutan Tech* 2011;21:230–6.

56. Jackson NR, Yao L, Tufano RP, Kandil EH. Safety of robotic thyroidectomy approaches: Meta-analysis and systematic review. *Head Neck* 2014;36:137–43.

57. Lee J, Chung WY. Current status of robotic thyroidectomy and neck dissection using a gasless transaxillary approach. *Curr Opin Oncol* 2012;24:7–15.

58. Lee S, Ryu HR, Park JH et al. Early surgical outcomes comparison between robotic and conventional open thyroid surgery for papillary thyroid microcarcinoma. *Surgery* 2012;151:724–30.

59. Lee JH, Nah KY, Soh EY, Chung WY. Comparison of endoscopic and robotic thyroidectomy. *Ann Surg Oncol* 2011;18:1439–46.

60. Lee S, Ryu HR, Park JH et al. Excellence in robotic thyroid surgery: A comparative study of robot-assisted versus conventional endoscopic thyroidectomy in papillary thyroid microcarcinoma patients. *Ann Surg* 2011;253:1060–6.

17

Video-assisted thyroid surgery

PAOLO MICCOLI AND GABRIELE MATERAZZI

INTRODUCTION

The first minimally invasive procedure ever performed in the neck area was the endoscopic parathyroidectomy carried out by Gagner in 1996 [1]. Parathyroid pathology seemed, in fact, very viable to be treated endoscopically; indeed, parathyroid adenomas are almost always benign, rarely does their volume exceeds 3 cm, and they do not present important vascular connections.

The success obtained by this and other similar accesses [2–4] convinced several surgeons to remove small thyroid nodules as well as parathyroid adenomas; in spite of the concern expressed by some endocrine surgeons, both endoscopic and video-assisted thyroidectomy soon became quite popular: this trend was expressed by the papers that appeared on surgical reviews [5–10].

Nowadays, minimally invasive video-assisted thyroidectomy (MIVAT) is one of the minimally invasive endoscopic techniques most widely performed all over the world [11–17] and represents the cosmetic alternative to endoscopic trans-axillary thyroidectomy (robot assisted or not) [18], which allows removal of the scar from the neck and treatment of large nodules, but it cannot be considered minimally invasive and is limited by costs [19–22].

MINIMALLY INVASIVE VIDEO-ASSISTED THYROIDECTOMY

This technique is characterized by the absence of any gas insufflation, and operative space is maintained by external retraction. It was first described in 1999 [8], and at that time, a short insufflation was used to create the operative space, but later on, a blunt dissection proved to be sufficient to create a good space between the thyroid and the strap muscles so as to rely only on external retraction. From that moment, more than 3000 procedures have been performed by the authors, the operation is routinely performed at the Department of Surgery of Pisa, and it was adopted by several surgical centers around the world.

INDICATIONS

A careful selection of the patients is of paramount importance to ensure a good outcome for this operation; the greatest limit is represented by the volume of the nodule and even more of the gland to be operated on. The lobe, in fact, has to be removed without disrupting its capsule because of the necessity of an accurate histologic evaluation, since these nodules are often suspect for carcinoma (either follicular of papillary). Other important limits are represented by the presence of adhesions that can make it difficult to recognize the most important structures, such as the recurrent nerve. That is why repeat surgery is considered a contraindication for this procedure, but great caution should also be addressed to thyroiditis. For this reason, an accurate evaluation of thyroid antibodies, characteristically increased in this disease, should be obtained before operating on these patients. Also, the preoperative ultrasonographic study should be the most accurate because it is important to correctly evaluate thyroid and nodule volume and because it can help to recognize echographic aspects of thyroiditis.

General indications might be summarized as follows:

1. Thyroid nodules less than 3.5 cm in largest diameter
2. Thyroid gland volume less than 25 mL, as estimated by ultrasound
3. Absence of thyroiditis
4. No previous neck surgery or irradiation
5. Benign disease (goiter, multinodular toxic goiter, or Graves' disease), follicular lesions, or "low-risk" papillary carcinoma

TECHNIQUE

The operation is generally performed with the patient under general anesthesia, but local anesthesia (deep bilateral cervical block) can also be used. It can be divided into four steps:

1. Preparation of the operative space. The patient, under general endotracheal anesthesia, is in the supine position with his neck not extended; hyperextension must be avoided because it would reduce the operative space. The skin is protected by means of a sterile film (Tegaderm˚). A 1.5 cm horizontal skin incision is performed 2 cm above the sternal notch in the central cervical area (Figure 17.1). Subcutaneous fat and platysma are carefully dissected so as to avoid any minimum bleeding. Two small retractors of the army–navy type (Figure 17.2) are used to expose the midline, which has to be incised for 2–3 cm on a bloodless plane.

   The blunt dissection of the thyroid lobe from the strap muscles is completely carried out through the skin incision by gentle retraction and using tiny spatulas.

   The same small retractors maintain the operative space in which a 30° 5 or 7 mm endoscope is inserted through the skin incision. From this moment on, the procedure is entirely endoscopic until the extraction of the affected lobe. Preparation of the thyrotracheal groove is completed under endoscopic vision by using the small (2 mm in diameter) instruments that are shown in Figure 17.3.

2. Ligature of the main thyroid vessels. Neither clips nor ligatures are currently used to achieve hemostasis. Since the beginning, the Harmonic Scalpel device (Ultracision˚) was utilized for all the vessels, but other energy devices using radiofrequency or bipolar technology have been introduced, and they can be utilized as

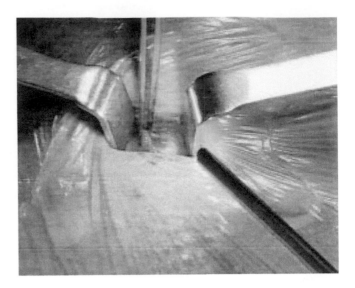

Figure 17.2 Two small retractors are used to expose the midline.

well. The first vessel to be sectioned is the middle vein, if present, or the small veins between the jugular vein and thyroid capsule. Their section allows a better exposure of the thyroid space. The upper pedicle is then prepared by retracting downward and medially the thyroid lobe (Figure 17.4). The spatula is used to retract the vessels laterally. This also allows the external branch of the superior laryngeal nerve to be easily identified during most procedures (Figure 17.5). Its injury can be avoided by keeping the inactive blade of Ultracision in the posterior position so as not to transmit heat to this delicate structure.

3. Visualization and dissection of the recurrent nerve and parathyroid glands. When retracting medially and lifting up the thyroid lobe by means of the retractors, the cervical fascia can be opened by gentle spatula retraction and the recurrent nerve appears in the groove between the trachea and thyroid. A good anatomical landmark for its visualization is the Zuckerkandl lobe of the thyroid. The superior parathyroid gland can be easily visualized, thanks to the endoscopic magnification, and dissected by Ultracision. Both of these structures must be carefully separated from the thyroid lobe before it is extracted (Figure 17.6).

4. Extraction of the lobe and resection. At this point in time the lobe is completely freed. The endoscope and the retractors can be removed, and the upper portion of the gland rotated and pulled out using conventional forceps. Gentle traction over the upper pole allows the thyroid lobe to be completely extracted (Figure 17.7). The operation is now conducted as in open surgery under direct vision. The lobe is freed from the trachea by dissecting Berry's ligament. It is very important to check the laryngeal nerve once again so as to avoid its injury before the final step. The isthmus is then dissected from the trachea and divided by means of Ultracision.

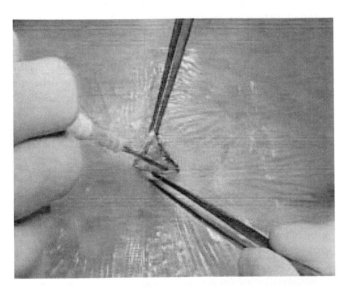

Figure 17.1 A 1.5 cm horizontal skin incision is performed 2 cm above the sternal notch.

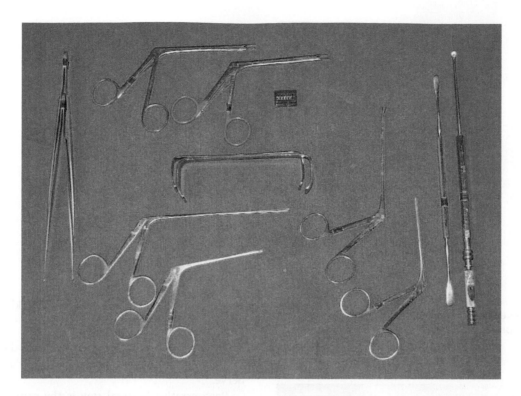

Figure 17.3 Instruments for MIVAT.

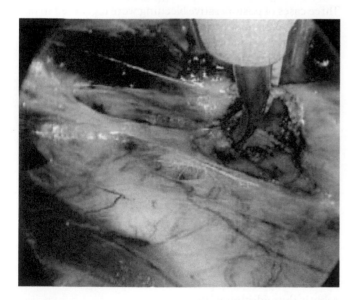

Figure 17.4 The upper pedicle is prepared and transected by Ultracision.

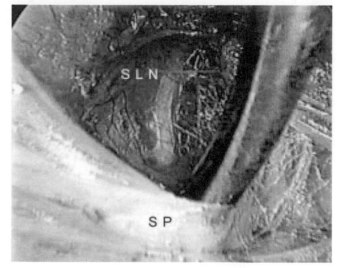

Figure 17.5 The external branch of the superior laryngeal nerve is easily visualized during section of the upper pedicle.

Drainage is not necessary. The midline is then approached by a single stitch; platysma is closed by a subcuticular readsorbable suture, and a cyanoachrilate sealant is used for the skin (Figure 17.8).

Surgical follow-up should include direct laryngoscopy to check vocal cord mobility and neck ultrasonography in all cases. Serum calcium measurement is obtained in those patients undergoing total thyroidectomy in order to evaluate their postoperative parathyroid function.

RESULTS

Our experience consists of more than 3000 patients operated on since 1998. The female-to-male ratio is 4:1. Lobectomy was carried out in 41.5% of patients, and total thyroidectomy in 58.5%.

The mean operative time of lobectomy is 38.3 [20–120] minutes, while total thyroidectomy was accomplished in 45.6 [30–130] minutes. Preoperative diagnosis was mainly

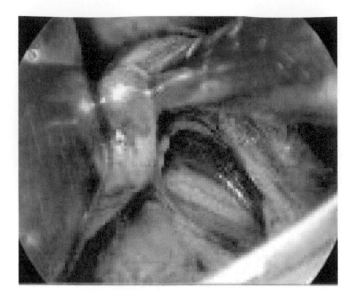

Figure 17.6 The endoscopic magnification allows a good visualization of parathyroid glands and the recurrent laryngeal nerve.

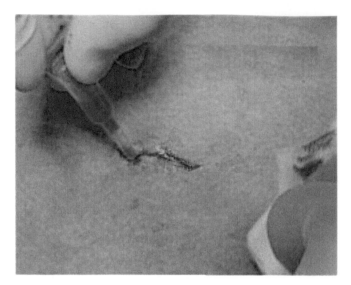

Figure 17.8 Sealant is used to close the skin.

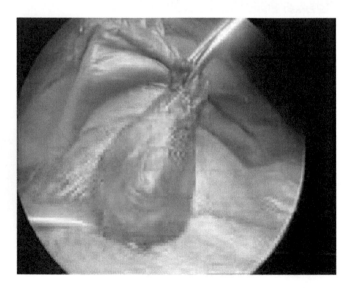

Figure 17.7 Gentle retraction over the upper pole allows the thyroid lobe to be completely extracted.

follicular nodule or low-risk papillary carcinoma (together representing more than 65% of the series); the remaining indications were Graves' disease, small multinodular goiter, toxic adenoma, and RET mutation gene carriers (undergoing prophylactic total thyroidectomy and level VI clearance).

Conversion to traditional cervicotomy was required in 2% of cases. The most frequent reasons for conversion are unexpected esophageal or tracheal invasion from a carcinoma, the presence of metastatic VI compartment lymph nodes, and finally, thyroiditis not revealed by preoperative workup. In a large series of 336 cases operated on with this technique and described inside a multicentric study [9], the first reason for conversion was in fact difficulty in lobe

dissection because it rendered uncertain the identification of the most important structures, such as the recurrent nerve.

Postoperative hospital stay is the same as in all other cases undergoing traditional surgery (overnight discharge). Three cases of postoperative bleeding were registered in our series. All patients were satisfied with the cosmetic results. In a prospective randomized study [10] on a limited series of patients comparing MIVAT with traditional thyroidectomy, we demonstrated that cosmetic results, evaluated by verbal response scale and numeric scale, as well as postoperative distress, were significantly better in patients undergoing MIVAT.

Successively, several publications from other authors showed benefits and advantages of MIVAT when dealing with postoperative pain and cosmetic results [23–28].

Nowadays, even after the advent of robot-assisted transaxillary thyroidectomy (RATT) (performed in Pisa since 2012), which is claimed to be the most cosmetic-friendly procedure when removing the thyroid gland, because it avoids any scar in the neck, MIVAT is still competitive as a cosmetic and minimally invasive procedure, as shown by our study recently performed, comparing MIVAT and robotic thyroidectomy [18].

One of the most controversial aspects in terms of indications is the opportunity to treat malignancies. MIVAT has shown to be very effective in the treatment of papillary carcinoma. Several studies were performed through the years, demonstrating that this minimally invasive technique is as safe and effective as traditional cervicotomy when dealing with low-risk papillary carcinoma [29–36].

When dealing with papillary carcinoma, MIVAT provides the same clearance at the thyroid bed level as the conventional technique, as clearly demonstrated in two different studies performed at the Department of Surgery in Pisa.

Table 17.1 Preoperative diagnosis

	N (%)
Follicular nodule	89 (36.9)
Papillary carcinoma	68 (28.3)
Multinodular goiter	44 (18.2)
Hürtle cell nodule	25 (10.3)
Toxic adenoma	11 (4.6)
Graves' disease	1 (0.4)
Toxic multinodular goiter	3 (1.2)
Total	241 (100%)

The first one is a prospective randomized study [37]: 35 patients with low-risk papillary carcinoma were allotted; 16 were operated on with MIVAT (group A) and 19 with conventional technique (group B). One month after surgery, the thyroglobulin (Tg) serum level was measured and a whole body scintigraphy (WBS) with I^{131} was performed in all patients. No statistically significant difference in the results between the two groups was found (Tg serum level was 5.3 ± 5.8 ng/L and 7.6 ± 21.7 ng/L and mean radioiodine uptake was $3.9 \pm 4.4\%$ and $4.6 \pm 6.7\%$, respectively, in groups A and B).

The second prospective study [36] involved 221 patients with a papillary carcinoma smaller than 30 mm, an ultrasound-estimated thyroid volume of less than 30 mL, and no ultrasound evidence of lymph node metastasis or thyroiditis. One hundred seventy-one patients were operated on with MIVAT (group A) and 50 with conventional technique (group B). After a mean follow-up of 3.6 ± 1.5 years (range 1–8 years, mean 5 years), there were no statistically significant differences between the two groups in terms of age, sex, and mean follow-up. No differences in serum Tg and thyroid-stimulating hormone levels and I^{131} neck uptake were observed between the two groups of patients (Table 17.1), and no statistical difference was found between cured and not cured PTC patients at the end of follow-up. The same rates of hypoparathyroidism and recurrent laryngeal nerve palsy were recorded.

These results after 5 years' follow-up clearly suggest that MIVAT is a safe and effective technique in the treatment of low- and intermediate-risk papillary carcinomas.

There is no doubt that low-risk papillary carcinomas constitute an ideal indication for MIVAT, but a good selection has to take into account the exact profile of possible lymph node involvement in the neck. In fact, although the completeness of a total thyroidectomy achievable with video-assisted procedures is beyond debate, the greatest caution should be taken when approaching a disease involving either metastatic lymph nodes or an extracapsular invasion of the gland. In these cases, an endoscopic approach might be inadequate to obtain a full clearance of the nodes or the complete removal of the neoplastic tissue (infiltration of the trachea or the esophagus). Again, an accurate echographic study is of paramount importance in order to select the right cases undergoing video-assisted surgery.

CONCLUSIONS

MIVAT has proved to be a safe procedure when performed in different surgical settings, and it has also proved to be a valid therapeutic option as long as indications are strictly followed, because some advantages in terms of cosmetic results and postoperative pain can be demonstrated. In the last 10 years, several minimally invasive approaches have been ideated, developed, and then standardized for the treatment of thyroid diseases, both benign and malignant. None of these different techniques, ranging from the "purely endoscopic" to the video-assisted approaches without CO_2 insufflation, are actually considered among the surgical community to be the best and most unique approach to be utilized, but MIVAT has been demonstrated to be easily reproducible in different settings and is also safely applicable to the treatment of low-risk thyroid malignancies.

RATT represents the cosmetic alternative to MIVAT, allowing the removal of scars from the neck. This robot-assisted procedure provides some advantages compared with MIVAT: the removal of large nodules (up to 6 cm), three-dimensional magnified endoscopic vision, and the ability to also perform lateral neck clearance in cases of metastatic papillary carcinoma. RATT has also some disadvantages compared with MIVAT: it is not as minimally invasive as the video-assisted technique, the operative time is necessarily longer, and costs are higher.

When dealing with satisfaction and cosmetic results, our study comparing RATT with MIVAT found that relocating the wound from the neck to a less visible area, such as the axilla, is not enough to meet patients' full expectations, probably because the axilla scar is still considered to be too long and its appearance is less likely to improve over time because it cannot be placed in a skin crease. Our results appear to be in agreement with the words of Q.Y. Duh, "For now … neck incisions … are here to stay" [38].

REFERENCES

1. Gagner M. Endoscopic parathyroidectomy [letter]. *Br J Surg* 1996;83:875.
2. Henry JF, Defechereux T, Gramatica L, de Boissezon C. Minimally invasive videoscopic parathyroidectomy by lateral approach. *Langenbecks Arch Surg* 1999;384:298–301.
3. Miccoli P, Bendinelli C, Vignali E et al. Endoscopic parathyroidectomy: Report of an initial experience. *Surgery* 1998;124:1077–80.
4. Miccoli P, Berti P, Raffaelli M, Conte M, Materazzi G, Galleri D. Minimally invasive video-assisted parathyroidectomy. *Am J Surg* 2001;181(6):567–70.

5. Shimizu K, Akira S, Jasmi AY et al. Video-assisted neck surgery: Endoscopic resection of thyroid tumors with a very minimal neck wound. *J Am Coll Surg* 1999;188:697–703.

6. Ohgami M, Ishii S, Ohmori T, Noga K, Furukawa T, Kitajima M. Scarless endoscopic thyroidectomy: Breast approach better cosmesis. *Surg Laparosc Endosc Percutan Tech* 2000;10:1–4.

7. Ikeda Y, Takami H, Sasaky Y, Kan S, Niimi M. Endoscopic neck surgery by the axillary approach. *J Am Coll Surg* 2000;191:849–51.

8. Miccoli P, Berti P, Conte M et al. Minimally invasive surgery for small thyroid nodules: Preliminary report. *J Endocrinol Invest* 1999;22:849–51.

9. Miccoli P, Bellantone R, Mourad M, Walz M, Raffaelli M, Berti P. Minimally invasive video-assisted thyroidectomy: Multiinstitutional experience. *World J Surg* 2002;26(8):972–5.

10. Miccoli P, Berti P, Raffaelli M, Materazzi G, Baldacci S, Rossi G. Comparison between minimally invasive video-assisted thyroidectomy and conventional thyroidectomy: A prospective randomized study. *Surgery* 2001;130(6):1039–43.

11. Kania R, Hammami H, Vérillaud B et al. Minimally invasive video-assisted thyroidectomy: Tips and pearls for the surgical technique. *Ann Otol Rhinol Laryngol* 2014;123(6):409–14.

12. Pisanu A, Podda M, Reccia I, Porceddu G, Uccheddu A. Systematic review with meta-analysis of prospective randomized trials comparing minimally invasive video-assisted thyroidectomy (MIVAT) and conventional thyroidectomy (CT). *Langenbecks Arch Surg* 2013;398(8):1057–68.

13. Barczyński M, Konturek A, Stopa M, Papier A, Nowak W. Minimally invasive video-assisted thyroidectomy: Seven-year experience with 240 cases. *Wideochir Inne Tech Malo Inwazyjne* 2012;7(3):175–80.

14. Pons Y, Vérillaud B, Blancal JP et al. Minimally invasive video-assisted thyroidectomy: Learning curve in terms of mean operative time and conversion and complication rates. *Head Neck* 2013;35(8):1078.

15. Minuto MN, Berti P, Miccoli M et al. Minimally invasive video-assisted thyroidectomy: An analysis of results and a revision of indications. *Surg Endosc* 2012;26(3):818–22.

16. Radford PD, Ferguson MS, Magill JC, Karthikesalingham AP, Alusi G. Meta-analysis of minimally invasive video-assisted thyroidectomy. *Laryngoscope* 2011;121(8):1675–81.

17. Linos D. Minimally invasive thyroidectomy: A comprehensive appraisal of existing techniques. *Surgery* 2011;150(1):17–24.

18. Materazzi G, Fregoli L, Manzini G, Baggiani A, Miccoli M, Miccoli P. Cosmetic result and overall satisfaction after minimally invasive video-assisted thyroidectomy (MIVAT) versus robot-assisted transaxillary thyroidectomy (RATT): A prospective randomized study. *World J Surg* 2014;38(6):1282–8.

19. Kwak HY, Kim HY, Lee HY et al. Robotic thyroidectomy using bilateral axillo-breast approach: Comparison of surgical results with open conventional thyroidectomy. *J Surg Oncol* 2015;111(2):141–5.

20. Shen H, Shan C, Qiu M. Systematic review and meta-analysis of transaxillary robotic thyroidectomy versus open thyroidectomy. *Surg Laparosc Endosc Percutan Tech* 2014;24(3):199–206.

21. Holsinger FC, Chung WY. Robotic thyroidectomy. *Otolaryngol Clin North Am* 2014;47(3):373–8.

22. Lee J, Chung WY. Robotic surgery for thyroid disease. *Eur Thyroid J* 2013;2(2):93–101.

23. Sahm M, Schwarz B, Schmidt S, Pross M, Lippert H. Long-term cosmetic results after minimally invasive video-assisted thyroidectomy. *Surg Endosc* 2011;25(10):3202–8.

24. Del Rio P, Arcuri MF, Pisani P, De Simone B, Sianesi M. Minimally invasive video-assisted thyroidectomy (MIVAT): What is the real advantage? *Langenbecks Arch Surg* 2010;395(4):323–6.

25. Barczyński M, Konturek A, Cichoń S. Minimally invasive video-assisted thyreoidectomy (MIVAT) with and without use of harmonic scalpel—A randomized study. *Langenbecks Arch Surg* 2008;393(5):647–54.

26. Del Rio P, Berti M, Sommaruga L, Arcuri MF, Cataldo S, Sianesi M. Pain after minimally invasive video-assisted and after minimally invasive open thyroidectomy—Results of a prospective outcome study. *Langenbecks Arch Surg* 2008;393(3):271–3.

27. Lombardi CP, Raffaelli M, Princi P, De Crea C, Bellantone R. Video-assisted thyroidectomy: Report of a 7-year experience in Rome. *Langenbecks Arch Surg* 2006;391(3):174–7.

28. Miccoli P, Berti P, Materazzi G, Minuto M, Barellini L. Minimally invasive video-assisted thyroidectomy: Five years of experience. *J Am Coll Surg* 2004;199(2):243–8.

29. Nenkov R, Radev R, Madjov R. Video-assisted thyroid resections in the treatment of papillary thyroid carcinoma. *Khirurgiia (Sofiia)* 2013;(2):15–9.

30. Gao W, Liu L, Ye G, Song L. Application of minimally invasive video-assisted technique in papillary thyroid microcarcinoma. *Surg Laparosc Endosc Percutan Tech* 2013;23(5):468–73.

31. Igarashi T, Shimizu K, Yakubouski S et al. Introduction and use of video-assisted endoscopic thyroidectomy for patients in Belarus affected by the Chernobyl nuclear disaster. *Asian J Endosc Surg* 2013;6(4):298–302.

32. DI JZ, Zhang HW, Han XD, Zhang P, Zheng Q, Wang Y. Minimally invasive video-assisted thyroidectomy for accidental papillary thyroid microcarcinoma: Comparison with conventional open thyroidectomy with 5 years follow-up. *Chin Med J (Engl)* 2011;124(20):3293–6.

33. Miccoli P, Materazzi G, Berti P. Minimally invasive thyroidectomy in the treatment of well differentiated thyroid cancers: Indications and limits. *Curr Opin Otolaryngol Head Neck Surg* 2010;18(2):114–8.

34. Wu CT, Yang LH, Kuo SJ. Comparison of video-assisted thyroidectomy and traditional thyroidectomy for the treatment of papillary thyroid carcinoma. *Surg Endosc* 2010;24(7):1658–62.

35. Del Rio P, Sommaruga L, Pisani P et al. Minimally invasive video-assisted thyroidectomy in differentiated thyroid cancer: A 1-year follow-up. *Surg Laparosc Endosc Percutan Tech* 2009;19(4):290–2.

36. Miccoli P, Pinchera A, Materazzi G et al. Surgical treatment of low- and intermediate-risk papillary thyroid cancer with minimally invasive video-assisted thyroidectomy. *J Clin Endocrinol Metab* 2009;94(5):1618–22.

37. Miccoli P, Elisei R, Materazzi G et al. Minimally invasive video-assisted thyroidectomy for papillary carcinoma: A prospective study of its completeness. *Surgery* 2002;132(6):1070–3.

38. QY Duh. Robot assisted endoscopic thyroidectomy: Has the time come to abandon neck incisions? *Ann Surg* 2011;253:1067–8.

18

Principles of thyroid cancer surgery and outcomes

JAMES Y. LIM AND WILLIAM B. INABNET III

INTRODUCTION

The incidence of thyroid cancer has steadily increased over the years. Although all histologic subtypes of thyroid cancer have increased, papillary thyroid cancer has had the greatest increase, from an annual incidence rate of 5.5 per 100,000 people in 1990 to 13.83 per 100,000 people in 2010 [1]. Thus, there is a growing need for expert thyroid surgeons. Thyroid surgery can be treacherous due to the proximity of important adjacent structures, such as the trachea, major blood vessels, and nerves. This chapter discusses the fundamental principles of thyroid surgery: hemostasis, capsular dissection, and preservation of the parathyroid glands and recurrent laryngeal nerves. In addition, outcomes of thyroid cancer are discussed in terms of both nonneoplastic and tumor variables.

PRINCIPLES OF THYROID SURGERY

Maintaining a bloodless field

The major principles of thyroid surgery are summarized in Table 18.1. As is the case in all surgical resections, one of the key steps of a thyroid lobectomy or total thyroidectomy is controlled devascularization of the organ. The thyroid is complicated because it has one of the richest blood supplies of any organ, with a number of blood vessels and plexus

(Figure 18.1). When thyroid surgeries were first attempted in the twelfth century, one of the major causes of death was due to the lack of ability to control the vasculature. It was not until the beginning of the twentieth century that the principles of safe and efficient thyroid surgery were established [2]. Paramount to these principles was that of maintaining a bloodless field by obtaining meticulous control of the vasculature. Not only is hemostasis important intraoperatively for careful dissection and identification of anatomy, but also it is important in preventing a postoperative emergency with the development of hematoma and airway compromise. Throughout the twentieth century, hemostasis was performed with the conventional clamp-tie technique with great success. As surgical technology has advanced, attempts to refine hemostatic techniques for thyroidectomies have similarly progressed. These techniques have ranged from vascular clips to monopolar and bipolar cautery. These traditional methods have several disadvantages. Suture ligation can be time-consuming and be limited by adequate space, as well as being susceptible to knot slippage. Vascular clips may interfere with future imaging and can also be prone to displacement. Monopolar and bipolar cautery can generate tremendous amounts of heat, up to 400°C, and can be dangerous when working around the parathyroid glands and laryngeal nerves.

Because of these disadvantages, two technologies used in other facets of surgery have also been adopted recently:

Table 18.1 Four major principles of thyroid surgery

- Maintaining a bloodless field
- Performing a capsular dissection
- Preserving the recurrent laryngeal and superior laryngeal nerves
- Preserving the parathyroid glands

the Ligasure vessel sealing device (small jaw hand piece) and Harmonic ultrasonic shears, originally developed for laparoscopic surgery. The Ligasure device achieves hemostasis by coagulating tissue through radiofrequency bipolar energy. Studies have shown the thermal spread of the Ligasure to be within 3 mm. The Harmonic ultrasonic shears employ ultrasound vibration at 55 kHz over a distance of 80 μM to create mechanical energy, not heat, to cause protein denaturation through cleavage of hydrogen bonds. Due to this principle, overall heat generation is kept to 60°C–80°C and collateral tissue injury is limited to approximately 2.2 mm or less. The added advantage of the Harmonic ultrasonic

shears over the Ligasure device is that they coagulate and cut tissue with the same instrument, allowing for more efficient dissection.

Studies comparing the Ligasure device and Harmonic scalpel with conventional techniques have concluded that there is no difference in complication rates, some stating decreased complications with the new technology. The consensus is that these newer technologies do not subject patients to any additional risks, with the overall benefit being a reduction in operative time, anywhere from 10 to 29 minutes on average. Even with the added cost of the new technologies, studies have shown that there is some cost benefit when factored in with the subtracted cost of decreased operative times.

The use of alternate hemostatic agents has also been studied. There have been increasing attempts to use a number of biosurgical agents designed to promote hemostasis in thyroid surgery, including oxidized regenerated cellulose, gelatin-compressed sponge, topical thrombin, and fibrin sealants. Although some studies have shown improved

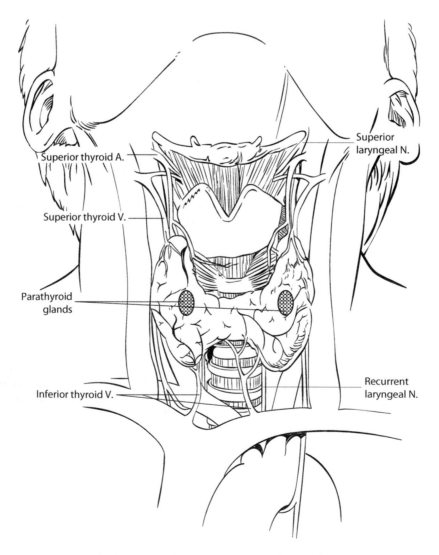

Figure 18.1 Anatomy of the central neck. A, artery; V, vein; N, nerve. (Adapted from Thawley SE et al. *Comprehensive Management of Head and Neck Tumors*, 2nd ed., W.B. Saunders Co., Philadelphia, 1999:1728–31.)

outcomes where these agents are used, most studies have shown that use of these agents led to worse outcomes. Surgical bleeding after a thyroidectomy is most likely due to surgical technique and not dependent on the use of hemostatic agents [3]. None of these newer hemostatic technologies replace meticulous surgical technique and finishing the procedure with a dry operative field.

Performing a capsular dissection

Capsular dissection has its roots in techniques that thyroid surgery pioneers such as Halsted first advocated in the early 1900s. In the 1970s, the standard approach was the lateral dissection, where the recurrent laryngeal nerve was first identified and dissected along its entire length up to the cricopharyngeus. After the nerve was dissected, all the tissue medial to the nerve was removed. There were several complications associated with this dissection approach. The blood supply to the parathyroid glands was very difficult to preserve with this manner of dissection. In addition, the extensive manipulation of the recurrent laryngeal nerve led to greater risk of neuropraxia [4].

The idea of capsular dissection was first popularized by Norman W. Thompson in 1973 by describing the development of a plane between the thyroid capsule and the inferior thyroid artery [4]. The technique has been best described as the thyroid lobe being medially retracted and elevated out of the wound, while the peripheral branches of the inferior thyroid artery lying on the capsule are individually ligated and divided (Figure 18.2). In this way, the dissection continues posteriorly along the thyroid capsule. The parathyroid glands are encountered during this dissection and preserved

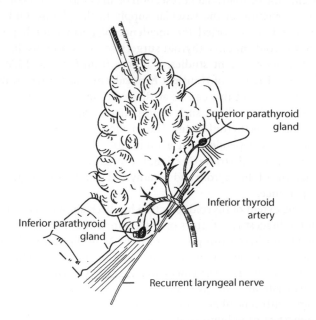

Figure 18.2 Capsular dissection ligating individual tertiary branches of the inferior thyroid artery while preserving the blood supply to both parathyroid glands. The dashed line indicates the plane of capsular dissection. (Adapted from Bliss RD et al. *World J. Surg.*, 24(8), 891–897, 2000.)

along with their blood supply and dissected off the thyroid. The recurrent laryngeal nerve can be encountered in this fashion at the region of the ligament of Berry. In this way, the nerve does not need to be dissected out along its entire length; instead, once it is free of the thyroid at this level, the dissection can continue medially along the thyroid gland and be removed off the surface of the trachea. Earlier dissection techniques recommended identifying the recurrent laryngeal nerve early in the thyroid dissection and visualizing the entire course of the nerve. In situations such as with advanced cancers, where the recurrent laryngeal nerve is difficult to identify, the recommendation is to identify the nerve at the thoracic inlet and trace it to the larynx in order to prevent injury. At the superior pole of the thyroid, the anterior and posterior branches of the superior thyroid vessels should be ligated as they course over the thyroid in order to prevent injury to the superior laryngeal nerve.

Looking at the results of one hospital utilizing this capsular dissection technique over a period of almost three decades, the incidence of permanent or major complications has remained extremely low. The incidence of permanent hypoparathyroidism was 0.3%, and that of permanent laryngeal nerve paralysis was 0.7% [5].

Preservation of the recurrent laryngeal and superior laryngeal nerves

Injury of the recurrent laryngeal nerves is a long recognized and potentially catastrophic complication of thyroid surgery. Injuring the nerve affects the abductors of the vocal cords, leading to symptoms ranging from hoarseness, if unilateral, to stridor and airway compromise in bilateral injuries. Routine recurrent laryngeal nerve visualization is considered the gold standard of care for the prevention of nerve injuries.

Thorough knowledge of the location of the recurrent laryngeal nerves on the left and right is paramount during thyroid dissection. Due to the principles of capsular dissection, the nerve is frequently encountered close to the ligament of Berry. The recurrent laryngeal nerve is at higher risk of injury in several types of thyroid surgeries: reoperations, cancer surgeries, and greater extents of thyroid surgery. Reoperations lead to scarring and distortion of planes, which leads to greater difficulty in identifying nerves, as well as placing them at greater risk of traction injury. Despite meticulous dissection, incidence of injuries is rare, but studies have shown the incidence of transient recurrent laryngeal nerve palsies can range from 0.4% to 12%. The risk of permanent injury in reoperations has been estimated from 2% to 30% [6,7]. Cancer surgeries also were found to have an increased risk of nerve injuries when compared with benign thyroid pathologies. In cancers, the thought is that the disease is locally advanced and involves the nerve or the tissue surrounding the nerve. One study had a rate of injury of 5.26% in malignant disease, compared with 0.7% in benign thyroid disease [8]. Finally, there have been studies showing that the training and experience of the surgeon has a role in nerve injuries as well, with one study showing a 0.72% rate of injury, compared with a 1.06% rate of injury in the less experienced group [6,9].

There is now good evidence to support the role of intraoperative identification of the recurrent laryngeal nerve in order to prevent injury. One review that looked at more than 12,000 operations found that the rate of nerve injury was 7.2% when not identified, compared with 1.2% in those cases where the nerve was identified. To that end, the use of intraoperative nerve monitoring has become increasingly accepted as an adjunct to visualization both to assist with nerve identification and to confirm nerve integrity. The intraoperative nerve monitoring works by documenting electromyographic (EMG) signals of elicited laryngeal muscle activity when the recurrent laryngeal nerve is stimulated either directly or indirectly [10]. The benefits of intraoperative nerve monitoring seem more apparent in reoperative thyroid surgery or advanced cancers. In addition, a benefit has been shown when nerve monitoring is used by surgeons who are considered low-volume thyroid surgeons, compared with more experienced thyroid surgeons [10]. Studies have been inconclusive, though, on the exact benefit of nerve monitoring compared with visualization alone, with several meta-analyses showing no statistical difference between the two groups when comparing the rate of recurrent laryngeal nerve palsies [7]. Because of this, there has yet to be universal acceptance of nerve monitoring during thyroid surgery, with a recent survey showing regular usage rates of 20%–40% [11].

Injury to the superior laryngeal nerve can be similarly devastating in certain patient populations. The external branch of the superior laryngeal nerve innervates the cricothyroid muscle and can potentially affect the vocal range of the patient. Unlike the recurrent laryngeal nerve, the superior laryngeal nerve tends to be avoided during thyroid surgery, with the thought that avoidance will prevent injury [4]. Studies have shown that complications affecting this nerve can be as high as 58% and are likely underreported due to the varying and subtle symptoms that patients may present with postoperatively [12]. Cadaveric studies have shown that approximately 70%–80% of the population should have a superior laryngeal nerve that is identifiable without intramuscular dissection of the pharyngeal constrictor muscle [13]. Classification systems are also in place to describe the various locations of the nerve, the most common being the Cernea classification system. Type 1 external branch superior laryngeal nerves are located well clear of the thyroid, more than 1 cm above the upper pole of the lobe, passing directly into the cricothyroid muscle. Type 2a nerves pass in the vicinity of the superior thyroid vessels as they enter the gland substance, and Type 2b nerves cross over the anterior surface of the thyroid lobe. This nerve should be routinely identified, as its path can come close to the superior pole vessels and be injured during this portion of the thyroidectomy (Cernea Types 2a and 2b). Intraoperative nerve monitoring has also been utilized in identifying this nerve. Several studies have shown that nerve monitoring consistently increased

the identification of the superior laryngeal nerve [14,15]. One recent study showed that of 357 nerves at risk, nerve monitoring-assisted dissection was able to identify the superior laryngeal nerve 97.2% of the time, as opposed to 85.7% of the time when using visualization alone [16]. Although identification of the nerve was able to be improved consistently using nerve monitoring, the difference in functional morbidity between the two patient groups is less clear and is something that needs to be further studied.

It is also important to keep in mind that not all voice changes after thyroidectomy are due to injuries to the superior or recurrent laryngeal nerves. Several studies have shown that after thyroidectomy, most of the voice alterations were not related to injuries of these nerves [17,18]. These alterations can be attributed to many different reasons other than nerve injury, such as trauma following endotracheal intubation, surgical trauma, modification of the vascular supply and venous drainage of the larynx, laryngotracheal fixation of the strap muscles with impairment of vertical movement, and a lesion of the perithyroidal plexus [14].

Preservation of the parathyroid glands

The proximity of the parathyroid glands to the thyroid gland requires careful dissection and identification to prevent the debilitating morbidity of permanent hypoparathyroidism after thyroid resection. Transient hypoparathyroidism can be problematic, as it may require an extended inpatient stay while symptoms of hypocalcemia are treated. Potential consequences of permanent hypoparathyroidism include calcification of the basal ganglia, cataract formation, and tetany. Hypoparathyroidism occurs after thyroid surgery due to accidental or inadvertent resection of all parathyroid glands or destruction of the vascular supply to the glands. Older studies have reported the incidence of permanent hypoparathyroidism after thyroid surgery to be as high as 46%, but in more recent studies, it ranges from 0.4% to 13.8% [19,20]. The rate of transient hypocalcemia is higher, from 2% to 53%, but this can be attributed to factors other than hypoparathyroidism, such as in patients who are operated on for hyperthyroid states. The incidence of hypoparathyroidism is dependent on a multitude of factors, such as the extent of thyroid resection, thorough knowledge of the anatomy of the thyroid and parathyroid glands, and surgeon experience.

The extent of thyroid resection has been shown to be one of the biggest risk factors of both transient and permanent hypoparathyroidism postoperatively. Multiple studies have shown that the extent of surgery is the greatest predictor of transient and permanent hypoparathyroidism on both univariate and multivariate analysis, with total thyroidectomy with central node dissection being associated with the highest rates of hypoparathyroidism. The extent of surgery was still significant even when surgical technique and experience were variables that were controlled during analysis [21,22]. The type of dissection and surgeon's experience are important, though, in that studies have shown decreased rates of hypoparathyroidism with capsular dissection, as well as when the surgeries are performed by high-volume endocrine surgeons.

One of the difficulties of preserving parathyroid function is the inability to accurately assess the viability of a parathyroid gland during surgery, as patients do not need all four glands to maintain parathyroid function. One study looking at the rate of inadvertent parathyroidectomies during thyroid surgery found that the rate was higher in reoperations, 20%, compared with primary thyroid procedures, 7.71%, but none of these patients developed either transient or permanent hypoparathyroidism [23]. Other studies have shown that the loss of at least two parathyroid glands is necessary before the risk of transient and permanent hypoparathyroidism occurs [20]. Techniques to evaluate parathyroid viability, such as using a scalpel to cut and observe bleeding from the parathyroid capsule, although encouraging, have not been validated through studies. Much of the assessment regarding parathyroid viability relies on a surgeon's experience. Apart from preservation of parathyroid glands *in situ* on initial dissection, the alternative is to reimplant devitalized parathyroid tissue. Autotransplantation has been shown to, overall, reduce the incidence of permanent hypoparathyroidism. Although some studies have seen no protective effect of autotransplantion on rates of hypoparathyroidism, others have seen decreased rates of hypoparathyroidism in those patients that were autotransplanted [24–28]. Rates of transient hypoparathyroidism seem not to be influenced by autotransplantation, likely because it takes several weeks for the devitalized parathyroid gland to integrate into the tissue [19,27]. The recommendation is to perform autotransplantation of any parathyroid glands that are identified and concerned to be nonviable. Some studies have shown that the perioperative parathyroid hormone level can be a good predictor of whether patients will require postoperative calcium supplementation and which patients are at risk for developing permanent hypoparathyroidism [29,30].

OUTCOMES: NONTUMOR VARIABLES

Nonneoplastic and tumor variable affecting outcome are summarized in Table 18.2. As each patient is an individual with a unique combination of variables when he or she presents, it is important to understand the prognostic features that can help predict how aggressively his or her thyroid cancer may behave. These variables are comprised of both patient characteristics and characteristics of the tumors themselves. There are other variables that have also been studied, but they have not been shown to have any correlation with thyroid cancer, such as body mass index, tobacco use, and alcohol use [31,32].

Age

Age of diagnosis has been well established as being a powerful predictor of death from thyroid cancer, with fatality

Table 18.2 Nonneoplastic and tumor variables affecting patient outcomes

Nonneoplastic variables
- Age
- Gender
- Race
- Surgeon volume

Tumor variables
- Genetics
- Histology
- Tumor size
- Multifocality
- Extrathyroidal extension

rates rising increasingly after the age of 40–45 in papillary and follicular thyroid cancers [33,34]. These findings have been validated looking at multiple large population-based studies, including the National Cancer Data Base (53,856 cases of thyroid cancer over a 10-year period) and the Surveillance, Epidemiology, and End Results (SEER) study (15,698 thyroid cancer cases over an 18-year period) [35]. Thyroid cancer is the only malignancy where age is factored into the staging criteria. The specific association between age and prognosis has not yet been clarified. Explanations range from the role of immune system decline with age to association with menopause in women. Studies have shown that there is an increased likelihood of radioiodine-resistant disease with age, and this likely plays a role in increased mortality rates.

Children presenting with differentiated thyroid cancers generally present with more extensive disease and mirror presentations often seen in adults above the age of 60. The prevalence of distant metastases at diagnosis, most commonly in the lung, is 20%–30% vs. 2% in adults [36]. In addition, multifocal disease is also more prevalent and is seen in about 40% of childhood papillary thyroid cancer cases. Children undergoing operative procedures on the thyroid also have higher complication rates than adults who had similar procedures [37]. Although the disease is more extensive upon initial presentation, 30-year survival rates in long-term follow-up range from 90% to 99% with differentiated thyroid cancers. In addition, mortality rates in children are more favorable than in adults [36,38]. Within the early adulthood population, between 20 and 44 years of age, the likelihood of thyroid cancer recurrence is lower and the incidence of radioiodine-resistant thyroid disease is lower as well [35].

Age over 45 has been recognized to be a poor prognostic factor for thyroid cancer and has been implemented in the staging system, but age over 60 years has been associated with a particularly poor prognosis in differentiated thyroid cancer. The worse prognosis is associated with more advanced presentations of the disease with larger tumors and more incidence of extrathyroidal extension [39]. Characteristics of the tumors in the elderly are also different in that the tumors have more aggressive features, such as prevalence of follicular histology, vascular invasion, and extracapsular extension. In addition, the elderly likely have a delayed presentation due to less active surveillance and present only when symptoms consistent with thyroid cancer, such as dysphagia, dyspnea, and hoarseness, appear. Once diagnosed, studies show that elderly patients are less likely to receive aggressive surgery or radioactive iodine treatment than similarly staged younger patients. Not undergoing these procedures was associated with worse survival rates. The management in this older population needs to be better evaluated, as initial results show that when appropriate treatment is received, there is improvement in long-term survival. Other factors that must be taken into consideration are the general condition of the patient, the number of comorbidities accumulated over the years, and the increasing likelihood of non-cancer-related death with or without treatment [40]. Studies have already shown that thyroid surgery in the elderly, patients over the age of 65, is associated with a substantially longer hospital stay and overall higher hospital costs than surgery performed on younger patients.

Gender

Gender has been identified to be a strong prognostic indicator of thyroid cancer aggressiveness. Although the recent increase in thyroid cancer incidence has occurred predominantly in women by a ratio of 3.5:1, men tend to present with more advanced stages and more aggressive tumors, and the estimated deaths were only 1.3 times higher in woman than men [41,42]. This predilection for women is still unexplained, although studies have suggested an association with estrogen and its metabolites and thyroid cancer [43,44]. According to the SEER database, women are more likely to have cancers confined to the thyroid and less likely to have lymph node involvement. Men are more likely to present with tumors larger than 4 cm, tumors with aggressive histopathology, lymph node involvement, and distant metastases [41,42]. Age of diagnosis in men is about 20 years later than in women, and men have twice the frequency of metastases at the time of diagnosis [45]. Mortality was greater in men than in women, 7.1% versus 3.5%, in all subtypes [41]. The difference in mortality is attributed to the fact that men tend to present with more advanced thyroid malignancies. When the disease is confined to the thyroid, there did not appear to be any survival difference between genders [42].

Race

Recent studies have shown that there are significant differences in outcomes in patients of different races with thyroid cancer [46–48]. Racial minorities (blacks, Hispanics, and Asians) have been found to present with more advanced differentiated thyroid cancers than the Caucasian population. Inherent biological differences of tumors found in racial minorities have been hypothesized, but as of yet, no specific genetic differences have been identified to account for the difference in outcomes. More importantly, disparities in socioeconomic status, environmental impacts, and access to health care seem to account for much of the differences in outcomes. Those with lower socioeconomic status consistently present with more advanced disease than those with a higher socioeconomic status. The overall incidence of thyroid cancer has been increasing in the Caucasian population, but with generally smaller tumors than in the black population. This increased incidence has been partly attributed to the likely increased access to care in the population, leading to a higher incidence of disease, but at an earlier stage. Regardless of socioeconomic status, biological differences are likely present. Studies have shown that black populations present with more advanced disease, even when socioeconomic status has been accounted for, and have worse survival than any other racial group. Conversely, Asian-Pacific Islanders and Hispanic populations seem to have a survival advantage. Further studies are required in order to further risk-stratify populations based on race [46].

Surgeon volume

Patient outcomes are also dependent on the experience of the performing surgeon. Starting with the initial operation, a recent study looking at patients with differentiated thyroid cancer showed that experienced surgeons are more likely to perform the initial appropriate operation and have a more complete initial resection than surgeons who perform <30 thyroid operations a year [49]. Completion thyroidectomies performed by high-volume surgeons were found to have much lower radioactive iodine uptake than those by low-volume thyroid surgeons, and so the completeness of resection is dependent on surgeon volume [49,50]. Studies have also shown that surgeons who perform a high volume of thyroid surgeries, defined as greater than 100 cases per year, have fewer complications than surgeons with less volume [47,48,51,52]. One study found that the complication rate for high-volume surgeons was 5.1% vs. 6.1%–8.6% for lower-volume surgeons. High-volume surgeons are also more likely to operate for thyroid malignancies, as well as perform more complicated neck dissections. This difference in complication rates holds true across all age groups as well; studies within pediatric populations have shown better outcomes when thyroid surgeries are performed by high-volume surgeons [37]. Surgeon experience was also associated with a decreased length of hospital stay, as well as lower hospital charges per patient [47].

OUTCOMES: TUMOR VARIABLES

Genetics

About 25% of medullary thyroid cancers are hereditary. The genetics of medullary thyroid cancers have been better characterized thus far and can present as a component of multiple endocrine neoplasia (MEN) type 2 or as a separate entity, familial medullary thyroid cancer. It is an aggressive cancer and is the leading cause of death in MEN 2A patients. Medullary thyroid cancer metastasizes early in its clinical course and is a difficult disease to manage, as it is resistant to both chemo- and radiotherapy. Hereditary medullary cancer is distinguished by a germline mutation in the *RET* proto-oncogene. This activating mutation is transmitted in an autosomal dominant fashion and predisposes these family members to C-cell hyperplasia at a very early age. The prognosis for these patients is dependent on the presence and spread of the medullary thyroid cancer and early diagnosis, and prophylactic thyroidectomy is recommended. As genetic testing becomes more advanced and specific *RET* mutations are becoming better characterized, the specific timeline of when to perform the thyroidectomy is becoming less clear. For example, *RET* mutations at codons 634 and 918 are associated with extremely early onset of disease, as early as 17 months of age [53]. *RET* mutations at codon 609 have been associated with a later onset of medullary thyroid cancer, with the youngest age of onset at 21, in a 38-member family tree [54]. Although the timeline of when to perform prophylactic thyroidectomy needs to be better elucidated for the specific *RET* mutation variants, it is paramount to understand that the patient's prognosis is dependent on the removal of the thyroid gland prior to disease metastasis.

Approximately 5% of nonmedullary thyroid cancers are hereditary in nature. These thyroid tumors can present as part of a larger hereditary cancer syndrome (familial adenomatous polyposis, Gardner's syndrome, Cowden's disease, Werner's syndrome, Carney's complex, and papillary renal neoplasia), and a subset of hereditary nonmedullary cancers have been identified in the population. This subset, named familial nonmedullary thyroid cancer (FNMTC), is defined as the presence of well-differentiated thyroid cancer in two or more first-degree relatives in the absence of other hereditary syndromes or environmental causes. The susceptibility gene for FNMTC has not been identified [55]. Families with these hereditary nonmedullary cancer syndromes have been advised to undergo more aggressive management of their thyroid disease, as studies have shown that it is associated with higher rates of multicentric tumors, higher rates of lymph node involvement, higher rates of extrathyroidal invasion, and shorter disease-free survival when compared with sporadic disease. One study identified 14 patients with FNMTC and found that the disease was multifocal in 93% and bilateral in 43%, compared with 20%–32% and 19% in the sporadic group. Another series identified the age of onset as being approximately 10 years earlier than sporadic cases, as well as having a higher likelihood of recurrence. Overall disease-free survival seemed to be worse in families that had more than three family members affected. Families with two or less members affected, though, had overall life expectancies similar to those of their unaffected family members. In addition, patients did worse when the hereditary nature of the cancer

had not been identified, implying that early treatment can improve survival [56].

More recently, the genetic landscape of papillary thyroid cancer was made clearer by the efforts of the Cancer Genome Atlas launched by the National Institutes of Health. The institute looked at almost 500 cases of papillary thyroid cancer and found a genetic lesion in more than 96% of the tumors. The most frequent mutations were in *BRAF* (~60%) and *RAS* (~13%). From these results, two subtypes of papillary thyroid cancer were able to be discerned. The papillary tumors that had a *BRAF*-type expression pattern had increased heterogeneity, more likely to be of the tall cell variant, and were less differentiated, whereas tumors that had a *RAS*-type expression pattern were well differentiated with a low likelihood of recurrence [57]. Although further investigation is required, it is easy to see how genetic investigations will continue to further modify our treatment approach to thyroid cancers in the future.

Histology

Almost 90% of thyroid cancers consist of well-differentiated variants of two histological subtypes, papillary and follicular thyroid cancers. In general, stage for stage, prognosis between the two is relatively similar. In both types, Stage I and Stage II disease is associated with a near 100% 5-year survival rate [58]. More than 80% of these cancers have a 20-year cause-specific mortality rate of <1% [59]. Of the remaining 20%, different subtypes within papillary and follicular types lead to worse prognosis. Within the papillary type, tall cell variant, columnar cell variant, and diffuse sclerosing variant are subtypes that are considered to be more aggressive histologies. Within the follicular type, subtypes include trabecular, insular, and solid tumors. These subtypes of follicular and papillary tumors are classified as being poorly differentiated thyroid cancers that are separate from anaplastic thyroid cancer. Their clinical behavior is intermediate between well-differentiated papillary or follicular tumors and anaplastic tumors [60]. Hürthle cell cancer is a separate variant of follicular cancer and also has a worse prognosis than well-differentiated follicular cancer. Hürthle cell carcinoma is associated with 5- and 10-year survival rates of 45%–96% and 45%–80%, respectively, whereas well-differentiated follicular thyroid cancer has survival rates from 82% to 92% and 67% to 90% [61]. Anaplastic thyroid cancer is the least common but most lethal thyroid cancer. It is thought to progress from existing papillary or follicular thyroid cancer. Patients have a median survival of 3–5 months primarily from local tumor invasion and tracheal compression [62].

A separate entity, derived from C-cells, is medullary thyroid cancer. The overall 10-year survival rate of patients with medullary cancer is about 80%. There appears to be no survival difference between hereditary or sporadic types of medullary cancer. Medullary thyroid cancer outcomes are overall worse when compared with well-differentiated papillary and follicular types once the tumor has spread, as the medullary cancer is not a candidate for radioactive iodine treatment [63].

Tumor size, multifocality, extrathyroidal extension, and lymph node invasion

Primary tumor size of well-differentiated papillary and follicular thyroid cancers has been associated with increased recurrence and mortality rates. One study following more than 1300 patients over a median of 15 years had zero deaths over that time period in treated patients with non-metastatic tumors less than 1.5 cm in size. The number of deaths increased incrementally as tumor size increased. One study calculated that a tumor size of more than 3 cm increased the risk of death nearly sixfold [33]. All the various prognostic scoring systems take size into account when risk-stratifying patients.

Papillary thyroid tumors have a propensity to present as multifocal tumors. Two separate theories to explain the multiple foci of tumors are that [1] these foci are independent tumors or [2] they are intrathyroidal metastases from the same original tumor. Either theory indicates an aggressive behavior of papillary thyroid cancer. Studies have shown that an increased number of tumor foci correlated with increased incidence of extrathyroidal extension, lymph node metastases, and the greatest risk of recurrence [64,65]. Extrathyroidal extension of papillary tumors is another finding with unclear significance. One study found that extrathyroidal extension was predictive of extranodal extension, which purports a worse prognosis [66]. Other studies have not seen any difference in survival when comparing tumors with extrathyroidal extension with those tumors without extension, although they have been significantly associated with larger tumors [67,68]. Types of lymph node invasion in medullary and papillary cancer are also being delineated, as more recent studies have shown that prognosis is different in patients with microscopic lymph node disease than that in patients with large-volume nodal metastases and extranodal extension. The recurrence rate for patients with less than five positive nodes was 4%, compared with patients with more than five positive nodes, 19% [69].

CONCLUSION

Thyroid surgery has evolved considerably over the years, with more recent changes involving the incorporation of new technologies, such as the nerve stimulator and ultrasonic shears. Improved techniques have reduced the risk of complications to the recurrent laryngeal nerves and parathyroid glands, as well as decreasing operative times and costs. Experience is very important, as studies have shown that the rate of complications is lowest in the hands of a high-volume thyroid surgeon. Finally, overall outcomes of thyroid cancer are very good, depending on the patient and tumor profile. Future therapies will be guided by all the current work being performed on understanding the genetics behind thyroid cancer.

REFERENCES

1. Callender GG, Carling T, Christison-Lagay E, Udelsman R. Surgery for thyroid cancer. *Endocrinol Metab Clin North Am* 2014;43(2):443–58.
2. Siperstein AE, Berber E, Morkoyun E. The use of the harmonic scalpel vs conventional knot tying for vessel ligation in thyroid surgery. *Arch Surg* 2002;137(2):137–42.
3. Amit M, Binenbaum Y, Cohen JT, Gil Z. Effectiveness of an oxidized cellulose patch hemostatic agent in thyroid surgery: A prospective, randomized, controlled study. *J Am Coll Surg* 2013;217(2):221–5.
4. Delbridge L. Total thyroidectomy: The evolution of surgical technique. *ANZ J Surg* 2003;73(9):761–8.
5. Bliss RD, Gauger PG, Delbridge LW. Surgeon's approach to the thyroid gland: Surgical anatomy and the importance of technique. *World J Surg* 2000;24(8):891–7.
6. Hayward NJ, Grodski S, Yeung M, Johnson WR, Serpell J. Recurrent laryngeal nerve injury in thyroid surgery: A review. *ANZ J Surg* 2013;83(1–2):15–21.
7. Pisanu A, Porceddu G, Podda M, Cois A, Uccheddu A. Systematic review with meta-analysis of studies comparing intraoperative neuromonitoring of recurrent laryngeal nerves versus visualization alone during thyroidectomy. *J Surg Res* 2014;188(1):152–61.
8. Lo CY, Kwok KF, Yuen PW. A prospective evaluation of recurrent laryngeal nerve paralysis during thyroidectomy. *Arch Surg* 2000;135(2):204–7.
9. Dralle H, Sekulla C, Haerting J et al. Risk factors of paralysis and functional outcome after recurrent laryngeal nerve monitoring in thyroid surgery. *Surgery* 2004;136(6):1310–22.
10. Dralle H, Sekulla C, Lorenz K, Brauckhoff M, Machens A, German ISG. Intraoperative monitoring of the recurrent laryngeal nerve in thyroid surgery. *World J Surg* 2008;32(7):1358–66.
11. Horne SK, Gal TJ, Brennan JA. Prevalence and patterns of intraoperative nerve monitoring for thyroidectomy. *Otolaryngol Head Neck Surg* 2007;136(6):952–6.
12. Barczynski M, Randolph GW, Cernea CR et al. External branch of the superior laryngeal nerve monitoring during thyroid and parathyroid surgery: International Neural Monitoring Study Group standards guideline statement. *Laryngoscope* 2013;123(Suppl 4):S1–14.
13. Lennquist S, Cahlin C, Smeds S. The superior laryngeal nerve in thyroid surgery. *Surgery* 1987;102(6):999–1008.
14. Inabnet WB, Murry T, Dhiman S, Aviv J, Lifante JC. Neuromonitoring of the external branch of the superior laryngeal nerve during minimally invasive thyroid surgery under local anesthesia: A prospective study of 10 patients. *Laryngoscope* 2009;119(3):597–601.

15. Barczynski M, Konturek A, Stopa M, Honowska A, Nowak W. Randomized controlled trial of visualization versus neuromonitoring of the external branch of the superior laryngeal nerve during thyroidectomy. *World J Surg* 2012;36(6):1340–7.

16. Glover AR, Norlen O, Gundara JS, Morris M, Sidhu SB. Use of the nerve integrity monitor during thyroid surgery aids identification of the external branch of the superior laryngeal nerve. *Ann Surg Oncol* 2015;22(6):1768–73.

17. Lombardi CP, Raffaelli M, D'Alatri L et al. Voice and swallowing changes after thyroidectomy in patients without inferior laryngeal nerve injuries. *Surgery* 2006;140(6):1026–32; discussion 1032–4.

18. Soylu L, Ozbas S, Uslu HY, Kocak S. The evaluation of the causes of subjective voice disturbances after thyroid surgery. *Am J Surg* 2007;194(3):317–22.

19. Lo CY. Parathyroid autotransplantation during thyroidectomy. *ANZ J Surg* 2002;72(12):902–7.

20. Thomusch O, Machens A, Sekulla C, Ukkat J, Brauckhoff M, Dralle H. The impact of surgical technique on postoperative hypoparathyroidism in bilateral thyroid surgery: A multivariate analysis of 5846 consecutive patients. *Surgery* 2003;133(2):180–5.

21. Cavicchi O, Piccin O, Caliceti U, De Cataldis A, Pasquali R, Ceroni AR. Transient hypoparathyroidism following thyroidectomy: A prospective study and multivariate analysis of 604 consecutive patients. *Otolaryngol Head Neck Surg* 2007;137(4):654–8.

22. Monacelli M, Lucchini R, Polistena A et al. Total thyroidectomy and central lymph node dissection. Experience of a referral centre for endocrine surgery. *G Chir* 2014;35(5–6):117–21.

23. Lin DT, Patel SG, Shaha AR, Singh B, Shah JP. Incidence of inadvertent parathyroid removal during thyroidectomy. *Laryngoscope* 2002;112(4):608–11.

24. Page C, Strunski V. Parathyroid risk in total thyroidectomy for bilateral, benign, multinodular goitre: Report of 351 surgical cases. *J Laryngol Otol* 2007;121(3):237–41.

25. Almquist M, Hallgrimsson P, Nordenstrom E, Bergenfelz A. Prediction of permanent hypoparathyroidism after total thyroidectomy. *World J Surg* 2014;38(10):2613–20.

26. Wei T, Li Z, Jin J et al. Autotransplantation of inferior parathyroid glands during central neck dissection for papillary thyroid carcinoma: A retrospective cohort study. *Int J Surg* 2014;12(12):1286–90.

27. Testini M, Rosato L, Avenia N et al. The impact of single parathyroid gland autotransplantation during thyroid surgery on postoperative hypoparathyroidism: A multicenter study. *Transpl Proc* 2007;39(1):225–30.

28. Karakas E, Osei-Agyemang T, Schlosser K et al. The impact of parathyroid gland autotransplantation during bilateral thyroid surgery for Graves' disease on postoperative hypocalcaemia. *Endocr Reg* 2008;42(2–3):39–44.

29. Quiros RM, Pesce CE, Wilhelm SM, Djuricin G, Prinz RA. Intraoperative parathyroid hormone levels in thyroid surgery are predictive of postoperative hypoparathyroidism and need for vitamin D supplementation. *Am J Surg* 2005;189(3):306–9.

30. Barczynski M, Cichon S, Konturek A, Cichon W. Applicability of intraoperative parathyroid hormone assay during total thyroidectomy as a guide for the surgeon to selective parathyroid tissue autotransplantation. *World J Surg* 2008;32(5):822–8.

31. Stansifer KJ, Guynan JF, Wachal BM, Smith RB. Modifiable risk factors and thyroid cancer. *Otolaryngol Head Neck Surg* 2015;152(3):432–7.

32. Kwon H, Kim M, Choi YM et al. Lack of associations between body mass index and clinical outcomes in patients with papillary thyroid carcinoma. *Endocrinol Metab* 2015;30(3):305–11.

33. Mazzaferri EL, Jhiang SM. Long-term impact of initial surgical and medical therapy on papillary and follicular thyroid cancer. *Am J Med* 1994;97(5):418–28.

34. Simpson WJ, McKinney SE, Carruthers JS, Gospodarowicz MK, Sutcliffe SB, Panzarella T. Papillary and follicular thyroid cancer. Prognostic factors in 1,578 patients. *Am J Med* 1987;83(3):479–88.

35. Haymart MR. Understanding the relationship between age and thyroid cancer. *Oncologist* 2009;14(3):216–21.

36. Rivkees SA, Mazzaferri EL, Verburg FA et al. The treatment of differentiated thyroid cancer in children: Emphasis on surgical approach and radioactive iodine therapy. *Endocr Rev* 2011;32(6):798–826.

37. Wang TS, Roman SA, Sosa JA. Predictors of outcomes following pediatric thyroid and parathyroid surgery. *Curr Opin Oncol* 2009;21(1):23–8.

38. O'Gorman CS, Hamilton J, Rachmiel M, Gupta A, Ngan BY, Daneman D. Thyroid cancer in childhood: A retrospective review of childhood course. *Thyroid* 2010;20(4):375–80.

39. Garg A, Chopra S, Ballal S, Soundararajan R, Bal CS. Differentiated thyroid cancer in patients over 60 years of age at presentation: A retrospective study of 438 patients. *J Geriatr Oncol* 2015;6(1):29–37.

40. Park HS, Roman SA, Sosa JA. Treatment patterns of aging Americans with differentiated thyroid cancer. *Cancer* 2010;116(1):20–30.

41. Mitchell I, Livingston EH, Chang AY et al. Trends in thyroid cancer demographics and surgical therapy in the United States. *Surgery* 2007;142(6):823–8; discussion 828 e821.

42. Nilubol N, Zhang L, Kebebew E. Multivariate analysis of the relationship between male sex, disease-specific survival, and features of tumor aggressiveness in thyroid cancer of follicular cell origin. *Thyroid* 2013;23(6):695–702.

43. Lee ML, Chen GG, Vlantis AC, Tse GM, Leung BC, van Hasselt CA. Induction of thyroid papillary carcinoma cell proliferation by estrogen is associated with an altered expression of Bcl-xL. *Cancer J* 2005;11(2):113–21.

44. Libutti SK. Understanding the role of gender in the incidence of thyroid cancer. *Cancer J* 2005;11(2):104–5.
45. Amdur RJ, Mazzaferri EL. *Essentials of Thyroid Cancer Management*. New York: Springer, 2005.
46. Harari A, Li N, Yeh MW. Racial and socioeconomic disparities in presentation and outcomes of well-differentiated thyroid cancer. *J Clin Endocrinol Metab* 2014;99(1):133–41.
47. Noureldine SI, Abbas A, Tufano RP et al. The impact of surgical volume on racial disparity in thyroid and parathyroid surgery. *Ann Surg Oncol* 2014;21(8):2733–9.
48. Hauch A, Al-Qurayshi Z, Friedlander P, Kandil E. Association of socioeconomic status, race, and ethnicity with outcomes of patients undergoing thyroid surgery. *JAMA Otolaryngol Head Neck Surg* 2014;140(12):1173–83.
49. Adkisson CD, Howell GM, McCoy KL et al. Surgeon volume and adequacy of thyroidectomy for differentiated thyroid cancer. *Surgery* 2014;156(6):1453–60.
50. Oltmann SC, Schneider DF, Leverson G, Sivashanmugam T, Chen H, Sippel RS. Radioactive iodine remnant uptake after completion thyroidectomy: Not such a complete cancer operation. *Ann Surg Oncol* 2014;21(4):1379–83.
51. Hauch A, Al-Qurayshi Z, Randolph G, Kandil E. Total thyroidectomy is associated with increased risk of complications for low- and high-volume surgeons. *Ann Surg Oncol* 2014;21(12):3844–52.
52. Sosa JA, Bowman HM, Tielsch JM, Powe NR, Gordon TA, Udelsman R. The importance of surgeon experience for clinical and economic outcomes from thyroidectomy. *Ann Surg* 1998;228(3):320–30.
53. Moore SW, Appfelstaedt J, Zaahl MG. Familial medullary carcinoma prevention, risk evaluation, and RET in children of families with MEN2. *J Pediatr Surg* 2007;42(2):326–32.
54. Calva D, O'Dorisio TM, Sue O'Dorisio M et al. When is prophylactic thyroidectomy indicated for patients with the RET codon 609 mutation? *Ann Surg Oncol* 2009;16(8):2237–44.
55. Vriens MR, Suh I, Moses W, Kebebew E. Clinical features and genetic predisposition to hereditary nonmedullary thyroid cancer. *Thyroid* 2009;19(12):1343–9.
56. Sippel RS, Caron NR, Clark OH. An evidence-based approach to familial nonmedullary thyroid cancer: Screening, clinical management, and follow-up. *World J Surg* 2007;31(5):924–33.
57. Santoro M, Melillo RM. Genetics: The genomic landscape of papillary thyroid carcinoma. *Nat Rev Endocrinol* 2015;11(3):133–4.
58. American Thyroid Association Guidelines Taskforce on Thyroid N, Differentiated Thyroid C, Cooper DS, Doherty GM et al. Revised American Thyroid Association management guidelines for patients with thyroid nodules and differentiated thyroid cancer. *Thyroid* 2009;19(11):1167–14.
59. Iyer NG, Shaha AR. Management of thyroid nodules and surgery for differentiated thyroid cancer. *Clin Oncol* 2010;22(6):405–12.
60. Volante M, Landolfi S, Chiusa L et al. Poorly differentiated carcinomas of the thyroid with trabecular, insular, and solid patterns: A clinicopathologic study of 183 patients. *Cancer* 2004;100(5):950–7.
61. Phitayakorn R, McHenry CR. Follicular and Hurthle cell carcinoma of the thyroid gland. *Surg Oncol Clin N Am* 2006;15(3):603–23.
62. Chiacchio S, Lorenzoni A, Boni G, Rubello D, Elisei R, Mariani G. Anaplastic thyroid cancer: Prevalence, diagnosis and treatment. *Minerva Endocrinol* 2008;33(4):341–57.
63. You YN, Lakhani V, Wells SA Jr, Moley JF. Medullary thyroid cancer. *Surg Oncol Clin N Am* 2006;15(3):639–60.
64. Qu N, Zhang L, Ji QH et al. Number of tumor foci predicts prognosis in papillary thyroid cancer. *BMC Cancer* 2014;14:914.
65. Kim HJ, Sohn SY, Jang HW, Kim SW, Chung JH. Multifocality, but not bilaterality, is a predictor of disease recurrence/persistence of papillary thyroid carcinoma. *World J Surg* 2013;37(2):376–84.
66. Clain JB, Scherl S, Dos Reis L et al. Extrathyroidal extension predicts extranodal extension in patients with positive lymph nodes: An important association that may affect clinical management. *Thyroid* 2014;24(6):951–7.
67. Ahn D, Sohn JH, Jeon JH, Jeong JY. Clinical impact of microscopic extrathyroidal extension in patients with papillary thyroid microcarcinoma treated with hemithyroidectomy. *J Endocrinol Invest* 2014;37(2):167–73.
68. Moon HJ, Kim EK, Chung WY, Yoon JH, Kwak JY. Minimal extrathyroidal extension in patients with papillary thyroid microcarcinoma: Is it a real prognostic factor? *Ann Surg Oncol* 2011;18(7):1916–23.
69. Randolph GW, Duh QY, Heller KS et al. The prognostic significance of nodal metastases from papillary thyroid carcinoma can be stratified based on the size and number of metastatic lymph nodes, as well as the presence of extranodal extension. *Thyroid* 2012;22(11):1144–52.

Parathyroids

19

Presentation of primary hyperparathyroidism

SHONNI J. SILVERBERG AND ANGELA L. CARRELLI

INTRODUCTION

Primary hyperparathyroidism (PHPT) is defined as hypercalcemia in the setting of a normal or elevated parathyroid hormone (PTH) level. PHPT is caused by excess PTH secretion from one or more of the parathyroid glands. It is estimated to affect as many as 1 in 500 to 1 in 1000 people [1].

The presentation of PHPT has evolved over the past 40 years, with new phenotypes of the disease increasingly recognized after the development of the multichannel biochemistry autoanalyzer in the 1960s. With this advance, serum calcium was included on routine laboratory testing, allowing for the detection of hypercalcemia in asymptomatic patients. Prior to the 1970s, patients with PHPT typically presented only after developing symptomatic disease. The symptoms of classical PHPT, often referred to as "bones, stones, and groans," included a specific bone disease known as osteitis fibrosa cystica, nephrolithiasis, and neuromuscular complaints. Today, these classic symptoms are uncommon. Osteitis fibrosa cystica is characterized radiologically by distal tapering of the clavicles, a "salt and pepper" appearance of the skull, brown tumors, and subperiosteal resorption of the distal phalanges [1]. In the United States, this skeletal disorder now affects less than 2% of patients with PHPT [2]. Similarly, nephrolithiasis previously affected about 50% of patients with PHPT, while today only about 15%–20% of patients have known stone disease [2]. Lastly, classic PHPT was associated with a characteristic neuromuscular syndrome that included symmetric

proximal muscle weakness and type 2 muscle fiber atrophy [2]. These symptoms would resolve following successful parathyroidectomy. This neuromuscular syndrome is rarely seen in modern-day PHPT [2].

TYPICAL PRESENT-DAY PRESENTATION AND EPIDEMIOLOGY

As mentioned above, approximately 15%–20% of patients in the United States today present with nephrolithiasis, while other symptoms of classical PHPT are rare. The most common presentation of PHPT in the United States today is described as "asymptomatic" PHPT [3]. Asymptomatic PHPT is defined as PHPT without the classic symptoms associated with hypercalcemia or PTH excess [4]. Most patients are diagnosed after they are noted to have mild hypercalcemia on routine labs. Women are more commonly affected than men, with a ratio of 3:1. The typical age at presentation is 50–60 years old, although PHPT can present at any age [2].

The incidence of PHPT appears to have changed over the past several decades. Epidemiologic studies from Rochester, Minnesota, found a significant increase in the incidence of PHPT in the early 1970s, which coincided with the use of the multichannel biochemistry autoanalyzer [5]. There was a subsequent decline in incidence from the 1980s through 2001 in the Rochester population. However, a recent epidemiologic study of a racially diverse population in Southern California found that the prevalence of PHPT tripled from

1995 to 2010, rising from 76 to 233 per 100,000 women and from 30 to 85 per 100,000 men [6]. This study also found differences in the incidence of PHPT based on race. The highest incidence of PHPT was found among blacks, followed by whites, with lower rates among Asians, Hispanics, and other races. In addition, incidence of PHPT in this population increased with age, rising from 12–24 per 100,000 in men and women younger than 50 years old up to 196 and 95 per 100,000 for women and men aged 70–79 years old, respectively [6].

PHYSICAL EXAM, BIOCHEMICAL AND IMAGING FEATURES OF PHPT

In patients with asymptomatic PHPT, the serum calcium is typically within 1 mg/dL of the upper limit of normal. PTH levels are either elevated or inappropriately normal. PTH may be measured either by second-generation assay, which measures whole PTH and retained carboxy-terminal fragments, or by the newer third-generation assays, which measure only the entire PTH 1-84 molecule. Current data do not support an advantage of one over another in the diagnosis of the disease, except in renal failure, in which retained fragments lead to an overestimation of PTH values using the second-generation PTH immunoradiometric assays [7]. Other lab findings may include low serum phosphorus, although the vast majority of patients have phosphorus levels that are within the lower end of the normal range. Hypercalciuria is relatively common: one-third of patients have hypercalciuria (defined as >250 mg/day for women and >300 mg/day for men) [1]. The creatinine clearance is usually normal. If a decline in creatinine clearance is noted, other causes would need to be ruled out prior to attributing this to PHPT [1]. Low vitamin D levels appear to be more common in PHPT than in the general population [8]. A study of 289 patients with PHPT found that 33% of subjects with PHPT had profound vitamin D deficiency (25-hydroxyvitamin D < 10 ng/mL) versus only 20% of control subjects. Similarly, 81% of PHPT subjects were vitamin D deficient (25-hydroxyvitamin D < 20 ng/mL), compared with only 60% of control subjects [8]. 1,25-Dihydroxyvitamin D levels are usually in the upper end of the normal range, with about one-third of patients having frankly elevated 1,25-dihdroxyvitamin D levels [2]. This pattern in vitamin D metabolites reflects the action of the excess PTH on the renal 1-alpha-hydroxylase enzyme, which converts 25-hydroxyvitamin D to 1,25-dihydroxyvitamin D.

The physical exam in patients with asymptomatic PHPT is generally normal. The enlarged parathyroid gland(s) are virtually never palpable on physical exam, except in patients with parathyroid cancer. Other physical findings seen in the past, such as band keratopathy, are mainly of historical interest.

Although osteitis fibrosa cystica is rarely seen today in the United States, the skeleton does remain a target organ in PHPT. The rate of fractures appears to be increased in modern-day PHPT [9,10]. For example, in a case–control

study of 150 patients with PHPT, there was an increased prevalence of vertebral fractures in patients with PHPT (37 out of 150 [24.6%] PHPT patients versus 12 out of 300 [4.0%] controls, $p < 0.0001$) [9]. In addition, a large cohort study of around 400 PHPT patients found an increased risk of vertebral, wrist, rib, and pelvic fractures [10].

In the absence of fracture, the bone disease associated with modern-day PHPT is not evident on plain X-ray, and instead is only detected on higher-order imaging. Using dual X-ray absorptiometry (DXA), the characteristic findings are relatively preserved bone mineral density (BMD) at trabecular sites, like the spine, and low BMD at cortical sites, in particular the distal one-third radius. These findings are due to the preferential catabolic action of PTH in cortical bone [11]. The preservation of bone at the spine on DXA imaging is discordant with the finding of increased vertebral fracture incidence. Evolving thought suggests that DXA may not be the best modality of assessing trabecular bone involvement in PHPT. Indeed, on high-resolution peripheral quantitative computed tomography (HRpQCT), an imaging technique that is able to resolve cortical and trabecular elements of bone, there is evidence of trabecular deficiencies, as well as cortical abnormalities, in PHPT (Figure 19.1) [3,12,13]. Data that similarly show trabecular abnormalities in PHPT are found using trabecular bone score analysis of lumbar spine DXA images [14]. Thus, we are coming to view mild PHPT as a disorder that has broad effects on the skeleton. Since vertebral fractures may not be obvious clinically, the new 2014 International Consensus Workshop Guidelines suggest that all patients with PHPT have vertebral imaging (X-ray or vertebral fracture assessment on DXA) to assess for compression fractures, and that those who have a fracture so documented be sent for surgery.

In asymptomatic PHPT, the kidney remains the organ most frequently affected by overt complications, primarily nephrolithiasis and nephrocalcinosis [3]. The presence of asymptomatic nephrolithiasis or nephrocalcinosis can be detected on renal imaging. The 2014 guidelines on the management of asymptomatic PHPT recommend routine renal imaging in patients at the time of presentation to evaluate for these potential complications (see the "Current Guidelines for Surgery" section) [3]. Data on the prevalence of subclinical nephrolithiasis or nephrocalcinosis in modern-day asymptomatic PHPT are limited. One retrospective

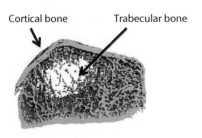

Cortical bone   Trabecular bone

Figure 19.1 HRpQCT images of the radius can distinguish between cortical and trabecular bone, and in PHPT shows evidence of trabecular bone loss.

chart review of asymptomatic patients with surgically proven PHPT reported a 7% prevalence of occult nephrolithiasis on renal imaging. This was significantly higher than the 1.6% prevalence of occult nephrolithiasis found in an age-matched control group having ultrasounds for other reasons [15]. There are no data on the incidence of nephrocalcinosis in PHPT, as no systematic studies assessing this end point have been reported.

NONCLASSICAL MANIFESTATIONS OF PHPT

It should be noted that the term *asymptomatic primary hyperparathyroidism* used today is to some extent controversial [16]. Much research has focused on whether these patients are truly asymptomatic. Nonclassical symptoms, in particular subclinical cardiovascular and neurocognitive disease, continue to undergo study and characterization.

Neuropsychological symptoms, quality of life, and cognition

Many patients with mild PHPT have neuropsychological and cognitive symptoms, including decreased concentration, depression and anxiety, fatigue, and weakness [16]. While the causal link between subtle neurocognitive symptoms and PHPT is not clear, both hypercalcemia and increased PTH levels have been proposed to be etiologic. Observational studies support a higher incidence of psychiatric complaints, predominantly depression and anxiety, in patients with PHPT [17–20]. In just one example, a case-control study investigating the prevalence of depression in PHPT found that clinically significant scores on depression questionnaire assessments were twice as common in patients with PHPT than in the control group of patients with surgical thyroid disease (31.4% vs. 15.3%, respectively, $p = 0.004$) [17]. Improvement in depression scores was greater in the PHPT patients who underwent parathyroidectomy in comparison to those not operated upon, and those in the thyroid surgery group.

Many studies have focused on quality of life symptoms among patients with PHPT. A specific measure of quality of life has been developed for patients with PHPT [21,22]. This questionnaire evaluates 13 nonspecific symptoms often reported in patients with PHPT, including feeling tired easily, being forgetful, and feeling weak. Based on the results, patients are given a parathyroidectomy assessment of symptoms (PAS) score, with a higher score indicating a patient is more symptomatic. Studies have shown improvement in PAS scores following successful parathyroidectomy [21,22]. Improvement in PAS score was not seen in a comparison group of patients undergoing surgery for nontoxic thyroid disease, suggesting that this score is specific to the symptomatology that may be seen in PHPT [21]. However, whether the enrolled PHPT patients met criteria for surgery, and would therefore be considered symptomatic, was not reported.

Although there are many observational studies reporting on neuropsychological manifestations of PHPT, high-level evidence from randomized controlled trials is available from only three studies of surgery vs. observation in mild PHPT. All used the same test vehicle, the well-validated SF-36, to measure quality of life, although some of the trials used additional investigative tools. In the first trial, 53 patients with mild PHPT were randomized to monitoring or parathyroidectomy [23]. It should be noted that only 19% of the eligible patients identified were enrolled in this study. At baseline, the quality of life in patients with mild PHPT was found to be similar to that reported in patients without PHPT. Patients who underwent parathyroidectomy had a statistically significant benefit compared with those monitored without surgery, in two of the nine quality of life domains assessed (social function and emotional problem). The psychological assessments revealed an improvement in two of the nine dimensions (anxiety and phobia) for patients undergoing surgery compared with those in the observation group. In a larger study, involving 191 patients with mild PHPT randomized to surgery or monitoring, patients with PHPT had significantly lower quality of life scores and more psychological symptoms at baseline compared with age- and sex-matched healthy controls [24]. However, no improvement was seen in these symptoms following parathyroidectomy compared with continued nonsurgical monitoring. In the third trial, 50 patients with mild PHPT were studied for 1 year following randomization to parathyroidectomy or observation [25]. At baseline, the quality of life and psychological scores were only minimally different compared with healthy controls. A significant difference in four quality of life measures was seen in the subjects who underwent parathyroidectomy compared with those monitored without surgery. Improvement was seen in bodily pain, general health, vitality, and mental health. Thus, all three randomized controlled trials demonstrated abnormalities in quality of life at baseline or improved quality of life after surgical cure. However, the data regarding specific quality of life and psychological symptom improvement in PHPT are conflicting, and the reversibility with parathyroidectomy is unpredictable if one looks across the three trials.

Studies have also addressed the effects of PHPT on cognitive function. Walker et al. conducted a case–control study involving 39 women with mild PHPT and 89 controls [18]. At baseline, patients with PHPT had lower scores on tests for verbal memory and nonverbal abstraction. Improvement was seen in nonverbal abstraction and some components of verbal memory following parathyroidectomy, so that they were indistinguishable from control values. However, the abnormalities and the improvement in these cognitive measures were not linearly associated with serum calcium or PTH levels. While several observational studies suggest an impact of PHPT on cognition, only one randomized controlled trial has addressed this issue [18,26–28]. Perrier et al. conducted a trial of 18 patients with asymptomatic PHPT randomized to surgery or observation [27]. Sleep and brain function were assessed using functional MRI at baseline,

6 weeks, and 6 months. While daytime sleepiness improved at 6 weeks in patients undergoing parathyroidectomy, no difference was seen at 6 months. In addition, no differences between groups over time were seen in neuropsychological testing results.

In summary, although patients with mild PHPT often have neuropsychological complaints, at this time specific workup for possible neurocognitive abnormalities is not recommended. In addition, after review of current data at the Fourth International Workshop on Asymptomatic Primary Hyperparathyroidism, it was concluded that the presence of these complaints should not constitute a stand-alone criterion for parathyroidectomy, given the lack of predictable improvement after surgery. This may change as more information is learned about the possible subclinical manifestations of asymptomatic PHPT [3].

Cardiovascular

PHPT was previously associated with increased mortality, in particular from cardiovascular causes [29,30]. However, the subjects described in these studies primarily had moderate to severe PHPT. The association between PHPT and increased mortality is not typically seen in current studies, likely reflecting the milder PHPT seen today. For example, in a large analysis of Swedish patients from 1965 to 1997, an increased risk of mortality, in particular from cardiovascular disease, was seen [31]. However, when only more recent cases were analyzed [1985–1997], no increase in mortality was seen. It is likely these patients had a milder form of PHPT. Similarly, in a study from Rochester, Minnesota, in 1998, overall survival was unchanged in patients with PHPT [32]. When compared with age- and gender-adjusted controls, the relative risk of death in patients with mild PHPT was 0.69 (95% confidence interval 0.57–0.83) [32]. One recent study from Scotland did find an increase in all-cause and cardiovascular mortality in mild PHPT, but based on the reported inclusion criteria used to identify PHPT, patients with other etiologies of hypercalcemia may have been included [33].

Hypertension (HTN) has often been associated with PHPT [34–36]. No direct link between PHPT and HTN has been identified. Some older observational studies, which describe patients with moderate to severe PHPT, suggested reversibility of HTN with parathyroidectomy, although this was not seen in all studies [34–36]. In modern-day PHPT, HTN does not appear to be reversed by parathyroidectomy. The one randomized controlled trial investigating this issue found no difference in blood pressure following parathyroidectomy or nonoperative observation [37]. One hundred sixteen patients with mild PHPT were randomized to observation or surgery and then followed for 2 years. No between-group differences in blood pressure were seen during this time. Overall, it does not appear that HTN is associated with modern-day PHPT, and surgery is not associated with the reversibility of HTN. Given the available data, the presence of HTN is not considered an indication

for parathyroidectomy. It should be noted that HTN may be associated with PHPT in the setting of MEN2A, when a pheochromocytoma is present (see the "Genetic Syndromes" section).

More recent research has focused on possible subclinical manifestations of PHPT, including valvular calcifications, left ventricular hypertrophy, carotid atherosclerosis, and vascular function [38–45]. However, there are limited data on subclinical manifestations in mild disease. For example, report of a relatively high incidence of aortic and mitral valve calcifications (54%) in a prospective study of patients with PHPT [39] was obtained in a cohort with a mean serum calcium of more than 12 mg/dL, which is significantly higher than typically seen in PHPT today. A case-control study of 51 patients with mild PHPT and 49 controls found an association between mild PHPT and subclinical aortic valve calcifications. Aortic valve calcification was predicted by PTH, but not serum calcium [38]. This cohort had no evidence of left ventricular hypertrophy but did have evidence of increased carotid stiffness and carotid intimal medial thickness, suggesting that the carotid vascular bed may be preferentially affected in mild PHPT. None of these findings reversed 2 years after parathyroidectomy [42].

Rheumatologic

In the past, PHPT was associated with rheumatologic disease, specifically gout and calcium pyrophosphate deposition disease. In addition, cure of PHPT was associated with the development of pseudogout. These manifestations are rarely seen today [46].

Gastrointestinal

Gastrointestinal manifestations were also common in classic PHPT, and are unusual today. While pancreatitis was a common concomitant of the very high serum calcium levels seen in classical disease, in a 2009 study of 684 patients with PHPT investigating the incidence of acute pancreatitis, only 10 patients (1.5%) developed acute pancreatitis. There was no significant difference in rate of development of acute pancreatitis compared with a control group (32 of 1364 patients, 2.3%) [47]. Peptic ulcer disease has also been epidemiologically linked to PHPT. In a series of 100 patients with PHPT, 16% had peptic ulcer disease [48]. About half of the patients had improvement in symptoms following parathyroidectomy. It should be noted that unlike pancreatitis in those with severe hypercalcemia, no clear causal link has been elucidated between peptic ulcer disease and PHPT. The exception to this is in patients with multiple endocrine neoplasia (MEN) type 1, as these patients can have Zollinger–Ellison syndrome (further discussed below).

PHPT is often thought to be associated with general gastrointestinal complaints. For example, in a study of 153 patients with PHPT from India, 80% had gastrointestinal complaints, most commonly abdominal pain (43%) or constipation (36%). However, these patients all had symptomatic disease, with mean serum calcium levels of 11.5 mg/dL and mean PTH of 735 pg/mL, levels that are significantly higher than in the typical patient with modern-day PHPT in Western countries. While significant elevations in serum calcium are associated with gastrointestinal symptoms, gastrointestinal disease is not considered part of the modern-day presentation of asymptomatic PHPT [16].

CURRENT GUIDELINES FOR SURGERY

Parathyroidectomy is recommended in all patients with symptomatic PHPT. The Fourth International Workshop on the Management of Asymptomatic Primary Hyperparathyroidism recently released updated guidelines on the indications for surgical management in patients with asymptomatic disease [3]. Most of these criteria reflect the severity of the underlying PHPT (serum calcium and skeletal or renal manifestations). One criterion that is unassociated with severity of disease is an age of <50 years. Evidence suggests that patients under the age of 50 have a far greater chance of disease progression than do their older counterparts with PHPT [49].

Patients with asymptomatic PHPT should be evaluated to see if they meet the current guidelines for surgical referral, shown in Table 19.1. These guidelines have changed since the first workshop in 1990, and are likely to continue to evolve as more is learned about the manifestations of asymptomatic PHPT. At this time, evaluation of patients with asymptomatic PHPT should include the following tests: measurement of biochemistries (including calcium, PTH, phosphorus, alkaline phosphatase, blood urea nitrogen [BUN], and creatinine), PTH, and 25-hydroxyvitamin D [4]. BMD should be assessed by DXA that includes measurements at the spine, hip and distal one-third radius.

Table 19.1 Fourth International Workshop on Asymptomatic Primary Hyperparathyroidism: Guidelines for recommending surgery

Measurement	Guideline
Biochemical	Serum calcium >1 mg/dL above upper limit of normal
Skeletal	A. BMD by DXA: T-score of <− 2.5 at any site
	B. Vertebral fracture (by X-ray, CT, MRI, or vertebral fracture assessment)
Renal	A. Creatinine clearance of <60 cm³/min
	B. 24-hour urinary calcium of >400 mg/day and increased stone risk by biochemical stone risk analysis
	C. Presence of nephrolithiasis or nephrocalcinosis on renal imaging (X-ray, CT, or ultrasound)
Age	<50 years old

Source: Adapted from Bilezikian JP et al. *J Clin Endocrinol Metab* 2014;99(10):3561–9.

Assessment for vertebral fractures is recommended, with either an X-ray or vertebral fracture assessment by DXA. Twenty-four-hour urine tests should include a urinary calcium determination to confirm the diagnosis of PHPT and to rule out familial hypocalciuric hypercalcemia (FHH). If the urinary calcium excretion is greater than 400 mg in 24 hours, a stone risk profile should be done to better characterize a patient's risk for nephrolithiasis, and parathyroidectomy should be considered in high-risk patients. Abdominal imaging to assess for asymptomatic nephrolithiasis or nephrocalcinosis should be done with X-ray, renal ultrasound, or a CT scan [4].

Of note, definitive treatment of PHPT with surgery is never an inappropriate choice, regardless of whether patients meet these surgical criteria. Patient and physician choice are important in this regard. Patients who are unwilling or unable to comply with regular follow-up for untreated PHPT should also be sent for surgery.

NORMOCALCEMIC PRIMARY HYPERPARATHYROIDISM

Normocalcemic PHPT is a variant of PHPT that has emerged as a clinical entity over the past decade. It was first formally addressed by the Third International Workshop on Asymptomatic Primary Hyperparathyroidism in 2008. Normocalcemic PHPT is defined as an elevated PTH with a normal serum total and ionized calcium. These patients are often identified during workup for metabolic bone disease, when a PTH level is measured despite normal serum calcium levels. A thorough search for secondary causes of hyperparathyroidism must be completed before this diagnosis can be applied. Assessment for secondary causes should include measurement of serum creatinine because chronic kidney disease can cause an elevated PTH. Evaluation must also include measurement of 25-hydroxyvitamin D, to rule out vitamin D deficiency, as vitamin D deficiency can lower serum calcium levels from the hypercalcemic into the normocalcemic range in PHPT. A 24-hour urinary calcium must be obtained to look for evidence of calcium malabsorption or hypercalciuria. In addition, the use of medications associated with hyperparathyroidism, like lithium and hydrochlorothiazide, should be investigated. If secondary causes are ruled out and persistent hyperparathyroidism with normal calcium levels confirmed, normocalcemic PHPT can be diagnosed. The Fourth International Workshop on the Management of Asymptomatic Primary Hyperparathyroidism proposed suggestions regarding the diagnosis of normocalcemic PHPT. The panel advised confirming an elevated PTH level by repeat measurement on at least two more occasions over a 3- to 6-month time period [7]. It should be noted that while hypercalcemic PHPT can be diagnosed in patients with normal PTH levels (it is abnormal for levels not to be suppressed in the presence of elevated serum calcium), the diagnosis of normocalcemic PHPT requires consistently elevated PTH levels.

Normocalcemic PHPT may affect 0.4%–3.1% of the population, based on screening studies of unselected, nonreferral populations [50]. It has been hypothesized that normocalcemic PHPT represents the initial phase in the biphasic development of PHPT. Patients initially present with normal calcium levels and elevated PTH levels, and then go on to develop PHPT when the serum calcium later rises [51,52]. This seems to be the case in some, but not all, patients. A longitudinal cohort study of 37 patients with normocalcemic PHPT found that 40% of patients developed additional evidence of PHPT over a median follow-up of 3 years. Seven of the 37 subjects (19%) developed hypercalcemia [53].

The surgical guidelines discussed above do not apply to normocalcemic PHPT, in part because of the limited data on the natural history of this disease, as well as its treatment. The largest study of bone densitometric response following parathyroidectomy in normocalcemic PHPT included 39 patients [54]. At 1 year after surgical cure, BMD in the normocalcemic PHPT patients showed small but significant improvement at the spine and hip, similar to the gains seen in a group of patients with hypercalcemic PHPT. A longitudinal cohort study that included 15 patients with normocalcemic PHPT found that 46% of patients had a BMD increase of at least 0.03 g/cm^2 at one site or more 1 year after parathyroidectomy [55]. However, the definition of normocalcemic PHPT was not clear, as some of the cohort had renal dysfunction (glomerular filtration rate [GFR] < 60) and urinary calcium results were not included. While these studies suggest a possible benefit to bone health in patients with normocalcemic PHPT following parathyroidectomy, the data remain limited. At this time, there are no evidence-based guidelines for management of normocalcemic PHPT. It is likely this will change as more information is learned about the clinical course of normocalcemic PHPT.

UNUSUAL PRESENTATIONS OF PHPT

Genetic syndromes

MULTIPLE ENDOCRINE NEOPLASIA

The majority of cases of PHPT are sporadic; however, PHPT can present as part of MEN syndromes type 1 and 2A. While these conditions are discussed in greater detail elsewhere in this book, they are briefly mentioned here. MEN1 is a rare disease with a prevalence of 2–3 per 100,000 [1]. It is characterized by PHPT, pituitary tumors, and pancreaticoduodenal endocrine tumors, like duodenal gastrinomas. PHPT is typically the first clinical manifestation of MEN1. In MEN1, the female-to-male ratio of patients with PHPT is about 1, unlike the female predominance seen in sporadic PHPT. In addition, patients with PHPT in the setting of MEN1 tend to present earlier than patients with sporadic PHPT, often in the second to fourth decade of life [1]. In MEN1, patients may have gastrinomas and Zollinger–Ellison syndrome. In this setting, PHPT can be associated with peptic ulcer disease.

MEN2A is characterized by PHPT, medullary thyroid cancer, and pheochromocytoma. PHPT tends to be present in about 20% of patients with MEN2A. PHPT in the setting of MEN2A is typically more mild and presents later than in MEN1 [1].

HYPERPARATHYROIDISM-JAW TUMOR SYNDROME

Hyperparathyroidism-jaw tumor syndrome is a rare autosomal dominant disorder [56]. This syndrome is associated with PHPT, ossifying jaw tumors of the maxilla and mandible, and renal cysts and tumors. The majority of patients present with PHPT. The PHPT associated with this syndrome is often associated with more severe hypercalcemia than in sporadic PHPT. In addition, there is a higher risk of parathyroid cancer, which occurs in 10%–15% of patients [56].

FAMILIAL ISOLATED PHPT

Familial isolated PHPT (FIHP) is PHPT that runs in a family, but is not associated with other tumors [56]. It is estimated to account for about 1% of cases of PHPT [57]. It is not clear if FIHP is a distinct genetic entity or instead a variant of MEN or hyperparathyroidism-jaw tumor syndrome [57]. For example, genetic analysis of several kindred with FIHP found four out of 11 families with FIHP had MEN1 gene mutations, which suggests they may have a variant form of MEN1 syndrome [57].

Parathyroid cancer

Parathyroid cancer is rare. It is typically estimated to account for less than 1% of cases of PHPT [58]. Unlike in benign PHPT, parathyroid cancer affects men and women in equal proportion. In addition, patients with parathyroid cancer tend to present at a younger age, often in their mid-40s. While the physical exam in patients with benign disease is usually unremarkable, in parathyroid cancer 30%–76% of patients have a palpable neck mass [59]. Patients present with signs and symptoms of hypercalcemia, including polydipsia, polyuria, muscle weakness, and nausea [58]. Serum calcium levels are typically above 14 mg/dL, with PTH levels between three and ten times the upper limit of normal [59]. The complications of hyperparathyroidism are more common and more severe than in PHPT. Approximately half of patients have kidney stones, and evidence of bone disease is seen on imaging in 34%–91% of patients with parathyroid cancer.

CONCLUSION

Modern-day PHPT typically presents as an asymptomatic disease diagnosed after mild hypercalcemia is noted on routine labs. The vast majority of cases of PHPT are sporadic. Management of asymptomatic PHPT at this time focuses on assessing for bone and renal complications. The nonclassical sequelae of PHPT, in particular regarding cardiovascular and neurocognitive disease, continue to be under investigation. Surgery remains the only option for cure of PHPT, and is recommended in all symptomatic patients. Many asymptomatic patients also meet criteria for surgery, and this list has recently been expanded to include asymptomatic vertebral fractures and asymptomatic renal calcifications (nephrolithiasis or nephrocalcinosis). Normocalcemic PHPT, a presentation of PHPT that has come to light in the past decade, is a condition whose natural history continues to be elucidated. The optimal management for this variant of PHPT is unknown at this time.

REFERENCES

1. Rosen CJ, American Society for Bone and Mineral Research. *Primer on the Metabolic Bone Diseases and Disorders of Mineral Metabolism.* 8th ed. Ames, IA: Wiley-Blackwell, 2013.

2. DeGroot LJ, Jameson JL. *Endocrinology: Adult and Pediatric.* 6th ed. Philadelphia: Saunders/Elsevier, 2010.

3. Silverberg SJ, Clarke BL, Peacock M et al. Current issues in the presentation of asymptomatic primary hyperparathyroidism: Proceedings of the Fourth International Workshop. *J Clin Endocrinol Metab* 2014;99(10):3580–94.

4. Bilezikian JP, Brandi ML, Eastell R et al. Guidelines for the management of asymptomatic primary hyperparathyroidism: summary statement from the Fourth International Workshop. *J Clin Endocrinol Metab* 2014;99(10):3561–9.

5. Wermers RA, Khosla S, Atkinson EJ et al. Incidence of primary hyperparathyroidism in Rochester, Minnesota, 1993–2001: An update on the changing epidemiology of the disease. *J Bone Miner Res* 2006;21(1):171–7.

6. Yeh MW, Ituarte PH, Zhou HC et al. Incidence and prevalence of primary hyperparathyroidism in a racially mixed population. *J Clin Endocrinol Metab* 2013;98(3):1122–9.

7. Eastell R, Brandi ML, Costa AG, D'Amour P, Shoback DM, Thakker RV. Diagnosis of asymptomatic primary hyperparathyroidism: Proceedings of the Fourth International Workshop. *J Clin Endocrinol Metab* 2014;99(10):3570–9.

8. Moosgaard B, Vestergaard P, Heickendorff L, Melsen F, Christiansen P, Mosekilde L. Vitamin D status, seasonal variations, parathyroid adenoma weight and bone mineral density in primary hyperparathyroidism. *Clin Endocrinol* 2005;63(5):506–13.

9. Vignali E, Viccica G, Diacinti D et al. Morphometric vertebral fractures in postmenopausal women with primary hyperparathyroidism. *J Clin Endocrinol Metab* 2009;94(7):2306–12.

10. Khosla S, Melton LJ 3rd, Wermers RA, Crowson CS, O'Fallon W, Riggs B. Primary hyperparathyroidism and the risk of fracture: A population-based study. *J Bone Miner Res* 1999;14(10):1700–7.

11. Silverberg SJ, Shane E, de la Cruz L et al. Skeletal disease in primary hyperparathyroidism. *J Bone Miner Res* 1989;4(3):283–91.

12. Hansen S, Beck Jensen JE, Rasmussen L, Hauge EM, Brixen K. Effects on bone geometry, density, and microarchitecture in the distal radius but not the tibia in women with primary hyperparathyroidism: A case-control study using HR-pQCT. *J Bone Miner Res* 2010;25(9):1941–7.

13. Vu TD, Wang XF, Wang Q et al. New insights into the effects of primary hyperparathyroidism on the cortical and trabecular compartments of bone. *Bone* 2013;55(1):57–63.

14. Silva BC, Boutroy S, Zhang C et al. Trabecular bone score (TBS)—A novel method to evaluate bone microarchitectural texture in patients with primary hyperparathyroidism. *J Clin Endocrinol Metab* 2013;98(5):1963–70.

15. Suh JM, Cronan JJ, Monchik JM. Primary hyperparathyroidism: Is there an increased prevalence of renal stone disease? *AJR Am J Roentgenol* 2008;191(3):908–11.

16. Walker MD, Rubin M, Silverberg SJ. Nontraditional manifestations of primary hyperparathyroidism. *J Clin Densitom* 2013;16(1):40–7.

17. Espiritu RP, Kearns AE, Vickers KS, Grant C, Ryu E, Wermers RA. Depression in primary hyperparathyroidism: Prevalence and benefit of surgery. *J Clin Endocrinol Metab* 2011;96(11):E1737–45.

18. Walker MD, McMahon DJ, Inabnet WB et al. Neuropsychological features in primary hyperparathyroidism: A prospective study. *J Clin Endocrinol Metab* 2009;94(6):1951–8.

19. Caillard C, Sebag F, Mathonnet M et al. Prospective evaluation of quality of life (SF-36v2) and nonspecific symptoms before and after cure of primary hyperparathyroidism (1-year follow-up). *Surgery* 2007;141(2):153–9; discussion 159–60.

20. Joborn C, Hetta J, Lind L, Rastad J, Akerstrom G, Ljunghall S. Self-rated psychiatric symptoms in patients operated on because of primary hyperparathyroidism and in patients with long-standing mild hypercalcemia. *Surgery* 1989;105(1):72–8.

21. Pasieka JL, Parsons LL. Prospective surgical outcome study of relief of symptoms following surgery in patients with primary hyperparathyroidism. *World J Surg* 1998;22(6):513–8; discussion 518–9.

22. Pasieka JL, Parsons LL, Demeure MJ et al. Patient-based surgical outcome tool demonstrating alleviation of symptoms following parathyroidectomy in patients with primary hyperparathyroidism. *World J Surg* 2002;26(8):942–9.

23. Rao DS, Phillips ER, Divine GW, Talpos GB. Randomized controlled clinical trial of surgery versus no surgery in patients with mild asymptomatic primary hyperparathyroidism. *J Clin Endocrinol Metab* 2004;89(11):5415–22.

24. Bollerslev J, Jansson S, Mollerup CL et al. Medical observation, compared with parathyroidectomy, for

asymptomatic primary hyperparathyroidism: A prospective, randomized trial. *J Clin Endocrinol Metab* 2007;92(5):1687–92.

25. Ambrogini E, Cetani F, Cianferotti L et al. Surgery or surveillance for mild asymptomatic primary hyperparathyroidism: A prospective, randomized clinical trial. *J Clin Endocrinol Metab* 2007;92(8):3114–21.

26. Babinska D, Barczynski M, Stefaniak T et al. Evaluation of selected cognitive functions before and after surgery for primary hyperparathyroidism. *Langenbecks Arch Surg* 2012;397(5):825–31.

27. Perrier ND, Balachandran D, Wefel JS et al. Prospective, randomized, controlled trial of parathyroidectomy versus observation in patients with "asymptomatic" primary hyperparathyroidism. *Surgery* 2009;146(6):1116–22.

28. Roman SA, Sosa JA, Pietrzak RH et al. The effects of serum calcium and parathyroid hormone changes on psychological and cognitive function in patients undergoing parathyroidectomy for primary hyperparathyroidism. *Ann Surg* 2011;253(1):131–7.

29. Hedback G, Tisell LE, Bengtsson BA, Hedman I, Oden A. Premature death in patients operated on for primary hyperparathyroidism. *World J Surg* 1990;14(6):829–35; discussion 836.

30. Ronni-Sivula H. Causes of death in patients previously operated on for primary hyperparathyroidism. *Ann Chir Gynaecol* 1985;74(1):13–8.

31. Nilsson IL, Yin L, Lundgren E, Rastad J, Ekbom A. Clinical presentation of primary hyperparathyroidism in Europe—Nationwide cohort analysis on mortality from nonmalignant causes. *J Bone Miner Res* 2002;17(Suppl 2):N68–74.

32. Wermers RA, Khosla S, Atkinson EJ et al. Survival after the diagnosis of hyperparathyroidism: A population-based study. *Am J Med* 1998;104(2):115–22.

33. Yu N, Donnan PT, Flynn RW et al. Increased mortality and morbidity in mild primary hyperparathyroid patients. The Parathyroid Epidemiology and Audit Research Study (PEARS). *Clin Endocrinol* 2010;73(1):30–4.

34. Lueg MC. Hypertension and primary hyperparathyroidism: A five-year case review. *South Med J* 1982;75(11):1371–4.

35. Nainby-Luxmoore JC, Langford HG, Nelson NC, Watson RL, Barnes TY. A case-comparison study of hypertension and hyperparathyroidism. *J Clin Endocrinol Metab* 1982;55(2):303–6.

36. Diamond TW, Botha JR, Wing J, Meyers AM, Kalk WJ. Parathyroid hypertension. A reversible disorder. *Arch Intern Med* 1986;146(9):1709–12.

37. Bollerslev J, Rosen T, Mollerup CL et al. Effect of surgery on cardiovascular risk factors in mild primary hyperparathyroidism. *J Clin Endocrinol Metab* 2009;94(7):2255–61.

38. Iwata S, Walker MD, Di Tullio MR et al. Aortic valve calcification in mild primary hyperparathyroidism. *J Clin Endocrinol Metab* 2012;97(1):132–7.

39. Stefenelli T, Abela C, Frank H et al. Cardiac abnormalities in patients with primary hyperparathyroidism: Implications for follow-up. *J Clin Endocrinol Metab* 1997;82(1):106–12.

40. Langle F, Abela C, Koller-Strametz J et al. Primary hyperparathyroidism and the heart: Cardiac abnormalities correlated to clinical and biochemical data. *World J Surg* 1994;18(4):619–24.

41. Walker MD, Fleischer JB, Di Tullio MR et al. Cardiac structure and diastolic function in mild primary hyperparathyroidism. *J Clin Endocrinol Metab* 2010;95(5):2172–9.

42. Walker MD, Rundek T, Homma S et al. Effect of parathyroidectomy on subclinical cardiovascular disease in mild primary hyperparathyroidism. *Eur J Endocrinol* 2012;167(2):277–85.

43. Lumachi F, Ermani M, Frego M et al. Intima-media thickness measurement of the carotid artery in patients with primary hyperparathyroidism. A prospective case-control study and long-term follow-up. *In Vivo* 2006;20(6B):887–90.

44. Kosch M, Hausberg M, Vormbrock K et al. Impaired flow-mediated vasodilation of the brachial artery in patients with primary hyperparathyroidism improves after parathyroidectomy. *Cardiovasc Res* 2000;47(4):813–8.

45. Carrelli AL, Walker MD, Di Tullio MR et al. Endothelial function in mild primary hyperparathyroidism. *Clin Endocrinol* 2013;78(2):204–9.

46. Rubin MR, Silverberg SJ. Rheumatic manifestations of primary hyperparathyroidism and parathyroid hormone therapy. *Curr Rheumatol Rep* 2002;4(2):179–85.

47. Khoo TK, Vege SS, Abu-Lebdeh HS, Ryu E, Nadeem S, Wermers RA. Acute pancreatitis in primary hyperparathyroidism: A population-based study. *J Clin Endocrinol Metab* 2009;94(6):2115–8.

48. Lafferty FW, Hubay CA. Primary hyperparathyroidism. A review of the long-term surgical and nonsurgical morbidities as a basis for a rational approach to treatment. *Arch Intern Med* 1989;149(4):789–96.

49. Silverberg SJ, Brown I, Bilezikian JP. Age as a criterion for surgery in primary hyperparathyroidism. *Am J Med* 2002;113(8):681–4.

50. Cusano NE, Maalouf NM, Wang PY et al. Normocalcemic hyperparathyroidism and hypoparathyroidism in two community-based non-referral populations. *J Clin Endocrinol Metab* 2013;98(7):2734–41.

51. Cusano NE, Silverberg SJ, Bilezikian JP. Normocalcemic primary hyperparathyroidism. *J Clin Densitom* 2013;16(1):33–9.

52. Rao DS, Wilson RJ, Kleerekoper M, Parfitt AM. Lack of biochemical progression or continuation of

accelerated bone loss in mild asymptomatic primary hyperparathyroidism: Evidence for biphasic disease course. *J Clin Endocrinol Metab* 1988;67(6):1294–8.

53. Lowe H, McMahon DJ, Rubin MR, Bilezikian JP, Silverberg SJ. Normocalcemic primary hyperparathyroidism: Further characterization of a new clinical phenotype. *J Clin Endocrinol Metab* 2007;92(8):3001–5.

54. Koumakis E, Souberbielle JC, Sarfati E et al. Bone mineral density evolution after successful parathyroidectomy in patients with normocalcemic primary hyperparathyroidism. *J Clin Endocrinol Metab* 2013;98(8):3213–20.

55. Koumakis E, Souberbielle JC, Payet J et al. Individual site-specific bone mineral density gain in normocalcemic primary hyperparathyroidism. *Osteoporos Int* 2014;25(7):1963–8.

56. Chen JD, Morrison C, Zhang C, Kahnoski K, Carpten JD, Teh BT. Hyperparathyroidism-jaw tumour syndrome. *J Intern Med* 2003;253(6):634–42.

57. Cetani F, Pardi E, Ambrogini E et al. Genetic analyses in familial isolated hyperparathyroidism: Implication for clinical assessment and surgical management. *Clin Endocrinol* 2006;64(2):146–52.

58. Marcocci C, Cetani F, Rubin MR, Silverberg SJ, Pinchera A, Bilezikian JP. Parathyroid carcinoma. *J Bone Miner Res* 2008;23(12):1869–80.

59. Shane E. Clinical review 122: Parathyroid carcinoma. *J Clin Endocrinol Metab* 2001;86(2):485–93.

20

Parathyroid ultrasound imaging

RICHARD S. HABER

UTILITY OF PARATHYROID ULTRASONOGRAPHY

The widespread use of minimally invasive surgical techniques for treating primary hyperparathyroidism has been made possible by the availability of preoperative imaging for localizing enlarged parathyroid glands. Parathyroid imaging methods include ultrasonography, radionuclide imaging with technetium-99m sestamibi, and more recently, four-dimensional computerized tomography based on the perfusion pattern over time. These imaging techniques are used to plan surgery in patients with biochemically confirmed primary hyperparathyroidism, 85%–90% of whom harbor a solitary parathyroid adenoma. However, the diagnosis of primary hyperparathyroidism should not be based on parathyroid imaging results, because the finding of a putative enlarged parathyroid gland with any imaging technique may represent a false-positive result.

Among the parathyroid imaging methods, ultrasonography is uniquely convenient and inexpensive [1]. With experience, surgeons can perform ultrasound examination for this purpose during an office evaluation, and recognition of the utility of this approach has led to its recommendation as the first-line method for parathyroid localization [1]. The superficial location of the parathyroid glands permits the utilization of high-frequency ultrasound transducers, since there is an inverse relationship between ultrasound frequency and depth of penetration. High-frequency ultrasound provides detailed images of enlarged parathyroid glands and their anatomic relationships, with excellent resolution of 1–2 mm. Moreover, ultrasonography is the best imaging test for coexisting thyroid disease, which may merit surgical attention at the time of parathyroid surgery.

In addition, there is no patient radiation exposure. All of these factors make ultrasonography an attractive front-line choice for parathyroid imaging [1,2], and in many cases, it may be the only imaging test that is required.

TECHNIQUE OF PARATHYROID ULTRASONOGRAPHY

Both linear and convex ultrasound transducers with a high-frequency range may be used. About 10 mHz is optimal for most examinations. Transducers with a smaller contact area ("footprint") facilitate movement over the contours of the neck.

Ultrasound examination of the anterior neck is best performed as a "real-time" examination, rather than by reviewing static images. The patient should be supine with the neck extended, which may be facilitated by placing a pad under the shoulders. Ultrasound transmission gel is applied to the skin and probe. With the probe oriented in the transverse plane, and beginning with the thyroid region on each side, the examiner moves the probe over the central compartment of the neck from the level of the clavicles to the hyoid bone, extending the examination laterally to the common carotid artery. About 1 cm of the upper mediastinum can be visualized by angling the probe inferiorly, deep to the head of the clavicle. Visualization of this area may be enhanced by asking the patient to swallow.

In the majority of patients with primary hyperparathyroidism, enlarged parathyroid glands are immediately apparent to experienced examiners. The precise location with respect to surrounding structures (thyroid and common carotid artery), the echogenicity, the depth, the shape, and the size in three dimensions should all be noted.

ULTRASONOGRAPHIC APPEARANCE AND LOCATION OF ENLARGED PARATHYROID GLANDS

Enlarged parathyroid glands typically appear as homogeneously hypoechoic structures, in sharp contrast to the hyperechoic thyroid tissue to which they are usually juxtaposed [1,3]. They are usually elongated in the longitudinal dimension, measuring 0.8–1.5 cm, and oval in shape with smooth borders. Less commonly, the echotexture is heterogeneous or partly cystic (anechoic) or the shape is lobulated. Normal parathyroid glands are only occasionally visualized by ultrasonography due to their small size. On color Doppler imaging, parathyroid adenomas show a typical unipolar vascular pattern and a "vascular arc" at the periphery, features that may help distinguish them from nonparathyroid structures with a similar ultrasonograhic appearance, such as lymph nodes and some thyroid nodules [4].

The inferior parathyroid glands are derived from the third branchial pouch. Inferior parathyroid adenomas (Figure 20.1) are usually found immediately adjacent to the lower pole of the thyroid, inferior, posterior, or lateral [1,3]. As a result of their embryologic migration with the thymus gland, they are often located ectopically in the thyrothymic ligament, thymus gland, or mediastinum outside the thymus gland, or occasionally above the superior parathyroid gland [1]. Ectopic inferior parathyroid glands thus lie at a variable inferior distance from the lower thyroid pole. Only the uppermost ectopic inferior parathyroid adenomas can be visualized by ultrasonography because of the acoustic shadow of the sternum. Their visualization is facilitated by orienting the ultrasound probe inferiorly from the lower neck.

Enlarged superior parathyroid glands (Figure 20.2), derived from the fourth branchial pouch, are usually found posterior and adjacent to the midportion of the upper thyroid lobe [1,3]. Less commonly, they are located posterior to the midthyroid or lower (in which case, they can be confused with inferior parathyroid glands), superior to the upper thyroid pole, or more posteriorly in the tracheoesophageal groove. The acoustic shadow of the tracheal cartilage limits the sensitivity of ultrasonography in the latter case.

Either the superior or inferior parathyroid glands may be intrathyroidal. Intrathyroidal parathyroid adenomas are easily detected by ultrasonography, since their hypoechoic appearance stands out against the surrounding hyperechoic normal thyroid tissue. However, their appearance is indistinguishable from that of a hypoechoic thyroid nodule. Because intrathyroidal parathyroid adenomas may not be evident during surgical exploration, their detection by ultrasonography can prevent unsuccessful surgery for hyperparathyroidism.

When only a single enlarged parathyroid gland is detected, a presumptive diagnosis of a solitary parathyroid adenoma is made. The finding of more than one putative enlarged gland suggests multigland parathyroid hyperplasia, or occasionally a double adenoma.

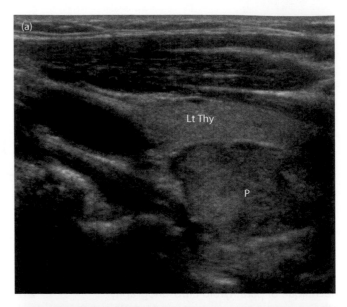

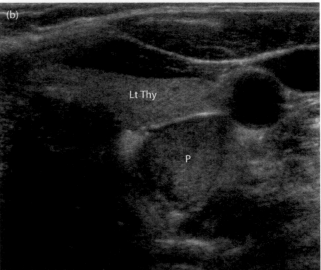

Figure 20.1 Parathyroid adenoma posterior to the left lower thyroid pole. Lt Thy, left thyroid lobe. P, parathyroid adenoma. **(a)** Longitudinal view. **(b)** Transverse view. Note the sharp contrast between the hyperechoic thyroid gland and the adjacent hypoechoic parathyroid adenoma, and the bright echo marking the posterior border of the thyroid gland. The dimensions of this parathyroid adenoma are 2.2 cm longitudinal × 1.3 cm anteroposterior × 1.6 cm transverse, a relatively large size.

DIAGNOSTIC WEAKNESSES OF PARATHYROID ULTRASONOGRAPHY

The major weakness of ultrasonography is the failure to localize enlarged parathyroid glands in some patients with primary hyperparathyroidism, since the sensitivity of the examination does not exceed 80% even in skilled hands [5,6]. Such false-negative results are in general more common in biochemically mild hyperparathyroidism or with parathyroid hyperplasia [7], both of which are associated with lesser degrees of gland enlargement. In addition, the presence of

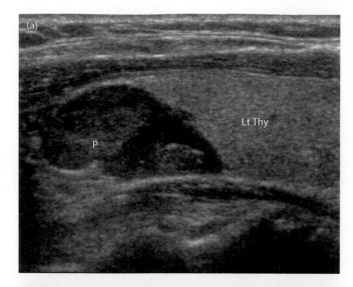

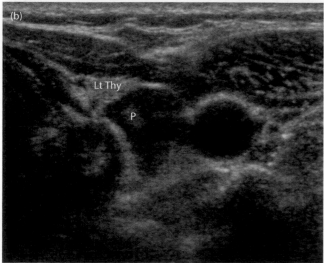

Figure 20.2 Parathyroid adenoma posterior to the left upper thyroid pole. Lt Thy, left thyroid lobe. P, parathyroid adenoma. (a) Longitudinal view. (b) Transverse view.

multinodular goiters decreases the sensitivity of parathyroid ultrasonography [7], probably because of diminished resolution posterior to large goiters. As discussed, false-negative examinations are inevitable for ectopic adenomas located in the acoustic shadows of bone (mediastinum) or of the trachea (paraesophageal region).

Ultrasonography may also yield false-positive results. First, apparently solitary parathyroid adenomas by ultrasonography may in fact represent multigland disease, and ultrasonography has poor sensitivity for diagnosing the presence of multigland parathyroid hyperplasia, as does radionuclide imaging with sestamibi [8,9]. Second, nonparathyroid anatomic structures may be mistaken for parathyroid adenomas. The hypoechoic appearance and elongated shape of cervical lymph nodes is similar to that of parathyroid adenomas, although the presence of linear hilar echoes in lymph nodes is a distinguishing feature. Autoimmune lymphocytic (Hashimoto's) thyroiditis, a

common condition in the general population, is associated with prominent perithyroidal lymphadenopathy, whose appearance and location are similar to those of enlarged parathyroid glands [4].

DIAGNOSTIC ACCURACY OF PARATHYROID ULTRASONOGRAPHY

The sensitivity of ultrasonography is 76%–79% [5,6]. The reliability of positive test results is high, with reported positive predictive values of 85%–100% based on anatomical findings at surgery [5]. In practice, the predictive value of positive findings varies according to the appearance and location of the putative enlarged gland. If the findings are highly typical and appear convincing to an experienced observer, the predictive value approaches 100%, but if the findings are atypical or ambiguous, then the predictive value is lower. In any case, the accuracy of the test is highly dependent on the skill and experience of the observer [10].

In comparison with technetium-99m sestamibi scintigraphy, ultrasonography is slightly less sensitive in several studies [10–13], which is attributable to the superior ability of sestamibi scanning to detect ectopic parathyroid adenomas, particularly in the mediastinum [11,14]. Of note, when the findings of ultrasonography and sestamibi scanning are concordant, the positive predictive value approaches 100% [11,15].

ULTRASOUND GUIDANCE FOR DIAGNOSTIC FINE-NEEDLE ASPIRATION

In cases where the nature of a putative enlarged parathyroid gland detected by ultrasonography is particularly uncertain based on appearance or location, the diagnosis can be confirmed biochemically by parathyroid hormone immunoassay on a fine-needle aspirate of the structure in question. The needle is placed under ultrasound guidance using techniques commonly employed for obtaining cytologic specimens from thyroid nodules. The aspirated material is diluted in 1 mL of saline for parathyroid hormone assay. True parathyroid adenomas usually yield unequivocally high levels by this technique [16].

Parathyroid fine-needle aspiration is not justified in routine situations in which ultrasonography alone has a high positive predictive value, and there has been concern that it may cause a local inflammatory reaction that makes surgery more difficult [17]. It is most useful in special circumstances, such as distinguishing intrathyroidal parathyroid adenomas from thyroid nodules, or in reoperation after unsuccessful parathyroid surgery.

DETECTION OF COEXISTING NODULAR THYROID DISEASE

Ultrasonography remains the best imaging test for nodular thyroid disease, and its ability to identify and characterize coexisting nodular thyroid disease in patients with hyperparathyroidism constitutes a significant advantage over other parathyroid imaging methods. Ultrasonography may show thyroid pathology in as many as 29%–51% of patients with primary hyperparathyroidism [18,19]. Although most thyroid nodules are benign, ultrasound-guided fine-needle aspiration cytology on selected nodules detected by ultrasonography permits the identification of coexisting thyroid cancer when present, which can then be treated surgically at the time of parathyroidectomy.

REFERENCES

1. Solorzano CC, Carneiro-Pla D. Minimizing cost and maximizing success in the preoperative localization strategy for primary hyperparathyroidism. *Surg Clin North Am* 2014;94:587–605.

2. Kunstman JW, Kirsch JD, Mahajan A, Udelsman R. Clinical review: Parathyroid localization and implications for clinical management. *J Clin Endocrinol Metab* 2013;98:902–12.

3. Johnson NA, Carty SE, Tubin ME. Parathyroid imaging. *Radiol Clin N Am* 2011;49:489–509.

4. Kamaya A, Quon A, Brooke Jeffrey R. Sonography of the abnormal parathyroid gland. *Ultrasound Q* 2006;22:253–62.

5. Cheung K, Wang TS, Farrokhyar F, Roman SA, Sosa JA. A meta-analysis of preoperative localization techniques for patients with primary hyperparathyroidism. *Ann Surg Oncol* 2012;19:577–83.

6. Ruda JM, Hollenbeak CS, Stack BC Jr. A systematic review of the diagnosis and treatment of primary hyperparathyroidism from 1995 to 2003. *Otolaryngol Head Neck Surg* 2005;132:359–72.

7. Berber E, Parikh RT, Ballem N, Garner CN, Milas M, Siperstein AE. Factors contributing to negative parathyroid localization: An analysis of 1000 patients. *Surgery* 2008;144:74–9.

8. Yip L, Pryma DA, Yim JH, Virji MA, Carty SE, Ogilvie JB. Can a lightbulb sestamibi SPECT accurately predict single-gland disease in sporadic primary hyperparathyroidism? *World J Surg* 2008;32:784–92.

9. Siperstein A, Berber E, Mackey R, Alghoul M, Wagner K, Milas M. Prospective evaluation of sestamibi scan, ultrasonography, and rapid PTH to predict the success of limited exploration for sporadic primary hyperparathyroidism. *Surgery* 2004;136:872–80.

10. Vitetta GM, Neri P, Chiecchio A et al. Role of ultrasonography in the management of patients with primary hyperparathyroidism: Retrospective comparison with technetium-99m sestamibi scintigraphy. *J Ultrasound* 2014;17:1–12.

11. Haber RS, Kim CK, Inabnet WB. Ultrasonography for preoperative localization of enlarged parathyroid glands in primary hyperparathyroidism: Comparison with (99m)technetium sestamibi scintigraphy. *Clin Endocrinol (Oxf)* 2002;57:241–9.

12. Lo C-Y, Lang BH, Chan WF, Kung AWC, Lam KSL. A prospective evaluation of preoperative localization by technetium-99m sestamibi scintigraphy and ultrasonography in primary hyperparathyroidism. *Am J Surg* 2007;193:155–9.

13. Bhansali A, Masoodi SR, Bhadada S, Mittal BR, Behra A, Singh P. Ultrasonography in detection of single and multiple abnormal parathyroid glands in primary hyperparathyroidism: Comparison with radionuclide scintigraphy and surgery. *Clin Endocrinol (Oxf)* 2006;65:340–5.

14. Barczynski M, Golkowski F, Konturek A et al. Technetium-99m-sestamibi subtraction scintigraphy vs. ultrasonography combined with a rapid parathyroid hormone assay in parathyroid aspirates in preoperative localization of parathyroid adenomas and in directing surgical approach. *Clin Endocrinol (Oxf)* 2006;65:106–13.

15. Lal G, Clark OH. Primary hyperparathyroidism: Controversies in surgical management. *Trends Endocrinol Metab* 2003;14:417–22.

16. Stephen AE, Milas M, Garner CN, Wagner KE, Siperstein AE. Use of surgeon-performed office ultrasound and parathyroid fine needle aspiration for complex parathyroid localization. *Surgery* 2005;138:1143–50.

17. Norman J, Politz D, Browarsky I. Diagnostic aspiration of parathyroid adenomas causes severe fibrosis complicating surgery and final histologic diagnosis. *Thyroid* 2007;17:1251–5.

18. Morita SY, Somervell H, Umbricht CB, Dackiw APB, Zeiger MA. Evaluation for concomitant thyroid nodules and primary hyperparathyroidism in patients undergoing parathyroidectomy or thyroidectomy. *Surgery* 2008;144:862–6.

19. Adler JT, Chen H, Schaefer S, Sippel RS. Does routine use of ultrasound result in additional thyroid procedures in patients with primary hyperparathyroidism? *J Am Coll Surg* 2010;211:536–9.

21

Parathyroid radionuclide imaging

JOSEF MACHAC

INTRODUCTION

This chapter reviews radionuclide imaging techniques used in parathyroid imaging, and the information obtained useful for management of primary hyperparathyroidism.

Primary hyperparathyroidism is defined as increased synthesis and release of parathyroid hormone (PTH), which results in an elevated serum calcium level and a decline in serum inorganic phosphate. The diagnosis is usually made as a result of an incidentally identified hypercalcemia by routine laboratory screening, followed by assay for serum PTH, with a higher than normal result. The clinical situation usually allows for the differentiation of primary versus secondary hyperparathyroidism. Radionuclide imaging is almost never used for the actual diagnosis of hyperparathyroidism. Patients referred for radionuclide imaging already come with that diagnosis.

The majority of cases of primary hyperparathyroidism (80%–90%) are due to a solitary parathyroid adenoma. Multigland hyperplasia and double adenomas account for about 10% of cases, while parathyroid carcinomas occur in only 1%–3% of cases of hyperparathyroidism [1].

Surgical resection is the primary mode of treatment, with an approximately 95% success rate of cure [2,3]. Unlike previously, when bilateral neck exploration was usually performed [4], selective minimally invasive laparoscopic surgery is the currently preferred approach [5], since the vast majority (87%) of patients with primary hyperparathyroidism have a solitary adenoma [6], which shortens operative and anesthesia time, decreases morbidity, and allows a shorter length of hospital stay. While the use of radionuclide parathyroid imaging was controversial at the time when bilateral neck exploration was routine, preoperative imaging, especially three-dimensional localization of the single adenoma, is the most important role of radionuclide imaging in surgical planning, which can help guide surgery with minimal invasiveness. The purpose of radionuclide parathyroid imaging, then, is to differentiate a single parathyroid adenoma from multiple adenomas or hyperplasia, and in adenoma localization for definitive surgical therapy [3].

Parathyroid radionuclide imaging is also indicated for localization of parathyroid tissues in patients with recurrent or persistent hyperparathyroidism. Because these patients have had one or more previous neck operations, reoperation is frequently more difficult. Also, ectopic parathyroid tissue is more prevalent in this population, making localization a challenge, with parathyroid scintigraphy providing helpful guidance [7].

The morphologic imaging methodologies, such as computed tomography (CT), ultrasound, and MRI, even though they feature good resolution, have a disadvantage in that they cannot easily distinguish functional parathyroid tissue from other types of tissue, resulting in a sensitivity of 50%–78% [3].

RADIONUCLIDE IMAGING TECHNIQUE

Initial methods

A succession of tumor imaging agents have been tried for radionuclide imaging, which show avidity for parathyroid tumors, such as cobalt-57 vitamin B12, selenium-75 methionine, and cesium-131 chloride. In the late 1970s, a promising agent was thallium-201, a cationic analog of potassium$^{(+1)}$, which is taken up by all metabolically active tissues, including the myocardium, muscle, glandular tissue, and a wide range of tumors. Such an agent is also taken up by the thyroid gland. The challenge was to distinguish parathyroid tissue from thyroid tissue. That was solved by dual-tracer imaging, combining thalium-201 imaging with thyroid imaging with technetium-99m (Tc-99m) pertechnetate, which is not taken up by parathyroid tissue. Uptake of thallium-201 in the vicinity of the thyroid gland, but no uptake of the Tc-99m pertechnetate, would indicate parathyroid tissue, by comparing the two images, aided by the technique of image subtraction [8]. The use of this technique in primary hyperparathyroidism yielded a sensitivity of 82% and diagnostic accuracy of 78% [9]. Since then, this technique has been superseded by Tc-99m sestamibi imaging because of greater accuracy and superior imaging resolution.

Single-tracer (Tc-99m sestamibi) double-phase imaging

Tc-99m sestamibi was introduced as an alternative to thallium-201 for myocardial perfusion imaging. This lipophilic radiotracer is taken up in the myocardium in proportion to blood flow. Cellular retention is related to mitochondrial metabolism and transmembrane potentials in the cytoplasmic reticulum and the mitochondria [10]. Tc-99m sestamibi is a substrate for transmembrane transporter P-glycoprotein (Pgp), incidentally found to be involved in multidrug resistance in many tumors. The degree of sestamibi retention or washout of sestamibi is related, at least in part, to the degree of Pgp expression in various tissues [11]. It has been shown that parathyroid adenomas have a large number of mitochondria in their cells. Tc-99m sestamibi is usually taken up more avidly in parathyroid adenomas than the surrounding thyroid parenchyma, and the washout from the parathyroid cells is slower than from the thyroid tissues [12].

The imaging of parathyroid adenomas, based on the differential washout principle, uses a single-isotope, double-phase protocol. The patient does not need any special preparation. Patients only need to remain still during image acquisition. Patients who are unable to remain immobilized during the study may require sedation. A single anterior pinhole collimator image or a magnified high-resolution parallel hole collimator image is obtained 10 minutes after intravenous injection of 20–25 mCi (740–1110 MBq) of Tc-99m sestamibi, and again at 1.5–2.5 hours [3]. Each image is taken approximately for 10 minutes. If the study is normal or inconclusive, and there is still retention of tracer in the thyroid, one may obtain an additional image at 3–4 hours after injection [3,13]. Additional anterior oblique planar images may be useful [3].

In addition, one obtains an image of the entire neck and chest, either as a single planar image with a parallel hole collimator or as part of a single-photon emission computed tomography (SPECT)-CT image of the neck and chest. With both methods, it is important to look for possible ectopic parathyroid tissue and, if possible, perform lesion localization with SPECT-CT. The mediastinal or chest planar or SPECT-CT imaging is obtained between the early and delayed neck images. Mediastinal images are particularly important before second operations in patients with persistent or recurrent disease because the likelihood of ectopic tissue is higher in this group [3].

As shown in Figure 21.1, the early sestamibi image (MIBI) shows uptake in the thyroid gland, as well as in the parathyroid adenoma, which shows persistence or at least slower washout of activity on the delayed sestamibi view, compared with the normal thyroid tissue. (It is also shown with an iodine-123 [I-123] image of the thyroid gland.) The result is that the parathyroid adenoma is progressively more pronounced against background and surrounding thyroid tissue, because of this differential washout.

The criterion of a positive study is one where the parathyroid–thyroid ratio becomes higher on delayed images. However, washout from the parathyroid adenoma compared with the thyroid uptake does vary. It may be similar to, or even faster than, washout from the thyroid, resulting in a focus seen on the early image that fades, or even disappears, on the delayed study. Hyperplastic parathyroid glands generally show faster washout than most adenomas and can be more difficult to detect [3].

In general, parathyroid adenomas larger than 500 mg can be identified scintigraphically with Tc-99m double-phase technique. Hyperplastic glands can also be frequently detected, but with less sensitivity than adenomas [3]. O'Doherty et al. compared Tc-99m sestamibi imaging with thallium-201 in the detection of parathyroid adenomas,

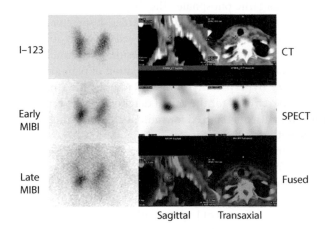

Figure 21.1 Classic parathyroid adenoma: The early MIBI image shows a prominent focus of increased uptake in the lower portion of the right lobe, which persists on the delayed MIBI image, while the rest of the thyroid uptake washes out. Also shown is an iodine-123 image which demonstrates uniform uptake. The SPECT-CT images show the focus located just posterior to the right thyroid lobe, consistent with an inferior parathyroid gland adenoma.

documented by surgical results [14]. In 57 subjects, there were 40 documented adenomas, 37 (92%) of which were localized by thallium-201, and 39 (97%) with Tc-99m sestamibi. Patients with hyperplastic glands, of which 29 (48%) were localized with thallium-201 and 32 (53%) with Tc-99m sestamibi. *In vitro* analysis of Tc-99m sestamibi and thallium-201 uptake in 20 patients showed that uptake of Tc-99 of sestamibi per gram of parathyroid tissue was greater than uptake per gram of thyroid tissue, which was not true for thallium-201. An early study by Taillefer et al. [13,15] in 23 patients, of which 21 had proven solitary parathyroid adenomas, showed a sensitivity of 90% on delayed sestamibi imaging and 70% on early sestamibi imaging. Additional, more recent studies showed an average sensitivity with Tc-99m sestamibi imaging of 90% [16].

When the thyroid gland is normal, with uniform uptake, the detection of parathyroid adenomas is straightforward with the sestamibi double-phase method. In the setting of a thyroid gland with one or multiple thyroid nodules, it becomes a challenge when one is trying to detect and localize a parathyroid adenoma. For that reason, dual-tracer imaging with I-123 or Tc-99m pertechnetate together with Tc-99m sestamibi can add additional accuracy.

Dual-tracer (I-123/Tc-99m pertechnetate + Tc-99m sestamibi) imaging

I-123, which has a half-life of 13 hours, emits a photon with energy of 159 keV, slightly different from the 140 keV emissions of Tc-99m. A total 200–600 μCi (7.5–22 MBq) of I-123 is administered orally prior to Tc-99m sestamibi imaging. Only a small dose of I-123 is used, due to the expense of I-123, compensated by the relatively high uptake of I-123 in the thyroid, with relatively high contrast. The I-123 scan is imaged 3–4 hours after administration, followed by Tc-99m sestamibi administration and imaging.

Instead of I-123 thyroid imaging, Tc-99m pertechnetate imaging can be performed either before or after the Tc-99m sestamibi images, provided that the dose of the first tracer is low, and the dose of the second tracer is at least five times higher, to avoid the two images from significantly affecting each other, since the two tracers share the same isotope with identical photon emissions. The administered activity of Tc-99m pertechnetate ranges from 2 to 10 mCi (74–370 MBq). Imaging is done 30 minutes after injection. Since Tc-99m pertechnetate is only trapped, its uptake in the thyroid gland is relatively low, with rapid washout after 30 minutes, which allows subsequent Tc-99m sestamibi imaging.

By combining the I-123 or Tc-99m pertechnetate images and the early and delayed Tc-99m sestamibi images with the same magnification and orientation, one can perform digital subtraction, or at least visual subtraction. In most cases, digital subtraction does not add additional accuracy, since all the information is contained in the unprocessed thyroid and sestamibi images. Some laboratories have used simultaneous dual-energy windows (159 keV for I-123 and 140 keV for Tc-99m sestamibi imaging) in order to eliminate error

due to patient motion and positioning differences [17]. Each image is taken for approximately 10 minutes. The resulting combination is shown in Figure 21.1.

The procedure should be explained to the patient, and the importance of preventing patient motion during the study, particularly important for the dual-isotope techniques when the subtraction method is used. Patients who are unable or unwilling to remain completely immobilized during the study may require sedation.

Patients with intact thyroid glands taking thyroid hormone supplementation should be instructed to withhold taking levothyroxine for about a week in advance of the study, if it is not contraindicated. It is not required that the patient become frankly hypothyroid, unlike hormone withdrawal for thyroid cancer imaging; only withdrawal long enough to remove the effects of thyroid hormone suppression is necessary. Patients who are shown to be taking thyroid hormone anyway on presentation should proceed to have only a single-isotope, double-phase Tc-99m sestamibi imaging study. If that shows clear-cut identification and localization of the parathyroid adenoma, then it is sufficient. If the single-isotope, double-phase study is not sufficient, then one may inject Tc-99m pertechnetate if the sestamibi has already washed out from the thyroid gland, or perform the thyroid imaging study on another day.

The combined sensitivity of dual-isotope subtraction imaging and double-phase sestamibi imaging protocols from pooled data from articles published in the 1990s was 87% for dual-isotope imaging and 73% for double-phase sestamibi imaging [18]. Nonetheless, single-tracer sestamibi, double-phase imaging is used in most centers, due to lower expense, simplicity, and less time required, despite the fact that subsequent additional studies show higher sensitivity for the combined dual-isotope, double-phase method [19–21]. The combined method also was shown to achieve a lower false-positive rate [20,21]. In our laboratory, we have found the combined dual-isotope and double-phase protocol to offer a slightly higher accuracy [22].

The use of the combined technique is further illustrated in Figure 21.2, which demonstrates a parathyroid adenoma plus a hyperfunctional thyroid nodule, which would have been misinterpreted as a second parathyroid adenoma if only a single-isotope, double-phase protocol had been used. Figure 21.3 shows a parathyroid adenoma in the setting of a multinodular gland, a particularly challenging situation for the single-tracer method. Figure 21.4 illustrates the finding of a double adenoma, easily detected with the combined technique. Figure 21.5 shows uniform uptake on either the I-123 or Tc-99m sestamibi scan, with uniform washout. Careful comparison of the I-123 and early sestamibi images shows excess sestamibi uptake at the lower portion of the right lobe, representing a mismatch, which turned out to be a small parathyroid adenoma, confirmed with an ultrasound and then histological examination on surgery.

It is not unusual to obtain a negative result. This does not mean that the patient does not have hyperparathyroidism. It means that either the parathyroid adenoma is too

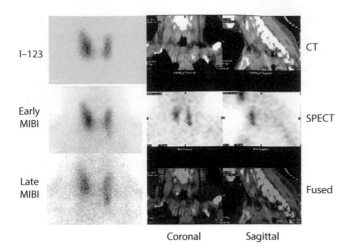

Figure 21.2 Parathyroid adenoma at the lower pole of the left thyroid lobe plus a nontoxic hyperfunctional thyroid nodule: A faint focus of activity is seen at the lower pole of the early MIBI image, not seen on the iodine-123 image, that becomes more prominent on the delayed MIBI image, further localized on the SPECT-CT images, consistent with a parathyroid adenoma. In addition, there is a focus of increased uptake in the mid-lower portion of the right lobe on both early MIBI and late MIBI images that might have been misinterpreted as a second parathyroid adenoma, were it not for the iodine-123 image, which showed it to be a nontoxic hyperfunctional nodule.

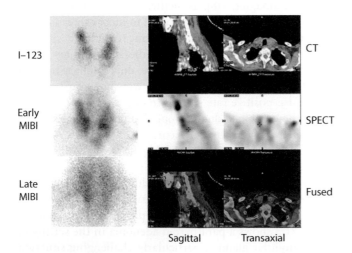

Figure 21.3 Parathyroid adenoma in the setting of a nodular thyroid: The iodine-123 image shows multiple foci of both increased and decreased uptake. The early MIBI image shows increased focal uptake in the middle of the right lobe, and middle of the left lobe, as well as mild uptake below the lower pole of the left lobe, and at the lower pole of the right lobe, corresponding to a hypofunctional area on the iodine-123 scan. The delayed MIBI image shows retention in only one region, the lower pole of the right lobe. This focus localizes inferior and quite posterior to the lower pole of the right lobe on the SPECT-CT images, raising the suspicion for a descended superior parathyroid.

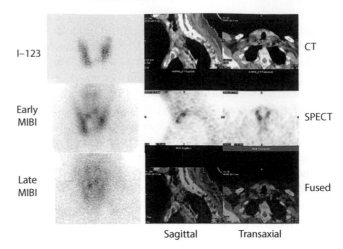

Figure 21.4 Double parathyroid adenomas: The iodine-123 image shows uniform uptake. The early MIBI image shows increased uptake in the middle of the left thyroid lobe, as well as two foci, each medial to upper portions of the right and left thyroid lobes, respectively. The latter two foci retain activity on the delayed MIBI image, while the activity from the thyroid washes out nearly completely. The SPECT-CT images only localize the right-sided focus, which is discretely posterior and medial to the upper portion of the right thyroid lobe.

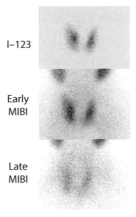

Figure 21.5 The iodine-123 study shows a normal thyroid gland. The early MIBI image shows uniform uptake, that uniformly washes out on the delayed MIBI image, seemingly negative. Careful comparison of the iodine-123 and early MIBI images shows excess MIBI uptake at the lower portion of the right lobe, representing a mismatch, which turned out to be a small parathyroid adenoma, confirmed with an ultrasound and then histological examination on surgery.

small to detect or it represents parathyroid hyperplasia. One must be sure to look carefully at the mediastinal or chest SPECT images for a possible ectopic adenoma. The clinician may obtain an ultrasound examination to try to detect parathyroid tissue, or follow up the patient and repeat the examination in 6–12 months. Another option is to perform a surgical exploration. If the parathyroid scan suggests a possible but not clear-cut adenoma, such as in Figure 21.5, this can be used to guide the surgeon to look for it in that

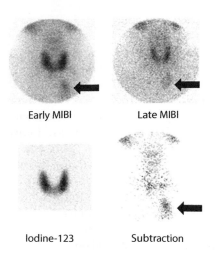

Early MIBI   Late MIBI

Iodine-123   Subtraction

Figure 21.6 Ectopic parathyroid adenoma: 26-year-old female patient with multiple physical and behavioral problems was found to have hypercalcemia. The parathyroid scan study shows uniform uptake in the iodine-123 image and the early MIBI image. The delayed image shows uniform washout from the thyroid gland. There is a focus of increased abnormal uptake on the early and late MIBI and subtraction images in the upper left chest, not present on the iodine-123 image, consistent with an ectopic parathyroid adenoma. The thoracic surgeon performed endoscopic surgery, 2 hours after the patient was injected pre-operatively with another dose of MIBI. The surgeon was unable to find the lesion until he used a gamma probe, which localized it within a portion of the thymus. A 1.0 cm lesion was found, with probe counts 10 times higher than background activity. At 20 min after resection with a partial thymectomy, the PTH level fell by 90%.

location. If confirmed, it may be removed. Intraoperative PTH assays allow the surgeon to determine if removal of that parathyroid gland results in an effective decrease in circulating PTH level. If not, the surgeon can proceed to explore on the other side. Situations like these undoubtedly represent a clinical challenge.

The dual-phase sestamibi images are also helpful in guiding the surgeon with an intraoperative handheld probe, both in the thyroid bed and elsewhere for ectopic glands, several hours after sestamibi injection, if it is documented that the parathyroid adenoma shows a high degree of retention on the delayed images. On the other hand, if the parathyroid adenoma shows rapid washout, then a sestamibi injection should be planned immediately before surgery, or even intraoperatively. Figure 21.6 illustrates an example of an ectopic parathyroid adenoma, where parathyroid scintigraphy was indispensable in locating the lesion and helping the surgeon find it intraoperatively, with a handheld gamma probe.

Tc-99m tetrofosmine imaging

It was subsequently demonstrated that Tc-99m tetrofosmine, a myocardial perfusion imaging agent with properties similar to those of Tc-99m sestamibi, also localizes in both functioning thyroid and parathyroid tissues, and can be used for parathyroid imaging. In contrast to Tc-99m sestamibi, with Tc-99m tetrofosmine there is no differential washout between thyroid and parathyroid tissue using the dual-isotope subtraction procedure. Therefore, Tc-99m tetrofosmine imaging must be used only in the setting of dual-tracer imaging, in conjunction with I-123 of Tc-99m pertechnetate thyroid imaging [23,24]. For that reason, use of Tc-99m tetrofosmine is not recommended if Tc-99m sestamibi is available [3].

SPECT-CT imaging

The most significant advance in the last 10–12 years in scintigraphic imaging in hyperparathyroidism has been the widespread availability and use of SPECT-CT, i.e., the combination of three-dimensional SPECT scintigraphy with CT imaging. CT imaging varies in quality from very low-dose, relatively poor-quality CT, through intermediate levels of quality, all the way to a full-fledged diagnostic CT. SPECT-CT imaging is usually performed between the early and delayed planar sestamibi imaging. It takes approximately 25 minutes. Its use is illustrated in Figures 21.1 through 21.4.

A disadvantage of a single SPECT acquisition is that by the time one acquires the study, the parathyroid adenoma may have already washed out, if featuring rapid washout, or to the contrary, there may not have been sufficient time for tracer localization in the adenoma, if it features slow late accumulation. Some laboratories acquire two SPECT-CT images, one at 10 minutes after injection and another at 1.5–2.5 hours later as a double-phase SPECT-CT study, without planar imaging. We prefer planar pinhole images, since pinhole imaging provides superior resolution compared with SPECT imaging, for detection, with SPECT imaging used to provide localization.

SPECT and SPECT-CT imaging have been markedly augmented recently by newer reconstruction techniques. As opposed to traditional filtered back-projection, iterative reconstruction has improved resolution while suppressing noise. Subsequently, novel "wide-beam" reconstruction techniques that incorporate the gamma camera-collimator resolution dependence on depth, and patient-specific internal attenuation and scatter characteristics, combined with the iterative reconstruction technique, have achieved superior resolution and noise suppression, greatly enhancing resolution or reducing acquisition times or reducing the administered patient radiotracer dosage [25,26].

EFFICACY OF RADIONUCLIDE PARATHYROID IMAGING

The sensitivity and specificity of parathyroid imaging, both single-tracer, dual-phase sestamibi, and the dual-isotope, double-phase technique, have already been discussed at some length. In the literature prior to the year 2000, the average sensitivity of multiple reports is reported as 90.7%, and the specificity 98.7% [6]. This should be qualified with caution since these studies involved a wide range of instrumentation types and a variety of techniques in their details, as well as a variety of patient types. In addition, the accuracy should be qualified with the requirement that not only the presence of an adenoma is determined, but also its location, and not just right and left sides of the thyroid bed versus ectopic locations, but also superior, middle, and inferior, anterior and posterior, thyroid beds, if the results are to be used to guide minimally invasive surgery, as well as for multiglandular disease. Whether SPECT improves sensitivity is debatable. Published results have been variable [27].

Double or multiple adenomas

Double adenomas occur in up to 12% of cases of primary hyperparathyroidism [28]. Double adenomas are bilateral in 55%–88% of cases (see Figure 21.4). Preoperative detection of double or multiple adenomas is not very reliable with any imaging technique. Tc-99m sestamibi imaging has less than 37% sensitivity for detection of all multiple adenomas [29–31].

Causes of false-positive studies

The interpretation of either sestamibi double-phase or dual-isotope, double-phase studies is straightforward when the thyroid uptake is uniform. Thyroid nodules are a common cause of false-positive studies. Most thyroid nodules show decreased uptake on the thyroid scan, if available, and increased uptake on the early sestamibi scan. Thyroid adenomas and carcinomas typically show washout in parallel with normal thyroid tissue, thus differentiating them from parathyroid adenomas (Figures 21.2 through 21.4), but variations exist, with thyroid nodules showing delayed retention, and parathyroid adenomas showing rapid washout. One can maintain accuracy by carefully paying attention to localization and relative washout rates.

Reactive cervical lymph nodes can represent false-positive findings [6]. Likewise, uptake in a portion of the right atrium, in the right parasternal region on planar views, which shows relatively increased uptake in as many as 40%–50% of subjects, can cause false-positive findings, and less frequently, uptake in the superoanterior portion of the right ventricle can cause misinterpretation as ectopic parathyroid tissue [32]. False positives can be seen in hyperplastic thymus, sarcoidosis, carcinoid tumor, and other malignant tumors of the thyroid and neighboring structures.

Sources of error include patient motion. When image subtraction is used, image misregistration may cause error. Careful examination of the original thyroid images (I-123 or Tc-99m pertechnetate) and sestamibi images helps resolve any discrepancies, since they contain all the relevant information.

False-negative studies

False-negative studies may occur when the parathyroid adenomas are smaller than 500 mg, with hyperplastic parathyroid glands, ectopic adenomas (the entire neck and chest should be imaged), and thyroid lesions, adenomas or carcinomas, which may be indistinguishable from parathyroid lesions, and parathyroid carcinomas, indistinguishable from other parathyroid lesions. Cystic adenomas, which comprise less than 9% of all parathyroid adenomas, have a smaller density of active tissue due to cystic degeneration and may not be visualized on scintigraphic studies [33]. A similar problem may be encountered with lipodenomas [34]. The case illustrated in Figure 21.5 would have represented a false-negative study had only a single-isotope, double-phase method been used.

Recently administered iodinated contrast agents may interfere with I-123 or Tc-99m pertechnetate uptake, thus decreasing the sensitivity of dual-isotope techniques. Concomitant administration of thyroid hormone, at doses that cause suppression of uptake, can interfere with this technique.

Previous thyroidectomy can pose a problem, causing disruption of local anatomy. Confusion will be introduced by the presence of unresected, unablated thyroid remnants. Further confusion may be caused when parathyroid glands have been transplanted to the arm. After autotransplantation, recurrent hyperparathyroidism occurs in approximately 14% of cases. A hyperfunctioning graft is demonstrated by ultrasound or Tc-99m sestamibi scintigraphy, if its presence is known [35].

CLINICAL USE OF RADIONUCLIDE PARATHYROID IMAGING

With improvement in sensitivity of parathyroid imaging with either single-isotope, double-phase Tc-99m sestamibi, or dual-isotope, dual-phase studies, along with localization with SPECT-CT imaging, parathyroid scintigraphy has become popular among surgeons preoperatively. This is aided by access to imaging data via hospital information technology, and wide-screen display monitors in the operating room. The question has shifted from an initial emphasis on accuracy of diagnosis to one of guiding the surgeon for a unilateral exploration, or minimally invasive parathyroidectomy. One challenge is the presence of multiple adenomas, which show decreased sensitivity with scintigraphy, which may be supplemented with ultrasound. Another challenge is proper identification of ectopic parathyroid adenomas, which are difficult to find by means other than scintigraphy [36].

SPECT-CT not only helps localize lesions with respect to the thyroid gland (Figures 21.1 through 21.4), but also helps localize the focus of sestamibi uptake with respect to other anatomical structures in the neck and chest. In the case of ectopic lesions, this is invaluable in helping to guide surgical resection. For adenomas located in the neck, one can sometimes see the enlarged gland directly on the CT scan.

Parathyroid adenomas demonstrate typical location of the glands in 80%–90% of cases. The inferior parathyroid glands have a more widespread localization, closely related to the migration of the thymus, inferior, posterior, or lateral to the lower [37] pole of the thyroid, accounting for most ectopic glands (see example in Figure 21.6). A superior parathyroid adenoma may have an abnormal superoposterior mediastinal position, such as retropharyngeal, retroesophageal, or paraesophageal location (see example in Figure 21.3). The frequency of ectopia for these glands is 39% of all ectopic glands, versus 61% for inferior gland adenomas. The more common ectopic inferior parathyroids are responsible for 10%–13% of all cases of hyperparathyroidism. The location of ectopic tissue ranges from the angle of the jaw to the mediastinum, thymus, aortopulmonary window, carotid bifurcation, carotid sheath, and pericardium [38].

SPECT-CT localization can help guide the surgical approach, aside from simple localization per se, left versus right and superior versus inferior location, and it can even distinguish inferior gland adenoma from a descended superior gland. In our laboratory, we [39] have found that the more posteriorly located (at the lower thyroid pole level) on the SPECT images the lesion is, the higher the probability of a descended superior retroesophageal solitary parathyroid adenoma (see example in Figure 21.3). This observation, if taken advantage of, can have a significant impact on the planned surgical route and potentially reduce the extent of exploratory dissection. In the mediastinum, accurate localization may assist in directing the surgical approach, such as median sternotomy versus left or right thoracotomy.

Norman et al. [40] studied 17 patients referred for persistent hyperparathydism following an unsuccessful neck exploration. All patients had sestamibi imaging preoperatively and intraoperatively, and were deemed at the time false positive. Nonetheless, after the surgery, all showed persistence of the abnormal focus. In all these patients, the parathyroid adenoma was successfully removed with guided minimally invasive surgery. Sestamibi imaging in patients with persistent or recurrent hyperparathyroidism appears to be useful in localizing previously unidentified parathyroid lesions in the neck or in ectopic locations in the chest, before a second operation [41–44].

One important impact of scintigraphic imaging, as mentioned above, is in decreasing operative time. In a summary of 15 articles in 753 patients, the average operative time for standard bilateral exploration was 109 ± 29 minutes, compared with 49 ± 5 minutes for a limited resection using sestamibi localization in three articles [6]. Norman et al. [45] reported surgery times of 127 minutes versus 90 minutes respectively. Hindie et al. [17] report the average surgery times reduced from 120 minutes to 90 minutes with guidance of sestamibi imaging. Gupta et al. [46] reported the total operative time of 49 ± 21 minutes for unilateral neck exploration guided by preoperative sestamibi imaging, compared with 103 ± 45 minutes for bilateral neck operation. An additional benefit is the potential use of local anesthesia versus general anesthesia, contributing to reduced costs, length of stay, and complications, albeit counterbalanced by the cost of PTH assays and ultrasound.

Intraoperative probe-guided localization

Some surgeons have found the use of an intraoperative handheld radiation probe useful in rapid localization of the parathyroid adenoma. Despite other imaging options, such as CT, MRI, and ultrasound, being available, scintigraphic guidance can be a useful tool in this application [47–49]. The patient is injected 2 hours before surgery, and the probe is used to detect the lesion, first by scanning before skin incision, and then after initial exploration [50,51]. Success is likely to be maximized when preoperative Tc-99m sestamibi imaging demonstrates a high degree of retention of Tc-99m sestamibi in the parathyroid adenoma on delayed imaging. Probe use is limited when the lesion shows rapid washout. Although there are individual instances of the usefulness, probe-directed localization of parathyroid adenomas, such as in the case of the ectopic parathyroid adenoma shown in Figure 21.6, probe-directed parathyroid surgery has not been widely adopted and has been abandoned by most high-volume endocrine surgeons.

UNRESOLVED ISSUES

There is clear consensus that Tc-99m sestamibi double-phase parathyroid imaging is superior to thallium-201 imaging [3]. Although dual-isotope, double-phase sestamibi imaging has been shown to yield superior accuracy compared with single-isotope, double-phase sestamibi imaging, there is no consensus on its use, after taking into account not only the standard measures of accuracy, but also cost, time of equipment usage, patient's time, and patient comfort. In our laboratory, we have continued to use the dual-isotope, dual-phase imaging whenever possible. Numerous published reports support the use of this technique for directing a minimally invasive unilateral neck exploration with or without intraoperative probe utilization.

The most difficult challenge to the detection and localization of parathyroid tissues is still posed by patients with multiple adenoma, hyperplastic parathyroid glands, recurrent or persistent hyperparathyroidism, and ectopic adenomas. Because these patients frequently have already had one or more previous neck operations, reoperation and reexploration is more difficult. With ectopic parathyroid tissue being more prevalent in this population, localization is a challenge for all parathyroid imaging.

Some surgeons and clinicians advocate the use of combined ultrasound and scintigraphy to enhance the detection accuracy of parathyroid adenomas, in the case of double adenomas, and use CT and MRI in the case of ectopic adenomas. While the combined use of multiple imaging modalities is comprehensive and likely to enhance overall accuracy, their routine combined use is not necessarily cost-effective for primary hyperparathyroidism; their use is probably justified in special challenging cases [52].

Positron emission tomography (PET) imaging has been investigated for detection and localization of parathyroid glands. The experience with ^{18}F-fluorodeoxyglucose (FDG) PET imaging has been mixed [53,54]. C-11 methionine PET has shown to be more promising than FDG. Sundin et al. reported in 32 patients a sensitivity of 85% for localization [55]. Beggs and Hain reported a sensitivity of 88% and specificity of 100% in 51 patients in whom other imaging modalities, including Tc-99m sestamibi, had failed [56]. Much additional work needs to be done to explore the usefulness of this novel methodology.

REFERENCES

1. Heath H III. Clinical spectrum of primary hyperparathyroidism: Evolution with changes in medical practice and technology. *J Bone Miner Res* 1991;6:S63–S70.
2. Wells SA Jr, Ashley SW. The parathyroid glands. In: Sabiston DC Jr, ed., *Textbook of Surgery: The Biological Basis of Modern Surgical Practice.* 14th ed. Philadelphia: WB Saunders Company, 1991:598–615.
3. Greenspan BS, Dillehay G, Intenzo C et al. SNM practice guideline for parathyroid scintigraphy 4.0. *J Nucl Med Technol* 2012;40:1–8.
4. Consensus Development Conference Panel. Diagnosis and management of asymptomatic primary hyperparathyroidism: Consensus development conference statement. *Ann Intern Med* 1991;114:593–7.
5. Assalia A, Inabnet WB. Endoscopic parathyroidectomy. *Otolaryngol Clin North Am* 2004;37:871–86.
6. Denham DW, Norman J. Cost-effectiveness of preoperative sestamibi scan for primary hyperparathyroidism is dependent solely upon the surgeon's choice of operative procedure. *J Am Coll Surg* 1998;186:293–305.
7. Majors JD, Burke GJ, Mansberger AR et al. Technetium Tc-99m sestamibi scan for localizing abnormal parathyroid glands after previous neck operations: Preliminary experience in reoperative cases. *South Med J* 1995;88:327–30.
8. Ferlin G, Borsato N, Camerani M et al. New perspectives in localizing enlarged parathyroids by technetium-thallium subtraction scan. *J Nucl Med* 1983;24:438–41.
9. Harty M, Swartz K, McClung M et al. Technetium-thallium scintiscanning for localization of parathyroid adenomas and hyperplasia. A re-appraisal. *Am J Surg* 1987;153:479–86.
10. Piwnica-Worms D, Kronauge JF, Chiu ML. Uptake and retention of hexakis (2-methoxyisobutyl isonitrile) technetium(I) in cultured chick myocardial cells. Mitochondrial and plasma membrane potential dependence. *Circulation* 1990;82:1826–38.
11. Piwnica-Worms D, Chiu ML, Bidding M, Kronauge JF, Kramer RA, Croop JM. Functional imaging of multidrug resistant P-glycoprotein with an organo-technetium complex. *Cancer Res* 1993;53:977–84.
12. Carpentier A, Jeannotte S, Verrault J et al. Preoperative localization of parathyroid lesions in hyperparathyroidism: Relationship between technetium-99m-MIBI and oxyphil cell count. *J Nucl Med* 1998;39:1441–4.
13. Taillefer R, Boucher Y, Potvin C et al. Detection and localization of parathyroid adenomas in patients with hyperparathyroidism using a single radionuclide imaging procedure with technetium-99m-sestamibi (double-phase study). *J Nucl Med* 1992;33:1801–7.
14. O'Doherty MJ, Kettle AJ, Wells P et al. Parathyroid imaging with technetium-99m-sestamibi: Preoperative localization and tissue uptake studies. *J Nucl Med* 1992;33:313–8.
15. Taillefer R, Lambert R, Essiambre R et al. Comparison between thallium-201, technetium-99m-sestamibi and technetium-99m-teboroxime planar myocardial perfusion imaging in detection of coronary artery disease. *J Nucl Med* 1992;33:1091–8.
16. Coakley AJ. Nuclear medicine and parathyroid surgery: A change in practice. *Nucl Med Commun* 2003;24:111–3.
17. Hindie E, Melliere D, Jeangillaume C, Perlemuter L, Galle P. Parathyroid imaging using double-window recording of technetium-99m-sestamibi and iodine-123. *J Nucl Med* 1998;39:1100–5.
18. McBiles M, Lambert AT, Core MG et al. Sestamibi parathyroid imaging. *Semin Nucl Med* 1995;25:221–34.
19. Chen CC, Skarulis MC, Fraker DL, Alexander R, Marx SJ, Spiegel AM. Technetim-99m-sestamibi imaging before reoperation for primary hyperparathyroidism. *J Nucl Med* 1995;36:2186–91.
20. Neumann DR, Esselstyn CB Jr, Go RT et al. Comparison of double-phase 99mTc-sestamibi with 123I-99mTc-sestamibi subtraction SPECT in hyperparathyroidism. *AJR AM J Roengenol* 1997;169:1671–4.
21. Chen CC, Holder LE, Scovill WA et al. Comparison of parathyroid imaging with technetium-99m pertechnetate/sestamibi substraction double phase technetium-99m-sestamibi and technetium-99m-sestamibi SPECT. *J Nucl Med* 1997;38:834–49.
22. Kim CK, Kim S, Krynyckyi BR et al. Efficacy of sestamibi parathyroid scintigraphy for directing surgical approaches based on modified interpretation criteria. *Clin Nucl Med* 2002;27:246–8.

23. Froeberg AC, Valkema R, Bonjer HU et al. Tc-99m tetrofosmin or Tc-99m sestamibi for double-phase parathyroid scintigraphy? *Eur J Nucl Med Mol Imaging* 2003;30:193–6.

24. Wakamatsu H, Noguchi S, Yamashita H et al. Technetium-99m tetrofosmin for parathyroid scintigraphy: A direct comparison with Tc-99m MIBI, Tl-201, MRI and US. *Eur J Nucl Med* 2001;28:1817–27.

25. Borges-Neto S, Pagnanelli RA, Shaw LK et al. Clinical results of a novel wide-beam reconstruction method for shortening scan time of Tc-99m cardiac SPECT perfusion studies. *J Nucl Cardiol* 2007;14:555–65.

26. Druz RS, Phillips LM, Chugkowski M et al. Wide-beam reconstruction half-time SPECT improves diagnostic certainty and preserved normalcy and accuracy: A quantitative perfusion analysis. *J Nucl Cardiol* 2011;18:52–61.

27. Nichols KJ, Thomas MB, Tronco GG et al. Optimizing the accuracy of preoperative parathyroid lesion localization. *Radiology* 2008;248:221–32.

28. Tazelman S, Shen W, Shaver JK. Double parathyroid adenomas: Clinical and biochemical characteristics before and after parathyroidectomy. *Ann Surg* 1993;218:300–9.

29. Clark OH, Duh QY. Primary hyperparathyroidism: A surgical perspective. *Endocrinol Metab Clin North Am* 1989;18:701–14.

30. McHenry CR, Lee K, Saadey J et al. Parathyroid localization with technetium-99m sestamibi: A prospective evaluation. *J Am Coll Surg* 1996;183:25–30.

31. Bergenfelz A, Tennvall J, Valdemarsson S et al. Sestamibi versus thallium subtraction scintigraphy in parathyroid localization: A prospective comparative study in patients with predominantly mild primary hyperparathyroidism. *Surgery* 1997;121:601–5.

32. Kim CK, Jung E, Youn M et al. A normal variant on thallium-201/Tc-99m MIBI whole body imaging: The superior right atrial wall (auricle) and superoanterior right ventricular wall are often seen as mediastinal lesions. *Clin Nucl Med* 2001;26:412–8.

33. Rogers LA, Fetter BF, Peete WPJ. Parathyroid cyst and cystic degeneration of parathyroid adenoma. *Arch Pathol* 1969;88:476–9.

34. Turner WJD, Baergen RN, Pelliteri PK et al. Parathyroid lipoadenoma: Case report and review of the literature. *Otolaryngol Head Neck Surg* 1996;114:313–6.

35. Lee VS, Spritzer CE, Coleman RE et al. Hyperparathyroidism in high-risk surgical patients: Evaluation with double-phase technetium-99m sestamibi imaging. *Radiology* 1995;197:627–33.

36. Oh SY, Kim S, Eskandar Y et al. Appearance of intrathymic parathyroid adenomas on pinhole sestamibi parathyroid imaging. *Clin Nucl Med* 2006;31:127–30.

37. Wang CA. The anatomic basis of parathyroid surgery. *Ann Surg* 1976;183:271–5.

38. Thomson NW, Eckhauser FE, Harness JK. The anatomy of primary hyperparathyroidism. *Surgery* 1982;92:814–21.

39. Kim SC, Kim S, Inabnet WB et al. Appearance of descended superior parathyroid adenoma on SPECT parathyroid imaging. *Clin Nucl Med* 2007;32:90–3.

40. Norman JG, Jaffray CE, Chheda H. The false-positive parathyroid sestamibi: A real or perceived problem and a case for radioguided parathyroidectomy. *Ann Surg* 2000;231:31–7.

41. Ishibashi M, Nishida H, Hiromatsu Y et al. Localization of ectopic parathyroid glands using technetium-99m sestamibi imaging: Comparison with magnetic resonance and computed tomographic imaging. *Eur J Nucl Med* 1997;24:197–201.

42. Cheung AH, Wheeler MS, Madanay LD et al. Multi-center sestamibi parathyroid imaging study in Hawaii. *Hawaii Med J* 1997;56:114–7.

43. Fayet P, Hoeffel C, Flla Y et al. Technetium-99m sestamibi scintigraphy, magnetic resonance imaging and venous blood sampling in persistent and recurrent hyperparathyroidism. *Br J Radiol* 1997;70:459–64.

44. Caixas A, Berna L, Hernandez A et al. Efficacy of preoperative diagnostic imaging localization of technetium 99m-sestamibi hyperparathyroidism. *Surgery* 1997;121:535–41.

45. Norman J, Chheda H, Farrell C. Minimally invasive parathyroidectomy for primary hyperparathyroidism: Decreasing operative time and potential complications while improving cosmetic results. *Am Surg* 1998;64:391–5.

46. Gupta VK, Yeh KA, Burke GJ et al. 99m-Technetium sestamibi localized solitary parathyroid adenoma as an indication for limited unilateral surgical exploration. *Am J Surg* 1998;176:409–12.

47. Casas AT, Burke GJ, Sathyanarayna et al. Prospective comparison of technetium-99m-setamibi/iodine-123 radionuclide scan versus high-resolution ultrasonography for the pre-operative localization of abnormal parathyroid glands in patients with previously unoperated primary hyperparathyroidism. *Am J Surg* 1993;166:369–73.

48. Light VL, McHenry CR, Jarjoura D et al. Prospective comparison of dual-phase technetium-99m-sestamibi scintigraphy and high resolution ultrasonography in the evaluation of abnormal parathyroid glands. *Am Surg* 1996;62:562–7.

49. Malhotra A, Silver CE, Deshpande V et al. Preoperative parathyroid localization with sestamibi. *Am J Surg* 1996;172:637–40.

50. Berland T, Smith SL, Huguet KL. Occult fifth gland intrathyroid adenoma identified by gamma probe. *Am Surg* 1005;71:264–6.

51. Ugur O, Bozkurt MF, Hamaloglu E et al. Clinicopathologic and radiopharmacokinetic factors affecting gamma probe-guided parathyroidectomy. *Arch Surg* 2004;139:1175–9.

52. Ruda JM, Stack BC Jr, Hollenbeak CS. The cost-effectiveness of sestamibi scanning compared to bilateral exploration for the treatment of primary hyperparathyroidism. *Otolaryngol Clin North Am* 2004;37:855–70.

53. Neumann DR, Esselstyn CB, MacIntyre WJ et al. Comparison of FDG-PET and sestamibi SPECT in primary hyperparathyroidism. *J Nucl Med* 1996;37:1809–15.

54. Melon PJ, Luxen, Hamoir E et al. Fluorine-18-fluorodeoxyglucose positron emission tomography for preoperative parathyroid imaging in primary hyperparathyroidism. *Eur J Nucl Med* 1995;22:556–8.

55. Sundin A, Johansson C, Hellman P et al. PET and Parathyroid, L-[carbon 11]methionine accumulation in hyperparathyroidism. *J Nucl Med* 1996;37:1766–70.

56. Beggs AD, Hain SF. Localization of parathyroid adenomas using C-11 methionine positron emission tomography. *Nucl Med Commun* 2005;26:133–6.

22

4D-CT for parathyroid localization

READE DE LEACY AND PUNEET S. PAWHA

INTRODUCTION

Minimally invasive (directed) parathyroidectomy (MIP) requires precise preoperative imaging localization of adenomas to be successful. This surgical technique has become the mainstay of surgical treatment for hyperparathyroidism, having been shown to be effective and associated with fewer complications than the classical bilateral cervical exploration (BCE) [1,2]. Further benefits include avoidance of both general anesthesia and overnight hospital admission, reducing the overall healthcare costs associated with the diagnosis and treatment of hyperparathyroidism [1].

Four-dimensional computed tomography (4D-CT) for parathyroid localization was first described in the surgical literature in 2006 [3]. It exploits the dynamic enhancement pattern of adenomatous parathyroid tissue, allowing identification of both eutopic and ectopic parathyroid adenomas. 4D-CT is both a sensitive and a specific test, which can reliably localize single parathroid adenomas to an anatomic quadrant and can often identify patients with multiglandular disease. The largest series published to date reported accurate lateralization of lesions in 86.3% of all cases in their cohort (including surgery-naïve and re-exploration patients) [4]. Its utility in identifying lesions in patients who have had previous surgery or radiotherapy and those with negative sestimibi or ultrasound examinations has also been demonstrated [4,5]. Studies have shown the cost-effectiveness of

4D-CT as a second-line imaging modality after ultrasound or nuclear medicine studies fail to localize a parathyroid lesion [6,7]. Initially, this modality was largely used as a problem-solving tool in patients where conventional parathyroid imaging methods had been inconclusive. As experience with this imaging examination has grown, some have begun to use 4D-CT as an initial localizing study [8].

IMAGING TECHNIQUE AND RELATIVE CONTRAINDICATIONS

Parathyroid 4D-CT is performed as a volumetric multiphase acquisition, typically from the level of the mandibular body superiorly to the level of the carina inferiorly. Combinations of two, three, or four imaging phases have been described [4,9–11], but in general, unenhanced, arterial, and delayed venous phase images are acquired. This technique provides adequate spatial resolution to anatomically localize small lesions in eutopic and ectopic locations and to determine the enhancement characteristic of each potential lesion in order to differentiate between parathyroid adenomas and their most common mimics—lymph nodes and adjacent thyroid tissue or nodules. The enhancement of each potential lesion may be quantified in terms of Hounsfield unit (HU) density (Figure 22.1) on each phase. The arterial phase may also be processed into a three-dimensional (3D) reconstruction to further demonstrate the location of the lesion (Figure 22.2).

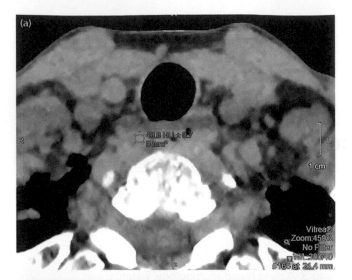

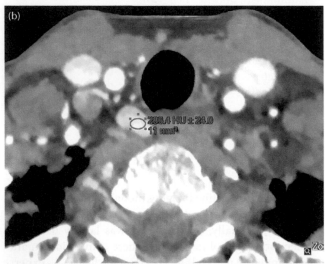

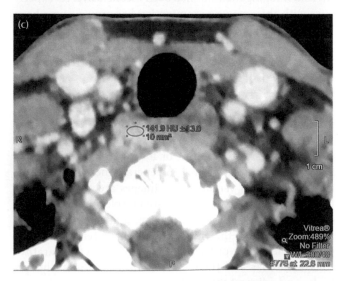

Figure 22.1 Right paraesophageal parathyroid adenoma with characteristic baseline attenuation, which is similar to skeletal muscle **(a)** on the initial noncontrast image. Both subjective assessment and Hounsfield unit values show robust enhancement in the arterial phase **(b)** with prominent washout in the delayed phase **(c)**.

In recent years, various techniques have become available to help reduce the radiation dose associated with CT scanning, including dose modulation and iterative reconstruction. Some recent studies have estimated that the effective dose for parathyroid 4D-CT is roughly 25% more than that of sestimibi scanning [12,13]. However, the radiation dose to the thyroid gland in particular is significantly higher for CT. For this reason, judicious use of 4D-CT is prudent, particularly in younger patients [12]. Utilizing currently available dose reduction techniques, significant steps can be taken to modify protocols and limit radiation exposure associated with this exam.

Prior anaphylactic reaction to iodinated contrast is an absolute contraindication to parathyroid 4D-CT, as this CT exam always requires intravenous contrast. Other allergic history may warrant premedication to reduce the risk of allergic reaction to contrast. Impaired renal function is a relative contraindication, and the decision to image with 4D-CT should be made on a case-by-case basis. In such patients, the benefits of preoperative localization should be balanced against the risk of contrast-induced nephropathy.

APPROACH TO INTERPRETATION

As with all diagnostic tests, a systematic approach to interpretation is required, and parathyroid 4D-CT is no exception. For the purposes of this chapter, we focus on lesion assessment with triple-phase 4D-CT, utilizing unenhanced, arterial, and delayed phases.

The principle underpinning multiphase CT imaging is that certain tissues and lesions can be differentiated by their patterns of dynamic enhancement, evaluating features such as "wash-in" and "washout." Parathyroid adenomas are similar in attenuation to muscle in the unenhanced phase, exhibit avid and rapid enhancement in the arterial phase, and typically demonstrate a degree of de-enhancment, or contrast washout, in the venous or delayed phases. This is in contrast to lymph nodes, which are also similar to muscle in attenuation in the unenhanced phase, but exhibit a more gradual progressive pattern of enhancement through the arterial and delayed phases. Exophytic thyroid tissue and some nodules are intrinsically hyperdense in the unenhanced phase due to the thyroid's inherent iodine content, allowing them to be differentiated from both parathyroid adenomas and lymph nodes.

The following is a stepwise approach to image interpretation.

Step 1. Identify potential lesions on the arterial phase

Parathyroid adenomas demonstrate their peak enhancement during the arterial phase [5,10]. It is for this reason that the arterial phase is the first that should be interrogated. Candidate lesions are typically avidly enhancing round or ovoid soft tissue nodules with lesion CT density

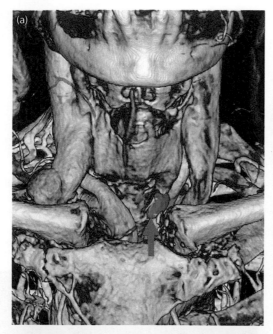

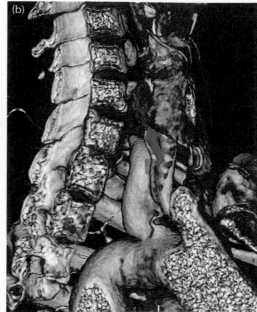

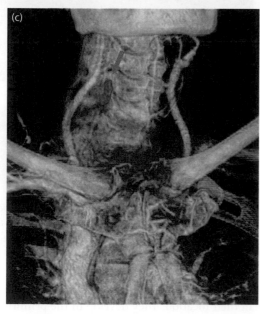

Figure 22.2 3D reformatted images (a–c) from three separate patients with surgically proven parathyroid adenomas (arrows). The raw source images may be processed into 3D reformats that may aid in surgical planning, giving an additional method of visualizing adjacent vascular structures, relations to other viscera, and the bony anatomy.

values of usually more than 100 HU (Figure 22.3). Normal lymph nodes typically demonstrate mild or no enhancement on the early postcontrast phase. The greatest difference in attenuation between parathyroid adenomas and lymph nodes is on the arterial phase. Exophytic thyroid tissue and some nodules will also enhance during the arterial phase, but can often be differentiated from parathyroid using the other available phases.

EUTOPIC GLANDS

Common or eutopic gland locations should be first assessed. The superior glands are usually found in a 2 cm diameter area, located approximately 1 cm above the intersection of the inferior thyroidal artery and recurrent laryngeal nerve, along the posterior aspect of the upper third of the thyroid (approximately 85% of cases) (Figure 22.4).

The inferior glands are more variable in location than the superior glands. In about 50% of cases, they are found within 1 cm inferior, lateral, or posterior to the lower pole of the thyroid. They are characteristically located anterior to the coronal plane of the recurrent laryngeal nerves, even when ectopic [14]. Supernumerary glands are present in up to 3%–13% of the population.

ECTOPIC GLANDS

It must be kept in mind when trying to localize parathyroid disease that up to 15%–20% of parathyroid glands are ectopically located [14,15]. Identifying these ectopic glands requires an understanding of the embryology of the parathyroid.

The superior glands arise from the endoderm of the fourth pharyngeal pouch and in general have less variation

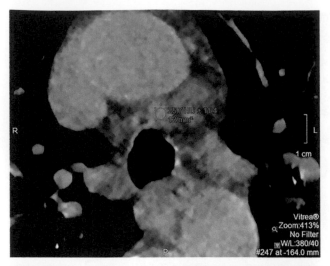

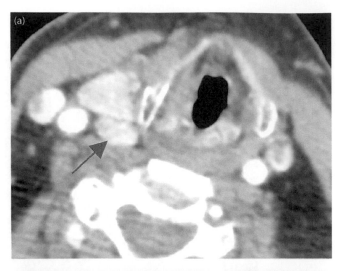

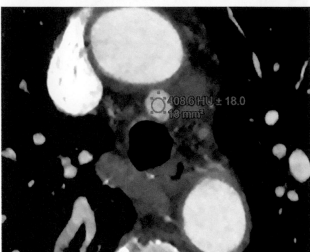

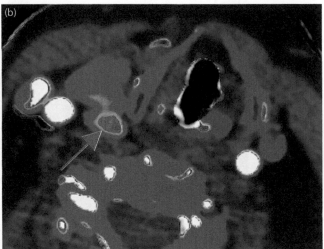

Figure 22.4 **(a)** Eutopic right superior gland parathyroid adenoma (arrow) located along the posterior aspect of the upper pole of the right lobe of thyroid. **(b)** Color map demonstrating a rapid rate of enhancement of the lesion in question.

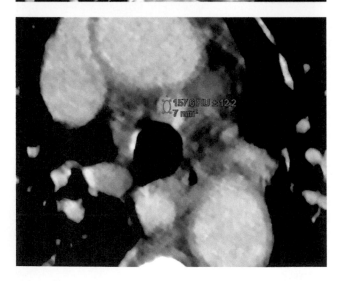

Figure 22.3 Ectopic parathyroid adenoma localized within the aortopulmonary window. Typical morphological features and enhancement characteristics can be seen with a well-demarcated, ovoid lesion that is isodense on the unenhanced phase. The lesion exhibits avid arterial enhancement and prominent washout in the delayed phase. Region of interest measurements show the Hounsfield units with standard deviations.

in their location. They develop in the primitive pharyngeal wall and attach to the thyroid gland accompanying it on its caudal migration. Ectopic superior parathyroid glands typically lie posterior to the coronal plane of the recurrent laryngeal nerves (Figure 22.5). Common locations for parathyroid adenomas include the paraesophageal regions and tracheoesophageal grooves.

The inferior glands arise from the endoderm of the third pharyngeal pouch and have a longer descent than the superior glands. The glands arise from a common origin with the thymus and descend along the thymopharyngeal duct, and in normal development separate from the thymus before it enters the mediastinum. Hence, ectopic inferior glands may be seen anywhere from the soft tissues at the level of the angle of the mandible to the pericardium, with a classic location being the anterior mediastinum (Figure 22.6) [14]. Most commonly,

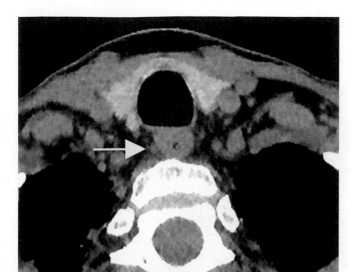

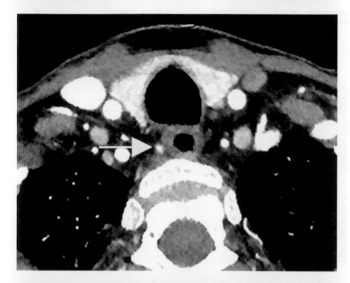

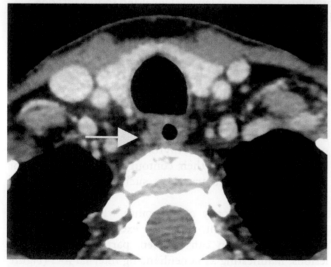

Figure 22.5 Small right-sided parathyroid adenoma (arrow), likely of the upper gland, localized to the posterior aspect of the right paraesophageal region, exhibiting typical enhancement kinetics.

however, ectopic inferior glands are found in the vicinity of the thyroid lower poles. In the younger population, the thymus must be carefully scrutinized, as the inferior glands can rest in any point along the course of the thyrothymic ligament, including within the thymus. They are rarely found superior to the intersection of the recurrent laryngeal nerve and the inferior thyroid artery.

Some uncommon ectopic locations for parathyroid adenomas include retroesophageal, above the level of the thyroid (usually retropharyngeal or parapharyngeal), within the carotid sheath, intrathyroidal, and along the pericardium (Figures 22.7 through 22.9).

In cases of supernumerary glands, the majority (60%–70%) are located inferior to the inferior pole of the thyroid gland, within the thyrothymic ligament. The remaining 30%–40% are located adjacent to the thyroid between the expected normal positions of the superior and inferior glands [14].

Step 2. Interrogate dynamic enhancement pattern of candidate lesions

Once potential lesions have been identified on the arterial phase, the remaining phases should be assessed to determine the lesions' density on the unenhanced acquisition and its overall enhancement kinetics. This may be done by subjective visual comparison of the three phases or by more quantitative means, obtaining Hounsfield unit values (Figure 22.1).

PARATHYROID ADENOMAS

Parathyroid adenomas characteristically demonstrate avid arterial phase enhancement, often with subsequent washout of contrast demonstrated on the delayed phase. They are less dense than the thyroid gland on the unenhanced acquisition (Figure 22.10).

THYROID

Thyroid tissue will normally be hyperdense on the unenhanced images due to its intrinsic iodine content, in contradistinction to parathyroid adenomas. This differentiation is the reason the noncontrast phase is obtained. Thyroid tissue will also typically show avid early enhancement like parathyroid adenomas, but may have less pronounced contrast washout on the delayed phase, which can in some cases aid in differentiation from parathyroid lesions (Figure 22.11).

Thyroid nodules are a heterogeneous group including thyroid adenomas, cysts, and other lesions, and have variable dynamic enhancement characteristics. That being said, most thyroid lesions will not follow the characteristic pattern seen with parathyroid adenomas, although there may be some overlap. In these problematic cases, it may be helpful to further interrogate the volumetric data set with varying reformatted planes to better determine whether the lesion is extrathyroidal.

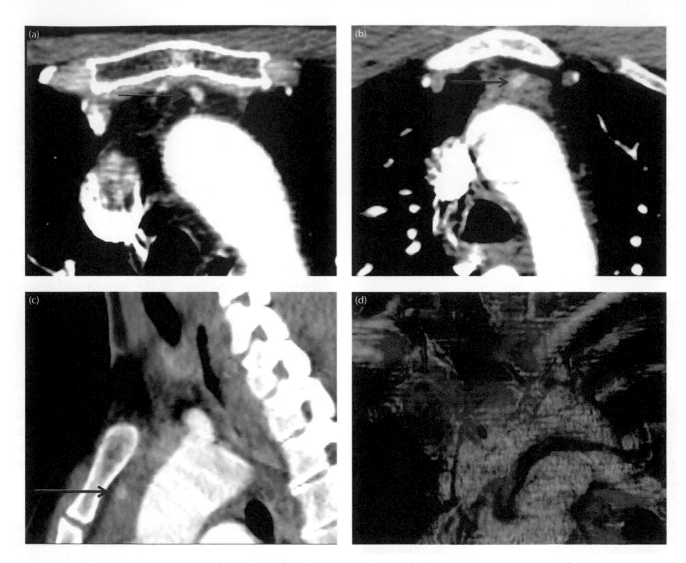

Figure 22.6 Two separate patients with ectopic inferior gland parathyroid adenomas (arrows) localized to the anterior mediastinum. Patient 1 **(a)** shows an avidly enhancing ectopic adenoma surrounded by anterior mediastinal fat on arterial phase imaging. Patient 2 **(b–d)** shows a similar avidly enhancing ectopic adenoma embedded within residual thymic tissue.

LYMPH NODES

Lymph nodes exhibit more gradual and less intense enhancement than parathyroid adenomas. They typically show only mild enhancement on the early postcontrast phase, and often increase in density by the delayed phase. There is usually no significant washout of contrast seen.

Step 3. Assess lesion morphology, variants, and ancillary features

CT allows us to assess various additional imaging characteristics of parathyroid lesions, including size and morphology. This information is relevant for the surgeon and the pathologist, but can also increase confidence in identifying the lesion correctly. Typical characteristics of parathyroid adenoma include

- Ovoid shape
- Sharply delineated margins
- Homogeneous enhancement

However, variation in shape is not uncommon. Other commonly encountered lesion shapes include teardrop, discoid, and elongated (Figure 22.12). Lesions typically have a sharply defined contour, which is not uncommonly gently lobulated. Occasionally, lesions may have more pronounced lobulations. Parathyroid adenomas also tend to be "soft" lesions, and their contour may be deformed or flattened by adjacent structures, such as the esophagus or vessels.

While the majority of adenomas will exhibit homogeneous enhancement, there are exceptions to the rule. Cystic degeneration can be seen, particularly in larger lesions, manifesting as nonenhancing internal foci (Figure 22.13). Hyperfunctioning parathyroid cysts have also been described, which demonstrate only thin peripheral, if any, enhancement. Intralesional calcification is uncommon, although its presence does not exclude the diagnosis.

Another imaging sign that can be used to increase confidence in diagnosis is the presence of a prominent feeding

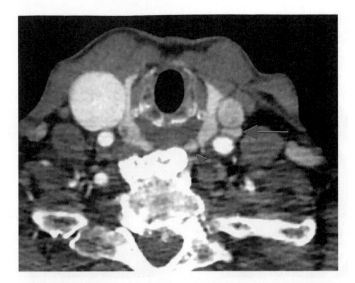

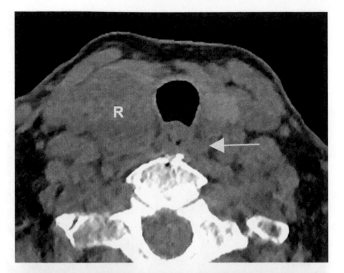

Figure 22.7 Ectopic parathyroid adenoma (arrow) interposed between the left common carotid artery and left internal jugular vein. The lesion is deformed by the adjacent vessels, reflecting the soft nature of these lesions. On surgery, the adenoma was found to be within the left carotid sheath. The patient also has a second smaller adenoma along the posteromedial aspect of the left thyroid lobe (arrowhead).

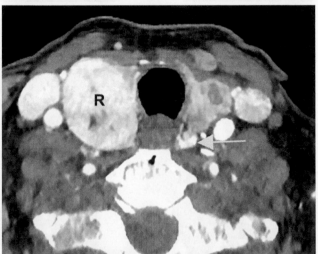

artery to the lesion, also known as the "polar vessel" sign (Figure 22.14) [15,16]. The feeding vessel is usually a branch that arises from the inferior thyroidal artery and enters the parathyroid adenoma at either of its poles (Figure 22.15). This vessel gives off perforating branches along the margin of the gland. This is in contrast to lymph nodes that characteristically have small hilar vessels.

Step 4. Do the findings make sense anatomically and clinically?

Reference should be made to any previous imaging and any history of previous parathyroid surgery. Previous operative notes may provide useful information if available, and can help the interpreting physician better direct his or her search. It is useful to know which glands have been previously removed in patients with prior surgery. In most cases, there should be one dominant candidate for parathyroid adenoma on the imaging study, since approximately 85% of cases of primary hyperparathyroidism result from a single hyperfunctioning gland. There are, of course, a minority of cases with multigland disease, and one should continue to search for additional possible lesions after a single lesion is localized. There should, however, only be one potential candidate to each quadrant.

CHALLENGES AND PITFALLS

Radiologists and clinicians need to be aware of the challenges and pitfalls associated with interpretation of parathyroid 4D-CT to ensure accuracy and reproducible results.

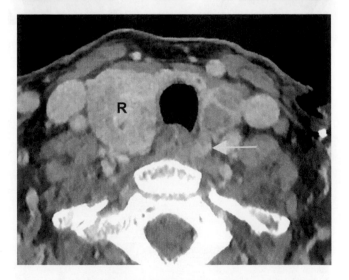

Figure 22.8 Multigland disease with a large right-sided intrathyroidal parathyroid adenoma (R), which is subtly hypodense compared with the adjacent normal thyroid tissue on noncontrast phase. There is also a smaller left lower gland adenoma (arrow) in a more characteristic location. Both lesions enhance greater than the remainder of the thyroid tissue on early postcontrast phase.

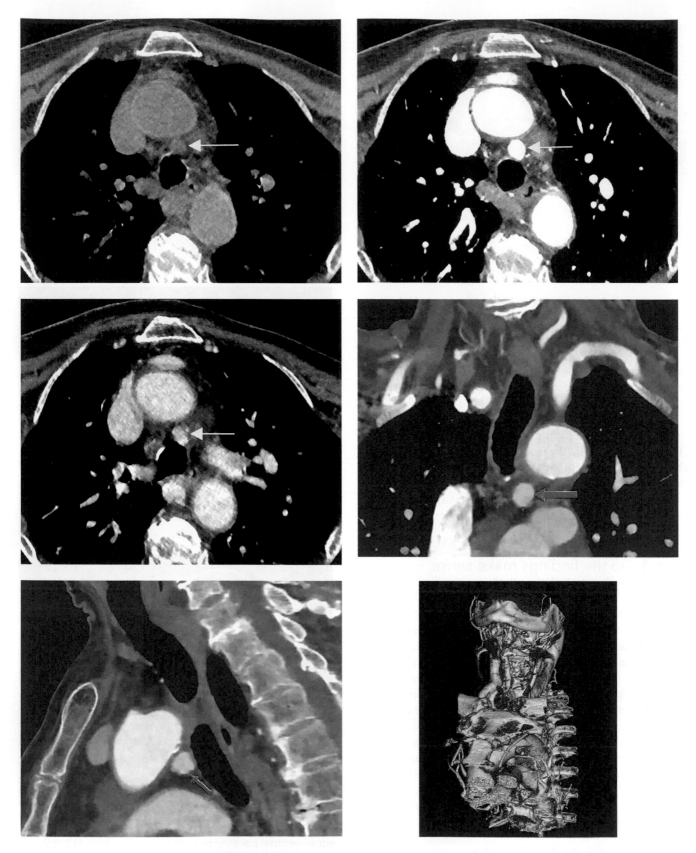

Figure 22.9 Ectopic inferior gland parathyroid adenoma (arrow) localized to the aortopulmonary window within the middle mediastinum. The lesion demonstrates characteristic morphology and enhancement kinetics.

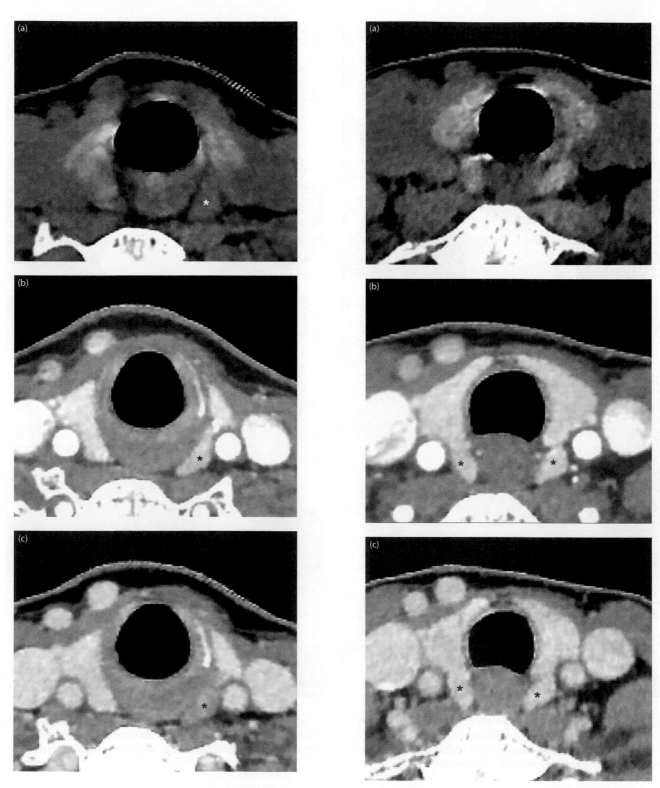

Figure 22.10 Left inferior gland eutopic parathyroid adenoma (*) with characteristic enhancement characteristics. On the arterial phase alone, this would be difficult to differentiate from exophytic thyroid tissue (as seen in Figure 22.12b). With dynamic CT scanning, one can see the lesion is hypodense compared with adjacent normal thyroid tissue on the unenhanced phase **(a)** due to the thyroid gland's inherent iodine content. The lesion enhances robustly in the arterial phase **(b)** and shows washout in the delayed phase **(c)**.

Figure 22.11 Bilateral lower lobe exophytic thyroid nodules and tissue (*). Both right and left potential lesions are isodense to the adjacent normal thyroid tissue on the unenhanced study **(a)**, indicating inherent iodine content. Both potential lesions also show identical patterns of enhancement to the adjacent thyroid gland in the arterial **(b)** and delayed **(c)** phases. On the arterial phase alone, these may be difficult to distinguish from parathyroid lesions (as in b), particularly on the left side.

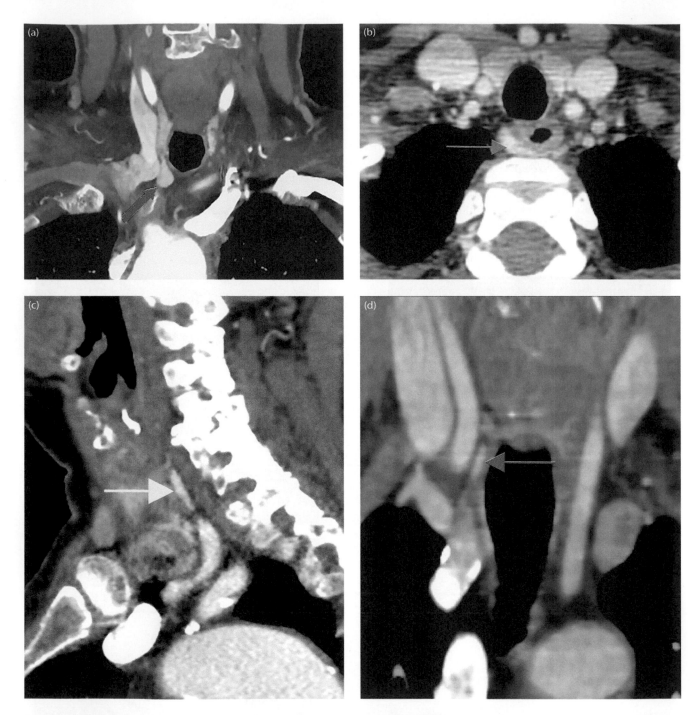

Figure 22.12 Commonly encountered variations in lesion shapes include teardrop **(a)**, discoid or plate-like **(c)**, or elongated or rod-like **(d and e)**. Less commonly encountered are lobulated lesions such as the bilobed adenoma shown in panels **(g and h)**. **(h)** Corresponding *ex vivo* lesion depicted in panel g showing good correlation between the imaging findings and the lesion's macroscopic appearance. *(Continued)*

These considerations may be broadly divided into patient-related and technical factors and limitations.

Patient factors

Taking steps to ensure that other nodules and normal structures are not misinterpreted as parathyroid adenomas, and vice versa, is essential. Various lesions may mimic an adenoma on a single phase, and for this reason, it is essential to assess all phases and, where appropriate, interrogate Hounsfield unit values for the target lesions.

Hyperenhancing abnormal lymph nodes can rarely mimic a parathyroid adenoma in the arterial phase, although they may not show the brisk contrast washout on delayed images typically seen with parathyroid adenoma. Lymph nodes will also more often demonstrate a

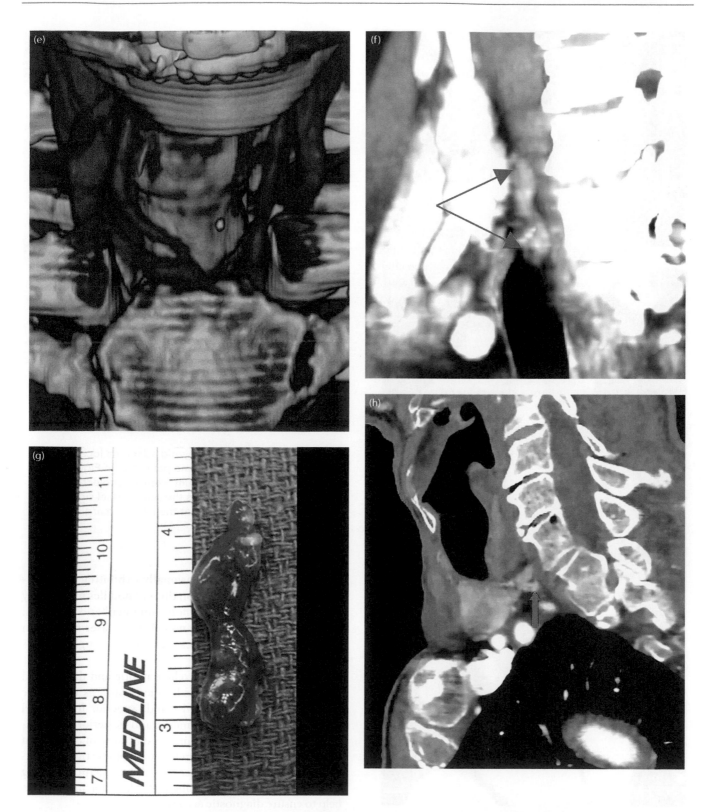

Figure 22.12 (Continued) Commonly encountered variations in lesion shapes include teardrop (a), discoid or plate-like (c), or elongated (c,d,e). Also depicted are less common bilobed (f,g) and curvilinear (h) morphologies. Panel (g) shows the corresponding *ex vivo* lesion seen in CT image (f), showing good correlation between the imaging findings and the lesion's macroscopic appearance.

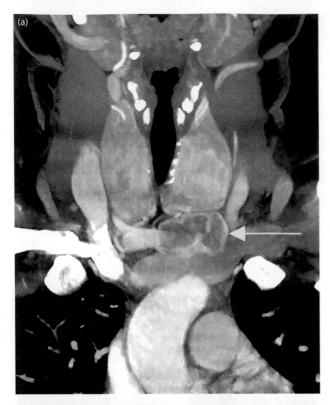

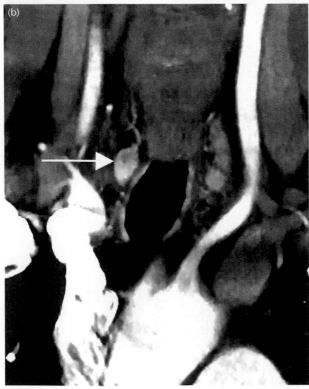

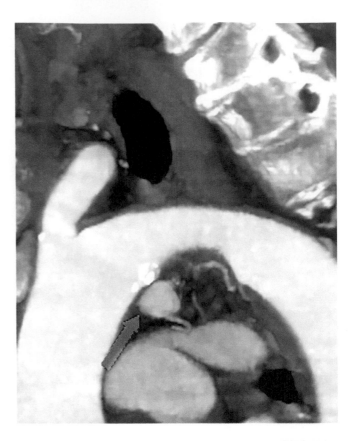

Figure 22.14 Ectopic parathyroid adenoma localized to the middle mediastinum (same patient as in Figure 22.10). This coronal oblique maximum intensity projection reformatted image demonstrates the polar vessel sign with a prominent feeding artery at the inferior margin of the lesion.

Figure 22.13 Two patients with inferior gland parathyroid adenomas (arrows), both of which demonstrate internal inhomogeneity and cystic change, manifested by hypoenhancement. The larger lesion **(a)** is predominantly cystic or necrotic, while the smaller lesion **(b)** contains a relatively small focus of internal cystic change. The lesion in panel b also demonstrates the characteristic polar vessel sign, which can be seen with parathyroid adenomas.

reniform morphology, occasionally exhibiting hilar vessels/pedicle. Low-attenuation thyroid nodules may closely resemble a parathyroid adenoma on unenhanced images. Assessment of the arterial and delayed phases may aid in differentiation between these lesions, although there is some overlap.

Care must be taken to exclude multigland disease and to assess uncommon ectopic locations, such as within the carotid sheath, undescended glands superior to the level of the thyroid, within the middle and posterior mediastinal compartments, and within the substance of the thyroid itself. Patients with large or multiple exophytic thyroid nodules and large goiters can pose a challenge. Again, following a stepwise approach and using a checklist for mimics can help to ensure diagnostic accuracy and reliability.

Technical factors

Technical factors common to cross-sectional imaging may affect the diagnostic quality of the scan regardless of the body part being investigated. Rigorous quality assurance is needed on the part of the imaging technician performing the study and the radiologist who establishes the scan

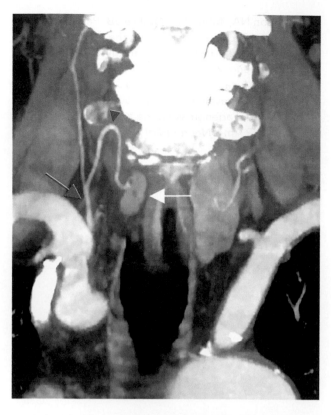

Figure 22.15 Coronal maximum intensity projection reformatted image shows arterial supply to a right inferior gland parathyroid adenoma (arrow) from the right inferior thyroidal artery, arising from the right thyrocervical trunk.

protocol and reads the examination. Optimal scan timing in relation to the intravenous contrast bolus may be affected by cardiovascular compromise. Beam-hardening artifact from a patient's shoulders can impair visualization of soft tissues at the root of the neck and lead to photon starvation, especially in larger patients. Patient positioning may help to ameliorate this issue. Patient movement and respiratory motion may also produce artifacts that can limit diagnostic quality. This has, however, become less of an issue with newer-generation CT scanners with multislice detectors and short scanning times.

CONCLUSION

4D-CT, performed for parathyroid localization, is a cross-sectional imaging technique that involves the consecutive acquisition of between two and four phases performed before and after the injection of contrast. It has been validated as a tool in the assessment of individuals with primary hyperparathyroidism and can be used in those who are either surgery-naïve or re-exploration patients. Radiologists should utilize currently available dose reduction techniques in scan protocols to limit radiation exposure. Radiologists and clinicians need to be aware of certain challenges and limitations of this technique to help ensure accurate and reproducible results.

REFERENCES

1. Udelsman R, Lin Z, Donovan P. The superiority of minimally invasive parathyroidectomy based on 1650 consecutive patients with primary hyperparathyroidism. *Ann Surg* 2011;253(3):585–91.
2. Kunstman JW, Udelsman R. Superiority of minimally invasive parathyroidectomy. *Adv Surg* 2012;46:171–89.
3. Rodgers SE, Hunter GJ, Hamberg LM et al. Improved preoperative planning for directed parathyroidectomy with 4-dimensional computed tomography. *Surgery* 2006;140(6):932–40; discussion 940–1.
4. Kelly HR, Hamberg LM, Hunter GJ. 4D-CT for preoperative localization of abnormal parathyroid glands in patients with hyperparathyroidism: Accuracy and ability to stratify patients by unilateral versus bilateral disease in surgery-naive and re-exploration patients. *AJNR Am J Neuroradiol* 2014;35(1):176–81.
5. Beland MD, Mayo-Smith WW, Grand DJ, Machan JT, Monchik JM. Dynamic MDCT for localization of occult parathyroid adenomas in 26 patients with primary hyperparathyroidism. *AJR Am J Roentgenol* 2011;196(1):61–5.
6. Wang TS, Cheung K, Farrokhyar F, Roman SA, Sosa JA. Would scan, but which scan? A cost-utility analysis to optimize preoperative imaging for primary hyperparathyroidism. *Surgery* 2011;150(6):1286–94.
7. Lubitz CC, Stephen AE, Hodin RA, Pandharipande P. Preoperative localization strategies for primary hyperparathyroidism: An economic analysis. *Ann Surg Oncol* 2012;19(13):4202–9.
8. Starker LF, Mahajan A, Bjorklund P, Sze G, Udelsman R, Carling T. 4D parathyroid CT as the initial localization study for patients with de novo primary hyperparathyroidism. *Ann Surg Oncol* 2011;18(6):1723–8.
9. Chazen JL, Gupta A, Dunning A, Phillips CD. Diagnostic accuracy of 4D-CT for parathyroid adenomas and hyperplasia. *AJNR Am J Neuroradiol* 2012;33(3):429–33.
10. Gafton AR, Glastonbury CM, Eastwood JD, Hoang JK. Parathyroid lesions: Characterization with dual-phase arterial and venous enhanced CT of the neck. *AJNR Am J Neuroradiol* 2012;33(5):949–52.
11. Hoang JK, Sung WK, Bahl M, Phillips CD. How to perform parathyroid 4D CT: Tips and traps for technique and interpretation. *Radiology* 2014;270(1):15–24.
12. Mahajan A, Starker LF, Ghita M, Udelsman R, Brink JA, Carling T. Parathyroid four-dimensional computed tomography: Evaluation of radiation dose exposure during preoperative localization of parathyroid tumors in primary hyperparathyroidism. *World J Surg* 2012;36(6):1335–9.

13. Madorin CA, Owen R, Coakley B et al. Comparison of radiation exposure and cost between dynamic computed tomography and sestamibi scintigraphy for preoperative localization of parathyroid lesions. *JAMA Surg* 2013;148(6):500–3.

14. Fancy T, Gallagher D 3rd, Hornig JD. Surgical anatomy of the thyroid and parathyroid glands. *Otolaryngol Clin North Am* 2010;43(2):221–7.

15. Johnson NA, Tublin ME, Ogilvie JB. Parathyroid imaging: Technique and role in the preoperative evaluation of primary hyperparathyroidism. *AJR Am J Roentgenol* 2007;188(6):1706–15.

16. Bahl M, Muzaffar M, Vij G, Sosa JA, Choudhury KR, Hoang JK. Prevalence of the polar vessel sign in parathyroid adenomas on the arterial phase of 4D CT. *AJNR Am J Neuroradiol* 2014;35(3):578–81.

23

Parathyroid surgery

RANDALL P. OWEN AND WENDY S. LIU

PATHOLOGY, PHYSIOLOGY, AND DIAGNOSIS

Hyperparathyroidism is typically diagnosed in the modern era by routine blood chemistry testing with a finding of hypercalcemia. An elevated intact parathyroid hormone (PTH) level generally confirms the diagnosis. Prior to the advent of the sequential multiple analyzer with computer (SMAC) in 1974, the diagnosis was generally made only when the examining physician detected a state of hypercalcemia based on findings such as severe osteoporosis and fractures, recurrent nephrolithiasis, or coma. Nowadays, patients rarely present initially with such symptoms. In fact, patients with early hyperparathyroidism may show borderline results, such as a high normal calcium and high normal PTH level. Although both of these levels may be in the normal range, a high normal PTH and a high normal (unsuppressed) calcium level are abnormal and generally represent the disease of hyperparathyroidism. A dilemma then arises as to whether patients with asymptomatic disease will benefit from surgery, and the equation of risk versus benefit demands a solution of clinical judgment with limited information on outcomes.

Differential diagnoses

It should be noted that the differential diagnosis of hypercalcemia also includes malignancy due to either a paraneoplastic syndrome from secretion of a PTH-like substance or bone destruction with calcium release. Whereas differentiating this from hyperparathyroidism was a common dilemma in the past, with the development of the intact PTH assay, it is now a rare quandary. It is extremely rare for a cancer—other than parathyroid cancer—to produce intact PTH. Generally, cancers produce partial PTH molecules, which cause hypercalcemia, but these are not usually cross-reactive with intact PTH on the modern assay.

The differential diagnosis of elevated PTH in the presence of a normal calcium level also includes vitamin D deficiency, which is now recognized as a very common disorder. With proper administration of vitamin D, the PTH level will most often return to within the normal range. For patients who have hyperparathyroidism and vitamin D deficiency, it is often prudent to give vitamin D preoperatively, as long as their calcium levels are not in a dangerously high range, in order to mitigate against hungry bone syndrome postoperatively.

Biochemical markers

Additional testing may be useful for patients whose calcium and PTH levels are borderline, to either confirm the diagnosis of hyperparathyroidism or determine the severity of end-organ manifestations. For example, an ionized calcium level may give a more accurate assessment of the physiologic calcium level in the bloodstream. Twenty-four-hour urine calcium should be done routinely to rule out the rare condition of familial hypercalcemic hypocalciuria, which is a relative contraindication to surgery [1]. A high urine calcium level may also help to measure the severity of hyperparathyroidism. Finally, bone densitometry is useful to determine the degree of bone loss and may help in determining the need for surgery. It should be noted, however, that bone density naturally decreases over time, thus the older the patient, the less useful the test becomes in determining the usefulness of surgery.

There are even a handful of publications suggesting that there are patients with normal calcium and normal PTH levels that have hyperparathyroidism [2]. These patients may present with kidney stones, osteoporosis, or neuropsychiatric manifestations but normal calcium and PTH levels, and yet, on exploration, parathyroid lesions may be found and removed, with intraoperative PTH levels decreasing by 50%. This suggests the possibility that certain individuals may have altered set points of their calcium and PTH levels. It remains to be determined whether this perspective is valid and will deliver appropriate outcomes for this very small group of patients.

SURGICAL INDICATIONS

Surgery for primary hyperparathyroidism carries a low risk of morbidity and mortality with a high probability of cure in experienced hands. Parathyroidectomy is clearly indicated for patients experiencing obvious sequelae of the disease, such as fractures, kidney stones, or coma, or end-organ damage such as severe osteoporosis. More controversial is the question of when to operate on an asymptomatic patient. The landmark study by Silverberg et al. [3] compared parathyroidectomy with observation or medical management in asymptomatic healthy patients under the age of 50. The study concluded that surgery was indicated because bone density scores were significantly better in the surgical arm at 10 years postenrollment. The rationale for studying patients 50 years and under was that these were young patients with many years left to live, and thus were at greater risk for developing complications of hyperparathyroidism, warranting consideration for surgical intervention. As a result, many endocrinologists and others have used the age of 50 as an arbitrary cutoff after which patients are not sent for surgical consultation. However, this should not be the case, because many patients over 50 still have a long life expectancy and the benefits of parathyroidectomy are not limited to bone density preservation. In fact, a more recent study by the group at Columbia showed an improvement in both bone density and quality of life measures in patients age 50–75 undergoing parathyroidectomy for mild asymptomatic disease [4].

For every surgical procedure, both the patient and surgeon must carefully consider whether the benefits of the operation outweigh the risks. In the past, when a standard parathyroidectomy consisted of a four-gland exploration under general anesthesia through a generous incision, an overnight hospital stay, and a significant risk of postoperative hypocalcemia, the risk side of the equation was weighty. However, now parathyroidectomy is possible under local anesthesia with sedation, through a minimal incision with confirmation of cure by rapid intraoperative PTH measurement. This significantly decreases the morbidity of the procedure, thereby reducing the overall risks and their influence in the decision for surgery [5]. Furthermore, it has become apparent that hyperparathyroidism often causes a variety of symptoms, such as neurocognitive dysfunction and bone and joint pain, which are often alleviated by parathyroidectomy, thus increasing the benefit side of the equation [6]. There is also some evidence that hyperparathyroidism may contribute to coronary and other vascular calcification [7]. However, recent guideline panels remain hesitant to include these lesser indications in their recommendations for surgery [8]. Nevertheless, as clinicians it is quite apparent that many patients who do not meet the guideline's criteria for surgery still benefit significantly from surgery with minimal morbidity.

PARATHYROID CARCINOMA (FIGURE 23.1)

Parathyroid cancer is rare, comprising 0.75%–0.9% of all cases of hyperparathyroidism [9,10]. Classically, parathyroid carcinoma presents as a rock-hard mass in the neck, along with biochemical signs of hyperparathyroidism, often with extremely high calcium levels. It may also present with invasion of surrounding structures, including the recurrent laryngeal nerve, with consequent vocal cord paralysis, or diffuse metastases. Once the diagnosis of hyperparathyroidism is established, further diagnostic testing should be obtained. A rock-hard mass in the neck should certainly raise the suspicion of a parathyroid or thyroid cancer, and an ultrasound and needle biopsy would be the first investigative step toward an expeditious diagnosis. Imaging with CT scan, ultrasound, and sestamibi nuclear scan may also be useful. Severe hypercalcemia should be treated with intravenous saline, diuretics, and if necessary, bisphosphonates or even hemodialysis. The calcium level should be optimized with medical management before surgery unless it is refractory to nonsurgical measures, in which case surgery should be performed expeditiously to lower the calcium level.

Histologic features of parathyroid carcinoma are elusive and often not present; therefore, the diagnosis is often made based on the surgeon's description of the adherence or local invasiveness of surrounding structures, necessitating sacrifice of the recurrent laryngeal nerve, strap muscles, thyroid lobe, or other surrounding structures. Recommended treatment is complete surgical resection of the tumor, as well as surrounding invaded structures and the ipsilateral thyroid lobe. Neurorrhaphy from the ansa cervicalis to the distal stump of the recurrent laryngeal nerve may be useful if the recurrent laryngeal nerve is sacrificed [11]. Postoperative radiation may be useful if gross disease is left behind or if aggressive histologic features are identified. There is no good

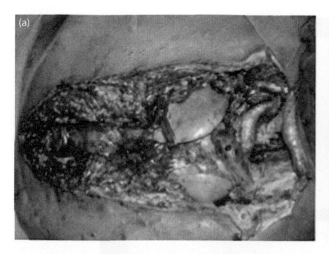
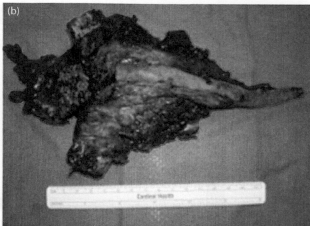

Figure 23.1 Sternectomy wound for parathyroid carcinoma **(a)** and pathological specimen **(b)**.

systemic treatment for parathyroid carcinoma. Prognosis is related to the presence of distant metastatic disease and, in the case of localized disease, the paramount importance of avoiding tumor rupture during the index operative resection of the parathyroid cancer [10]. Patients can be followed with serial PTH measurements and can be effectively treated by lowering their PTH with repeat operations for both primary and metastatic disease.

IMAGING TECHNIQUES

The three most commonly used imaging studies for preoperative parathyroid localization are ultrasound, sestamibi nuclear scintigraphy, and four-dimensional computed tomography (4D-CT) scan, with all three valid for use in properly selected patients. A recent meta-analysis showed sensitivity and positive predictive values of 76% and 93% for ultrasound, 79% and 91% for sestamibi, and 89% and 94% for CT, respectively [12]. All three studies are useful depending on the manner in which they are carried out and interpreted, and any or all can be an aide to the surgeon in performing

expeditious and minimally invasive surgery. However, the adage that the best way to localize a parathyroid lesion is to localize a good parathyroid surgeon still holds true [13].

Sestamibi radioisotope nuclear scans (Figures 23.2 and 23.3)

The usefulness of sestamibi radioisotope nuclear scans in locating parathyroid lesions was discovered by chance [14] in about 1989. While performing a sestamibi radioisotope nuclear scan for cardiac function assessment, it was found that there was a high concentration of radiotracer in the neck. This was subsequently correlated to the presence of a parathyroid lesion. Since then, sestamibi parathyroid scans have become one of the mainstays of preoperative imaging in hyperparathyroidism. It is hypothesized that sestamibi is preferentially taken up by both cardiac and parathyroid tissue because both are rich in mitochondria.

In the authors' experience, the utility of sestamibi scans greatly depends on the experience of the institution performing the scan and its procedural technique. There are

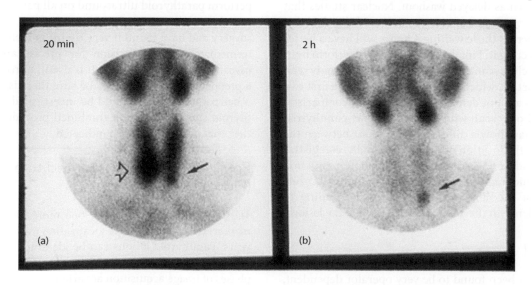

Figure 23.2 Technetium-99m sestamibi scan for thyroid adenoma **(a)** and parathyroid adenoma **(b)**.

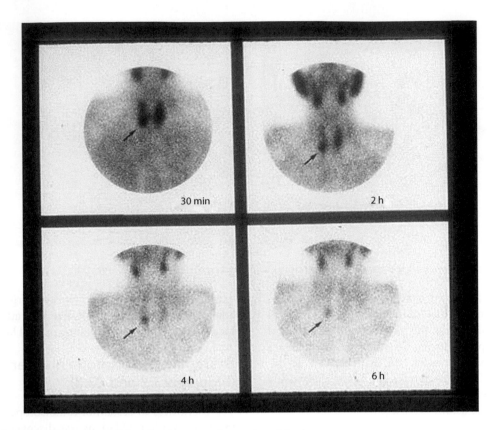

Figure 23.3 Technetium-99m sestamibi—classic case of parathyroid adenoma.

three scan characteristics of a parathyroid lesion. First is initial hyperconcentration. The radiotracer is initially taken up by normally functioning thyroid tissue, as well as by abnormally enlarged and hyperfunctioning parathyroid glands. Sometimes, the parathyroid lesion shows up very bright in comparison with the thyroid tissue on the initial scan and its location is obvious. However, often the parathyroid and thyroid scan will display similar brightness initially, but as the tracer washes out of the thyroid sooner than in the parathyroid lesion, it gives rise to the second characteristic, known as delayed washout. Nuclear studies that only wait for 1 or 2 hours after injection may fail to find this difference, whereas those waiting 4 hours will have a better chance of detecting it. Finally, the best studies perform both a sestamibi nuclear scan and a concurrent thyroid-only scan with pertechnetate, which is very helpful when the first two characteristics are not definitive. This allows a comparison of the thyroid-only scan with the thyroid-plus-parathyroid scan, which may show a difference in contour between the two, revealing the location of the lesion. Finally, coregistration with low-dose CT scanning (single-photon emission computed tomography [SPECT]) allows more accurate localization of the abnormality on the scan, leading to greater confidence in the anatomical location of the lesion.

Ultrasound

Ultrasound has been found to be very operator dependent, with less reliable sensitivities and positive predictive values

than sestamibi nuclear scanning. However, as surgeon-performed ultrasound has become more common, the use of ultrasound has risen dramatically [15]. Surgeons are able to perform a high volume of these studies over a short period of time, both in the office and in the operating room, and correlate these findings immediately to what is found during the procedure. Thus, the usefulness of learning and using this technique for immediate application is obvious. Further, it requires no preparation, injections, or intravenous lines, imparts no radiation, and is low cost. The authors perform parathyroid ultrasound on all patients undergoing parathyroidectomy in the operating room before starting surgery and have found it very useful in identifying lesions immediately before incision for precise and minimally invasive parathyroidectomy. It is useful to routinely obtain a preoperative ultrasound to be sure there is no thyroid or other pathology that should be investigated prior to parathyroid surgery in case a combined procedure addressing the other pathology is also indicated.

Four-dimensional computed tomography (Figure 23.4)

4D-CT scanning has become one more tool in the armamentarium of preoperative localization over the past several years. Parathyroid lesions can be identified by a unique set of characteristics relative to other structures by using several phases of image acquisition at various times before and after intravenous injection of contrast. Analysis of the radiation

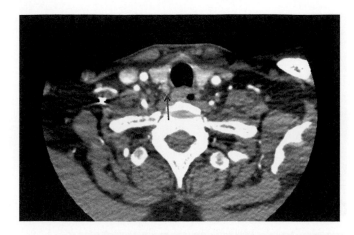

Figure 23.4 New parathyroid protocol dynamic CT (at Mount Sinai Hospital).

dose of our low-radiation protocol 4D-CT scans at Mount Sinai compared with the sestamibi nuclear scans showed them to be roughly equivalent [16]. Another advantage of CT over sestamibi is that it only takes 15 minutes to complete the study, as opposed to 4+ hours for a good-quality sestamibi scan. This axial imaging technique may also reveal lesions in deep and unusual locations inaccessible to ultrasound, as well as nonparathyroid pathology. Finally, the anatomic localization information afforded by this modality is considerably more detailed and accurate than that from nuclear scans.

SURGICAL MANAGEMENT

In past decades, parathyroidectomy involved a four-gland exploration through a generous cervical incision under general anesthesia. Typically, patients stayed in the hospital for 1–3 days postoperatively for pain management, as well as for monitoring of hypocalcemia. Imaging techniques were limited and intraoperative PTH assay was not available. This led patients and referring doctors to a sober view of parathyroid surgery with limited indications for referral. However, this all changed with the development of new technologies and techniques over the past 20 years.

Ninety percent of primary hyperparathyroidism is caused by a single adenoma [9]. Intraoperative rapid PTH assay has allowed the measurement of PTH immediately after excision of a parathyroid lesion, providing real-time data to confirm cure of hyperparathyroidism [17]. Imaging has also improved, with dual-isotope nuclear scans, detailed parathyroid protocol CT scans, and surgeon-performed ultrasound, giving more complete localizing information [12,14–16]. These technological advances have led to the common practice of focused parathyroidectomy, or single-gland excision, followed by biochemical confirmation of PTH decrease, obviating the need for visualization of all four glands. This has increased the opportunity for development of more minimally invasive techniques, such as smaller and more precisely placed incisions, the avoidance of general anesthesia, decreased pain, and decreased length of stay [5].

The criteria for what is considered an adequate decrease of PTH after excision of the lesion varies from a 50% drop of PTH from baseline (Miami criteria) to a drop of PTH into the normal range, or both [18,19]. The stricter the criteria, the more likely the patient is cured, but the possibility of an unnecessary contralateral exploration also increases. There is also controversy questioning whether focused parathyroid surgery is valid at all, with some arguing that four-gland exploration should still be performed in every patient. The authors who recommend and routinely perform traditional four-gland parathyroid exploration have concluded that the rate of cure remains higher, with no substantial increase in complications or morbidity [20,21]. However, there is strong sentiment from the majority of leading parathyroid surgeons that unilateral parathyroid surgery should not be abandoned [22]. Whichever technique is utilized, the goals of the surgery remain the same, namely, to normalize parathyroid physiology and avoid complications.

Single-gland exploration (Figure 23.5)

In the focused or single-gland technique, a smaller incision is made, approximately 1.5–3 cm in length. In experienced hands, this can be done under light sedation with local anesthesia injected in the skin and subcutaneous tissue. Some advocate the use of a regional block, which probably decreases the possibility of the patient feeling pain or discomfort during the surgery. However, complications of the block itself can also occur, such as prolonged anesthesia of the brachial plexus, phrenic, or accessory nerves, or seizure due to injection of the carotid artery. The authors routinely perform an on-table ultrasound to confirm the location of the lesion, as well as to identify any second lesions or thyroid or other neck pathology that may impact the operation. Upon opening the skin, the median raphe is opened and the strap muscles elevated off the thyroid lobe on the side of the lesion. A search is undertaken in the area identified as suspicious for the lesion on preoperative imaging. Often, the lesion is quickly identified, easily dissected free from surrounding tissues, its blood supply clipped and cut, and it is then removed. Frozen section can be very useful to confirm the finding of the parathyroid lesion, and to obtain a weight documenting that it is abnormal in size (normal weight is 35–65 mg). Intraoperative PTH assay should be sent before surgery begins (some argue before anesthesia is induced, as there are reports of elevated PTH after induction of anesthesia [23]) and then at the time of lesion excision. PTH levels should then be sent at 5-minute intervals thereafter until criteria for cure are obtained. Manipulation of the lesion can cause increases in PTH, which is useful to know when comparing subsequent levels to determine whether the patient is cured.

Four-gland exploration

Another controversy is whether the other gland on the side of the lesion should be visualized and biopsied. Doing so does

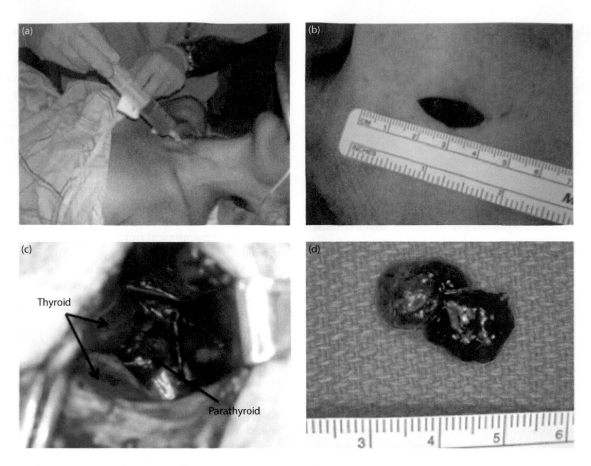

Figure 23.5 Upper panels demonstrate the operative technique for parathyroid surgery with subcutaneous injection of local anesthetic **(a)** and skin incision approximately 1.5–3 cm in length **(b)**. Lower panels show visualization of the thyroid and parathyroid glands **(c)** and the parathyroid lesion excised from a patient with hyperparathyroidism **(d)**.

not generally add any time to the operation since it takes between 15 and 30 minutes to obtain definitive data from intraoperative PTH and frozen section. If the local anesthesia or block and sedation are adequate, then any additional discomfort due to further exploration should be minimal. Identifying the other parathyroid gland on the same side as the lesion can yield valuable information, particularly if the PTH does not decrease to a satisfactory level. In that case, if a normal gland has been identified and proven to be parathyroid by frozen section, then the surgeon can rule out four-gland hyperplasia as the cause for hyperparathyroidism. Thus, the diagnosis must be a double adenoma involving a contralateral gland. If a second lesion is found on the same side and is removed, a drop in the PTH indicates cure, whereas a persistently high PTH indicates the diagnosis of four-gland hyperplasia. Finally, if the patient is considered cured at the time of the index operation but hyperparathyroidism recurs later, then the information that the surgeon identified two glands on one side allows subsequent surgery to focus primarily on the contralateral side. It is not a good argument that frozen section may harm, devascularize, or devitalize the gland, as a properly done biopsy on the opposite side of the vascular pedicle will rarely compromise its blood supply, and furthermore, even if the gland were to be devitalized, the chance that would have a clinical impact is minimal, given that the two contralateral glands most likely do not need to be explored.

Some surgeons insist that the recurrent laryngeal nerve should be visualized at every parathyroid operation. However, unlike in thyroid surgery, the nerve does not appose the gland along a great length, but in most cases only a short distance and sometimes not at all. Further, the parathyroid gland or lesion is typically very mobile, such that dissection, which circumscribes the parathyroid, generally isolates the vascular pedicle, which then can be easily clipped. By avoiding routine visualization of the nerve, the risk of nerve damage due to dissection is minimized. There are times when a parathyroid lesion is massive or there is thyroid pathology, and then nerve dissection is required. Given the decreased need for nerve dissection in parathyroid surgery versus thyroid surgery, it is the authors' practice only to use nerve monitoring in redo parathyroid surgery or in cases where difficulty and an extensive exploration are anticipated.

Surgical techniques for lesions difficult to locate

Despite advances in imaging techniques, there are times when a parathyroid lesion is difficult to locate, and Dr. John

Doppman's oft-quoted statement remains true: "The best way to localize a parathyroid lesion is to localize a good parathyroid surgeon" [13]. All imaging modalities available are limited in their ability to accurately depict multigland disease [9]. This is one reason intraoperative PTH measurement is so valuable. In most cases, one lesion is identified on preoperative imaging, a focused exploration and excision of that one lesion is performed, and an intraoperative PTH is sent for confirmation. In the 10% of cases with multigland disease, the PTH will not fall to within the appropriate range, thus prompting the surgeon to search for the other pathological gland or glands. However, as there is more often no imaging to help the surgeon find these additional lesions, it is important to know the common and uncommon locations of the parathyroid glands.

The superior parathyroid glands are commonly located posterior and sometimes lateral to the upper pole of the thyroid gland. They are generally found superior to the inferior thyroid artery and posterolateral to the recurrent laryngeal nerve. However, it is not uncommon to see the blood supply of a superior parathyroid originate from this area, but for the gland itself to have descended and rest below the inferior thyroid artery. Thus, to determine whether an inferiorly located gland is truly superior or inferior, it is important to delineate the relationship between the blood supply, inferior thyroid artery, and recurrent laryngeal nerve, as well as to identify the other parathyroid gland.

The inferior parathyroid gland commonly rests inferior and posterior to the inferior pole of the thyroid gland. However, the inferior gland location is more variable than the superior gland location, and ectopic glands are most commonly the inferior. This is thought to be because the inferior gland originates embryologically from the third branchial pouch, which descends from the upper carotid sheath region all the way down to the thymus and anterior mediastinum. Thus, an ectopic (inferior) parathyroid lesion can be located anywhere along this developmental pathway. However, it should be noted that most of the time a missing gland is quite close to the usual location, but is simply being missed by the surgeon. Therefore, after perusal of the area surrounding the inferior pole, the next step should be widening the exploration to include the paratracheal region, as well as dissecting the recurrent laryngeal nerve and the inferior thyroid artery. This helps to delineate the anatomy thoroughly and identify a parathyroid lesion that often rests along one of these structures. Next, the depth (posteriorly) of the exploration is important, as my mentor Dr. Carl Silver always said, "Your exploration is not complete until you've reached the prevertebral fascia." Truly, I have found many lesions, even in reoperations, resting posteriorly, not previously identified simply because the first surgeon did not explore deeply or posteriorly enough and thus failed. If the patient has a large thyroid gland, it may also be useful to transect the superior pole of the ipsilateral thyroid lobe to allow for more thorough exploration, especially if it is the superior

gland that is missing. If these maneuvers fail to produce the offending lesion, the next most common location for the lesion is the cervical thymus, which can be removed without consequence. It may be useful to take a minute to search through the thymic tissue removed to see if a parathyroid lesion can be identified, and to wait and send another intraoperative PTH level after excision of the thymus to confirm whether cure has been achieved. If not, continued exploration should include the carotid sheath from the clavicle to the mandible, retrotracheal and retroesophageal regions, and the anterior mediastinum as much as allowed through the cervical incision. If the PTH level remains high despite all of these maneuvers, there is one final action to consider: removing the thyroid lobe. It is uncommon for a parathyroid lesion to rest completely within the thyroid lobe, but it can happen, and I have cured at least one patient of hyperparathyroidism by removing a thyroid lobe with an embedded parathyroid lesion. In these situations, on-table ultrasound can again be useful, as a completely normal-appearing thyroid is unlikely to harbor a lesion, whereas a lobe with some nodules or abnormalities may. Lobectomy should only be done if only one gland has been found on the ipsilateral side and two glands have been found on the contralateral side. I prefer to confirm these findings by frozen section biopsy before proceeding with thyroid lobectomy. Once three glands have been confirmed, one may then consider removing the thyroid lobe contralateral to the side on which two glands were confirmed. Again, intraoperative PTH can then be measured to assess for cure.

It is contraindicated to proceed to sternal split and further mediastinal exploration without imaging confirmation first. Therefore, if all of the above maneuvers have been completed and the patient remains uncured, then the operation should be terminated. Another quotation from Dr. Silver is "You will not cure every patient with hyperparathyroidism at the first operation." In the case of an operative failure, postoperative biochemical testing should be done to confirm the persistence of hyperparathyroidism and its level. The surgeon should double-check that there is no possibility the patient has familial hypercalcemic hypocalciuria. If hyperparathyroidism persists, then it is generally reasonable to proceed with imaging tests such as a parathyroid protocol chest CT scan and a sestamibi nuclear scan. These may be particularly useful if one lesion has been removed or if the thymus or part of the thyroid has been removed. If these tests are unrevealing, then a femoral vein catheterization with sampling of PTH from all of the great vessels of the chest and neck is performed, further localizing the region from which the highest level of PTH is emanating. Identifying the area of highest PTH may help when reviewing the radiologic studies to search for possible lesions. Finally, if the vein catheterization indicates the lesion is in the mediastinum but cross-sectional imaging is not revelatory, then sternotomy with total thymectomy is the most appropriate next step and will often be curative.

PERIOPERATIVE MANAGEMENT

With the advent of minimally invasive methods for parathyroid surgery, it is now feasible to discharge patients home on the same day of surgery, shortly after the procedure. Although general anesthesia in itself does not necessitate an overnight stay, lower doses of anesthetic medications and avoidance of inhaled anesthesia decrease the probability of severe nausea and vomiting, as well as other complications, such as damage to teeth or larynges. Thus, the avoidance of general anesthesia by using either generous infiltration of local anesthetics or the administration of a deep or superficial cervical plexus block often facilitates an ambulatory procedure. The focused approach to parathyroidectomy in which only one gland is identified and removed, or perhaps at most one side of the neck is explored, often allows for a smaller incision and a more limited surgical field within that wound, leading to less postoperative pain and swelling, again facilitating the possibility of early discharge. Finally, with the use of intraoperative PTH, the knowledge that the patient is cured is secured by the end of the procedure, allowing a very satisfying explanation to the patient that he or she no longer has the disease and that no further exploration is needed. If the PTH is profoundly low at this point, the surgeon may be prompted to prescribe prophylactic calcium and vitamin D supplementation, thereby avoiding hypocalcemia in the early postoperative period. Conversely, if the PTH is not profoundly low, the surgeon may be more comfortable discharging the patient with little or no supplementation. Since in most of these surgeries two or more parathyroid glands remain untouched, the patient's secretion of PTH should at least be to a level that does not risk dangerous hypocalcemia.

In patients who require a four-gland exploration due to multigland disease, known preoperatively, discovered intraoperatively, or because preoperative imaging was unrevealing and therefore a four-gland exploration was planned, postoperative hypocalcemia is a much more common phenomenon. If a single gland or two glands are excised and the remaining glands are biopsied to prove that they are in fact parathyroid glands, their blood supply may be compromised and the patient may therefore become hypoparathyroid.

Four gland parathyroidectomy

If a patient has four-gland hyperplasia, there are two standard options for treatment. The first is four-gland parathyroidectomy with reimplantation of parathyroid tissue into the forearm. (Traditionally, this has been done in the brachioradialis muscle, but more recent series have described implanting in the subcutaneous tissues with similar rates of graft success [24].) This procedure leaves the patient with no intact functioning parathyroid tissue immediately after the procedure, and therefore the parathyroid level will be zero. The parathyroid tissue graft is placed in the forearm because it is recognized that this is abnormal tissue prone to grow, causing recurrence of hyperparathyroidism.

This is much easier to deal with in the forearm by excising additional parathyroid tissue through a small incision under local anesthesia, as opposed to reentering a scarred neck with the possibility of injuring the recurrent laryngeal nerve and more difficulty in finding any recurring lesion. Furthermore, in the case of recurrent disease, one may differentiate between hyperparathyroidism due to the graft in the arm and a recurrence in the neck by drawing blood from the ipsilateral antecubital fossa and comparing it to blood drawn from the contralateral arm. If the PTH is equally elevated in both samples, then it is due to neck pathology. If the arm with the graft is considerably higher, then the disease has recurred in the graft. Postoperatively from the original procedure of four-gland parathyroidectomy, the patient will have no PTH in the bloodstream for 2–8 weeks, during which time massive doses of calcium with vitamin D must be administered to avoid profound hypocalcemia. The authors generally use a dose of 3.0 µg of calcitriol and 2500 mg of calcium carbonate in the recovery room, followed by 1–3 µg of calcitriol and 1500 mg three times daily of calcium carbonate daily.

Three-and-one-half-gland parathyroidectomy

The alternative procedure to four-gland parathyroidectomy is three-and-one-half-gland parathyroidectomy. In this case, the most normal-appearing parathyroid gland is identified, with only half of the gland removed. If this strategy is planned, then all four glands should first be visualized before deciding which one to bisect and leave partially in place. Once the decision is made, the gland to be partially left should be divided first to determine the viability of the gland before removing the other three. It should be marked with a long stitch and metal clips in case of the need for re-exploration and removal. A detailed operative report describing the location of the gland and its proximity to the recurrent laryngeal nerve should also be noted. A copy of the report should be given to the patient in case a second surgeon operates at a future date. The advantage of this approach is that it allows the patient to retain some continuously functioning parathyroid tissue so that much less supplemental calcium and vitamin D are needed. While there is a risk that the gland may devascularize, leaving the patient with no functioning parathyroid tissue, it is also possible that a forearm graft will not work, so this possible disadvantage exists with both approaches.

Cryopreservation of parathyroid tissue to allow for the possibility of future autotransplantation has been utilized at some centers with limited success. The practice of cryopreservation is, however, questionable, as it is a very labor-intensive undertaking, with some risk and liability due to the long-term storage of human specimens with generally no obvious means of funding [25].

Patients who have had four-gland or three-and-one-half-gland parathyroidectomies should be admitted to the hospital for postoperative calcium monitoring and management.

Many will not have stable calcium levels initially, requiring the administration of intravenous calcium. Once the calcium level is stabilized on a postoperative regimen of calcium and calcitriol, the patient may be discharged.

Renal failure patients with hyperparathyroidism almost always have four-gland hyperplasia, and four-gland explorations should be planned. Further discussion of renal hyperparathyroidism is beyond the scope of this chapter, but readers are referred to the author's review article on the subject [26].

Redo parathyroid surgery

Patients referred for recurrent or persistent hyperparathyroidism after a prior parathyroid exploration present a uniquely challenging situation. The chief risks of parathyroid surgery, namely, hypocalcemia and recurrent nerve injury, are much higher in redo parathyroid surgery.

The increased risk of nerve injury is due to scar tissue on the nerve from prior surgery, making identification, dissection, and preservation of the nerve more difficult. Whereas the use of intraoperative nerve monitoring is of very limited value in primary parathyroid operations, it may be particularly useful in the case of redo parathyroid surgery, as it may aid in both finding the nerve and identifying its course, thus preventing injury [27]. It may also guide the surgeon in the extent of exploration that is required. For instance, if the recurrent nerve on the first side explored presents a difficult dissection and it is found that the nerve signal is lost, then it may be prudent to delay exploration of the contralateral side to avoid the catastrophic complication of bilateral vocal cord paralysis, leading to airway compromise. Given these considerations, it is critical to examine the larynx preoperatively in a patient who has had prior thyroid or parathyroid surgery—even if the voice is normal—to be sure there is no vocal cord paresis or paralysis. Some patients can compensate very well after unilateral vocal cord paralysis, such that the patient or clinician may not realize that there is a nerve injury unless laryngeal visualization is performed. If the larynx is not examined preoperatively, then the operating surgeon assumes all risk of subsequent laryngeal dysfunction, which may or may not have been his or her complication. More importantly, if unilateral vocal cord paresis or paralysis is not known preoperatively and the contralateral nerve is injured, then a very unwelcome complication of airway compromise, or at least severe impairment of the voice, will likely occur.

COMPLICATIONS

The most common complications of parathyroid surgery are hypocalcemia and recurrent laryngeal nerve injury resulting in voice change and hoarseness.

Hypocalcemia

The cause of hypocalcemia is that insufficient normal-functioning parathyroid tissue has been left in the patient.

This is generally due to either parathyroidectomy for four-gland hyperplasia or removal of remaining parathyroid tissue in a redo operation after a failed primary operation or after recurrence of hyperparathyroidism. It is also possible for hypoparathyroidism to be caused by four-gland exploration with removal of one or more glands and biopsy of other glands compromising their viability. This is one reason to consider single-gland exploration over four-gland exploration.

Hypocalcemia is more common in reoperations because one or more parathyroid glands may have previously been removed or biopsied, and despite proper review of previous operative and pathology reports, it may not be entirely clear what exactly was done during the prior operation. Therefore, removing or performing a biopsy on additional parathyroid tissue may sacrifice critical remaining functional glands, resulting in hypoparathyroidism and hypocalcemia. For this reason, intraoperative PTH monitoring is extremely useful in reoperative parathyroid surgery. If parathyroid tissue is found and removed in such a case, some of this tissue should always be preserved on the surgical field until the final PTH levels are obtained. If the levels are undetectable at the end of the procedure, then some parathyroid tissue should be reimplanted. If the parathyroid tissue is thought to be normal, then it can be reimplanted into the sterno-cleidomastoid muscle. If it is thought to be abnormal, then it should implanted into the forearm for easy access in case it grows further and must be re-excised at a later date. This almost guarantees at least some parathyroid tissue to produce PTH, thereby reducing the chance of severe hypoparathyroidism, which leads to the need for enormous doses of calcium and vitamin D supplementation, as well as abnormal bone physiology.

Recurrent laryngeal nerve injury

Injury to the recurrent laryngeal nerve should be a rare event in parathyroid surgery, much less than in thyroid surgery, as opposed to thyroid surgery, because parathyroid lesions are usually extremely mobile and do not usually adhere to the nerve. Many parathyroid surgeons do not routinely find and dissect the recurrent laryngeal nerve because the dissection itself may be riskier than surgery in which the nerve is simply avoided. Knowledge of the location of the nerve is obviously critical, and the course should be dissected if there is any concern that the nerve might be nearby or require dissection to separate it safely from a less mobile parathyroid lesion.

Nerve transection results in a paralyzed ipsilateral vocal cord, which in most cases will result in a hoarse, breathy, and weak voice. Occasionally, a single vocal cord paralysis may also affect the patient's ability to breathe, particularly if there are other respiratory comorbidities. Bilateral vocal cord injury and paralysis almost always cause airway obstruction necessitating tracheostomy and therefore should be strictly avoided.

If the recurrent laryngeal nerve is transected during a parathyroidectomy, then a primary repair is the optimal course of action [11]. Tone will usually return to the nerve approximately 6 months after neurorrhaphy, generally resulting in an improvement in voice quality. Alternatively, a laryngologist may offer a range of treatments, from voice therapy to injection of a substance to bulk up the vocal cord, or even an open surgical procedure to place a Teflon strut, creating a rigid midline cord against which the other cord can appose, thus restoring the voice.

Other complications

One interesting complication of parathyroidectomy that seems to be more common when done under local anesthesia with sedation, as opposed to under general endotracheal anesthesia, is pneumothorax [28,29]. While the exact mechanism is unclear, it is thought to be due to increased intrathoracic pressure and rupture of an apical pleural bleb during surgery. It may sometimes be observed to resolve spontaneously, but otherwise is easily remedied by tube thoracostomy. The important thing is to recognize it and treat it as necessary.

Other rarer complications are of course possible, such as injury to any number of surrounding structures, including the carotid artery, jugular vein, vagus nerve, sympathetic trunk, trachea, thyroid, or pleura. However, these complications are truly rare in the hands of an experienced parathyroid surgeon.

CONCLUSION

Parathyroid surgery has evolved considerably over the past two decades. The use of advanced preoperative imaging and intraoperative rapid PTH assay have given rise to the option of minimally invasive and focused approaches to curing patients with this disease. However, knowledge of the anatomy, surgical experience, and clinical judgment remain critical to properly carrying out these often challenging operations in a safe and effective manner.

REFERENCES

1. Schwartz S, Futran N. Hypercalcemic hypocalciuria: A critical differential diagnosis for hyperparathyroidism. *Otolaryngol Clin North Am* 2004;37:887–96.
2. Wallace L, Parikh R, Ross LJ et al. The phenotype of primary hyperparathyroidism with normal parathyroid hormone levels: How low can parathyroid hormone go? *Surgery* 2011;150:1102–12.
3. Silverberg S, Shane E, Jacobs T, Siris E, Bilezikian J. A 10-year prospective study of primary hyperparathyroidism with or without parathyroid surgery. *N Engl J Med* 1999;341:1249–55.
4. Ambrogini E, Cetani F, Cianferotti L et al. Surgery or surveillance for mild asymptomatic primary hyperparathyroidism: A prospective, randomized clinical trial. *J Clin Endocrinol Metabol* 2007;92:3114–21.
5. Udelsman R. Six hundred fifty-six consecutive explorations for primary hyperparathyroidism. *Ann Surg* 2002;235:665–72.
6. Pasieka J, Parsons L, Demeure M et al. Patient-based surgical outcome tool demonstrating alleviation of symptoms following parathyroidectomy in patients with primary hyperparathyroidism. *World J Surg* 2002;26:942–9.
7. Walker M, Silverberg S. Cardiovascular aspects of primary hyperparathyroidism. *J Endocrinol Invest* 2008;31:925–31.
8. Bilezikian J, Khan A, Potts J. Guidelines for the management of asymptomatic primary hyperparathyroidism: Summary statement from the third international workshop. *J Clin Endocrinol Metabol* 2009;94:335–9.
9. Ruda J, Hollenbeak C, Stack B Jr. A systematic review of the diagnosis and treatment of primary hyperparathyroidism from 1995 to 2003. *Otolaryngol Head Neck Surg* 2005;132:359–72.
10. Villar-del-Moral J, Jiménez-García A, Salvador-Egea P et al. Prognostic factors and staging systems in parathyroid cancer: A multicenter cohort study. *Surgery* 2014;156:1132–44.
11. Miyauchi A, Inoue H, Tomoda C et al. Improvement in phonation after reconstruction of the recurrent laryngeal nerve in patients with thyroid cancer invading the nerve. *Surgery* 2009;146:1056–62.
12. Cheung K, Wang T, Farrokhyar F, Roman S, Sosa J. A meta-analysis of preoperative localization techniques for patients with primary hyperparathyroidism. *Ann Surgical Oncol* 2011;19:577–83.
13. Doppman J, Hammond W. Localization of parathyroid adenoma. *N Engl J Med* 1969;281:1248–49.
14. Malhotra A, Silver C, Deshpande V, Freeman L. Preoperative parathyroid localization with sestamibi. *Am J Surg* 1996;172:637–40.
15. Bumpous J, Randolph G. The expanding utility of office-based ultrasound for the head and neck surgeon. *Ultrasound Clin* 2012;7:191–5.
16. Madorin C, Owen R, Coakley B et al. Comparison of radiation exposure and cost between dynamic computed tomography and sestamibi scintigraphy for preoperative localization of parathyroid lesions. *JAMA Surg* 2013;148:500.
17. Irvin G, Deriso G. A new, practical intraoperative parathyroid hormone assay. *Am J Surg* 1994;168:466–8.
18. Lombardi C, Raffaelli M, Traini E et al. Intraoperative PTH monitoring during parathyroidectomy: The need for stricter criteria to detect multiglandular disease. *Langenbecks Arch Surg* 2008;393:639–45.
19. Carneiro D, Solorzano C, Nader M, Ramirez M, Irvin G. Comparison of intraoperative iPTH assay (QPTH) criteria in guiding parathyroidectomy: Which criterion is the most accurate? *Surgery* 2003;134:973–9.

20. Mazzaglia P, Milas M, Berber E, Siperstein A, Monchik J. Normalization of 2-week postoperative parathyroid hormone values in patients with primary hyperparathyroidism: Four-gland exploration compared to focused-approach surgery. *World J Surg* 2010;34:1318–24.

21. Norman J, Lopez J, Politz D. Abandoning unilateral parathyroidectomy: Why we reversed our position after 15,000 parathyroid operations. *J Am Coll Surg* 2012;214:260–9.

22. Hodin R, Angelos P, Carty S et al. No need to abandon unilateral parathyroid surgery. *J Am Coll Surg* 2012;215:297.

23. Hong J, Morris L, Park E, Ituarte P, Lee C, Yeh M. Transient increases in intraoperative parathyroid levels related to anesthetic technique. *Surgery* 2011;150:1069–75.

24. Conzo G, Della Pietra C, Tartaglia E et al. Long-term function of parathyroid subcutaneous autoimplantation after presumed total parathyroidectomy in the treatment of secondary hyperparathyroidism: A clinical retrospective study. *Int J Surg* 2014;12:165–9.

25. Shepet K, Alhefdhi A, Usedom R, Sippel R, Chen H. Parathyroid cryopreservation after parathyroidectomy: A worthwhile practice? *Ann Surg Oncol* 2013;20:2256–60.

26. Madorin C, Owen R, Fraser W et al. The surgical management of renal hyperparathyroidism. *Eur Arch Otorhinolaryngol* 2014;269:1565–76.

27. Snyder S, Sigmond B, Lairmore T, Govednik-Horny C, Janicek A, Jupiter D. The long-term impact of routine intraoperative nerve monitoring during thyroid and parathyroid surgery. *Surgery* 2013;154:704–13.

28. Guerrero M, Wray C, Kee S, Frenzel J, Perrier N. Minimally invasive parathyroidectomy complicated by pneumothoraces: A report of 4 cases. *J Surg Educ* 2007;64:101–7.

29. Slater B, Inabnet W. Pneumothorax: An uncommon complication of minimally invasive parathyroidectomy. *Surg Laparosc Endosc Percutan Tech* 2005;15:38–40.

24

Reoperation for hyperparathyroidism

MASHA J. LIVHITS AND MICHAEL W. YEH

INTRODUCTION

Some of the earliest, best-chronicled cases of primary hyperparathyroidism (PHPT) were patients who suffered from persistent or recurrent disease. One of the first operations was performed by Dr. Felix Mandl on Albert Ghane, a Viennese tram car conductor who presented with a femur fracture and advanced osteitis fibrosa cystica [1]. Mr Ghane was initially thought to be cured, but he developed a recurrence 6 years later and ultimately died of uncontrolled hypercalcemia. A similar early case was Captain Charles Martell, a U.S. merchant mariner who developed multiple bone fractures and recurrent kidney stones [2]. Captain Martell underwent six failed parathyroid explorations in the United States before a mediastinal adenoma was found during sternotomy by Drs. Edward Churchill and Oliver Cope.

The vast majority of patients (92%) with PHPT are now cured after their initial operation [3]. A number of factors have led to the improved surgical success, including a thorough understanding of the embryology and anatomy of the parathyroid glands, preoperative localization, and intraoperative parathyroid hormone (PTH) monitoring. Advanced age, low or medium hospital volume, and negative preoperative localization remain risk factors for failed parathyroidectomy [3].

Perioperative risks are significantly higher with reoperative surgery; therefore, all attempts should be made to achieve a cure at the time of initial operation. Regardless, a minority of patients will continue to have persistent or recurrent disease. These patients remain at risk for the metabolic complications related to hypercalcemia and may be eligible for reoperative parathyroidectomy. A thoughtful approach is necessary to determine which patients are appropriate candidates for reoperation, and to plan the surgical approach. Advances in preoperative localization have improved the chances of success while limiting operative risks.

BURDEN OF DISEASE

The incidence of PHPT has tripled in the past decade. PHPT now affects 1 in 400 women and 1 in 1200 men [4]. However, only 28% of patients with PHPT currently undergo surgery [5]. This amounts to an estimated 150,000 parathyroidectomies performed annually in the United States alone [6]. Given that only 12% of patients with persistent or recurrent PHPT currently undergo reoperative parathyroidectomy, there are approximately 1000 such cases performed in the United States per year [3].

In reports by expert centers, the success rate of initial surgery is >95% regardless of surgical technique (limited versus four-gland exploration) [7]. In a recent population-level study, patients treated at high-volume centers (hospitals performing ≥100 total parathyroidectomies over a 15-year time period) were noted to experience durable eucalcemia more often than those treated at low- and medium-volume centers. Patients with negative preoperative localization who underwent surgery at low-volume centers had the lowest surgical success rate (79.5%) [3].

ETIOLOGY OF HYPERPARATHYROIDISM OCCURRING AFTER INITIAL PARATHYROIDECTOMY

Persistent hyperparathyroidism

Persistent hyperparathyroidism (HPT) is defined by an increased serum calcium level occurring within 6 months of parathyroidectomy. Approximately two-thirds of patients who are not durably cured after initial parathyroidectomy have persistent disease, with the remainder having recurrent disease, that is, an increased serum calcium level occurring more than 6 months after initial parathyroidectomy (described further below) [3]. The 6-month time point distinguishing between persistent and recurrent PHPT is arbitrary and determined by convention rather than having a true physiologic basis. Having said that, the underlying causes of persistent and recurrent PHPT are not entirely overlapping and thus merit discussion.

When persistent PHPT was initially described in the literature, most cases were attributed to unrecognized multigland hyperplasia [8,9]. However, these reports were from individual high-volume surgeons. As experience with parathyroidectomy has grown and broadened, the most common reason for failed parathyroidectomy has emerged to be a missed parathyroid adenoma [10]. Other causes of persistent PHPT include incomplete resection of an adenoma, failure to identify a second adenoma, or inadequate subtotal parathyroidectomy for four-gland hyperplasia.

Recurrent hyperparathyroidism

From our experience, we have learned that recurrent PHPT most commonly arises when a single, dominant hyperfunctioning gland is removed in a patient with underlying multigland hyperplasia. Over time, subordinate hyperfunctioning glands may become disinhibited, eventually leading to hypercalcemia. A less common cause of recurrent PHPT is overgrowth of the parathyroid remnant that is left after a subtotal parathyroidectomy. Familial HPT cases have a significant risk of recurrence due to the intrinsic genetic abnormality in all of the parathyroid tissue. Patients with multiple endocrine neoplasia type 1 (MEN-1) have recurrence in at least one-third of cases [8].

Other rare causes of recurrent HPT include parathyroid carcinoma and parathyromatosis. Parathyroid carcinoma is rare, occurring in less than 1% of cases of PHPT [11]. A major risk factor is hyperparathyroidism-jaw tumor syndrome, which carries a 15% rate of parathyroid carcinoma [12]. Treatment involves excision with *en bloc* resection of any locally invaded adjacent tissue. Recurrence rates are as high as 50%–60% in cases of incomplete resection, but recurrence is common even after resection of all gross disease [13]. In cases of benign adenoma, intraoperative violation of the tumor capsule can result in spillage of parathyroid tissue and miliary regrowth of parathyroid tissue in the operative field (within muscle, fat, or soft tissue), known as parathyromatosis [14].

Location of missed parathyroid adenoma

The most common cause of persistent PHPT after parathyroidectomy is a missed adenoma in the normal location. This occurs in approximately 65% of failed cases [10,15,16]. In our experience and that of other high-volume centers, the most common locations of missed adenomas, in order of decreasing frequency, are (1) posterior and adjacent to the esophagus (embryologically superior glands); (2) within the thymus or thyrothymic tract, including extension into the anterior mediastinum (embryologically inferior glands); (3) intrathyroidal; (4) within the carotid sheath; and (5) undescended in the high cervical position (Figure 24.1) [17–19]. Although the term *ectopic* frequently appears in the literature concerning reoperative parathyroidectomy, no standard definition of the term exists. Hence, for the purposes of this chapter, the locations of missed parathyroid adenomas are described only in specific anatomic terms.

Classification of reoperative parathyroidectomy

Reoperative cases can be divided into two groups: those with a prior failed parathyroidectomy and those with a prior nonparathyroid neck operation (commonly thyroidectomy or anterior cervical approach for spinal surgery). Most published series of reoperative parathyroidectomy include both groups. The difficulty of reoperative parathyroidectomy arises from two distinct factors: scarring from prior surgery and adverse selection. Adverse selection refers to the removal of anatomically straightforward cases from the population through successful initial surgery, leaving a disproportionately high number of anatomically complex cases in the reoperative pool. In our opinion, adverse selection is the greatest contributor to the difficulty of reoperative parathyroidectomy. Indeed, in some cases of previous nonparathyroid neck surgery, such as previous thyroid lobectomy contralateral to a positively imaged adenoma, subsequent parathyroidectomy is actually made easier via a reduction in the number of potential operative targets. We have found that scar tissue, although unpleasant, can generally be managed with persistence and careful technique, whereas adverse selection is more difficult to overcome. Therefore, we believe that patients with prior nonparathyroid neck surgery should not be included in the reoperative group, as they dilute the sample with technically less challenging cases.

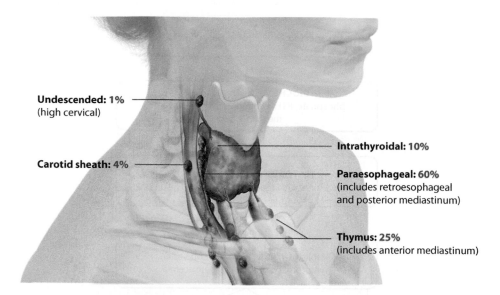

Undescended: 1%
(high cervical)

Carotid sheath: 4%

Intrathyroidal: 10%

Paraesophageal: 60%
(includes retroesophageal
and posterior mediastinum)

Thymus: 25%
(includes anterior mediastinum)

Figure 24.1 Location and frequency of parathyroid adenomas found during reoperation.

PREOPERATIVE EVALUATION

The evaluation of patients for reoperative parathyroidecomy comprises biochemical, clinical, and radiographic steps, as depicted in Figure 24.2.

Biochemical confirmation

Any patient who is suspected of having persistent or recurrent PHPT must first undergo laboratory testing to confirm the diagnosis biochemically. In brief, our practice is to complete a battery of tests (total and ionized serum calcium, phosphate, intact PTH, 25-hydroxy vitamin D, and creatinine), which are repeated in 2–3 weeks in equivocal cases. A 24-hour urine calcium collection is helpful in ruling out familial hypocalciuric hypercalcemia (FHH). Patients should have clear evidence of elevated calcium and inappropriate PTH excess to secure the diagnosis. Secondary causes of HPT should be considered, including vitamin D deficiency, renal insufficiency, and gastrointestinal abnormalities such as malabsorption or prior bariatric surgery.

Review of clinical history

A thorough personal and family history should be taken to rule out rare causes of hypercalcemia. A personal history of malignancy may suggest paraneoplastic hypercalcemia, most commonly caused by excess production of parathyroid hormone-related protein (PTHrp). Patients with a family history of hypercalcemia may have FHH, which generally presents with mild asymptomatic hypercalcemia and hypocalciuria. Other familial hyperparathyroid disorders include MEN-1, MEN-2A, and hyperparathyroidism-jaw tumor syndrome. Identification of familial HPT is important to guide operative management, screening for associated conditions, and genetic testing of family members.

Review of prior operative history

Prior operative reports should be reviewed to help guide the reoperation. Depending on the initial surgical approach (central versus lateral and focused versus four-gland exploration), a strategy can be developed to start in an area of less scarring. However, operative reports must be viewed with an appropriate amount of skepticism, as they are often fraught with misperception by the initial operating surgeon. By definition, cases of persistent PHPT arise from inadequate initial surgery; i.e., a misjudgment must have taken place in order to necessitate a reoperation. The surgeon planning the reoperation must be wary of accepting false assumptions and not take for granted any subjective observations not substantiated by objective evidence.

We have found that unless the initial surgeon has considerable experience with parathyroidectomy, the operative report may be of considerably less value than the pathology report. The pathology report can provide unequivocal evidence of parathyroid tissue that has been removed or biopsied. We routinely obtain outside pathology slides, as many samples of parathyroid tissue reported elsewhere to be hypercellular are ultimately found to contain only normal parathyroid tissue upon review by our expert pathologists.

Evaluation of vocal cord function

An evaluation of vocal cord function should be considered prior to reoperation. This can help to establish the perioperative risks, and may raise the threshold for surgery (i.e., in a patient with a nerve injury on the contralateral side to the planned reexploration). Direct laryngoscopy is performed routinely by some surgeons, while others take a selective approach based on clinical findings of hoarseness or weak cough.

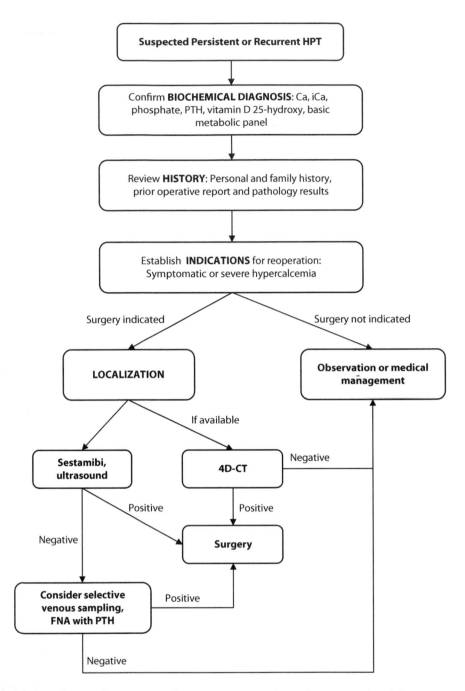

Figure 24.2 Algorithm for workup and treatment of recurrent or persistent hyperparathyroidism.

INDICATIONS FOR REOPERATIVE PARATHYROIDECTOMY

Once the diagnosis of persistent or recurrent PHPT is established biochemically, a decision is made jointly by the surgeon, patient, and referring endocrinologist of whether to embark on a reoperation. The surgical indications for initial and reoperative parathyroidectomy are the same, and include symptomatic hypercalcemia (nephrolithiasis or bone disease), severe hypercalcemia (serum calcium > 11.5 mg/dL), and osteoporosis. However, as a general rule, a greater degree of biochemical or clinical disease

severity is warranted to justify taking on the elevated risks of reoperative surgery.

As an increasing proportion of patients are identified through routine laboratory testing, the role of initial surgery for asymptomatic PHPT to prevent ongoing bone loss has expanded [20]. However, patients who are asymptomatic or minimally symptomatic may not be appropriate candidates for a reoperation, particularly if they do not have osteoporosis. The ideal candidate for reoperative parathyroidectomy has severe disease and a clear target on imaging. Patients without severe disease or who have negative preoperative localization should generally not be offered surgery.

LOCALIZATION STUDIES

Imaging studies are a critical step and must be performed prior to operative exploration. It is ideal, although in our opinion not absolutely necessary, to have two positive concordant imaging studies prior to reoperation, to decrease the need for bilateral neck exploration and maximize the chance of successful surgery. Noninvasive studies include ultrasound, technetium 99m sestamibi, computed tomography (CT), and MRI. Four-dimensional computed tomography (4D-CT) is a novel and highly sensitive imaging technique that is particularly helpful in planning reoperations. Invasive studies include selective venous sampling and ultrasound-guided PTH aspiration.

Ultrasound

It has been our practice to rely heavily on ultrasound for initial parathyroid surgery. The sensitivity for identifying abnormal parathyroid glands is between 57% and 74% [10,16]. Surgeon-performed ultrasound may be even more accurate (up to 86% sensitivity and 96% specificity) and helpful in preoperative planning [21,22].

In the reoperative setting, however, ultrasound is confounded by the presence of postoperative changes, inflammation, and reactive lymphadenopathy early in the postoperative course. In general, unless the patient is in distress from hypercalcemia, we recommend waiting at least 6 months from the time of the initial operation to perform an ultrasound. Ultrasound is highly operator dependent, which is one of its main limitations. It cannot detect mediastinal parathyroid adenomas or glands that are very posteriorly located in a patient with a deep neck. The accuracy of ultrasound diminishes in the presence of multiple thyroid nodules. It is most useful in the reoperative setting to guide aspiration of an intrathyroidal nodule for PTH measurement. Otherwise, it cannot be used as the sole study to direct a reoperation.

Technetium 99M sestamibi

Sestamibi scans have a slightly higher sensitivity (77%–85%) compared with ultrasound in identifying abnormal parathyroid glands [10]. This can be increased further by the addition of single-photon emission CT (SPECT-MIBI). Sestamibi scans are particularly helpful in ruling out a mediastinal adenoma, given the lack of background tracer uptake in that area. The drawbacks of this modality are the increased cost of the scan and necessity for radioisotope administration.

Prior to the advent of 4D-CT, sestamibi scans were the principal imaging modality used for persistent or recurrent HPT. Because most centers require two positive localization studies prior to reoperative parathyroidetomy, a negative sestamibi scan was sufficient to preclude a substantial number of patients from surgery. In our experience, 4D-CT

has increased the number of patients who are candidates for reoperation.

Other noninvasive imaging modalities

The combined sensitivity and specificity of ultrasound and sestamibi are higher than either study alone. When they are concordant, the accuracy is close to 95% [23]. If both studies are negative or the results are discordant, further localization is necessary prior to pursuing reoperation. MRI and conventional CT scans have moderate sensitivity for localizing abnormal parathyroid glands (67% and 48%, respectively) and are generally not that useful [16].

4D parathyroid CT

The new frontier in parathyroid imaging has been the development of the 4D-CT scan [24]. Helical scanning is performed through the neck and mediastinum, and the images are reconstructed as contiguous 1 mm slices in the axial, coronal, and sagittal planes. This provides anatomical detail to identify the parathyroid gland with respect to adjacent structures. Noncontrast images are obtained first, followed by administration of intravenous contrast. Two additional sets of images are then obtained (arterial phase and venous phase). The fourth dimension provides perfusion data over time. The characteristic enhancement pattern of a parathyroid adenoma includes low attenuation on the noncontrast phase, peak enhancement on the arterial phase, and washout of contrast on the delayed (venous) phase (Figures 24.3 and 24.4). 4D-CT provides anatomic and functional information, differentiating normal from abnormal parathyroid glands. The cost and radiation dose are only slightly higher than those of a sestamibi scan.

At our institution, 4D-CT has become the primary and sole imaging modality for patients with persistent or recurrent PHPT. The current practice represents the culmination of a 2-year development process. The first year consisted of developing the protocol and refining technical aspects such as patient positioning, contrast dose and timing, and radiation dose. During the second year, we validated and improved our results through a continual feedback process between the surgical team and the single, experienced radiologist who reads all of our 4D-CT scans. During this time, our execution and interpretation of the images significantly improved. A commitment to quality control, process improvement, and effective interdisciplinary communication is a prerequisite for any institution planning to develop a parathyroid 4D-CT program.

With 4D-CT, we have increased our eligibility for reoperative parathyroidectomy to 95%. We have found a very high surgical concordance with imaging results in reoperative cases (90%) [25]. Other groups have reported sensitivities of up to 88% for 4D-CT [26]. Parathyroid hyperplasia can be detected by 4D-CT in up to 80% of cases [25]. We have

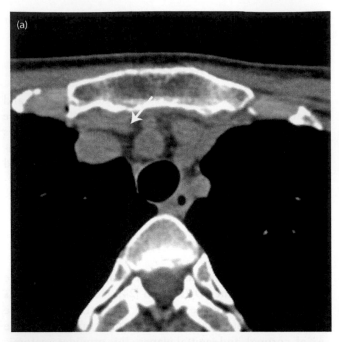

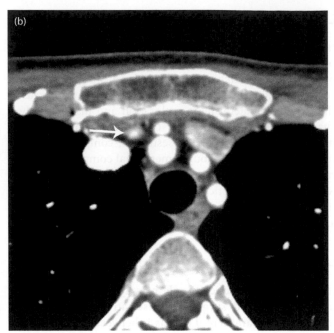

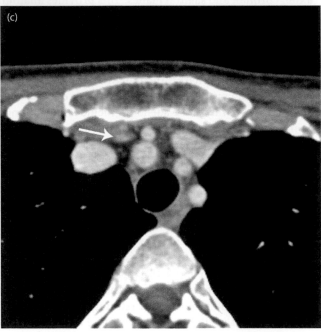

Figure 24.3 4D-CT enhancement pattern of parathyroid adenoma, located in mediastinum. **(a)** Axial noncontrast phase shows a small low-density nodule anterolateral to the brachiocephalic artery (arrow). **(b)** Axial arterial phase shows intense enhancement of this nodule. **(c)** Axial venous phase shows decreased density compared with panel b, reflecting contrast washout typical of a parathyroid adenoma.

been able to detect abnormal parathyroid glands as small as 6 mm. In the past, patients with missed hyperplasia would not have been candidates for surgery, as most, if not all, would have negative sestamibi scans and no gradient on selective venous sampling. Now, these patients can often be correctly identified preoperatively and cured with a bilateral neck exploration and creation of a subtotal parathyroidectomy. In patients undergoing evaluation for reoperative parathyroidectomy at institutions without 4D-CT, consideration should be given for referral to a center with a dedicated 4D-CT program, especially if other imaging tests have been negative.

Invasive imaging modalities

With the advent of 4D-CT, the need for invasive studies has diminished. However, if all noninvasive studies are negative or discordant but the patient has strong indications for reoperative parathyroidectomy, invasive modalities can be utilized. Currently, the most useful of these is ultrasound-guided fine-needle aspiration (FNA) with PTH measurement, which we employ principally for the evaluation of thyroid nodules suspected of being intrathyroidal parathyroid adenomas by virtue of their homogeneously hypoechoic appearance on ultrasound and location in characteristic

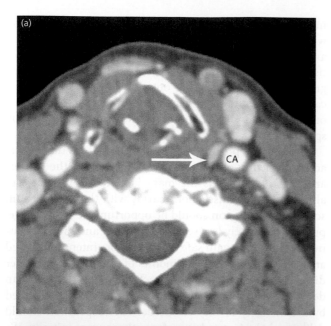

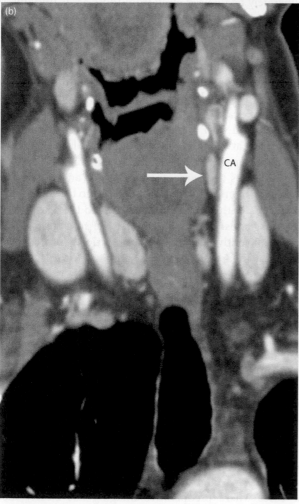

Figure 24.4 4D-CT images of parathyroid adenoma, located within carotid sheath. CA, common carotid artery. (a) Axial arterial phase shows enhancement of carotid sheath parathyroid adenoma. (b) Coronal arterial phase shows enhancement of the same adenoma.

positions for superior or inferior glands. The FNA material is washed out with 1 cc of normal saline and typically yields a binary result: either a value in the thousands (pg/mL) that clinches the presence of abnormal parathyroid tissue or a single-digit result that is negative. Cervical arteriography deserves mention for historical reasons but is seldom used today. Selective venous sampling with measurement of PTH levels in bilateral small neck blood vessels can direct the laterality of exploration. However, the utility of selective venous sampling is limited by a low rate of concordance with surgical findings, presumably due to altered venous anatomy [27].

NONOPERATIVE THERAPY

Surgery provides the best chance of a permanent cure in both initial and persistent or recurrent HPT. However, some patients may have unacceptably high perioperative risks due to medical comorbidities, while others may refuse surgery. The alternatives to reoperation include pharmacologic therapy: estrogens, raloxifene, bisphosphonates, calcitonin, and cinacalcet. Although cinacalcet reduces serum calcium levels in >60% of patients with PHPT, there is no evidence that bone mineral density (BMD) improves in these patients [28].

Angiographic and ethanol ablation of parathyroid adenomas have been described in limited case series with suboptimal results. The role of angiographic ablation is generally limited to patients with mediastinal adenomas who have prohibitive operative risks [29]. Ethanol ablation can be utilized for patients with multiple prior operations who may have excessive perioperative risks due to scarring. With the improvement in parathyroid imaging, there are almost no indications for these procedures. They expose the patient to the rare complication of parathyromatosis and increase scarring in the event that a reoperation is later attempted. Patients with mild disease and no significant skeletal manifestations can reasonably be observed. Patients with indications for treatment should be offered surgery if possible.

SURGICAL TECHNIQUE

A thorough knowledge of the embryology and anatomy of the parathyroid glands is critical for a successful reoperation. Ideally, a focused exploration is planned based on preoperative localization. A key determinant of the safety and success of reoperation is the severity of scarring, which cannot be determined by any imaging modality of which we are aware. Whenever possible, we postpone reoperations for at least 6 months after initial surgery to allow for the most intense period of scarring to subside. The most difficult type of scar tissue is laminar scar tissue, which completely obliterates tissue planes. We have noted that the worst scarring occurs in cases complicated by postoperative hematoma after initial surgery, presumably due to widespread inflammation in the central neck. Since scarring cannot be predicted, the surgeon must exercise good judgment intraoperatively by keeping the indications for surgery closely in mind. In other words, the surgeon should be prepared to cease operating if there is excessive risk to vascular structures or nerves, especially if the indication for surgery is not life threatening. If a thorough exploration of the target territory identified by imaging fails to reveal abnormal parathyroid tissue, strong consideration should be given to stop the operation and perform further workup rather than embarking on further blind exploration.

The incision should be made to allow for optimal exposure. Sometimes, the operation can be performed through the same cervical incision that was used for the initial surgery. However, the surgeon should not hesitate to make a new incision, since part of the reason for a failed initial operation can be poor exposure (most often an incision placed too low with respect to the cricoid cartilage). Most reoperations are performed through a standard anterior approach. The surgeon may be assisted by transverse division of the strap muscles to aid exposure.

In cases where the initial operation was performed via an anterior approach and imaging is adequate to direct a focused reoperation, a lateral approach can be utilized to minimize operating in a scarred field. This is performed by mobilizing the medial border of the sternocleidomastoid muscle away from the lateral border of the strap muscles. The carotid sheath is then retracted laterally, exposing the thyroid gland and parathyroid-bearing regions of the central neck. This approach can facilitate identification of the recurrent laryngeal nerve (RLN) in an unscarred field, and is particularly useful for posteriorly located, paraesophageal adenomas.

The most important initial operative milestone during re-exploration is to achieve orientation. This can be very difficult in the reoperative neck due to scarring and distorted anatomy. We utilize the cricoid cartilage as an essential early landmark for orientation. Identification of the readily palpable cricoid cartilage orients the surgeon in both the lateral–medial and cephalocaudad dimensions. We have noted that achieving cephalocaudad orientation can be particularly challenging in patients with prior thyroid resection, as the presence of the thyroid gland normally serves as an important orienting cue. Proceeding inferiorly from the cricoid, it is generally straightforward to dissect out the airway in the midline, which we usually do with electrocautery. The trachea is the most resilient anatomic structure in the central neck (even when it is injured, it is almost always readily reparable), and thus represents an early "anchor" for the surgeon in gaining some degree of forward traction in a hostile operative field.

The second step is to become oriented to the carotid sheath, which can be identified through palpation of the carotid pulse. The carotid sheath is opened, at first vertically down on the common carotid artery and then medial to it, exposing the carotid artery with caution. Care must be taken to avoid getting into a subadventitial plane while dissecting out the carotid artery, which can predispose it to

injury with resulting hemorrhage. Most often, the surgeon will find that the carotid sheath was previously undissected and offers virgin territory. If the surgeon encounters scar tissue at this stage, the dissection must proceed with even greater caution. Dissecting out the medial aspect of the carotid artery allows for gentle lateral traction to be placed on the carotid sheath, exposing the parathyroid-bearing space.

The third step is identification of the RLN. This is best accomplished in an "outside-in" fashion using the trachea and carotid sheath as the main landmarks. We perform almost all of this dissection sharply with the Metzenbaum scissors. The surgeon should be opportunistic at this stage, pursuing relatively less scarred areas first and then exploiting these areas to gain safe access to more intensely scarred areas as necessary. These windows of opportunity for safer dissection are individual for each case. The surgeon can deduce where the bulk of the initial surgery was performed by the intensity of the scar tissue. The reoperation should deliberately be focused away from those areas initially. We often accomplish this by starting very inferiorly in the neck and identifying the RLN at the level of the thoracic inlet, and then tracing it superiorly into the scarred field.

Aside from these points, the strategy for reoperative parathyroidectomy is based on the same embryologic principles as the initial operation. The superior parathyroid glands are located posterolateral to the RLN and are usually associated with the inferior thyroid artery, which runs transversely at the level of the cricoid cartilage. Due to the frequency of paraesophageal missed adenomas, it is imperative to access the paraesophageal space and prevertebral fascia by dissecting sufficiently posterior to the inferior thyroid artery, both superior and inferior to the artery. Many superior glands are missed because the surgeon has failed to go sufficiently deep to find a posteriorly located gland. Indeed, at this stage of the case we often "break through" to unscarred territory and discover a posteriorly located adenoma in the paraesophageal space that has not been previously dissected. Superior glands may also be within the carotid sheath, undescended (above the superior pole of the thyroid), or intrathyroidal (requiring enucleation or some degree of thyroid resection).

The inferior parathyroid glands are located anteromedial to the RLN and are usually associated with the inferior pole thyroid veins running into the thyrothymic tract. Inferior glands are commonly associated with the thymus, but may also be undescended, within the carotid sheath, or intrathyroidal. Most mediastinal glands are located in the anterior superior mediastinum and can be removed through a cervical incision. Median sternotomy or thoracoscopy is reserved for cases where preoperative imaging has clearly localized a mediastinal adenoma that is not accessible from the neck. Supernumerary glands are found in 13% of patients in autopsy series, and have been reported in up to 30% of patients with PHPT [30]. This should be suspected if four normal glands have been histopathologically documented in a patient with biochemically confirmed PHPT.

A number of intraoperative adjuncts may be helpful when there is difficulty locating a parathyroid gland. Intraoperative ultrasound may identify abnormal parathyroid glands that were not previously detected, including intrathyroidal glands [18]. Ultrasound-guided methylene blue dye injection has been described with good success in small series [31]. Frozen section is best utilized to confirm that parathyroid tissue has been excised when a single target was identified preoperatively, and scarring prevents positive identification by gross visual inspection alone. Bilateral internal jugular vein sampling for PTH can establish a gradient between the left and right neck and help lateralize an operation. When a parathyroid gland cannot be found but has been localized to one side, ipsilateral inferior thyroid artery ligation can be attempted to infarct the gland. Radioguided gamma probe has been described to help locate and confirm removal of the abnormal gland, but with no clear evidence of improved success [32]. Intraoperative PTH monitoring is highly accurate and may increase the cure rate of reoperation [32,33].

PERIOPERATIVE COMPLICATIONS

The risks of parathyroidectomy, namely, RLN injury and permanent hypocalcemia, are higher when performed in a reoperative field. The rate of hoarseness from temporary unilateral nerve injury has been reported to be between 6% and 8%, compared with 2%–5% for an initial parathyroidectomy [30,34]. Despite the difficulty in identifying the anatomy in a scarred field, permanent nerve injury is rare. It occurs in approximately 1% of cases in published series from high-volume surgeons (range 0.4%–4%), compared with 0.5% for the initial surgery [17,18]. Regardless, the surgical strategy during reoperation is usually unilateral in accordance with positive preoperative localization to avoid the risk of endangering both nerves, which can necessitate a tracheostomy. Intraoperative nerve monitoring has not been shown to prevent nerve injury, and its use is surgeon specific [35].

The rate of permanent hypocalcemia may be as high as 5%–8%, compared with 1% for initial parathyroidectomy [34]. In rare cases, the prior operation has resulted in removal of all normal parathyroid tissue. The possibility of permanent hypoparathyroidism after reoperation must be considered and discussed with the patient during preoperative counseling. In cases where it is suspected that the patient may have no residual parathyroid tissue after reoperation, cryopreservation should be considered. Other risks of surgery (neck hematoma or infection) should occur in less than 1% of cases.

OUTCOMES OF REOPERATION

In experienced hands, the success of reoperative parathyroidectomy is 80%–95% (Table 24.1), as defined by continuous eucalcemia for 6 months after surgery. The rate of success is largely dependent on the underlying pathology

Table 24.1 Success rates for reoperative parathyroidectomy

Author (reference)	No. of patients	% cured
Wang [37]	112	91
Brennan [38]	175	90
Grant [39]	157	89
Levin [40]	81	91
Cheung [41]	83	86
Rothmund [42]	70	96
Carty [43]	206	95
Järhult [44]	93	82
Rodriquez [45]	152	93
Shen [19]	102	95
Jaskowiak [17]	222	97
Mariette [30]	38	92
Rotstein [46]	28	85
Thompson [47]	124	88
Irvin [33]	33	94
Udelsman [10]	130	95
Hessman [48]	144	93
Yen [16]	39	92
Powell [18]	163	92
Silberfein [15]	54	93
Cham [25]	90	87

and surgeon experience. Experienced, high-volume centers have demonstrated success rates up to 97% in modern series of cases of missed adenomas [17,10,36]. Series that include patients with multigland disease have lower success rates of 86%–96%. Most published series include patients with prior nonparathyroid surgery, which may artificially inflate the success rate. Patients with positive preoperative localization are also more likely to be cured.

CONCLUSIONS

Although relatively uncommon, persistent and recurrent PHPT continue to be significant clinical problems. Despite the high cure rate of initial parathyroidectomy, the frequency of reoperative parathyroidectomy does not appear to be declining over time on the population level [49], suggesting that endocrine surgeons will need to carry out these very difficult operations for the foreseeable future. Improvements in preoperative localization have facilitated the surgical care of these patients. 4D-CT has been the greatest incremental advance in reoperative parathyroidectomy. In our experience, it has displaced the use of other imaging modalities and increased eligibility for surgery (Figure 24.2). 4D-CT has enhanced our ability to perform safe, efficient reoperations with a high cure rate. It has also allowed us to identify and cure patients with missed hyperplasia, who previously were not candidates for surgery.

An important caveat is that all of these reoperative cases need to be performed by high-volume centers due to the increased risks involved and significant potential for a second failed operation. Although these cases remain challenging, careful development of surgical strategy and adherence to the above-mentioned technical principles contribute to the safety and success of reoperation.

REFERENCES

1. Mandl F. Hyperparathyroidism; a review of historical developments and the present state of knowledge on the subject. *Surgery* 1947;21(3):394–440.

2. Bauer W, Federman DD. Hyperparathyroidism epitomized: The case of Captain Charles E. Martell. *Metabolism* 1962;11:21–9.

3. Yeh MW, Wiseman JE, Chu SD et al. Population-level predictors of persistent hyperparathyroidism. *Surgery* 2011;150(6):1113–9.

4. Yeh MW, Ituarte PH, Zhou HC et al. Incidence and prevalence of primary hyperparathyroidism in a racially mixed population. *J Clin Endocrinol Metab* 2013;98(3):1122–9.

5. Yeh MW, Wiseman JE, Ituarte PH et al. Surgery for primary hyperparathyroidism: Are the consensus guidelines being followed? *Ann Surg* 2012;255(6):1179–83.

6. Sosa JA, Wang TS, Yeo HL et al. The maturation of a specialty: Workforce projections for endocrine surgery. *Surgery* 2007;142(6):876–83.

7. Udelsman R. Six hundred fifty-six consecutive explorations for primary hyperparathyroidism. *Ann Surg* 2002;235(5):665–70; discussion 670–2.

8. Clark OH, Way LW, Hunt TK. Recurrent hyperparathyroidism. *Ann Surg* 1976;184(4):391–402.

9. Haff RC, Ballinger WF. Causes of recurrent hypercalcemia after parathyroidectomy for primary hyperparathyroidism. *Ann Surg* 1971;173(6):884–91.

10. Udelsman R, Donovan PI. Remedial parathyroid surgery: Changing trends in 130 consecutive cases. *Ann Surg* 2006;244(3):471–9.

11. Al-Kurd A, Mekel M, Mazeh H. Parathyroid carcinoma. *Surg Oncol* 2014;23(2):107–14.

12. Carpten JD, Robbins CM, Villablanca A et al. HRPT2, encoding parafibromin, is mutated in hyperparathyroidism-jaw tumor syndrome. *Nat Genet* 2002;32(4):676–80.

13. Kebebew E, Arici C, Duh QY, Clark OH. Localization and reoperation results for persistent and recurrent parathyroid carcinoma. *Arch Surg* 2001;136(8):878–85.

14. Shen WT. Parathyromatosis and parathyroid cancer. *Cancer Treat Res* 2010;153:105–16.

15. Silberfein EJ, Bao R, Lopez A et al. Reoperative parathyroidectomy: Location of missed glands based on a contemporary nomenclature system. *Arch Surg* 2010;145(11):1065–8.

16. Yen TW, Wang TS, Doffek KM, Krzywda EA, Wilson SD. Reoperative parathyroidectomy: An algorithm for imaging and monitoring of intraoperative parathyroid hormone levels that results in a successful focused approach. *Surgery* 2008;144(4):611–9; discussion 619–21.

17. Jaskowiak N, Norton JA, Alexander HR et al. A prospective trial evaluating a standard approach to reoperation for missed parathyroid adenoma. *Ann Surg* 1996;224(3):308–20; discussion 320–1.

18. Powell AC, Alexander HR, Chang R et al. Reoperation for parathyroid adenoma: A contemporary experience. *Surgery* 2009;146(6):1144–55.

19. Shen W, Düren M, Morita E et al. Reoperation for persistent or recurrent primary hyperparathyroidism. *Arch Surg* 1996;131(8):861–7; discussion 867–9.

20. Bilezikian JP, Khan AA, Potts JT, Third International Workshop on the Management of Asymptomatic Primary Hyperthyroidism. Guidelines for the management of asymptomatic primary hyperparathyroidism: Summary statement from the third international workshop. *J Clin Endocrinol Metab* 2009;94(2):335–9.

21. Hughes DT, Sorensen MJ, Miller BS, Cohen MS, Gauger PG. The biochemical severity of primary hyperparathyroidism correlates with the localization accuracy of sestamibi and surgeon-performed ultrasound. *J Am Coll Surg* 2014;219:1010–19.

22. Schenk WG, Hanks JB, Smith PW. Surgeon-performed ultrasound for primary hyperparathyroidism. *Am Surg* 2013;79(7):681–5.

23. Prasannan S, Davies G, Bochner M, Kollias J, Malycha P. Minimally invasive parathyroidectomy using surgeon-performed ultrasound and sestamibi. *ANZ J Surg* 2007;77(9):774–7.

24. Rodgers SE, Hunter GJ, Hamberg LM et al. Improved preoperative planning for directed parathyroidectomy with 4-dimensional computed tomography. *Surgery* 2006;140(6):932–40; discussion 940–1.

25. Cham S, Sepahdari AR, Hall KE, Yeh MW, Harari A. Dynamic parathyroid computed tomography (4DCT) facilitates reoperative parathyroidectomy and enables cure of missed hyperplasia. *Ann Surg Oncol* 2014;22(11):3537–42.

26. Mortenson MM, Evans DB, Lee JE et al. Parathyroid exploration in the reoperative neck: Improved preoperative localization with 4D-computed tomography. *J Am Coll Surg* 2008;206(5):888–95; discussion 895–6.

27. Morris LF, Loh C, Ro K et al. Non-super-selective venous sampling for persistent hyperparathyroidism using a systemic hypocalcemic challenge. *J Vasc Interv Radiol* 2012;23(9):1191–9.

28. Marcocci C, Bollerslev J, Khan AA, Shoback DM. Medical management of primary hyperparathyroidism: Proceedings of the fourth international workshop on the management of asymptomatic primary hyperparathyroidism. *J Clin Endocrinol Metab* 2014;99(10):3607–18.

29. McIntyre RC, Kumpe DA, Liechty RD. Reexploration and angiographic ablation for hyperparathyroidism. *Arch Surg* 1994;129(5):499–503; discussion 494–5.

30. Mariette C, Pellissier L, Combemale F, Quievreux JL, Carnaille B, Proye C. Reoperation for persistent or recurrent primary hyperparathyroidism. *Langenbecks Arch Surg* 1998;383(2):174–9.

31. Candell L, Campbell MJ, Shen WT, Gosnell JE, Clark OH, Duh QY. Ultrasound-guided methylene blue dye injection for parathyroid localization in the reoperative neck. *World J Surg* 2014;38(1):88–91.

32. Chen H, Mack E, Starling JR. A comprehensive evaluation of perioperative adjuncts during minimally invasive parathyroidectomy: Which is most reliable? *Ann Surg* 2005;242(3):375–80; discussion 380–3.

33. Irvin GL, Molinari AS, Figueroa C, Carneiro DM. Improved success rate in reoperative parathyroidectomy with intraoperative PTH assay. *Ann Surg* 1999;229(6):874–8; discussion 878–9.

34. Patow CA, Norton JA, Brennan MF. Vocal cord paralysis and reoperative parathyroidectomy. A prospective study. *Ann Surg* 1986;203(3):282–5.

35. Pisanu A, Porceddu G, Podda M, Cois A, Uccheddu A. Systematic review with meta-analysis of studies comparing intraoperative neuromonitoring of recurrent laryngeal nerves versus visualization alone during thyroidectomy. *J Surg Res* 2014;188(1):152–61.

36. Prescott JD, Udelsman R. Remedial operation for primary hyperparathyroidism. *World J Surg* 2009;33(11):2324–34.

37. Wang CA. Parathyroid re-exploration. A clinical and pathological study of 112 cases. *Ann Surg* 1977 Aug;186(2):140–5.

38. Brennan MF, Norton JA. Reoperation for persistent and recurrent hyperparathyroidism. *Ann Surg* 1985;201(1):40–4.

39. Grant CS, van Heerden JA, Charboneau JW, James EM, Reading CC. Clinical management of persistent and/or recurrent primary hyperparathyroidism. *World J Surg* 1986;10(4):555–65.

40. Levin KE, Clark OH. The reasons for failure in parathyroid operations. *Arch Surg* 1989;124(8):911–4; discussion 914–5.

41. Cheung PS, Borgstrom A, Thompson NW. Strategy in reoperative surgery for hyperparathyroidism. *Arch Surg* 1989;124(6):676–80.

42. Rothmund M, Wagner PK, Seesko H, Zielke A. Lessons from reoperations in 55 patients with primary hyperparathyroidism [in German]. *Dtsch Med Wochenschr* 1990;115(42):1579–85.

43. Carty SE, Norton JA. Management of patients with persistent or recurrent primary hyperparathyroidism. *World J Surg* 1991;15(6):716–23.

44. Järhult J, Nordenström J, Perbeck L. Reoperation for suspected primary hyperparathyroidism. *Br J Surg* 1993;80(4):453–6.

45. Rodriquez JM, Tezelman S, Siperstein AE et al. Localization procedures in patients with persistent or recurrent hyperparathyroidism. *Arch Surg* 1994;129(8):870–5.

46. Rotstein L, Irish J, Gullane P, Keller MA, Sniderman K. Reoperative parathyroidectomy in the era of localization technology. *Head Neck* 1998;20(6):535–9.

47. Thompson GB, Grant CS, Perrier ND et al. Reoperative parathyroid surgery in the era of sestamibi scanning and intraoperative parathyroid hormone monitoring. *Arch Surg* 1999;134(7):699–704; discussion 704–5.

48. Hessman O, Stålberg P, Sundin A et al. High success rate of parathyroid reoperation may be achieved with improved localization diagnosis. *World J Surg* 2008;32(5):774–81; discussion 782–3.

49. Abdulla AG, Ituarte PH, Harari A, Wu JX, Yeh MW. Trends in the frequency and quality of parathyroid surgery: Analysis of 17,082 cases over 10 years. *Ann Surg* 2015;261(4):746–50.

Adrenals

Adrenals

25

Adrenocortical function, adrenal insufficiency

GILLIAN M. GODDARD AND ALICE C. LEVINE

Proper function of the adrenal cortex is essential for the maintenance of all tissues and organs. Both hyper- and hypofunction can be life threatening. Understanding the etiology, treatment, and management of adrenal cortical disease is particularly critical in the perioperative management of patients.

ADRENAL CORTICAL INSUFFICIENCY

Adrenal insufficiency (AI) commonly refers to the deficient production of the adrenal cortical hormones cortisol, aldosterone, and adrenal androgens. AI is divided by etiology into primary and secondary. *Primary insufficiency,* which is due to destruction of all cells of the adrenal cortex, presents with signs and symptoms of both mineralocorticoid and glucocorticoid deficiency and requires replacement of both. In contrast, secondary adrenal cortical insufficiency is due to lack of adrenocorticotropic hormone (ACTH) stimulation, and since aldosterone is primarily regulated by the renin–angiotensin system and *not* ACTH, patients with secondary adrenal cortical insufficiency *only* require glucocorticoid replacement. This is an important distinction, as patients with primary adrenal cortical insufficiency are more severely deficient, and the lack of mineralocorticoid renders them more prone to electrolyte abnormalities (low sodium and high potassium), as well as hypotension and cardiovascular collapse. *Secondary adrenal cortical insufficiency,* which is generally due to lack of ACTH or suppression of the entire hypothalamic–pituitary–adrenal (HPA) axis, often from long-term exogenous glucocorticoids or their equivalent, can also be severe in the setting of stress when glucocorticoid requirements are increased.

ETIOLOGY OF ADRENAL CORTICAL INSUFFICIENCY

The most common cause of primary AI in developed countries is autoimmune destruction of the adrenal cortex, often referred to as Addison's disease. It may occur alone or in association with other autoimmune disorders, as in autoimmune polyglandular syndrome types 1 and 2. In undeveloped areas, infectious causes such as tuberculosis are the most common cause of primary AI. HIV-related causes of primary insufficiency are increasingly common. Additionally, many medications can lead to primary insufficiency [1] (Table 25.1).

Iatrogenic causes are the most frequent etiology of secondary AI. Medications such as exogenous steroids suppress ACTH production, leading to atrophy of the zona fasciculata that produces cortisol. Abrupt withdrawal of exogenous steroids is the most common cause of AI. As little as 5 mg of prednisone or the equivalent taken daily for longer than 3 weeks can lead to secondary insufficiency. Of note, all steroid hormones and their receptors are quite structurally similar, and therefore when pharmacologic doses of nonglucocorticoid steroids are given (i.e., the progestational agent, megestrol acetate, given for AIDS wasting), there can be suppression of the HPA glucocorticoid axis, resulting in prolonged AI and the need for stress dose glucocorticoids perioperatively [2] (Table 25.1).

SIGNS AND SYMPTOMS

In the nonstressed state, signs and symptoms of AI may be very vague and nonspecific, such as fatigue and weakness. The majority of patients with complete primary AI will

Table 25.1 Medications that may cause adrenal insufficiency

Mechanism	Medication
Primary Adrenal Insufficiency	
Inhibit cortisol synthesis	Aminoglutethimide
	Trilostane
	Ketoconazole
	Fluconazole
	Etomidate
Activate cortisol metabolism	Phenobarbital
	Phenytoin
	Rifampin
	Troglitazone
Secondary Adrenal Insufficiency	
Suppress CRH and ACTH	Exogenous glucocorticoids
	Opioids
	Megesterol acetate
	Medroxyprogesterone acetate
	Fluticasone
	Ketorolactromethamine
Induce peripheral cortisol resistance	Mifepristone
	Chlorpromazine
	Imipramine

exhibit a true anorexia, and will report weight loss even in the nonstressed state. Signs and symptoms of severe adrenal cortical insufficiency more likely occur in the setting of stress (i.e., surgery) and include nausea, vomiting, muscle aches and weakness, anorexia, and hypotension.

In addition, patients with primary AI may demonstrate orthostatic hypotension, hyponatremia, and hyperkalemia due to the concomitant mineralocorticoid deficiency. Elevations in ACTH levels in primary AI can also lead to skin hyperpigmentation [3].

Acute AI, or adrenal crisis, presents as persistent hypotension or shock that is out of proportion to the concurrent illness. Other presenting features include fever, abdominal pain, altered mental status, and electrolyte disturbances, but these symptoms may be nonspecific. If adrenal crisis is suspected in an unstable patient, immediate initiation of stress dose steroids is necessary. Of note, severe, acute AI with hypotension and electrolyte imbalance is most often seen in patients with primary AI who have *both* glucocorticoid and mineralocorticoid deficiency.

DIAGNOSING ADRENAL INSUFFICIENCY

Diagnosing adrenal insufficiency in unstressed patients

In the unstressed state, cortisol is secreted in a circadian rhythm with peak levels in the early morning (between 0600

and 0800) and the lowest levels around midnight (2400) [4]. Cortisol circulates in the serum bound to the proteins cortisol binding globulin (CBG) and albumin, and only the free fraction of cortisol in the serum is biologically active [5]. Multiple factors modulate cortisol levels, including older age, low-serum protein levels (CBG and albumin), and stress. Many drugs can cause suppression of steroid levels without overt signs or symptoms of AI in the unstressed patient that may be uncovered in the hospitalized setting [1].

A baseline morning cortisol level drawn between 0600 and 0800 may be used as an initial screening test for an unstressed patient (Figure 25.1).

The cosyntropin stimulation test is the most widely used test for the diagnosis of AI. The cosyntropin test uses synthetic ACTH injected intravenously to stimulate the adrenal gland to produce cortisol. Peak cortisol levels occur between 30 and 60 minutes after ACTH injection. This test can be performed at any time of day and is generally easy and safe [6,7] (Figure 25.1).

Distinguishing primary AI versus secondary AI can be difficult, but in general, patients with primary AI will have high levels of ACTH and low levels of the mineralocorticoid aldosterone. Patients with secondary AI generally have low or inappropriately normal levels of ACTH with no aldosterone deficiency.

Diagnosing adrenal insufficiency in stressed or critically ill patients

Although previous reports indicated that critically ill patients without any impairment in their adrenal cortical axis should have a random total cortisol level of >35 µg/dL [8], a greater understanding of the dynamics of cortisol secretion and binding during stress has called into question some of the older dogma regarding testing and the interpretation of results in stressed patients [9,10]. In the setting of critical illness, the two major binding proteins for cortisol in serum, CBG and albumin, decrease, thus leading to lower *total* cortisol levels but *higher* percentage free, active cortisol. Furthermore, a low cortisol response to corticotrophin stimulation does not necessarily reflect "relative AI" in this setting, since cortisol production in critically ill patients is not subnormal and free cortisol levels are often increased due to constitutive activation of the hypothalamic–pituitary corticotropin-releasing hormone (CRH)-ACTH axis. Therefore, in the stressed state, measurements of free cortisol in serum would be optimal. Unfortunately, there are no convenient, rapid free cortisol assays available. *If there is a high index of suspicion of AI, or pre-existing AI, in a surgical patient, total and free cortisol levels should be sent, and while awaiting results, stress dose steroids should be initiated.*

TREATMENT OF ADRENAL CORTICAL INSUFFICIENCY

In the *nonstressed state*, patients with AI will require 15–30 mg of hydrocortisone orally or the equivalent per

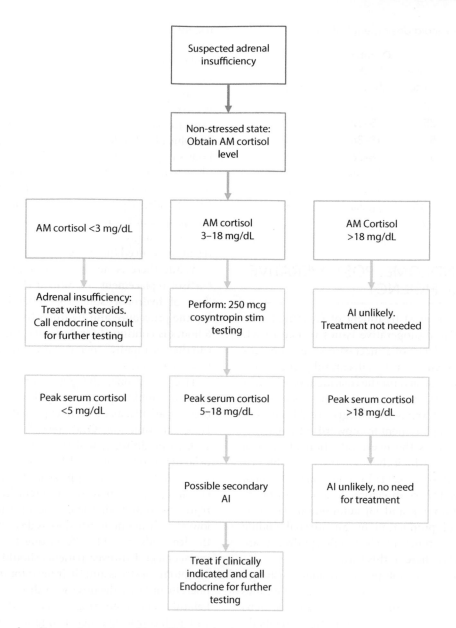

Figure 25.1 Algorithm for diagnosing adrenal insufficiency in the nonstressed state.

day. The precise formulation of glucocorticoid replacement given varies according to patient preference, lifestyle, and the estimated need for acute vs. chronic replacement therapy. If it is anticipated that the HPA axis will return with time, it is preferable to utilize a short-acting glucocorticoid such as hydrocortisone, to allow for recovery. Patients with primary AI require mineralocorticoid replacement with fludrocortisone as well. In cases of moderate illness, such as fever, patients require two to three times their usual daily dose of glucocorticoid replacement.

Surgical procedures place a significant stress on the body. When AI is present, it is important to provide appropriate perioperative supplementation of cortisol when surgical procedures are planned. Of note, when any degree of AI is suspected, or if there is a history of glucocorticoid or other steroid hormone use in the months prior to surgery,

it is always safer to give stress dose glucocorticoids on call to the operating room, and then continue for 24 hours postoperatively, rather than run the risk of having the patient develop AI in the perioperative period [11]. In the past, very high doses of steroids, the equivalent of 300 mg of hydrocortisone per 24 hours, were given intra- and postoperatively. More recent studies suggest that this may not be necessary and may be harmful to patients [12]. Doses of 25–50 mg intravenous (IV) hydrocortisone every 6 hours are adequate to provide both glucocorticoid and mineralocorticoid replacement during stress. If the stress glucocorticoid given is dexamethasone (no mineralocorticoid activity even at high doses) in a patient with primary AI during stress, mineralocorticoid replacement with florinef must be continued (see Table 25.2 for glucocorticoid dosing equivalents).

Table 25.2 Glucocorticoid dosing equivalents

	Dose (mg)	Duration of action (hours)	Mineralo-corticoid activity (Y/N)
Hydrocortisone	20	8–12	Y
Cortisone acetate	25	8–12	Y
Prednisone	5	18–36	Y
Prednisolone	5	18–36	Y
Methylprednisolone	4	18–36	Y
Triamcinolone	4	18–36	N
Dexamethasone	0.75	36–54	N
Betamethasone	0.6	36–54	N

CUSHING'S SYNDROME: POSTOPERATIVE ADRENAL INSUFFICIENCY

Patients undergoing surgical treatment of Cushing's syndrome pose particular postoperative issues related to AI. Postoperative AI is evidence of a successful surgical procedure in these patients. Given this goal, careful preoperative planning should be performed for the treatment of AI. Most patients with Cushing's syndrome that are successfully treated surgically will develop some degree of AI, necessitating glucocorticoid replacement for upwards of 1 year.

Cushing's syndrome is the overproduction of cortisol by the adrenal cortex, of which there are three possible etiologies: [1] oversecretion of ACTH by a pituitary adenoma, [2] production of ACTH by an ectopic lesion (most often, the source is lung tumors), and [3] autonomous (ACTH-independent) cortisol production by an adrenal nodule or nodules. All three types of Cushing's syndrome are addressed in detail elsewhere in this text.

Increasingly, a new phenotype of adrenal Cushing's is being recognized—*mild hypercortisolism*, sometimes referred to as subclinical Cushing's syndrome. Autonomous cortisol production is not as robust, and thus patients do not typically develop the classical features of Cushing's syndrome. However, they may develop metabolic derangements, such as obesity, hyperglycemia or diabetes mellitus, lipid abnormalities, and osteoporosis [13]. Data from recent literature suggest that any degree of mild hypercortisolism over time is particularly deleterious to the cardiovascular system [14,15].

In adrenal Cushing's, the autonomous production of cortisol by an adrenal nodule or nodules suppresses the production of cortisol by the normal adrenal tissue. Often, the contralateral gland is atrophic [16].

Careful perioperative dosing of supplemental steroids is imperative when surgical resection of an adrenal nodule or nodules that are oversecreting cortisol is planned. All patients with adrenal nodules should have a 1 mg dexamethasone suppression test preoperatively, even if no signs or symptoms of Cushing's are noted. Failure to suppress morning cortisol to <1.8 µg/dL after 1 mg of dexamethasone the night before with adequate serum dexamethasone levels for

test interpretation should alert the surgeon that mild hypercortisolism may exist and should trigger some glucocorticoid replacement postoperatively. We recommend the use of high-dose cortisol during and immediately after unilateral adrenalectomy in patients with suspected hypercortisolism undergoing adrenalectomy. The surgery itself is a significant stress to the patient, and furthermore, the contralateral atrophic gland is dormant and is not capable of meeting the body's requirements for cortisol. Additionally, the patient is likely to have transient primary AI for many months following unilateral adrenalectomy if hypercortisolism was noted prior to adrenalectomy, requiring steroid supplementation for upwards of a year of more. Recent literature suggests that even mild degrees of hypercortisolism preoperatively will result in the need for exogenous glucocorticoid therapy [17].

While there is no validated approach to perioperative cortisol replacement, we utilize the following strategy. A dose of hydrocortisone 25–50 mg is administered during the procedure and hydrocortisone 25–50 mg IV every 6 hours is continued for 24 hours postoperatively. Patients can then be rapidly tapered to an oral hydrocortisone maintenance regimen.

Hydrocortisone, the glucocorticoid with the shortest half-life, should be used for supplementation in this population of patients, as they are expected to regain endogenous HPA axis function. Oral steroids with a longer half-life, such as prednisone, will suppress the HPA axis, possibly delaying recovery of the HPA axis.

A patient-centered approach should be employed that encourages patients to try different hydrocortisone dosing regimens to find what works best for them. In general, the lowest daily maintenance dose is desirable, as this will cause the least adverse side effects due to glucocorticoid over-replacement. However, patients should be alert to signs and symptoms of stress and their need for increased dosing, and liberally increase the dose according to their symptoms. It is helpful to check morning cortisol and ACTH levels after the patient has held hydrocortisone for 24 hours to gauge the degree of recovery of the HPA axis.

Even after daily cortisol replacement is discontinued, patients may continue to require exogenous steroid replacement during times of stress.

CONGENITAL ADRENAL HYPERPLASIA

Genetic diseases in which cortisol production is compromised due to mutations in genes encoding either the enzymes responsible for steroid hormone synthesis or their cofactors are termed congenital adrenal hyperplasia (CAH). Bilateral enlargement of the adrenal cortex occurs due to the low cortisol levels and lack of negative feedback on ACTH, with increased ACTH secretion that stimulates both adrenal cortical growth and steroid hormone production. The most common form of CAH is 21-hydroxylase deficiency, and it exists in both a "classic" (severe) and a "nonclassic" (mild) form. In the perioperative period, the nonclassic, mild form is only important if the patient was receiving glucocorticoid therapy prior to the surgery. However, the classic form of 21-hydroxylase deficiency may have several relevant features that must be addressed in surgical patients.

First and foremost, in classic 21-hydroxylase deficiency, there is cortisol insufficiency, so these patients require stress dose glucocorticoids perioperatively. Second, in some mutations, there is a combined deficiency of both glucocorticoids and mineralocorticoids, so that *unless* a glucocorticoid replacement is utilized that has sufficient mineralocorticoid activity in the perioperative period (i.e., hydrocortisone at doses exceeding 50 mg/day), a mineralocorticoid such as florinef must be added. Finally, untreated, classic, severe 21-hydroxylase deficiency is associated with chronic enlargement of the adrenal glands and an increased prevalence of adrenal tumors, including massive myelolipomas. Males with classic 21-hydroxylase deficiency also commonly develop testicular adrenal rest tumors (TARTs) [10–20].

SUMMARY

It is essential to identify patients with AI prior to any planned surgery and develop a perioperative treatment protocol. Although primary AI is a relatively rare disorder, secondary deficiency, particularly due to the use of exogenous steroids, is not unusual. Finally, in patients undergoing surgery for adrenal adenomas or carcinomas, there is a high incidence of mild hypercortisolism that can result in postoperative AI.

REFERENCES

1. Bornstein SR. Predisposing factors for adrenal insufficiency. *N Engl J Med.* 2009;360:2328–39.
2. Mann M, Koller E, Murgo A, Malozowsky S, Bacsanyi J, Leinung M. Glucocorticoidlike activity of megestrol: A summary of Food and Drug Administration experience and a review of the literature. *Arch Intern Med* 1997;157:1651–56.
3. Arlt W, Allolio B. Adrenal insufficiency. *Lancet* 2003;361:1881–93.
4. Lennernas H, Skrtic S, Johannsson G. Replacement therapy of oral hydrocortisone in adrenal insufficiency: The influence of gastrointestinal factors. *Expert Opin Drug Metab Toxicol* 2008;4:749–58.
5. Maxime V, Lesur O, Annane D. Adrenal insufficiency in septic shock. *Clin Chest Med* 2009;30:17–27.
6. Kronenberg HM. Glucocorticoid deficiency. In: Kronenberg HM, Melmed S, Polonsky KS, Larsen PR, eds., *Williams Textbook of Endocrinology.* 11th ed, pp. 519–20. Philadelphia: Saunders Elsevier, 2008.
7. Neary N, Nieman L. Adrenal insufficiency: Etiology, diagnosis and treatment. *Curr Opin Endocrinol Diabetes Obes* 2010;17:217–23.
8. Cooper MS, Stewart PM. Corticosteroid deficiency in acutely ill patients. *N Engl J Med* 2003;348:727–34.
9. Boonen E, Vervenne H, Meersseman P et al. Reduced cortisol metabolism during critical illness. *New Engl J Med* 2013;368:1477–88.
10. Arafah BM. Hypothalamic pituitary adrenal function during critical illness: Limitations of current assessment methods. *J Clin Endocrinol Metab* 2006;91:3725–45.
11. Salem M, Tainsh RE, Bromberg J, Loriaux DL, Chernow B. Perioperative glucocorticoid coverage: A reassessment 42 years after emergence of a problem. *Ann Surg* 1994;219:416–25.
12. Crown A, Lightman S. Why is the management of glucocorticoid deficiency still controversial: A review of the literature. *Clin Endocrinol* 2005;63:483–92.
13. Chiodini I. Diagnosis and treatment of subclinical hypercortisolism. *J Clin Endocrinol Metab* 2011;96:1223–36.
14. DiDalmazi G, Vincennati V, Garelli S et al. Cardiovascular events and mortality in patients with adrenal incidentalomas that are either non-secreting or associated with intermediate phenotype or subclinical Cushing's syndrome: A 15-year retrospective study. *Lancet Diab Endocrinol* 2014;2:396–405.
15. Morelli V, Reimondo G, Giordano R et al. Long-term follow-up in adrenal incidentalomas: An Italian multicenter study. *J Clin Endocrinol Metab* 2014;99:827–34.
16. Lindsay JR, Neiman LK. Differential diagnosis and imaging in Cushing's syndrome. *Endocrinol Metab Clin N Am* 2005;34:403–21.
17. DiDalmazi G, Berr CM, Fassnacht M, Beuschlein F, Reincke M. Adrenal function after adrenalectomy for subclinical hypercortisolism and Cushing's syndrome: A systematic review of the literature. *J Clin Endocrinol Metab* 2014;99:2637–45.
18. Ravichandran R, Lafferty F, McGinniss MJ, Taylor HC. Congenital adrenal hyperplasia presenting as a massive adrenal incidentaloma in the sixth decade of life: Report of two patients with 21-hydroxylase deficiency. *J Clin Endocrinol Metab* 1996;81;1776–79.
19. Finkielstein GP, Kim MS, Sinaii N et al. Clinical characteristics of a cohort of 244 patients with congenital adrenal hyperplasia. *J Clin Endocrinol Metab* 2012;97:4429–38.
20. Nermoen I, Rorvik J, Homedal SH et al. High frequency of adrenal myelolipomas and testicular adrenal rest tumours in adult Norwegian patients with classical congenital adrenal hyperplasia because of 21-hydroxylase deficiency. *Clin Endocrinol (Oxf)* 2011;75:753–9.

26

Surgical pathology of the adrenal gland

G. KENNETH HAINES III

THE NORMAL ADRENAL GLAND

The adrenals are paired retroperitoneal organs, pyramidal on the right, crescentic on the left, located superior and medial to the kidneys. The weight of the adrenal gland varies with age and physiologic conditions. Each gland weighs approximately 10 g in a healthy newborn, dropping to 5 g by 2 weeks of age due to the rapid degeneration of the provisional or fetal cortex. The combined adrenal weights in adults can vary significantly with physiologic stress. One manifestation of this is the difference in weight between surgical specimens (4 g) and autopsy cases (6 g) [1].

On cross section, the adrenal cortex is approximately 1 mm in thickness, and consists of a thick golden-yellow layer overlying a thin brown layer. In the head and body of the adrenal, the cortex overlies a gray core (medulla) (Figure 26.1).

The adrenal cortex is divided histologically into three functionally and morphologically distinct zones (Figure 26.2). Located immediately beneath the capsule, the *zona glomerulosa* consists of scattered clusters of small, compact aldosterone-producing cells. Grossly visible as a thick yellow band (due to its high steroid lipid [cholesterol]), the *zona fasciculata* consists of columns of large foamy or clear cells. This layer is the major site of cortisol production. The *zona reticularis* is visible as a dark brown line, immediately beneath the fasciculate. In contrast to the large clear cells of the fasiculata, the reticularis is composed of smaller (compact) cells with eosinophilic cytoplasm, arranged in short cords. Intracytoplasmic lipofuscin pigment is prominent in cells in the innermost portion of the reticularis. While primarily the site of androgen production, these cells are also capable of producing cortisol.

The medulla appears grossly as a solid gray core, up to 2 mm in thickness, generally limited to the head and body of the adrenal. It is grossly and microscopically sharply demarcated from the cortex (Figure 26.3). The medullary cells (pheochromocytes) are pleomorphic in both nuclear and cytologic details. The nucleus may be large or small, round to elliptical. Larger nuclei often have a prominent nucleolus, while smaller nuclei may be condensed and hyperchromatic. The cytoplasm is most often basophilic, but may be eosinophilic or vacuolated. Cell membranes are often indistinct. The medulla is organized into small clusters of cells, more apparent when the peripherally located sustentacular cells are highlighted by s100 immunostain. Clusters of cortical cells are frequently found within the medulla (Figure 26.4).

ADRENAL CORTICAL PATHOLOGY

Nonneoplastic

ADRENAL HETEROTOPIA

It is not uncommon for microscopic nests of adrenal cortical tissue to be seen external to the adrenal capsule (Figure 26.5). Larger collections of adrenal tissue located in aberrant sites are referred to as adrenal heterotopia. Such ectopic tissue is most commonly found in the retroperitoneal adipose tissue adjacent to the adrenal, but may also be seen within or adjacent to the ovary, testis, kidney, liver, or other sites. Due to differences in embryonic development and migration, medullary elements are not found within ectopic sites away from the celiac plexus. The ectopic cortical tissue responds to physiologic signals, and may be affected by the

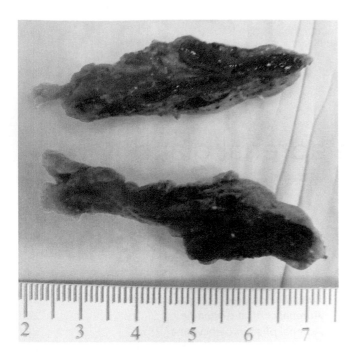

Figure 26.1 Normal adrenal gland. Gross photograph showing serial sections of the adrenal gland, with adjacent adipose tissue. Note the golden-yellow cortex with an inner brown core.

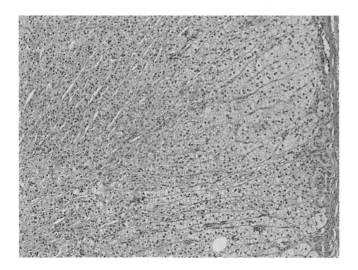

Figure 26.2 Normal adrenal gland. The adrenal cortex is divided into three zones. The outermost zone (right side, beneath capsule) is the discontinuous zona glomerulosa. The foamy cells underneath comprise the zona fasiculata. The anastomosing cords of light pink cells are the zona reticularis. Hematoxylin and eosin (H&E), 100×.

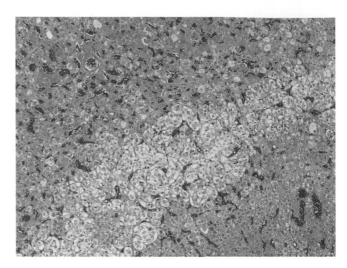

Figure 26.3 Normal adrenal gland. The medulla (central) appears sharply demarcated from the cortex, due to differential staining of cortical and medullary cells. H&E, 400×.

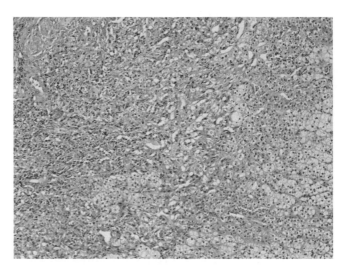

Figure 26.4 Despite its apparent demarcation, nests of cortical cells (light staining cells) are commonly found within the medulla. H&E, 100×.

same processes seen within the normally positioned gland. This is most evident in the hyperplasia seen with adrenocorticotropic hormone (ACTH) excess (e.g., Cushing syndrome and congenital adrenal hyperplasia [CAH]) [2].

ADRENAL CYTOMEGALY

Markedly enlarged (up to 150 um) and pleomorphic adrenal cortical cells may be seen focally or diffusely within the adrenal cortex of infants (Figure 26.6). Generally affecting the provisional or fetal cortex, these most often regress without clinical significance. A subset of cases are associated with specific syndromes (e.g., Beckwith–Weidemann, trisomy 13, and trisomy 18) or other clinical settings (fetal hemolysis) [3,4].

ADRENAL CORTICAL HYPERPLASIA

Hyperplasia of the adrenal cortex occurs in a number of disorders that can be divided into ACTH-dependent and ACTH-independent groups. The ACTH-dependent hyperplasias are further divided into primary and secondary categories, depending on whether the specific defect in the cortisol–ACTH feedback loop is located within or outside of the adrenal gland. CAH, the prototypical example of a

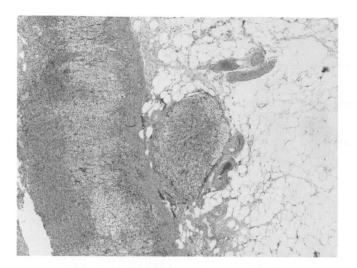

Figure 26.5 It is not uncommon for adrenal cortical tissue to extend outside of the adrenal capsule. H&E, 40×.

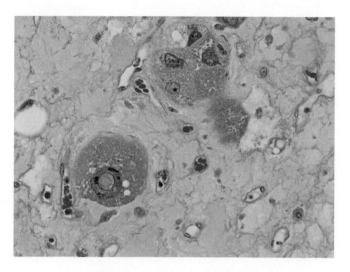

Figure 26.6 Adrenal cytomegaly is most often found within the provisional (fetal) cortex of newborns. Some cases are associated with specific syndromes, but most cases regress without clinical impact. H&E, 400×.

primary ACTH-dependent cortical hyperplasia, results from a mutation in any of the genes (e.g., 21-hydroxylase, 11-β-hydroxylase, 3β-hydroxysteroid dehydrogenase, and 17α-hydroxylase) necessary for adrenal steroid hormone production (Figure 26.7). A mutation in the 21-hydroxylase gene is the most common of these, resulting in deficient cortisol and aldosterone production, with compensatory overproduction of androgens [5–7] These disorders often have distinct biochemical profiles, and variable clinical signs and symptoms, dependent on the specific defect.

As expected with chronically elevated ACTH levels, the adrenal glands are typically bilaterally enlarged, with diffusely expanded zona fasicularis and reticulatum (Figure 26.8). The cortical enlargement may be asymmetric, and in up to a fifth of cases, distinct cortical nodules may be apparent (Figure 26.9) [1]. Identification of a hyperplastic cortex

between the nodules on histologic examination helps classify the process as an ACTH-dependent hyperplasia.

Secondary hyperplasia results from the abnormal production of ACTH. This most commonly involves a pituitary lesion (adenoma or microadenoma), but in about 15% of cases, the excessive ACTH is produced ectopically by a tumor elsewhere in the body (e.g., small cell carcinoma of the lung), or as a physiologic response to chronic stress.

In secondary hyperplasia, the cortical hyperplasia is most often diffuse, bilateral, and symmetric, with glands weighing on average 15 g each.

Hyperplasia of the adrenal cortex may also occur in the absence of excess systemic ACTH. These so-called "ACTH-independent pathways" can produce grossly visible (macronodular, >1 cm) or microscopic (micronodular, <1 cm) hyperplastic cortical nodules.

ACTH-independent macronodular cortical hyperplasia (AIMAH), perhaps better referred to as primary macronodular adrenal hyperplasia, can be caused by aberrant receptors for hormones other than ACTH (such as gastric inhibitory polypeptide [GIP]), mutations in G proteins (McCune–Albright syndrome), or mutations in the multiple endocrine neoplasia type 1 (MEN1) gene, among others [8]. Clusters of steroidogenic cells within the adrenal respond to this aberrant signaling by producing corticotropin (ACTH), which acts locally to stimulate cortical hyperplasia [8,9].

The adrenal glands are often distorted by large nodules up to 5 cm in diameter (Figure 26.10). As the nodules may be unilateral or metachronous, a neoplastic process is often a consideration.

In contrast to the enlarged adrenals seen in the hyperplastic conditions discussed above, the adrenal glands are often of grossly normal size in *ACTH-independent micronodular hyperplasia*. Multiple small nodules, often pigmented, are scattered within an otherwise atrophic cortex. The nodules are composed of large cells with eosinophilic cytoplasm, with or without prominent brown granular pigment. Grossly pigmented cases are referred to as *primary pigmented nodular adrenal cortical disease* (PPNAD), a subset of which may be associated with the Carney complex [10].

Adrenal neoplasms

ADRENAL CORTICAL ADENOMAS

The distinction between a cortical nodule and an adenoma is not always clear.

Autopsy studies have shown small cortical nodules, usually multiple, to be present in more than half of all cases. A single distinct nodule (defined somewhat arbitrarily as an adenoma) is less common, found in 2%–5% of autopsies [1]. Such incidental adrenal masses (incidentalomas) are increasingly being found on imaging studies (computed tomography [CT] and MRI), particularly in the elderly. While the majority represent *nonfunctional adrenal cortical adenomas*, particularly when less than 4 cm and under 50 g, other tumors (e.g., adrenal cortical carcinoma, pheochromocytoma, and metastatic carcinoma or melanoma) must

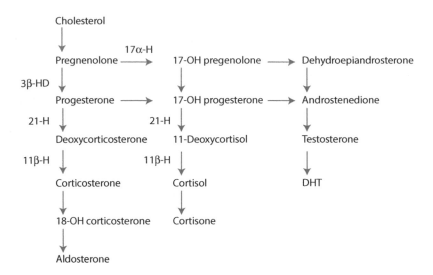

Figure 26.7 Simplified schematic of adrenal cortical steroid synthetic pathways. 3β-HD, 3β-hydroxysteroid dehydrogenase; 11β-H, 11β-hydroxylase; 17α-H, 17α-hydroxylase; 21-H, 21-hydroxylase; DHT, dihydrotestosterone.

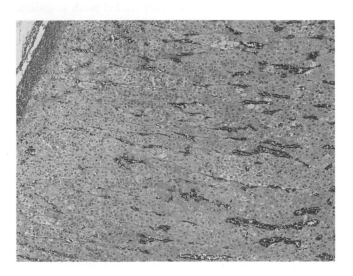

Figure 26.8 Adrenal cortical hyperplasia. The adrenal glands from this 30-year-old with Cushing's syndrome weighed a combined 79 g. Note the expanded zona fasicularis comprising the bulk of the cortex. H&E, 200×.

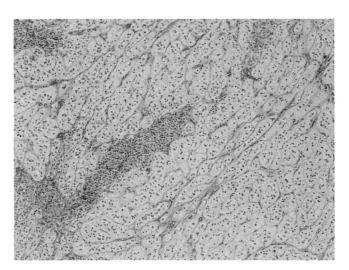

Figure 26.10 Primary macronodular adrenal hyperplasia. The grossly visible nodules are composed primarily of large cortical cells with clear or foamy cytoplasm. Note the clusters of smaller cells with eosinophilic cytoplasm, interspersed within the hyperplastic tissue. H&E, 40×.

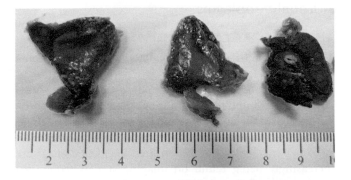

Figure 26.9 Adrenal cortical hyperplasia. The left adrenal gland from this patient with Cushing's disease weighed 18 g. Note the dominant nodule as well as additional smaller nodules in the cortex. The right adrenal was similarly enlarged.

be considered. Thorough clinical, radiologic, and hormonal evaluation is thus critical for appropriate management of the lesion.

Adrenal cortical adenomas are circumscribed lesions, with or without a discrete capsule. Most are composed of large steroid lipid rich (cholesterol) clear cells, smaller (compact) cells with eosinophilic cytoplasm, or a mixture (Figures 26.11 and 26.12). The architectural features vary, with fascicles, short cords, and small or large nests being common. A reticulin stain highlights a regular network of supporting collagen fibers surrounding the nests, similar to that seen in the nonneoplastic cortex (Figure 26.13). Metaplastic (myeloid and lipomatous) and degenerative changes, including fibrosis, cystic change, and hemorrhage, are not uncommon in larger lesions, and by themselves are

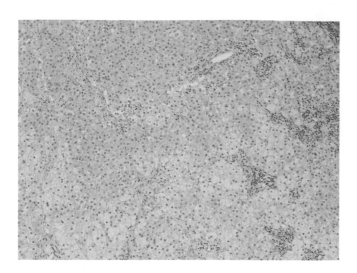

Figure 26.11 Adrenal cortical adenoma. Most adenomas, regardless of the presence or absence of hormone production, are composed of large clear to foamy cells, compact eosinophilic cells, or a combination. Aggregates of lymphoid cells, as seen here, are a common finding. H&E, 100×.

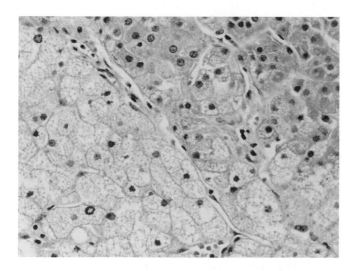

Figure 26.12 Adrenal cortical adenoma. Higher magnification demonstrates the larger clear cells and smaller eosinophilic cortical cells. H&E, 400×.

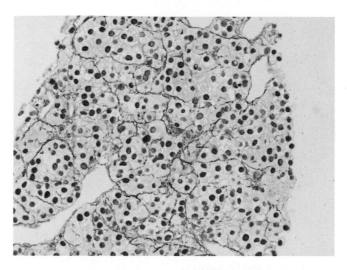

Figure 26.13 Adrenal cortical adenoma. Reticulin stain highlights a regular pattern of nests. This pattern is often disrupted in adrenocortical carcinomas. Reticulin, 200×.

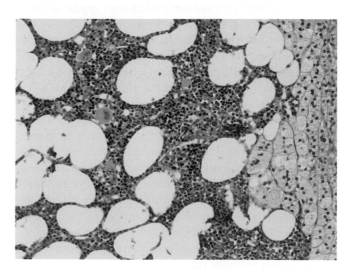

Figure 26.14 Adrenal cortical adenoma with myeloid metaplasia, resembling bone marrow. Note the large multinucleated megakaryocytes. H&E, 200×.

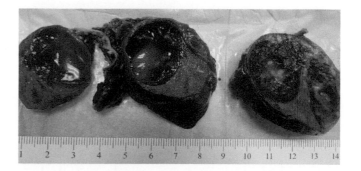

Figure 26.15 Adrenal cortical adenoma. This clinically nonfunctioning cortical adenoma shows cystic degeneration, a common occurrence in both benign and malignant adrenal tumors.

not worrisome for aggressive clinical behavior (Figures 26.14 through 26.16). As in most endocrine organs, larger cells with enlarged, smudgy hyperchromatic nuclei or a prominent nucleolus may be seen individually or in small clusters. This "endocrine atypia" is also not indicative of malignancy. Mitotic figures should be absent or rare, and invasion into adjacent tissue is not seen in an adenoma. Such features are more typical of adrenal cortical carcinoma, and are discussed more thoroughly below. The adjacent nonneoplastic adrenal cortex is often atrophic in cortisol-producing (functional) adenomas, but otherwise which hormones, if any, produced cannot be determined by evaluation of an adenoma's architectural or cytologic features.

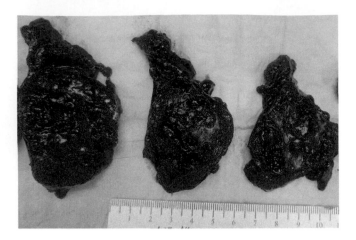

Figure 26.16 Adrenal cortical adenoma with extensive hemorrhage and fibrosis.

FUNCTIONING ADRENAL CORTICAL ADENOMAS

Conn syndrome is a unilateral lesion (adenoma). Upon excision, aldosterone-producing adenomas appear as well-circumscribed bright "canary yellow" masses, usually less than 3 cm in size (Figure 26.17). Many glands removed for a presumed adenoma in fact contain multiple hyperplastic cortical nodules, making a subtotal adrenalectomy a suboptimal treatment option [11]. Somatic mutations in KCNJ5, a potassium channel gene, or others related to calcium transport, are commonly found in aldosterone-producing adenomas and have been identified in these multinodular glands, typically within the dominant nodule [12]. Histologically, adenomas or hyperplastic nodules may be arranged in short cords or nests, resembling the zona glomerulosa, but more often show a zonal pattern with a central area of large steroid lipid cells surrounded peripherally by eosinophilic compact cells (Figures 26.18 and 26.19). Laminated eosinophilic inclusions (*spironolactone bodies*) may be seen within the cytoplasm of tumor cells.

Cortisol-producing adenomas, a cause of Cushing syndrome, are circumscribed yellow to golden masses, generally less than 4 cm and under 50 g (Figure 26.20). They

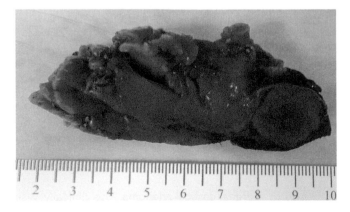

Figure 26.17 Aldosterone-producing adrenal cortical adenomas typically have a "canary yellow" color.

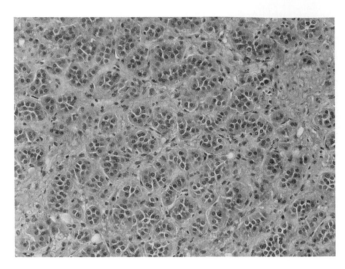

Figure 26.18 Aldosterone-producing adrenal cortical adenomas may resemble the zona glomerulosa, with short cords and rounded nests of compact eosinophilic cells. H&E, 200×.

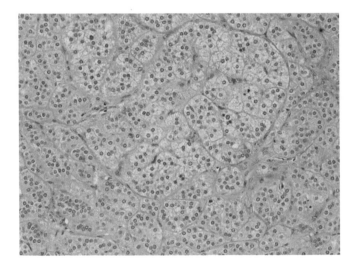

Figure 26.19 Central nests of steroid lipid cells surrounded by a peripheral rim of compact eosinophilic cells are another pattern commonly seen in aldosterone-producing adenomas. H&E, 200×.

tend to have a sharp but unencapsulated pushing border, and are arranged in nests or longer fasicles. They generally are comprised of a mixture of large vacuolated lipid-rich clear cells and smaller compact eosinophilic cells (Figure 26.21). A mutation in the catalytic subunit of cAMP-dependent protein kinase A (PKRACA) has recently been described in up to 50% of cortisol-producing cortical adenomas [13].

Sex steroid-producing adenomas are uncommon, accounting for less than 5% of all adrenal cortical adenomas [14,15]. As a group, they are larger than other functional adenomas, weighing an average of 475 g (testosterone producing) to 1000 g (estrogen producing). Their size, in combination with the frequent presence of hemorrhage or foci of

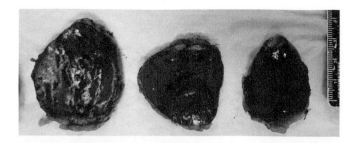

Figure 26.20 Cortisol-producing adrenal cortical adenomas often have a golden-yellow to orange cut surface.

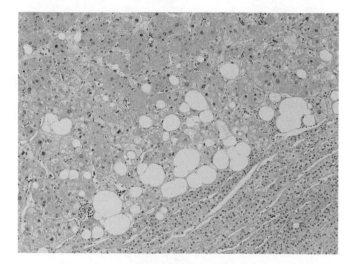

Figure 26.21 This cortisol-producing adrenal cortical adenoma shows a mixture of small pale staining cells (bottom) surrounding a nodule of larger eosinophilic cells with moderate nuclear pleomorphism. Note the focus of lipomatous change. H&E, 100×.

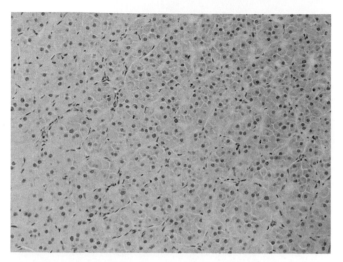

Figure 26.22 Oncocytomas of the adrenal gland are histologically similar to those found in the kidney or salivary gland. This one shows trabeculae of moderately sized cortical cells with granular eosinophilic cytoplasm and round nuclei, often with a prominent nucleolus. Adrenal oncocytoma. H&E, 200×.

and demonstrating necrosis or capsular or sinusoidal (i.e., small vessels lacking smooth muscle) invasion is placed in a "borderline" or "uncertain malignant potential" category. Tumors lacking any of these features are classified as benign [16–18].

ADRENAL CORTICAL CARCINOMA

Adrenal cortical carcinomas are rare tumors, comprising only 3% of endocrine tumors. They may occur sporadically or be syndromic (Beckwith–Weideman, Li–Fraumeni, MEN1, Carney complex, and others) [19,20]. Cases show a bimodal distribution, with peaks in the seventh decade and a smaller peak in early childhood. The tumors may present as a mass lesion causing flank pain, but more frequently are identified due to manifestations of cortisol, aldosterone, androgen, or estrogen overproduction. The tumors are often large at time of presentation, averaging 12 cm and more than 200 g (Figure 26.23). Up to 40% of cases have demonstrable metastatic disease (liver, lungs, lymph nodes, and bone) at the time of diagnosis.

Histologically, malignancy may be readily apparent, with frequent typical and atypical mitotic figures, and invasion into large veins or surrounding structures (Figures 26.24 through 26.28). At other times, distinction from a benign cortical adenoma may be virtually impossible. A number of pathologic and clinicopathologic systems have been devised to assist in making this distinction. No single feature (other than metastasis) is diagnostic of carcinoma, and each system can misclassify an individual tumor. The two most common purely histopathologic systems are those devised by Weiss and Van Slooten (Table 26.1) [21–23]. In the current modification of the Weiss system, the presence of three or more of the nine features correlates with malignancy. In the Van Slooten system, seven histologic criteria are differentially

necrosis, invariably raises the possibility of carcinoma. The tumor is composed of compact eosinophilic cells arranged in short anastomosing cords, similar to the zona reticularis. Adequate sampling of the capsule and interface with adjacent tissue is critical, as benign tumors are well circumscribed and often encapsulated, in contrast to the invasive front often found in carcinoma.

Adrenal cortical oncocytoma is a form of nonfunctioning adenoma that deserves special attention, as application of traditional criteria risks misclassifying a biologically benign neoplasm as malignant. Oncocytomas are often large (mean 8.5 cm, 200 g), well circumscribed, and often encapsulated. Like oncocytomas in other organs, the tumor has a mahogany-brown cut surface. The tumor is composed of large polygonal cells with abundant mitochondrial-rich granular eosinophilic cytoplasm, in a nested or sheet-like arrangement (Figure 26.22). The cells have a large nucleus with prominent nucleolus. Using the Lin–Weiss–Bisceglia criteria, oncocytic tumors are defined as malignant if they show more than five mitotic figures per 50 high-power fields (hpf), any atypical mitotic figures, or invasion into veins. Any tumor larger than 10 cm, greater than 200 g,

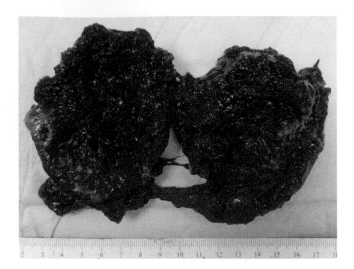

Figure 26.23 Adrenal cortical carcinomas are often large masses with overt invasion into adipose tissue or adjacent structures. Note areas of hemorrhage and cystic degeneration in this tumor. A rim of residual adrenal cortex is seen compressed along the bottom of the tumor.

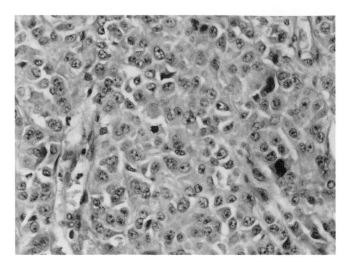

Figure 26.25 Adrenocortical carcinoma with moderately pleomorphic cells with a high nucleus-to-cytoplasmic ratio and readily apparent mitotic activity. H&E, 400×.

Figure 26.24 Adrenocortical carcinoma showing sheets of variably sized eosinophilic cells. H&E, 100×.

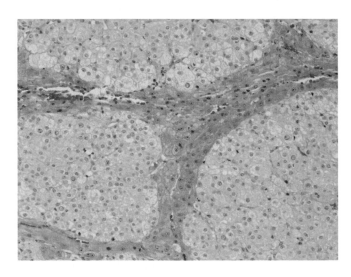

Figure 26.26 Some adrenocortical carcinomas are composed of relatively bland cells. This photomicrograph shows nests of pale pink tumor cells metastatic to the liver (dark pink cells surrounding the nests). H&E, 200×.

weighted, with a score of >8 correlating with malignancy. Other investigators utilize both clinical and histopathologic factors in their assessment of malignant potential [24,25]. Other systems have been proposed, to refine prognostication, address unique tumor types (e.g., oncocytic tumors) or specific patient populations (e.g., pediatric cases), emphasize other histologic features (e.g., disruption of the reticulin framework), or analyze aberrant expression patterns of microRNAs (e.g., MiR483-3p) or other biomarkers [16,26,27].

ADRENAL PHEOCHROMOCYTOMA

Whereas the adrenal cortex arises from coelomic epithelium adjacent to the gonadal ridge, the adrenal medulla derives from neuroectodermal precursors in the sympathetic chain. These catecholamine-producing cells (pheochromocytes) are often termed *chromaffin cells* due to the ability of chromium salts to oxidize catecholamines, particularly noradrenaline, into a brown pigment that can be visualized grossly or microscopically. The medulla is usually limited to the medial-most portions of the adrenal (head and body). Grossly identifiable medullary tissue within the adrenal tail and alae raises the possibility of medullary hyperplasia, as may be seen in the setting of MEN2A and ME2B [28].

Pheochromocytoma is a neoplasm of the medullary chromaffin cells. Similar-appearing tumors found outside of the adrenal (extra-adrenal pheochromocytoma) are termed "paraganglioma." These latter tumors are usually of sympathetic origin, and are therefore nonchromaffin lesions.

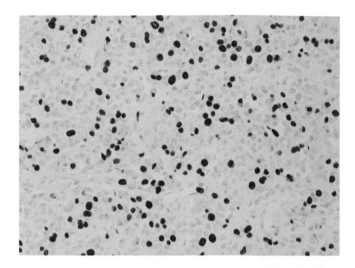

Figure 26.27 Adrenocortical carcinoma. This tumor demonstrates high proliferative activity, with many tumor cell nuclei staining for ki-67. MIB-1 immunostain, 200×.

Table 26.1 Comparison of the Weiss and Van Slooten criteria for identification of malignant potential within adrenal cortical tumors

Weiss system	Van Slooten system
High nuclear grade	≥2 mitoses/10 hpf (9.0)
>5 mitoses/50 hpf	Extensive hemorrhage, necrosis, fibrosis (5.7)
Atypical mitoic figures	Abnormal nucleoli (4.1)
<25% clear cell component	Vascular or capsular invasion (3.3)
Diffuse architecture in >1/3	Nuclear hyperchromasia (2.6)
Necrosis	Significant nuclear atypia (2.1)
Venous invasion	Loss of normal structure (1.6)
Sinusoidal invasion	
Capsular invasion	
Malignant potential: ≥3	**Malignant potential: >8**

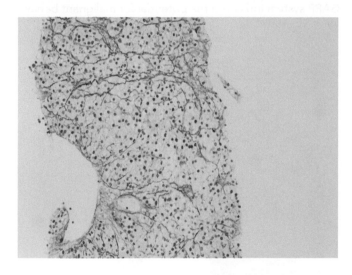

Figure 26.28 Adrenocortical carcinoma. The normal uniform nested pattern evident on reticulin stain is often disrupted in adrenocortical carcinomas. Reticulin, 400×.

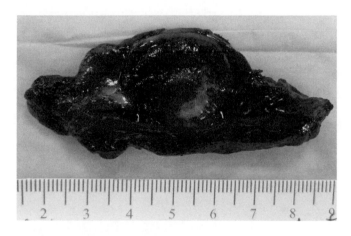

Figure 26.29 Adrenal gland with 2.5 cm pheochromocytoma. The red-brown to gray color is distinct from the yellow or golden color found in most cortical neoplasms.

With advances in molecular and genetic analysis, up to 40% of pheochromocytomas and paragangliomas demonstrate a germline mutation. Over 10 genes have been implicated, including RET (MEN2A or MEN2B), VHL (von Hippel–Lindau), NF1 (neurofibromatosis type 1), and SDHx genes (hereditary paraganglioma–pheochromocytoma syndromes) [29,30]. As mutations in the succinate dehydrogenase B (SDHB) gene have been associated with an increased risk for metastasis or aggressive clinical behavior, routine use of immunohistochemical stains for SDHB has been advocated as a useful screening test to identify patients for further genetic testing. SDHB protein expression is lost with mutations in any of the four SDHx genes, necessitating further testing to identify the specific mutation in an individual patient [31–33].

Pheochromocytoma can be grossly distinguished from adrenal cortical neoplasms, as it forms a tan to gray mass, in contrast to the yellow or orange appearance of cortical tumors (Figure 26.29). Pheochromocytomas are usually solid, although larger tumors may undergo cystic degeneration. Microscopically, a nested pattern likened to a ball of cells (zellballen) is characteristic (Figure 26.30). The tumor is composed predominantly of small pleomorphic cells (chief cells) with clear, amphophilic, or basophilic cytoplasm. The nuclei may be round or spindled, with small or large nucleoli, or may be markedly hyperchromatic. Flattened s100-positive sustentacular cells are frequently identified surrounding the nests (Figure 26.31).

Whether hereditary or sporadic, prediction of the biologic behavior of these neoplasms is difficult. The only definitive criterion for malignancy is the presence of metastasis to a site normally devoid of paraganglia. In

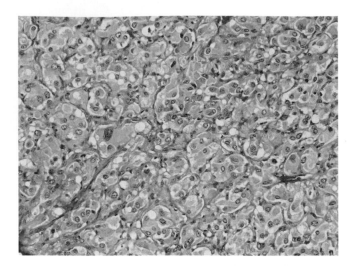

Figure 26.30 This pheochromocytoma shows a distinct nested pattern termed zellballen, with polygonal cells with abundant amphophilic cytoplasm and pleomorphic nuclei, surrounded by smaller spindled (sustentacular) cells. H&E, 200×.

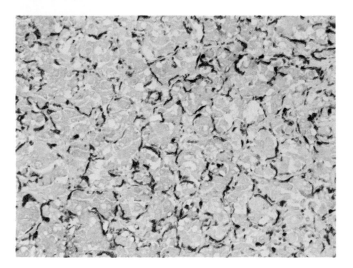

Figure 26.31 Immunostain for s100 protein labels the sustentacular cells, highlighting the characteristic nested architecture. s100 immunostain, 200×.

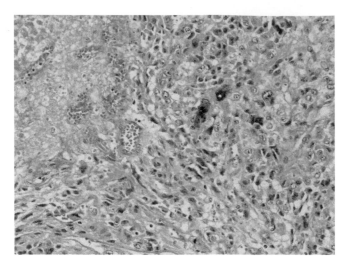

Figure 26.32 This pheochromocytoma invaded adjacent adipose tissue and blood vessels. On histologic examination, tumoral necrosis (left upper), marked nuclear pleomorphism with hyperchromasia, and frequent mitotic figures were apparent. Application of either the PASS or GAPP system indicated the potential for malignant behavior. H&E, 400×.

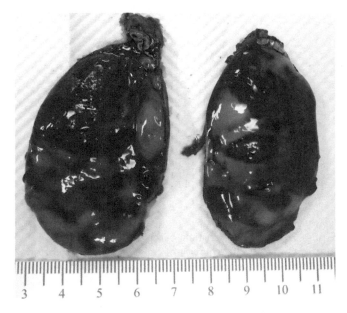

Figure 26.33 This NB appears as a soft fleshy mass with areas of hemorrhage. Note residual adrenal tissue at the top of the mass.

the fashion of the Weiss scoring system for adrenal cortical tumors, in 2002 Thompson published the pheochromocytoma of the adrenal gland scaled score (PASS) to predict the likelihood of malignant behavior [34]. Eight items (diffuse growth pattern, tumoral necrosis, cellularity, monotony, spindle cells, >3 mf/10 hpf, atypical mitosis, and extension into adipose tissue) were each assigned 2 points. Four other features (vascular invasion, capsular invasion, marked nuclear pleomorphism, and hyperchromasia) were scored as 1 point apiece. A total score of ≥4 denoted a potential for aggressive behavior (Figure 26.32). Subsequent studies have questioned its utility in practice [35]. A different grading system (grading system for adrenal pheochromocytoma and paraganglioma [GAPP]) has been proposed, evaluating similar histologic features as the PASS system, but also including ki-67 as a marker of cellular proliferation, and determination of the catecholamine produced [36].

NEUROBLASTOMA/GANGLIONEUROBLASTOMA

Neuroblastoma (NB) is the fourth most common malignant tumor in early childhood, with half of all cases detected by age 2 (including those detected prenatally) and 85% by age 5. At least half of all cases arise in the abdomen, predominantly within the adrenal gland (Figure 26.33).

Two-thirds of cases have metastatic disease at time of presentation [37].

Histologically, NB falls into the broad category of "small blue cell tumors," being composed of cells somewhat larger than lymphocytes, with a nucleus surrounded by very little cytoplasm (Figure 26.34). Rings of tumor cell nuclei surrounding a core of neuropil (*Homer Wright rosette*) may occasionally be present (Figure 26.35). Larger cells with abundant amphophilic cytoplasm and an eccentric nucleus, often with prominent nucleolus, indicate ganglionic differentiation (*ganglioneuroblastoma*). Extensive ganglionic differentiation is usually accompanied by the production of a fibrillar stroma with spindled nuclei resembling Schwann cells. The International Neuroblastoma Pathology Committee (INPC) classifies NBs (based on pretreatment biopsy or resection) as [1] "undifferentiated

NB" or [2] "poorly differentiated NB" if they have minimal Schwannian-type stroma and either no or <5% ganglionic cell differentiation, respectively, and [3] "differentiating NB" with >5% ganglionic differentiation but less than 50% Schwannian-type stroma. Tumors with greater amounts of Schwannian-type stroma are categorized as [4] "nodular ganglioneuroblastoma" if grossly visible nodules of NB are present, or [5] "intermixed ganglioneuroblastoma" if the NB component is microscopic.

A mitotic–karyorrhectic index (MKI) is calculated for the NBs by counting the number of mitotic figures plus apoptotic (karyorrhectic) cells per 5000 tumor cells, and is classified as low (<100), intermediate (100–200), or high (>200). In combination with the patient age, the histologic classification and MKI are used to place the tumor into favorable or unfavorable histologic categories [38].

In brief, favorable cases are limited to poorly differentiated NB with low or intermediate MKI and age of <18 months, and differentiating NB with either an intermediate MKI and age of <18 months, or low MKI and age of <5 years. The unfavorable categories include all undifferentiated NB, all NB with a high MKI, and the remaining NB not falling into the above favorable histology categories.

Additional features used for prognostic assessment include N-myc amplification, amplification or mutation of ALK, DNA index, and chromosomal abnormalities (numerical or segmental) [37]. MicroRNA expression profiles and next-generation sequencing approaches may provide additional independent prognostic information [39,40].

GANGLIONEUROMA

Ganglioneuroma represents the most differentiated end of the spectrum of neuroblastic tumors [41,42]. This benign lesion is composed of spindled Schwann cells with a variable number of scattered or clustered ganglion cells, in a fibrotic stroma (Figure 26.36). More than a quarter of these

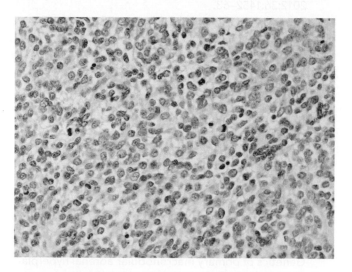

Figure 26.34 NB is a prototypical small blue cell tumor. Note frequent mitotic figures and apoptotic bodies. The number of either per 5000 cells counted constitutes the MKI. H&E, 400×.

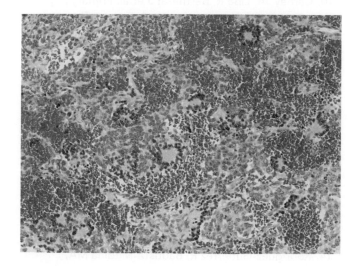

Figure 26.35 The ring-like arrangement of nuclei around an acellular zone of pink fibrillar material constitutes a Homer Wright (pseudo)rosette. H&E, 200×.

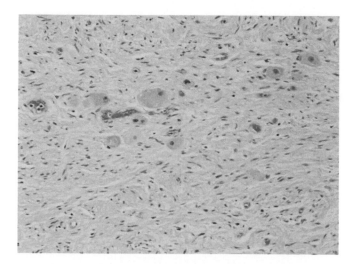

Figure 26.36 Ganglioneuromas are benign tumors composed of mature ganglion cells set in a spindled stroma containing Schwann cells. H&E, 200×.

tumors arise in the adrenal gland, but they may also occur in the adjacent retroperitoneum or elsewhere.

Composite tumors (pheochromocytoma plus a related tumor) are occasionally seen. The second component is most often a ganglioneuroma (Figures 26.37 and 26.38), but may be a ganglioneuroblastoma or rarely a NB or malignant peripheral nerve sheath tumor (MPNST) [43].While the latter is an aggressive tumor, NBs and ganglioneuroblastomas arising as a component of a composite tumor often follow an indolent clinical course.

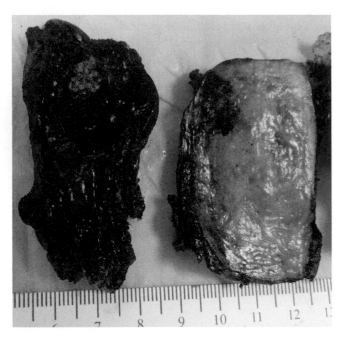

Figure 26.37 Gross photograph of a composite tumor consisting of a pheochromocytoma (red-brown solid mass, left side) plus a ganglioneuroma (solid tan mass, right side).

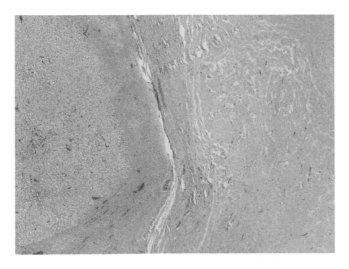

Figure 26.38 The pheochromocytoma (left side) is sharply demarcated from the ganglioneuroma (right side) in this composite tumor. H&E, 20×.

REFERENCES

1. McNicol AM. Diagnostic and molecular aspects of adrenal cortical tumors. *Semin Diagn Pathol* 2013;30:197–206.
2. Claahsen-van der Grinten HL, Kuthio K, Otten BJ et al. An adrenal rest tumor in the perirenal region in a patient with congenital adrenal hyperplasia due to congenital 3beta-hydroxysteroid dehydrogenase deficiency. *Eur J Endocrinol* 2008;159:489–91.
3. Carney JA, Ho J, Kitsuda K et al. Massive neonatal adrenal enlargement due to cytomegaly, persistence of the transient cortex, and hyperplasia of the permanent cortex: Findings in Cushing syndrome associated with hemihypertrophy. *Am J Surg Pathol* 2012;36:1452–63.
4. Taweevisit M, Atikankul T, Thorner PS. Histologic changes in the adrenal gland reflect fetal distress in hydrops fetalis. *Pediatr Dev Pathol* 2014;17:190–7.
5. Auchus RJ. The classic and nonclassic congenital adrenal hyperplasias. *Endocr Pract* 2015;21:383–9.
6. Concolino P, Mello E, Zuppi C et al. Molecular diagnosis of congenital adrenal hyperplasia due to 21-hydroxylase deficiency: An update of new CYP2A2 mutations. *Clin Chem Lab Med* 2010;48:1057–62.
7. Yoo Y, Chang MS, Lee J et al. Genotype-phenotype correlation in 27 pediatric patients in congenital adrenal hyperplasia due to 21-hydroxylase deficiency in a single center. *Ann Pediatr Endocrinol Metab* 2013;18:128–34.
8. Fragosol MCBV, Alencar GA, Lerario AM et al. Genetics of primary macronodular adrenal hyperplasia. *J Endocrinol* 2015;224:R31–43.
9. Louiset E, Duparc C, Young J et al. Intraadrenal corticotropin in bilateral macronodular adrenal hyperplasia. *N Engl J Med* 2013;369:2115–25.
10. Carney JA, Libé R, Bertherat J et al. Primary pigmented nodular adrenocortical disease: The original 4 cases revisited after 30 years for follow-up, new investigations, and molecular genetic findings. *Am J Surg Pathol* 2014;38:1266–73.
11. Weisbrod AB, Webb RC, Mathur A et al. Adrenal histologic findings show no difference in clinical presentation and outcome in primary hyperaldosteronism. *Ann Surg Oncol* 2013;20:753–58.
12. Dekkers T, Meer MT, Lenders JWM et al. Adrenal nodularity and somatic mutations in primary aldosteronism: One node is the culprit? *J Clin Endocrinol Metab* 2014;99:E1341–51.
13. Sato Y, Maekawa S, Ishii R et al. Recurrent somatic mutations underlie corticotropin-independent Cushing's syndrome. *Science* 2014;344:917–20.
14. Rodriguez-Gutiérrez R, Bautista-Medina MA, Teniente-Sanchez AE et al. Pure androgen-secreting adrenal adenoma associated with resistant hypertension. *Case Rep Endocrinol* 2013;2013:356086.

15. Mitschke H, Saeger W, Breustedt HJ. Feminizing adrenocortical tumor. Histological and ultrastructural study. *Virchows Arch A Pathol Anat Histol* 1978;377:301–9.

16. Duregon E, Volante M, Cappia S et al. Oncocytic adrenocortical tumors: Diagnostic algorithm and mitochondrial DNA profile in 27 cases. *Am J Surg Pathol* 2011;35:1882–93.

17. Wong DD, Spagnolo DV, Bisceglia M et al. Oncocytic adrenocortical neoplasms—A clinicopathologic study of 13 new cases emphasizing the importance of their recognition. *Hum Pathol* 2011;42:489–99.

18. Mearini L, Del Dordo R, Costantini E et al. Adrenal oncocytic neoplasm: A systematic review. *Urol Int* 2013;91:125–33.

19. Erickson LA, Rivera M, Zhang J. Adrenocortical carcinoma: Review and update. *Adv Anat Pathol* 2014;21:151–9.

20. Else T, Kim AC, Sabolch A et al. Adrenocortical carcinoma. *Endocr Rev* 2014;35:282–326.

21. Weiss LM. Comparative histologic study of 43 metastasizing and nonmetastasizing adrenocortical tumors. *Am J Surg Pathol* 1984;8:163–9.

22. Van Slooten H, Schaberg A, Smeenk D et al. Morphologic characteristics of benign and malignant adrenocortical tumors. *Cancer* 1985;55:766–73.

23. Van't Sant HP, Bouvy ND, Kazemier G et al. The prognostic value of two different histopathologic scoring systems for adrenocortical carcinomas. *Histopathology* 2007;51:239–45.

24. Hough AJ, Hollifield JW, Page DL et al. Prognostic factors in adrenal cortical tumors. A mathematical analysis of clinical and morphologic data. *Am J Clin Pathol* 1979;72:390–9.

25. Lau SK, Weiss LM. The Weiss system for evaluating adrenocortical neoplasms: 25 years later. *Hum Pathol* 2009;40:757–68.

26. Volante M, Bollito E, Sperone P et al. Clinicopathologic study of a series of 92 adrenocortical carcinomas: From a proposal of simplified diagnostic algorithm to prognostic stratification. *Histopathology* 2009;55:535–43.

27. Wang C, Sun Y, Wu H et al. Distinguishing adrenal cortical carcinomas and adenomas: A study of clinicopathological features and biomarkers. *Histopathology* 2014;64:567–76.

28. Korpershoek E, Petri B-J, Post E et al. Adrenal medullary hyperplasia is a precursor lesion for pheochromocytoma in MEN2 syndrome. *Neoplasia* 2014;16:868–73.

29. Gimenez-Roqueplo AP, Dahia PL, Robledo M. An update on the genetics of paraganglioma, pheochromocytoma, and associated hereditary syndromes. *Horm Metab Res* 2012;44:328–33.

30. Dahia PLM. Pheochromocytoma and paraganglioma pathogenesis: Learning from genetic heterogeneity. *Nat Rev Cancer* 2014;14:108–19.

31. Gimenez-Roqueplo AP, Favier J, Rustin P et al. Mutations in the SDHB gene are associated with extra-adrenal and/or malignant phaeochromocytomas. *Cancer Res* 003;63:5615–21.

32. Castelblanco E, Santacana M, Valls J et al. Usefulness of negative and weak-diffuse pattern of SDHB immunostaining in assessment of SDH mutations in paragangliomas and pheochromocytomas. *Endocr Pathol* 2013;24:199–205.

33. Pai R, Manipadam MT, Singh P et al. Usefulness of succinate dehydrogenase B (SDHB) immunohistochemistry in guiding mutational screening among patients with pheochromocytoma-paraganglioma syndromes. *APMIS* 2014;122:1130–35.

34. Thompson, LDR. Pheochromocytoma of the adrenal gland scaled score (PASS) to separate benign from malignant neoplasms: A clinicopathologic and immunophenotypic study of 100 cases. *Am J Surg Pathol* 2002;26:551–66.

35. Mlika M, Kourda N, Zorgati MM et al. Prognostic value of pheochromocytoma of the adrenal gland scaled score (PASS score) tests to separate benign from malignant neoplasms. *Tunis Med* 2013;91:209–15.

36. Kimura N, Takayanagi R, Takizawa N et al. Pathologic grading for predicting metastasis in phaeochromocytoma and paraganglioma. *Endocr Relat Cancer* 2014;21:405–14.

37. Irwin MS, Park JR. Neuroblastoma: Paradigm for precision medicine. *Pediatr Clin N Am* 2015;62:225–56.

38. Shimada H, Ambros IM, Dehner LP et al. The international neuroblastoma pathology classification (the Shimada system). *Cancer* 1999;86:364–72.

39. De Preter K, Mestdagh P, Vermeulen J et al. miRNA expression profiling enables risk stratification in archived and fresh neuroblastoma tumor samples. *Clin Cancer Res* 2011;17:7684–92.

40. Stricker TP, Morales La Madrid A, Chlenski A et al. Validation of a prognostic multi-gene signature in high-risk neuroblastoma using the high throughput digital NanoString nCounter™ system. *Mol Oncol* 2014;8:669–78.

41. Shawa H, Elsayes KM, Javadi S et al. Adrenal ganglioneuroma: Features and outcomes of 27 cases at a referral cancer centre. *Clin Endocrinol (Oxf)* 2014;80:342–7.

42. Rondeau G, Nolet S, Latour M et al. Clinical and biochemical features of seven adult adrenal ganglioneuromas. *J Clin Endocrinol Metab* 2010;95:3118–25.

43. Khan AN, Solomon SS, Childress RD. Composite pheochromocytoma-ganglioneuroma: A rare experiment of nature. *Endocr Pract* 2010;16:291–9.

27

Imaging of the adrenal glands

ERIC J. WILCK

INTRODUCTION

Technological improvements in cross-sectional imaging continue to better define adrenal anatomy and improve characterization of adrenal lesions. Multidetector computed tomography (CT) scanners can produce submillimeter axial slice thickness, and these data are then used to generate a volumetric data set. Images can then be reconstructed in any orientation with isotropic resolution, where resolution is equal in all three dimensions. As the number of CT detectors has increased and the rotation time of the X-ray tube has decreased, scan times have been dramatically diminished to a few seconds. At the same time, newer scanners can accomplish this with a reduced radiation dose by utilizing a technique termed iterative reconstruction. When CT images are acquired using a lower radiation dose, there is a greater amount of image noise present. Iterative reconstruction is an algorithm used to reconstruct two-dimensional (2D) and three-dimensional (3D) images that are relatively insensitive to noise compared with traditional reconstruction techniques. It produces an optimal image, even when the acquired data are incomplete, as occurs in the setting of metal artifact.

Indeterminate nodules that used to be detected on conventional contrast-enhanced CT exams often required follow-up with either unenhanced CT or chemical shift MRI. Recent implementation of dual-energy CT scanners provides the potential to have a virtual noncontrast scan from a single-phase intravenous (IV) contrast-enhanced study [1]. A dual-energy CT scanner will have either two separate X-ray sources or a single X-ray tube that is able to rapidly switch tube voltage between two different values during the scan, so that a scan is obtained at two separate peak energies. During postprocessing, differences in X-ray interaction at the different energy levels allow the scanner to decompose materials based on its specific attenuation profile. A virtual noncontrast scan is accomplished by mathematically subtracting iodine or minimizing its effects in image reconstruction, which then approximates unenhanced images. The ability to classify a lesion on a single-phase contrast-enhanced CT has the potential to both reduce patient radiation dose and reduce medical costs.

MRI scanners have also seen technological improvements that reduce imaging time and improve quality. Parallel imaging techniques have been developed that acquire data simultaneously from different locations, significantly reducing scan times. A reduction in scan time allows patients to better hold their breath during breath-hold sequences, which decreases respiratory motion artifact. This is particularly valuable during dynamic contrast-enhanced scans. Rodacki et al. [2] used early dynamic serial contrast-enhanced MRI to improve characterization of adrenal tumors when combined with traditional MRI techniques.

Newer sequences such as diffusion MRI, which were originally utilized for brain imaging, are now being applied to abdominal imaging. Initial reports of diffusion analysis of adrenal lesions, however, have been disappointing. Studies have found no difference in apparent diffusion coefficient (ADC) values between benign and malignant lesions [3,4]. Magnetic resonance (MR) spectroscopy is a technique that looks at the chemical composition of tissue and shows promise in distinguishing between adrenal lesions.

Choline–creatine, choline–lipid, and lipid–creatine ratios have been used to distinguish adenomas and pheochromocytomas from carcinomas and metastases with high sensitivity and specificity [5]. There are also newer sequences that separate water and fat signal and allow quantification of these elements. At this time, it is uncertain if these newer sequences will have any role in evaluation of the adrenal glands.

IMAGING OF THE NORMAL ADRENAL

The adrenal glands are located in the retroperitoneum, paraspinal, and subphrenic. They have a thin inverted V or Y shape and are composed of medial and lateral limbs that join at the crus. The crus or body of the right adrenal lies partially dorsal to the inferior vena cava. Identifying the left adrenal can sometimes be challenging because the left adrenal can be difficult to separate from the pancreatic tail, the splenic or renal vessels, and the aorta. Although there are no size criteria to distinguish a normal from abnormal gland, the thickness of each limb is typically a few millimeters in diameter. Both adrenal glands are easier to identify when the periadrenal and perinephric adipose tissue, both covered by Gerota's fascia, are generous. Infrequently, nonadrenal conditions can mimic the appearance of an adrenal mass at imaging. An accessory spleen, upper pole renal cyst, or posterior gastric diverticulum may be confused with a left adrenal lesion. An exophytic liver lesion may be confused with a right adrenal tumor. Multiplanar imaging is crucial in these cases to make the correct diagnosis. Vascular structures such as varices and splenic or renal artery aneurysms can also be misinterpreted as an adrenal lesion on nonenhanced images, but usually become apparent after the IV administration of contrast material.

On noncontrast CT, the adrenal glands show a soft tissue density similar to that of the adjacent kidney, measuring approximately 40–50 Hounsfield units (HU). On MRI, the adrenals demonstrate intermediate to low signal intensity on T1- and T2-weighted sequences. The normal gland enhances homogeneously following IV contrast administration.

There is a variable appearance to the normal adrenal gland. An interesting study by Benitah et al. [6] evaluated 197 patients with lung cancer and no focal adrenal mass. They reported that the normal adrenals were smoothly enlarged at CT (both limbs > 6 mm) in 11%–18% of patients and nodular in 18%–23%. These patients had no greater risk of developing adrenal metastases at follow-up. Bilateral diffuse, micro- or macronodular hyperplasia, on the other hand, is due to unregulated production of adrenocorticotropic hormone (ACTH). This is often due to a pituitary adenoma, although a variety of other tumors, such as neurogenic lung carcinoma and bronchopulmonary, thymic, pancreatic, prostatic, adrenal medullary, and other neuroendocrine neoplasms, may also secrete ACTH. In women with pituitary-dependent Cushing's syndrome, 70% have bilateral diffuse, micro- or macronodular hyperplasia. Primary aldosteronism, or Conn syndrome, is due to excess aldosterone production by the adrenal glands and may be caused by aldosterone hypersecretion by bilateral adrenal hyperplasia or a unilateral cortical adenoma.

The increasing use of imaging in the population has led to the increasing detection of asymptomatic adrenal lesions. Incidental adrenal nodules are present in approximately 4%–6% of all abdominal CT examinations in patients with no known malignancy or endocrine abnormality. In patients imaged for a known malignancy, the incidence of an adrenal nodule increased to 9%–13%, although only 26%–36% of these lesions are metastatic [7]. Most adrenal masses are nonfunctioning cortical adenomas even in patients with known extra-adrenal malignancy.

Morphologic features of an adrenal mass can also be helpful in characterization, although most features are not specific enough and there is sufficient overlap between lesions such that the appearance alone may be inadequate to determine if a lesion is benign or malignant. Larger lesions, greater than 4 cm, are more likely to be malignant. Adenomas tend to have a smooth contour, while large malignant lesions tend to have an irregular border. Multicentric adrenal lesions are usually adenomatous hyperplasia and associated with benignity. Size stability indicates benignity, and any lesion that increases more than 1 cm in 1 year raises suspicion of malignancy. Adenomas and myelolipomas can increase in size but do so very slowly. A large area of necrosis within a lesion signifies malignancy, although a complex cyst can occasionally be confused with a necrotic mass. Initial contrast enhancement has little value in characterizing a solid adrenal mass since both benign and malignant lesions will demonstrate heterogeneous enhancement.

LESIONS OF THE ADRENAL CORTEX

Adenoma

Nonfunctioning adenomas are usually detected as an incidental finding in patients undergoing imaging studies that are performed for unrelated reasons. Although most are small in size, occasionally they are large enough to cause pain or compression of adjacent structures. The incidence of adenomas increases with age, as well as in certain inherited disorders, such as multiple endocrine neoplasia type 1 and the Carney complex [8]. Typically, adenomas are clinically silent, but their detection can lead to further imaging characterization or hormonal evaluation. About 70% of adrenal adenomas contain significant intracellular steroid lipid (i.e., cholesterol, a precursor to steroid hormones) or lipid to allow characterization by unenhanced CT adrenal densitometry. The high intracellular lipid content lowers the CT density of most adenomas. Korobkin et al. [9,10] showed a linear inverse relationship between lipid concentration and CT attenuation on unenhanced CT images. Almost all nonadenomatous lesions have low intracellular lipid and higher CT attenuation values. In clinical practice, 10 HU is the most widely used threshold value for the diagnosis of a lipid-rich adenoma (Figure 27.1). At this level, a meta-analysis by

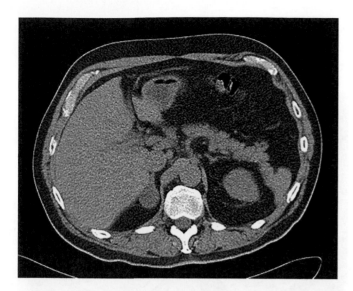

Figure 27.1 Noncontrast CT scan demonstrating a 2.0 cm right adrenal nodule with a density measurement of less than 10 HU.

Boland et al. [11] determined that a noncontrast CT density measurement would have a sensitivity of 71%, and a specificity of 98% to distinguish a benign adenoma from a nonadenomatous lesion. Unfortunately, up to 30% of adenomas are lipid poor and have attenuation values greater than 10 HU on unenhanced CT scans.

Since most standard CT scans are obtained after IV contrast, unenhanced attenuation measurements are often unavailable. While many adrenal lesions enhance rapidly following IV contrast administration, adenomas show a rapid loss of contrast on delayed images termed "contrast washout" (Figure 27.2). This is true for both lipid-rich and lipid-poor adenomas. Washout CT characterizes lipid-poor adenomas with a sensitivity of almost 100% [12,13,14]. A CT adrenal protocol typically includes a noncontrast scan, a contrast-enhanced scan, and a 15-minute delayed scan. Using density measurements from these three scans, an absolute percentage washout can be calculated for an adrenal nodule (Figure 27.3). An absolute percentage washout of 60% or greater has a reported sensitivity of 86%–88% and a specificity of 92%–96% for the diagnosis of an adenoma. When an adrenal nodule is found as an incidental finding during a CT scan, noncontrast images may not be available. In this case, a relative contrast washout can be calculated utilizing a contrast-enhanced and delayed scan (Figure 27.4). After 15 minutes, a relative percentage washout of 40% or greater has a reported sensitivity of 96% and a specificity of 100% for the diagnosis of an adenoma [15–17]. Malignant lesions enhance rapidly but usually show a slower washout of contrast due to leakage of contrast through tumor vessels.

The accuracy of MRI in the differentiation between benign and malignant adrenal tumors has been extensively reported. MR evaluation of an adenoma utilizes chemical shift imaging, which is a variation of a T1 gradient echo

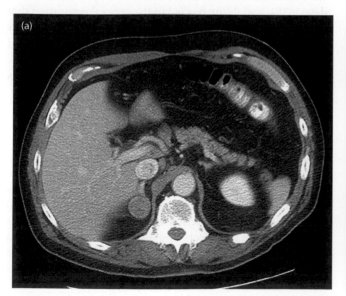
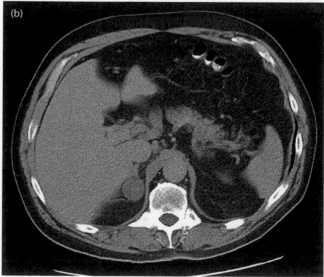

Figure 27.2 **(a)** A postcontrast image demonstrates enhancement of the right adrenal nodule. **(b)** A delay scan performed 15 minutes after injection demonstrates contrast washout. Using noncontrast, postcontrast, and delayed density measurements, an absolute percentage washout can be calculated.

Absolute percentage washout = (Enhanced HU – Delayed HU)/(Enhanced HU – Noncontrast HU) × 100

Figure 27.3 Formula for calculating absolute percentage washout.

$$\text{Relative percentage washout} = (\text{Enhanced HU} - \text{Delayed HU})/(\text{Enhanced HU}) \times 100$$

Figure 27.4 Formula for calculating relative percentage washout.

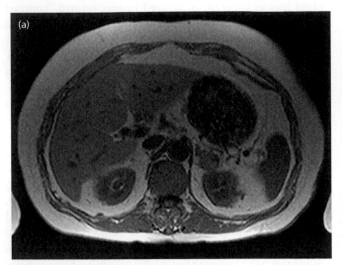 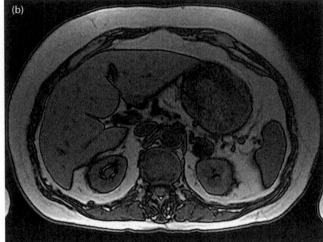

Figure 27.5 Axial in-phase **(a)** and out-of-phase **(b)** image of a left adrenal adenoma. Note a large portion of the nodule loses signal on the out-of-phase image, consistent with an adenoma.

sequence. The chemical shift sequence exploits the difference in rotational frequencies of protons that exist in water and lipid. Two sets of images are obtained simultaneously that differ only in TE (echo time). One set is termed "in phase," where the radiofrequency signals from fat and water are additive. The other set is termed "out of phase," where the signals from fat and water are at opposite points in their frequency cycle. If fat and water coexist in the same voxel (volume element) on an out-of-phase sequence, their signal cancels out and does not contribute to the MR image. Adrenal adenomas characteristically lose signal and thereby appear decreased in density on out-of-phase images (Figure 27.5). Loss of signal on opposed phase images compared with in-phase images has been shown to correlate with CT density measurements and histology findings [18,19]. It is possible to measure the loss of signal and quantitatively compare it with adjacent structures such as the spleen or psoas muscle, which do not typically demonstrate signal loss on this sequence. Studies have shown that qualitative assessment by experienced observers is as effective as quantitative measures to differentiate adenomas from nonadenomas [20,21].

Lipid-poor adenomas have a low lipid-to-water proton ratio, and their signal intensity is unchanged on out-of-phase images. These lesions therefore cannot be characterized by chemical shift imaging and are considered indeterminate, although many will prove to be adenomas. In addition, there are other benign and malignant adrenal lesions that can exhibit high lipid content that might mimic lipid-rich adenomas.

There are no imaging features to distinguish between a functional and nonfunctional adenoma. Patients with primary aldosteronism may have bilateral adrenal hyperexcretion from adrenal hyperplasia or a unilateral aldosteronoma. They could also have unilateral excretion from hyperplasia. A nonfunctional adenoma can coexist in the setting of bilateral or unilateral adrenal hyperplasia. Functional adenomas can also be small and difficult to detect. This variability has led to the general realization that CT or MRI can be an unreliable screening test in patients with syndromes of adrenocortical excess. In order to avoid inappropriate surgery, these patients should undergo adrenal vein sampling to determine if the overproduction is unilateral or bilateral [22].

Carcinoma

Primary adrenal cortical carcinoma (ACC) is an uncommon malignancy that usually presents as a large mass, with the majority of lesions measuring more than 6 cm [23]. Patients may present with a palpable mass, pain, or gastrointestinal symptoms. Approximately half of these tumors are functioning and can be detected by the manifestations of excess hormone production. These functional tumors tend to be detected earlier and at a small size [24,25]. Cushing's syndrome is most frequent, followed by virilization and feminization. These lesions are heterogeneous due to hemorrhage and necrosis. Calcification can be seen in approximately 30% of cases. ACC can contain foci of intracytoplasmic lipid, which could potentially cause them to be falsely diagnosed as an adenoma on MRI. After contrast administration, adrenocortical carcinomas enhance heterogeneously so that washout values will vary, depending on which part of the mass is sampled (Figure 27.6). Typically, there is a

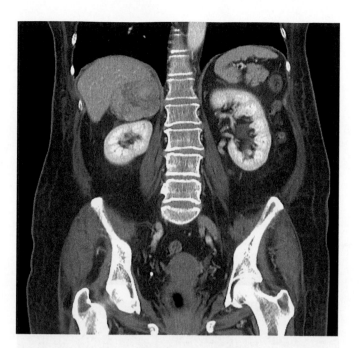

Figure 27.6 Postcontrast coronal CT image of a 64-year-old female with a 7.5 × 5.3 cm heterogeneously enhancing right adrenal mass proven to be an adrenocortical carcinoma.

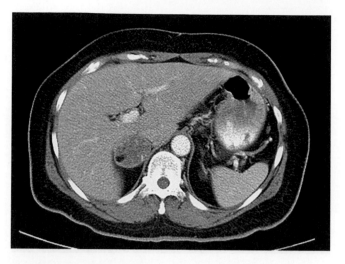

Figure 27.7 Axial CT image of a right adrenal myelolipoma. This particular lesion is predominantly solid but does have a discrete focus of macroscopic fat sufficient to make the correct diagnosis.

relative percent washout of less than 40% [26]. The large size and heterogeneity, however, are more reliable indicators of malignancy. Invasion of the IVC is a well-known complication and more common on the right. Metastatic disease is most frequent to the liver, lung, and lymph nodes, as well as direct tumor invasion.

Myelolipoma

A myelolipoma is a benign tumor composed of hematopoietic tissue and mature adipose. They are relatively uncommon, well-defined lesions that are functionally inactive. These tumors are usually detected incidentally, but if there are symptoms, they are generally due to mass effect, tumor necrosis, or hemorrhage. The key to diagnosis is the detection of macroscopic fat on either CT or MRI. CT and MRI show a well-defined mass with variable quantities of fat and soft tissue (Figure 27.7). A typical isolated lesion will have a fat content in the range of 50%–90%, with an average size of 10 cm [27]. The majority will have a pseudocapsule, and calcification occurs in 24% of lesions. Areas of low density within the lesion on CT will be similar to adjacent retroperitoneal fat.

Infrequently, these tumors can arise from an extra-adrenal location. There are a number of other adrenal tumors that have been reported to demonstrate macroscopic fat. These include adrenocortical adenoma, pheochromocytoma, adrenocortical carcinoma, and metastatic adenocarcinoma [28,29].

LESIONS OF THE ADRENAL MEDULLA

Pheochromocytoma

Although patients with pheochromocytoma may present with hypertension, palpitations, headache, diaphoresis, and flushing, 10% of patients are asymptomatic. In patients with incidentally discovered pheochromocytoma, 53% have hypertension [30]. The diagnosis is made clinically by measuring metanephrines (i.e., metanephrine plus normetanephrine) and parent catacholamines. Urinary catecholamines and their metabolites, metanephrines, vanillyl-mandelic acid (VMA), and homovanillic acid (HVA), are rarely used because of low sensitivity and specificity. Pheochromocytomas are associated with a number of syndromes, including multiple endocrine neoplasia type 2, von Hippel–Lindau syndrome, neurofibromatosis, tuberous sclerosis, and Sturge–Weber syndrome (Figure 27.8). Extra-adrenal pheochromocytoma can occur anywhere along the sympathetic chain, with the periadrenal, the para-aortic, and the ureterocystic junction being common locations. Familial paraganglioma is associated with parasympathetic tumors at the carotid bifurcation or glomus jugulare at the base of the skull. Carney's triad is a constellation of extra-adrenal pheochromocytoma, gastrointestinal stromal tumor (GIST) of the stomach, and pulmonary chondroma.

Pheochromocytomas tend to be larger than cortical adenomas, and nonsecretory lesions are usually detected at a larger size than functional masses. Approximately 10%–15% of pheochromocytomas are malignant [31]. On CT and MRI, pheochromocytomas have a variable appearance. On noncontrast MRI, they are usually isointense or hypointense to liver on T1 and hyperintense on T2. They typically demonstrate intense enhancement, but lesions containing hemorrhage or necrosis will have heterogeneous

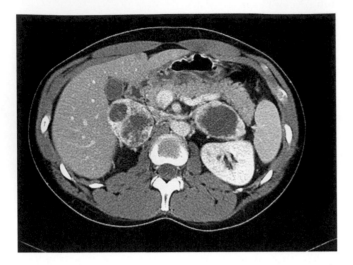

Figure 27.8 A patient with von Hippel–Lindau syndrome with bilateral adrenal pheochromocytoma.

attenuation. There can also be areas of intracellular fat and cystic degeneration that will result in decreased density. A subset of pheochromocytoma is cystic with thick enhancing walls (Figure 27.9). These lesions are less likely to be symptomatic due to lower levels of biochemical excretion [32].

LESIONS THAT CAN INVOLVE BOTH THE CORTEX AND MEDULLA

Collision tumor

A collision tumor is formed by the coexistence of two lesions of different pathologies, for example, a metastasis to a pre-existing cortical adenoma. Collision tumors can have atypical appearances, such as an adenoma–myelolipoma, which may present with a hormonal syndrome yet demonstrate intratumoral macroscopic fat.

Lymphoma

Lymphoma uncommonly arises as a primary adrenal tumor. When it occurs secondarily, it frequently is bilateral. Paling and Williamson [33] reported that 4% of patients with non-Hodgkin's lymphoma had secondary adrenal involvement, and 43% of these cases were bilateral. The imaging appearance is variable and includes both a discrete mass and an infiltrative, poorly defined appearance. Positron emission tomography (PET)-CT has been found valuable in the treatment of adrenal lymphoma, since the degree of PET activity tends to parallel other involved areas.

Metastases

The adrenal glands are a common site of metastatic disease. Adrenal metastases are most commonly from lung and breast carcinoma, and rarely from gastric, esophageal, hepatobiliary, pancreatic, colon, or renal origin. The imaging appearances of adrenal metastases are nonspecific. Larger

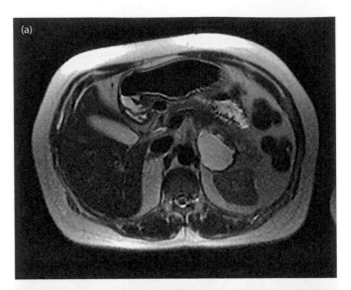

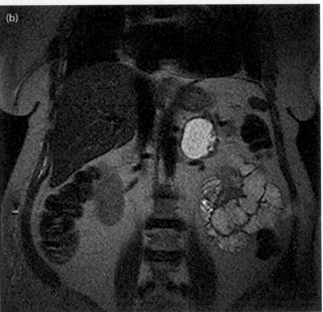

Figure 27.9 Axial (a) and coronal (b) T2 MR images of a cystic left adrenal pheochromocytoma. Note the eccentric nodular wall thickening in this predominantly cystic lesion.

lesions may show central necrosis or areas of hemorrhage. Metastases can be hypervascular, especially from renal cell carcinoma. After contrast administration, metastases usually demonstrate slower washout at delayed imaging than adenomas (absolute percentage washout of <60% and relative percentage washout of <40%). A metastasis should be considered if the patient is more than 60 years old, or the lesion is larger than 4 cm or has significantly increased in size within 1 year. Adrenal metastases can develop several years after the occurrence of the primary tumor.

Hemorrhage

Spontaneous adrenal hemorrhage often occurs in patients with sepsis, renal vein thrombosis, anticoagulation, or

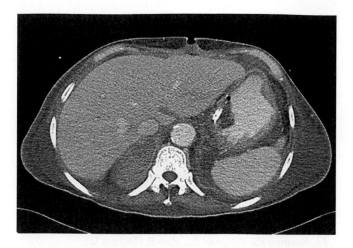

Figure 27.10 Mixed attenuation right adrenal lesion on CT in a postoperative patient with sepsis. This lesion was not present on a preoperative scan compatible with acute adrenal hemorrhage.

underlying adrenal mass. Adrenal hemorrhage is more common in neonates than in older children or adults, which may be due to the trauma of delivery, asphyxia, septicemia, or abnormal clotting factors. Hemorrhage more commonly involves the right than the left adrenal, and is bilateral in only approximately 10% of neonates. Adrenal hemorrhage may occur in up to 25% of severely traumatized adult patients with a higher rate of bilateral involvement of 20%. On CT, acute hematoma initially has a high density of 50–90 HU, which will gradually decrease over time (Figure 27.10). The MR appearance will vary depending on the stage of hemoglobin degradation. Serial imaging usually demonstrates an evolving lesion that changes in signal intensity over time. Most adrenal hematomas will eventually resorb, but some may liquefy and persist as an adrenal pseudocyst, or calcify.

Cyst

Adrenal cysts are occasionally identified as an incidental finding on an imaging examination. Although most are asymptomatic and benign, large cysts may present with abdominal pain, gastrointestinal symptoms, or a palpable mass. Cysts can be classified by histologic types: endothelial cysts, epithelial cysts, pseudocysts, and parasitic cysts [34]. Endothelial cysts are usually unilateral with a thin-wall, purely fluid internal composition, with no soft tissue component or internal enhancement. Pseudocysts have a wall composed of dense, fibrous connective tissue and may result from pancreatitis, cystic degeneration of a neoplasm, trauma, disseminated infection, adrenal infarction, or hemorrhage. Epithelial cysts are rare and thought to arise from displaced urogenital tissue, since the normal adrenal does not contain any true follicular cells. Most parasitic adrenal cysts are echinococcal in origin. Echinococcal calcified cysts contain nonviable scolices. These cysts have thick walls, with or without calcification, and can be associated with eosinophilia. Although small simple cysts can be

managed conservatively with surveillance, any functional, malignant, or benign lesion more than 5 cm in diameter deserves surgical treatment [35].

CONCLUSION

Adrenal lesions as a group comprise a wide variety of etiologies and overlapping features. Evaluation of these lesions requires identifying characteristics such as size, contour, unilateral or bilateral distribution, CT washout values or MR signal changes, and the presence of calcification, fat, or hemorrhage [36,37]. Although much progress has been made in characterizing adrenal lesions by imaging techniques, some lesions remain indeterminate. Complex clinical algorithms have been published to guide the workup of an incidentally discovered adrenal nodule [38]. When a lesion defies accurate characterization, surgical excision, percutaneous needle biopsy, or short-term follow-up evaluation may be necessary as the next step in patient management [39]. Percutaneous intervention (biopsy) or angioembolization in pheochromocytoma should be done with preintervention alpha-adrenergic blockade, anesthesia, and available IV alpha- and beta-adrenergic blocker.

REFERENCES

1. Glazer D, Maturen K, Kaza R et al. Adrenal incidentaloma triage with single-source (fast-kilovoltage switch) dual-energy CT. AJR Am J Roentgenol 2014;203:329–35.
2. Rodacki K, Ramalho M, Dale BM et al. Combined chemical shift imaging with early dynamic serial gadolinium-enhanced MRI in the characterization of adrenal lesion. AJR Am J Roentgenol 2014;203:99–106.
3. Tsushima Y, Takahashi-Taketomi A, Endo K. Diagnostic utility of diffusion-weighted MR imaging and apparent diffusion coefficient value for the diagnosis of adrenal tumors. J Magn Reson Imaging 2009;29:112–17.
4. Miller FH, Wang Y, McCarthy RJ et al. Utility of diffusion-weighted MRI in characterization of adrenal lesions. AJR Am J Roentgenol 2010;194:459W179–85.
5. Faria JF, Goldman SM, Szejnfeld J et al. Adrenal masses: Characterization with in vivo proton MR spectroscopy—Initial experience. Radiology 2007;245:788–97.
6. Benitah N, Yeh BM, Qayyum A, Williams G, Breiman RS, Coakley FV. Minor morphologic abnormalities of adrenal glands at CT: Prognostic importance in patients with lung cancer. Radiology 2005;235(2):517–22.
7. Blake MA, Cronin CG, Boland GW. Adrenal imaging. AJR Am J Roentgenol 2010;194:1450–60.
8. Kloos RT, Gross MD, Francis IR, Korobkin M, Shapiro B. Incidentally discovered adrenal masses. Endocr Rev 1995;16(4):460–84.

9. Korobkin M, Giordano TJ, Brodeur FJ et al. Adrenal adenomas: Relationship between histologic lipid and CT and MR findings. *Radiology* 1996;200:743–7.

10. Korobkin M, Brodeur FJ, Yutzy GG et al. Differentiation of adrenal adenomas from nonadenomas using CT attenuation values. *Am J Roentgenol* 1996;166:531–6.

11. Boland GW, Lee MJ, Gazelle GS et al. Characterization of adrenal masses using unenhanced CT: An analysis of the CT literature. *AJR Am J Roentgenol* 1998;171:201–4.

12. Caoili EM, Korobkin M, Francis IR, Cohan RH, Dunnick NR. Delayed enhanced CT of lipid-poor adrenal adenomas. *AJR Am J Roentgenol* 2000;175:1411–5.

13. Pena CS, Boland GW, Hahn PF, Lee MJ, Mueller PR. Characterization of indeterminate (lipid-poor) adrenal masses: Use of washout characteristics at contrast-enhanced CT. *Radiology* 2000;217:789–802.

14. Park BK, Kim CK, Kim B, Lee JH. Comparison of delayed enhanced CT and chemical shift MR for evaluating hyperattenuating incidental adrenal masses. *Radiology* 2007;243:760–5.

15. Caoili EM, Kroobkin M, Francis IR et al. Adrenal masses: Characterization with combined unenhanced and delayed CT. *Radiology* 2002;222:629–33.

16. Korobkin M, Brodeur FJ, Francis IR, Quint LE, Dunnick NR, Londy F. CT time-attenuation wash-out curves of adrenal adenomas and nonadenomas. *AJR Am J Roentgenol* 1998;170(3):747–52.

17. Korobkin M, Brodeur FJ, Francis IR, Quint LE, Dunnick NR, Goodsitt M. Delayed enhanced CT for differentiation of benign from malignant adrenal masses. *Radiology* 1996;200(3):737–42.

18. Outwater EK, Siegelman ES, Huang AB, Birnbaum BA. Adrenal masses: Correlation between CT attenuation values and chemical shift ratio at MR imaging with in-phase and opposed-phase sequences. *Radiology* 1996;200(3):749–52.

19. Korobkin M, Giordano TJ, Brodeur FJ et al. Adrenal adenomas: Relationship between histologic lipid and CT and MR findings. *Radiology* 1996;200(3):743–7.

20. Mayo-Smith WW, Lee MJ, McNicholas MM, Hahn PF, Boland GW, Saini S. Characterization of adrenal masses (<5 cm) by use of chemical shift MR imaging: Observer performance versus quantitative measures. *AJR Am J Roentgenol* 1995;165(1):91–5.

21. Korobkin M, Lombardi TJ, Aisen AM et al. Characterization of adrenal masses with chemical shift and gadolinium-enhanced MR imaging. *Radiology* 1995;197(2):411–8.

22. Daunt N. Adrenal vein sampling: How to make it quick, easy, and successful. *Radiographics* 2005;25:S143–58.

23. Wajchenberg BL, Albergaria Pereira MA, Medonca BB et al. Adrenocortical carcinoma: Clinical and laboratory observations. *Cancer* 2000;88(4):711–36.

24. Ng L, Libertino JM. Adrenocortical carcinoma: Diagnosis, evaluation and treatment. *J Urol* 2003;169(1):5–11.

25. Slattery JM, Blake MA, Kalra MK et al. Adrenocortical carcinoma: Contrast washout characteristics on CT. *AJR Am J Roentgenol* 2006;187(1):W21–4.

26. Fishman EK, Deutch BM, Hartman DS, Goldman SM, Zerhouni EA, Siegelman SS. Primary adrenocortical carcinoma: CT evaluation with clinical correlation. *AJR Am J Roentgenol* 1987;148(3):531–5.

27. Kenney PJ, Wagner BJ, Rao P, Heffess CS. Myelolipoma: CT and pathologic features. *Radiology* 1998;208(1):87–95.

28. Yamada T, Ishibashi T, Saito H et al. Non-functioning adrenocortical adenomas containing fat components. *Clin Radiol* 2002;57(11):1034–43.

29. Heye S, Woestenborghs H, Van Kerkhove F, Oyen R. Adrenocortical carcinoma with fat inclusion: Case report. *Abdom Imaging* 2005;30(5):641–3.

30. Motta-Ramirez GA, Remer EM, Herts BR, Gill IS, Hamrahian AH. Comparison of CT findings in asymptomatic and incidentally discovered pheochromocytomas. *AJR Am J Roentgenol* 2005;185(3):684–8.

31. Blake MA, Kalra MK, Maher MM et al. Pheochromocytoma: An imaging chameleon. *Radiographics* 2004;24(Suppl 1):S87–99.

32. Andreoni C, Krebs RK, Bruna PC. Cystic phaeochromocytoma is a distinctive subgroup with special clinical, imaging and histological features that might mislead the diagnosis. *BJU Int* 2008;101(3):345–50.

33. Paling MR, Williamson BR. Adrenal involvement in non-Hodgkin lymphoma. *AJR Am J Roentgenol* 1983;141(2):303–5.

34. Chien HP, Chang YS, Hsu PS et al. Adrenal cystic lesions: A clinicopathological analysis of 25 cases with proposed histogenesis and review of the literature. *Endocr Pathol* 2008;19:274–81.

35. Wedmid A, Palese M. Diagnosis and treatment of the adrenal cyst. *Curr Urol Rep* 2010;11:44–50.

36. Dunnick NR. Adrenal imaging: Current status. *AJR Am J Roentgenol* 1990;154:927–36.

37. Johnson PT, Horton KM, Fishman EK. Adrenal mass imaging with multidetector CT: Pathologic conditions, pearls, and pitfalls. *Radiographics* 2009;29:1333–51.

38. Berland LL, Silverman SG, Gore RM et al. Managing incidental findings on abdominal CT: White paper of the ACR Incidental Findings Committee. *JACR* 2010;7(10):754–73.

39. Copeland PM. The incidentally discovered adrenal mass. *Ann Surg* 1984;199(1):116–22.

28

Adrenal vein sampling for diagnosis and localization of aldosteronoma

VIVEK V. PATIL AND ROBERT A. LOOKSTEIN

INTRODUCTION

Adrenal vein sampling is a valuable tool in the diagnosis and localization of aldosterone-secreting tumors in patients with clinically suspected primary hyperaldosteronism. Accurate identification of unilateral aldosterone-producing adrenal adenomas is critical because surgical resection of such lesions may be offered to this subset of patients. Key factors in successful adrenal vein sampling include proper patient selection and adherence to standardized technique.

BACKGROUND

First described in 1967 by Melby and colleagues, adrenal vein sampling has been in use for decades for the preoperative localization of aldosterone-secreting tumors [1]. The need for adrenal vein sampling arises from the inaccuracy of imaging modalities such as computed tomography (CT) to accurately distinguish unilateral from bilateral disease [2,3]. The classification of disease as unilateral or bilateral is clinically significant because primary hyperaldosteronism may be due to bilateral idiopathic hyperaldosteronism (IHA), which is treated medically, or unilateral aldosterone-producing adenoma (APA), which is treated with adrenalectomy.

In one study of 62 patients comparing CT with adrenal vein sampling, CT was inaccurate or provided no additional information in 68% of patients [4]. Another study found CT to localize adenomas in only 50% of histologically proven cases [5]. Therefore, despite advancement in CT imaging techniques, adrenal vein sampling remains an integral part of the evaluation of patients with primary hyperaldosteronism.

MRI EVALUATION

The role of MRI, as with CT, in patients with primary hyperaldosteronism is to exclude certain diagnoses, which would clearly warrant surgery and thus obviate the need for adrenal vein sampling. For example, a patient with MRI findings compatible with adrenal pheochromocytoma or adrenocortical carcinoma would not require adrenal vein sampling. Pheochromocytoma on MRI is classically hypervascular and hyperintense on T2-weighted imaging, although atypical imaging findings may also be seen [6]. Adrenal cortical carcinoma may present clinically with hyperaldosteronism and is suspected when imaging reveals a large (>4 cm) adrenal mass or signs of aggressiveness, such as necrosis or tumor extension [7–9].

PATIENT SELECTION AND PREPARATION

Primary hyperaldosteronism has been reported to account for 10%–11% of patients referred to hypertension specialists, and may be suspected clinically in patients presenting with hypertension and hypokalemia [10,11]. An abnormally elevated aldosterone–renin ratio utilizing plasma renin activity measurement has been described in the literature as a biochemical screening test for primary hyperaldosteronism, and is routinely used for this purpose at the authors' institution [12].

According to the 2014 American Heart Association expert consensus statement on adrenal vein sampling, patients with primary hyperaldosteronism should undergo adrenal vein sampling when adrenalectomy is considered, with the following exceptions:

- Patients of age <40 years with marked primary hyperaldosteronism and a clear unilateral adrenal adenoma and a normal contralateral adrenal gland on CT
- Patients at unacceptable high risk of surgery (due to age or comorbidities)
- Patients suspected of having adrenocortical carcinoma
- Patients with proven familial hyperaldosteronism (FH-I or FH-III) [13]

To identify the above scenarios and to aid in procedure planning, a CT study is routinely obtained before adrenal vein sampling at the authors' institution.

Patient preparation includes correction of hypokalemia before the procedure in order to avoid false-negative results due to hypokalemia decreasing aldosterone secretion via the feedback loop. Similarly, antihypertensive medications that may interfere with the renin–angiotensin system should be discontinued. Mineralocorticoid receptor antagonists such as spironolactone should be discontinued at least 4 weeks before the study in order to decrease the risk of elevated renin levels stimulating the contralateral gland, thereby decreasing sensitivity of the study [13]. Some authors have suggested measuring plasma renin activity after discontinuation of mineralocorticoid receptor antagonists to ensure a plasma renin activity of <1 ng/mL/h [11].

PROCEDURE TECHNICAL CONSIDERATIONS

Adrenal vein sampling may be performed on an outpatient basis in the interventional radiology suite. Bilateral common femoral vein access is obtained utilizing ultrasound guidance, thereby allowing for simultaneous sampling of right and left adrenal vein blood. Although single-access sequential catheterization of the right and left adrenal veins has been described, simultaneous catheterization is preferred to minimize variation given the pulsatile nature of cortisol and aldosterone secretion [13]. Plasma cortisol and aldosterone are measured from each sample (right adrenal vein, left adrenal vein, and infrarenal inferior vena cava [IVC]).

Pharmacologic stimulation via administration of cosyntropin (adrenocorticotropic hormone [ACTH] analog) at a rate of 50 μg/h starting 30 minutes before sampling or as a 250 μg bolus is recommended by the American Heart Association consensus guidelines. The stimulation serves to increase the selectivity index (SI), decrease stress-related fluctuation, and increase aldosterone secretion from adenomas (Table 28.1) [13].

Table 28.1 ACTH administration during adrenal vein sampling

Benefits	Administration protocol
Increase SI	Infusion of 50 μg/h starting 30 minutes before sampling (preferred) or 250 μg bolus
Decrease fluctuation in aldosterone secretion	
Increase aldosterone secretion by adenoma	

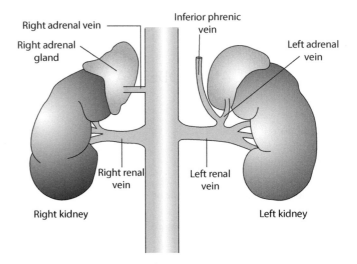

Figure 28.1 Adrenal vein anatomy. (Adapted from Monticone S et al. *Lancet Diabetes Endocrinol* 2015;3:296–303.)

Knowledge of adrenal vein anatomy and variations therein helps facilitate successful catheterization (Figure 28.1). Each adrenal gland commonly has one central draining vein. In conventional anatomy, the right central vein drains into the IVC and the left central vein joins with the inferior phrenic vein to drain into the left renal vein [14]. Variations are rare and include multiplicity of draining veins, as well as altered sites of drainage. A right adrenal vein that drains into a hepatic vein is possible [15]. Several anatomic variations have been described with regard to the left adrenal vein in cadaveric studies, including direct drainage into the left renal vein or IVC [14]. Once catheterized, retrograde venography via a gentle injection of contrast is performed to confirm position (Figure 28.2).

PATIENT SAFETY

Adrenal vein sampling is a relatively safe procedure. In the Adrenal Vein Sampling International Study (AVIS) registry of 2604 cases from 20 institutions, the overall rate of adrenal vein rupture was 0.61%. The rate of adrenal vein rupture was inversely correlated with a given institution and practitioner's adrenal vein sampling volume [16]. Gentle hand injection of contrast is recommended to minimize the risk of this complication. Other possible complications include arterial

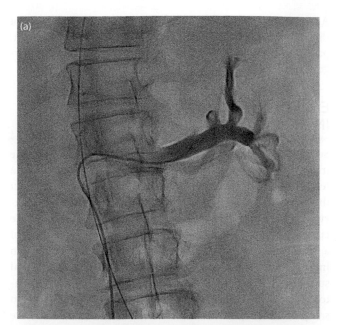

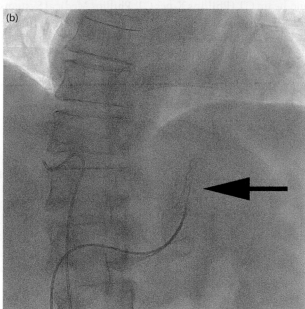

Figure 28.2 Left adrenal vein catheterization. Initial access into the left renal vein is obtained with a Simmons catheter **(a)** and subsequently the left adrenal vein. Retrograde venography opacifies the left adrenal vein (arrow), confirming successful catheterization **(b)**.

puncture, vagal reaction, transient increase in serum creatinine, allergic reaction, and infection [17].

INTERPRETATION OF ADRENAL VEIN SAMPLING DATA

The SI and laterality index (LI) are calculated to describe the results of an adrenal vein sampling study. SI is essentially a measure of the cortisol step-up between blood from the infrarenal IVC and blood from a catheterized adrenal vein. SI is a metric used to describe the operator's successful catheterization of the target adrenal vein with minimal dilution. The formula for SI is plasma cortisol concentration in the sampled adrenal vein divided by the plasma cortisol concentration of the infrarenal IVC (see Table 28.2) [18]. Although there is great heterogeneity in SI threshold values used worldwide, the American Heart Association expert consensus guidelines state the SI should be greater than or equal to 2 under basal conditions and greater than or equal to 3 after ACTH. Studies with SI values below these thresholds indicate poor selectivity of catheterization and should be regarded as nondiagnostic [13].

LI is the ratio of aldosterone/cortisol of dominant gland to aldosterone/cortisol of contralateral gland. The dominant gland is the side (right or left) with the higher aldosterone-to-cortisol ratio. Calculation of LI is reviewed in Table 28.2. Although there are no randomized controlled trials to determine optimal LI threshold values, there are several observational studies [19,20]. The guidelines suggest using an LI threshold of 2 for basal protocols and 4 for adrenal vein sampling done with cosyntropin stimulation [13]. LI values greater than or equal to these thresholds are diagnostic of unilateral aldosterone excess.

LIMITATIONS OF ADRENAL VEIN SAMPLING

Adrenal vein sampling is a technically challenging procedure. In a recent retrospective review of 343 adrenal vein sampling procedures performed at a high-volume center, Trerotola and colleagues reported a 3.5% failure rate. Failure was right-sided in 57% of their cases and left-sided in 29%, with the remainder being bilateral or due to laboratory error. A common cause of left-sided failure is dilution of sample.

Table 28.2 Interpretation of adrenal vein sampling

	Formula	Significance	Threshold values
Sensitivity index	$\dfrac{PCC_{adrenal\ vein}}{PCC_{IVC}}$	Higher SI indicates successful selective catheterization of the adrenal vein	SI ≥ 2 basal or SI ≥ 3 post-ACTH
Laterality index	$\dfrac{\dfrac{PAC_{dominant\ gland}}{PCC_{dominant\ gland}}}{\dfrac{PAC_{contralateral\ gland}}{PCC_{contralateral\ gland}}}$	Higher LI (>2) indicates unilateral aldosterone excess	

Note: PCC, plasma cortisol concentration; PAC, plasma aldosterone concentration.

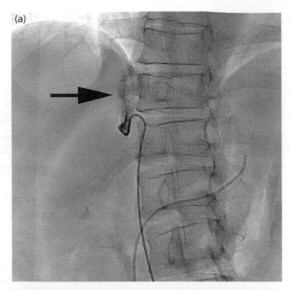

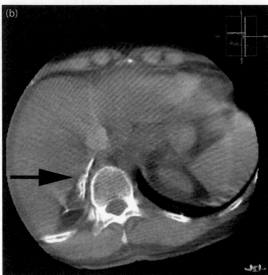

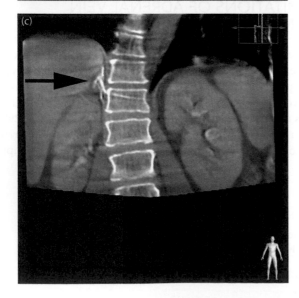

Figure 28.3 Intraprocedure cone-beam CT. Conventional retrograde venography **(a)** demonstrates opacification of the right adrenal gland (arrow). Axial **(b)** and coronal **(c)** cone-beam CT confirms successful catheterization.

A common cause of right-sided failure is misidentification of the adrenal vein [17]. In the event of a nondiagnostic result, patients may be offered repeat adrenal vein sampling if surgery is still being considered [21].

EMERGING TECHNOLOGIES IN INTERVENTIONAL ENDOCRINOLOGY

Successful catheterization of the right adrenal vein is the most challenging aspect of adrenal vein sampling from a technical standpoint. As mentioned previously, the direct drainage of the right central vein into the IVC makes catheterization difficult. When the operator believes he or she is in the vein, retrograde venography via slow injection of a small volume of contrast is used to confirm location. An increasingly available technology on modern interventional suites known as cone-beam CT may offer improved operator confidence of successful catheterization in adrenal vein sampling [22,23]. At the author's institution, intraprocedure cone-beam CT (Phillips X-per CT, Phillips Medical Systems, Bothell, Washington) is performed routinely on every adrenal vein sampling case in order to confirm catheter position, in addition to the traditional biochemical assessment via the SI. The cone-beam CT images are acquired during retrograde venography, thereby confirming proper catheter placement (Figure 28.3).

CONCLUSION

Despite advances in CT and MRI, adrenal vein sampling remains a key component in the evaluation of patients with clinically suspected primary hyperaldosteronism. Successful adrenal vein sampling is achieved with proper patient selection and adherence to standardized technique. Emerging technology such as intraprocedure cone-beam CT may help interventional radiologists gain confidence in performing adrenal vein sampling.

REFERENCES

1. Melby JC, Spark RF, Dale SL, Egdahl RH, Kahn PC. Diagnosis and localization of aldosterone-producing adenomas by percutaneous bilateral adrenal vein catheterization. *Prog Clin Cancer* 1970;4:175–84.
2. Doppman JL, Gill JR Jr, Miller DL et al. Distinction between hyperaldosteronism due to bilateral hyperplasia and unilateral aldosteronoma: Reliability of CT. *Radiology* 1992;184:677–82.
3. Oh EM, Lee KE, Yoon K, Kim SY, Kim HC, Youn YK. Value of adrenal venous sampling for lesion localization in primary aldosteronism. *World J Surg* 2012;36:2522–7.
4. Magill SB, Raff H, Shaker JL et al. Comparison of adrenal vein sampling and computed tomography in the differentiation of primary aldosteronism. *J Clin Endocrinol Metab* 2001;86:1066–71.

5. Harper R, Ferrett CG, McKnight JA et al. Accuracy of CT scanning and adrenal vein sampling in the pre-operative localization of aldosterone-secreting adrenal adenomas. *QJM* 1999;92:643–50.

6. Blake MA, Kalra MK, Maher MM et al. Pheochromocytoma: An imaging chameleon. *Radiographics* 2004;24(Suppl 1):S87–99.

7. Sturgeon C, Shen WT, Clark OH, Duh QY, Kebebew E. Risk assessment in 457 adrenal cortical carcinomas: How much does tumor size predict the likelihood of malignancy? *J Am Coll Surg* 2006;202:423–30.

8. Zhang HM, Perrier ND, Grubbs EG et al. CT features and quantification of the characteristics of adreno-cortical carcinomas on unenhanced and contrast-enhanced studies. *Clin Radiol* 2012;67:38–46.

9. Lattin GE Jr, Sturgill ED, Tujo CA et al. From the radiologic pathology archives: Adrenal tumors and tumor-like conditions in the adult: Radiologic-pathologic correlation. *Radiographics* 2014;34:805–29.

10. Rossi GP, Bernini G, Caliumi C et al. A prospective study of the prevalence of primary aldosteronism in 1,125 hypertensive patients. *J Am Coll Cardiol* 2006;48:2293–300.

11. Monticone S, Viola A, Rossato D et al. Adrenal vein sampling in primary aldosteronism: Towards a standardised protocol. *Lancet Diabetes Endocrinol* 2015;3:296–303.

12. Rossi GP, Barisa M, Belfiore A et al. The aldosterone-renin ratio based on the plasma renin activity and the direct renin assay for diagnosing aldosterone-producing adenoma. *J Hypertens* 2010;28:1892–9.

13. Rossi GP, Auchus RJ, Brown M et al. An expert consensus statement on use of adrenal vein sampling for the subtyping of primary aldosteronism. *Hypertension* 2014;63:151–60.

14. Cesmebasi A, Du Plessis M, Iannatuono M, Shah S, Tubbs RS, Loukas M. A review of the anatomy and clinical significance of adrenal veins. *Clin Anat* 2014;27:1253–63.

15. Daunt N. Adrenal vein sampling: How to make it quick, easy, and successful. *Radiographics* 2005;25(Suppl 1):S143–58.

16. Rossi GP, Barisa M, Allolio B et al. The Adrenal Vein Sampling International Study (AVIS) for identifying the major subtypes of primary aldosteronism. *J Clin Endocrinol Metab* 2012;97:1606–14.

17. Trerotola SO, Asmar M, Yan Y, Fraker DL, Cohen DL. Failure mode analysis in adrenal vein sampling: A single-center experience. *J Vasc Interv Radiol* 2014;25:1611–9.

18. Rossi GP, Pitter G, Bernante P, Motta R, Feltrin G, Miotto D. Adrenal vein sampling for primary aldosteronism: The assessment of selectivity and lateral-ization of aldosterone excess baseline and after adrenocorticotropic hormone (ACTH) stimulation. *J Hypertens* 2008;26:989–97.

19. Ishidoya S, Kaiho Y, Ito A et al. Single-center outcome of laparoscopic unilateral adrenalectomy for patients with primary aldosteronism: Lateralizing disease using results of adrenal venous sampling. *Urology* 2011;78:68–73.

20. Mulatero P, Bertello C, Sukor N et al. Impact of different diagnostic criteria during adrenal vein sampling on reproducibility of subtype diagnosis in patients with primary aldosteronism. *Hypertension* 2010;55:667–73.

21. Bouhanick B, Delchier MC, Fauvel J, Rousseau H, Amar J, Chamontin B. Is it useful to repeat an adrenal venous sampling in patients with primary hyperaldosteronism? *Ann Cardiol Angeiol* 2014;63:23–7.

22. Georgiades CS, Hong K, Geschwind JF et al. Adjunctive use of C-arm CT may eliminate technical failure in adrenal vein sampling. *J Vasc Interv Radiol* 2007;18:1102–5.

23. Plank C, Wolf F, Langenberger H, Loewe C, Schoder M, Lammer J. Adrenal venous sampling using Dyna-CT—A practical guide. *Eur J Radiol* 2012;81:2304–7.

29

Cushing's syndrome, cortical carcinoma, and estrogen- and androgen-secreting tumors

ALEXANDER STARK AND O. JOE HINES

CUSHING'S SYNDROME

Described famously in 1932 by Harvey Cushing as "pituitary basophilism," Cushing's syndrome refers to the clinical constellation of obesity, diabetes, arterial hypertension, muscular weakness, and adrenal hyperplasia [1]. An elevated serum cortisol is the *sine qua non* of Cushing's syndrome. Conversely, symptomatic patients with physiologic hypercortisolism are often described as having "pseudo-Cushing's syndrome" [2]. All signs and symptoms of Cushing's syndrome result directly or indirectly from prolonged exposure to excess cortisol. While the full-blown syndrome is unmistakable, the large spectrum of disease and its protean manifestations dictate that Cushing's syndrome must be considered in the differential diagnosis for many diverse and nonspecific clinical manifestations.

Epidemiology and etiology

As defined by excess hypercortisolism of any etiology, the true incidence of Cushing's syndrome has been difficult to accurately determine. Glucocorticoids continue to be a mainstay of therapy for many immunologic, allergic, and malignant diseases; accordingly, exogenous administration of these drugs is the most common cause of Cushing's syndrome in the population. The vast number of patients taking these medications, and the varying degrees to which they are symptomatic, contributes to the difficulty in determining the true incidence of Cushing's syndrome.

Endogenous hypercortisolism, however, is a rare phenomenon. The reported incidence ranges from 0.7 to 3 per million per year, with an estimated prevalence of about 39 per million [3–5]. A reported female predominance exists, with a ratio ranging widely from 3–15:1 [3,4,6,7]. More recent data suggests Cushing's syndrome may be far more common in certain patient populations. In screening studies of obese patients with type 2 diabetes, the reported prevalence of Cushing's syndrome is 2%–5%. In these patients, their metabolic disorder improved after treatment of an underlying Cushing's syndrome [5,8–11]. This suggests that the true incidence of endogenous hypercortisolism is under-reported when patients are screened based on clinical suspicion alone, and that more frequent screening of such populations may be warranted [5,11].

The term *Cushing's syndrome* is used to signify hypercortisolism of any etiology. Often misused, the term *Cushing's disease* is given specifically to hypercortisolism secondary to an adrenocorticotropic hormone (ACTH)-secreting pituitary microadenoma. Of all endogenous causes of Cushing's syndrome, ACTH-dependent hypercortisolism constitutes 80%–85%; of these, Cushing's disease is by far the most common, representing up to 80% of ACTH-dependent cases. The remaining 20% are predominantly the result of ectopic ACTH secretion [12,13]. The latter is most commonly a paraneoplastic syndrome associated with small cell carcinoma of the lung, but may be seen in association with intestinal and bronchial carcinoid tumors and an endocrine tumor of any tissue origin, and has been reported in numerous other carcinomas. Ectopic secretion of corticotropin-releasing hormone (CRH) is a rare cause of ACTH-dependent hypercortisolism [6,12].

So-called ACTH-independent causes of hypercortisolism are predominantly adrenal in origin. The most common of these is a unilateral, cortisol-producing adrenal adenoma, followed by adrenal cortical carcinoma. Very rare causes of adrenal hypercortisolism include bilateral macronodular adrenal hyperplasia (BMAH) (distinct from the bilateral adrenal hyperplasia that results from ACTH hypersecretion) and primary pigmented nodular adrenocortical adrenal hyperplasia [6,14]. Finally, causes of physiologic hypercortisolism include pregnancy, major depression, alcohol dependence, morbid obesity, physical stress, malnutrition, and chronic intense exercise [15].

Clinical features and prognosis

Chronic exposure to excessive glucocorticoids manifests itself in myriad nonspecific physical and metabolic changes. Physically, the patient with Cushing's syndrome will most commonly gain weight in a truncal distribution and display a combination of acne, hirsutism, thin skin, facial plethora, facial rounding ("moon facies"), and increased fat in the dorsal neck and supraclavicular area ("dorsal hump"). The physical finding most specific for Cushing's syndrome is abdominal striae, particularly if large (>1 cm wide) and reddish-purple in color [16–18]. A more in-depth evaluation may reveal easy bruising, poor wound healing, early-onset osteoporosis, menstrual irregularity, impaired glucose tolerance, and hypertension. In combination with some of the above findings, proximal muscle weakness is

particularly suggestive of Cushing's syndrome [2,17,19]. Patients must be monitored carefully for an increased risk of developing cardiovascular and atherosclerotic disease, diabetes, pathologic fractures, early cognitive decline, and mood disorders [20].

Untreated, patients with Cushing's syndrome have a grave prognosis, with 5-year mortality in early studies as high as 50% [21]. More recent data demonstrates that patients with poorly controlled disease have a standard mortality ratio (SMR) between 4 and 9, indicating a risk of death at least four times greater than that of the average population. Death occurs mainly as a result of cardiovascular or infectious processes [4,22]. Achievement of eucortisolism has been shown to reduce SMR to baseline in one cohort study; however, data is conflicting whether morbidity and mortality truly return to population baseline [15,20,23]. Some studies demonstrate reduced cardiovascular risk after surgery; however, multiple studies have shown persistent elevated myocardial risk greater than 5 years after surgery for disease [20,24,25].

Diagnosis of Cushing's syndrome

As described above, the signs and symptoms of Cushing's syndrome have considerable overlap with common conditions in the general population, and varying populations are at risk. This, in combination with the clear morbidity and mortality associated with uncontrolled disease, dictates that an evidence-based, systematic, and reproducible method for diagnosis should be followed. Initial screening tests should be highly sensitive and followed by confirmatory tests with higher specificity. In 2008, the Endocrine Society issued a set of evidence-based guidelines for practitioners to follow in establishing the diagnosis of Cushing's syndrome (Figure 29.1).

In general, the first step is to rule out exogenous glucocorticoid ingestion by history. This is followed by confirmation of hypercortisolism. Physiologic hypercortisolism—aka pseudo-Cushing's syndrome—may be indicated by a history of polycystic ovary syndrome, severe stress or infection, chronic alcoholism, long-standing major depression, and morbid obesity. The diagnosis of Cushing's syndrome is made once confirmed hypercortisolism is found to be pathologic in nature. Initial tests recommended by the Endocrine Society include the urine free cortisol (UFC), late-night salivary cortisol, 1 mg (low-dose) overnight dexamethasone suppression test (DST), and 2-day low-dose DST. Tests not recommended include the random serum cortisol or ACTH, urinary 17-ketosteroids, an insulin tolerance test, the loperamide test, and any specific test reserved for the diagnosis of a *cause* of hypercortisolism [15].

The measurement of UFC has been widely used since the 1970s as an initial screening test for patients clinically suspected to have Cushing's syndrome [26]. A complete 24-hour urine collection specimen is provided by the patient, which is screened for appropriate volume and urinary creatinine in addition to cortisol [2,15]. The reference range depends

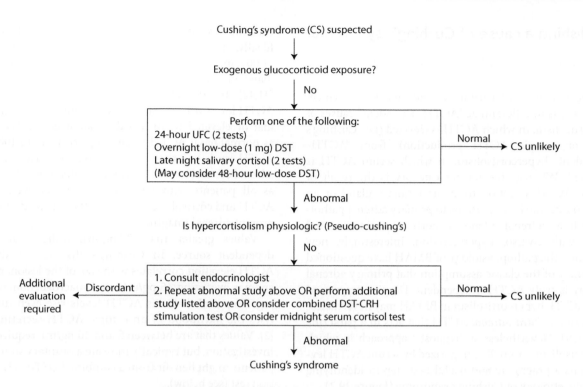

Figure 29.1 Algorithm adaptation of the 2008 Endocrine Society Clinical Practice Guidelines for the diagnosis of Cushing's syndrome (Adapted from Nieman LK et al. *J Clin Endocrinol Metab* 2008;93(5):1526–40.)

on the specific assay used, typically radioimmunoassay (RIA) or high-performance liquid chromatography. Assays of UFC in an outpatient setting can offer sensitivities up to 100%, with specificity up to 98% depending on the cutoff [27]. Current evidence supports using all values above the upper limit of normal to identify a "positive" result, achieving the desired sensitivity at the expense of a higher false-positive rate [15,28,29]. As 11%–15% of patients with Cushing's syndrome may have normal results in one of four UFC samples, it is recommended to perform the test twice in all patients. False negatives are rare, but may occur in patients with very mild disease or in patients with cyclical disease [15,30].

Late-night salivary cortisol is an increasingly used and convenient method for detecting hypercortisolism with high sensitivity and specificity. The test operates on the following premises: (1) cortisol levels reach their normal circadian nadir around midnight; (2) in patients with Cushing's syndrome, alteration in cortisol circadian rhythms is common, and may be the most sensitive finding of the disease [31]; and (3) salivary cortisol has been shown to accurately reflect serum cortisol, obviating the need for late-night blood draws in many patients [15,32]. Patients collect a saliva sample on two separate evenings near midnight, which can be stored at room temperature. Late-night salivary cortisol has a reported sensitivity and specificity between 90% and 100% [31,33–35]. False positives can occur with significant tobacco use, with steroid-containing lotions, or in patients that work night shifts or are otherwise prevented from normal sleep–wake cycles (i.e., insomnia and depression) and thereby have altered circadian rhythms [15].

Low-dose DST is another highly sensitive screening test commonly used. One milligram of dexamethasone is administered near midnight, and serum cortisol is measured between 8 and 9 hours later. In normal patients, the administration of exogenous glucocorticoid suppresses ACTH and cortisol through a negative-feedback loop; in all causes of endogenous hypercortisolism, this suppression fails [6]. When measured by RIA, a plasma cortisol level of 5 µg/dL (140 nmol/L) is considered a failure to suppress [36,37]. This results in a specificity of 95%; lowering the cutoff to 1.8 µg/dL (50 nmol/L) achieves a sensitivity of 95% at a specificity of 80% and is currently the recommended level [38]. Alternatively, this test may be administered in a 48-hour, 2 mg/day format; while preferred by some experts, this format does not appear to have a diagnostic advantage over the shorter version [29].

The Endocrine Society Clinical Practice Guidelines recommend that any patient with a positive screening test undergo repeat testing. Additional confirmatory tests, such as midnight serum cortisol level or the combined low-dose DST and CRH stimulation test, may also be used. The latter operates on the principle that while dexamethasone will suppress cortisol secretion in all patients without Cushing's syndrome, a small proportion of patients with pituitary Cushing's disease will also suppress. Simultaneous CRH administration will result in an immediate increase in ACTH and cortisol in patients with Cushing's disease, but not in normal patients, who will continue to suppress cortisol secretion [15]. Patients with concordant positive results can be confirmed to have Cushing's syndrome, provided no physiologic hypercortisolism is suspected.

Establishing a cause of Cushing's syndrome

ACTH-DEPENDENT VERSUS ACTH-INDEPENDENT CUSHING'S SYNDROME

After the diagnosis of Cushing's syndrome is confirmed, the first step is to differentiate "ACTH-dependent" causes of hypercortisolism, in which ACTH is elevated (i.e., Cushing's disease or ectopic ACTH production), from "ACTH-independent" hypercortisolism, in which serum ACTH is suppressed. Whereas the former category is the result of excessive ACTH secretion from the pituitary gland or an ectopic source, the latter pertains to primary adrenal pathology—such as adrenal adenoma, cortical carcinoma, and BMAH—with cortisol hypersecretion. Interestingly, new insights into the pathophysiology of BMAH have questioned the accuracy of the classic assumption that primary adrenal pathology is truly ACTH independent. Despite suppressed *plasma* ACTH, hypercortisolism in BMAH may nevertheless be the result of *intra-adrenal* ACTH that acts in a paracrine fashion [39]. Nevertheless, a diagnostic approach in which hypercortisolism is initially categorized by serum ACTH levels remains a pragmatic and useful first step in identifying the specific etiology of Cushing's syndrome (Figure 29.2).

ACTH ASSAY

The simplest and most effective method of distinguishing between ACTH-independent and ACTH-dependent Cushing's syndrome remains a plasma ACTH assay [40]. Ideally, plasma ACTH should be measured between 11:00 p.m. and 2:00 a.m., as this time should reflect its circadian nadir; in practice, ACTH is often measured at any time [41,42]. In adrenal or ACTH-independent cases, plasma ACTH levels will be suppressed, whereas levels will be normal or elevated in ACTH-dependent cases. Accordingly, as normal basal ACTH levels range from 10 to 100 pg/mL, ACTH levels less than 5 pg/mL are indicative of primary adrenal cortisol hypersecretion. Results should be repeated, as all patients with Cushing's syndrome have episodic ACTH and cortisol secretion [43]. If confirmed, this should prompt adrenal imaging.

Values greater than 20 pg/mL indicate an ACTH-dependent source. In Cushing's disease, the degree of ACTH elevation correlates with size of the lesion, microadenomas averaging 45 pg/mL, and macroadenomas averaging 136 pg/mL [44]. As ACTH levels rise even further, so rises the likelihood of an ectopic ACTH-secreting tumor [2]. Values that are between 5 and 20 pg/mL require further investigation, but typically indicate a pituitary source; these patients might benefit from a combined DST-CRH stimulation test (see below).

HIGH-DOSE DEXAMETHASONE SUPPRESSION TEST

Whereas in Cushing's disease pituitary corticotroph cells retain a degree of responsiveness to negative feedback from

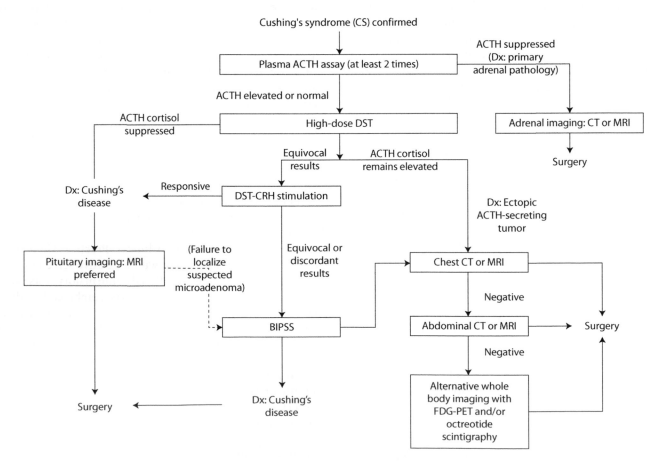

Figure 29.2 Algorithm for the identification and localization of the cause of Cushing's syndrome. Dx, diagnosis.

serum cortisol, ACTH-secreting tumors have no such feedback mechanism [6,45]. Thus, the high-dose DST is an effective method in separating Cushing's disease from ectopic ACTH production, in which there is a failure to suppress ACTH and cortisol. Traditionally a 48-hour test involving UFC collection, a frequently performed alternative involves administration of 8 mg of dexamethasone at 11:00 p.m. followed by an 8:00 a.m. collection of cortisol or ACTH [46]. The 48-hour test has a sensitivity and specificity of 69% and 100%, respectively, for the identification of an ACTH-secreting pituitary lesion [47]. Despite a reported 81% sensitivity and 67% specificity, the shorter test is preferred by many authors for ease of administration; follow-up testing is required for equivocal results [48].

CORTICOTROPIN-RELEASING HORMONE STIMULATION TEST

Pituitary adenomas express CRH receptors and remain responsive to stimulation by CRH [49]. The CRH stimulation test is therefore another tool to distinguish Cushing's disease from ectopic ACTH secretion. Meta-analysis of published series has established criteria for a positive result after CRH stimulation as an increase of more than 50% of plasma ACTH or greater than 20% of plasma cortisol. These cutoffs result in a sensitivity of 86% and 91%, and a specificity of 95% and 95% for ACTH and cortisol levels, respectively [26]. If both high-dose DST and CRH stimulation tests indicate Cushing's disease, then the diagnosis is ensured; any discordant results should prompt further investigation with inferior petrosal sinus sampling [50,51].

BILATERAL INFERIOR PETROSAL SINUS SAMPLING

Simultaneous, bilateral inferior petrosal sinus sampling (BIPSS) has been described as the most accurate and reliable method of distinguishing a pituitary from ectopic source of ACTH production, with some experts advocating for its routine use in such patients [52–54]. As the venous drainage of the pituitary is the petrosal sinuses via the cavernous sinuses, BIPSS can establish the diagnosis of pituitary ACTH hypersecretion by directly measuring a central-to-peripheral ACTH gradient. This is performed by simultaneously measuring serum ACTH in bilateral petrosal sinuses and in a peripheral vein at a basal level, and then at set intervals after CRH administration. BIPSS requires significant operator expertise, but in such hands, successful access to the petrosal sinuses via femoral vein catheterization can be achieved in 90% of cases [55].

A central-to-peripheral gradient of >2 at baseline and >3 after CRH stimulation is diagnostic of a pituitary source with a sensitivity of 96% and 100%, with much higher gradients often seen [6,53]. Pooled data from 14 studies indicates an overall sensitivity and specificity of 95% and 93% [56]. By calculating a right versus left petrosal sinus ACTH ratio, BIPSS can also be used to localize a pituitary adenoma to the precise pituitary lobe with an accuracy of up to 71% [53]. BIPSS has been shown to be equivalent or even superior to magnetic resonance imaging (MRI) for localization

of pituitary adenomas in some series, and may be considered for this purpose when MRI resolution is inadequate to detect a suspected microadenoma [57]. A recent prospective trial of 501 patients with confirmed adenomas found that BIPSS correctly identified a pituitary lesion in 98%, and the positive predictive value for lateralization was 69% [58]. Most experts advise against BIPSS as an initial procedure solely for tumor localization, however, for reasons of cost and potential morbidity. The risk of cerebrovascular accident or other neurologic complication is less than 1%, but devastating. Other complications, including inguinal hematoma and venous thromboembolism, are similarly rare [59,60].

Localization by imaging

PITUITARY GLAND

Patients diagnosed with ACTH-dependent Cushing's syndrome typically undergo imaging of the pituitary gland, as a pituitary microadenoma is the most common responsible etiology. Such imaging should be undertaken only when the diagnosis is highly suspected; 10% of the population will have an incidental pituitary adenoma on MRI, and the overall prevalence of pituitary adenomas in the population may be as high as 17% [61]. MRI with and without gadolinium enhancement is more sensitive than computed tomography (CT); however, sensitivity may only be 50%–60% [62,63]. The main benefit of MRI is typically in the diagnosis of lesions 6 mm or greater, and in preoperative anatomical survey [56]. A positive MRI typically shows a hypodense pituitary lesion that typically fails to enhance with gadolinium; however, 5% *do* take up gadolinium, necessitating a precontrast phase to increase overall sensitivity [64]. In patients with a lesion of >6 mm and a concordant biochemical profile, no further workup is indicated. A recent study shows that a positive MRI has an 86% positive predictive value for correctly localizing the lesion; however, older studies document as little as 52% correlation between imaging and operative findings [65]. Finally, in cases where Cushing's disease is confirmed by either a positive MRI or BIPSS, a positive MRI may increase the likelihood that a patient will be able to undergo selective adenomectomy versus a subtotal hypophysectomy. However, therapeutic success, complication rate, and recurrence rate are not affected [66].

ADRENAL GLAND

Patients with Cushing's syndrome with suppressed serum ACTH should directly undergo dedicated adrenal imaging to identify an adrenal source. In identification of an adrenal mass, both MRI and CT have sensitivity greater than 95%; however, thin-section CT is recommended as first line based on cost (Figure 29.3). Differentiating adenoma from adenocarcinoma via CT is highly accurate, with frequently reported 100% sensitivity and 98% specificity [67–69]. MRI may be useful in differentiating benign from malignant disease when CT cannot [70]. CT is also useful in the diagnosis of adrenal hyperplasia, as seen in BMAH.

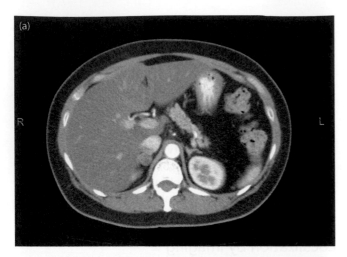

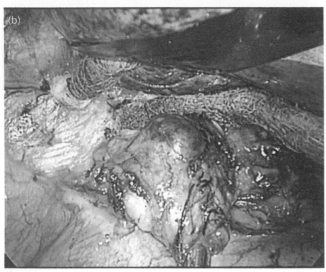

Figure 29.3 (a) A 1.6 cm, benign-appearing right adrenal mass identified on CT abdomen in a patient with ACTH-independent Cushing's syndrome. **(b)** Intraoperative image of this mass taken at time of laparoscopic adrenalectomy. Final pathology identified a 9.2 g adrenal cortical tumor without evidence of invasion consistent with a benign adrenal adenoma.

ECTOPIC ACTH-SECRETING TUMORS

After initial testing identifies ACTH-dependent Cushing's syndrome with a negative DST, a search for an ectopic ACTH-secreting tumor should commence. While older studies indicate that the most common cause of ectopic ACTH secretion is small cell carcinoma of the lung, newer series find an increasing amount of pulmonary carcinoids and other occult neuroendocrine tumors [13,18]. Thus, imaging of the chest with CT or MRI should be performed first. Imaging of the abdomen can be performed if no culprit is found. The overall sensitivity of CT and MRI is low (53% and 37%, respectively) [71], and in a recent series, the source of ectopic ACTH remained unknown in 19% of patients [13]. Other modalities, such as octreotide-analog scintigraphy and ^{18}F-fluorodeoxyglucose positron emission tomography (FDG-PET), may aid in the diagnosis of an ectopic

source of ACTH, although they do not in themselves have a sensitivity advantage over CT and MRI [71]. When negative, scintigraphy is useful in identifying false positives on CT or MRI; however, it should not be used as a sole modality due to a high false-positive rate [72].

Surgical management of Cushing's syndrome

The treatment of choice for both ACTH-dependent and ACTH-independent causes of Cushing's syndrome is surgery with curative intent. The underlying etiology dictates whether the initial operation will be directed at the pituitary gland, adrenal glands, or source of ectopic ACTH secretion. In all cases, bilateral adrenalectomy can be performed as definitive therapy, guaranteeing a cure but requiring life-long glucocorticoid supplementation and the risk of developing Nelson's syndrome [73,74].

APPROACH TO THE PITUITARY GLAND: TRANSSPHENOIDAL ADENOMECTOMY

In patients with Cushing's disease caused by a circumscribed microadenoma, transsphenoidal selective adenomectomy is the surgery of choice [19]. If unable to identify the lesion, then a subtotal hypophysectomy—85%–90% resection—is recommended [2]. Fortunately, at institutions where the technology is available, advances in intraoperative MRI (iMRI) are allowing for better and immediate identification of missed or residual tumor at the time of operation [75,76]. The total remission rate after transsphenoidal surgery is approximately 80%–90% for microadenomas, but likely lower for macroadenomas despite one recent study demonstrating a 92% initial remission [23,73,77,78]. A meta-analysis combining results for micro- and macroadenomas found a 79% overall initial remission rate [79].

The main criterion for cure after transsphenoidal surgery is an undetectable postoperative plasma cortisol level [80]. Patients with a postoperative cortisol of less than 50 nmol/L have the highest long-term remission rates, between 85% and 100% [80–82]. A relapse after initial surgery is defined as the recurrence of clinical and biochemical signs of Cushing's syndrome more than 6 months after surgery. The cure rate after reoperation for remission has been documented at 55% at a single tertiary referral center, but ranges between 22% and 64% in the literature [83–85]. The risk of pan-hypopituitarism is significantly increased after reoperative transsphenoidal surgery. Thus, in the absence of residual pituitary tumor on MRI, the second-line treatment for recurrent Cushing's syndrome after transsphenoidal surgery is irradiation, which can achieve remission in 83% [86]. Irradiation is a first-line therapy only in children, in whom it can achieve an 85% initial remission rate [87].

Transsphenoidal exploration of the sella has traditionally been via a sublabial or endonasal approach, utilizing a surgical microscope. Complications are rare but include cerebrospinal fluid (CSF) leak, transient diabetes insipidus, and neurologic injury; patients with Cushing's are particularly susceptible to deep venous thrombosis [88,89]. More recently, an endoscopic approach has gained widespread adoption [75,90]. Benefits include a wider field of vision, increased tumor resection potential, decreased operative time, decreased length of stay, and increased patient satisfaction [91,92]. Meta-analyses have found initial remission rates in Cushing's disease between 75% and 81% after endoscopic approach [93,94]. Data is conflicting regarding the relative risk of complications when compared with microsurgical transsphenoidal surgery [95,96].

APPROACH TO THE ADRENAL GLAND: LAPAROSCOPIC ADRENALECTOMY

In Cushing's disease, a bilateral adrenalectomy may be performed in patients without cure after transsphenoidal surgery and irradiation [19]. A laparoscopic approach is unequivocally favored over an open approach due to shorter average hospital stays and lower complication rates [97]. It has been demonstrated to be an effective and definitive treatment for hypercortisolism in Cushing's syndrome [74,98]. Lifelong substitution of glucocorticoids and mineralocorticoids is required, and the risk of Nelson's syndrome—pituitary tumor, elevated ACTH, and dark pigmentation—is reported to be between 10% and 25% [73].

When Cushing's syndrome arises from primary adrenal pathology, the treatment is likewise adrenalectomy. For BMAH and primary pigmented nodular adrenocortical adrenal hyperplasia, laparoscopic bilateral adrenalectomy is recommended. If the cause of hypercortisolism is a unilateral adrenal adenoma or carcinoma, then a unilateral adrenalectomy is recommended [2]. After unilateral adrenalectomy, glucocorticoid substitution is only required until the endogenous hypothalamic–pituitary–adrenal (HPA) recovers [99].

APPROACH TO ECTOPIC SOURCE OF ACTH

For Cushing's syndrome resulting from paraneoplastic and ectopic secretion of ACTH, resection of the culprit tumor with curative intent is the treatment of choice. As the risk of malignancy is high, proper oncologic resection is typically required for tumors of the lung, thymus, pancreas, and gastrointestinal tract. In unresectable cases, palliative bilateral adrenalectomy may be performed to control hypercortisolism; likewise, medical therapy may be attempted.

Medical treatment of Cushing's syndrome

As mentioned above, the primary treatment of hypercortisolism in Cushing's syndrome is surgical. Indications for medical therapy include management of hypercortisolism when surgery cannot be performed, preoperative control of hypercortisolism, failure of surgery and irradiation, and treatment of occult ectopic ACTH syndrome. Medications used in the treatment of Cushing's syndrome fall into the following broad categories: adrenal enzyme inhibitors, adrenolytic agents, drugs that target the pituitary gland, and glucocorticoid receptor antagonists. Response to medical therapy is typically obtained by measuring changes in UFC.

ADRENAL ENZYME INHIBITORS AND ADRENOLYTIC AGENTS

Ketoconazole is an antifungal that inhibits the first step in steroid biosynthesis and can be administered at relatively low doses; therefore, it is a frequently used adrenal enzyme inhibitor in Cushing's syndrome [100,101]. Treatment with 600–800 mg/day may keep the UFC values within upper normal levels [102]. A recent systematic review notes the response rate in Cushing's syndrome ranges from 53% to 88% in low-quality, retrospective studies [103]. Although rare, use of ketoconazole comes with a reported risk of devastating hepatoxicity [104]. Conversely, metapyrone inhibits the final step in steroid biosynthesis. Response rates range from 57% to 75% in the literature [103], but side effects related to androgen excess, such as hirsutism and acne, may limit its use [105].

Mitotane is the only adrenolytic agent commonly used, and its mechanism of action in reducing plasma cortisol appears to be multifactorial [106]. Primarily used in the treatment of adrenal cortical carcinoma, it can be used as a medical adrenalectomy in patients with Cushing's syndrome. The rationale for use is supported by a low level of evidence, derived from small retrospective studies in which the reported response rate ranges from 59% to 70% [103,107].

PITUITARY GLAND

Many drugs that target the HPA axis and have been used in Cushing's disease are now known to be ineffective, such as bromocriptine, cypropheptadine, and valproic acid [108–110]. Pasireotide is a somatostatin analog that binds to multiple somatostatin receptors and directly blocks the release of ACTH from the pituitary gland. The response rate in Cushing's disease to monotherapy with pasireotide ranges from 17% to 19%, and is supported by high-quality data, including a randomized, double-blind study [111]. The main side effect is a risk of hypoglycemia. Cabergoline is a dopamine receptor agonist with a response rate in Cushing's disease that ranges from 25% to 50% in prospective studies [103]. Combination therapy may be more effective, with one study reporting a 53% response rate with the combination of pasireotide and cabergoline, and an 88% response rate when ketoconazole is added as a third agent [111].

GLUCOCORTICOID RECEPTOR ANTAGONISTS

Of these, mifepristone is the first clinically available glucocorticoid antagonist with affinity for adrenal ACTH receptors when given at high doses. Mifepristone has been studied in a limited fashion, the most compelling data coming from a prospective trial of patients with hypertension or diabetes as a result of Cushing's syndrome [112]. As a result, mifepristone is approved for the control of blood pressure and hypertension in Cushing's syndrome not amenable or refractory to surgery [103].

CORTICAL CARCINOMA

Adrenocortical carcinoma (ACC) is an exceedingly rare and highly aggressive disease, with a reported incidence of between 0.7 and 2 cases per million persons, and it is estimated to account for 0.2% of annual cancer deaths in the United States. Surveillance, Epidemiology, and End Results (SEER) data, data from the German registry, and data from the Netherlands indicate a median age of diagnosis of between 46 and 55 years [113–115]. Some published series demonstrate an additional peak in the first decade, suggesting a bimodal distribution [116,117]. Children with localized ACC appear to have a better prognosis than adults, in whom ACC is associated with a more aggressive phenotype and poorer prognosis [118–120]. Overall, there appears to be a slight female predominance, but data is mixed [121–123]. Historically, only 30% of cases are confined to the adrenal gland at the time of diagnosis [124].

Environmental risk factors for ACC are largely unknown, with one study suggesting a correlation with smoking in men and contraceptives in women [125]. Estrogens may play a role in the pathogenesis of ACC, as epidemiologic data suggests a relative increase in ACC diagnosis during pregnancy [121,126]. Evidence is mounting for a strong genetic component in the development of ACC. Loss of heterozygosity on chromosome 11p, 13q, or 17p may play a role [127,128]. The majority of evidence indicates a central role of the tumor suppressor p53 in the pathogenesis of ACC [129–131]. Childhood ACC is a core malignancy of Li–Fraumeni syndrome, in which there is a germline mutation of p53 [132]; this is the underlying genetic cause in 50%–80% of childhood ACC [133,134]. In southern Brazil, a highly prevalent p53 mutation with low penetrance contributes to significantly increased local incidence of ACC in children [135]. However, the prevalence of germline p53 mutations in adults with ACC is estimated to be between 3% and 7% [136,137], and despite being associated with other hereditary cancer syndromes (Lynch syndrome, MEN1, and Beckwith–Wiedemann), this indicates ACC is a primarily sporadic malignancy in adults [115]. Recently, the Wnt/β-catenin pathway and IGF-2 signaling pathway have been confirmed active in ACC [138]. Although a stepwise progression model from adenoma to carcinoma has been proposed and advocated, the molecular mechanisms for sporadic ACC remain largely unknown [139,140].

Clinical presentation

ACC typically presents in one of three clinical scenarios: [1] as a functional tumor with signs and symptoms of hormone excess, [2] as a nonfunctional (or subclinically functional) tumor with nonspecific symptoms secondary to mass effect or tumor growth, and [3] as an incidentally discovered tumor on imaging obtained for another health-related issue [115].

A review of the literature reveals that approximately 40%–60% of ACC cases present with signs and symptoms

of hormone hypersecretion [120,121,126,141,142]. The number of tumors found to be secretory upon laboratory investigation is as high as 80% [143]. Functional tumors result in symptoms related to the hormone secreted: cortisol leads to Cushing's syndrome (see the "Clinical Features and Prognosis" section), androgens to virilization, estrogens to feminization, and mixed Cushing–virilization/feminization is seen when multiple hormones are secreted. Epidemiologically, functional tumors are more likely to be found in women and patients less than 30 years of age [116,117]. Depending on the series, the most common presentation of functional ACC is Cushing's syndrome or a mixed Cushing–virilization syndrome [121,144–146]. Children most commonly present with virilization [122], whereas in adult males, the frequency of isolated hyperandrogenism may be under-reported as a result of subtle physical findings. In the majority of series, estrogen and mineralocorticoid secretion are both uncommon [146–148]. Hypertension is a common symptom in ACC, either by direct hormone effect or by local tumor effect on the renal vasculature, resulting in activation of the renin–angiotensin system [149,150]. Rarely, so-called "Anderson's syndrome" arises from IGF-2-mediated hypoglycemia [151].

Nonfunctional ACC represents approximately 40% of cases, arising with relative frequency in adult males but rare in children [118,119]. These tumors often present with non-specific complaints secondary to tumor growth, including abdominal or flank pain, palpable abdominal mass, early satiety, weight loss, weakness, anorexia, and nausea and vomiting [121,152,153]. Abdominal complaints are likely as common as endocrine syndromes in ACC, as Kendrick et al. reported that 48% of all patients presented with abdominal pain versus 47% with various endocrine syndromes [154].

Finally, clinically inapparent adrenal masses are common in the population, with a prevalence of 2% on autopsy studies. Cross-sectional imaging identifies many of these incidentally, the majority being benign adenomas. The risk of an ACC masquerading as an incidentaloma increases with the size of the lesion, from 2% if less than 4 cm to 25% if greater than 6 cm [155]. Of all cases of ACC, an estimated 20%–30% may come to clinical attention incidentally [115].

Diagnosis and preoperative studies

When the diagnosis of ACC is suspected, a comprehensive hormonal and imaging workup must be performed prior to definitive therapy. In addition to providing a diagnosis, a methodical workup will guide perioperative medical management, surgical planning, and selection of postoperative adjuvant therapy.

HORMONAL EVALUATION

In 2005, the European Network for the Study of Adrenal Tumors (ENSAT) put forth guidelines for the hormonal evaluation of all suspected ACC, for the following reasons: (1) to diagnosis steroid excess and confirm adrenal origin, (2) because certain patterns of steroid excess are highly suggestive of malignancy, (3) to become aware of cortisol secretion such that postoperative adrenal insufficiency can be expected and managed, and (4) to identify hormones that may be useful as tumor markers for postoperative surveillance [156]. In general, high levels of estradiol in males, high levels of serum dehydroepiandrosterone sulfate (DHEAS), and secretion of a large amount of steroid precursors are suggestive of malignancy [143]. Due to inefficient steroidogenesis, ACC may spill large amounts of steroid precursors even in the setting of relatively normal serum hormone levels. Not measured through traditional means, the use of high-sensitivity gas chromatography–mass spectrometry in 24-hour urine samples of patients with suspected lesions can identify these with a high degree of sensitivity ("urine steroid metabolomics") [157].

Prior to surgery, ENSAT also recommends checking plasma metanephrines or urinary metanephrines and catecholamines to rule out pheochromocytoma, as the perioperative management of such tumors is delicate and requires diligent planning.

DIAGNOSTIC IMAGING

The widespread use of cross-sectional imaging identifies a large number of incidental adrenal masses, with an estimated 1%–2% prevalence in the population [158]. Differentiating between benign adenomas and ACC is the primary task in the workup of an incidentaloma or otherwise suspicious adrenal mass. Unequivocally, dedicated adrenal imaging with CT or MRI should first be obtained. More recently, FDG-PET has become increasingly utilized in this task. Ultrasonography no longer has a primary role in the diagnosis and staging of ACC. Adrenal cortical scintigraphy represents another modality that, although still used occasionally as an adjunct in specific cases, has little additional value over CT, MRI, or PET [138]. Imaging of the chest should be obtained simultaneously, as the presence of

metastasis is diagnostic of malignancy [159]. ACC preferentially metastasizes to the liver (85%), followed by the lung (60%), bone (10%), and lymph nodes (10%) [116].

By imaging criteria, several features of adrenal masses are suspicious for ACC. These include size greater than 4 cm, irregular margins, central necrosis or hemorrhage, heterogeneous contrast enhancement, and tumor invasion or extension into nearby structures [70,160,161]. ACCs are typically large, averaging 9 cm, with 70% of tumors reported to be larger than 6 cm [159]. Inferior vena cava (IVC) invasion may be present in 9%–19% of cases [147]. Conversely, benign masses tend to be smaller, display homogeneous enhancement, and have sharp borders (Figure 29.4) [116,162,163]. After logistic regression, Hussain et al. found a tumor size of >4 cm and heterogeneous enhancement to be most predictive of malignancy [164].

Computed tomography

CT performed with a thin-cut, adrenal-specific protocol is considered the first-line imaging modality for the diagnosis of adrenal tumors. Tumors as small as 0.5 cm can be detected [165]. The typical appearance of ACC on unenhanced CT is that of a large, inhomogeneous suprarenal mass [160]. As ACCs are typically lipid poor and adenomas lipid rich, ACCs generally display a higher CT density (Hounsfield units [HU]). One meta-analysis found that using a simple threshold of 10 HU, unenhanced CT has a sensitivity and specificity of 71% and 98% in identifying a benign adrenal adenoma [67]. No known case of ACC in the literature has been documented with an HU of less than 13 [138]. Intravenous contrast is given to differentiate ACC from lipid-poor adenomas; ACCs reliably retain contrast, demonstrating an enhancement washout of less than 50% at 10 minutes. One study using this criterion accurately differentiated adenoma from ACC with greater than 98% accuracy [166]. To achieve superior accuracy in diagnosing

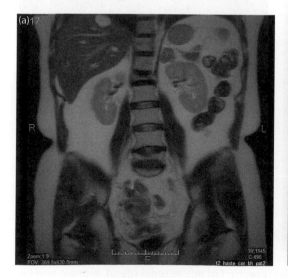
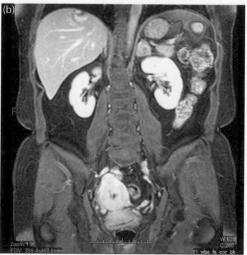

Figure 29.4 An incidentally found, 2.5 cm left-sided adrenal adenoma with typical benign features on (a) T2-weighted MRI and (b) T1-weighted MRI. Subsequent biochemical analysis documented hypercortisolemia with failure to suppress after low-dose DST.

ACC, experts recommend using CT with delayed contrast and criteria that include less than 50% washout and density of >35 HU after 10–15 minutes [70,138,167].

Magnetic resonance imaging

MRI improves adrenal imaging through the specific tissue characteristic of adrenal tissue on T1- and T2-weighted images [168]. Normal adrenal tissues appear darker than surrounding adipose tissue on both T1 and T2 images. The typical appearance of ACC on MRI is heterogeneous in signal intensity. When compared with liver parenchyma, ACC is typically iso- or hypointense on T1 images, while characteristically hyperintense on T2 images [169]. Intravenous gadolinium helps differentiate ACC from adenoma, as the former demonstrates strong enhancement and slow washout in comparison with the mild enhancement and quick washout typical of adenomas [170–173].

Chemical shift imaging (CSI) is the mainstay of MRI evaluation of solid adrenal lesions. CSI appears to be equal to CT for the differentiation of incidental adrenal lesions, with a sensitivity of 81%–100% versus 94%–100%, respectively [172,174–176]. MRI has been demonstrated superior to CT in identifying invasion of the IVC (Figure 29.5) [177,178]. In selecting MRI versus CT, the familiarity and preference of the local institution should be solicited.

¹⁸F-fluorodeoxyglucose positron emission tomography

Malignant adrenal masses may have increased metabolic activity and will demonstrate increased FDG uptake. When FDG-PET is combined with CT (PET/CT), the sensitivity and specificity for identifying a malignant adrenal mass are 100% and 87%–97%, respectively [179,180]. However, PET/CT cannot differentiate ACC from metastases, lymphoma, pheochromocytoma, or metabolically active benign tissues (infection or postoperative changes) [181]. PET/CT may provide helpful diagnostic information when CT or MRI is inconclusive, and is used frequently for evaluation of local recurrence or for development of metastases.

Pathology

Historically, it has been challenging to differentiate benign and malignant adrenal tumors by histopathology. Upon gross examination, tumor weight, capsular and vascular invasion, and hemorrhage are considered. Known as the "Weiss score," the following microscopic criteria for ACC were proposed in 1984: (1) high nuclear grade, (2) mitotic rate of >5 per 50 high-power fields, (3) atypical mitotic figures, (4) clear cells comprising 25% or less of the tumor, (5) diffuse architecture present in >33% of tumor, (6) necrosis, (7) vascular invasion, (8) sinusoidal invasion, and (9) capsular invasion. Adrenal tumors with three or more of the above criteria are considered malignant [182]. The prognostic value has been validated in numerous studies, with patients having three or fewer of the above markers having near 100% 5-year survival, as opposed to 62% in patients with more than three. Mitotic rate and atypical mitoses are the most significant in predicting survival in patients with and without metastatic disease [183–187]. There has been concern over the difficulty, as well as the risk of interobserver variability inherent in the Weiss system. A modified Weiss system with five of the above variables—selected after regression analysis and for a high degree of interobserver agreement—has since been validated [188,189]. A number of other, simplified algorithms have been proposed in order to improve the reproducibility of pathologic diagnosis [138].

(a)

(b)

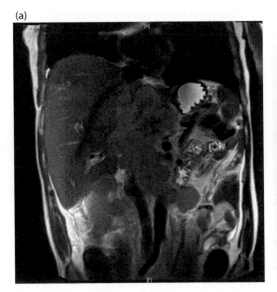 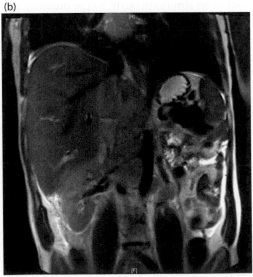

Figure 29.5 Recurrent ACC in a patient with previous *en bloc* resection of left adrenal gland, kidney, and left renal vein tumor thrombus. **(a)** Coronal T2-weighted MRI demonstrating tumor encasement of aorta and IVC invasion. **(b)** More posterior cut demonstrating tumor thrombus in the IVC extending to the level of the confluence with the hepatic veins, as well as encasement of the right renal artery.

Immunohistochemistry is becoming increasingly useful in determining the diagnosis and prognosis of ACC. Steroidogenic factor-1 (SF-1) has become the marker of choice for determining adrenal origin of a tumor with high sensitivity and specificity. Furthermore, it has been shown to be a stage-independent predictor of prognosis [190,191]. Quantification of proliferation marker Ki67 has recently been demonstrated as a significant prognostic indicator. In two large ENSAT trials, Ki67 was strongly predictive of both recurrence risk after R0 resection and risk of death in patients with unresectable disease.

STAGING AND PROGNOSIS

The first staging criterion for ACC was put forth by the International Union Against Cancer (UICC), which was reiterated in the 2010 seventh edition of the American Joint Committee on Cancer (AJCC) *Staging Manual* (Table 29.1) [192]. Historically, most patients presented with advanced disease: stage I, 2%; stage II, 19%; stage III, 18%; and stage IV, 61% [193]. Newer series indicate that patients are now presenting most commonly with stage II disease [126,145,154]. Furthermore, prognosis may be improving for patients with stage II disease [194]. Due to the rarity of the disease, survival has varied greatly in the literature, with many large series reporting an approximately 38% 5-year survival (Table 29.2) [114,121,124,126,141,146,154,195,196].

Concern over the adequacy of the above UICC/AJCC staging systems has arisen. An in-depth review of the German ACC database found that UICC staging predicted prognosis, but did so inadequately. Disease-specific survival (DSS) was not significantly different between stages II and III, and there was a significant difference in survival between stage IV patients with metastasis and those without metastasis [197]. The resulting ENSAT staging system, in which stage IV is reserved for patients with metastatic disease only, has since been validated as prognostically superior to the UICC system (Table 29.1) [198]. Using ENSAT staging, 5-year stage-dependent survivals are 81%, 61%, 51%, and 13%, for stages I, II, III, and IV, respectively [197].

The most significant factors on prognosis are stage and completeness of resection [121,122,126,146,147,184,186]. Tumor grade is a significant, stage-independent predictor of prognosis; accordingly, proposed modifications to staging include the addition of tumor grade. Miller et al. found a statistically significant difference in overall and recurrence-free survival between ENSAT stage II patients with low-grade tumors and those with high-grade tumors; the Ann Arbor modification therefore adjusts low-grade stage II and III down [199]. Ki67 is another marker of tumor biology that some advocate for inclusion in staging [138,200]. Cortisol secretion has been linked to poor prognosis in one study, but in the majority of studies, functional status has no effect on prognosis [121,146,150,153,201].

Treatment

Due to the low incidence of disease, the majority of evidence for the optimal treatment of ACC continues to be retrospective and nonrandomized in nature. Complete R0 surgical resection (R0 = complete microscopic resection, R1 = residual microscopic disease, R2 = residual macroscopic disease) remains the treatment of choice and determines prognosis. Historically, complete resection has yielded 5-year survival rates between 38% and 62%, in comparison with a 0%–9% 5-year survival seen when tumor is left behind [120,123,142,149,202]. Mitotane is used routinely as adjuvant therapy in patients with risk of recurrence, although data on its efficacy continues to be mixed. Adjuvant external beam radiotherapy is used primarily to control or prevent local recurrence after R1 resection. Other chemotherapy agents have been investigated both in an adjuvant setting

Table 29.1 Staging of adrenocortical carcinoma

TNM	TNM staging criteria
T1	Tumor ≤ 5 cm, no extra-adrenal invasion
T2	Tumor > 5 cm, no extra-adrenal invasion
T3	Tumor of any size with local invasion, but without invasion of adjacent organs
T4	Tumor of any size with local invasion
N0	No positive regional lymph nodes
N1	Positive regional lymph nodes
M0	No distant metastasis
M1	Distant metastatic disease

Stage	AJCC	ENSAT
I	T1N0M0	T1N0M0
II	T2N0M0	T2N0M0
III	T1N1M0, T2N1M0, T3N0M0	T1N1M0, T2N1M0, T3N0M0, T3N1M0, T4N0M0, T4N1M0
IV	T3N1M0, T4N0M0, T4N1M0, any T, any NM1	Any T, any NM1

Table 29.2 5-Year survival rates for adrenocortical carcinoma

Author (reference)	Year published	Patients (N)	5-Year survival (%)	Time period	Data source
Bilimoria et al. [114]	2008	3982	38.6	1985–2005	National database (NCDB-ACS)
Paton et al. [195]	2006	602	38	1988–2002	National database (SEER-NCI)
Abiven et al. [146]	2006	202	37	1963–2003	Single institution (France)
Vassilopoulou-Sellin and Schultz [141]	2001	139	60	1980–2001	Single institution (MDA)
Kendrick et al. [154]	2001	58	37	1980–1996	Single institution (Mayo)
Icard et al. [126]	2001	253	38	1978–1997	Multiple institutions (France)
Schulick and Brennan [196]	1999	113	37	n/a	Single institution (MSK)
Luton et al. [121]	1990	105	22	1963–1987	Single institution (France)

Note: NCDB, National Cancer Data Base; ACS, American College of Surgeons; NCI, National Cancer Institute; MDA, MD Anderson; MSK, Memorial Sloan Kettering.

and as primary therapy in cases of unresectability; their role in therapy is less well defined.

SURGERY

Open adrenalectomy via a subcostal, thoracoabdominal, or abdominal midline incision is the gold standard and remains the treatment of choice for stage I–III ACC. A standardized approach to achieve R0 resection has been proposed [203]. For all tumors, an ipsilateral adrenalectomy and locoregional lymph node dissection should be performed, including the renal hilum nodes, celiac nodes, para-aortic nodes, and paracaval nodes. Performance of a locoregional lymph node dissection has been shown to improve staging and decrease risk of recurrence and disease-related death [203,204]. In stage III disease, radical tumor resection should be attempted. If tumor thrombus extends into the IVC, an aggressive attempt to extract the thrombus should be made, as relatively low perioperative mortality and long disease-free survival can be achieved [205–208]. Right-sided lesions more commonly involve the IVC; left-sided lesions commonly invade the left renal vein and thereby the IVC. Successful resection of ACC involving the IVC from either side can be performed successfully [203]. If local invasion of surrounding structures occurs, an *en bloc* resection should be performed, performing nephrectomy, splenectomy, or liver resection as necessary. All efforts should be made to avoid rupturing the tumor capsule [206,209]. For incompletely resectable tumors, the role of tumor debulking remains controversial, as most patients survive less than 12 months after surgery [142,149,210,211]. In stage IV disease, limited data supports a survival advantage when complete R0 resection can be obtained, regardless of the location of metastatic disease [212].

Recurrence rates are high, even after R0 resection. Kendrick et al. saw a 73% recurrence rate with a median time to recurrence of 17 months [154]. More recent series from MD Anderson and the Mayo Clinic demonstrate 50% and 74% recurrence rates after R0 resection, respectively [213,214]. Surgery for recurrence has been firmly established to improve survival on the basis of retrospective

series, with an improved median survival of 29 versus 11 months [196,215–217]. In a recent study, surgery for recurrence was associated with overall survivals of 82%, 67%, and 30% at 1, 2, and 5 years, respectively. This was significantly better than the group treated with adjuvant therapy alone, in whom 1-, 2-, and 5-year survivals were 26%, 13%, and 0%, respectively. Among patients that underwent surgery, those that achieved R0 for recurrence and had an initial disease-free interval greater than 6 months had a distinct survival advantage [213].

As laparoscopic adrenalectomy has become the standard of care for the operative management of benign diseases of the adrenal gland, there has recently been debate about the appropriateness of a laparoscopic approach to ACC. Overall, the quality of data is low and based on retrospective, nonrandomized series. A number have reported higher rates of positive margins, intraoperative tumor spillage, and recurrence with laparoscopic adrenalectomy [218–222]. Conversely, some studies have documented equivalency in terms of overall and recurrence-free survival [223–225]. Expert opinion has achieved consensus that the open approach should be undertaken when tumors are large (>10 cm), invading adjacent organs, or thought likely to involve lymph nodes. Some advocate for laparoscopy when tumors are <10 cm and appear to be confined to the adrenal gland [143]. High-quality randomized trials are needed.

Finally, surgeon and institutional experience may play a role in patient outcomes. A recent series out of Italy compared high-volume centers (>10 cases per year) with low-volume centers; despite routinely operating on larger tumors, high-volume centers documented longer recurrence-free survival and lower risk of recurrence than low-volume centers. This was achieved through a higher rate of lymph node dissection, *en bloc* multiorgan resection, and adjuvant therapy [226]. A recent study of the National Cancer Data Base in the United States found that patients treated at high-volume centers were more likely to receive radical resection, regional lymphadenectomy, and adjuvant mitotane, but overall survival was not affected [227]. In the Netherlands, patients with ENSAT stages I–III that were operated on in hospitals with expertise in ACC had improved 5-year survival (63% versus 42%) when compared with patients treated in centers without expertise [228].

MITOTANE

Mitotane (o,p'-DDD) is an adrenal-specific agent that inhibits corticoid biosynthesis and causes mitochondrial and cell death [106,229]. In low doses, the effect is primarily suppression of adrenal corticoid secretion, whereas in doses greater than 3 g per day, there is a marked cytotoxic effect. Frequent side effects, such as nausea, vomiting, anorexia, diarrhea, lethargy, somnolence, rash, and dose-dependent hepatotoxicity are seen and limit patient compliance [230,231]. Drug levels must be monitored carefully when taking mitotane to avoid toxicity. Mitotane has been demonstrated effective when used as a primary maintenance therapy in patients with metastatic or unresectable ACC, with repeatedly documented tumor regression [121,152,153,230]. Whether a response to mitotane results in a survival benefit to patients has been debated over the past few decades.

Several studies have shown a median survival of 6.5 months after primary mitotane therapy, which is not significantly altered from the natural history of ACC [228,230,231].

Currently, the most common use of mitotane is in the adjuvant setting. The best evidence in support of adjuvant mitotane comes from a recent large, multi-institutional retrospective analysis of German and Italian patients. Terzolo et al. reported that patients who received adjuvant mitotane experienced a median survival of 42 months, compared with 10 months (Italian) and 25 months (German) in the control cohorts. Multivariate analysis demonstrated a significant improvement in recurrence-free survival with adjuvant mitotane, and an overall recurrence rate of 49% [232]. In contrast, a more recent study from MD Anderson found an identical recurrence rate and recurrence-free survival after surgery alone, calling into question the adequacy of resection in Terzolo et al. [214].

An international consensus panel has recommended adjuvant mitotane for cases of ACC in which there is a question of incomplete resection (R1 or R2), or in cases where the proliferation index is high (Ki67 positive in >10% of cells). They also concluded that adjuvant mitotane is not required if the following requirements are met: R0 resection, stage I or II, and low proliferation index [233].

CHEMOTHERAPY AS PRIMARY THERAPY

The experience with cytotoxic chemotherapy in ACC is limited. In patients that are not candidates for definitive resection and cannot tolerate mitotane, the agents cisplatin, cyclophosphamide, doxorubicin, 5-fluorouracil, and combinations thereof have led to partial response or disease stabilization [117,234,235]. The Berruti protocol—a combination of mitotane, etoposide, doxorubicin, and cisplatin (EDP)—was established after a prospective trial of 72 inoperable patients with ACC achieved a 49% response rate. Of those patients, 10 became eligible for radical resection of residual disease posttreatment; these patients had significantly improved survival when compared with partial and nonresponders [236]. The combination of mitotane and streptozotocin generated interest as a potential primary regimen after demonstrating efficacy in the adjuvant setting [237]. To investigate the above, the FIRM-ACT trial randomized 304 patients with advanced ACC to first-line therapy with mitotane plus EDP or mitotane plus streptozotocin. Patients receiving mitotane plus EDP demonstrated significantly higher response rates (23% versus 9%) and progression-free survival (5.0 versus 2.1 months). There was no difference in overall survival (14.8 versus 12.0 months) [238].

The use of monoclonal antibodies and other novel agents for targeted therapy remains limited. Bevacizumab, an anti-vascular endothelial growth factor (VEGF) monoclonal antibody, has produced disappointing preliminary results in clinical trials. Sunitinib is an anti-VEGF tyrosine kinase inhibitor that has shown promise. Other investigational agents include monoclonal antibodies against IGF-2 and IGF-1R, as well as inhibitors of mammalian target of rapamycin (mTOR) [138].

RADIOTHERAPY

External beam radiotherapy has been considered largely ineffective in the treatment of ACC [116,121,239,240]. Although numbers are small and results somewhat mixed, retrospective series do support a role for adjuvant radiotherapy in reducing the risk of local recurrence. In one study, patients that received adjuvant radiotherapy had a 4.7 magnitude reduction in the risk of local failure [241]. In another, the probability of being recurrence-free at 5 years was 79% versus 12% in patients with and without adjuvant radiotherapy, respectively [242]. In patients with advanced disease and in need of palliation, a recent review found that 57% had a favorable response to radiotherapy [243]. Currently, experts recommend adjuvant radiotherapy for select patients with R1 or R2 resection, and for palliation in patients with symptoms related to disease burden.

RADIOFREQUENCY ABLATION

For tumors less than 5 cm, there is limited evidence that radiofrequency ablation (RFA) may provide short-term local control in patients that are unresectable or have metastatic disease. No effect on overall survival has been demonstrated [244,245].

ESTROGEN- AND ANDROGEN-SECRETING TUMORS

Both benign and malignant adrenal tumors can present with signs and symptoms of sex steroid excess. As a general rule, the diagnosis of androgen-secreting tumors in males and estrogen-secreting tumors in females is challenging as a result of the subtle and nonspecific nature of presenting symptoms. However, the converse is not necessarily true, as feminization in males and virilization in females can present on a spectrum from subtle to overt. If an adrenal tumor is suspected to be the source of sex steroid excess, the workup should follow the steps outlined above to investigate the possibility of cortical carcinoma. In most cases, tumor resection is the treatment of choice, although mild symptoms arising from benign lesions may be treated medically.

Androgen-secreting tumors

Androgen-producing tumors of the adrenal gland cause the symptomatology of sex steroid excess. Prepubertal males present with isosexual precocious puberty, leading to penile enlargement, androgen-dependent hair development, deepening of the voice, and secondary sexual characteristics. For prepubertal females, heterosexual precocious puberty is manifested by acne, hirsutism, and clitoromegaly. For prepubertal patients of both sexes, hyperandrogenism can lead to accelerated growth but premature skeletal maturation, resulting ultimately in less than expected adult height. The clinical manifestations in adult males are minimal and may include early hair loss and acne. In adult females, the spectrum of presentation may include arrest of menarche, hirsutism, acne, male pattern baldness, infertility, and frank virilization [246]. Alternative causes of hyperandrogenism, such as polycystic ovary syndrome, congenital adrenal hyperplasia, tumors of the testicle and ovary, and exogenous androgen use, must always be considered and evaluated if appropriate.

Androgen-secreting adrenal adenomas are rare; androgen secretion is relatively more common in ACC but nevertheless rare. The diagnostic evaluation of a suspected androgen-secreting tumor begins with measurement of plasma DHEA, DHEAS, androstenedione, testosterone, and urinary 17-ketosteroids. Rarely, an adrenal adenoma will secrete only testosterone. The degree of hyperandrogenism is typically greater with ACC, particularly DHEA and DHEAS, and there may be associated hypercortisolemia. Failure of adrenal androgens to suppress after administration of high-dose dexamethasone is consistent with an adrenal origin; however, this does not distinguish between benign and malignant lesions [247,248] Dedicated adrenal imaging should be obtained to evaluate for malignancy, as described previously (Figure 29.6).

For both benign and malignant androgen-secreting tumors of the adrenal gland, the definitive and preferred treatment is surgical. In most cases, the approach will be open, as the risk of malignancy is high; only lesions that behave and are radiographically consistent with adenomas should be approached laparoscopically. When mild, medical therapy for hyperandrogenism includes steroid synthesis inhibitors and androgen antagonists. In the mildest cases, control of acne and hirsutism can be achieved superficially.

Estrogen-secreting tumors

Signs of estrogen excess in males include a loss of libido, gynecomastia, and increased hair in a female distribution. In females, signs are subtle and may be represented solely as menstrual irregularity in many patients. A typical laboratory

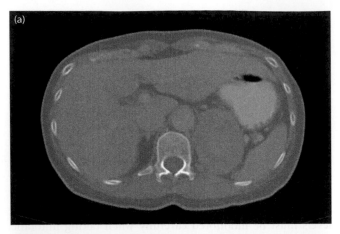

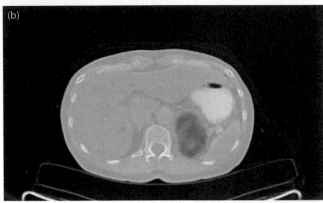

Figure 29.6 (a) CT and (b) corresponding PET/CT image of a large, left-sided 6.8 cm adrenal mass identified in a patient with hirsutism and virilization. The size, PET positivity, and confirmed biochemical androgen excess are highly suspicious for malignancy.

profile consists of elevated serum estrone, 11-deoxycortisol, androstenedione, and urinary 17-ketosteroids that fail to suppress with dexamethasone. In females, it is imperative to rule out an ovarian source.

Estrogen-secreting adrenal tumors are very rare and highly associated with carcinoma. In a large French series of 801 adrenalectomies, only three patients were found to have had a "feminizing" tumor with estradiol hypersecretion and elevated 17-OH progesterone: all were carcinoma. They estimate that such tumors comprise 1%–2% of all ACC [249]. Given the high likelihood of malignancy, radical surgical excision is the treatment of choice.

REFERENCES

1. Cushing H. The basophil adenomas of the pituitary body and their clinical manifestations (pituitary basophilism). 1932. *Obesity Res* 1994;2(5):486–508.
2. Orth DN. Cushing's syndrome. *N Engl J Med* 1995;332(12):791–803.
3. Etxabe J, Vazquez JA. Morbidity and mortality in Cushing's disease: An epidemiological approach. *Clin Endocrinol* 1994;40(4):479–84.

4. Lindholm J, Juul S, Jorgensen JO et al. Incidence and late prognosis of Cushing's syndrome: A population-based study. *J Clin Endocrinol Metab* 2001;86(1):117–23.

5. Newell-Price J, Bertagna X, Grossman AB, Nieman LK. Cushing's syndrome. *Lancet* 13 2006;367(9522):1605–17.

6. Newell-Price J, Trainer P, Besser M, Grossman A. The diagnosis and differential diagnosis of Cushing's syndrome and pseudo-Cushing's states. *Endocr Rev* 1998;19(5):647–72.

7. Steffensen C, Bak AM, Rubeck KZ, Jorgensen JO. Epidemiology of Cushing's syndrome. *Neuroendocrinology* 2010;92(Suppl 1):1–5.

8. Catargi B, Rigalleau V, Poussin A et al. Occult Cushing's syndrome in type-2 diabetes. *J Clin Endocrinol Metab* 2003;88(12):5808–13.

9. Leibowitz G, Tsur A, Chayen SD et al. Pre-clinical Cushing's syndrome: An unexpected frequent cause of poor glycaemic control in obese diabetic patients. *Clin Endocrinol* 1996;44(6):717–22.

10. Contreras LN, Cardoso E, Lozano MP, Pozzo J, Pagano P, Claus-Hermbeg H. Detection of preclinical Cushing's syndrome in overweight type 2 diabetic patients [in Spanish]. *Medicina* 2000;60(3):326–30.

11. Terzolo M, Reimondo G, Chiodini I et al. Screening of Cushing's syndrome in outpatients with type 2 diabetes: Results of a prospective multicentric study in Italy. *J Clin Endocrinol Metab* 2012;97(10):3467–75.

12. Isidori AM, Kaltsas GA, Pozza C et al. The ectopic adrenocorticotropin syndrome: Clinical features, diagnosis, management, and long-term follow-up. *J Clin Endocrinol Metab* 2006;91(2):371–7.

13. Ilias I, Torpy DJ, Pacak K, Mullen N, Wesley RA, Nieman LK. Cushing's syndrome due to ectopic corticotropin secretion: Twenty years' experience at the National Institutes of Health. *J Clin Endocrinol Metab* 2005;90(8):4955–62.

14. Lacroix A, Ndiaye N, Tremblay J, Hamet P. Ectopic and abnormal hormone receptors in adrenal Cushing's syndrome. *Endocr Rev* 2001;22(1):75–110.

15. Nieman LK, Biller BM, Findling JW et al. The diagnosis of Cushing's syndrome: An Endocrine Society Clinical Practice Guideline. *J Clin Endocrinol Metab* 2008;93(5):1526–40.

16. Katayama M, Nomura K, Ujihara M, Obara T, Demura H. Age-dependent decline in cortisol levels and clinical manifestations in patients with ACTH-independent Cushing's syndrome. *Clin Endocrinol* 1998;49(3):311–6.

17. Ross EJ, Linch DC. Cushing's syndrome—Killing disease: Discriminatory value of signs and symptoms aiding early diagnosis. *Lancet* 1982;2(8299):646–9.

18. Newell-Price J, Grossman A. Diagnosis and management of Cushing's syndrome. *Lancet* 1999;353(9170):2087–8.

19. Boscaro M, Barzon L, Fallo F, Sonino N. Cushing's syndrome. *Lancet* 2001;357(9258):783–91.

20. Valassi E, Crespo I, Santos A, Webb SM. Clinical consequences of Cushing's syndrome. *Pituitary* 2012;15(3):319–29.

21. Plotz CM, Knowlton AI, Ragan C. The natural history of Cushing's syndrome. *Am J Med* 1952;13(5):597–614.

22. Ntali G, Asimakopoulou A, Siamatras T et al. Mortality in Cushing's syndrome: Systematic analysis of a large series with prolonged follow-up. *Eur J Endocrinol* 2013;169(5):715–23.

23. Swearingen B, Biller BM, Barker FG 2nd et al. Long-term mortality after transsphenoidal surgery for Cushing disease. *Ann Intern Med* 1999;130(10):821–4.

24. Terzolo M, Allasino B, Pia A et al. Surgical remission of Cushing's syndrome reduces cardiovascular risk. *Eur J Endocrinol* 2014;171(1):127–36.

25. Dekkers OM, Horvath-Puho E, Jorgensen JO et al. Multisystem morbidity and mortality in Cushing's syndrome: A cohort study. *J Clin Endocrinol Metab* 2013;98(6):2277–84.

26. Kaye TB, Crapo L. The Cushing syndrome: An update on diagnostic tests. *Ann Intern Med* 1990;112(6):434–44.

27. Mengden T, Hubmann P, Muller J, Greminger P, Vetter W. Urinary free cortisol versus 17-hydroxy-corticosteroids: A comparative study of their diagnostic value in Cushing's syndrome. *Clin Invest* 1992;70(7):545–8.

28. Pecori Giraldi F, Ambrogio AG, De Martin M, Fatti LM, Scacchi M, Cavagnini F. Specificity of first-line tests for the diagnosis of Cushing's syndrome: Assessment in a large series. *J Clin Endocrinol Metab* 2007;92(11):4123–9.

29. Elamin MB, Murad MH, Mullan R et al. Accuracy of diagnostic tests for Cushing's syndrome: A systematic review and metaanalyses. *J Clin Endocrinol Metab* 2008;93(5):1553–62.

30. Nieman L. The sensitivity of the urine free cortisol measurement as a screening test for Cushing's syndrome. *Programs Abstr Endocr Soc 72nd Annu Meet* 1990;1990:822.

31. Raff H, Findling JW. A physiologic approach to diagnosis of the Cushing syndrome. *Ann Intern Med* 2003;138(12):980–91.

32. Dorn LD, Lucke JF, Loucks TL, Berga SL. Salivary cortisol reflects serum cortisol: Analysis of circadian profiles. *Ann Clin Biochem* 2007;44(Pt 3): 281–4.

33. Laudat MH, Cerdas S, Fournier C, Guiban D, Guilhaume B, Luton JP. Salivary cortisol measurement: A practical approach to assess pituitary-adrenal function. *J Clin Endocrinol Metab* 1988;66(2):343–8.

34. Gafni RI, Papanicolaou DA, Nieman LK. Nighttime salivary cortisol measurement as a simple, non-invasive, outpatient screening test for Cushing's syndrome in children and adolescents. *J Pediatr* 2000;137(1):30–5.

35 Papanicolaou DA, Mullen N, Kyrou I, Nieman LK. Nighttime salivary cortisol: A useful test for the diagnosis of Cushing's syndrome. *J Clin Endocrinol Metab* 2002;87(10):4515–21.

36. Nugent CA, Nichols T, Tyler FH. Diagnosis of Cushing's syndrome; single dose dexamethasone suppression test. *Arch Intern Med* 1965;116:172–6.

37. Nieman LK, Ilias I. Evaluation and treatment of Cushing's syndrome. *Am J Med* 2005;118(12):1340–6.

38. Wood PJ, Barth JH, Freedman DB, Perry L, Sheridan B. Evidence for the low dose dexamethasone suppression test to screen for Cushing's syndrome—Recommendations for a protocol for biochemistry laboratories. *Ann Clin Biochem* 1997;34(Pt 3):222–9.

39. Louiset E, Duparc C, Young J et al. Intraadrenal corticotropin in bilateral macronodular adrenal hyperplasia. *N Engl J Med* 2013;369(22):2115–25.

40. Invitti C, Pecori Giraldi F, de Martin M, Cavagnini F. Diagnosis and management of Cushing's syndrome: Results of an Italian multicentre study. Study Group of the Italian Society of Endocrinology on the Pathophysiology of the Hypothalamic-Pituitary-Adrenal Axis. *J Clin Endocrinol Metab* 1999;84(2):440–8.

41. Weitzman ED, Fukushima D, Nogeire C, Roffwarg H, Gallagher TF, Hellman L. Twenty-four hour pattern of the episodic secretion of cortisol in normal subjects. *J Clin Endocrinol Metab* 1971;33(1):14–22.

42. Meier CA, Biller BM. Clinical and biochemical evaluation of Cushing's syndrome. *Endocrinol Metab Clin North Am* 1997;26(4):741–62.

43. Van Cauter E, Refetoff S. Evidence for two subtypes of Cushing's disease based on the analysis of episodic cortisol secretion. *N Engl J Med* 1985;312(21):1343–9.

44. Woo YS, Isidori AM, Wat WZ et al. Clinical and biochemical characteristics of adrenocorticotropin-secreting macroadenomas. *J Clin Endocrinol Metab* 2005;90(8):4963–9.

45. Liddle GW. Tests of pituitary-adrenal suppressibility in the diagnosis of Cushing's syndrome. *J Clin Endocrinol Metab* 1960;20:1539–60.

46. Dichek HL, Nieman LK, Oldfield EH, Pass HI, Malley JD, Cutler GB Jr. A comparison of the standard high dose dexamethasone suppression test and the overnight 8-mg dexamethasone suppression test for the differential diagnosis of adrenocorticotropin-dependent Cushing's syndrome. *J Clin Endocrinol Metab* 1994;78(2):418–22.

47. Flack MR, Oldfield EH, Cutler GB Jr et al. Urine free cortisol in the high-dose dexamethasone suppression test for the differential diagnosis of the Cushing syndrome. *Ann Intern Med* 1992;116(3):211–7.

48. Aron DC, Raff H, Findling JW. Effectiveness versus efficacy: The limited value in clinical practice of high dose dexamethasone suppression testing in the differential diagnosis of adrenocorticotropin-dependent Cushing's syndrome. *J Clin Endocrinol Metab* 1997;82(6):1780–5.

49. Chrousos GP, Schuermeyer TH, Doppman J et al. NIH conference. Clinical applications of corticotropin-releasing factor. *Ann Intern Med* 1985;102(3):344–58.

50. Hermus AR, Pieters GF, Pesman GJ, Smals AG, Benraad TJ, Kloppenborg PW. The corticotropin-releasing-hormone test versus the high-dose dexamethasone test in the differential diagnosis of Cushing's syndrome. *Lancet* 1986;2(8506):540–4.

51. Nieman LK, Chrousos GP, Oldfield EH, Avgerinos PC, Cutler GB Jr, Loriaux DL. The ovine corticotropin-releasing hormone stimulation test and the dexamethasone suppression test in the differential diagnosis of Cushing's syndrome. *Ann Intern Med* 1986;105(6):862–7.

52. Findling JW, Kehoe ME, Shaker JL, Raff H. Routine inferior petrosal sinus sampling in the differential diagnosis of adrenocorticotropin (ACTH)-dependent Cushing's syndrome: Early recognition of the occult ectopic ACTH syndrome. *J Clin Endocrinol Metab* 1991;73(2):408–13.

53. Oldfield EH, Doppman JL, Nieman LK et al. Petrosal sinus sampling with and without corticotropin-releasing hormone for the differential diagnosis of Cushing's syndrome. *N Engl J Med* 1991;325(13):897–905.

54. Findling JW, Raff H. Diagnosis and differential diagnosis of Cushing's syndrome. *Endocrinol Metab Clin North Am* 2001;30(3):729–47.

55. Kaltsas GA, Giannulis MG, Newell-Price JD et al. A critical analysis of the value of simultaneous inferior petrosal sinus sampling in Cushing's disease and the occult ectopic adrenocorticotropin syndrome. *J Clin Endocrinol Metab* 1999;84(2):487–92.

56. Nieman L. Establishing the cause of Cushing's syndrome. Waltham, MA: UpToDate. http://www.uptodate.com/contents/establishing-the-cause-of-cushings-syndrome (accessed July 27, 2014).

57. Booth GL, Redelmeier DA, Grosman H, Kovacs K, Smyth HS, Ezzat S. Improved diagnostic accuracy of inferior petrosal sinus sampling over imaging for localizing pituitary pathology in patients with Cushing's disease. *J Clin Endocrinol Metab* 1998;83(7):2291–95.

58. Wind JJ, Lonser RR, Nieman LK, DeVroom HL, Chang R, Oldfield EH. The lateralization accuracy of inferior petrosal sinus sampling in 501 patients with Cushing's disease. *J Clin Endocrinol Metab* 2013;98(6):2285–93.

59. Gandhi CD, Meyer SA, Patel AB, Johnson DM, Post KD. Neurologic complications of inferior petrosal sinus sampling. *AJNR Am J Neuroradiol* 2008;29(4):760–5.

60. Miller DL, Doppman JL, Peterman SB, Nieman LK, Oldfield EH, Chang R. Neurologic complications of petrosal sinus sampling. *Radiology* 1992;185(1):143–7.

61. Ezzat S, Asa SL, Couldwell WT et al. The prevalence of pituitary adenomas: A systematic review. *Cancer* 2004;101(3):613–9.

62. Hall WA, Luciano MG, Doppman JL, Patronas NJ, Oldfield EH. Pituitary magnetic resonance imaging in normal human volunteers: Occult adenomas in the general population. *Ann Intern Med* 1994;120(10):817–20.

63. Newton DR, Dillon WP, Norman D, Newton TH, Wilson CB. Gd-DTPA-enhanced MR imaging of pituitary adenomas. *AJNR Am J Neuroradiol* 1989;10(5):949–54.

64. Findling JW, Doppman JL. Biochemical and radiologic diagnosis of Cushing's syndrome. *Endocrinol Metab Clin North Am* 1994;23(3):511–37.

65. Buchfelder M, Nistor R, Fahlbusch R, Huk WJ. The accuracy of CT and MR evaluation of the sella turcica for detection of adrenocorticotropic hormone-secreting adenomas in Cushing disease. *AJNR Am J Neuroradiol* 1993;14(5):1183–90.

66. Salenave S, Gatta B, Pecheur S et al. Pituitary magnetic resonance imaging findings do not influence surgical outcome in adrenocorticotropin-secreting microadenomas. *J Clin Endocrinol Metab* 2004;89(7):3371–6.

67. Blake MA, Kalra MK, Sweeney AT et al. Distinguishing benign from malignant adrenal masses: Multi-detector row CT protocol with 10-minute delay. *Radiology* 2006;238(2):578–85.

68. Fig LM, Gross MD, Shapiro B et al. Adrenal localization in the adrenocorticotropic hormone-independent Cushing syndrome. *Ann Intern Med* 1988;109(7):547–53.

69. Dunnick NR, Schaner EG, Doppman JL, Strott CA, Gill JR, Javadpour N. Computed tomography in adrenal tumors. *AJR Am J Roentgenol* 1979;132(1):43–6.

70. Ilias I, Sahdev A, Reznek RH, Grossman AB, Pacak K. The optimal imaging of adrenal tumours: A comparison of different methods. *Endocr Relat Cancer* 2007;14(3):587–99.

71. Pacak K, Ilias I, Chen CC, Carrasquillo JA, Whatley M, Nieman LK. The role of [(18)F]fluorodeoxyglucose positron emission tomography and [(111)In]-diethylenetriaminepentaacetate-D-Phe-pentetreotide scintigraphy in the localization of ectopic adrenocorticotropin-secreting tumors causing Cushing's syndrome. *J Clin Endocrinol Metab* 2004;89(5):2214–21.

72. Torpy DJ, Chen CC, Mullen N et al. Lack of utility of ^{111}In-pentetreotide scintigraphy in localizing ectopic ACTH producing tumors: Follow-up of 18 patients. *J Clin Endocrinol Metab* 1999;84(4):1186–92.

73. Sonino N, Zielezny M, Fava GA, Fallo F, Boscaro M. Risk factors and long-term outcome in pituitary-dependent Cushing's disease. *J Clin Endocrinol Metab* 1996;81(7):2647–52.

74. Osswald A, Plomer E, Dimopoulou C et al. Favorable long-term outcomes of bilateral adrenalectomy in Cushing's disease. *Eur J Endocrinol* 2014;171(2):209–15.

75. Swearingen B. Update on pituitary surgery. *J Clin Endocrinol Metab* 2012;97(4):1073–81.

76. Martin CH, Schwartz R, Jolesz F, Black PM. Transsphenoidal resection of pituitary adenomas in an intraoperative MRI unit. *Pituitary* 1999;2(2):155–62.

77. Mampalam TJ, Tyrrell JB, Wilson CB. Transsphenoidal microsurgery for Cushing disease. A report of 216 cases. *Ann Intern Med* 1988;109(6):487–93.

78. Fomekong E, Maiter D, Grandin C, Raftopoulos C. Outcome of transsphenoidal surgery for Cushing's disease: A high remission rate in ACTH-secreting macroadenomas. *Clin Neurol Neurosurg* 2009;111(5):442–9.

79. Kelly DF. Transsphenoidal surgery for Cushing's disease: A review of success rates, remission predictors, management of failed surgery, and Nelson's syndrome. *Neurosurg Focus* 2007;23(3):E5.

80. Estrada J, Garcia-Uria J, Lamas C et al. The complete normalization of the adrenocortical function as the criterion of cure after transsphenoidal surgery for Cushing's disease. *J Clin Endocrinol Metab* 2001;86(12):5695–99.

81. Yap LB, Turner HE, Adams CB, Wass JA. Undetectable postoperative cortisol does not always predict long-term remission in Cushing's disease: A single centre audit. *Clin Endocrinol* 2002;56(1):25–31.

82. Newell-Price J. Transsphenoidal surgery for Cushing's disease: Defining cure and following outcome. *Clin Endocrinol* 2002;56(1):19–21.

83. Porterfield JR, Thompson GB, Young WF Jr et al. Surgery for Cushing's syndrome: An historical review and recent ten-year experience. *World J Surg* 2008;32(5):659–77.

84. Ram Z, Nieman LK, Cutler GB Jr, Chrousos GP, Doppman JL, Oldfield EH. Early repeat surgery for persistent Cushing's disease. *J Neurosurg* 1994;80(1):37–45.

85. Patil CG, Veeravagu A, Prevedello DM, Katznelson L, Vance ML, Laws ER Jr. Outcomes after repeat transsphenoidal surgery for recurrent Cushing's disease. *Neurosurgery* 2008;63(2):266–70; discussion 270–1.

86. Estrada J, Boronat M, Mielgo M et al. The long-term outcome of pituitary irradiation after unsuccessful transsphenoidal surgery in Cushing's disease. *N Engl J Med* 1997;336(3):172–7.

87. Jennings AS, Liddle GW, Orth DN. Results of treating childhood Cushing's disease with pituitary irradiation. *N Engl J Med* 1977;297(18):957–62.

88. Semple PL, Laws ER Jr. Complications in a contemporary series of patients who underwent transsphenoidal surgery for Cushing's disease. *J Neurosurg* 1999;91(2):175–9.

89. Nemergut EC, Zuo Z, Jane JA Jr, Laws ER Jr. Predictors of diabetes insipidus after transsphenoidal surgery: A review of 881 patients. *J Neurosurg* 2005;103(3):448–54.

90. Jankowski R, Auque J, Simon C, Marchal JC, Hepner H, Wayoff M. Endoscopic pituitary tumor surgery. *Laryngoscope* 1992;102(2):198–202.

91. Atkinson JL, Young WF Jr, Meyer FB et al. Sublabial transseptal vs transnasal combined endoscopic microsurgery in patients with Cushing disease and MRI-depicted microadenomas. *Mayo Clin Proc* 2008;83(5):550–3.

92. McLaughlin N, Eisenberg AA, Cohan P, Chaloner CB, Kelly DF. Value of endoscopy for maximizing tumor removal in endonasal transsphenoidal pituitary adenoma surgery. *J Neurosurg* 2013;118(3):613–20.

93. Tabaee A, Anand VK, Barron Y et al. Endoscopic pituitary surgery: A systematic review and meta-analysis. *J Neurosurg* 2009;111(3):545–54.

94. Dorward NL. Endocrine outcomes in endoscopic pituitary surgery: A literature review. *Acta Neurochir* 2010;152(8):1275–9.

95. Berker M, Hazer DB, Yucel T et al. Complications of endoscopic surgery of the pituitary adenomas: Analysis of 570 patients and review of the literature. *Pituitary* 2012;15(3):288–300.

96. Ammirati M, Wei L, Ciric I. Short-term outcome of endoscopic versus microscopic pituitary adenoma surgery: A systematic review and meta-analysis. *J Neurol Neurosurg Psychiatry* 2013;84(8):843–9.

97. Henry JF, Defechereux T, Raffaelli M, Lubrano D, Gramatica L. Complications of laparoscopic adrenalectomy: Results of 169 consecutive procedures. *World J Surg* 2000;24(11):1342–6.

98. Chow JT, Thompson GB, Grant CS, Farley DR, Richards ML, Young WF Jr. Bilateral laparoscopic adrenalectomy for corticotrophin-dependent Cushing's syndrome: A review of the Mayo Clinic experience. *Clin Endocrinol* 2008;68(4):513–9.

99. Doherty GM, Nieman LK, Cutler GB Jr, Chrousos GP, Norton JA. Time to recovery of the hypothalamic-pituitary-adrenal axis after curative resection of adrenal tumors in patients with Cushing's syndrome. *Surgery* 1990;108(6):1085–90.

100. Chou SC, Lin JD. Long-term effects of ketoconazole in the treatment of residual or recurrent Cushing's disease. *Endocr J* 2000;47(4):401–6.

101. Sonino N, Boscaro M, Paoletta A, Mantero F, Ziliotto D. Ketoconazole treatment in Cushing's syndrome: Experience in 34 patients. *Clin Endocrinol* 1991;35(4):347–52.

102. Sonino N. The use of ketoconazole as an inhibitor of steroid production. *N Engl J Med* 1987;317(13):812–8.

103. Gadelha MR, Vieira Neto L. Efficacy of medical treatment in Cushing's disease: A systematic review. *Clin Endocrinol* 2014;80(1):1–2.

104. McCance DR, Ritchie CM, Sheridan B, Atkinson AB. Acute hypoadrenalism and hepatotoxicity after treatment with ketoconazole. *Lancet* 1987;1(8532):573.

105. Verhelst JA, Trainer PJ, Howlett TA et al. Short and long-term responses to metyrapone in the medical management of 91 patients with Cushing's syndrome. *Clin Endocrinol* 1991;35(2):169–78.

106. Luton JP, Mahoudeau JA, Bouchard P et al. Treatment of Cushing's disease by O,p'DDD. Survey of 62 cases. *N Engl J Med* 1979;300(9):459–64.

107. Schteingart DE, Tsao HS, Taylor CI, McKenzie A, Victoria R, Therrien BA. Sustained remission of Cushing's disease with mitotane and pituitary irradiation. *Ann Intern Med* 1980;92(5):613–9.

108. Invitti C, De Martin M, Danesi L, Cavagnini F. Effect of injectable bromocriptine in patients with Cushing's disease. *Exp Clin Endocrinol Diabetes* 1995;103(4):266–71.

109. van Waveren Hogervorst CO, Koppeschaar HP, Zelissen PM, Lips CJ, Garcia BM. Cortisol secretory patterns in Cushing's disease and response to cyproheptadine treatment. *J Clin Endocrinol Metab* 1996;81(2):652–5.

110. Colao A, Pivonello R, Tripodi FS et al. Failure of long-term therapy with sodium valproate in Cushing's disease. *J Endocrinol Invest* 1997;20(7):387–92.

111. Feelders RA, de Bruin C, Pereira AM et al. Pasireotide alone or with cabergoline and ketoconazole in Cushing's disease. *N Engl J Med* 2010;362(19):1846–8.

112. Fleseriu M, Biller BM, Findling JW et al. Mifepristone, a glucocorticoid receptor antagonist, produces clinical and metabolic benefits in patients with Cushing's syndrome. *J Clin Endocrinol Metab* 2012;97(6):2039–49.

113. Kerkhofs TM, Verhoeven RH, Van der Zwan JM et al. Adrenocortical carcinoma: A population-based study on incidence and survival in the Netherlands since 1993. *Eur J Cancer* 2013;49(11):2579–86.

114. Bilimoria KY, Shen WT, Elaraj D et al. Adrenocortical carcinoma in the United States: Treatment utilization and prognostic factors. *Cancer* 2008;113(11):3130–6.

115. Else T, Kim AC, Sabolch A et al. Adrenocortical carcinoma. *Endocr Rev* 2014;35(2):282–326.

116. Wajchenberg BL, Albergaria Pereira MA, Medonca BB et al. Adrenocortical carcinoma: Clinical and laboratory observations. *Cancer* 2000;88(4):711–36.

117. Wooten MD, King DK. Adrenal cortical carcinoma. Epidemiology and treatment with mitotane and a review of the literature. *Cancer* 1993;72(11):3145–55.

118. Mendonca BB, Lucon AM, Menezes CA et al. Clinical, hormonal and pathological findings in a comparative study of adrenocortical neoplasms in childhood and adulthood. *J Urol* 1995;154(6):2004–9.

119. Sabbaga CC, Avilla SG, Schulz C, Garbers JC, Blucher D. Adrenocortical carcinoma in children: Clinical aspects and prognosis. *J Pediatr Surg* 1993;28(6):841–3.

120. Pommier RF, Brennan MF. An eleven-year experience with adrenocortical carcinoma. *Surgery* 1992;112(6):963–70; discussion 970–1.

121. Luton JP, Cerdas S, Billaud L et al. Clinical features of adrenocortical carcinoma, prognostic factors, and the effect of mitotane therapy. *N Engl J Med* 1990;322(17):1195–201.

122. Michalkiewicz E, Sandrini R, Figueiredo B et al. Clinical and outcome characteristics of children with adrenocortical tumors: A report from the International Pediatric Adrenocortical Tumor Registry. *J Clin Oncol* 2004;22(5):838–45.

123. Soreide JA, Brabrand K, Thoresen SO. Adrenal cortical carcinoma in Norway, 1970–1984. *World J Surg* 1992;16(4):663–7; discussion 668.

124. Fassnacht MAB. Epidemiology of adrenocortical carcinoma. In: Hammer GD, Else T, eds., *Adrenocortical Carcinoma: Basic Science and Clinical Concepts.* New York: Springer, 2010:23–29.

125. Hsing AW, Nam JM, Co Chien HT, McLaughlin JK, Fraumeni JF Jr. Risk factors for adrenal cancer: An exploratory study. *Int J Cancer* 1996;65(4):432–6.

126. Icard P, Goudet P, Charpenay C et al. Adrenocortical carcinomas: Surgical trends and results of a 253-patient series from the French Association of Endocrine Surgeons study group. *World J Surg* 2001;25(7):891–7.

127. Henry I, Grandjouan S, Couillin P et al. Tumor-specific loss of 11p15.5 alleles in del11p13 Wilms tumor and in familial adrenocortical carcinoma. *Proc Natl Acad Sci USA* 1989;86(9):3247–51.

128. Yano T, Linehan M, Anglard P et al. Genetic changes in human adrenocortical carcinomas. *J Natl Cancer Inst* 1989;81(7):518–23.

129. McNicol AM, Nolan CE, Struthers AJ, Farquharson MA, Hermans J, Haak HR. Expression of p53 in adrenocortical tumours: Clinicopathological correlations. *J Pathol* 1997;181(2):146–52.

130. Ohgaki H, Kleihues P, Heitz PU. p53 mutations in sporadic adrenocortical tumors. *Int J Cancer* 1993;54(3):408–10.

131. Reincke M, Karl M, Travis WH et al. p53 mutations in human adrenocortical neoplasms: Immunohistochemical and molecular studies. *J Clin Endocrinol Metab* 1994;78(3):790–4.

132. Chompret A, Brugieres L, Ronsin M et al. P53 germline mutations in childhood cancers and cancer risk for carrier individuals. *Br J Cancer* 2000;82(12):1932–7.

133. Wagner J, Portwine C, Rabin K, Leclerc JM, Narod SA, Malkin D. High frequency of germline p53 mutations in childhood adrenocortical cancer. *J Natl Cancer Inst* 1994;86(22):1707–10.

134. Rodriguez-Galindo C, Figueiredo BC, Zambetti GP, Ribeiro RC. Biology, clinical characteristics, and management of adrenocortical tumors in children. *Pediatr Blood Cancer* 2005;45(3):265–73.

135. Custodio G, Parise GA, Kiesel Filho N et al. Impact of neonatal screening and surveillance for the TP53 R337H mutation on early detection of childhood adrenocortical tumors. *J Clin Oncol* 2013;31(20):2619–26.

136. Raymond VM, Else T, Everett JN, Long JM, Gruber SB, Hammer GD. Prevalence of germline TP53 mutations in a prospective series of unselected patients with adrenocortical carcinoma. *J Clin Endocrinol Metab* 2013;98(1):E119–25.

137. Herrmann LJ, Heinze B, Fassnacht M et al. TP53 germline mutations in adult patients with adrenocortical carcinoma. *J Clin Endocrinol Metab* 2012;97(3):E476–85.

138. Fassnacht M, Kroiss M, Allolio B. Update in adrenocortical carcinoma. *J Clin Endocrinol Metab* 2013;98(12):4551–64.

139. Hamwi GJ, Serbin RA, Kruger FA. Does adrenocortical hyperplasia result in adrenocortical carcinoma. *N Engl J Med* 1957;257(24):1153–7.

140. Koch CA, Pacak K, Chrousos GP. The molecular pathogenesis of hereditary and sporadic adrenocortical and adrenomedullary tumors. *J Clin Endocrinol Metab* 2002;87(12):5367–84.

141. Vassilopoulou-Sellin R, Schultz PN. Adrenocortical carcinoma. Clinical outcome at the end of the 20th century. *Cancer* 2001;92(5):1113–21.

142. Crucitti F, Bellantone R, Ferrante A, Boscherini M, Crucitti P. The Italian Registry for Adrenal Cortical Carcinoma: Analysis of a multiinstitutional series of 129 patients. The ACC Italian Registry Study Group. *Surgery* 1996;119(2):161–70.

143. Allolio B, Fassnacht M. Clinical review: Adrenocortical carcinoma: Clinical update. *J Clin Endocrinol Metab* 2006;91(6):2027–37.

144. Cohn K, Gottesman L, Brennan M. Adrenocortical carcinoma. *Surgery* 1986;100(6):1170–7.

145. Ayala-Ramirez M, Jasim S, Feng L et al. Adrenocortical carcinoma: Clinical outcomes and prognosis of 330 patients at a tertiary care center. *Eur J Endocrinol* 2013;169(6):891–9.

146. Abiven G, Coste J, Groussin L et al. Clinical and biological features in the prognosis of adrenocortical cancer: Poor outcome of cortisol-secreting tumors in a series of 202 consecutive patients. *J Clin Endocrinol Metab* 2006;91(7):2650–5.

147. Ng L, Libertino JM. Adrenocortical carcinoma: Diagnosis, evaluation and treatment. *J Urol* 2003;169(1):5–11.

148. Brooks RV, Felix-Davies D, Lee MR, Robertson PW. Hyperaldosteronism from adrenal carcinoma. *Br Med J* 1972;1(5794):220–1.

149. Zografos GC, Driscoll DL, Karakousis CP, Huben RP. Adrenal adenocarcinoma: A review of 53 cases. *J Surg Oncol* 1994;55(3):160–4.

150. Hutter AM Jr, Kayhoe DE. Adrenal cortical carcinoma. Clinical features of 138 patients. *Am J Med* 1966;41(4):572–80.

151. Zapf J, Futo E, Peter M, Froesch ER. Can "big" insulin-like growth factor II in serum of tumor patients account for the development of extrapancreatic tumor hypoglycemia? *J Clin Invest* 1992;90(6):2574–84.

152. Venkatesh S, Hickey RC, Sellin RV, Fernandez JF, Samaan NA. Adrenal cortical carcinoma. *Cancer* 1989;64(3):765–9.

153. Henley DJ, van Heerden JA, Grant CS, Carney JA, Carpenter PC. Adrenal cortical carcinoma—A continuing challenge. *Surgery* 1983;94(6):926–31.

154. Kendrick ML, Lloyd R, Erickson L et al. Adrenocortical carcinoma: Surgical progress or status quo? *Arch Surg (Chicago, Ill.: 1960)* 2001;136(5):543–9.

155. Grumbach MM, Biller BM, Braunstein GD et al. Management of the clinically inapparent adrenal mass ("incidentaloma"). *Ann Intern Med* 2003;138(5):424–9.

156. Fassnacht M, Allolio B. Clinical management of adrenocortical carcinoma. *Best Pract Res Clin Endocrinol Metab* 2009;23(2):273–89.

157. Arlt W, Biehl M, Taylor AE et al. Urine steroid metabolomics as a biomarker tool for detecting malignancy in adrenal tumors. *J Clin Endocrinol Metab* 2011;96(12):3775–84.

158. Glazer GM, Woolsey EJ, Borrello J et al. Adrenal tissue characterization using MR imaging. *Radiology* 1986;158(1):73–9.

159. Fishman EK, Deutch BM, Hartman DS, Goldman SM, Zerhouni EA, Siegelman SS. Primary adrenocortical carcinoma: CT evaluation with clinical correlation. *AJR Am J Roentgenol* 1987;148(3):531–5.

160. Bharwani N, Rockall AG, Sahdev A et al. Adrenocortical carcinoma: The range of appearances on CT and MRI. *AJR Am J Roentgenol* 2011;196(6):W706–14.

161. Rockall AG, Babar SA, Sohaib SA et al. CT and MR imaging of the adrenal glands in ACTH-independent Cushing syndrome. *Radiographics* 2004;24(2):435–52.

162. Davis PL, Hricak H, Bradley WG Jr. Magnetic resonance imaging of the adrenal glands. *Radiol Clin North Am* 1984;22(4):891–5.

163. Krestin GP, Freidmann G, Fishbach R, Neufang KF, Allolio B. Evaluation of adrenal masses in oncologic patients: Dynamic contrast-enhanced MR vs CT. *J Comput Assist Tomogr* 1991;15(1):104–10.

164. Hussain S, Belldegrun A, Seltzer SE, Richie JP, Gittes RF, Abrams HL. Differentiation of malignant from benign adrenal masses: Predictive indices on computed tomography. *AJR Am J Roentgenol* 1985;144(1):61–5.

165. Schultz CL, Haaga JR, Fletcher BD, Alfidi RJ, Schultz MA. Magnetic resonance imaging of the adrenal glands: A comparison with computed tomography. *AJR Am J Roentgenol* 1984;143(6):1235–40.

166. Pena CS, Boland GW, Hahn PF, Lee MJ, Mueller PR. Characterization of indeterminate (lipid-poor) adrenal masses: Use of washout characteristics at contrast-enhanced CT. *Radiology* 2000;217(3):798–802.

167. Park BK, Kim CK, Kim B, Lee JH. Comparison of delayed enhanced CT and chemical shift MR for evaluating hyperattenuating incidental adrenal masses. *Radiology* 2007;243(3):760–5.

168. Chang A, Glazer HS, Lee JK, Ling D, Heiken JP. Adrenal gland: MR imaging. *Radiology* 1987;163(1):123–8.

169. Schlund JF, Kenney PJ, Brown ED, Ascher SM, Brown JJ, Semelka RC. Adrenocortical carcinoma: MR imaging appearance with current techniques. *J Magn Reson Imaging* 1995;5(2):171–4.

170. Doppman JL, Reinig JW, Dwyer AJ et al. Differentiation of adrenal masses by magnetic resonance imaging. *Surgery* 1987;102(6):1018–26.

171. Korobkin M, Lombardi TJ, Aisen AM et al. Characterization of adrenal masses with chemical shift and gadolinium-enhanced MR imaging. *Radiology* 1995;197(2):411–8.

172. Outwater EK, Siegelman ES, Radecki PD, Piccoli CW, Mitchell DG. Distinction between benign and malignant adrenal masses: Value of T1-weighted chemical-shift MR imaging. *AJR Am J Roentgenol* 1995;165(3):579–83.

173. Reinig JW, Stutley JE, Leonhardt CM, Spicer KM, Margolis M, Caldwell CB. Differentiation of adrenal masses with MR imaging: Comparison of techniques. *Radiology* 1994;192(1):41–6.

174. Blake MA, Cronin CG, Boland GW. Adrenal imaging. *AJR Am J Roentgenol* 2010;194(6):1450–60.

175. Israel GM, Korobkin M, Wang C, Hecht EN, Krinsky GA. Comparison of unenhanced CT and chemical shift MRI in evaluating lipid-rich adrenal adenomas. *AJR Am J Roentgenol* 2004;183(1):215–9.

176. Haider MA, Ghai S, Jhaveri K, Lockwood G. Chemical shift MR imaging of hyperattenuating (>10 HU) adrenal masses: Does it still have a role? *Radiology* 2004;231(3):711–6.

177. Hricak H, Amparo E, Fisher MR, Crooks L, Higgins CB. Abdominal venous system: Assessment using MR. *Radiology* 1985;156(2):415–22.

178. Soler R, Rodriguez E, Lopez MF, Marini M. MR imaging in inferior vena cava thrombosis. *Eur J Radiol* 1995;19(2):101–7.

179. Groussin L, Bonardel G, Silvera S et al. 18F-Fluorodeoxyglucose positron emission tomography for the diagnosis of adrenocortical tumors: A prospective study in 77 operated patients. *J Clin Endocrinol Metab* 2009;94(5):1713–22.

180. Boland GW, Blake MA, Holalkere NS, Hahn PF. PET/CT for the characterization of adrenal masses in patients with cancer: Qualitative versus quantitative accuracy in 150 consecutive patients. *AJR Am J Roentgenol* 2009;192(4):956–62.

181. Sundin A. Imaging of adrenal masses with emphasis on adrenocortical tumors. *Theranostics* 2012;2(5):516–22.

182. Weiss LM, Medeiros LJ, Vickery AL Jr. Pathologic features of prognostic significance in adrenocortical carcinoma. *Am J Surg Pathol* 1989;13(3):202–6.

183. Lau SK, Weiss LM. The Weiss system for evaluating adrenocortical neoplasms: 25 years later. *Hum Pathol* 2009;40(6):757–68.

184. Lucon AM, Pereira MA, Mendonca BB, Zerbini MC, Saldanha LB, Arap S. Adrenocortical tumors: Results of treatment and study of Weiss's score as a prognostic factor. *Rev Hosp Clin* 2002;57(6):251–6.

185. Gicquel C, Bertagna X, Gaston V et al. Molecular markers and long-term recurrences in a large cohort of patients with sporadic adrenocortical tumors. *Cancer Res* 2001;61(18):6762–7.

186. Stojadinovic A, Ghossein RA, Hoos A et al. Adrenocortical carcinoma: Clinical, morphologic, and molecular characterization. *J Clin Oncol* 2002;20(4):941–50.

187. Assie G, Antoni G, Tissier F et al. Prognostic parameters of metastatic adrenocortical carcinoma. *J Clin Endocrinol Metab* 2007;92(1):148–54.

188. Aubert S, Wacrenier A, Leroy X et al. Weiss system revisited: A clinicopathologic and immunohistochemical study of 49 adrenocortical tumors. *Am J Surg Pathol* 2002;26(12):1612–9.

189. van't Sant HP, Bouvy ND, Kazemier G et al. The prognostic value of two different histopathological scoring systems for adrenocortical carcinomas. *Histopathology* 2007;51(2):239–45.

190. Sbiera S, Schmull S, Assie G et al. High diagnostic and prognostic value of steroidogenic factor-1 expression in adrenal tumors. *J Clin Endocrinol Metab* 2010;95(10):E161–171.

191. Duregon E, Volante M, Giorcelli J, Terzolo M, Lalli E, Papotti M. Diagnostic and prognostic role of steroidogenic factor 1 in adrenocortical carcinoma: A validation study focusing on clinical and pathologic correlates. *Hum Pathol* 2013;44(5):822–8.

192. Adrenal. In: Edge S, Byrd DR, Compton CC, Fritz AG, Greene FL, Trotti A, eds., *AJCC Cancer Staging Manual.* 7th ed. New York: Springer, 2010, pp. 585–90.

193. Jaques DP, Brennan MF. Tumors of the adrenal cortex. In: Cameron J, ed., *Current Surgical Therapy.* Toronto: BC, Decker, 1989:435–44.

194. Fassnacht M, Johanssen S, Fenske W et al. Improved survival in patients with stage II adrenocortical carcinoma followed up prospectively by specialized centers. *J Clin Endocrinol Metab* 2010;95(11):4925–32.

195. Paton BL, Novitsky YW, Zerey M et al. Outcomes of adrenal cortical carcinoma in the United States. *Surgery* 2006;140(6):914–20; discussion 919–20.

196. Schulick RD, Brennan MF. Long-term survival after complete resection and repeat resection in patients with adrenocortical carcinoma. *Ann Surg Oncol* 1999;6(8):719–26.

197. Fassnacht M, Johanssen S, Quinkler M et al. Limited prognostic value of the 2004 International Union Against Cancer staging classification for adrenocortical carcinoma: Proposal for a revised TNM classification. *Cancer* 2009;115(2):243–50.

198. Lughezzani G, Sun M, Perrotte P et al. The European Network for the Study of Adrenal Tumors staging system is prognostically superior to the International Union Against Cancer-staging system: A North American validation. *Eur J Cancer* 2010;46(4):713–9.

199. Miller BS, Gauger PG, Hammer GD, Giordano TJ, Doherty GM. Proposal for modification of the ENSAT staging system for adrenocortical carcinoma using tumor grade. *Langenbecks Arch Surg* 2010;395(7):955–61.

200. King DR, Lack EE. Adrenal cortical carcinoma: A clinical and pathologic study of 49 cases. *Cancer* 1979;44(1):239–44.

201. Bertagna X, Bertagna C, Laudat MH, Husson JM, Girard F, Luton JP. Pituitary-adrenal response to the antiglucocorticoid action of RU 486 in Cushing's syndrome. *J Clin Endocrinol Metab* 1986;63(3):639–43.

202. Haak HR, Hermans J, van de Velde CJ et al. Optimal treatment of adrenocortical carcinoma with mitotane: Results in a consecutive series of 96 patients. *Br J Cancer* 1994;69(5):947–51.

203. Gaujoux S, Brennan MF. Recommendation for standardized surgical management of primary adrenocortical carcinoma. *Surgery* 2012;152(1):123–32.

204. Reibetanz J, Jurowich C, Erdogan I et al. Impact of lymphadenectomy on the oncologic outcome of patients with adrenocortical carcinoma. *Ann Surg* 2012;255(2):363–9.

205. Geelhoed GW, Dunnick NR, Doppman JL. Management of intravenous extensions of endocrine tumors and prognosis after surgical treatment. *Am J Surg* 1980;139(6):844–8.

206. Mihai R, Iacobone M, Makay O et al. Outcome of operation in patients with adrenocortical cancer invading the inferior vena cava—A European Society of Endocrine Surgeons (ESES) survey. *Langenbecks Arch Surg* 2012;397(2):225–31.

207. Mingoli A, Nardacchione F, Sgarzini G, Marzano M, Ciccarone F, Modini C. Inferior vena cava involvement by a left side adrenocortical carcinoma: Operative and prognostic considerations. *Anticancer Res* 1996;16(5B):3197–200.

208. Chiche L, Dousset B, Kieffer E, Chapuis Y. Adrenocortical carcinoma extending into the inferior vena cava: Presentation of a 15-patient series and review of the literature. *Surgery* 2006;139(1):15–27.

209. Dackiw AP, Lee JE, Gagel RF, Evans DB. Adrenal cortical carcinoma. *World J Surg* 2001;25(7):914–26.

210. Grondal S, Cedermark B, Eriksson B et al. Adrenocortical carcinoma. A retrospective study of a rare tumor with a poor prognosis. *Eur J Surg Oncol* 1990;16(6):500–6.

211. Icard P, Louvel A, Chapuis Y. Survival rates and prognostic factors in adrenocortical carcinoma. *World J Surg* 1992;16(4):753–8.

212. Dy BM, Strajina V, Cayo AK et al. Surgical resection of synchronously metastatic adrenocortical cancer. *Ann Surg Oncol* 2015;22(1):146–51.

213. Dy BM, Wise KB, Richards ML et al. Operative intervention for recurrent adrenocortical cancer. *Surgery* 2013;154(6):1292–9; discussion 1299.

214. Grubbs EG, Callender GG, Xing Y et al. Recurrence of adrenal cortical carcinoma following resection: Surgery alone can achieve results equal to surgery plus mitotane. *Ann Surg Oncol* 2010;17(1):263–70.

215. Schteingart DE, Doherty GM, Gauger PG et al. Management of patients with adrenal cancer: Recommendations of an international consensus conference. *Endocr Relat Cancer* 2005;12(3):667–80.

216. Bellantone R, Ferrante A, Boscherini M et al. Role of reoperation in recurrence of adrenal cortical carcinoma: Results from 188 cases collected in the Italian National Registry for Adrenal Cortical Carcinoma. *Surgery* 1997;122(6):1212–8.

217. Jensen JC, Pass HI, Sindelar WF, Norton JA. Recurrent or metastatic disease in select patients with adrenocortical carcinoma. Aggressive resection vs chemotherapy. *Arch Surg (Chicago, Ill.:1960)* 1991;126(4):457–61.

218. Gonzalez RJ, Shapiro S, Sarlis N et al. Laparoscopic resection of adrenal cortical carcinoma: A cautionary note. *Surgery* 2005;138(6):1078–85; discussion 1085–6.

219. Cobb WS, Kercher KW, Sing RF, Heniford BT. Laparoscopic adrenalectomy for malignancy. *Am J Surg* 2005;189(4):405–11.

220. Miller BS, Ammori JB, Gauger PG, Broome JT, Hammer GD, Doherty GM. Laparoscopic resection is inappropriate in patients with known or suspected adrenocortical carcinoma. *World J Surg* 2010;34(6):1380–5.

221. Miller BS, Gauger PG, Hammer GD, Doherty GM. Resection of adrenocortical carcinoma is less complete and local recurrence occurs sooner and more often after laparoscopic adrenalectomy than after open adrenalectomy. *Surgery* 2012;152(6):1150–7.

222. Mir MC, Klink JC, Guillotreau J et al. Comparative outcomes of laparoscopic and open adrenalectomy for adrenocortical carcinoma: Single, high-volume center experience. *Ann Surg Oncol* 2013;20(5):1456–61.

223. Porpiglia F, Fiori C, Daffara F et al. Retrospective evaluation of the outcome of open versus laparoscopic adrenalectomy for stage I and II adrenocortical cancer. *Eur Urol* 2010;57(5):873–8.

224. Brix D, Allolio B, Fenske W et al. Laparoscopic versus open adrenalectomy for adrenocortical carcinoma: Surgical and oncologic outcome in 152 patients. *Eur Urol* 2010;58(4):609–15.

225. Lombardi CP, Raffaelli M, De Crea C et al. Open versus endoscopic adrenalectomy in the treatment of localized (stage I/II) adrenocortical carcinoma: Results of a multiinstitutional Italian survey. *Surgery* 2012;152(6):1158–64.

226. Lombardi CP, Raffaelli M, Boniardi M et al. Adrenocortical carcinoma: Effect of hospital volume on patient outcome. *Langenbecks Arch Surg* 2012;397(2):201–7.

227. Gratian L, Pura J, Dinan M et al. Treatment patterns and outcomes for patients with adrenocortical carcinoma associated with hospital case volume in the United States. *Ann Surg Oncol* 2014;21(11):3509–14.

228. Kerkhofs TM, Verhoeven RH, Bonjer HJ et al. Surgery for adrenocortical carcinoma in the Netherlands: Analysis of the national cancer registry data. *Eur J Endocrinol* 2013;169(1):83–9.

229. Schteingart DE. Cushing's syndrome. *Endocrinol Metab Clin North Am* 1989;18(2):311–38.

230. Lubitz JA, Freeman L, Okun R. Mitotane use in inoperable adrenal cortical carcinoma. *JAMA* 1973;223(10):1109–12.

231. Hutter AM Jr, Kayhoe DE. Adrenal cortical carcinoma. Results of treatment with o,p'DDD in 138 patients. *Am J Med* 1966;41(4):581–92.

232. Terzolo M, Angeli A, Fassnacht M et al. Adjuvant mitotane treatment for adrenocortical carcinoma. *N Engl J Med* 2007;356(23):2372–80.

233. Berruti A, Fassnacht M, Baudin E et al. Adjuvant therapy in patients with adrenocortical carcinoma: A position of an international panel. *J Clin Oncol* 2010;28(23):e401–402; author reply e403.

234. Kasperlik-Zaluska AA, Migdalska BM, Zgliczynski S, Makowska AM. Adrenocortical carcinoma. A clinical study and treatment results of 52 patients. *Cancer* 1995;75(10):2587–91.

235. Schlumberger M, Ostronoff M, Bellaiche M, Rougier P, Droz JP, Parmentier C. 5-Fluorouracil, doxorubicin, and cisplatin regimen in adrenal cortical carcinoma. *Cancer* 1988;61(8):1492–94.

236. Berruti A, Terzolo M, Sperone P et al. Etoposide, doxorubicin and cisplatin plus mitotane in the treatment of advanced adrenocortical carcinoma: A large prospective phase II trial. *Endocr Relat Cancer* 2005;12(3):657–66.

237. Khan TS, Imam H, Juhlin C et al. Streptozocin and o,p'DDD in the treatment of adrenocortical cancer patients: Long-term survival in its adjuvant use. *Ann Oncol* 2000;11(10):1281–7.

238. Fassnacht M, Terzolo M, Allolio B et al. Combination chemotherapy in advanced adrenocortical carcinoma. *N Engl J Med* 2012;366(23):2189–97.

239. Bodie B, Novick AC, Pontes JE et al. The Cleveland Clinic experience with adrenal cortical carcinoma. *J Urol* 1989;141(2):257–60.

240. Schteingart DE, Motazedi A, Noonan RA, Thompson NW. Treatment of adrenal carcinomas. *Arch Surg (Chicago, Ill.: 1960)* 1982;117(9):1142–6.

241. Sabolch A, Feng M, Griffith K, Hammer G, Doherty G, Ben-Josef E. Adjuvant and definitive radiotherapy for adrenocortical carcinoma. *Int J Radiat Oncol Biol Physics* 2011;80(5):1477–84.

242. Fassnacht M, Hahner S, Polat B et al. Efficacy of adjuvant radiotherapy of the tumor bed on local recurrence of adrenocortical carcinoma. *J Clin Endocrinol Metab* 2006;91(11):4501–4.

243. Polat B, Fassnacht M, Pfreundner L et al. Radiotherapy in adrenocortical carcinoma. *Cancer* 2009;115(13):2816–23.

244. Wood BJ, Abraham J, Hvizda JL, Alexander HR, Fojo T. Radiofrequency ablation of adrenal tumors and adrenocortical carcinoma metastases. *Cancer* 2003;97(3):554–60.

245. Mayo-Smith WW, Dupuy DE. Adrenal neoplasms: CT-guided radiofrequency ablation—Preliminary results. *Radiology* 2004;231(1):225–30.

246. Chrousos GP. Adrenal hyperandrogenism. Waltham, MA: UpToDate. http://www.uptodate.com/contents/adrenal-hyperandrogenism (accessed August 30, 2014).

247. Tsigos CKT, Chrousos GP. Adrenal disease. In: Moore WT, Eastman RC, eds., *Diagnostic Endocrinology*. Philadelphia: Decker, 1996, pp. 125–56.

248. Derksen J, Nagesser SK, Meinders AE, Haak HR, van de Velde CJ. Identification of virilizing adrenal tumors in hirsute women. *N Engl J Med* 1994;331(15):968–73.

249. Moreno S, Guillermo M, Decoulx M, Dewailly D, Bresson R, Proye C. Feminizing adreno-cortical carcinomas in male adults. A dire prognosis. Three cases in a series of 801 adrenalectomies and review of the literature. *Ann Endocrinol* 2006;67(1):32–8.

30

Primary aldosteronism

MIHAIL ZILBERMINT AND CONSTANTINE A. STRATAKIS

INTRODUCTION

Primary aldosteronism (PA) describes a number of conditions, all characterized by excess production of aldosterone. Dr. Jerome Conn described the phenomenon of hypertension and hypokalemia in the 1950s, improving after resection of an adrenocortical adenoma [1]. He suggested that this clinical picture was due to overproduction of aldosterone by the adrenal adenoma. Today, this constellation of findings bears Dr. Conn's name and is known as Conn's syndrome. While PA is often due to an adrenal adenoma, other causes have since been identified; aldosterone-producing adrenal hyperplasia, in particular, has been recognized as a genetic disorder and is now divided into three types: familial hyperaldosteronism (FH) types I–III. Genetic causes have also been discovered in the past decade for both adenoma and hyperplasia.

PA is a relatively common and, most importantly, potentially treatable cause of secondary hypertension. Therefore, it is crucial to recognize the syndrome, confirm the diagnosis, and provide a surgical cure to the appropriate individuals in order to prevent poor cardiovascular outcomes of hyperaldosteronism [2]. This chapter reviews the basics of physiology and epidemiology, describes important clinical features, summarizes diagnostic methods, and provides guidance in choosing an appropriate treatment option of PA [3].

PHYSIOLOGICAL MECHANISM OF ALDOSTERONE SECRETION

Control of aldosterone secretion

Aldosterone is a mineralocorticoid hormone, produced in the outer layer of the adrenal cortex (zona glomerulosa). Its main effects include sodium and fluid retention, via the exchange of potassium and hydrogen ions in the distal convoluted tubule of the kidney, resulting in increased intravascular volume (hypertension), hypokalemia, and metabolic alkalosis. A number of aldosterone precursors, including deoxycorticosterone and 18-hydroxycorticosterone, have some mineralocorticoid activity, and their hypersecretion in various disorders may yield features of mineralocorticoid hypertension.

Aldosterone participates in blood volume and serum potassium homeostasis; these physiologic parameters feed back to regulate aldosterone secretion by the zona glomerulosa of the adrenal cortex [4]. Hypokalemia and hypervolemia suppress aldosterone secretion, whereas blood volume depletion or an increase in serum potassium levels stimulates it.

Aldosterone secretion is regulated mostly by the renin–angiotensin system and potassium levels, and minimally by adrenocorticotropic hormone (ACTH). In the case of PA, aldosterone overproduction is independent of the

Table 30.1 Common causes and potential treatment of primary aldosteronism

Causes of primary aldosteronism	Treatment strategy
Aldosterone-producing adenoma	Unilateral adrenalectomy
	+/− MR antagonists
Bilateral adrenal hyperplasia (idiopathic hyperaldosteronism)	MR antagonists
Aldosterone-producing adrenocortical carcinoma	Unilateral adrenalectomy, tumor removal
	+/− MR antagonists
FH type I (GRA)	Dexamethasone
FH type II (non-GRA)	Unilateral adrenalectomy
	+/− MR antagonists
FH type III (germline KCNJ5 mutation)	Bilateral adrenalectomy
	+/− MR antagonists

Note: MR, mineralocorticoid receptor.

juxtaglomerular apparatus and robust aldosterone secretion suppresses production of renin.

ACTH regulates aldosterone secretion almost exclusively in the case of glucocorticoid-remediable aldosteronism (GRA), also known as FH type I (see also the "Familial Hyperaldosteronism Type I" section). A fusion of ACTH-dependent 11β-hydroxylase gene (CYP11B1) promoter to the coding sequence of the aldosterone-producing gene (CYP11B2) is the cause of FH type I, allowing for ACTH stimulation to lead to increased aldosterone overproduction [5–10]. Other types of aldosterone hypersecretion have a different pathophysiology. The diagnosis and treatment depend on the pathophysiology of PA (Table 30.1) [11–15].

Aldosterone biosynthesis

Aldosterone is synthesized from cholesterol in a series of well-described biosynthetic steps [16–19]. The first four steps are also involved in the synthesis of cortisol, and the last two are unique to aldosterone (Figure 30.1). The product of the CYP11B2 gene (8q21-q22) is responsible for all steps, those that require 11β-hydroxylase, 18-hydroxylase, and 18-hydroxydehydrogenase activities [20].

Aldosterone acts on the distal renal tubules, sweat glands, large intestine epithelium, and salivary glands via, the aldosterone-specific mineralocorticoid receptor (MR) [21]. The MR exhibits similar affinity for aldosterone and glucocorticoids, whereas distal renal tubular receptors are protected from the effects of cortisol by 11β-hydroxysteroid dehydrogenase (which converts cortisol to cortisone) [22,23]. Patients with Cushing syndrome (cortisol excess) often present with hypokalemia, hypertension, and adrenal nodularity, which can be confused with PA.

PRIMARY ALDOSTERONISM

Epidemiology

According to a recent Centers for Disease Control report, the overall age-adjusted prevalence of hypertension among U.S. adults was 28.6% in 2009–2010 [24]. PA is a common cause of hypertension, although it is not often recognized. It may account for up to 10%–15% of hypertensive patients, especially in those who have resistant hypertension [25–32]. It used to be thought that PA is a rare condition. This was likely due to screening and identification of cases with hypokalemia only. Normokalemic hypertension may be a more common presentation of PA, while up to 37% of patients may have low potassium [30]. PA is often diagnosed in middle-age adults, is more common in women, and is rare in children [3].

Clinical features

Patients usually are referred for evaluation of long-standing hypertension with or without hypokalemia. Some describe their hypertension refractory to multiple medications (two to four), while a number of patients report improvement in their symptoms after initiation of drug therapy that includes one of the MR antagonists (spironolactone or eplerenone). Nonspecific symptoms, such as headaches, muscle cramps,

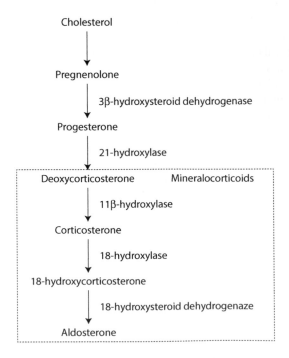

Figure 30.1 Aldosterone biosynthesis pathway.

Table 30.2 Common genetic causes of primary aldosteronism

Genetic alteration	Condition
CYP11B1/CYP11B2	FH type I
CYP11B1	
CYP11B2	
Somatic KCNJ5 mutation	FH type II
Locus 7p22	
Germline KCNJ5 mutation	FH type III

weakness, fatigue, polyuria, and edema of lower extremities, are common.

Importantly, hyperaldosteronism carries high cardiovascular risk, leading to left ventricular hypertrophy, stroke, and myocardial infarction [33–35]. Cardiac and cerebrovascular outcomes could be improved after treatment of hyperaldosteronism [2].

Other metabolic effects of PA include glucose intolerance [34,36] and increased weight. The exact mechanism is not clear, but it can be due to impairment of insulin secretion by hypokalemia or mild cosecretion of corticosteroids by some adrenal tumors [37].

Causes and genetics

The most common causes of PA are bilateral adrenal hyperplasia (60%) and aldosterone-producing adenomas (APAs) (30%) [30,38,39]. The remaining 10% are various genetic conditions [40–48] (Table 30.2).

Other conditions may present as secondary hyperaldosteronism or aldosterone excess-like disorders (apparent mineralocorticoid excess) and have to be differentiated from PA (Table 30.3). These disorders are not the focus of the chapter and are discussed elsewhere in this book [49–60].

DIAGNOSIS OF PRIMARY ALDOSTERONISM

Screening

Given that PA has a relatively high prevalence, we advise active screening of patients with hypertension in stages II

and III, particularly those whose hypertension is associated with drug resistance [13,26,31,61,62], adrenal incidentalomas [63–65], hypokalemia, or a strong family history, particularly at young age. First-degree relatives of patients with familial hypertension should also be screened [13].

The plasma aldosterone-to-renin ratio (ARR) is a simple and reliable screening method of PA [4,66–69]. The test was described in 1981 and has been validated in large series and at many centers. As aldosterone level rises, plasma renin activity (PRA) falls because of sodium retention. This negative feedback response occurs when aldosterone secretion is supraphysiologic [3].

Renin assays to document PRA should be sensitive to measure levels as low as 0.2–0.3 ng/mL × h (32). ARR > 20 is usually considered a positive test. Some institutions are using different cutoffs, such as 15 or 30. This depends on the particular aldosterone and renin assay and usage of conventional units. ARR has its own limitations, and can be quite variable. A single normal ARR may not exclude PA [68]. Medications, such as eplerenone, spironolactone, amiloride, triamterene, and some potassium-wasting diuretics, can markedly affect ARR, and should be discontinued for at least 2–6 weeks prior to case detection. Importantly, β-blockers can reduce PRA levels, leading to falsely increased ARR [13].

There are five medications that have a minimal effect on plasma aldosterone and renin level: verapamil, hydralazine, prazosin, doxazosin, and terazosin. These agents can be safely used to control blood pressure during the case detection and case confirmation [13,70].

We also suggest screening all patients with hypertension and adrenal lesions for pheochromocytoma. This condition may present with symptoms such as sweating, flushing, heart palpitation and adrenal nodule(s). Plasma and urinary catecholamines and metanephrines should be measured (see Chapter 32).

Confirmatory tests

All positive ARRs have to be confirmed with one of the four confirmatory tests, listed in Table 30.4. In our institution, most patients undergo both saline suppression and oral sodium loading tests. These tests should be administered

Table 30.3 Causes of secondary hyperaldosteronism and aldosterone excess-like disorders

Aldosterone excess-like disorders	Secondary hyperaldosteronism
Congenital adrenal hyperplasia	Renovascular hypertension
11β-hydroxylase deficiency	Reninoma
17α-hydroxylase deficiency	Edema (e.g., congestive heart failure)
Primary glucocorticoid resistance	Pregnancy
Apparent mineralocorticoid excess	
Deoxycorticosterone-secreting tumor	
Liddle's syndrome	
Licorice ingestion	
Carbenoxolone (derived from licorice root)	

Table 30.4 Confirmatory tests for primary aldosteronism

Test	Procedure	Interpretation	Notes
Saline suppression test	Patients lay supine for 1 hour prior to procedure and for 4 hours during the infusion of 2 L of intravenous 0.9% normal saline (500 mL/h). Baseline STAT potassium level is drawn and hypokalemia is treated prior to saline infusion. Baseline aldosterone, renin, and potassium levels are checked at time zero and 4 hours. We suggest taking vital signs during the test.	Plasma aldosterone at 4 hours of >10 ng/dL makes the diagnosis of PA likely. Levels of <5 ng/dL probably indicate a negative test. Levels between 5 and 10 ng/dL are borderline.	This test requires an admission to an ambulatory center. Should be avoided in patients with severe hypokalemia, cardiac arrhythmia, and uncontrolled hypertension.
Oral sodium loading test	Patients take 2 g of sodium tablets three times daily with meals for 3 days. Urinary sodium and aldosterone are measured in the 24-hour urine collection from the morning of day 3 until the morning of day 4.	Urine sodium should be >200 mmol/day to verify compliance with the procedure. Urinary aldosterone of >12–14 µg/24 h makes the diagnosis of PA highly likely. Levels of <10 µg/24 h are unlikely to indicate PA.	
Captopril challenge test	Patients sit or stand for at least 1 hour, and then intake 25–50 mg of captopril. Plasma, aldosterone, and cortisol are drawn at 0, 1, or 2 hours after medication intake, while the patient remains seated.	Captopril suppresses aldosterone under normal conditions. Patients with PA still have elevated plasma aldosterone and suppressed renin.	Not commonly used, given a high number of false-negative results.
Fludrocortisone suppression test	Patients receive fludrocortisone 0.1 mg every 6 hours for 4 days, along with potassium supplements (every 6 hours to keep serum potassium level around 4 mmol/L), slow-release sodium chloride tablets (30 mmol three times daily with meals), and sufficient dietary salt (to keep a urinary sodium excretion rate of at least 3 mmol/kg of body weight). On the fourth day, the plasma cortisol level is measured at 7:00 a.m. and 10:00 a.m., and aldosterone and renin are measured at 10:00 a.m., in the seated position.	Upright plasma aldosterone of >6 ng/dL on the fourth day at 10:00 a.m. confirms PA. Plasma renin should be <1 ng/mL × h.	May require hospitalization for 4 days for frequent potassium checks.

Note: Review medication list prior to the testing. Make sure that spironolactone and eplerenone have been discontinued for at least 4–6 weeks prior to the testing.

with caution in patients with congestive heart failure or uncontrolled hypertension [13,26,45,71–78].

Imaging studies

Dedicated adrenal computed tomogram (CT) is a helpful imaging method in diagnosing APAs with a sensitivity of 70% (Figure 30.2). A third of adrenal nodules are <1 cm, and may not be clearly visualized on the CT scan. Adrenal glands of patients with idiopathic hyperaldosteronism may show some adrenal hyperplasia, or may look normal. Aldosterone-producing carcinomas are usually large and have suspicious features on CT scan [65,79]. Adrenal incidentalomas are common (particularly in older patients), and the presence of nonfunctioning adrenal adenomas may confuse the practitioner because they are almost indistinguishable on CT from APAs [13]. Concordance between CT and adrenal venous sampling (AVS) could be as low as 54% [80,81]. Thus,

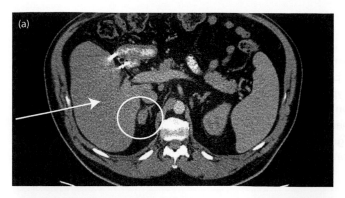

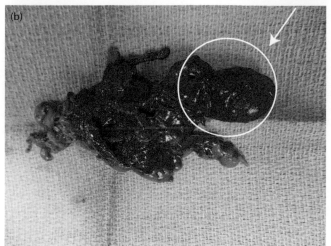

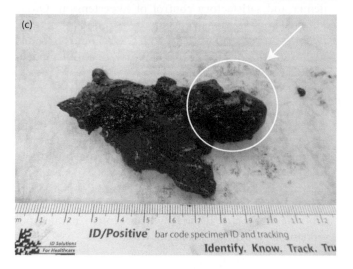

Figure 30.2 APA in a 62-year-old male patient with PA. **(a)** Adrenal CT. **(b and c)** Gross pathology. The arrow points to the adenoma.

lateralizing surgical decisions should not be done routinely based only on the results of CT, with the exception perhaps of patients below the fourth decade of life. Magnetic resonance imaging (MRI) of the adrenals may be inferior to CT because of less adrenal-specific resolution. MRI may also be complicated by motion in the retroperitoneal area; however, MRI could be justified in patients with iodine allergy or chronic kidney disease, or in children (Figure 30.3).

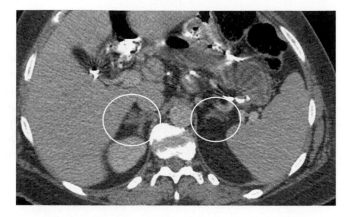

Figure 30.3 Bilateral adrenal hyperplasia (idiopathic hyperaldosteronism) in a 39-year-old female. AVS confirmed bilateral aldosterone production. Currently treated with spironolactone 100 mg/day with satisfactory control of hypertension. Adrenal CT.

Adrenal venous sampling

AVS is the gold standard diagnostic or lateralization study of PA [82]. However, it is expensive and invasive, requires considerable skill, and should be performed at centers with extensive experience. AVS is both sensitive (95%) and specific (100%) in identifying unilateral overproduction of aldosterone [81,83]. One of the biggest challenges of the procedure is the ability to successfully catheterize the right adrenal vein because of its anatomical location (usually empties directly into the inferior vena cava, rather than the renal vein). The procedure success rate depends on the radiologist's experience and may vary (74%–96%) [80,81,84]. The complication rate at experienced centers is <2.5% [81]. AVS is discussed in detail in Chapter 28.

Other forms of primary aldosteronism

FAMILIAL HYPERALDOSTERONISM TYPE I (GLUCOCORTICOID-REMEDIABLE ALDOSTERONISM)

FH type I or GRA is a rare, mostly autosomal dominant (occasionally sporadic) disorder, causing less than 1% of PA (Table 30.1) [85]. The key finding is early onset of severe and resistant hypertension, sometimes accompanied by hemorrhagic strokes [86,87]. The GRA can be excluded with a 4-day dexamethasone suppression test (0.5 mg administered every 6 hours). Plasma aldosterone and renin are measured at baseline, at days 2 and 4. Non-GRA patients respond with decreased levels of aldosterone by approximately 50% and return to baseline levels by day 4. In the case of GRA, aldosterone levels remain suppressed. Urinary levels of 18-hydroxycortisol (>100 nmol/L) and 18-oxocortisol may also be elevated, although sometimes this is misleading [3,88]. Most cases of GRA are caused by a fusion of the ACTH-dependent 11β-hydroxylase gene (*CYP11B1*) promoter to the coding sequence of the aldosterone-producing

Table 30.5 Preoperative and postoperative management of primary aldosteronism

Preoperative management	Postoperative management
Blood pressure control	Plasma aldosterone and renin activity, serum potassium level, creatinine
• Verapamil	Discontinue potassium supplements
• Hydralazine	Adjust antihypertensive therapy (usually patients still require at least one
• Prazosin	medication)
• Doxazosin	Diet with liberal sodium intake
• Terazosin	Check for signs of adrenal insufficiency (in case of glucocorticoid
Correction of hypokalemia	cosecretion) and renal failure
Consider transthoracic 2D echocardiogram	

gene (*CYP11B2*), allowing for ACTH to exclusively control aldosterone secretion [5–10]. Genetic testing via polymerase chain reaction techniques is widely available and should be considered the first step in the confirmatory workup of the selected population [13,86,87].

FAMILIAL HYPERALDOSTERONISM TYPE II (NON-GLUCOCORTICOID-REMEDIABLE ALDOSTERONISM)

FH type II or non-GRA is an autosomal dominant disorder, and appears to be clinically and biochemically indistinguishable from APA or bilateral adrenal hyperplasia. It can be unilateral and bilateral and appears to be genetically heterogeneous, one of its loci mapping to chromosome 7 (7p22) [48,89].

FAMILIAL HYPERALDOSTERONISM TYPE III

FH type III is rare disorder, likely due mostly to a few germline *KCNJ5* gene mutations; patients with germline *KCNJ5* defects need bilateral adrenalectomy if their blood pressure is not controlled by medications. So far, five germline mutations in the *KCNJ5* gene have been identified and characterized in patients with FH type III [90,91].

TREATMENT

Surgical

Patients with unilateral APA and carcinoma and unilateral adrenal hyperplasia (FH type II) should be offered surgery. Patients who undergo unilateral adrenalectomy show a great improvement in hypertension (30%–60%) and hypokalemia [92,93]. Some older patients may have coexisting primary hypertension (formerly essential hypertension), which may be associated with refractory hypertension even after adrenalectomy. Today, laparoscopic adrenalectomy is the standard of care and should be performed by an experienced surgeon [94,95]. It is associated with fewer complications and shorter hospital stays. This technique is discussed elsewhere in this book.

Perioperative care is summarized in Table 30.5. Notably, we suggest discontinuing MR antagonists (e.g., eplerenone and spironolactone) prior to the surgery and substituting them with antihypertensive agents, mentioned in the "Diagnosis of Primary Aldosteronism" section (Table 30.5). This is important in preventing postoperative hyperkalemia and transient postoperative hypoaldosteronism. There is some evidence that prevalence of chronic kidney disease in PA may be increased after treatment [96]; therefore, kidney function should be closely monitored postoperatively.

Medical

Medical therapy is the treatment of choice for patients with bilateral adrenal hyperplasia or glucocorticoid-remediable hyperaldosteronism [13]. Spironolactone (100–400 mg/day) or eplerenone (25–100 mg/day) can usually lead to normokalemia and satisfactory control of hypertension. Often, additional antihypertensive agents are required for optimal blood pressure control. Patients with GRA should be treated with dexamethasone (0.125–0.25 mg/day) or another glucocorticoid equivalent.

ACKNOWLEDGMENTS

This work was supported by the Intramural Research Program of the Eunice Kennedy Shriver National Institute of Child Health and Human Development (NICHD), National Institutes of Health (NIH). We thank Diane Cooper, MSLS, NIH Library, for providing assistance in writing this manuscript. We thank Drs. Elena Belyavskaya and Charalampos Lysikatos for providing assistance with figures.

REFERENCES

1. Conn JW. Primary aldosteronism. *J Lab Clin Med* 1955;45(4):661–4.
2. Rossi GP, Sacchetto A, Visentin P et al. Changes in left ventricular anatomy and function in hypertension and primary aldosteronism. *Hypertension* 1996;27(5):1039–45.
3. Stergiopoulos SG, Torpy DJ, Stratakis CA. Primary aldosteronism. In: *Endocrine Surgery*. Boca Raton, FL: CRC Press, 2003.
4. Torpy DJ, Stratakis CA, Chrousos GP. Hyper- and hypoaldosteronism. *Vitam Horm* 1999;57:177–216.

5. Lifton RP, Dluhy RG, Powers M, Ulick S, Lalouel JM. The molecular basis of glucocorticoid-remediable aldosteronism, a Mendelian cause of human hypertension. *Trans Assoc Am Physicians* 1992;105:64–71.

6. Lifton RP, Dluhy RG, Powers M et al. Hereditary hypertension caused by chimaeric gene duplications and ectopic expression of aldosterone synthase. *Nat Genet* 1992;2(1):66–74.

7. Lifton RP, Dluhy RG, Powers M et al. A chimaeric 11 beta-hydroxylase/aldosterone synthase gene causes glucocorticoid-remediable aldosteronism and human hypertension. *Nature* 1992;355(6357):262–5.

8. DiNorcia, J. and Lee, J.A. Primary Hyperaldosteronism. In: Hubbard J, Inabnet WB, Lo C-Y, eds., *Endocrine Surgery: Principles and Practice*, pp. 365–77. London: Springer-Verlag London, 2009.

9. Rich GM, Ulick S, Cook S, Wang JZ, Lifton RP, Dluhy RG. Glucocorticoid-remediable aldosteronism in a large kindred: Clinical spectrum and diagnosis using a characteristic biochemical phenotype. *Ann Intern Med* 1992;116(10):813–20.

10. Jonsson JR, Klemm SA, Tunny TJ, Stowasser M, Gordon RD. A new genetic test for familial hyperaldosteronism type I aids in the detection of curable hypertension. *Biochem Biophys Res Commun* 1995;207(2):565–71.

11. Irony I, Kater CE, Biglieri EG, Shackleton CH. Correctable subsets of primary aldosteronism. Primary adrenal hyperplasia and renin responsive adenoma. *Am J Hypertens* 1990;3(7):576–82.

12. Ganguly A. Primary aldosteronism. *N Engl J Med* 1998;339(25):1828–34.

13. Funder JW, Carey RM, Fardella C et al. Case detection, diagnosis, and treatment of patients with primary aldosteronism: An Endocrine Society Clinical Practice Guideline. *J Clin Endocrinol Metab* 2008;93(9):3266–81.

14. Sutherland DJ, Ruse JL, Laidlaw JC. Hypertension, increased aldosterone secretion and low plasma renin activity relieved by dexamethasone. *Can Med Assoc J* 1966;95(22):1109–19.

15. Pascoe L, Jeunemaitre X, Lebrethon MC et al. Glucocorticoid-suppressible hyperaldosteronism and adrenal tumors occurring in a single French pedigree. *J Clin Invest* 1995;96(5):2236–46.

16. Muller J, Lauber M. Regulation of aldosterone biosynthesis: A continual challenge. *Am J Hypertens* 1991;4(3 Pt 1):280–2.

17. Muller J. Final steps of aldosterone biosynthesis: Molecular solution of a physiological problem. *J Steroid Biochem Mol Biol* 1993;45(1–3):153–9.

18. Curnow KM, Tusie-Luna MT, Pascoe L et al. The product of the CYP11B2 gene is required for aldosterone biosynthesis in the human adrenal cortex. *Mol Endocrinol* 1991;5(10):1513–22.

19. Russell DW, White PC. Four is not more than two. *Am J Hum Genet* 1995;57(5):1002–5.

20. Martinez-Aguayo A, Fardella C. Genetics of hypertensive syndrome. *Horm Res* 2009;71(5):253–9.

21. Funder JW. Aldosterone and mineralocorticoid receptors: Orphan questions. *Kidney Int* 2000;57(4):1358–63.

22. Sheppard KE, Funder JW. Equivalent affinity of aldosterone and corticosterone for type I receptors in kidney and hippocampus: Direct binding studies. *J Steroid Biochem* 1987;28(6):737–42.

23. Funder JW. Apparent mineralocorticoid excess. *Endocrinol Metab Clin North Am* 1995;24(3):613–21.

24. Yoon SS, Burt V, Louis T, Carroll MD. Hypertension among adults in the United States, 2009–2010. Hyattsville, MD: National Center for Health Statistics, 2012.

25. Fardella CE, Mosso L, Gómez-Sánchez C et al. Primary hyperaldosteronism in essential hypertensives: Prevalence, biochemical profile, and molecular biology. *J Clin Endocrinol Metab* 2000;85(5):1863–7.

26. Gordon RD, Stowasser M, Tunny TJ, Klemm SA, Rutherford JC. High incidence of primary aldosteronism in 199 patients referred with hypertension. *Clin Exp Pharmacol Physiol* 1994;21(4):315–8.

27. Grim CE, Weinberger MH, Higgins JT, Kramer NJ. Diagnosis of secondary forms of hypertension. A comprehensive protocol. *JAMA* 1977;237(13):1331–5.

28. Hamlet SM, Tunny TJ, Woodland E, Gordon RD. Is aldosterone/renin ratio useful to screen a hypertensive population for primary aldosteronism? *Clin Exp Pharmacol Physiol* 1985;12(3):249–52.

29. Young WF. Primary aldosteronism: Renaissance of a syndrome. *Clin Endocrinol (Oxf)* 2007;66(5):607–18.

30. Mulatero P, Stowasser M, Loh KC et al. Increased diagnosis of primary aldosteronism, including surgically correctable forms, in centers from five continents. *J Clin Endocrinol Metab* 2004;89(3):1045–50.

31. Douma S, Petidis K, Doumas M et al. Prevalence of primary hyperaldosteronism in resistant hypertension: A retrospective observational study. *Lancet* 2008;371(9628):1921–6.

32. Mosso L, Carvajal C, Gonzalez A et al. Primary aldosteronism and hypertensive disease. *Hypertension* 2003;42(2):161–5.

33. Milliez P, Girerd X, Plouin PF, Blacher J, Safar ME, Mourad JJ. Evidence for an increased rate of cardiovascular events in patients with primary aldosteronism. *J Am Coll Cardiol* 2005;45(8):1243–8.

34. Giacchetti G, Ronconi V, Turchi F et al. Aldosterone as a key mediator of the cardiometabolic syndrome in primary aldosteronism: An observational study. *J Hypertens* 2007;25(1):177–86.

35. Rossi G, Boscaro M, Ronconi V, Funder JW. Aldosterone as a cardiovascular risk factor. *Trends Endocrinol Metab* 2005;16(3):104–7.

36. Giacchetti G, Sechi LA, Rilli S, Carey RM. The renin-angiotensin-aldosterone system, glucose metabolism and diabetes. *Trends Endocrinol Metab* 2005;16(3):120–6.

37. Tunny TJ, Klemm SA, Gordon RD. Some aldosterone-producing adrenal tumours also secrete cortisol, but present clinically as primary aldosteronism. *Clin Exp Pharmacol Physiol* 1990;17(3):167–71.

38. Schirpenbach C, Reincke M. Primary aldosteronism: Current knowledge and controversies in Conn's syndrome. *Nat Clin Pract Endocrinol Metab* 2007;3(3):220–7.

39. Funder JW. Genetics of primary aldosteronism. *Front Horm Res* 2014;43:70–8.

40. Torpy DJ, Stratakis CA, Gordon RD. Linkage analysis of familial hyperaldosteronism type II—Absence of linkage to the gene encoding the angiotensin II receptor type 1. *J Clin Endocrinol Metab* 1998;83(3):1046.

41. Xekouki P, Hatch MM, Lin L et al. KCNJ5 mutations in the National Institutes of Health cohort of patients with primary hyperaldosteronism: An infrequent genetic cause of Conn's syndrome. *Endocr Relat Cancer* 2012;19(3):255–60.

42. Choi M, Scholl UI, Yue P et al. K+ channel mutations in adrenal aldosterone-producing adenomas and hereditary hypertension. *Science* 2011;331(6018):768–72.

43. Stowasser M, Gordon RD, Tunny TJ, Klemm SA, Finn WL, Krek AL. Familial hyperaldosteronism type II: Five families with a new variety of primary aldosteronism. *Clin Exp Pharmacol Physiol* 1992;19(5):319–22.

44. Gordon RD, Klemm SA, Tunny TJ, Stowasser M. Primary aldosteronism: Hypertension with a genetic basis. *Lancet* 1992;340(8812):159–61.

45. Gordon RD, Stowasser M, Klemm SA, Tunny TJ. Primary aldosteronism—Some genetic, morphological, and biochemical aspects of subtypes. *Steroids* 1995;60(1):35–41.

46. Taymans SE, Pack S, Pak E, Torpy DJ, Zhuang Z, Stratakis CA. Human CYP11B2 (aldosterone synthase) maps to chromosome 8q24.3. *J Clin Endocrinol Metab* 1998;83(3):1033–6.

47. Torpy DJ, Gordon RD, Lin JP et al. Familial hyperaldosteronism type II: Description of a large kindred and exclusion of the aldosterone synthase (CYP11B2) gene. *J Clin Endocrinol Metab* 1998;83(9):3214–8.

48. Lafferty AR, Torpy DJ, Stowasser M et al. A novel genetic locus for low renin hypertension: Familial hyperaldosteronism type II maps to chromosome 7 (7p22). *J Med Genet* 2000;37(11):831–5.

49. Kotchen TA, Lytton B, Morrow LB, Mulrow PJ, Shutkin PM, Stansel HC. Angiotensin and aldosterone in renovascular hypertension. *Arch Intern Med* 1970;125(2):265–72.

50. Cheung KL, Lafayette RA. Renal physiology of pregnancy. *Adv Chronic Kidney Dis* 2013;20(3):209–14.

51. Conn JW, Cohen EL, Lucas CP et al. Primary reninism. Hypertension, hyperreninemia, and secondary aldosteronism due to renin-producing juxtaglomerular cell tumors. *Arch Intern Med* 1972;130(5):682–96.

52. Dzau VJ, Colucci WS, Hollenberg NK, Williams GH. Relation of the renin-angiotensin-aldosterone system to clinical state in congestive heart failure. *Circulation* 1981;63(3):645–51.

53. Cerame BI, New MI. Hormonal hypertension in children: 11beta-Hydroxylase deficiency and apparent mineralocorticoid excess. *J Pediatr Endocrinol Metab* 2000;13(9):1537–47.

54. Miller WL. Steroid 17alpha-hydroxylase deficiency—Not rare everywhere. *J Clin Endocrinol Metab* 2004;89(1):40–2.

55. Charmandari E, Kino T, Ichijo T, Chrousos GP. Generalized glucocorticoid resistance: Clinical aspects, molecular mechanisms, and implications of a rare genetic disorder. *J Clin Endocrinol Metab* 2008;93(5):1563–72.

56. Dave-Sharma S, Wilson RC, Harbison MD et al. Examination of genotype and phenotype relationships in 14 patients with apparent mineralocorticoid excess. *J Clin Endocrinol Metab* 1998;83(7):2244–54.

57. Irony I, Biglieri EG, Perloff D, Rubinoff H. Pathophysiology of deoxycorticosterone-secreting adrenal tumors. *J Clin Endocrinol Metab* 1987;65(5):836–40.

58. Palmer BF, Alpern RJ. Liddle's syndrome. *Am J Med* 1998;104(3):301–9.

59. Farese RV Jr, Biglieri EG, Shackleton CH, Irony I, Gomez-Fontes R. Licorice-induced hypermineralocorticoidism. *N Engl J Med* 1991;325(17):1223–7.

60. Ullian ME, Hazen-Martin DJ, Walsh LG, Davda RK, Egan BM. Carbenoxolone damages endothelium and enhances vasoconstrictor action in aortic rings. *Hypertension* 1996;27(6):1346–52.

61. Benchetrit S, Bernheim J, Podjarny E. Normokalemic hyperaldosteronism in patients with resistant hypertension. *Isr Med Assoc J* 2002;4(1):17–20.

62. Calhoun DA, Nishizaka MK, Zaman MA, Thakkar RB, Weissmann P. Hyperaldosteronism among black and white subjects with resistant hypertension. *Hypertension* 2002;40(6):892–6.

63. Nieman LK. Approach to the patient with an adrenal incidentaloma. *J Clin Endocrinol Metab* 2010;95(9):4106–13.

64. Aso Y, Homma Y. A survey on incidental adrenal tumors in Japan. *J Urol* 1992;147(6):1478–81.

65. Mantero F, Terzolo M, Arnaldi G et al. A survey on adrenal incidentaloma in Italy. Study Group on Adrenal Tumors of the Italian Society of Endocrinology. *J Clin Endocrinol Metab* 2000;85(2):637–44.

66. Schwartz GL, Turner ST. Screening for primary aldosteronism in essential hypertension: Diagnostic accuracy of the ratio of plasma aldosterone concentration to plasma renin activity. *Clin Chem* 2005;51(2):386–94.

67. Montori VM, Young WF Jr. Use of plasma aldosterone concentration-to-plasma renin activity ratio as a screening test for primary aldosteronism. A systematic review of the literature. *Endocrinol Metab Clin North Am* 2002;31(3):619–32.

68. Tanabe A, Naruse M, Takagi S, Tsuchiya K, Imaki T, Takano K. Variability in the renin/aldosterone profile under random and standardized sampling conditions in primary aldosteronism. *J Clin Endocrinol Metab* 2003;88(6):2489–94.

69. Hiramatsu K, Yamada T, Yukimura Y et al. A screening test to identify aldosterone-producing adenoma by measuring plasma renin activity. Results in hypertensive patients. *Arch Intern Med* 1981;141(12):1589–93.

70. Mulatero P, Rabbia F, Milan A et al. Drug effects on aldosterone/plasma renin activity ratio in primary aldosteronism. *Hypertension* 2002;40(6):897–902.

71. Giacchetti G, Ronconi V, Lucarelli G, Boscaro M, Mantero F. Analysis of screening and confirmatory tests in the diagnosis of primary aldosteronism: Need for a standardized protocol. *J Hypertens* 2006;24(4):737–45.

72. Rossi GP, Belfiore A, Bernini G et al. Prospective evaluation of the saline infusion test for excluding primary aldosteronism due to aldosterone-producing adenoma. *J Hypertens* 2007;25(7):1433–42.

73. Kem DC, Weinberger MH, Mayes DM, Nugent CA. Saline suppression of plasma aldosterone in hypertension. *Arch Intern Med* 1971;128(3):380–6.

74. Mantero F, Fallo F, Opocher G, Armanini D, Boscaro M, Scaroni C. Effect of angiotensin II and converting enzyme inhibitor (captopril) on blood pressure, plasma renin activity and aldosterone in primary aldosteronism. *Clin Sci (Lond)* 1981;61(Suppl 7):289s–93s.

75. Agharazii M, Douville P, Grose JH, Lebel M. Captopril suppression versus salt loading in confirming primary aldosteronism. *Hypertension* 2001;37(6):1440–3.

76. Rossi GP, Belfiore A, Bernini G et al. Comparison of the captopril and the saline infusion test for excluding aldosterone-producing adenoma. *Hypertension* 2007;50(2):424–31.

77. Mulatero P, Bertello C, Garrone C et al. Captopril test can give misleading results in patients with suspect primary aldosteronism. *Hypertension* 2007;50(2):e26–7.

78. Gordon RD. Mineralocorticoid hypertension. *Lancet* 1994;344(8917):240–3.

79. Young WF Jr. Clinical practice. The incidentally discovered adrenal mass. *N Engl J Med* 2007;356(6):601–10.

80. Nwariaku FE, Miller BS, Auchus R et al. Primary hyperaldosteronism: Effect of adrenal vein sampling on surgical outcome. *Arch Surg* 2006;141(5):497–502; discussion 502–3.

81. Young WF, Stanson AW, Thompson GB, Grant CS, Farley DR, van Heerden JA. Role for adrenal venous sampling in primary aldosteronism. *Surgery* 2004;136(6):1227–35.

82. Doppman JL, Gill JR Jr. Hyperaldosteronism: Sampling the adrenal veins. *Radiology* 1996;198(2):309–12.

83. Dunnick NR, Doppman JL, Mills SR, Gill JR Jr. Preoperative diagnosis and localization of aldosteronomas by measurement of corticosteroids in adrenal venous blood. *Radiology* 1979;133(2):331–3.

84. Daunt N. Adrenal vein sampling: How to make it quick, easy, and successful. *Radiographics* 2005;25(Suppl 1):S143–58.

85. McMahon GT, Dluhy RG. Glucocorticoid-remediable aldosteronism. *Cardiol Rev* 2004;12(1):44–8.

86. Dluhy RG, Anderson B, Harlin B, Ingelfinger J, Lifton R. Glucocorticoid-remediable aldosteronism is associated with severe hypertension in early childhood. *J Pediatr* 2001;138(5):715–20.

87. Litchfield WR, Anderson BF, Weiss RJ, Lifton RP, Dluhy RG. Intracranial aneurysm and hemorrhagic stroke in glucocorticoid-remediable aldosteronism. *Hypertension* 1998;31(1 Pt 2):445–50.

88. Fardella CE, Pinto M, Mosso L, Gomez-Sanchez C, Jalil J, Montero J. Genetic study of patients with dexamethasone-suppressible aldosteronism without the chimeric CYP11B1/CYP11B2 gene. *J Clin Endocrinol Metab* 2001;86(10):4805–7.

89. So A, Duffy DL, Gordon RD et al. Familial hyperaldosteronism type II is linked to the chromosome 7p22 region but also shows predicted heterogeneity. *J Hypertens* 2005;23(8):1477–84.

90. Mulatero P, Monticone S, Rainey WE, Veglio F, Williams TA. Role of KCNJ5 in familial and sporadic primary aldosteronism. *Nat Rev Endocrinol* 2013;9(2):104–12.

91. Monticone S, Hattangady NG, Penton D et al. A novel Y152C KCNJ5 mutation responsible for familial hyperaldosteronism type III. *J Clin Endocrinol Metab* 2013;98(11):E1861–5.

92. Meyer A, Brabant G, Behrend M. Long-term follow-up after adrenalectomy for primary aldosteronism. *World J Surg* 2005;29(2):155–9.

93. Sawka AM, Young WF, Thompson GB et al. Primary aldosteronism: Factors associated with normalization of blood pressure after surgery. *Ann Intern Med* 2001;135(4):258–61.

94. Young WF Jr. Primary aldosteronism—Treatment options. *Growth Horm IGF Res* 2003;13(Suppl A):S102–8.

95. Young WF Jr. Minireview: Primary aldosteronism—changing concepts in diagnosis and treatment. *Endocrinology* 2003;144(6):2208–13.

96. Iwakura Y, Morimoto R, Kudo M et al. Predictors of decreasing glomerular filtration rate and prevalence of chronic kidney disease after treatment of primary aldosteronism: Renal outcome of 213 cases. *J Clin Endocrinol Metab* 2014;99(5):1593–8.

Neuroblastoma

MARCUS M. MALEK

BACKGROUND

Neuroblastoma is an embryonal tumor of the sympathetic nervous system that arises from neural crest cells. It is the most common solid extracranial malignancy of childhood and the most common malignant tumor of infants. Most cases occur under 1 year of age, with a median age of detection of 22 months. Neuroblastoma accounts for 8% of all childhood cancers diagnosed under 15 years of age and has been showing an increasing incidence. There are about 700 new cases annually in the United States. Fifteen percent of pediatric cancer deaths can be attributed to neuroblastoma, which is a disproportionately high mortality compared with the incidence. This can be explained by the poor survival in the high-risk group. Low- and intermediate-risk groups, on the other hand, have an excellent survival, leading to a push to decrease intensity of therapy for these groups. With less therapy, the low and intermediate groups have still had excellent outcomes. There is a slight male preponderance in neuroblastoma, with a male-to-female ratio of 1.3:1.

The presentation of neuroblastoma is variable, but it will most often present with a palpable mass. Stage IV disease can present with fever, weight loss, and significant systemic illness. If there are metastases to bone, anemia from marrow involvement may be the presenting symptom. Bone pain may occur when there is cortical bone involvement. A rare finding that may be the presenting symptom of neuroblastoma is opsoclonus–myoclonus. This finding consists of horizontal nystagmus and clonic movements of the extremity. Opsoclonus–myoclonus occurs secondary to antibodies that form against the tumor that cross-react and cause opsoclonus, myoclonus, ataxia, and sleep disturbance. It is important to counsel families that even if the child is able to achieve remission, these symptoms remain because the antibodies will still exist. Therapeutic benefit has been described with steroids, intravenous immunoglobulin, cyclophosphamide, azathioprine, and rituximab [1].

Periorbital ecchymoses and proptosis result from metastatic disease to the bones of the orbit. These findings may be the presenting signs of metastatic neuroblastoma.

Neuroblastoma can arise from anywhere in the body, along the migration of neural crest cells or where they ultimately reside during development. This includes the posterior mediastinum, the pelvis (arising from the organ of Zuckerkandl), the retroperitoneum, and the adrenal gland. The retroperitoneum, specifically the adrenal gland, accounts for a majority of the disease; however, about 20% will develop in the mediastinum.

DIAGNOSTIC TESTING

The diagnosis of neuroblastoma should be considered in any child with an abdominal mass. Once the tumor is suspected, the workup will include blood and urine testing, bone marrow biopsy, imaging including computed tomography (CT) or MRI, and methyl-iodo-benzylguanidine (MIBG) scan. Laboratory testing for confirmation should include urinary catecholamine levels, CBC to look for anemia, and a serum ferritin. Serum ferritin levels often correlate with disease severity, whereby elevated ferritin levels of >150 are seen with high-risk disease [2]. A CT scan or MRI from the head to pelvis is important to identify the primary tumor, as well as any metastatic disease, if present. A critical factor to consider when evaluating the primary tumor is its relationship to the major vasculature. The International Neuroblastoma Risk Group (INRG) staging system utilizes a list of image-defined risk factors (IDRFs) to standardize communication about the tumor. Although not currently used by the Children's Oncology Group (COG) for planning therapy, the INRG may also be utilized as a guide for treatment and as a staging system. COG is currently investigating the use of IDRFs for this purpose [3] (Table 31.1). Assessment of the bone marrow via bone marrow biopsy is also important for defining the extent of disease. MIBG scan is an excellent study for identifying the primary tumor and metastatic sites of disease. Although an MIBG scan will identify bone marrow disease, a bone scan will be required to visualize cortical bone disease.

At completion of the workup, the patient will be designated as having either locoregional or stage IV disease. If the disease is locoregional, it is up to the surgeon's discretion to decide if the disease is amenable to a gross total resection (GTR) up front, or if the first operation should be a limited biopsy. As we review the risk groups, we will demonstrate that this decision will change the stage and therefore the risk grouping, which in turn will decide what further therapy, if any, will be required. If the patient has stage IV disease, the patient has systemic disease and the most important primary goal is to obtain tissue to confirm diagnosis so that chemotherapy can be initiated as soon as possible. Although the diagnosis can be confirmed based on catecholamines and bone marrow biopsy alone, it is important to biopsy the tumor for biological studies that require at least 1 cm^3 of tissue (*MYCN* and ALK). Core biopsies are acceptable but not recommended because multiple passes would be required to obtain the 1 cm^3 required, and it may be tougher to do adequate studies. In the rare case where the patient has stage IV disease and a GTR requires little more effort than the biopsy, it can be considered up front, but any attempt at a more complete resection should not increase morbidity in any way that would delay the start of chemotherapy. After initial surgery and review by pathology, a stage and risk designation can be assigned. This will determine therapy and prognosis [4] (Tables 31.2 and 31.3).

The prognosis is based on both clinical and biological factors. The clinical factors are tumor stage and patient age. The biological factors are *MYCN* amplification, tumor histology, and DNA ploidy. By far the most important of the biological factors is the *MYCN* status. The combination of these factors will assign a risk group, which will dictate therapy and prognosis.

RISK FACTORS

Age

It is well established that patients diagnosed in infancy have a better prognosis [5]. Schmidt et al. in 2005 reviewed all stage IV patients from Children's Cancer Group (CCG) protocols 321P2 (1986–1991) and 3891 (1991–1996), looking specifically at patients diagnosed in the second year of life to compare the group diagnosed between 12 and 18 months with those diagnosed between 18 and 24 months. They found a significantly improved event-free survival (EFS) and overall survival (OS) in patients diagnosed before 18 months [6]. Based on this observation, age less than 18 months is considered a positive prognostic factor and has a dramatic impact on risk grouping. For example, patients with stage IV tumors and favorable biology who are younger than 18 months old are actually considered intermediate risk, whereas the same patient diagnosed at older than 18 months is considered high risk.

Stage

Staging of neuroblastoma is based on the degree of surgical resection (Table 31.2). The downside to this staging system is that the degree of resection is determined not only by the tumor, but also by the result of surgery, and therefore is more difficult to standardize. In an effort to make the staging more uniform, IDRFs are now being used to assess tumors prior to any therapy (Table 31.1). Staging based on IDRFs will allow for more uniform preoperative staging,

Table 31.1 Image defined risk factors by body location

Objective surgical risk factors for primary resection of localized neuroblastoma

Neck

1. Tumor encasing major vessel(s) (e.g., carotid artery, vertebral artery, internal jugular vein)
2. Tumor extending to base of skull
3. Tumor compressing the trachea
4. Tumor encasing the brachial plexus

Thorax

1. Tumor encasing major vessel(s) (e.g., subclavian vessels, aorta, superior vena cava)
2. Tumor compressing the trachea or principal bronchi
3. Lower mediastinal tumor, infiltrating the costo-vertebral junction between T9 and T12 (may involve the artery of Adamkiewicz perfusing the lower spinal cord)

Abdomen

1. Tumor infiltrating the porta hepatis and/or the hepatoduodenal ligament
2. Tumor encasing the origin of the celiac axis, and/or the superior mesenteric artery
3. Tumor invading one or both renal pedicles
4. Tumor encasing the aorta and/or vena cava
5. Tumor encasing the iliac vessels
6. Pelvic tumor crossing the sciatic notch

Source: Data from Davidoff AM. *Semin Pediatr Surg* 2012; 21:2–14.

Table 31.2 International Neuroblastoma Staging System

1	Localized tumor with complete gross excision, with or without microscopic residual disease; representative ipsilateral lymph nodes negative for tumor microscopically (nodes attached to and removed with primary tumor may be positive).
2A	Localized tumor with incomplete gross excision; representative ipsilateral nonadherent lymph nodes negative for tumor microscopically.
2B	Localized tumor with or without complete gross excision, with ipsilateral nonadherent lymph nodes positive for tumor. Enlarged contralateral lymph nodes must be negative microscopically.
3	Unresectable unilateral tumor infiltrating across the midline,[a] with or without regional lymph node involvement; or localized unilateral tumor with contralateral regional lymph node involvement; or midline tumor with bilateral extension by infiltration (unresectable) or by lymph node involvement
4	Any primary tumor with dissemination to distant lymph nodes, bone marrow, bone, liver, skin and/or other organs (except as defined for stage 4[S])
4S	Localized primary tumor (as defined for stage 1 and 2[A], or 2[B]), with dissemination limited to skin, liver and/or bone marrow[b] (limited to infants <1 year of age).

Source: Data from Davidoff AM. *Semin Pediatr Surg* 2012;21:2–14.
Note: The MIBG scan (if performed) should be negative in the marrow.
[a] The midline is defined as the vertebral column. Tumors originating on one side and crossing the midline must infiltrate to or beyond the opposite side of the vertebral column.
[b] Marrow involvement in stage 4(S) should be minimal, that is, <10% of total nucleated cells identified as malignant on bone marrow biopsy or on marrow aspirate. More extensive marrow involvement would be considered stage.

Table 31.3 Children's Oncology Group risk stratification for children with neuroblastoma

Risk stratification	INSS stage	Age	Biology
Low			
Group 1			
	1	Any	Any
	2A/2B (>50% resected)	Any	MYCN-NA, any histology/ploidy
	4S	<365 days	MYCN-NA, FH, DI > 1
Intermediate			
Group 2			
	2A/2B (<50% resected or Bx only)	0–12 years	MYCN-NA, any histology/ploidy[a]
	3	<365 days	MYCN-NA, FH, DI > 1[a]
	3	>365 days – 12 years	MYCN-NA, FH[a]
	4S (symptomatic)	<365 days	MYCN-NA, FH, DI > 1[a]
Group 3			
	3	<365 days	MYCN-NA, either UH or DI = 1[a]
	4	<365 days	MYCN-NA, FH, DI > 1[a]
	4S	<365 days	MYCN-NA, either UH or DI = 1[a]; or unknown biology
Group 4			
	4	<365 days	MYCN-NA, either DI = 1 or UH
	3	365 – < 547 days	MYCN-NA, UH, any ploidy
	4	365 – < 547 days	MYCN-NA, FH, DI > 1
High			
	2A/2B, 3, 4, 4S	Any	MYCN-amplified, any histology/ploidy
	3	>547 days	MYCN-NA, UH, any ploidy
	4	365 – >547 days	MYCN-NA, UH or DI = 1
	4	>547 days	Any

Source: Data from Davidoff AM. *Semin Pediatr Surg* 2012;21:2–14.
Note: DI, DNA index; FH, favorable histology; *MYCN*-NA, *MYCN* not amplified; UH, unfavorable histology.
[a] If tumor contains chromosomal 1p LOH or unb11qLOH, or if data are missing, treatment assignment is upgraded to next group.

which in combination with other clinical and biological factors will assign a risk group that then will direct therapy. Primary tumors are considered L1 if they have no evidence of IDRFs and L2 if IDRFs are present (Table 31.1). Patients with metastatic disease are considered to have stage M disease. Patients that would have been considered stage IV-S in the INSS are now considered stage M-S in the INRG staging system.

The downside of image-defined risk grouping is that a tumor with IDRFs may still be eligible for up-front resection, particularly for a surgeon with a high level of comfort with aggressive neuroblastoma. Clearly, there are advantages to both staging systems, and the COG is currently studying the benefits of using IDRFs.

MYCN

In neuroblastoma, the tumor behavior is very dependent on its biology. The clearest example of this is the aggressive nature of tumors that show *MYCN* amplification. *MYCN* amplification is defined by greater than 10 copies of the gene per cell. *MYCN* resides on the distal short arm of chromosome 2 (2p24). About 25% of primary neuroblastomas demonstrate *MYCN* amplification. Some patients that would otherwise be considered to have low-risk disease can be upgraded to high-risk disease simply by the presence of *MYCN* amplification in the primary tumor (i.e., stage IIA tumor in a baby less than 18 months old).

The histopathology of neuroblastoma, as defined by the International Neuroblastoma Pathology Classification (INPC) system, also known as the Shimada classification, also plays a role in determining how aggressive the tumor is [7]. The Shimada classification evaluates the tumor specimen, before treatment, for the amount of Schwannian stroma, the degree of neuroblastic maturation, and the mitosis–karyorrhexis index. Combining these features with patient age, the Shimada classification determines whether the histology is favorable or unfavorable, which has an effect on risk grouping and prognosis. The Shimada classification also places the tumor into one of four subtypes of neurogenic tumors. Neuroblastoma is stroma poor, ganglioneuroma is stroma dominant, and ganglioneuroblastoma can be either intermixed or nodular, both of which are stroma rich, with the nodular type having some areas that are stroma poor.

TREATMENT

Treatment for neuroblastoma is dependent on the risk group of the patient. As previously described, the risk group of the patient is determined on the patient age at diagnosis, the biology of the tumor (*MYCN*, DNA ploidy, and histology), and the stage of the tumor (Table 31.3).

Low-risk disease

Patients with low-risk disease have an excellent prognosis, with a 95%–100% EFS. These patients typically require surgical resection alone, followed by observation. These patients do so well that a recent COG study looked to identify a subset of patients that would require observation alone. This group was selected in part due to the excellent outcomes of patients with low-risk disease, in addition to a Japanese screening program that identified adrenal tumors in the perinatal period and followed them. The screening program led to a higher incidence of diagnosing neuroblastoma, but there was a very high rate of spontaneous regression, and despite the increased incidence found with the screening program, there was no change seen in the rate of mortality from neuroblastoma [8–10].

The COG perinatal neuroblastoma study (ANBL00P2), published in 2012, established that observation with serial imaging is all that is required for a subset of patients diagnosed prenatally or under the age of 6 months. The tumor should be localized to the adrenal gland as identified on cross-sectional imaging and MIBG scan. A baseline ultrasound is also done at the same time, so that the tumor can be followed with ultrasound. To be eligible for observation, the tumor must have a volume of less than 16 mL (about a 3 cm sphere) if completely solid, and less than 64 mL (about a 5 cm sphere) if at least 25% cystic. Patients are removed from observation if they show a greater than 50% increase in tumor size or homovanillic acid (HVA) and vanillylmandelic acid (VMA) levels that increase by more than 50% and remain elevated for 12 weeks. The results of this study showed that 81% of enrolled patients were spared a resection. OS was 100% with an EFS of 95%. The events were progression of neuroblastoma in two patients and two adrenal cortical neoplasms. All four cases necessitated surgery, but all survived [11].

The encouraging results of the perinatal neuroblastoma study have led the COG to open protocol ANBL1232, which is currently enrolling patients. This study will examine expanding the criteria for observation.

Infants with stage IV-S disease represent a very interesting subset of patients with neuroblastoma because although they have metastatic disease, their disease is typically nonaggressive. These infants have a localized tumor with metastases limited to skin, liver, and bone marrow. Less than 10% of the bone marrow should be involved, which means the bone marrow must be negative on MIBG scan. A greater degree of bone marrow involvement would upstage the infant to stage IV disease. Diagnostic workup should proceed as with any other stage of neuroblastoma, but the primary tumor usually does not need to be biopsied, as the diagnosis can be confirmed on bone marrow biopsy and lab testing. If skin lesions are present, these blue-gray lesions (Figure 31.1) are also usually biopsied, as they are very easily accessible [12]. Most patients are asymptomatic and will require only observation with supportive care. Some infants may develop organ dysfunction from the mass effect of the primary tumor or metastases. These patients should receive chemotherapy to control the symptoms, with surgery reserved for abdominal compartment syndrome, or to decompress the spinal cord, if necessary. Resection of the

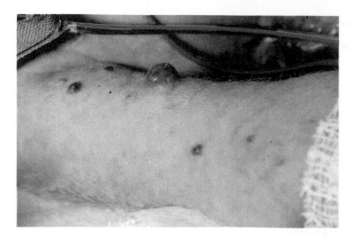

Figure 31.1 Typical blueberry skin lesion in stage IV-S neuroblastoma. (Reprinted from Auckland District Health Board, Neuroblastoma, 2011, http://www.adhb. govt.nz/newborn/TeachingResources/Dermatology/ Neuroblastoma/Neuroblastoma.jpg.)

primary has not been associated with improved outcomes [13–15]. Infants in the first month of life can potentially deteriorate quickly, so chemotherapy should be considered in this very young group as well. About 8%–10% of infants with stage IV-S disease are *MYCN* amplified. These infants are considered to have high-risk disease and receive multimodal therapy as any other high-risk patient.

Intermediate-risk disease

Intermediate-risk disease also has an excellent prognosis, with an EFS of at least 85%–90%. This group will typically receive chemotherapy before or after resection. If up-front resection appears difficult, a biopsy is obtained and chemotherapy is given. After chemotherapy, a GTR of all residual disease should be performed. The most common chemotherapy regimen for intermediate-risk disease includes cyclophosphamide, etoposide, doxorubicin, and carboplatin [16].

High-risk disease

As we discussed, the survival for low- and intermediate-risk neuroblastoma is excellent. We have seen these patients do so well that most of the recent COG efforts have been directed toward minimizing therapy for these patients. Secondary to these efforts, we have seen more patients meet criteria for observation with no treatment. Unfortunately, patients with high-risk disease have a significantly worse prognosis. Despite massive efforts by pediatric oncologists, pediatric surgeons, and the COG, the survival for high-risk neuroblastoma is still only around 50% [17]. These efforts have not been without benefit, as reported survival was previously closer to 10%–30%. This observed survival improvement can be attributed to multiple factors, including more aggressive surgery to obtain a GTR, hematopoietic stem cell transplant (HSCT), antibody therapy, and

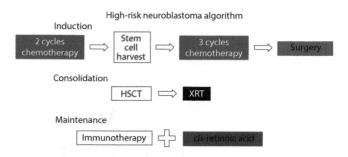

Figure 31.2 General treatment algorithm for high-risk neuroblastoma. XRT, external beam radiation therapy.

cis-retinoic acid. Each patient's treatment algorithm will be slightly different, but the general treatment algorithm can be seen in Figure 31.2.

INDUCTION

Induction includes chemotherapy and surgery. After several cycles of chemotherapy, the tumor will usually shrink significantly. In the case of retroperitoneal neuroblastoma, despite a good response, the tumor will typically still remain intimately involved with the aorta or the inferior vena cava and its visceral branches. The goal of surgery should be to obtain a GTR, which can be defined as the removal of all visible and palpable tumor from the primary site and regional lymphatics. The role of a GTR in high-risk neuroblastoma has been an issue of debate for many years, but at present, a GTR is the standard of care. In fact, all high-risk COG protocols include a GTR as part of induction therapy. A large review of the Memorial Sloan Kettering Cancer Center (MSKCC) experience clearly demonstrated a lower probability of local progression (Figure 31.3), as well as an

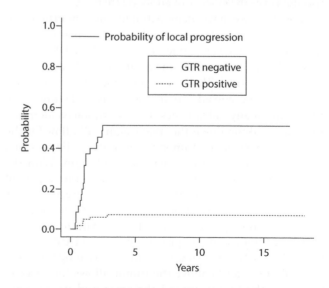

Figure 31.3 The probability of local progression in patients undergoing GTR compared with those who do not (*p* < 0.01). Gray's test was used to compare probabilities of local progression. (Reprinted with permission from La Quaglia MP et al. *J Pediatr Surg* 2004;39:412–417.)

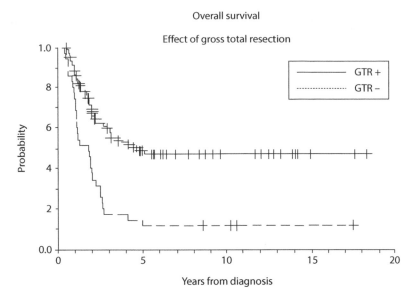

Overall survival

Effect of gross total resection

Figure 31.4 The OS rate of patients undergoing GTR compared with those who do not ($p < 0.01$). The Kaplan–Meier probability distributions were compared using the log-rank test. (Reprinted with permission from La Quaglia MP et al. *J Pediatr Surg* 2004;39:412–417.)

OS benefit (Figure 31.4) for patients undergoing a GTR, compared with those that underwent a less than complete resection [18].

Another study by Adkins and the CCG in 2004 showed that patients that underwent a complete resection also demonstrated an improved 5-year EFS without a significant difference in the complication rate [19]. Studies by the International Society of Paediatric Oncology Europe Neuroblastoma (SIOPEN) have demonstrated the benefit of GTR for neuroblastoma as well [20]. In addition to the survival benefit, we believe that reducing the tumor burden also improves the efficacy of antibody therapy.

Now that we have demonstrated the importance of a GTR, it is important to emphasize the planning and approach to these very difficult tumors. To safely remove tumor that is encasing the major abdominal vasculature, exposure is critical. That is why a thoracoabdominal incision should be considered in these cases (Figure 31.5). There are many advantages to the thoracoabdominal approach. Taking down the diaphragm will allow for the superior aspect of the tumor to be more easily accessed without having to work under the diaphragm. With the diaphragm open, the chest cavity now becomes a part of your working space, again allowing you greater access to the tumor. The lateral position places the aorta in the forefront of the operative field, allowing you to control it above the tumor, and also providing excellent access to the visceral branches, which are usually encased by the mass. Control of the aorta above the tumor allows the surgeon to bivalve the tumor around the aorta and its branches to protect those vessels. This approach also allows you to easily work behind the kidney and renal vessels, where you almost invariably find a significant amount of tumor (Figure 31.6).

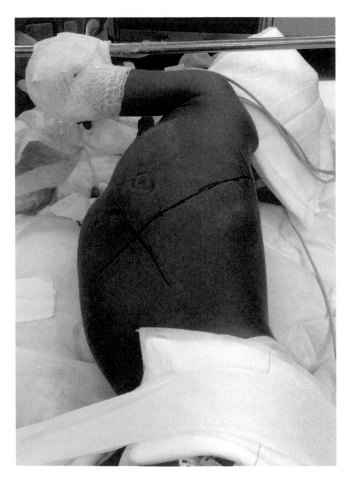

Figure 31.5 Thoracoabdominal incision. In addition to the axillary roll, a bump is placed under the contralateral costal margin to open the rib spaces.

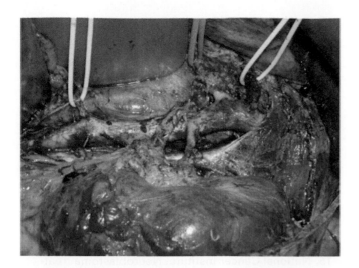

Figure 31.6 Exposure of aorta, celiac artery, superior mesenteric artery, inferior mesenteric artery, and renal vessels after dissection of tumor through a thoracoabdominal incision. (Reprinted with permission from Qureshi SS, Patil VP. *J Pediatr Surg* 2012;47:694–9.)

Thoracoabdominal incisions are well tolerated in children, and the recovery time is similar to that of a laparotomy. A chest tube is obviously required, but this usually can be removed within the first two or three postoperative days. The expected length of stay is about 7–10 days.

As previously discussed, the complication rate for GTR is not any higher than that for less complete resections [19]. Renal loss is among the worst complications, and is a risk because the renal vessels are almost invariably encased in the tumor. It is important to note, however, that renal loss can certainly be avoided and should be a rare event. In fact, renal loss was only identified in 5/141 patients (3.5%) in the MSKCC experience [18]. The exposure from a thoracoabdominal incision and the ability to work both in front of and behind the kidney provides the best chance to remove all tumor from the renal vessels and ureter without injury.

Chylous ascites is not uncommon but is rarely significant. High-volume chylous ascites can be avoided with liberal use of surgical clips.

Diarrhea is frequently observed after GTR, and can be seen in as many as 17%–30% of patients. The mechanism leading to diarrhea is unclear. It is hypothesized that disruption of the sympathetic nerve supply may attenuate the inhibition of peristalsis, while disruption of parasympathetic nerve fibers may lead to poor motility and bacterial overgrowth. A disturbance in gut hormone activity caused by disruption of autonomic fibers could also be a contributing factor [22].

CONSOLIDATION

After surgery, usually one or more cycles of chemotherapy are given, which completes induction. Consolidation begins with myeloablative chemotherapy and HSCT. The stem cells given are actually harvested from the patient during induction, typically after the second cycle of chemotherapy. Very

intense chemotherapy is given to eradicate minimal residual disease, but the bone marrow is also significantly affected. Autologous stem cells are given to repopulate the bone marrow after the myeloablative chemotherapy [16]. The benefit of HSCT has been demonstrated in several large randomized controlled studies. Collectively, the studies have shown a 3-year EFS in the HSCT group of 31%–47%, compared with a 3-year EFS in the conventional chemotherapy group of 22%–31% [23–25].

In 1999, Matthay and the CCG [23] published their series of 379 patients that were randomized to receive myeloablative chemotherapy with HSCT or continuation of standard chemotherapy, with a second randomization to either receive *cis*-retinoic acid or not. The results of this study showed a significant difference in EFS for each randomization. In 2009, Matthay and the COG again published on the long-term follow-up for these patients, which continued to show a significantly improved EFS for both myeloablative chemotherapy with HSCT and maintenance therapy with *cis*-retinoic acid.

The next treatment strategy in the consolidation phase is radiation therapy. Radiation is aimed at the primary tumor site and any area that is persistently MIBG positive. Radiation can be given before, during, or after myeloablative therapy; however, it is typically given after due to concern that radiation may have a negative effect on stem cell engraftment. Radiation may also be aimed at sites of metastatic disease, but this is determined on an individual case basis.

MAINTENANCE

A lot of progress has been made in the maintenance phase of high-risk neuroblastoma treatment. Differentiation therapy with *cis*-retinoic and immunotherapy are the critical elements of the maintenance phase.

As mentioned previously, multiple studies have shown that differentiation therapy with *cis*-retinoic acid has an independent effect on increasing OS and EFS in high-risk neuroblastoma. In fact, when looking at patients that receive HSCT, those that also received *cis*-retinoic acid during the maintenance phase of therapy had a 59% OS, compared with only 41% in those that did not receive *cis*-retinoic acid [23,25].

Immunotherapy is given along with differentiation therapy. Antibodies have been developed to target GD2, which is present on the surface of neuroblastoma cells, and targeted therapy against this receptor has been shown to have a significant effect on survival, with a 2-year EFS of 66% vs. 46% in the group that received standard therapy without immunotherapy. It is important to note that patients can have fairly significant systemic responses to the immunotherapy and should be monitored closely during infusion [26,27].

NEW TREATMENT STRATEGIES

MIBG therapy utilizes the excellent uptake of the radiotracer to deliver radioactive ^{131}I-MIBG or ^{125}I-MIBG. Currently, its use is limited to patients with refractory tumors; however, in this subset, MIBG therapy has shown some promise with response rates approaching 33% [28]. In addition to treating refractory tumors, a recent study has shown a trend toward increased OS in older patients with neuroblastoma treated with MIBG therapy and in ultra-high-risk neuroblastoma, which are those with expected survival of less than 15% [29].

Multiple other modalities are currently under study, including angiogenesis inhibition, ALK inhibition, tyrosine kinase inhibition, tubulin binding agents, and epigenetic targeting.

REFERENCES

1. Pike M. Opsoclonus-myoclonus syndrome. *Handb Clin Neurol* 2013;112:1209–11.
2. Lau L. Neuroblastoma: A single institution's experience with 128 children and an evaluation of clinical and biological prognostic factors. *Pediatr Hematol Oncol* 2002l;19:79–89.
3. Monclair T, Brodeur GM, Ambros PF et al. The International Neuroblastoma Risk Group (INRG) staging system: An INRG task force report. *J Clin Oncol* 2009;27:298–303.
4. Davidoff AM. Neuroblastoma. *Semin Pediatr Surg* 2012;21:2–14.
5. Schmidt ML, Lal A, Seeger RC et al. Favorable prognosis for patients 12–18 months of age with stage 4 nonamplified MYCN neuroblastoma: A Children's Cancer Group study. *J Clin Oncol* 2005;23:6474–80.
6. Schmidt ML, Lukens JN, Seeger RC et al. Biological factors determine prognosis in infants with stage IV neuroblastoma: A prospective Children's Cancer Group study. *J Clin Oncol* 2000;18:1260–8.
7. Shimada H, Ambros IM, Dehner LP et al. The international neuroblastoma pathology classification (the Shimada system). *Cancer* 1999;86(2):364–72.
8. Yamamoto K, Hanada R, Kikuchi A et al. Spontaneous regression of localized neuroblastoma detected by mass screening. *J Clin Oncol* 1998;16:1265–9.
9. Yoneda A, Oue T, Imura K et al. Observation of untreated patients with neuroblastoma detected by mass screening: A "wait and see" pilot study. *Med Pediatr Oncol* 2001;36:160–2.
10. Oue T, Inoue M, Yoneda A et al. Profile of neuroblastoma detected by mass screening, resected after observation without treatment: Results of the wait and see pilot study. *J Pediatr Surg* 2005;40:359–63.
11. Nuchtern JG, London WB, Barnewolt CE et al. A prospective study of expectant observation as primary therapy for neuroblastoma in young infants: A Children's Oncology Group study. *Ann Surg* 2012;256:573–80.
12. Auckland District Health Board. Neuroblastoma. 2011. http://www.adhb.govt.nz/newborn/TeachingResources/Dermatology/Neuroblastoma/Neuroblastoma.jpg.
13. Guglielmi M, De Bernardi B, Rizzo A et al. Resection of primary tumor at diagnosis in stage IV-S neuroblastoma: Does it affect the clinical course? *J Clin Oncol* 1996;14:1537–44.
14. Katzenstein HM, Bowman LC, Brodeur GM et al. Prognostic significance of age, MYCN oncogene amplification, tumor cell ploidy, and histology in 110 infants with stage D(S) neuroblastoma: The Pediatric Oncology Group experience—A Pediatric Oncology Group study. *J Clin Oncol* 1998;16:2007–17.
15. Nickerson HJ, Matthay KK, Seeger RC et al. Favorable biology and outcome of stage IV-S neuroblastoma with supportive care or minimal therapy: A Children's Cancer Group study. *J Clin Oncol* 2000;18:477–86.
16. National Cancer Institute. Neuroblastoma treatment. 2014. http://www.cancer.gov/cancertopics/pdq/treatment/neuroblastoma/HealthProfessional.
17. Maris JM. Recent advances in neuroblastoma. *N Engl J Med* 2010;362(23):2202–11.
18. La Quaglia MP, Kushner BH, Su W et al. The impact of gross total resection on local control and survival in high-risk neuroblastoma. *J Pediatr Surg* 2004;39:412–417.
19. Adkins ES, Sawin R, Gerbing RB, London WB, Matthay KK, Haase GM. Efficacy of complete resection for high-risk neuroblastoma: A Children's Cancer Group study. *J Pediatr Surg* 2004;39:931–6.
20. Kohler JA, Rubie H, Castel V et al. Treatment of children over the age of one year with unresectable localized neuroblastoma without MYCN amplification: Results of the SIOPEN study. *Eur J Cancer* 2013;49:3671–9.
21. Qureshi SS, Patil VP. Feasibility and safety of thoracoabdominal approach in children for resection of upper abdominal neuroblastoma. *J Pediatr Surg* 2012;47:694–9.
22. Rees H, Markley MA, Kiely EM, Pierro A, Pritchard J. Diarrhea after resection of advanced abdominal neuroblastoma: A common management problem. *Surgery* 1998;123:568–72.
23. Matthay KK, Villablanca JG, Seeger RC et al. Treatment of high-risk neuroblastoma with intensive chemotherapy, radiotherapy, autologous bone marrow transplantation, and 13-cis-retinoic acid. Children's Cancer Group. *N Engl J Med* 1999;341:1165–73.
24. Berthold F, Boos J, Burdach S et al. Myeloablative megatherapy with autologous stem-cell rescue versus oral maintenance chemotherapy as consolidation treatment in patients with high-risk neuroblastoma: A randomised controlled trial. *Lancet Oncol* 2005;6:649–58.
25. Matthay KK, Reynolds CP, Seeger RC et al. Long-term results for children with high-risk neuroblastoma treated on a randomized trial of myeloablative

therapy followed by 13-cis-retinoic acid: A Children's Oncology Group study. *J Clin Oncol* 2009;27:1007–13.

26. Yu AL, Gilman AL, Ozkaynak MF et al. Anti-GD2 antibody with GM-CSF, interleukin-2, and isotretinoin for neuroblastoma. *N Engl J Med* 2010;363:1324–34.

27. Cheung NK, Cheung IY, Kushner BH et al. Murine anti-GD2 monoclonal antibody 3F8 combined with granulocyte-macrophage colony-stimulating factor and 13-cis-retinoic acid in high-risk patients with stage 4 neuroblastoma in first remission. *J Clin Oncol* 2012;30:3264–70.

28. Lashford LS, Lewis IJ, Fielding SL et al. Phase I/II study of iodine131 metaiodobenzylguanidine in chemoresistant neuroblastoma: A United Kingdom children's cancer study group investigation. *J Clin Oncol* 1992;10:1889–96.

29. Polishchuk AL, DuBois SG, Haas-Kogan DA, Hawkins R, Matthay KK. Response, survival, and toxicity after iodine-131-metaiodobenzylguanidine therapy for neuroblastoma in preadolescents, adolescents, and adults. *Cancer* 2011;117:4286–93.

32

Pheochromocytoma

DAVID S. PERTSEMLIDIS

OVERVIEW

Dual adrenergic systems

The adrenal medulla and the sympathoneural extra-adrenal paraganglia comprise the adrenergic sympathoadrenal neuroendocrine system. The two adrenergic components have common characteristics, but also major differences. The common embryologic ancestry from the neural crest, the secretion of catecholamines, and the potential to produce "ectopic" neuropeptide or amine hormones are identical. The presence of the enzyme phenylethanolamine-N-methyl-tranferase in the adrenal medulla converts norepinephrine to epinephrine, facilitating the biochemical distinction between paraganglioma and adrenal pheochromocytoma. The separate anatomic locations, the genomic difference, the high frequency of multiple paragangliomas, the young age, and the more aggressive tumor biology are the major differences, in comparison with adrenal pheochromocytoma (Table 32.1).

Neuroendocrine system and neoplasms

During organogenesis, the neural crest stem cells migrate to numerous endocrine organs from the hypothalamus to the prostate, urinary bladder, and skin, where they are differentiated to synthesize neuropeptide and amine (catecholamines, serotonin, and histamine) hormones. Whereas adrenal pheochromocytomas are confined anatomically to the glands, the paragangliomas can be found along the sympathetic chain, mostly in the abdomen and about 2% in the neck and mediastinum. Pheochromocytomas arising from the adrenal medulla or the sympathetic ganglia retain the stem cell potential of producing ectopic neuropeptides or amines, i.e., adrenocortical hormone (ACTH), vasoactive intestinal polypeptide (VIP), parathormone, calcitonin, and other neuroendocrine hormones. Pheochromocytomas originate mostly from the adrenal medulla and 10%–15% from the sympathetic ganglia.

Clinical manifestations

The clinical expressions are paroxysmal or sustained hypertension, headaches, palpitations, excessive sweating, and numerous other symptoms unrelated to the hyperadrenergic state. The triad of headache, palpitations, and hyperhidrosis is less than 30%. For atypical presentations, if diagnosed late or undiagnosed, the outcomes can be catastrophic. Myocardial infarction with patent coronary arteries; grand mal seizures with normal encephalography;

Table 32.1 Overview of the common and dissimilar biology and neoplasia between adrenal medulla and sympathoneural ganglia

Adrenomedullary sympathoneural neuroendocrine adrenergic system		
Characteristics	**Adrenomedulla**	**Sympathoneural ganglia**
Embryology	Neural crest	Neural crest
Anatomy	Adrenals	Sympathoneural ganglia
Age group	Mid-40s	Young
Genetics	RET proto-oncogene	SDHB and SDHD subunits
Tumor multiplicity	Rare	Common
Secretion	Norepinephrine, epinephrine	Norepinephrine
Ectopic secretion	Neuropeptides + amines	Neuropeptides + amines
Malignant potential	Very low	High
Associations	Inherited multicancer syndromes	Parasympathetic paragangliomas

Note: Common are embryology, orthotopic, and ectopic (stem cell) hormonal secretions; uncommon characteristics are in anatomy, age of neoplastic expression, genomic differences (RET proto-oncogene for adrenal medullary and succinyl-dehydrogenase subunits B and D for sympathoneural tumor expression), aggressive tumor biology, and associations with inherited syndromes.

stroke with patent carotid arteries, absent uncontrolled hypertension or ruptured brain aneurysm; Type II diabetes mellitus in young nonobese; diabetes insipidus; and dilating cardiomyopathy with normal coronary arteries, no alcoholism, chronic hypertension, or viral myocarditis should raise strong suspicion of pheochromocytoma.

Inherited associations

There are a variety of associations of pheochromocytoma with inherited cancer syndromes [1–6]. Multiple endocrine neoplasia (MEN 2A and 2B) is generally linked to medullary thyroid carcinoma (MTC) and hyperparathyroidism. In MEN 2B, hyperparathyroidism is virtually absent.

Pheochromocytomas associated with inherited neoplasia syndromes are commonly bilateral adrenal or in multicentric paragangliomas. MEN 2A and 2B have germline mutations in the RET proto-oncogene and are expressed in C-cell thyroid medullary hyperplasia or carcinoma and primary parathyroid hyperplasia, which is absent in MEN 2B.

Hirschsprung's disease, caused by mutations in the RET proto-oncogene, and the cutaneous lichen amyloidosis have mutations in codon 634, the signature of MEN 2A.

In the neurocutaneous syndromes, von Hippel–Lindau (VHL) is composed of hemangioblastomas of the retina, brain, and spinal cord; bilateral multicentric renal cancer; serous cystadenoma of the pancreas; and epididymal and endolymphatic cysts. About 20% of pheochromocytomas are associated with the VHL syndrome.

Von Recklinghausen neurofibromatosis Type 1 (NF 1), especially with hypertension or duodenal carcinoid, is linked to pheochromocytoma in 4%–15%. The Sturge–Weber and tuberous sclerosis syndromes are rarely associated with pheochromocytoma. Von Recklinghausen NF 1 mutations arise from the NF tumor suppressor gene at chromosome 17q11. The VHL tumor suppressor gene is located in chromosome 3p25-26.

Familial paraganglioma

The familial paraganglioma (PGL 1) syndrome arises from the sympathetic adrenergic ganglia, including the organ of Zuckerkandl. It is associated with parasympathetic paraganglia, i.e., the carotid body (chemodectoma), which produce acetylcholine and catecholamines (dopamine and norepinephrine). The carotid body parasympathetic paraganglion originates from the neural crest and is located anatomically at the carotid bifurcation. The carotid body protects organs from hypoxic damage by releasing neurotransmitters. Carotid body tumors are 85% sporadic and 15% familial.

The gene mutations of the succinate dehydrogenase (SDHB and SDHD) have been documented in the diad of Carney–Stratakis syndrome, composed of gastrointestinal stromal tumor (GIST) sarcoma of the stomach and pheochromocytoma [7]. There are no identifiable gene mutations in Carney's triad syndrome, composed of paraganglioma, GIST tumor, and pulmonary chondroma.

The rare Beckwith–Wiedemann syndrome (BWS) is composed of body hemihypertrophy, nesidioblastosis, Wilms' tumor of the kidneys, and pheochromocytoma. The BWS gene is located on chromosome 11p15.5.

Biochemical diagnosis and imaging localization

Clinical suspicion of pheochromocytoma must be followed by biochemical testing with plasma and, if needed, urinary catecholamines and their metabolites, always collected in the absence of physical or emotional stress and medications causing spurious elevation or suppression.

Anatomic localization is achieved by highly sensitive conventional noninvasive computed tomography (CT) and magnetic resonance imaging (MRI). Dual recognition of anatomic location and hormonal function is made possible

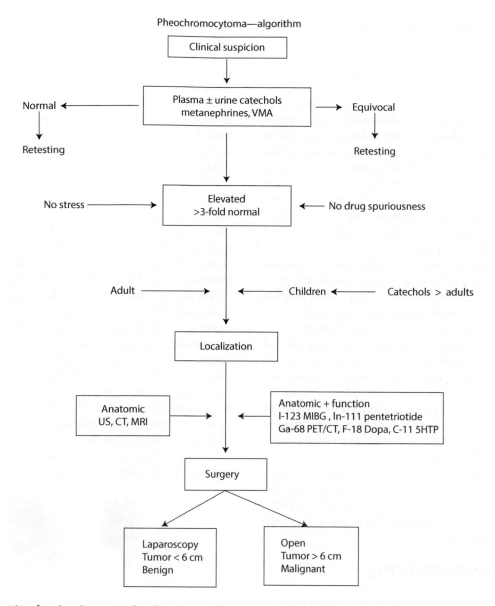

Pheochromocytoma—algorithm

Figure 32.1 Algorithm for the diagnosis, localization, and treatment of pheochromocytoma.

through receptor-based radiolabeled or metabolic-based scintigraphies.

In the perioperative period, control of arterial pressure and cardiac rhythm is based first on alpha- and beta-adrenergic blockers. Surgical intervention, laparoscopic or open, should be considered urgent. Surgical mortality should be close to zero (Figure 32.1).

HISTORICAL LANDMARKS

The name *pheochromocytoma* was derived from the Greek Φαϊός, meaning brown, chroma color, and Κϋϯϯωμα, meaning tumor [8,9]. In 1946, von Euler discovered the neurotransmitter property of norepinephrine that led to the pathophysiologic characterization of pheochromocytoma, and earned the Nobel Prize in 1970 [8]. Armstrong, in 1956, and Axelrod, in 1957, identified the urinary catecholamine

metabolites, vanillylmandelic acid (VMA), and metanephrines. Prior to these discoveries, one-third to half of pheochromocytomas were discovered at autopsy [10].

Gitlow et al., from our institution, extended the clinical–biochemical diagnosis of pheochromocytoma [10–12]. Lenders et al. [13], in 1995, and Eisenhofer et al. [14], in 1999, perfected the plasma assays of catecholamines and metanephrines, offering greater sensitivity and specificity in comparison with the urinary catecholamines and their metabolites.

Aside from the assays of parent hormones and their metabolites, plasma, and tissue antigens against the cytoplasmic neurosecretory granules, which are present in functioning and silent neuroendocrine tumors, provide diagnostic value.

Conventional imaging offers anatomic detection of high sensitivity, and the receptor-based isotopic imaging offers dual recognition of anatomic location and function of high sensitivity and specificity.

PREVALENCE AND DISTRIBUTION

The prevalence is less than 0.5% in hypertensive adults, but 10-fold higher in hypertensive adolescents and children because of greater likelihood of inherited disease [15,16]. In von Recklinghausen NF 1 and VHL, pheochromocytoma occurs in up to 8% and 20% of such patients, respectively [4,5,17,18]. However, patients with NF 1 and coexisting hypertension [19] or duodenal carcinoids [20] have a substantially greater prevalence, approaching 15%, of pheochromocytoma. Close to 40% of patients with MEN 2A and 2B harbor a pheochromocytoma [21].

Pheochromocytoma is neither gender nor race specific and can occur at any age. Sporadic tumors commonly present in the third and fourth decades of life, while familial disease is manifested one decade earlier. In sporadic cases, usually a single pheochromocytoma arises from the adrenal medulla, almost never coexisting with extra-adrenal tumors. In the inherited syndromes, however, bilateral adrenal disease, synchronous or metachronous, approaches more than 80%. Multicentricity of extra-adrenal tumors is found in 30%. Medullary hyperplasia (diffuse or nodular) or multiple subcentimeter tumors are commonly identified in both the involved ipsilateral and normal-appearing contralateral glands. Finally, extra-adrenal tumors do not coexist with adrenal pheochromocytomas, have a higher predisposition to malignancy, and affect mostly young patients. The absence of coexistence of adrenal and extra-adrenal pheochromocytomas is understandable since they are genetically different syndromes.

CLINICAL MANIFESTATIONS

Pheochromocytoma is a capricious neoplasm with nonspecific phenotype and can therefore be difficult to diagnose clinically. Hypertension is almost always present and may be constant, rather than paroxysmal, in one-third to one-half of patients. Paroxysmal hypertensive crises may be so fleeting that they frequently escape detection. In a small minority of MEN 2A and 2B patients and those with predominantly epinephrine-secreting adrenal tumors, paroxysmal cardiac arrhythmia may be the presenting symptom.

Excess catecholamines affect a plurality of target organs, thus inducing a wide spectrum of symptoms that are often inseparable from those of a variety of common illnesses. In the broad constellation of symptoms, the triad of paroxysmal headaches, palpitations, and excess sweating is present in 30% of adults. In children, profuse sweating is a common manifestation, often ignored due to the infrequent use of blood pressure measurements. Some unusual clinical features are transient ischemic cerebral events, (stroke or grand mal seizures), cardiomyopathy, gastrointestinal crises, and Type II diabetes mellitus or insipidus. Severe constipation or pseudo-obstruction may be the initial manifestation [22],

and secretory diarrhea from elaboration of VIP or calcitonin by pheochromocytoma has been reported [23–26].

Paroxysmal events are usually precipitated by physical or emotional stress, which induce a flux of catecholamines from the expanded storage in the cytoplasmic neurosecretory granules of the sympathetic neurons and adrenal medulla. Despite common misconceptions, stress-induced neural stimulation does not cause release of catecholamines directly from the tumor, as no innervation exists. In fact, only direct mechanical pressure by blunt abdominal trauma, deep abdominal palpation, certain body postures, vigorous application of the ultrasound probe, retrograde adrenal venography, and intraoperative manipulation can cause sudden release of catecholamine by the tumor. An analogy to the compression-induced flux of catecholamines is the induction of symptoms during micturition in pheochromocytomas located in the wall of the urinary bladder.

Physical stigmata, seen mostly in inherited syndromes associated with pheochromocytoma, facilitate the recognition of the disease. Cutaneous NF 1, café-au-lait pigmentations, and Lisch nodules of the eye, especially with coexisting hypertension, should raise strong suspicion of pheochomocytoma (Figure 32.2). Visible neuromas of the oral mucosa, tongue, and conjunctiva and marfanoid habitus are indicative of MEN 2B (Figure 32.3). Loss of vision or of an eye from retinal angiomas or angioblastomas should alert the physician to possible existence of VHL disease.

Family history is a reliable source of information that may lead to discovery of pheochromocytoma or coexisting

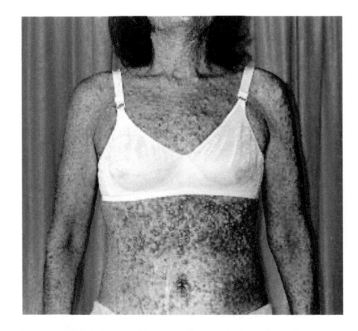

Figure 32.2 Inherited NF 1 with coexisting pheochromocytoma of the right adrenal, resected through open transperitoneal approach at age 27. She returned 21 years later with a gastrinoma that was treated with distal pancreatectomy. Her father died following resection of a unilateral adrenal pheochromocytoma elsewhere, and autopsy revealed medullary hyperplasia of the remaining adrenal.

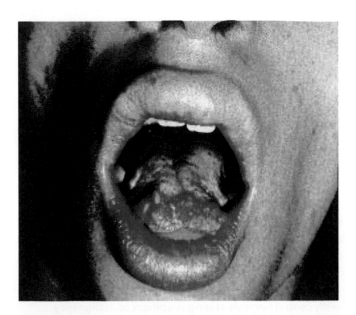

Figure 32.3 Oral and lingual mucosal neuromas in a patient with MEN 2B. (Photograph provided by Dr. Donald Bergman, endocrinologist at the Mount Sinai Hospital of New York.)

but silent cancer syndromes. Sudden death of a parent or sibling at a young age, premature myocardial infarction or cardiomyopathy [27], endocrine surgery, and colorectal operation for Hirschsprung's disease, ganglioneuromatosis, or megacolon [22] are important leads in directing diagnostic investigations.

Offspring of parents harboring germline mutations of the autosomal dominant RET proto-oncogene mapped to chromosome 10 (10q11.2), the VHL tumor suppressor gene mapped to chromosome 3 (3p25-26), or the NF 1 gene mapped to chromosome 17 (17q11.2) are at high risk for developing pheochromocytoma and other syndromic components. About 40% of all pheochromocytomas are discovered by screening families with MEN 2A and 2B or neurocutaneous syndromes, especially VHL and NF 1. Phenotypic and genetic screening and surveillance are important because pheochromcytoma may be the first expression in about one-third to one-half of affected kindred in MEN 2A and 2B and VHL families [28]. Family history of surgery for carotid body tumor, glomus jugulare, or other paragangliomas should initiate the search for extra-adrenal pheochromocytoma and screening for the presence of mutations of the genes for SDHD and SDHB, which encode mitochondrial enzymes involved in oxidative phosphorylation [29].

A history of gastrointestinal GIST tumor and pulmonary chondroma should alert the physician to possible coexistence of extra-adrenal pheochromocytoma. This trial was described by Carney in 1976 [30], and later chromosome 1 was identified, but no germline mutations. The dual coexistence of GIST tumors and paragangliomas, but no pulmonary chondroma, is inherited by autosomal dominance, and germline mutations in SDHB, SDHC, and SDHD genes (Carney–Stratakis syndrome) [7]. Germline mutations in

SDHB, SDHC, and SDHD genes are identical to those of familial paraganglioma syndrome. Other neurocutaneous syndromes that may be associated with pheochromocytoma are tuberous sclerosis and the Sturge–Weber syndrome. In tuberous sclerosis, visible angiofibromas distributed in a butterfly pattern on the cheeks, chin, and forehead coexist with malformations of tumors of the central nervous system. In the Sturge–Weber encephalotrigeminal angiomatosis, there are visible cavernous hemangiomas along the distribution of the trigeminal nerve in association with hemangiomas of the leptomeninges.

Catecholamine-induced dilating but reversible cardiomyopathy has remained obscure among endocrinologists, endocrine surgeons, and even cardiologists. In our experience with 244 operations for pheochromocytoma, 13% presented with atypical expressions: cardiomyopathy treated with heart transplant, pulmonary edema during surgery unrelated to pheochromocytoma, and cerebrovascular events ranging from ischemic attack to grand mal seizures. In extra-adrenal pheochromocytoma (paraganglioma), the association of carotid body tumor (chemodectoma) and glomus jugulare at the base of the skull is not uncommon. Imaging should be routine to include the neck and base of the skull. In MEN 2A and 2B, the usual multiorgan neoplasia, the metachronous clinical expression is 80%, making annual biochemical and imaging testing obligatory until the full spectrum of the components is treated, realizing that the intervals of clinical expression may range from 6 months to 10 years.

BIOCHEMICAL DIAGNOSIS

Once clinical suspicion of pheochromocytoma is raised, treatment with oral long-acting alpha- and beta-adrenergic blockers should be started and testing should be initiated under standardized, unstressed conditions. Physical or emotional stress from illness, surgery, or trauma will raise the concentrations of catecholamines and their metabolites in the plasma and urine [10,11,31].

All medications should be screened, and those known to falsely elevate or suppress the catecholamines or their metabolite concentrations in the plasma or urine should be stopped for at least 1 week. Phenoxybenzamine and tricyclic antidepressants are major causes of false-positive elevation of norepinephrine and its metabolites [32]. Labetalol, one of the frequently used antihypertensive drugs, interferes with catecholamine and metanephrine assays and should be stopped 1 week before sampling plasma or urine [33]. Acetaminophen interferes with the analytical method of plasma normetanephrine assay and should be stopped several days before blood is collected [33]. Metoclopramide raises the arterial pressure, through catecholamine hypersecretion, and may cause death. Alpha-methyl-DOPA, monoaminooxidase (MAO) inhibitors, amphetamine (phenylephrine, pseudoephedrine, and phenylpropalamine), cocaine, and calcium antagonists may interfere with assays of the parent catecholamines and their metanephrines in the plasma and urine [33]. Dietary caffeic acid, a catechol ingredient in natural and decaffeinated coffee, and its metabolite dihydrocaffeic acid interfere with assays of plasma catecholamines [33].

Provocative or suppressive tests with histamine, glucagon, or phentolamine may cause severe parosyxmal rise or fall of the arterial pressure, resulting in stroke, myocardial infarction, or even death. Given the precision of current biochemical testing, these unnecessary provocative manipulations are strictly contraindicated. Patients should be fasting and resting in a quiet environment, and collection of blood should not be started until 10–15 minutes after venipuncture. Urine 24-hour collections or random samples of urine, preferably 50 mL of the first concentrated morning specimen, are sufficient. The results are expressed in micrograms of the catecholamine metabolite per milligram of urinary creatinine. The assays of these stable urinary metabolites are valid even in the presence of renal dysfunction [10,11].

CONVENTIONAL AND ISOTOPIC IMAGING

Ultrasound

Interposition of gastric, duodenal, and colonic gas may cause limitations, but modern equipment and an experienced ultrasonographer can detect subcentimeter tumors [34]. Adequate adrenergic blockade offers prophylaxis from hypertensive crisis or cardiac arrhythmia from compression of the abdomen by the ultrasound probe.

Computed tomography and magnetic resonance imaging

Multiplanar CT and modern MRI techniques permit localization of adrenal and extra-adrenal subcentimeter tumors in the neck, mediastinum, abdomen, and pelvis with a sensitivity of 90%–95%. Distinction between benign and malignant pheochromocytomas is based on size, confluent necrosis, disruption of the capsule, invasion of adjacent organs, or regional enlarged lymph nodes [35] (Figure 32.4). Prophylaxis against induction of a crisis from intravenous contrast is necessary and is accomplished with oral alpha- and beta-adrenergic blockade [36,37].

MRI offers additional confirmation of specificity through enhancement on T-2 images (Figure 32.5a and b). T-2 enhancement is not pathognomonic for pheochromocytoma because adrenocortical malignancy has a similar property. Therefore, T-2 enhancement must be correlated with clinical and biochemical information.

Receptor-based isotopic imaging

Neuroendocrine neoplasms express receptors to somatostatin (subtypes 2 and 5) and catecholamines.

CT and MRI fail to screen the whole body and offer no information on functional status of the tumor. Molecular

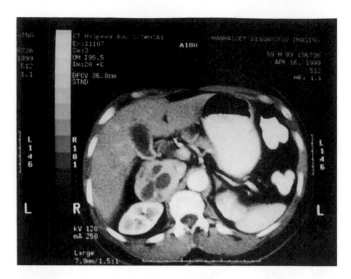

Figure 32.4 Large right adrenal pheochromocytoma with central necrosis raising suspicion of malignancy. Pathologic examination revealed invasion of the capsule indicative of a malignant tumor.

scintigraphy examines the entire body and identifies the functional properties of neuroendocrine neoplasms.

Uptake of the labeled tracers by the catecholamine and somatostatin receptors relies on the adequacy of cytoplasmic neurosecretory granules in the tumor cells. Meta-iodo-benzylguanidine (MIBG) scintigraphy is superior in detecting small extra-adrenal tumors and metastases from malignant pheochromocytoma. The sensitivity and specificity of MIBG tracer ranges from 87% to 94% [31,38]. The sensitivity of pentetriotide scintigraphy for pheochromocytoma ranges from 60% to 90%. New positron emission tomography (PET) scanning with Ga-68-labeled tracers and F-18-DOPA and C-11-5HTP is promising high sensitivity. I-123 or I-131 MIBG tracer, a norepinephrine analog, uptake has a limited sensitivity of 50% by gastrointestinal neuroendocrine tumors.

Fluorodeoxyglucose-18 (FDG) PET imaging for pheochromocytoma does not depend on catecholamine uptake or adequacy of cytoplasmic neurosecretory granules in the tumor, but on proliferative activity and the number of viable tumor cells. The sensitivity of FDG is lower than that of MIBG and pentetrioscan. PET-F-18-DOPA is linked to precursors of catecholamines in poorly differentiated malignant pheochromocytomas.

Percutaneous biopsy

The temptation to perform percutaneous CT-guided needle biopsy in suspected, but not proven, pheochromocytomas should be avoided due to risk of inducing a crisis. In exceptional cases, such as patients with prohibitive surgical risk and equivocal diagnostic test results, percutaneous fine-needle aspiration should only be performed under adequate adrenergic blockade and a standby anesthesiologist.

The plurality of available conventional noninvasive and isotopic imaging methods has improved the precision of

(a) 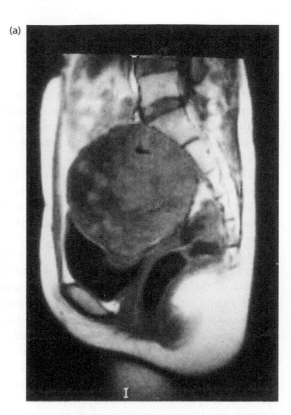 (b)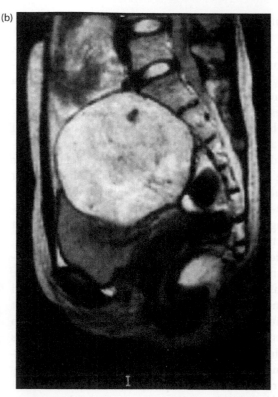

Figures 32.5 Large pelvic pheochromocytoma with change of signal intensity from T-1 to T-2 MRI images. These imaging features are strongly suggestive but not pathognomonic for pheochromocytoma.

anatomic localization and the definition of functional status of both benign and malignant tumors.

PERIOPERIATIVE MANAGEMENT

Ambulatory preoperative care

Once the diagnosis of pheochromocytoma is established by biochemical parameters, alpha-adrenergic blockade should be initiated. Only after this blockade has restored normotension can beta-adrenergic inhibition be used to treat compensatory tachycardia. This sequence should never be reversed, since beta-adrenergic blockade alone inhibits beta-receptor-mediated vasodilation, allowing unopposed alpha-receptor stimulation and potentially inducing a hypertensive crisis. In the majority of patients, nonselective or selective alpha-blockade alone is sufficient, reserving beta-antagonism for patients who develop significant tachycardia. Recent studies argue for the use of oral calcium channel blockade alone for the preoperative management of pheochromocytoma [39].

Phenoxybenzamine, a long-acting, nonselective oral alpha-blocker, is the drug of choice for ambulatory management. An initial dose of 10 mg twice daily is used with progressive increases until normotension is achieved and paroxysmal symptoms are eliminated or minimized. Usually 30–40 mg/day, divided in three or four doses, is sufficient, although higher doses may be necessary. Prazocin, a selective alpha-receptor inhibitor, can be used at doses of 1–2 mg three times daily [40]. Oral phentolamine, a short-acting

alpha-receptor antagonist, has a variable absorption and is therefore unsuitable for therapy in the ambulatory setting. Similarly, tyrosine hydroxylase inhibition with metyrosine is not useful in the management of benign pheochromocytoma because Parkinsonian symptoms may occur due to depletion of dopamine. Oral beta-receptor inhibition or calcium channel blockade can be achieved with a variety of selective and nonselective medications. Small doses of metoprolol or atenolol usually provide adequate restoration of eurhythmia.

The debate over the need for expansion of the circulating blood volume in the preoperative phase is plagued by basic misconception. The notion that patients with pheochromocytoma are hypovolemic [41] is not valid. Measurements of plasma and red cell volumes in these patients have proven to be within the normal range [42], and in fact, pheochromocytoma patients are hypervolemic relative to the capacity of the constricted vascular system. Attempts to expand the circulating volume with prolonged preoperative adrenergic blockade do not prevent intraoperative cardiovascular crises and the hypotension that follows tumor removal [43]. The proposed 4- to 6-week delay for volume expansion serves only to increase the time period during which these patients are at continued risk from physical or emotional stress-induced paroxysmal crises. The surgical treatment of pheochromocytoma must be expeditious and should be performed immediately after diagnosis and localization. The appropriate timing of volume restoration is immediately after tumor removal.

In-hospital preoperative preparation

In an era when the practice of surgery has, by necessity, shifted from the inpatient to the outpatient setting, the safest setting for immediate preoperative management of a pheochromocytoma patient remains the critical care unit. The highest priority is optimal control of the arterial pressure and heart rate in a monitored setting. The choice of drugs for adrenergic inhibition is a matter of personal preference and institutional idiosyncrasy rather than scientific reasoning. The spectrum of pharmacologic management includes alpha-blockade, combined alpha- and beta-blockade, short- or long-acting antagonists, and powerful vasodilating agents such as nitroprusside, whose action is not mediated through adrenergic receptors.

The selection of the short-acting alpha-blocker phentolamine combined with the beta-receptor antagonist esmolol, permits easy minute-to-minute titration of the doses needed to attain normotension and cardiac eurhythmia. The short half-life and virtual absence of toxicity render these two medications highly desirable. The required infusion rates of these drugs are proportional to the levels of excess catecholamines in the plasma and tissue and the sensitivity of adrenergic receptors. The preoperative requirements of alpha- and beta-blockers permit an estimate of the amounts needed during induction of anesthesia, endotracheal intubation, and intraoperative manipulation of the tumor [44].

In the surgical intensive care unit, continuous intravenous infusion of phentolamine should be started at 10 mg/h, with incremental rates every 5–10 minutes until normotension is achieved. Usually, a mean infusion rate of 30–35 mg/h is sufficient, but the requirements may range from 10 to 100 mg/h. Aside from normotension, the two other criteria for sufficiency of alpha-blockade are a mild compensatory sinus tachycardia and nasal stuffiness. The solutions should be freshly prepared and contain 1 mg/mL of phentolamine per milliliter of glucose/water. The concentration for intraoperative use should be two- to threefold higher to rapidly control intraoperative hypertensive events [45].

Continuous intravenous infusion of esmolol is started after the development of sinus tachycardia from adequate alpha-receptor blockade. The esmolol concentration should be 10 mg/mL of esmolol in glucose/water. The infusion rate should be started at 25 mg/h, with incremental titration until normal sinus rhythm is attained. The mean infusion rate is 150 mg/h. Labetalol, with combined long-acting beta- and intermediate alpha-activity at a ratio of 7:1, offers the advantage of a single drug that can be used orally or intravenously [45]. Despite this 7:1 ratio of beta- to alpha-activity, the rapid onset of alpha-blockade makes labetalol a useful drug in the perioperative period. Nitroprusside, a potent vasodilator and smooth muscle relaxant, should always be available in the perioperative setting for limited use during episodes when adrenergic blockade proves ineffective [40]. Prolonged infusion rates greater than 2 µg/kg/min generate cyanide faster than the body can dispose, leading to toxicity and potential fatality [40].

The availability of phentolamine was suddenly stopped because the production by the manufacturer was drastically reduced. The future is unpredictable, but there is hope that access to this drug will be restored. After 4½ decades of relying on this short-acting, nontoxic alpha-blocker to perform 244 operations for pheochromocytoma, we used continuous intravenous calcium channel blocker in the last six cases with success. An infusion rate of 5–6 mg/h of nicardipine proved successful.

The advantages of continuous intravenous use of short-acting adrenergic blockers are easy titration, rapid onset of action, negligible toxicity, and the restoration of physiologic hemodynamic and cardiac parameters within minutes after stopping the drugs [45]. Bolus injections of alpha- or beta-receptor blockers may produce extreme fluctuations of arterial pressure and heart rate and should be avoided. Although the titration of intravenous infusion rates of short-acting antiadrenergic medications requires greater effort and subtlety, especially during surgery, they are superior to the "simplicity" of drugs with sustained action. The rapid control of intraoperative hypertensive or arrhythmic episodes, the quick return of physiologic indices, and the surgeon's ability to judge the completeness of tumor removal are powerful reasons for the preferential use of the continuous intravenous infusion of short-acting catecholamine antagonists.

Intraoperative management

Patients should arrive in the operating room after a day's preparation in the critical care unit with appropriate monitors and well-controlled arterial pressure and heart rate with intravenous phentolamine and esmolol. All of the needed solutions must be freshly prepared and available in the operating room for immediate infusion through dedicated venous access. Delay in the control of a crisis, even for a few moments, may cause serious morbidity or death.

Phentolamine and esmolol solutions with concentrations of 2 and 10 mg/mL in glucose/water, respectively, should be continuously infused at an appropriate rate. A sodium nitroprusside solution of 0.2 mg/mL (50 mg in 250 mL) glucose/water should be available for brief use only to control paroxysmal hypertension that is not responsive to intravenous phentolamine. The solution should be protected from light using aluminum foil or other opaque material; however, there is no need to cover the infusion chamber or tubing. A norepinephrine solution of 16 µg/mL (8 mg in 500 mL) of glucose/water should be ready for infusion in case of hypotension that is unresponsive to discontinuation of phentolamine and rapid volume infusion.

Surgery should not commence until normal adrenergic steady state is reached. Anesthetic induction and endotracheal intubation should be performed under optimal pharmacologic protection to minimize critical hypertension or arrhythmia. Continuous intravenous infusion of phentolamine and esmolol or nicardipine should be adjusted, when needed, to control hypertensive or arrhythmic events

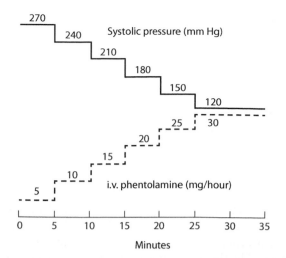

Figure 32.6 Intraoperative continuous intravenous infusion of phentolamine used to treat a hypertensive crisis during mobilization of a sizable adrenal pheochromocytoma. Bolus injections of phentolamine cause inevitable rapid fall of arterial pressure, creating a vicious cycle between norepinephrine and phentolamine infusions. Cautious increments and gradual reduction of phentolamine have led to good outcomes.

during unavoidable tumor manipulation in the course of mobilization and resection (Figure 32.6).

The choice of inhalational anesthetic and muscle relaxants is no longer an issue of debate. Our experience and that of others [40] have demonstrated no correlation between the anesthetic agent used and the incidence of cardiovascular events. The primary determinants of the safe conduct of anesthesia and of successful surgical outcome are the adequacy of adrenoreceptor blockade and the maintenance of sufficient anesthetic depth.

Surgical approaches

The choice between minimally invasive and traditional open surgery is a matter of the surgeon's experience, the limitations imposed by tumor size, suspicion of malignancy, adequacy of exposure, and patient comorbidities. Patients with recent cardiac failure or intracranial hemorrhage may be at greater surgical risk with minimally invasive surgery, compared with open techniques, because pneumoperitoneum lowers venous return to the heart and increases intracranial pressure [46]. Small, benign, adrenal pheochromocytomas can be safely resected by laparoscopic transperitoneal or retroperitoneal approaches, while tumors larger than 7 cm and with imaging features suggestive of malignancy should be accessed by open techniques. The open transperitoneal anterior approach offers excellent exposure for complete exploration, easier control of bleeding, and resection of large invasive tumors or multiple extra-adrenal pheochromocytomas. Minimally invasive techniques offer quick recovery, less adhesion formation, and superior cosmetic results.

The concern that the pressure of pneumoperitoneum may induce flux of catecholamines by the tumor has been dispelled by clinical observations and assays of plasma catecholamines during minimally invasive adrenalectomy for pheochromocytoma.

The approach to extra-adrenal abdominal pheochromocytomas depends on anatomic location, size, and multiplicity of the tumors. The deep retroperitoneal location; proximity to the aorta, cava, iliac vessels, or ureters; and potential malignancy, dictate caution in employing a laparoscopic approach.

Patients with left adrenal pheochromocytomas, especially large ones, should have preoperative antipneumococcal and meningococcal vaccinations because of the small likelihood of incidental splenectomy (1%–2%). Knowledge of bilateral renal function with contrast-enhanced CT is essential because large or malignant pheochromocytomas may be difficult to resect completely without nephrectomy due to inseparable blood supply or direct invasion of the kidney. Informed consent should also be obtained from patients with large, vascular, invasive tumors, where nephrectomy may become necessary for oncologic or vascular anatomic reasons. Cleansing of the colon is desirable but not necessary, but antibiotic prophylaxis should be routine. Stress doses of cortisol are needed if bilateral synchronous adrenalectomy is planned, with or without orthotopic preservation or heterotopic autotransplantation of pure acrenocortical tissue.

Early ligation of the main adrenal vein has been proposed to minimize hypertensive and arrhythmic events during dissection around the tumor. This concept ignores the presence of numerous emissary veins connecting the central vein with the pericapsular venous plexus and renal capsular veins. Easier exposure, isolation, and ligation of the main adrenal veins, especially the short right, are facilitated greatly by dissection along the less vascular lateral planes first. Access to the planes along the renal vein on the left and inferior vena cava on the right is made easier with gentle retraction of the mobilized gland. The late ligation of main venous outflow protects the gland from hemorrhage, especially when the inferior phrenic arterial branch is divided. Delaying ligation and division of the inferior phrenic arterial branch at the apex avoids obscuring the main veins, when the body of the gland slides downward [47,48].

Figure 32.7 demonstrates the anatomy of the main adrenal veins. The right adrenal is partially retrocaval, and the main vein is very short; as a result, isolation for stapling and division is difficult. The distance between the junction of the renal vein and the cava is 6–7 cm. The left main adrenal vein is long, about 2–3 cm, and the junction with the inferior phrenic vein is usually close to the adrenal lining. Stapling of the inferior phrenic vein proximal to the junction with the main adrenal vein makes it easier to staple the main vein below or above the junction.

Complete removal of the tumor is followed by fall of systolic arterial pressure to less than 90 mmHg. This hypotension can be corrected within minutes by stopping the short-acting alpha-receptor blocker (phentolamine) and rapidly infusing 2–3 L of crystalloid. Infusion of

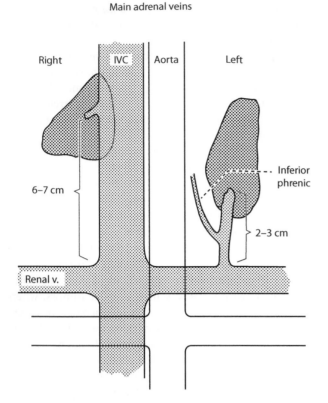

Main adrenal veins

Figure 32.7 The main adrenal veins are depicted here to demonstrate the anatomic differences. A third of the right adrenal gland is retrocaval, and the main vein is short (about 1–1.5 cm). The adrenal vein enters the inferior vena cava about 6–7 cm from the renocaval junction. The left main adrenal vein joins the branch of the inferior phrenic vein, entering above the renal–adrenal venous junction. After ligation and division of the inferior phrenic, the length of the main adrenal vein is about 2–3 cm.

norepinephrine to restore normotension should be avoided, as it prolongs undesirable vasoconstriction.

HEREDITARY PHEOCHROMOCYTOMA

Pheochromocytoma is linked genetically to other syndromes of multiple neoplasms, almost always of Mendellian autosomal dominance. Associations with MEN 2A and 2B, neurocutaneous syndromes (especially VHL and NF 1), and familial paraganglioma have been well documented [1,3–6,17–22,29,49].

Inherited pheochromocytoma is clinically expressed one decade earlier than sporadic. About 20% of all pheochromocytomas are discovered by prospective screening of families. In families with MEN 2A and 2B, synchronous and metachronous adrenal pheochromocytomas are bilateral and multicentric in 80% and 60% of VHL syndromes [28]. The multicentricity of tumors in each adrenal suggests pathogenesis from precursor diffuse or nodular hyperplasia.

In a recent retrospective genetic study of 271 patients labeled as nonsyndromic (sporadic) pheochromocytoma,

66 (24%) were found to have mutations. Of those, 30 had mutations of the VHL gene, 13 of the RET proto-oncogene, 12 of the SDHB gene, and 11 of the SDHD gene. Patients with multiple extra-adrenal pheochromocytomas presented at age 18 or younger and were highly likely to have mutations of the SDHB and SDHD genes [29]. This study indicates that the prevalence of inherited pheochromocytoma is far greater than once thought.

Multiple endocrine neoplasia Type 2

MEN 2 is a cancer syndrome affecting organs derived from the neuroectoderm. The previous narrow definition of MEN 2A, which included MTC or thyroid C-cell hyperplasia, pheochromcytoma, and hyperparathyroidism, has been broadened by the international RET Mutation Consortium [3]. The MEN 2B phenotype was defined as the constellation of MTC with pheochromocytoma, usually without parathyroid disease, and characteristic clinical abnormalities (mucosal neuromas, marfanoid constitution, and intestinal ganglioneuromatosis). The susceptibility gene for MEN 2 has been traced to chromosome 10 (10q11.2) [3].

In MEN syndromes, the full expression of the phenotype occurs sequentially, rather than simultaneously. In MEN 2A, only 20% of patients will present with clinical manifestation of all components. Prospective screening and long-term surveillance are therefore imperative to detect asymptomatic family members and the clinical or biochemical development of latent, subclinical components.

The prevalence of pheochromocytoma in MEN 2A and 2B families is about 40% [29]. It originates from the adrenals, is bilateral (synchronous or metachronous) in 80% of MEN 2A (Figure 32.8, Table 32.2) [45], and is rarely malignant [28]. Multiple tumors or medullary hyperplasia (diffuse or nodular) are commonly present in the ipsilateral-involved and contralateral adrenal, which may appear normal on imaging.

Members with only familial medullary thyroid cancer and absence of other MEN 2 components are classified with MEN 2 because of genetic overlapping with MEN 2A. The North American and European Endocrinology Societies decided to categorize such families as MEN 2 after identifying 10 members per family with only medullary thyroid cancer. The precise recognition of such families implies no need of continued surveillance. The biology of medullary thyroid cancer in those families is less aggressive and begins later in life, in comparison with MEN 2A and 2B.

The distribution of the three components is as follows: MEN 2A is the most common (60%), MEN 2B is the most aggressive (5%), and familial medullary cancer is the most benign (35%).

The alarming report by Carney et al. in 1976 [50] that MEN 2 patients are at higher risk for malignancy proved incorrect. Subsequent larger series of MEN 2 and VHL patients did not verify the high risk for malignant pheochromocytoma in

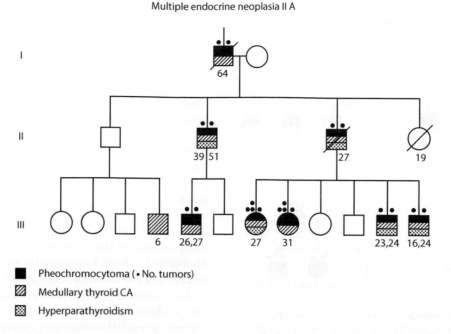

Multiple endocrine neoplasia II A

■ Pheochromocytoma (• No. tumors)
▨ Medullary thyroid CA
▩ Hyperparathyroidism

Figure 32.8 Family tree of three generations of MEN 2A. The grandfather in the first generation died at age 64, having inherited MTC and bilateral adrenal pheochromocytomas. The cause of death was unknown. In the second generation, a 19-year-old girl died suddenly, most likely from unknown cause. Two men inherited bilateral adrenal pheochromocytomas (one metachronous), MTC, and hyperparathyroidism. One died at age 27 from thyroid cancer. In the third generation, five of 12 had bilateral adrenal (two multicentric) pheochromocyomas, six had medullary thyroid cancer, and three had hyperparathyroidism. Three pheochromocytomas were metachronous (1–8 years); none died from pheochromocytoma.

Table 32.2 Our personal experience with inherited pheochromocytoma

	Patients (n)	Mean Age (years)	Bilateral (n)	Mean follow up (months)
MEN 2A	18	31	15	88
VHL/NF-1	18	24	12	118
Pheo only	2	31	1	25
PGLI	2	22	0	205
All diagnoses	40	28	28	89

Note: The 18 MEN 2A and 18 VHL/NF-1 families make up the majority of the inherited cases. All MEN 2A and VHL/NF-1 had bilateral adrenalectomies (10 metachronous). The remaining two with bilateral adrenalectomies did not have associations with multiple cancer syndromes. Two with familial paraganglioma each had multiple extra-adrenal tumors, and they were young.

such families [21,28,51]. As a result, the recommendation for prophylactic removal of the contralateral normal-appearing gland to prevent malignancy is no longer tenable.

Intestinal manifestations of MEN 2A include Hirschsprung's disease and ganglioneuromatosis. Familial Hirschsprung's disease can be autosomal dominant or recessive. Linkage to the chromosomal region containing the RET proto-oncogene has been documented [3]. A recent study revealed that some patients with MEN 2A develop Hirschsprung's disease, and kindred with MEN 2B develop intestinal neuromas and megacolon [22]. Six of eight patients

with Hirschsprung's disease among 83 MEN 2A families had surgery for aganglionosis 2–23 years prior to the diagnosis of MEN 2A. Almost all 28 patients with MEN 2B had gastrointestinal symptoms, but only one-third had surgery (colectomy, colostomy, or pull-through 1–30 years prior to the MEN 2B diagnosis) [22]. Although this study was conducted with questionnaires and had only a 59% response, it has promoted awareness of the expanding spectrum of MEN manifestations and the need for prospective screening for MEN in children with intestinal manifestations.

Association with neurocutaneous syndromes

Pheochromocytoma can be genetically linked to neurocutaneous syndromes, also known as phacomatoses, which are inherited by autosomal dominance. In VHL disease, pheochromocytoma occurs in about 20% of family members (Figure 32.9) [5,18,51]. Genetic linkage analysis showed that the gene responsible for VHL is located on the short arm of chromosome 3, within the region of 3p25-26 [52]. The incidence of VHL disease is approximately 1:36,000. The spectrum of VHL-associated neoplasms also includes hemangioblastoma of the central nervous system, spinal cord, and retina; renal cell carcinoma (usually multicentric and bilateral); renal and pancreatic cysts; cystic or solid lesions of the liver, spleen, epididymis, ovary, and endolymphatic sac; and pancreatic neuroendocrine tumors [5,51–53]. Of 256 VHL patients screened by history, physical

Pheochromocytoma and von Hippel's disease

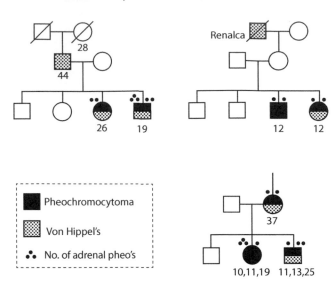

Figure 32.9 In four generations of inherited pheochromocytomas associated with VHL syndrome. Seven of 21 members inherited pheochromocytoma, 5 bilateral adrenal, 2 unilateral, and 3 multicentric. Seven inherited renal carcinomas. Six had pheochromocytomas as teenagers. Six had metachronous pheochromocytoma, four with an early interval of 1 year.

examination, and genotyping and imaging studies, 30 (12%) had pancreatic neuroendocrine tumors [49].

The incidence of NF 1 is 1:3000, and pheochromocytoma is found in 4%–15% of those patients with coexisting hypertension or duodenal carcinoids [4,19,20,54]. The NF 1 gene has been localized on chromosome 17 (17q11.2) [54].

Pheochromocytoma is rarely associated with two subtypes of neurocutaneous syndromes, the Sturge–Weber syndrome and tuberous sclerosis. The former is also known as encephalotrigeminal syndrome and is characterized by cavernous hemangioma along the facial distribution of the trigeminal nerve and venous hemangiomas of the leptomeninges. The syndrome of tuberous sclerosis comprises hypopigmented skin lesions; angiofibromas distributed in a butterfly configuration over the cheeks, chin, and forehead; and tumors of the central venous system.

Familial paraganglioma syndrome

The genotype of the familial paraganglioma syndrome has been recently defined through discovery of mutations in the genes of succinate dehydrogenase subunit D (SDHD) and succinate dehydrogenase subunit B (SDHB) encoding mitochondrial enzymes involved in oxidative phosphorylation [6,29]. The familial paraganglioma Type 1 syndrome comprises extra-adrenal pheochromocytoma and parasympathetic tumors of the carotid body, aortic arch, and jugulotympanic region.

The term *functioning paraganglioma* is synonymous with *extra-adrenal pheochromocytoma*. These tumors originate

from the system of paraganglia, which extends from the base of the skull to the pelvis and include the jugulotympanic, vagal, carotid body, laryngeal, aorticopulmonary, and visceroautonomic regions [55]. The incidence of extra-adrenal tumors is 15%–22% of all pheochromocytomas [56,57], with anatomic predilection to the periadrenal regions. Extra-adrenal pheochromocytomas rarely coexist with primary adrenal tumors, sporadic or familial. Eighty-five percent of extra-adrenal pheochromocytomas are located in the abdomen [58], in anatomic regions defined as superior para-aortic, inferior para-aortic, and pelvic (Figures 32.10 and 32.11) [59]. The superior para-aortic region includes the periadrenal and renal perihilar sites, and the inferior para-aortic includes the inferior perinephric and iliac artery regions. The urinary bladder paragangliomas are classified separately because of their characteristic symptomatology [60]. Multiplicity is high, ranging between 15% and 30% overall, and is higher in children [15,16,56–59].

Extra-adrenal pheochromocytomas secrete norepinephrine exclusively, because they lack the cortisol-sensitive enzyme phenylethanolamine-N-methyltransferase, which catalyzes norepinephrine to epinephrine. Localization and surgical treatment of extra-adrenal tumors is more difficult than that of primary adrenal pheochromocytomas. The small size and multiplicity are often difficult to detect, and confusion with enlarged lymph nodes is not unusual. The best imaging is I-123 MIBG scintigraphy, which offers total body scanning and detection of subcentimeter metastatic tumors.

Extra-adrenal pheochromocytomas are the most aggressive of the adult sympathoadrenal tumors and should be considered malignant and approached accordingly, whether in the abdomen, chest, or neck. Multifocal disease does not have a higher rate of malignancy than solitary tumors. The reported incidence of malignancy in tumors arising from the organ of Zuckerkandl is 22% [60], and up to 15% in those originating from the urinary bladder [61]. The deep retroperitoneal location, often between the cava and aorta, the close proximity to the origin of the inferior mesenteric vessels in Zuckerkandl tumors, and the malignant propensity may not make these neoplasms suitable for laparoscopic approach (Figure 32.10a and b).

MALIGNANT PHEOCHROMOCYTOMA

Primary adrenal pheochromocytoma, whether sporadic or familial, carries a risk of malignancy of about 5%, whereas extra-adrenal origin is associated with a 5- to 10-fold higher risk [28,58,62,63]. In our experience and that of others, one-half of all malignant pheochromocytomas arise from extra-adrenal sites [45,58,63–65]. Other than extra-adrenal origin, there is no identifiable risk factor in the genesis of malignancy (Figure 32.11).

Markedly elevated serum chromogranin A and high excretion of urinary homovanillic acid (HVA) in adults are suggestive of malignant pheochromocytoma. Large size with confluent necrosis, local invasion, and distant

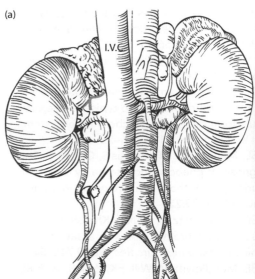

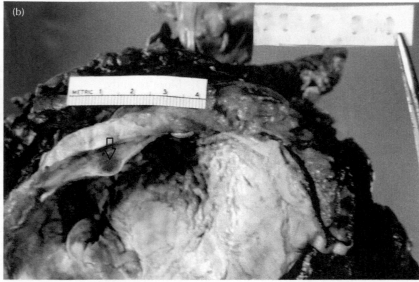

Figure 32.10 **(a, b)** A 13-year-old girl had pheochromocytoma of the superior mediastinum, 1 pharyngeal and 13 abdominal extra-adrenal pheochromocytomas (10 were para-aortic, 2 in the urinary bladder, and 1 in the vagina). The mediastinal and five para-aortic tumors were resected successfully. The patient died at age 19 from massive carotid bleeding following resection of the pharyngeal pheochromocytoma by an otolaryngology team. The adrenal glands were normal at autopsy.

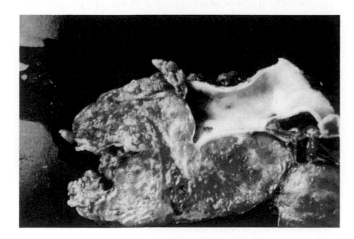

Figure 32.11 Malignant extra-adrenal para-aortic tumor invading the inferior vena cava. The patient had three operations for removal of extra-adrenal pheochromocytomas, the first at age 13. The involved infrarenal cava was resected, and an interposition vein graft was used. The patient died at the age of 39 from metastatic and locally recurrent disease.

metastases are the hallmarks of malignant disease. The histology of the primary tumor by light microscopy does not permit distinction between benign and malignant tumors. The natural history of malignant pheochromocytoma cannot be predicted by morphologic or histochemical features of the primary or metastatic tumors. The typically slow growth of malignant pheochromocytomas favors aggressive surgical debulking and management with antihypertensive and antiarrhythmic medications. Overall, a 50% 5-year survival with advanced disease is not unusual [45,58,62,64–68].

Reduction in tumor size, serum tumor markers, catecholamine hypersecretion, and clinical improvement have been difficult to achieve with chemotherapy and conventional radiotherapy.

In a small sample of 14 patients, combination chemotherapy with cyclophosphamide, vincristine, and dacarbazine yielded complete and partial biochemical and clinical responses in 79% and 57%, respectively, with a median duration of 21–22 months [69].

Following diagnostic avid uptake of the isotope, intravenous radiotherapy has been recently reported. I-131 MIBG is taken up and concentrated by 85%–90% of pheochromocytomas and metastases, enabling delivery of selective therapeutic radiation [70]. More than 100 patients have been treated with I-131 MIBG at several medical centers, with doses ranging from 100 to more than 500 mCi in single or multiple sessions [71]. The radionuclide is also concentrated in the sympathetic neurons and adrenal medulla, but there were no adverse effects on the sympathoadrenal system. Partial remission was reflected in reduction of tumor size and improved function in one-third of the patients. Complete remissions were rare, and recurrence or progression was observed within 2 years. The only serious side effect was transient bone marrow depression.

PHEOCHROMOCYTOMA AND PREGNANCY

Hypertension and pre-eclampsia, common during gestation; the limitations in biochemical diagnosis and localization; the risk of exposure to ionizing radiation; and the unknown effects of adrenergic blockade on the fetus during the first two trimesters have magnified the challenges in pregnancy.

Prior to the 1970s, unrecognized pheochromocytoma before or during pregnancy, during delivery, and in the early postpartum recovery carried a mortality rate of about 50% for the fetus and the mother [72,73]. More recently, improved recognition, localization, and management have resulted in drastic reduction of maternal mortality to 17% overall and 1% if the diagnosis was made antepartum [74]. In a review of 139 patients by Harper et al. [74], the correct diagnosis was made before delivery in only about one-half of the cases.

The normal range of concentrations of catecholamines and their metabolites in the plasma and urine during pregnancy has not been adequately studied, even though Freier and Thompson found that they are not affected by pregnancy. Imaging of the abdomen is limited to ultrasonography and MRI, as I-123 MIBG and CT are contraindicated because of unknown consequences to the fetus.

The surgical strategies are determined by the obstetrician, endocrine physician, surgeon, and mother. Uncontrolled hypertension at any stage is an indication for immediate surgical intervention. After completion of organogenesis at about 24 weeks, adrenergic blockade is no longer contraindicated, and pregnancy can be continued with adequate pharmacologic control in the second trimester; the risk of spontaneous abortion is low, and laparoscopic or open surgery is apparently safe [75]. The synchronous caesarian delivery and resection of the pheochromocytoma is the safest surgical option.

REFERENCES

1. Curley SA, Lott ST, Luca JW, Frazier ML, Killary AM. Surgical decision-making affected by clinical and genetic screening of a novel kindred with von Hippel-Lindau disease and pancreatic islet cell tumors. *Ann Surg* 1998;227:229–35.
2. Sipple JH. The association of pheochromocytoma with carcinoma of the thyroid gland. *Am J Med* 1961;31:163–6.
3. Eng C. The RET proto-oncogene in multiple endocrine neoplasias type 2 and Hirschsprung's disease. *N Engl J Med* 1996;335:943–51.
4. Ricardi VM. Neurofibromatosis: Past, present, and future. *N Engl J Med* 1991;324:1283–5.
5. Couch V, Lindor N, Karnes PS, Michels VV. Von Hippel-Lindau disease. *Mayo Clin Proc* 2000;75:265–72.
6. Arguiar RCT, Cox G, Pomeroy SL, Dahia RLM. Analysis of the SDHD gene, the susceptibility gene for familial paraganglioma syndrome (PGLI) in pheochromocytoma. *J Clin Endocrinol Metab* 2001;86:2890–4.
7. Stratakis CA, Carney JA. The triad of paragangliomas, gastric stromal tumors and pulmonary chondromas (Carney's triad) and the dyad of paragangliomas and gastric stromal sarcomas (Carney-Stratakis syndrome): Molecular genetics and clinical implications. *J Int Med* 2009;266:43–52.
8. Manger W, Gifford RW Jr. *Pheochromocytoma*. New York: Springer Verlag, 1977.
9. Pick L. Das ganglioma embryonale sympathicum (sympathoma embryonale), eine typische boesartige geschwulstform des sympathisches nervensystem. *Berl Klin Wochenschr* 1912;49:16–22.
10. Gitlow SE, Mendlowitz M, Khassis S, Cohen G, Sha J. The diagnosis of pheochromocytoma by determination of urinary 3-methoxy-4-hydroxy-mandelic acid. *J Clin Invest* 1960;39:221–6.
11. Gitlow SE, Mendlowitz M, Kruk E, Khassis S. Diagnosis of pheochromocytoma by assay of catecholamine metabolites. *Circ Res* 1961;9:746–54.
12. Gitlow SE, Mendlowitz M, Wilk EK, Wilk S, Wolf RL, Bertani LM. Excretion of catecholamine metabolites by normal children. *J Lab Clin Invest* 1968;72:612–20.
13. Lenders JWM, Keiser HR, Goldstein DS et al. Plasma metanephrines in the diagnosis of pheochromocytoma. *Ann Intern Med* 1995;123:101–9.
14. Eisenhofer G, Lenders JWM, Linehan WM et al. Plasma normetanephrine and metanephrine for detecting pheochromocytoma in von Hippel-Lindau disease and multiple endocrine neoplasia type 2. *N Engl J Med* 1999;340:1872–9.
15. Hume DM. Pheochromocytoma in the adult and in the child. *Am J Surg* 1960;99:458–96.
16. Stackpole RH, Melicow MM, Uson AC. Pheochromocytoma in children: Report of 9 cases and review of the first 100 published cases with follow-up studies. *J Pediatr* 1963;63:315–30.
17. Lamiell JM, Salazar FG, Hsia YE. Von Hippel-Lindau disease affecting 43 members of a single kindred. *Medicine (Baltimore)* 1989;68:1–29.
18. Maher ER, Yates ER, Harries R. Clinical features and natural history of von Hippel-Lindau disease. *Q J Med* 1990;77:1151–63.
19. Kalff V, Shapiro B, Lloyd R et al. The spectrum of pheochromocytoma in hypertensive patients with neurofibromatosis. *Arch Intern Med* 1982;142:2092–8.
20. Griffiths DFR, Williams GT, Williams ED. Duodenal carcinoid tumors, pheochromocytoma and neurofibromatosis; islet cell tumors, pheochromocytoma and von Hippel-Lindau complex: two distinctive neuroendocrine syndromes. *Q J Med* 1987;245:769–89.
21. Howe JR, Norton JA, Wells SA Jr. Prevalence of pheochromocytoma and hyperparathyroidism in multiple endocrine neoplasia type 2A: Results of long-term follow-up. *Surgery* 1993;114:1070–7.
22. Cohen MA, Phay JE, DeBenedetti MK et al. Gastrointestinal manifestations of multiple endocrine neoplasia type 2. Presented at 113th Annual Session of the Southern Surgical Association, Hot Springs, VA, December 2–5, 2001.

23. Trump DL, Livingston JN, Brylin DB. Watery diarrhea syndrome in an adult with ganglioneuroma-pheochromocytoma: Identification of vasoactive intestinal polypeptide, calcitonin and catecholamines and assessment of their biologic activity. *Cancer* 1977;40:15–26.

24. Sackel SG, Manson JE, Hazawi SJ, Burakof R. Watery diarrhea syndrome due to an adrenal pheochromocytoma secreting vasoactive intestinal polypeptide. *Dig Dis Sci* 1985;30:1201–7.

25. Fisher BM, MacPhee GJA, Davies DL et al. A case of watery diarrhea syndrome due to an adrenal pheochromocytoma secreting vasoactive intestinal polypeptide with coincidental autoimmune thyroid disease. *Acta Endocrinol* 1987;114:340–4.

26. Herrera MF, Stone E, Deitel M, Asa SL. Pheochromocytoma producing multiple vasoactive peptides. *Arch Surg* 1992;127:105–8.

27. Wilkenfeld C, Cohen M, Lansman SL et al. Heart transplantation for end-stage cardiomyopathy caused by an occult pheochromocytoma. *J Heart Lung Transpl* 1992;11:363–6.

28. Inabnet WB, Caragliano P, Pertsemlidis D. Pheochromocytoma: Inherited associations, bilaterality and cortex preservation. *Surgery* 2000;128(6):1007–1.

29. Neumann HPH, Bausch B, McWjinney SR et al. Germline mutations in nonsyndromic pheochromocytoma. *N Engl J Med* 2002;346:1459–70.

30. Carney JA, Sheps SG, Gordon H. The triad of gastric leiomyosarcoma, functioning extra-adrenal paraganglioma and pulmonary chondroma. *N Engl J Med* 1977;296:1517–8.

31. Pertsemlidis D, Gitlow SE, Siegel W, Kark AE. Pheochromocytoma: 1) Specificity of laboratory diagnostic tests. 2) Safeguards during operative removal. *Ann Surg* 1969;169:376–85.

32. Lenders JWM, Pacak K, Walther MM et al. Biochemical diagnosis of pheochromocytoma. *JAMA* 2002;287:1427–34.

33. Young WF Jr. Pheochromocytoma and primary aldosteronism: Diagnostic approaches. *Endocrinol Metab Clin North Am* 1997;26(4):801–27.

34. Yeh HC. Ultrasonography of normal adrenal glands and small adrenal masses. *AJR Am J Roentgenol* 1980;1135:1167–77.

35. Korobkin M, Brodeur FJ, Francis IR et al. Delayed enhanced CT for differentiation of benign from malignant adrenal masses. *Radiology* 1996;200:737–42.

36. Raisanen J, Shapiro B, Glazer GM et al. Plasma catecholamines in pheochromocytoma: Effect of urographic contrast media. *AJR Am J Roentgenol* 1984;143:43–6.

37. Mukherjee JJ, Peppercorn PD, Reznek RH et al. Pheochromocytoma: Effect of nonionic contrast medium in CT on circulating catecholamine levels. *Radiology* 1997;202:227–31.

38. Seregni B, Chiti A, Bombardieri E. Radionuclide imaging of neuroendocrine tunours: Biological basis and diagnostic results. *Eur J Nucl Med* 1998;25:639–58.

39. Proye C, Thevenin D, Cecat P et al. Exclusive use of calcium channel blockers in preoperative and intraoperative control of pheochromocytomas: Hemodynamics and free catecholamine assays in ten consecutive patients. *Surgery* 1989;106(1067):1149–54.

40. Boutros AR, Bravo EL, Zanettin G, Straffon RA. Perioperative management of 63 patients with pheochromocytoma. *Cleve Clin J Med* 1990;57:613–7.

41. Johns VJ, Brunjes S. Pheochromocytoma. *Am J Cardiol* 1962;9:120–5.

42. Sjoerdsma A, Engelman K, Waldmann TA, Cooperman LH, Hammond WG. Pheochromocytoma: Current concepts of diagnosis and treatment; combined clinical staff conference at the National Institutes of Health. *Ann Intern Med* 1996;65:1302–6.

43. Newell KA, Prinz RA, Brooks MH et al. Plasma catecholamine changes during excision of pheochromocytoma. *Surgery* 1988;104:1064–73.

44. Gabrielson G, Guffin A, Kaplan J, Pertsemlidis D, Iberti T. Continuous intravenous infusions of phentolamine and esmolol for preoperative and intraoperative adrenergic blockade in patients with pheochromocytoma. *J Cardiothorac Anesthes* 1987;6:554–8.

45. Pertsemlidis D. Laparoscopic versus open adrenalectomy in pheochromocytoma. In: Bruch HP, Koeckerling F, Bouchard R, Schug-Pass C, eds., *New Aspects of High Technology in Medicine*. Bologna: Monduzzi Editore, 2000:65–74.

46. Rosenthal RJ, Friedman RL, Phillips EJ. Intra-abdominal pressure, intracranial pressure and hemodynamics. In: Rosenthal RJ, Friedman RL, Phillips EH, eds., *Pathophysiology of Pneumoperitoneum*. Berlin: Springer Verlag, 1998:85–98.

47. Mitty HA, Yeh HC. *Radiology of the Adrenals with Sonography and CT*. Philadelphia: Saunders Company, 1982.

48. Pertsemlidis D. Minimal access versus open adrenalectomy. *Surg Endosc* 1995;9:384–6.

49. Libutti SK, Choyke PL, Bartlett DL et al. Pancreatic neuroendocrine tumors associated with von Hippel-Lindau disease: Diagnostic and management recommendations. *Surgery* 1998;124(6):1153–9.

50. Carney JA, Sizemore GW, Sheps SG. Adrenal medullary disease in multiple endocrine neoplasia type 2: Pheochromocytoma and its precursors. *Am J Clin Pathol* 1976;66:279.

51. Neumann HPH, Berger DP, Sigmund G et al. Pheochromocytoma, multiple endocrine neoplasia type 2 and von Hippel-Lindau disease. *N Engl J Med* 1993;329:1531–8.

52. Latif F, Tory K, Gnaza J et al. Identification of the von Hippel-Lindau disease tumor suppressor gene. *Science* 1993;260:1317–20.

53. Curley SA, Lott ST, Luca JW et al. Surgical decision making affected by clinical and genetic screening of a novel kindred with von Hippel-Lindau disease and pancreatic islet cell tumors. *Ann Surg* 1998;227:229–35.

54. Walther MM, Herring J, Enquist E et al. von Recklinghausen's disease and pheochromocytoma. *J Urol* 1999;162:1582–6.

55. Lack EE. *Pathology of Adrenal and Extra-Adrenal Paraganglia*. Philadelphia: WB Saunders, 1994:1–14.

56. Moulton JS. CT of adrenal glands. *Semin Roentgenol* 1988;23:299.

57. Stenstroem G, Svaerdsudd K. Pheochromocytoma in children 1958–81: An analysis of the National Cancer Registry. *Acta Med Scand* 1986;220:225.

58. Melicow MM. One-hundred cases of pheochromocytoma (107 tumors) at the Columbia-Presbyterian Medical Center 1926–1976; a clinicopathological analysis. *Cancer* 1977;40:1987–2004.

59. Fries JG, Chamberlin JA. Extra-adrenal pheochromocytoma; literature review and report of a cervical pheochromocytoma. *Surgery* 1968;63:268–79.

60. Glenn F, Gray GF. Functional tumors of the organ of Zuckerkandl. *Ann Surg* 1976;183:578–86.

61. Khan O, Williams G, Chisholm GD, Welbourn RB. Pheochromocytoma of the bladder. *J R Soc Med* 1982;75:17–20.

62. Scott HW Jr, Halter SA. Oncologic aspects of pheochromocytoma; the importance of follow-up. *Surgery* 1984;96:1061–6.

63. van Heerden JA, Sizemore GW, Carney JA et al. Surgical management of the adrenal glands in the multiple endocrine neoplasia 2 syndrome. *World J Surg* 1984;8:612.

64. Mahoney EM, Harrison JH. Malignant pheochromocytoma; clinical course and treatment. *J Urol* 1977;118:225–9.

65. Sclafani LM, Woodruff JM, Brennan MF. Extra-adrenal retroperitoneal paragangliomas; natural history and response to treatment. *Surgery* 1990;108:1124–30.

66. Thompson JW, Allo MD, Shapiro B et al. Extra-adrenal and metastatic pheochromocytoma; the role of I-131 meta-iodobenzylguanidine (I-131 MIBG) in localization and management. *World J Surg* 1984;8:605–11.

67. Hayes WS, Davidson AJ, Grimley PM et al. Extra-adrenal retroperitoneal paraganglioma; clinical, pathological and CT findings. *AJR Am J Roentgenol* 1990;155:1247–50.

68. van Heerden JA, Sheps BH, Sheedy PF et al. Pheochromocytoma: Current status and changing trends. *Surgery* 1982;91:367–73.

69. Averbuch SD, Steakly CS, Young RC et al. Malignant pheochromocytoma: Effective treatment with a combination of cyclophosphamide, vincristine and dacarbazine. *Ann Intern Med* 1988;109:267–73.

70. Shapiro B, Copp JE, Sissan JC et al. Iodine-131 metaiodobenzylguanidine for the locating of suspected pheochromocytoma: Experience in 400 cases. *J Nucl Med* 1985;26:576–85.

71. Sisson JC. Radiopharmaceutical treatment of pheochromocytoma. *Ann NY Acad Sci* 2002;970:54–60.

72. Schenker JG, Chowers I. Pheochromocytoma and pregnancy. *Obstet Gynecol Surg* 1971;26:739–46.

73. Schenker JG, Granat M. Pheochromocytoma and pregnancy—An updated appraisal. *Aust NZ J Obstet Gynaecol* 1982;22:1–10.

74. Harper MA, Murnaghan GA, Kennedy L et al. Pheochromocytoma in pregnancy: Five cases and a review of the literature. *Br J Obstet Gynaecol* 1989;996:594–606.

75. Brunt LM. Phaeochromocytoma in pregnancy. *Br J Surg* 2001;88:481–483.

33

Adrenal incidentalomas

DAVID C. ARON, ALEXIS K. OKOH, AND EREN BERBER

INTRODUCTION

The discovery of an adrenal mass in the course of abdominal imaging performed for other reasons, "adrenal incidentaloma," is a common clinical problem that poses a challenging management dilemma [1–4]. This dilemma arises because while most incidentalomas will be clinically insignificant (benign and hormonally inactive adenomas) and pose no risk to a patient's health, there may be some lesions that do carry a significant risk, either because of their hormonal activity or because of their malignant histology. The challenge is to recognize and treat these few, while leaving the others alone. As imaging techniques improve and their use becomes more widespread, we can expect to encounter this challenge more frequently. Over the years, myriad approaches have been recommended related to diagnosis and management. Controversies remain and practice varies [5–15].

MAGNITUDE OF THE PROBLEM

Incidentaloma is not so much a disease entity as it is a finding that may or may not represent disease [9]. What is the magnitude of this management dilemma? The question is difficult to answer, in part due to lack of standard definitions and in part due to variability in methods and circumstances of detection. Although there is disagreement, most authors agree on the fact that an adrenal incidentaloma is a mass discovered by imaging done for reasons other than suspected adrenal pathology. Differences of opinion exist about exclusion criteria, such as the known presence of extra-adrenal cancer. It is arguable to call something an incidentaloma when the complaints that prompt the imaging, although not initially suspected to be related to adrenal pathology, later turn out to be caused by the adrenal mass. The prevalence of incidentaloma, however defined, will vary depending upon the circumstances under which these lesions are detected, both the methods of detection and the reasons for the imaging study. For example, the prevalence of clinically inapparent adrenal masses found at autopsy is about 2.1%, but "clinically inapparent" is in the eye of the beholder. Prevalence estimates range from about 0.1% for general health screening with ultrasound, to 0.4%–1.9% among patients evaluated for nonendocrinologic complaints, to more than 4% among patients who have had a previous cancer diagnosis [9]. Prevalence on abdominal computed tomography (CT) scans can exceed 10%, but such estimates are affected by selection bias. The prevalence of adrenal incidentalomas increases with age.

The differential diagnosis of an incidentally discovered mass is extensive (Table 33.1), but most are nonsecreting cortical adenomas. In a recent systematic review that combined studies using the broadest definitions, adenomas accounted for 41%, metastases 19%, adrenocortical carcinoma 10%, myelolipoma 9%, and pheochromocytoma 8%, with other,

Table 33.1 Differential diagnosis of an incidentally discovered adrenal mass

Adrenal cortical tumors
- Adenoma[a]
- Carcinoma[a]
- Nodular hyperplasia[a]

Adrenal medullary tumors
- Pheochromocytoma[a]
- Ganglioneuroma/neuroblastoma[a]

Other adrenal tumors
- Myelolipoma
- Metastases
- Miscellaneous, e.g., hamartoma, teratoma, lipoma, and hemangioma

Infections, granulomas, and infiltrations
- Abscess
- Amyloidosis
- Fungal infection, e.g., histoplasmosis, coccidiomycosis, blastomycosis, and tuberculosis
- Sarcoidosis
- Cytomegalovirus

Cysts and pseudocysts
- Parasitic
- Endothelial
- Degenerative adenomas

Congenital adrenal hyperplasia[a]

Hemorrhage

Pseudoadrenal masses
- Splenic, pancreatic, and renal lesions
- Vascular lesions (especially aneurysms and tortuous splenic veins)
- Technical artifacts

[a] Potentially functional.

mostly benign lesions comprising the remainder [9,16,17]. The distribution of diagnoses will change as other inclusion and exclusion criteria are applied, i.e., metastases becoming far less common if patients with known extra-adrenal cancer are excluded. The distribution of etiologies varies by size of the lesion; larger tumors are more likely to be malignant than smaller ones. Among lesions larger than 6 cm, adrenal carcinomas comprised 25% and metastases 18%, while adenomas accounted for only 18% [9]. When bilateral adrenal masses are found, which occurs in about 10%–15%, several diagnoses are more likely. These include metastatic disease, congenital adrenal hyperplasia, lymphoma, infection (e.g., tuberculosis or fungal), hemorrhage, adrenocorticotropic hormone (ACTH)-dependent Cushing's syndrome, pheochromocytoma, amyloidosis, and infiltrative disease of the adrenal glands. Incidental adrenal enlargement (defined as an adrenal body of >10 mm or limb of >5 mm) was found in 11.3% in a retrospective review of CT scans, but that finding was mentioned on contemporaneous reports by the radiologist in fewer than 15% of those cases [18].

DEMOGRAPHICS AND GENETIC RISK FACTORS

The prevalence of adrenal incidentalomas identified at autopsy increases from less than 1% among individuals less than 30 years of age to about 7% in those 70 years of age or older [9]. There appear to be no gender differences in prevalence from autopsy studies or general health exams. Patients with clinical features associated with functioning adrenal lesions (e.g., primary hyperaldosteronism, pheochromocytoma, Cushing's syndrome, and virilization) are more likely to have adrenal tumors. Although in many cases these features are subtle and do not prompt early diagnosis, whether one should consider these lesions to be "incidental" or serendipitous is a matter of dispute.

Although the molecular pathogenesis of adrenal tumors has not been elucidated, these mechanisms are under active investigation [19–21]. A variety of rare genetic syndromes predispose to adrenocortical tumors. These include Beckwith–Wiedemann, Li–Fraumeni, multiple endocrine neoplasia (MEN) 1, Carney complex, and McCune–Albright syndromes [22]. Similarly, some syndromes predispose to adrenomedullary tumors: MEN 2, von Hippel–Lindau disease, and neurofibromatosis type 1. Because of their rarity and obvious clinical characteristics, they are not diagnosed after the finding of an incidentaloma. Nevertheless, some of the molecular targets for these syndromes have been isolated. Understanding these targets may be relevant to the more typical sporadic adrenal incidentaloma and lead to better diagnostic, therapeutic, and preventive measures. For example, overexpression of the insulin-like growth factor II (IGF-II) gene has been associated with the tumors of the Beckwith–Wiedemann syndrome. Germline mutations in the p53 tumor suppressor gene contribute to the high cancer risk (breast carcinoma, soft tissue and bone sarcoma, brain tumor, leukemia, and adrenocortical carcinoma) in the autosomal dominant Li–Fraumeni syndrome. Adrenal cancer is a very unusual presentation of this unusual syndrome. Abnormalities in the RET-2 proto-oncogene have been associated with pheochromocytoma in MEN 2 [19]. More recently, genetic studies have moved from specific target genes to genome-wide expression profiling and other techniques that allow identification of specific tumor subgroups with distinct patterns of markers, activation of molecular pathways, and clinical behavior [19]. Thus, while the risks for developing an adrenal mass remain to be elucidated, the major risk factor for discovery is clear—undergoing an imaging procedure that includes the abdomen.

CLINICAL FEATURES: CLASSIC AND SUBTLE PHENOTYPIC EXPRESSIONS

A patient with an incidental adrenal mass is susceptible to three types of adverse outcomes: morbidity (endocrinologic or oncologic, or both), mortality, and anxiety from knowing about a tumor that might cause problems in the future [23,24]. Hypersecretion of glucocorticoids, mineralocorticoids, or sex steroids, or catecholamines, produces clinical syndromes, each associated with morbidity and premature mortality if left untreated. The clinical features associated with Cushing's syndrome, primary hyperaldosteronism, virilization, and pheochromocytoma are addressed in other chapters in this volume and elsewhere. More germane to the management of patients with adrenal incidentalomas is the potential morbidity and mortality of autonomous hormone secretion without clear clinical features, especially subclinical autonomous cortisol secretion and "silent" pheochromocytoma.

Subclinical autonomous glucocorticoid hypersecretion (SAGH), sometimes misleadingly termed "subclinical Cushing's syndrome," has been found in 5%–20% of patients with adrenal incidentalomas [25–29]. This autonomous hypersecretion is subtle and may be transient. Variation in prevalence relates to, among other things, lack of standardized criteria for the diagnosis [9,30,31]. Yet, although by definition overt Cushing's syndrome must be absent, these patients have a high prevalence of obesity, hypertension, and diabetes and insulin resistance [32–36]. Use of the glucocorticoid receptor blocker in such patients has reduced insulin resistance [37]. Abnormalities in bone turnover and bone mass have been reported [9,38–42]. Tauchmanova et al. used the criteria of the National Italian Group on Adrenal Tumors in a study to assess cardiovascular risk factors in patients with SAGH. In addition to the absence of clinical signs of cortisol excess, these include two abnormalities in the regulation of the hypothalamic–pituitary–adrenal axis: failure to suppress serum cortisol to less than 83 nmol/L (3 μg/dL) by a 2 mg dexamethasone suppression test and the combination of a low ACTH, high urinary free cortisol, and diminished response to corticotropin-releasing hormone [43]. This study involved 28 consecutive patients and 100 age-, sex-, and body mass index-matched controls. They found that systolic and diastolic blood pressures were higher in patients, as were fasting glucose, insulin, total cholesterol, and triglycerides. In addition to elevated insulin resistance, the patients had increased waist-to-hip ratios and high frequencies of hypertension (61%), lipid abnormalities (71%), and impaired glucose tolerance or diabetes (64%); 85% had multiple cardiovascular risk factors. Evidence of cardiovascular disease was present in a high proportion of patients based on clinical evidence, electrocardiogram, or carotid ultrasound examination. There is increasing evidence of impact of SAGH on long-term morbidity [29,44]. These metabolic abnormalities may improve after removal of the adrenal incidentaloma. In the continuum from normal cortisol–ACTH feedback to autonomous cortisol production, the stage at which cortisol autonomy results in clinical morbidity is not clear [29,44]. Tsagarakis et al. performed a dexamethasone suppression test in 61 patients with incidentally detected adrenal masses. In a *post hoc* analysis patients were divided into three groups: patients with a post dexamethasone level of cortisol of >70 nmol/L (group A, $n = 19$), 30–70 nmol/L (group B, $n = 27$), and <30 nmol/L (group C, $n = 15$) [45]. Group A patients had significantly higher cholesterol and triglyceride

concentrations than group C patients. The hypersecretion of cortisol may be reflected in the occurrence of adrenal insufficiency after removal of an adrenal incidentaloma and in the amelioration of metabolic syndrome following incidentaloma resection (see below) [30,46].

Although the classic features of pheochromocytoma are well known, many patients lack those features and the diagnosis is often missed or delayed [47]. Among patients with adrenal incidentalomas, the frequency of pheochromocytoma varies widely; in most series of incidentalomas, pheochromocytomas account for ≤10% [9,48–50]. Among patients referred to the Mayo Clinic for management of adrenal pheochromocytoma, 10% were discovered in the course of evaluation for adrenal incidentalomas [50]. These silent pheochromocytomas may also be lethal [47]. Hormonal testing for urinary or plasma metanephrines counts among the most reliable tests, with both sensitivity and specificity of around 95% [51].

The most feared diagnostic possibility for an adrenal incidentaloma is adrenal cancer, which has a mean survival of approximately 18 months and 5-year survival of approximately 16%; the clinical manifestations of this disorder are addressed in other chapters in this volume and elsewhere [52–56]. Mercifully, clinically diagnosed cases are rare; the incidence of adrenal carcinoma in general is approximately 0.5–2.0 cases per million population per year [53]. However, the relative frequency of adrenal cancer varies considerably among adrenal incidentaloma series: 4.2% in the whole National Italian Study Group (AI-SIE) series, but 25% in another study [57–59]. The reasons for the differences among adrenal incidentaloma series and between adrenal incidentaloma series and population estimates are unclear. With the increased detection of incidentalomas and their surgical removal, it might be anticipated that the adrenal cancer would be detected at an earlier stage. Although some single-site studies have suggested as much, a larger national sample found no differences across four equal time quartiles from 1973 to 2000 [60]. Adrenal cancers can be functional or nonfunctional; most are probably functional, although the steroids synthesized may have low biological activity. Adrenal cancers may also cause Cushing's syndrome, virilizing syndromes, or a mixed Cushing–virilizing syndrome. Estrogen-secreting tumors causing feminization are rare, as are aldosterone-secreting carcinomas.

The adrenal glands are highly vascular organs, and therefore common sites of metastases from extra-adrenal malignancy. In patients with a history of malignant disease, metastases are the most common cause of an incidental adrenal mass, regardless of size, accounting for 48% of all incidentalomas in these patients [61–63]. Carcinomas of the lung, breast, kidney, and gastrointestinal tract, and melanoma or lymphoma constitute the most common sources of adrenal metastases [9]. In fact, of those who die of epithelial malignancies, adrenal metastases are found in 25%–75%. The source of the primary malignancy usually is known when an adrenal incidentaloma is discovered; metastatic cancer presenting as an isolated true adrenal incidentaloma is distinctly unusual. Although adrenal metastases are generally bilateral and larger than 3 cm, they may be unilateral and small.

Finally, the unknown is also a concern. Anxiety for both patient and physician stemming from the knowledge about the presence of a mass of uncertain importance is not a trivial concern [64]. All of these findings suggest a benefit of presymptomatic diagnosis for individual patients. However, at the population level the health risk posed by adrenal incidentalomas (in patients without known malignancy), although real, is small because of the low prevalence of clinically significant tumors with hormonal activity or malignant potential, and the more common presence of a nonfunctional adrenal incidentaloma.

BIOCHEMICAL DIAGNOSIS

Established algorithms exist for the diagnosis of hormonally active adrenal lesions [52,65–68]. When patients present with signs or symptoms of these disorders, diagnostic evaluation can proceed apace. However, when patients have few or no signs of a particular disorder, the evaluation is more challenging. Diagnostic test performance characteristics in such patients in actual practice are not known, but they will be less accurate than in patients with clinically apparent disease [69]. Test sensitivity is likely to be lower than in the study population from which the original characteristics were derived (spectrum bias); test specificity is also likely to be lower. Moreover, the absence of gold standards for the diagnosis makes assessment of test characteristics problematic. Finally, predictive value is dependent upon the prevalence of disease. Even a test with high sensitivity and specificity will, when used to detect a rare condition, falsely identify many nonaffected individuals as having the disease. Notwithstanding these limitations, a few studies have evaluated test performance [9]. For example, two studies have used unilateral uptake on [131]beta-iodo-methylnorcholesterol (NP-59) (radioiodinated cholesterol) scintigraphy as the indicator of autonomous activity of the incidentaloma [70]. No single biochemical test was found to discriminate reliably between unilateral and bilateral uptake on scintigraphy. Bardet et al. [70] found that low 8:00 a.m. dehydroepiandrosterone sulfate, low 8:00 a.m. ACTH, basal urinary free cortisol, unsuppressed 8:00 a.m. serum cortisol after overnight 1 mg dexamethasone suppression, unsuppressed day 2 serum cortisol, and unsuppressed day 2 urinary free cortisol after low-dose dexamethasone suppression had low sensitivity (0%–50%) and moderate specificity (79%–94%) to differentiate unilateral from bilateral scintigraphy uptake. In contrast, Valli et al. found that unsuppressed 8:00 a.m. cortisol after overnight dexamethasone suppression had 100% sensitivity and 67% specificity to predict unilateral uptake [71]. Studies of diagnosis of catecholamine excess and primary hyperaldosteronism reveal similar problems in sensitivity and specificity [48]. Recently, the use of late-night salivary cortisol as a screening test has been evaluated in adrenal incidentalomas and found to have high sensitivity, although results for specificity were mixed [72,73].

The optimal strategy for biochemical evaluation of a patient with an incidentally discovered adrenal mass is unclear and remains controversial. Nevertheless, systematic screening may reduce the number of unnecessary surgeries. Musella et al. conducted a retrospective study of the value of preoperative workup in the assessment of adrenal incidentalomas in 282 consecutive laparoscopic adrenalectomies [74]. Patients who had preoperative evaluation were compared with those who did not receive that evaluation. The evaluation consisted of a 1 mg dexamethasone suppression test, serum potassium, plasma renin and aldosterone, and fractionated metanephrines. They concluded that the unnecessary number of adrenalectomies performed in understudied patients, causing higher morbidity, was not associated with a higher detection rate of primary adrenocortical cancer [74]. Regardless of the approach used, it should be tailored to what is available; tests should be chosen based on their performance characteristics in the laboratories and radiology suites where they are actually performed [75].

MOLECULAR MARKERS

A variety of tissue molecular markers have been used to distinguish malignant from benign adrenal tumors and determine prognosis. These include mutant p53, the proliferation-associated antigen Ki67 protein, loss of heterozygosity at the 17p13 and 11p15 loci, and overexpression of the IGF-II gene and other IGF system products, such as IGF binding protein 2 (IGFBP-2). Serum levels of IGFBP-2 have been assessed as a tumor marker [76]. Boulle et al. found no significant difference in plasma IGFBP-2 concentration between healthy controls and patients with complete remission or localized tumors [76]. In contrast, patients with metastatic disease had significantly higher IGFBP-2 plasma levels than the control group ($p < 0.001$). IGFBP-2 levels in patients with metastatic disease were inversely correlated with survival ($R2 = 0.308$; $p = 0.0026$). However, the overall sensitivity and specificity of this test were low; five patients (17.8%) with metastatic tumors had normal IGFBP-2 levels and two patients (13.3%) in complete remission had high plasma IGFBP-2 levels, limiting its value in diagnosis and follow-up of adrenocortical carcinoma.

IMAGING FOR ADRENAL INCIDENTALOMA

While usually discovered on CT, various imaging methods have been used and advocated for the assessment of adrenal incidentaloma [6,77–81]. They can be subdivided into purely morphological methods, on the one hand, and function-based imaging methods, on the other. Examples of the first category are ultrasonography, CT scanning, and magnetic resonance imaging (MRI), while meta-iodobenzylguanidine (MIBG) and NP59 scanning are well-known examples of the latter. The relevance of ultrasonography for adrenal incidentaloma is mainly in its role for detection. As ultrasound scanning is widely used for the assessment of gall bladder pathology, most ultrasound-detected incidentalomas are located in the right adrenal gland. For the diagnostic evaluation of adrenal incidentaloma ultrasound is of limited use [82–84]. It provides some information about the malignant or benign nature of a mass, but none about its functional status; ultrasound data may provide indirect evidence for or against malignancy. Large diameter (as opposed to small), solidity (as opposed to cystic nature), and rapid diameter increase (as opposed to slow growth) can be assessed by ultrasound, and may be used as indicators of malignancy. However, both CT and MRI outperform ultrasound in their ability to diagnose malignancy. The use of ultrasound as a means for following adrenal masses over time has not been extensively studied, although its lack of radiation makes ultrasound a potentially attractive modality.

CT has been used in the assessment of adrenal incidentaloma both to detect malignancy (i.e., to identify those incidentalomas that should be treated) and to identify adenoma (i.e., to identify those insignificant incidentalomas where treatment is not necessary). Large size, irregular shapes, vague contour, invasion into surrounding structures, and high signal intensity have all been used to identify malignancy [85]. Large tumor size has traditionally been one of the diagnostic hallmarks of adrenal incidentaloma; however, only 25% of adrenal incidentalomas greater than 6 cm harbor malignancy [86–88]. In one retrospective study of 210 incidentalomas, a cutoff size of 5 cm yielded a sensitivity of 93% and a specificity of 64% for determining malignancy [58]. Hence, in addition to an absolute tumor size greater than 4–6 cm, any increase in tumor growth over a 6-month period should also trigger the suspicion of malignancy. High signal intensity can be expressed in either so-called Hounsfield units (with an intensity higher than 10 or 20 units being used as diagnostic threshold) or ratio of signal lesion to signal fat (SL/SF) (with above 1.5 suggesting malignancy). Analysis of the German Adrenal Carcinoma Registry found that a threshold of >13 Hounsfield units detected all of the cancerous lesions [85]. The threshold used determines the sensitivity and specificity of the test. At low threshold, sensitivity for malignancy is around 0.9 and specificity around 0.4 [89]. Higher thresholds lead to better specificity (around 0.9), but at the cost of lower sensitivity (0.55). Different techniques have been introduced, e.g., assessing contrast washout on CT and chemical shift MRI. Although individual studies and techniques vary, CT and MRI generally have fairly high sensitivity for detection of adrenal cancer in an incidentally discovered adrenal mass, but specificity is more variable [89]. In addition, radiological technique is not only procedure dependent, but also operator dependent [75]. There are many recent reviews of adrenal radiology; examples of CT and MRI of adrenal incidentalomas are shown in Figures 33.1 through 33.5; Figure 33.6 demonstrates the correlation between radiological findings and anatomical findings at surgery.

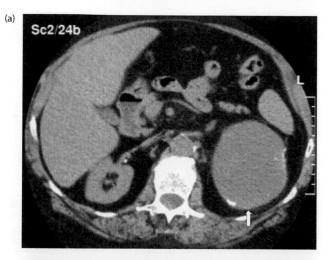

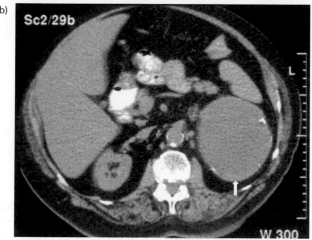

Figure 33.1 Patient B, female, 79 years old, with large mass in the left adrenal region (11 cm cystic incidentaloma), first seen at ultrasound examination for suspected gallstones. Because of the low suspicion of malignancy and no hormonal activity, physician and patient agreed on follow-up without surgery. The mass was stable over a 2-year period. (a) CT scan showing 11 × 10 × 9.5 cm cystic incidentaloma. (b) CT 2 years later: mass stable at 10.5 × 9 cm.

Of the function-based isotope imaging studies, the two most frequently used are ^{131}I or ^{123}I-labeled MIBG and NP-59 [90]. MIBG is mainly used to detect pheochromocytoma, while NP-59 has claimed to assess adrenal hormonal function, as well as to differentiate between benign and malignant adrenal tumors. MIBG has the advantage over CT or MRI in that it provides a whole body image with the administration of one tracer dose. As pheochromocytoma may occur bilaterally, and its occurrence is not confined to the periadrenal region (especially in the case of malignant pheochromocytoma with metastases), MIBG may be used for whole body screening on pheochromocytoma. For pheochromocytoma detection, MIBG has a sensitivity and specificity of around 87% and 95%, respectively [89]. Positive and negative MIBG results therefore change the prior probability of pheochromocytoma in adrenal

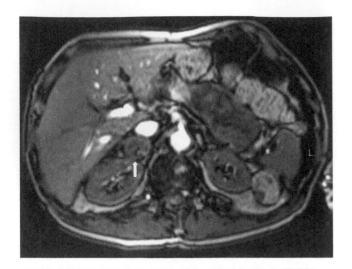

Figure 33.2 Patient K, male, 75 years old, with multiple sclerosis and a 3 cm adrenal mass first seen at imaging for neurological assessment. He was normotensive, and urinary catecholamines were not increased. MRI shows a 3 cm mass in the right adrenal gland (arrow), with fluid level, possibly necrosis, not typical for pheochromocytoma, but cystic pheochromocytoma could not be excluded. A 5 × 3 cm pheochromocytoma was removed laparoscopically. The blood pressure was 150/80 without medication. Final diagnosis: asymptomatic pheochromocytoma.

incidentaloma from 3.5% to around 40% and 0.5%, respectively. Scanning with NP-59 has been advocated as a means to assess adrenal masses [90]. On the basis of concordant or discordant imaging activity, NP-59 has been claimed to help in the identification of adrenocortical cancer, or in identifying hormonally active benign adenomas [90,91]. However, the limited availability of NP59 has kept its use confined to a few centers.

The use of positron emission tomography (PET) scans in diagnosis of adrenal incidentalomas has increased markedly in recent years [92–101]. A meta-analysis of combination PET/CT reports revealed that ¹⁸F-fluorodeoxyglucose (FDG) PET was highly sensitive and specific for differentiating malignant from benign adrenal disease. Diagnostic accuracy was not influenced by the type of imaging device (PET vs. PET/CT), but specificity was dependent on the clinical status (cancer vs. no cancer) [93]. Thus, PET scanning may be particularly useful in patients with known malignancies. PET scanning may also identify functional lesions that would suggest the need for surgery [92]. Finally, CT-guided adrenal biopsy can be performed. However, this procedure is useful primarily in identifying malignancies metastatic to the adrenal; its use in diagnosis of adrenal carcinoma is limited at best [102]. If a biopsy is planned, it is wise to exclude the possibility of pheochromocytoma beforehand [103], In fact, the 2002 National Institutes of Health consensus panel on the management of adrenal incidentaloma strongly discouraged the use of fine-needle aspiration biopsy for the workup of adrenal masses, until the

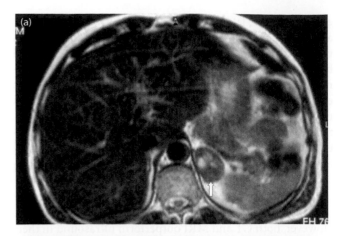

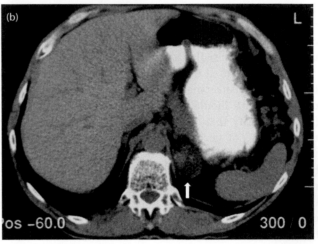

Figure 33.3 Patient D, male, 48 years old, with hypertension and marginally elevated 24-hour urinary cortisol excretion. **(a)** MRI: 4 × 3 cm adrenal mass (arrow), no specific characteristics, but consistent with an adenoma. **(b)** CT 1 year later: 3 × 4.5 cm mass (arrow). At laparoscopic adrenalectomy, an 8 × 5 × 2 cm adenoma was removed. Conclusion: probable SAGH.

patient has conclusive biochemical proof of the absence of pheochromocytoma or another type of functioning tumor [30,104].

DIAGNOSTIC STRATEGIES FOR ADRENAL INCIDENTALOMAS

Adrenal incidentaloma is a typical illustration of the fact that incidental findings, by their nature, pose a considerable threat of overdiagnosis and overtreatment [105]. However, some adrenal incidentalomas are clinically significant, and inadvertently leaving them alone might damage the patient's health, not to mention the doctor's professional status. Therefore, detection of an incidentaloma creates a situation where a decision concerning its management has to be made. Such a decision may range from a most conservative "leave alone" to a most aggressive "take the adrenal gland out straight away," preceded or not by additional biochemical or radiological assessment. Ideally, this decision is

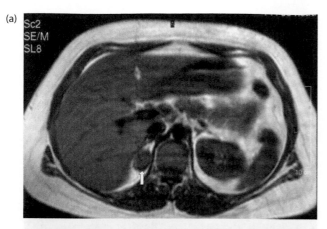

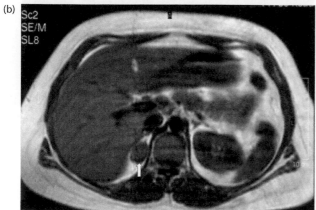

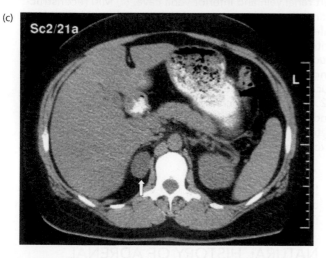

Figure 33.4 Patient S, female, 37 years old, with hypertension and adrenal mass first seen at ultrasound imaging for dyspepsia. **(a)** MRI (T1-weighted imaging): 3 cm mass in right adrenal gland (arrow). **(b)** MRI (T2-weighted imaging): 3 cm mass in right adrenal gland (arrow); no elevated signal intensity. **(c)** CT: 3.3 × 2.5 cm mass (arrow), 17–20 Hounsfield units, possible cortical adenoma. Laboratory data showed marginally elevated urinary norepinephrine and dopamine, normal vanillylmandelic acid, and marginally elevated cortisol excretion. A dexamethasone suppression test showed inadequate suppression. At laparoscopic adrenalectomy, a radical excision of an adenoma was performed. Final diagnosis: SAGH.

based on a careful weighing of the risks and benefits of each diagnostic and therapeutic step [90].

Many different strategies have been devised to deal with adrenal incidentaloma [1,10,11,106–109]. Unfortunately, in a study of guideline quality using the Appraisal of Guidelines Research and Evaluation II (AGREE-II) tool and the Institute of Medicine (IOM) criteria, Shen et al. found that none of the selected guidelines were satisfactory in all aspects [110]. Notwithstanding their shortcomings, most strategies are guided by the aim to elucidate at least two concerns:

1. Assessment of function: Could the incidentaloma, in spite of its not being detected on the basis of clinical signs and symptoms, still be hormonally active and thereby pose a threat to the patient's health?
2. Assessment of histological nature: Could the incidentaloma itself be a malignant tumor, which, if left alone, will continue to grow and metastasize?

The first concern is the reason that all strategies have some form of hormone assessment, focused on either the adrenal medulla (searching for pheochromocytoma) or the adrenal cortex (searching for subclinical Cushing, aldosteronoma, or sex hormone hyperactivity), or both. The second concern is less easily dealt with, as cytology is notoriously less reliable in the differentiation between benign or malignant primary adrenal tumors than for the detection of metastases from extra-adrenal origin in oncology patients [111].

There are numerous specific strategies for hormonal assessment, but most advocate hormonal assessment for pheochromocytoma or autonomous cortisol secretion; assessment for hyperaldosteronism should be undertaken in hypertensive patients. These strategies also vary somewhat in the specific screening tests recommended. Similarly, CT, especially unenhanced with contrast, is generally considered the best procedure to identify a cortical adenoma since lesions of <10 Hounsfield units are benign, though some recommend higher thresholds. CT with contrast and assessment of washout is considered most appropriate when baseline attenuation value is higher. Follow-up could then be used as a means to monitor change in functional activity, or as a way to differentiate between malignant and benign lesions on the basis of increase in diameter over time [112–114]. For biochemical testing, the most commonly recommended studies include a low-dose (1 or 2 mg) dexamethasone suppression test, plasma or urine fractionated metaphrines, and for patients with hypertension, plasma renin and aldosterone.

Differences between strategies can be traced to three main reasons: (1) differences in the use of empirical data to assess the probability of different disorders being present; (2) differences in assumptions about diagnostic and therapeutic effectiveness, again traceable to available empirical evidence; and (3) differences in the importance placed on various outcomes. The first two relate to the quality and validity of the information used. Therefore, differences may be reduced or

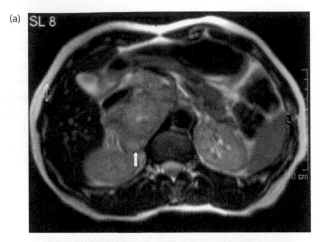

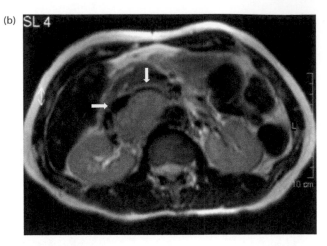

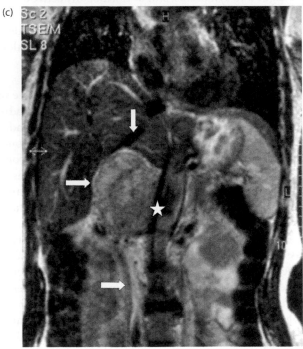

Figure 33.5 Patient T, female, 52 years old, with hypertension (180/110), nonspecific chest pain, and upper abdominal discomfort, for which imaging was performed. (a) MRI (T2-weighted imaging): large 11 × 8 mass in right (peri-)adrenal region (arrow) with low signal intensity. No intravascular growth or other signs of malignancy. (b) MRI (T2-weighted imaging): arrows indicate the close relationship between the mass and the left renal vein and inferior vena cava. (c) MRI reconstruction in frontal plane. Arrows indicate relationship with inferior vena cava. The star indicates the aorta. Urinary catecholamines were elevated. Attempt at surgery; introduction of anesthesia had to be terminated because of uncontrollably elevated blood pressure. Two weeks later: successful extended transabdominal adrenalectomy, 12 × 8 × 5 cm pheochromocytoma with local perineural and intravascular growth. Final diagnosis: pheochromocytoma; malignancy cannot be excluded, but patient in excellent health 2 years after surgery.

eliminated by using methods from evidence-based medicine to identify the correct underlying information. The third cause is not so easily solved, as it relates to judgment, not evidence. Examples of judgmental issues are the weight that is assigned to missing a relevant disorder, to short- or long-term morbidity and mortality, to life expectancy and quality of life, etc. Even the term *relevant* may be defined in different ways, pertaining to either "posing a severe risk to the patient" or "where outcome can be affected by diagnosis and treatment." An adrenal metastasis is relevant in the first sense, but may be considered less relevant or even irrelevant in the second sense, because of the impossibility of influencing the poor prognosis. For such judgmental differences, there are no universal right or wrong answers. The rise of evidence-based medicine has emphasized the quality, transparency, and accountability about the information we use in standard practice [69]. It is equally valuable to reveal how choices are guided by value judgments concerning process and outcome

[89]. The combination of best evidence and careful patient-centered value judgment is the key to good clinical practice for adrenal incidentaloma.

NATURAL HISTORY OF ADRENAL INCIDENTALOMA

There have been several prospective studies of patients with adrenal incidentalomas to determine their natural history and the risk that such lesions developed hormonal hypersecretion or malignancy after initial detection. Among the earliest was that of Barzon et al. [112]. Of 246 consecutive patients with adrenal incidentaloma, 91 underwent surgery. Of the remaining patients, a group of 75 (52 females and 23 males, median age 56 years, range 19–77 years) with incidentally discovered asymptomatic adrenal masses (60 unilateral and 15 bilateral, median diameter 2.5 cm, range 1.0–5.6 cm) were followed for at least 2 years after

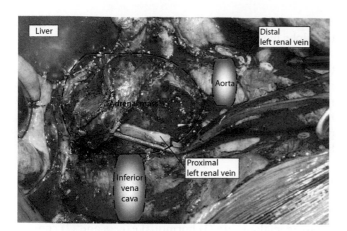

Figure 33.6 Patient T. Intraoperative view (as seen from the right ventral side) of a large adrenal incidentaloma extending from the right adrenal gland behind the inferior vena. The tumor has its maximum diameter between the aorta and the inferior vena cava, pressing these two apart and thereby stretching the left adrenal vein and artery. To gain better access to the tumor, the right colon was mobilized upward, and the left adrenal vein was divided between clamps (with reanastomosis at the end of the operation). Histology demonstrated a pheochromocytoma with angioinvasive and perineural growth.

diagnosis (median 4 years, range 2–10 years). During follow-up, no patients developed malignancy. The estimated cumulative risks to develop mass enlargement and hyperfunction were 8% and 4%, respectively, after 1 year; 18% and 9.5% after 5 years; and 22.8% and 9.5% after 10 years. They concluded that subtle hormonal abnormalities were risk factors for mass size increase [112]. A Swedish multisite study by Bülow et al. involved 229 patients in prospective follow-up (median time 25 months, range 3–108 months) [115]. During the follow-up period, an increase in incidentaloma size of ≥0.5 cm was reported in 17 (7.4%) and of ≥1.0 cm was reported in 12 (5.2%) of the 229 patients. A decrease in size was seen in 12 patients (5.2%). A hypersecreting tumor was found in 2% of the hormonally investigated patients, but no cases of primary adrenal malignancy were observed. Operation was undertaken in 11 patients based on size increase or suspicion of hypersecretion [115]. Vassilatou et al. found similar results, but noted that autonomous hypersecretion (of cortisol) could be intermittent [116]. A major limitation of all of these studies is their exclusion of patients in whom initial testing prompted surgery. The natural history of SAGH remains somewhat uncertain. Barzon et al. found a rate of progression from SAGH to overt Cushing's syndrome in 12.5% of patients at 1 year of follow-up [112]. In one cohort study that followed 12 SAGH patients for a mean period of 25.5 months without surgery, none of the patients progressed to overt Cushing's syndrome; however, some moderate worsening of biochemical indices of the disease was observed, thus suggesting mild disease progression [112]. In fact,

progressively increased patterns of SAGH are associated with worse metabolic and cardiovascular outcomes [44].

There is one (small) randomized trial [117]. Over a 15-year period, 45 SAGH patients were randomly selected to undergo surgery ($n = 23$) or conservative management ($n = 22$) [117]. All surgical procedures were laparoscopic adrenalectomies performed by the same surgeon. All patients were followed up (mean 7.7 years, range 2–17 years) clinically by two experienced endocrinologists 6 and 12 months after surgery and then yearly, or yearly after joining the trial, particularly monitoring diabetes mellitus (DM), arterial hypertension, hyperlipidemia, obesity, and osteoporosis. All 23 patients in the surgical arm had elective surgery. Another three patients randomly assigned to conservative management crossed over to the surgical group due to an increasing adrenal mass of >3.5 cm. In the surgical group, diabetes normalized or improved in 62.5% of patients (5 of 8), hypertension in 67% (12 of 18), hyperlipidemia in 37.5% (3 of 8), and obesity in 50% (3 of 6). No changes in bone parameters were seen after surgery in patients with osteoporosis. On the other hand, some worsening of DM, hypertension, and hyperlipidemia was noted in conservatively managed patients. They concluded that laparoscopic adrenalectomy performed by skilled surgeons appears more beneficial than conservative management for SAGH [117]. When cardiovascular risk factors cannot be controlled medically, surgery is reasonable [10]. For other patients, especially given the small size of the randomized controlled trial, the jury is still out.

SURGERY FOR ADRENAL INCIDENTALOMA

Surgery offers the most direct solution to the diagnostic–therapeutic dilemma of an adrenal incidentaloma: taking out the mass and the adrenal gland both answers the diagnostic question and may offer cure for a disorder that needed treatment. The fact that diagnosis may be uncertain at the time of actual treatment makes surgery for adrenal incidentaloma different from surgery for a nonincidentaloma adrenal mass. Therefore, before surgery is undertaken, careful planning is needed with respect to preoperative, intraoperative, and postoperative management. In addition, as in many other procedures, there is a learning curve and experience is important; high-volume surgeons tend to have lower complication rates than low-volume surgeons [118]. Preoperative management issues include decisions about hormonal blocking of a suspected pheochromocytoma or of adrenocortical hyperfunction. Concerning intraoperative care, a choice must be made for a laparoscopic, robotic, or open surgical approach, depending on both the size and the suspected nature of the incidentaloma. Postoperative management includes anticipating the consequences of the reduction in stress hormone levels that follows pheochromocytoma extirpation, or the consequences of hormone withdrawal in the case of clinical or SAGH.

PREOPERATIVE MANAGEMENT

Preoperative evaluation of patients for surgery mainly aims at ruling out the presence or absence of adrenocortical or adrenomedullary hyperfunction. An appropriate preoperative preparation of patients is essential to prevent complications. This includes a thorough biochemical evaluation of the hypothalamic–pituitary–adrenal axis and the correction of electrolyte abnormalities in patients with adrenocortical hyperfunction before surgery. Ruling out SAGH is important, as hyperfunction of the involved gland, apart from the long-term risks it may pose, might suppress the contralateral adrenal gland and thereby expose the patient to the risk of adrenal crisis after adrenalectomy [30]. Diagnostic strategies are discussed above. Patients with significant and long-lasting Cushing's syndrome could be significantly deconditioned. These patients need significant attention to optimally prepare them for their adrenal surgery. However, these cases should not have come to surgical attention because of incidentalomas, but more properly should have been identified based on clinical grounds.

Pheochromocytoma presence, especially if unnoticed and not managed adequately by blockage of the adrenergic system, may increase perioperative risk [53,119,120]. Certainty about pheochromocytoma status is not always easily obtained. Even if careful history taking reveals no pheochromocytoma triad (headache, palpitations, and diaphoresis) and if physical examination demonstrates normotension, this clinical information is insufficient proof of pheochromocytoma absence [119]. Patients suspected of having pheochromocytomas need to be prepared to undergo surgery by alpha blockade. The classic agent used is phenoxybenzamine, with some groups also advocating calcium channel blockers or other agents. In a retrospective comparison of two institutions (Mayo Clinic and Cleveland Clinic) with differing approaches to preoperative preparation of patients who underwent laparoscopic removal of pheochromocytomas [120], Mayo Clinic predominantly used the long-lasting nonselective alpha(1,2) antagonist phenoxybenzamine, and Cleveland Clinic predominantly used selective alpha(1) blockade with doxazosin, terazosin, or prazosin. Intraoperatively, patients at Cleveland Clinic had a greater maximal systolic blood pressure (209 ± 44 mmHg versus 187 ± 30 mmHg, $p = 0.011$) and had received a greater amount of intravenous crystalloid (median 5000, interquartile range 3400–6400, versus median 2977, interquartile range 2000–3139; $p < 0.010$) and colloid (median 1000, interquartile range 500–1000, versus median 0, interquartile range 0–0; $p < 0.001$). At Mayo Clinic, more patients had received phenylephrine (56.0% versus 27.0%, $p = 0.009$). No differences were found in the postoperative surgical outcomes, and the hospital stay was comparable between the two groups. Either option should be used for at least 3 weeks before surgery to prevent hypertensive crisis during adrenalectomy. These patients also need to be optimally hydrated preoperatively, as preoperative alpha blockade will shrink their blood volume.

A good assessment of the size and imaging characteristics of the mass is warranted before any surgical resection is performed. This can give an insight into the nature of the tumor and potential surgical challenges, although all imaging procedures have their limitations. Finally, the cardiac, pulmonary, and nutritional status of the patients must also be considered, as in any preoperative evaluation.

INDICATIONS FOR SURGERY

The two main indications for surgery to remove an adrenal incidentaloma are (1) hormonal excess and (2) concern about the possibility of an adrenal carcinoma, most often based on size of the lesion. When a lesion is overtly hyperfunctioning, the decision is relatively straightforward. Biochemical evidence of pheochromocytoma is a sufficient indication for removal even if clinically silent; the future risk of adverse outcomes is too high. The issue of surgery for subclinical autonomous cortisol secretion is more controversial and will be addressed separately below. Risk of adrenal carcinoma is generally size dependent, and various experts have reported a tumor size range from 3 to 5 cm as an indication for surgical resection. The most commonly quoted size is 4 cm; however, since both CT and MRI can underestimate final pathologic adrenal size by up to 40%, some clinicians suspect an increased risk of malignancy in tumors of >3 cm [121,122]. In tumors of <4 cm, the risk of primary adrenal cortical carcinoma (ACC) is ~2%, and 6% in patients with tumors of 4–6 cm [105,124]. An increase in risk to more than 25% is reported in tumors of >6 cm. The most recent guidelines have been suggested by American Association of Clinical Endocrinologists (AACE) and the American Association of Endocrine Surgeons (AAES) [15]. These guidelines recommend surgery for those tumors larger than 4 cm. In addition to the size, suspicious features on imaging, such as irregular borders, heterogeneity, high density on noncontrast imaging, local invasion, and lymphadenopathy, should also lead to surgery, irrespective of the size. As the prognosis is best if ACC is resected early, it is very important to have a high suspicion for ACC with these worrisome features [123,124]. These patients should also have a CT of the lungs performed preoperatively to rule out metastatic disease.

OPERATIVE TECHNIQUES

Several operative approaches to the adrenal gland exist; however, due to the lack of prospective randomized trials, the advantages of one approach over the other are not clearly outlined. Most comparative studies are retrospective, which results in notable selection bias. In the past decade, however, there have been dramatic changes in adrenal surgery, with the introduction of laparoscopic adenalectomy techniques by Gagner and associates in 1992 [123,125,126].

Laparoscopic surgery has revolutionized adrenal surgery by decreasing morbidity and accelerating the return to full activity after operation. Recently, the potential benefits of a robotic platform over conventional laparoscopy for resection of adrenal masses, in terms of both visualization of the operative field with three-dimensional optics and more precise, less cumbersome dissection with tremor-minimizing wristed instruments, have also been reported.

Laparoscopic

Since its initial description by Gagner and associates in 1992, multiple minimally invasive approaches to the adrenal gland have been developed. The small size of the adrenal gland, the benign nature of most adrenal tumors, and the difficulty of exposure with open methods have made this gland particularly amenable to laparoscopic surgery. Laparoscopy provides a magnified view of the operative field, allowing the precise identification of small vessels and more precise dissection with less blood loss, so that transfusion is rare. There have been numerous reports in the literature establishing the safety, efficacy, and cost-effectiveness of laparoscopic adrenalectomy [127–129]. For example, reported morbidity of laparoscopic adrenalectomy for pheochromocytoma ranges from 0% to 21% [130–132]. Most clinical concerns stem from reports of hypertensive crises, rare patient deaths, and intra-abdominal tumor spillage as a result of fine-needle aspiration biopsy of an unsuspected pheochromocytoma [133].

Because the incision, rather than the internal dissection, affects the pain and recovery after surgery, laparoscopic adrenal surgery has resulted in a decrease in wound complications, less postoperative pain, a shorter hospital stay, and rapid return to normal activity [126,128,134,135]. Laparoscopic surgery is regarded as the gold standard for the removal of benign adrenal lesions. It is performed under endotracheal general anesthesia via either the lateral transabdominal approach or the posterior retroperitoneoscopic approach.

The lateral approach requires the lateral recumbent position for the patients with ports placed in a subcostal position (Figures 33.7 and 33.8). Full mobilization of the liver or spleen enables improved visualization of and access to the adrenal gland. Bleeding is minimized as a result of the increased insufflation pressure. With this approach, a decrease in pain and a faster return of gastrointestinal function have been suggested by some clinicians. The posterior retroperitoneoscopic approach has been particularly recommended for bilateral adrenalectomy, as it does not require the repositioning of patients during the operation. It obviates the need for extensive lysis of intra-abdominal adhesions in patients who have previously undergone upper abdominal surgery. A shortcoming of this approach includes anesthetic considerations associated with prone positioning, and for adrenal glands situated anteriorly on the kidney and near the renal hilum, resection may be technically difficult [136,137].

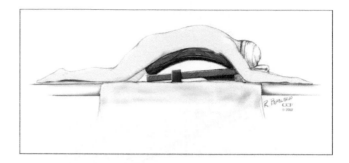

Figure 33.7 Patient positioning for a posterior retroperitoneal adrenalectomy. The patient is taken to the operating room and general endotracheal anesthesia is induced on the gurney. The patient is then flipped onto the operating table with the chest and abdomen supported laterally by a Wilson frame or parallel bolsters. (Reprinted from *Oper. Tech. Gen. Surg.*, 4, Berber, E and Siperstein AE, 331–337, 2002, with permission from Elsevier.)

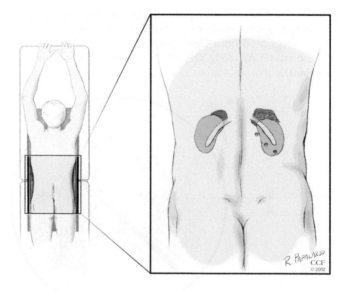

Figure 33.8 Trocar entry. The procedure is performed with three incisions placed below the 12th rib. (Reprinted from *Oper. Tech. Gen. Surg.*, 4, Berber, E and Siperstein AE, 331–337, 2002, with permission from Elsevier.)

Figures 33.7 through 33.11 illustrate basic steps for patient positioning, trocar entry, creation of a potential space, laparoscopic ultrasound, and dissection.

Although technically more demanding, the posterior technique provides more direct access to the adrenal gland by minimizing intra-abdominal dissection. Our current indications for the posterior technique include tumors less than 6 cm in size, bilateral tumors, and patients with a history of multiple previous abdominal surgeries. The lateral transabdominal approach is more suitable for larger tumors.

Robotic

Current indications for robotic adrenalectomy are similar to those for the laparoscopic approach, and include all

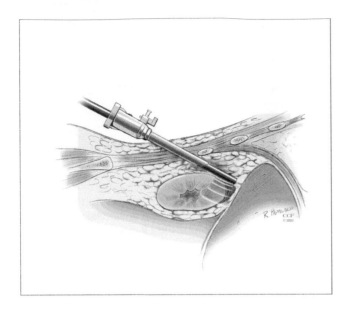

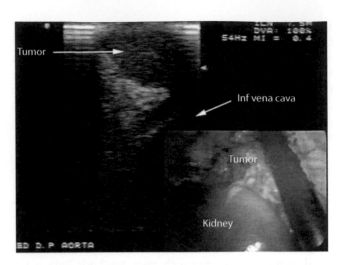

Figure 33.9 Creation of a potential space. The retroperitoneal space is created using a balloon trocar and insufflated. (Reprinted from *Oper. Tech. Gen. Surg.*, 4, Berber, E and Siperstein AE, 331–337, 2002, with permission from Elsevier.)

Figure 33.10 Laparoscopic ultrasound. Laparoscopic ultrasound is used to identify the adrenal mass and establish its relationship with surrounding structures. (Reprinted from *Oper. Tech. Gen. Surg.*, 4, Berber, E and Siperstein AE, 331–337, 2002, with permission from Elsevier.)

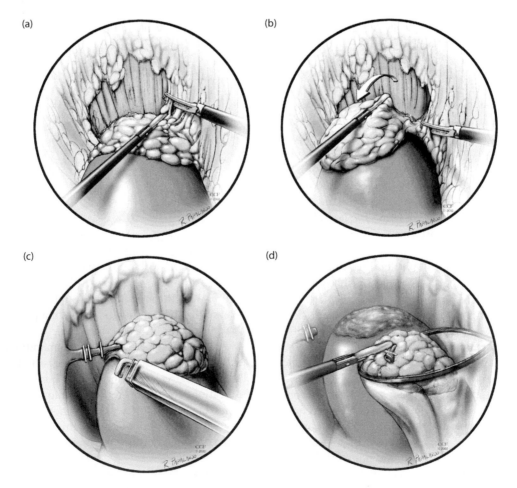

Figure 33.11 Dissection. **(a)** The adrenal dissection is started superiorly and laterally. **(b)** An energy device can be used to divide the periadrenal attachments. **(c)** The adrenal vein is taken last, using metallic clips. **(d)** Then the specimen is placed inside a specimen bag and removed. (Reprinted from *Oper. Tech. Gen. Surg.*, 4, Berber, E and Siperstein AE, 331–337, 2002, with permission from Elsevier.)

benign functional adrenal tumors, nonfunctional tumors of ≥4 cm, and those demonstrating significant growth on follow-up CT scan, as well as adrenal metastases in selected patients with soft tissue or solid-organ primary tumors, usually in the setting of mono- or oligometastatic disease [15,138,139]. Robotic adrenalectomy is currently performed via either a lateral transperitoneal or a posterior retroperitoneal approach. Patient selection for a particular technique should take into consideration the underlying endocrinopathy, body habitus, tumor bilaterality, and type and extent of previous surgery [140].

Operative outcomes of robotic adrenalectomy are similar to those of standard laparoscopic surgery. For example, the robotic technique has been shown to be efficient for the resection of pheochromocytoma even for tumors greater than 5 cm. We previously reported perioperative outcome results similar to those of our laparoscopic adrenalectomy–pheochromocytoma group. There was no morbidity or mortality in the robotic group; however, morbidity was 10% ($p = 0.041$) and mortality 2.5% in the laparoscopic group [141].

Although the indications for a posterior versus lateral procedure have not been completely defined in the literature, the posterior approach may not be suitable for larger tumors (e.g., tumors > 6 cm) considering the relatively limited confines of the retroperitoneal space, and enhanced risk of malignancy. In this same manner, patients with impairment of access to the retroperitoneum, such as those with a small space between the 12th rib and iliac crest (>4 cm), or with a long distance between the skin and Gerota's facia (>7 cm), should also be considered for an alternative approach [142,143]. On the contrary, the larger working space and the familiarity of landmarks associated with the lateral technique make it more favorable for larger, unilateral tumors, in which there is a small retroperitoneal space or previous retroperitoneal kidney surgery. It also offers a lesser burden in the event that conversion to an open transperitoneal approach is required. In our institution, we prefer lateral transabdominal adrenalectomy for tumors of >6 cm. If the tumor size is <6 cm, the distance between the skin and Gerota's space is not long (generally <7 cm) and the 12th rib is rostral to the renal hilum, and we carry out the posterior retroperitoneal technique. Whether to use the robotic or laparoscopic approach depends on the preference of the surgeon. There are no level 1 data that compare robotic to laparoscopic adrenalectomy. The benefits of the robot seem to include more precise dissection, stable surgical platform, and three-dimensional visualization. One concern against robotic surgery is the additional cost.

POSTOPERATIVE CARE

As with any major operation, general postoperative problems may arise, such as bleeding, wound infection, or respiratory problems. In patients with Cushing's, wound complications are more likely to occur than in those without. Specific problems, related to the nature of the adrenal incidentaloma, may arise in hormonally active disorders, being either cortical or medullary tumors. After removal of pheochromocytoma, chronically present vasoconstriction will give way to relative vasodilatation, and thus will cause hypotension or overt hypovolemic shock. Replacement of intravascular volume should be performed under the guide of central venous pressure and urine production in an intensive or intermediate care setting. In most cases, fluid balance and hemodynamic stability can be restored within 24 hours, with no need for further specific support or monitoring. Steroid-producing tumors (in the case of either subclinical or clinical Cushing's syndrome) present a different picture. Removal of the hyperactive ipsilateral gland will leave only the suppressed contralateral adrenal gland to take care of cortical adrenal function. To prevent an adrenal crisis from occurring in such situations, intra- and postoperative substitution with glucocorticoid is necessary and should be continued for as long as it may take the other gland to fully restore adrenal cortical function. This may take up to a year or more in many cases [30]. No matter what combination of preoperative testing is done, it might still not be possible to document cortisol oversecretion in some patients (subclinical Cushing's). A practice what helps identify these patients is checking their postoperative day 1 cortisol levels. Those patients with low levels should be started on steroids and assessed in follow-up for the recovery of the pituitary–adrenal axis.

Prognosis

The long-term prognosis and outcomes of incidentally discovered adrenal masses in this current era of evidence-based medicine remain uncertain. Management of these tumors is therefore limited to the empirically accepted clinical protocols. Surveillance and resection are the two clinical options that address the question of the long-term effects of incidentally identified adrenal masses. Prognosis, follow-up, and outcomes of surgically treated adenomas with clinically evident catecholamine, cortisol, or aldosterone excess appear to be reasonably good.

Patients with incidentally discovered aldosterone-producing tumors that are treated and followed in a systematic fashion have a high rate of successful disease and blood pressure control. Notwithstanding a required long-term follow-up in a smaller number of these patients, at least 72% of this patient group may ultimately be safely discharged to the community with controlled blood pressures [144]. Of note is the fact that without any antihypertensive medication, the majority of patients are unable to maintain normal blood pressure [145–148]. This can be associated with the long-standing hypertension with remodeling of the vascular system [149–151]. Nevertheless, resection of the mass, when possible, has been shown to allow for faster normalization of blood pressure and final discharge. Also, an early diagnosis has been shown to be predictive of achieving normokalemia and reducing the need for antihypertensive drugs [152]. Recently, an aldosteronoma resolution score has been proposed to predict outcome after surgery based on duration of hypertension and preoperative medication [153]. The longest follow-up data in patients with aldosterone-producing tumors to date were published by Catena et al. [149]. Over a study period of 7.4 years, the authors were able to show that aldosteronoma patients could be treated surgically or medically to blood pressure levels similar to those achievable in essential hypertension. Although some other published studies do exist, they are limited by their smaller cohorts, comprising 24–52 patients; shorter duration of follow-up (76–86 months); and lack of medically treated comparison groups or standardized postoperative blood pressure treatment targets [114,146,154].

Issues surrounding SAGH are more problematic. Postoperative adrenal insufficiency may occur. A systematic review including 13 retrospective, 14 prospective, and 1 randomized controlled trial (level 1 evidence) found that the prevalence of postoperative adrenal insufficiency was 65.3% in 248 patients with subclinical hypercortisolism and 99.7% in 377 patients with Cushing's syndrome. Patients with subclinical hypercortisolism were reclassified according to the following diagnostic criteria: subjects defined by pathological dexamethasone test only, and those defined by the dexamethasone test with one or two additional criteria. They were compared with patients who had clinically apparent Cushing's syndrome. The prevalence of adrenal insufficiency after adrenalectomy was 51.4%, 60.6%, 91.3%, and 99.7%, respectively, with no significant difference between the two latter groups. The test with the best compromise between sensitivity (64%) and specificity (81%) in predicting adrenal insufficiency was the midnight serum cortisol [30]. Some studies have shown amelioration of the biochemical abnormalities and cardiovascular risk factors associated with SAGH, as well as some comorbidies, such as diabetes and hypertension [43,155–158]. However, there are many uncertainties surrounding the impact [159]. First, obesity, hypertension, type 2 diabetes, dyslipidemia, and osteoporosis are more common among those with incidentalomas, regardless of adrenal function. More surprising, perhaps, is that some patients have amelioration of their comorbidities regardless of adrenal function. Second, most studies are retrospective and involve relatively small numbers and limited lengths of follow-up. Conflicting findings may relate not only to diagnostic difficulties in general, but also to the fact that SAGH may be intermittent [159]. In their study of guidelines, Shen et al. found considerable differences in the recommendations for managing SAGH and suggested that the differences were derived from citation selection bias, evidence interpretation bias, differences in the composition of the guidelines' workgroups, and the omission of guidelines for updating and externally reviewing the recommendations [110].

The prognosis of incidentally found tumors that histopathologically turn out to be consistent with adrenocortical carcinoma is certainly dependent on an accurate diagnosis; thus, the pathologic criteria employed preoperative clinical, biochemical, and imaging characteristics.

Although survival of these patients has been associated with intraoperative findings and the surgical technique, prognosis has remained unchanged over the past 20 years. The median survival is 2 years for all patients, with an unadjusted 5-year overall survival of approximately 40% for those individuals with surgically resectable disease [160,161]. The application of laparoscopic adrenalectomy in the setting of ACC has been highly controversial, with concerns over inadequate resection and resulting suboptimal patient outcomes. Relative to the open technique, early descriptive and more recent multi-institutional studies have described potential increased rates of tumor fragmentation, margin positivity, and peritoneal carcinomatosis after laparoscopic adrenalectomy for patients with histopathologically diagnosed ACC [162–165]. Similarly, a multi-institutional study from the MD Anderson Cancer Center, which included 302 patients with European Network for the Study of Adrenal Tumors stage I–III ACC, reported an increased risk of multifocal peritoneal carcinomatosis in the 46 patients who received laparoscopic adrenalectomy at an outside institution relative to those receiving conventional open adrenalectomy at either an outside or the index institution. Moreover, open surgical resection was independently associated with increased recurrence-free and overall survival in a multivariate analysis adjusted for tumor stage [166].

Although widely accepted as the gold standard of care, laparoscopic adrenalectomy for pheochromocytoma does not guarantee long-term cure [167]. After initial resection, a local recurrence rate ranging between 0.05% and 3% over a follow-up period of 1–21 years has been reported by previous studies [168,169]. This has been associated with reasons such as initial tumor spillage, incomplete resection, or the presence of an accessory tissue, and emphasizes the need for diligence during laparoscopic cases to completely remove all adrenal tissue and not fracture the gland during resection. Counseling of all patients undergoing resection of pheochromocytoma about disease recurrence is therefore warranted, and a careful annual follow-up should be encouraged.

For those patients found to have adrenal gland metastases, prognosis is defined by the primary tumor—histology, grade, stage, and site. Approximately 25% of masses greater than 6 cm in diameter are ACCs, and these patients have very poor clinical outcomes. Among a large series of studies of adrenal cancer (usually not presenting as incidentalomas), 5-year survival ranged from 19% to 62%, with a median of 34% [9]. There is some evidence suggesting that surgical extirpation of adrenal cancer at stage I or II may improve the survival rate.

The few cost-effectiveness analyses have not settled the issues of how to deal with the individual patient [170–172]. A strategy of observation also has impacts. For example, Muth et al. conducted a retrospective study of 2-year follow-up involving 145 patients with nonfunctioning, benign adrenal incidentalomas, of whom 111 (77%) responded to surveys [64,117]. Of the respondents, 77% reported that the adrenal incidentaloma diagnosis had caused them to be worried, although <20% had thought about the lesion often during the follow-up period; only 3% had felt that it had a large impact on their current daily life, but 10% reported a negative impact on their health-related quality of life [64]. These findings indicate the need for tailored counseling in individual patients to ameliorate negative impacts of follow-up [64].

FOLLOW-UP

Much of the controversy surrounding management of adrenal incidentalomas involves what to do with patients who do not undergo surgery at the time of their identification. Here, the evidence base is far weaker. The natural history of hormonally inactive incidentalomas is relatively benign; subsequent development of clinical adrenal carcinoma seems to be a rare event. Nevertheless, follow-up CT scan is often recommended [108]. For example, the NIH statement suggested that patients whose lesions were not removed should have a follow-up CT at 6–12 months and repeat only if the lesion is increasing in size [11]. Others have recommended more frequent CTs [15,173]. For example, AACE/AAES guidelines recommend reevaluation at 3–6 months and then annually for 1–2 years [15]. A contrary view was offered by Cawood et al. [8]. They used estimates of the ionizing radiation exposure of the average recommended CT and calculated the chance of the radiation itself causing fatal cancer. They found that their estimate of a 1 in 430–2170 chance of such a cancer was similar to the chance of developing adrenal malignancy during 3-year follow-up of adrenal incidentaloma [8]. Needless to say, this article has sparked controversy. Because of the potential lethality of adrenal carcinoma, a single follow-up CT at 3–6 months is prudent. Patients with low-density lesions (<10 Hounsfield units) and those with clear diagnoses of simple cysts or myelolipomas may need no follow-up CT at all [3,109].

In addition to the concern about increase in lesion size, hormone overproduction may occur after initial evaluation; up to 20% of patients develop hormone overproduction, which is less likely in tumors smaller than 3 cm. The risk that a tumor will become hormonally active appears to plateau after 3–4 years. Thus, it has been suggested that hormonal evaluation be carried out annually for ~4 years. Cawood et al. made estimates of false-positive rates for hormonal tests and concluded that current recommendations for evaluation of adrenal incidentaloma are likely to result in significant costs, both financial and emotional [8]. The controversy continues.

SUMMARY AND CONCLUSIONS

The optimal strategy for evaluation of a patient with an incidentally discovered adrenal mass remains controversial. The quality of the data upon which such decisions are made remains imperfect, to say the least. We lack the randomized (or even nonrandomized) trials that would go a long way toward resolving the controversies. Even in the unlikely event that such trials were carried out, they would take years to yield results. Moreover, individual preferences are likely to be critical in such decision making. Review of the literature supports the view that such patients are at somewhat increased risk of morbidity and mortality, and this implies a benefit of early diagnosis for at least some of the disorders. Our ability to accurately determine clinically those at increased risk among the vast majority who are not at increased risk is poor. We therefore rely on biochemical and radiological diagnostic tests, which have their own limitations. Subjecting patients to unnecessary testing and treatment carries its own set of risks. The diagnostic process itself may contribute considerable anxiety and expense and, if invasive, cause pain and other morbidity. The harm that occurs as false-positive results are pursued has been termed the "cascade effect." We must avoid the pitfalls of overestimation of disease prevalence and of the benefits of therapy resulting from advances in diagnostic imaging. In the meantime, we must use our best clinical judgment based upon the best-available evidence to ensure that we maximize the benefit to those patients with adrenal incidentalomas who have clinically significant adrenal disorders, and minimize the harm to those who do not.

REFERENCES

1. Aron D, Terzolo M, Cawood TJ. Adrenal incidentalomas. *Best Pract Res Clin Endocrinol Metab* 2012;26:69–82.
2. Aron DE. Endocrine incidentalomas. *Endocrinol Metab Clin North Am* 2000;29:1–238.
3. Berland L, Silverman S, Gore R et al. Managing incidental findings on abdominal CT: White paper of the ACR Incidental Findings Committee. *Am Coll Radiol* 2010;7:754–3.
4. Lumberas B, Donat L, Hernández-Aguado I. Incidental findings in imaging diagnostic tests: A systematic review. *Br J Radiol* 2010;83:279–89.
5. Zeiger MA, Thompson GB, Duh Q et al. American Association of Clinical Endocrinologists and American Association of Endocrine Surgeons medical guidelines for the management of adrenal incidentalomas: Executive summary of recommendations. *Endocr Pract* 2009;15:450–3.
6. Paterson F, Theodoraki A, Amajuoyi A, Bouloux PM, Maclachlan J, Khoo B. Radiology reporting of adrenal incidentalomas—Who requires further testing? *Clin Med* 2014;14:16–21.
7. Berland LL, Silverman SG, Megibow AJ, Mayo-Smith WW. ACR members' response to white paper on the management of incidental abdominal CT findings. *J Am Coll Radiol* 2014;11:30–5.
8. Cawood TJ, Hunt PJ, O'Shea D, Cole D, Soule S. Recommended evaluation of adrenal incidentalomas is costly, has high false-positive rates and confers

a risk of fatal cancer that is similar to the risk of the adrenal lesion becoming malignant; time for a rethink? *Eur J Endocrinol* 2009;161:513–27.

9. Lau J, Balk E, Rothberg M et al. *Management of Clinically Inapparent Adrenal Mass.* Evidence Report/Technology Assessment, no. 56. Rockville, MD: Agency for Healthcare Research and Quality, 2002.

10. Nieman L. Approach to the patient with an adrenal incidentaloma. *J Clin Endocrinol Metab* 2010;95:4106–3.

11. NIH Consensus Panel. NIH State of the Science Conference on Management of the Clinically Inapparent Adrenal Mass. 2002. https://consensus.nih.gov/2002/2002AdrenalIncidentalomasos021main.htm (accessed 12/2/2016).

12. Kannan S, Remer EM, Hamrahian AH. Evaluation of patients with adrenal incidentalomas. *Curr Opin Endocrinol Diabetes Obes* 2013;20:161–9.

13. Davenport E, Lang Ping NP, Wilson M, Reid A, Aspinall S. Adrenal incidentalomas: Management in British district general hospitals. *Postgrad Med J* 2014;90:365–9.

14. Wickramarachchi BN, Meyer-Rochow GY, McAnulty K, Conaglen JV, Elston MS. Adherence to adrenal incidentaloma guidelines is influenced by radiology report recommendations. *ANZ J Surg* 2016;86:483–6.

15. Zeiger MA, Thompson GB, Duh QY et al. The American Association of Clinical Endocrinologists and American Association of Endocrine Surgeons medical guidelines for the management of adrenal incidentalomas. *Endocr Pract* 2009;15(Suppl 1):1–20.

16. Sebastiano C, Zhao X, Deng FM, Das K. Cystic lesions of the adrenal gland: Our experience over the last 20 years. *Hum Pathol* 2013;44:1797–803.

17. Gershuni VM, Bittner JG, Moley JF, Brunt LM. Adrenal myelolipoma: Operative indications and outcomes. *J Laparoendosc Adv Surg Tech A* 2014;24:8–12.

18. Tang YZ, Bharwani N, Micco M, Akker S, Rockall AG, Sahdev A. The prevalence of incidentally detected adrenal enlargement on CT. *Clin Radiol* 2014;69:e37–42.

19. Lerario AM, Moraitis A, Hammer GD. Genetics and epigenetics of adrenocortical tumors. *Mol Cell Endocrinol* 2014;386:67–84.

20. Patel D, Boufraqech M, Jain M et al. MiR-34a and miR-483-5p are candidate serum biomarkers for adrenocortical tumors. *Surgery* 2013;154:1224–8.

21. Damjanovic SS, Antic JA, Ilic BB et al. Glucocorticoid receptor and molecular chaperones in the pathogenesis of adrenal incidentalomas: Potential role of reduced sensitivity to glucocorticoids. *Mol Med* 2012;18:1456–5.

22. Gatta-Cherifi B, Chabre O, Murat A et al. Adrenal involvement in MEN1. Analysis of 715 cases from the Groupe d'etude des Tumeurs Endocrines database. *Eur J Endocrinol* 2012;166:268–79.

23. Aron D, Terzolo M, Cawood TJ. Adrenal incidentalomas. *Best Pract Res Clin Endocrinol Metab* 2012;26:69–82.

24. Nawar R, Aron D. Adrenal incidentalomas—A continuing management dilemma. *Endocr Relat Cancer* 2005;12:585–98.

25. Piaditis G, Kaltsas G, Androulakis I et al. High prevalence of autonomous cortisol and aldosterone secretion from adrenal adenomas. *Clin Endocrinol* 2009;71:772–8.

26. Reimondo G, Allasino B, Bovio S et al. Pros and cons of dexamethasone suppression test for screening of subclinical Cushing's syndrome in patients with adrenal incidentalomas. *J Endocrinol Invest* 2011;34:e1–5.

27. Sippel R, Chen H. Subclinical Cushing's syndrome in adrenal incidentalomas. *Surg Clin North Am* 2004;84:875–85.

28. De LM, Cozzolino A, Colao A, Pivonello R. Subclinical Cushing's syndrome. *Best Pract Res Clin Endocrinol Metab* 2012;26:497–505.

29. Di Dalmazi G, Vicennati V, Garelli S et al. Cardiovascular events and mortality in patients with adrenal incidentalomas that are either non-secreting or associated with intermediate phenotype or subclinical Cushing's syndrome: A 15-year retrospective study. *Lancet Diabetes Endocrinol* 2014;2:396–405.

30. Di Dalmazi G, Berr C, Fassnacht M, Beuschlein F, Reincke M. Adrenal function after adrenalectomy for subclinical hypercortisolism and Cushing's syndrome: A systematic review of the literature. *J Clin Endicrinol Metab* 2014;99:2637–45.

31. Akehi Y, Kawate H, Murase K et al. Proposed diagnostic criteria for subclinical Cushing's syndrome associated with adrenal incidentaloma. *Endocr J* 2013;60:903–12.

32. Terzolo M, Pia A, Ali A et al. Adrenal incidentaloma: A new cause of the metabolic syndrome? *J Clin Endicrinol Metab* 2008;87:998–1003.

33. Oki Y, Hashimoto K, Hirata Y et al. Development and validation of a 0.5 mg dexamethasone suppression test as an initial screening test for the diagnosis of ACTH-dependent Cushing's syndrome. *Endocr J* 2009;56:897–904.

34. Giordano R, Guaraldi F, Berardelli R et al. Glucose metabolism in patients with subclinical Cushing's syndrome. *Endocrine* 2012;41:415–23.

35. Ivovic M, Marina LV, Vujovic S et al. Nondiabetic patients with either subclinical Cushing's or non-functional adrenal incidentalomas have lower insulin sensitivity than healthy controls: Clinical implication. *Metabolism* 2013;62:786–92.

36. Debono M, Prema A, Hughes TJ, Bull M, Ross RJ, Newell-Price J. Visceral fat accumulation and post-dexamethasone serum cortisol levels in patients with adrenal incidentaloma. *J Clin Endocrinol Metab* 2013;98:2381–91.

37. Debono M, Chadarevian R, Eastell R, Ross RJ, Newell-Price J. Mifepristone reduces insulin resistance in patient volunteers with adrenal incidentalomas that secrete low levels of cortisol: A pilot study. *PLoS One* 2013;8:e60984.

38. Eller-Vainicher C, Morelli V, Salcuni AS et al. Accuracy of several parameters of hypothalamic-pituitary-adrenal axis activity in predicting before surgery the metabolic effects of the removal of an adrenal incidentaloma. *Eur J Endocrinol* 2010;163:925–35.

39. Chiondini I, Guglielmi G, Battista C et al. Spinal volumetric bone mineral density and vertebral fractures in female patients with adrenal incidentalomas: The effects of subclinical hypercortisolism and gonadal status. *J Clin Endicrinol Metab* 2004;89:2237–41.

40. Francucci C, Caudarella R, Rillis S, Fiscaletti P, Ceccoli L, Boscaro M. Adrenal incidentaloma: Effects on bone metabolism. *J Endocrinol Invest* 2008;31:48–52.

41. Hadjidakia D, Tsagarakis S, Roboti C et al. Does subclinical hypercortisolism adversely affect the bone mineral density of patients with adrenal incidentalomas? *Clin Endocrinol (Oxf)* 2003;58:72–7.

42. Tauchmanova L, Rossi R, Nuzzo V et al. Bone loss determined by quantitative ultrasonometry correlates inversely with disease activity in patients with endogenous glucocorticoid excess due to adrenal mass. *Eur J Endocrinol* 2001;145:241–7.

43. Tauchmanova L, Rossi R, Biondi B et al. Patients with subclinical Cushing's syndrome due to adrenal adenoma have increased cardiovascular risk. *J Clin Endicrinol Metab* 2002;87:4872–78.

44. Di Dalmazi G, Vicennati V, Rinaldi E et al. Progressively increased patterns of subclinical cortisol hypersecretion in adrenal incidentalomas differently predict major metabolic and cardiovascular outcomes: A large cross-sectional study. *Eur J Endocrinol* 2012;166:669–77.

45. Tsagarakis S, Roboti C, Kokkoris P, Vasiliou V, Alevizaki C, Thalassinos N. Elevated post-dexamethasone suppression cortisol concentrations correlate with hormonal alterations of the hypothalamo-pituitary adrenal axis in patients with adrenal incidentalomas. *Clin Endocrinol (Oxf)* 1998;49:165–71.

46. Iacobone M, Citton M, Viel G et al. Adrenalectomy may improve cardiovascular and metabolic impairment and ameliorate quality of life in patients with adrenal incidentalomas and subclinical Cushing's syndrome. *Surgery* 2012;152:991–7.

47. Prejbisz A, Lenders JW, Eisenhofer G, Januszewicz A. Mortality associated with phaeochromocytoma. *Horm Metab Res* 2013;45:154–8.

48. Haissaguerre M, Courel M, Caron P et al. Normotensive incidentally discovered pheochromocytomas display specific biochemical, cellular, and molecular characteristics. *J Clin Endocrinol Metab* 2013;98:4346–54.

49. Wachtel H, Cerullo I, Bartlett EK et al. Clinicopathologic characteristics of incidentally identified pheochromocytoma. *Ann Surg Oncol* 2015;22:132–8.

50. Young W Jr. Management approaches to adrenal incidentalomas. A view from Rochester, Minnesota. *Endocrinol Metab Clin North Am* 2000;29:159–85.

51. Lenders JW, Duh Q, Eisenhofer G et al. Pheochromocytoma and paraganglioma: An Endocrine Society Clinical Practice Guideline. *J Clin Endocrinol Metab* 2014;99:1915–42.

52. Bourdeau I, MacKenzie-Feder J, Lacroix A. Recent advances in adrenocortical carcinoma in adults. *Curr Opin Endocrinol Diabetes Obes* 2013;20:192–7.

53. Fassnacht M, Libe R, Kroiss M, Allolio B. Adrenocortical carcinoma: A clinician's update. *Nat Rev Endocrinol* 2011;7:323–5.

54. Fassnacht M, Kroiss M, Allolio B. Update in adrenocortical carcinoma. *J Clin Endocrinol Metab* 2013;98:4551–64.

55. Stratakis CA. Adrenal cancer in 2013: Time to individualize treatment for adrenocortical cancer? *Nat Rev Endocrinol* 2014;10:76–8.

56. Kerkhofs T, Verhoeven R, Van der Zwan J et al. Adrenocortical carcinoma: A population-based study on incidence and survival in the Netherlands since 1993. *Eur J Cancer* 2013;49:2579–86.

57. Mantero F, Terzolo M, Arnaldi G et al. A survey on adrenal incidentaloma in Italy. Study group on adrenal tumors of the Italian Society of Endocrinology. *J Clin Endocrinol Metab* 2000;85:637–44.

58. Terzolo M, Ali A, Osella G, Mazza E. Prevalence of adrenal carcinoma among incidentally discovered adrenal masses. A retrospective study from 1989 to 1994. Gruppo Piemontese Incidentalomi Surrenalici. *Arch Surg* 1997;132:914–9.

59. Allan BJ, Thorson CM, Van Haren RM, Parikh PP, Lew JI. Risk of concomitant malignancy in hyperfunctioning adrenal incidentalomas. *J Surg Res* 2013;184:241–6.

60. Kebebew E, Reiff E, Duh Q, Clark O, McMillian A. Extent of disease at presentation and outcome for adrenocortical carcinoma: Have we made progress? *World J Surg* 2006;30:872–8.

61. McLean K, Lilienfeld H, Caracciolo JT, Hoffe S, Tourtelot JB, Carter WB. Management of isolated adrenal lesions in cancer patients. *Cancer Control* 2011;18:113–26.

62. Frilling A, Tecklenborg K, Weber F et al. Importance of adrenal incidentaloma in patients with a history of malignancy. *Surgery* 2004;136:1289–96.

63. Bradley CT, Strong VE. Surgical management of adrenal metastases. *J Surg Oncol* 2014;109:31–5.

64. Muth A, Taft C, Hammarstedt L, Bjorneld L, Hellstrom M, Wangberg B. Patient-reported impacts of a conservative management programme for the clinically inapparent adrenal mass. *Endocrine* 2013;44:228–36.

65. Nieman L, Biller B, Findling J et al. The diagnosis of Cushing's syndrome: An Endocrine Society Clinical Practice Guideline. *J Clin Endocrinol Metab* 2008;93:1526–40.

66. Tabarin A, Bardet S, Bertherat J et al. Exploration and management of adrenal incidentalomas. French Society of Endocrinology Consensus. *Ann Endocrinol (Paris)* 2008;69:487–500.

67. Legro R, Arslanian S, Ehrmann D et al. Diagnosis and treatment of polycystic ovary syndrome: An Endocrine Society Clinical Practice Guideline. *J Clin Endocrinol Metab* 2013;98:4565–92.

68. Funder J, Carey R, Fardella C et al. Case detection, diagnosis, and treatment of patients with primary aldosteronism: An Endocrine Society Clinical Practice Guideline. *J Clin Endocrinol Metab* 2008;93:3266–81.

69. Aron D. Evidence-based endocrinology & clinical epidemiology. In: Gardner D, Shoback D, eds., *Greenspan's Basic and Clinical Endocrinology*. 9th ed. New York: McGraw Hill, 2011;47–64.

70. Bardet S, Rohmer V, Murat A et al. 131I-6 Beta-iodomethylnorcholesterol scintigraphy: An assessment of its role in the investigation of adrenocortical incidentalomas. *Clin Endocrinol (Oxf)* 1996;44:587–96.

71. Valli N, Catargi B, Ronci N et al. Biochemical screening for subclinical cortisol-secreting adenomas amongst adrenal incidentalomas. *Eur J Endocrinol* 2001;144:401–8.

72. Ceccato F, Barbot M, Zilio M et al. Performance of salivary cortisol in the diagnosis of Cushing's syndrome, adrenal incidentaloma, and adrenal insufficiency. *Eur J Endocrinol* 2013;169:31–6.

73. Tateishi Y, Kouyama R, Mihara M, Doi M, Yoshimoto T, Hirata Y. Evaluation of salivary cortisol measurements for the diagnosis of subclinical Cushing's syndrome. *Endocr J* 2012;59:283–9.

74. Musella M, Conzo G, Milone M et al. Preoperative workup in the assessment of adrenal incidentalomas: Outcome from 282 consecutive laparoscopic adrenalectomies. *BMC Surg* 2013;13:57.

75. Hammarstedt L, Thilander-Klang A, Muth A, Wangberg B, Oden A, Hellstrom M. Adrenal lesions: Variability in attenuation over time, between scanners, and between observers. *Acta Radiol* 2013;54:817–26.

76. Boulle N, Baudin E, Gicquel C et al. Evaluation of plasma insulin-like growth factor binding protein-2 as a marker for adrenocortical tumors. *Eur J Endocrinol* 2001;144:29–36.

77. Boland G. Adrenal imaging: Why, when, what, and how? Part 2. What technique? *AJR Am J Roentgenol* 2011;196:W1–5.

78. Boland G. Adrenal imaging: Why, when, what, and how? Part 3. The algorithmic approach to definitive characterization of the adrenal incidentaloma. *AJR Am J Roentgenol* 2011;196:W109–11.

79. Boland G. Adrenal imaging: Why, when, what, and how? Part 1. Why and when to image? *AJR Am J Roentgenol* 2010;195:W377–81.

80. Choyke P. ACR Committee on Appropriateness Criteria. ACR appropriateness criteria on incidentally discovered adrenal mass. *J Am Coll Radiol* 2006;3:498–504.

81. Taffel M, Haji-Momenian S, Nikolaidis P, Miller F. Adrenal imaging: A comprehensive review. *Radiol Clin North Am* 2012;50:219–43.

82. Friedrich-Rust M, Glasemann T, Polta A et al. Differentiation between benign and malignant adrenal mass using contrast-enhanced ultrasound. *Ultraschall Med* 2011;32:460–71.

83. Kim K, Kim J, Choi H, Kim M, Lee J, Cho K. Sonography of the adrenal glands in the adult. *J Clin Ultrasound* 2012;40:357–63.

84. Suzuki Y, Sasagawa, Suzuki H, Izumi T, Kaneko H, Nakada T. The role of ultrasonography in the detection of adrenal masses: Comparison with computed tomography and magnetic resonance imaging. *Int Urol Nephrol* 2001;32:303–6.

85. Petersenn S, Richter P, Broemel T et al. CT criteria for adrenal cancer—Analysis of the German ACC Registry. *Exp Clin Endocrinol Diabetes* 2013;121.

86. Angeli A, Osella G, Ali A, Terzolo M. Adrenal incidentaloma: An overview of clinical and epidemiological data from the National Italian Study Group. *Horm Res* 1997;47:279–83.

87. Mantero F, Terzolo M, Arnaldi G et al. A survey on adrenal incidentaloma in Italy. Study group on adrenal tumors of the Italian Society of Endocrinology. *J Clin Endocrinol Metab* 2000;85:637–44.

88. Zhang HM, Perrier ND, Grubbs EG et al. CT features and quantification of the characteristics of adrenocortical carcinomas on unenhanced and contrast-enhanced studies. *Clin Radiol* 2012;67:38–46.

89. Kievit J, Haak H. Diagnosis and treatment of adrenal incidentaloma. A cost-effectiveness analysis. *Endocrinol Metab Clin North Am* 2000;29:69–90.

90. Kurtaran A, Traub T, Shapiro B. Scintigraphic imaging of the adrenal glands. *Eur J Radiol* 2002;41:123–30.

91. Ricciato MP, Di Donna V, Perotti G, Pontecorvi A, Bellantone R, Corsello SM. The role of adrenal scintigraphy in the diagnosis of subclinical Cushing's syndrome and the prediction of post-surgical hypoadrenalism. *World J Surg* 2014;38:1328–35.

92. Ansquer C, Scigliano S, Mirallié E et al. 18F-FDG PET/CT in the characterization and surgical decision concerning adrenal masses: A prospective multicentre evaluation. *Eur J Nucl Mol Imaging* 2010;37:1678.

93. Boland G, Dwamena B, Sangwaiya MJ et al. Characterization of adrenal masses by using FDG PET: A systematic review and meta-analysis of diagnostic test performance. *Radiology* 2011;259:117–26.

94. Deandreis D, Leboulleux S, Caramella C, Schlumberger M, Baudin E. FDG PET in the management of patients with adrenal masses and adrenal carcinoma. *Horm Cancer* 2011;2:354–62.

95. Dong A, Cui Y, Wang Y, Zuo C, Bai Y. ^{18}F-FDG PET/CT of adrenal lesions. *AJR Am J Roentgenol* 2014;203:245–52.

96. Jana S, Zhang T, Milstein D, Isasi C, Blaufox M. FDG-PET and CT characterization of adrenal lesions in cancer patients. *Eur J Nucl Mol Imaging* 2006;33:29–35.

97. Kim YI, Cheon GJ, Paeng JC et al. Total lesion glycolysis as the best 18F-FDG PET/CT parameter in differentiating intermediate-high risk adrenal incidentaloma. *Nucl Med Commun* 2014;35:606–12.

98. Santhanam P, Oakley C. Pet imaging of the adrenal gland—Utility and pitfalls. *Endocr Pract* 2014;20:375–7.

99. Sharma P, Singh H, Dhull VS et al. Adrenal masses of varied etiology: Anatomical and molecular imaging features on PET-CT. *Clin Nucl Med* 2014;39:251–60.

100. Takanami K, Kaneta T, Morimoto R et al. Characterization of lipid-rich adrenal tumors by FDG PET/CT: Are they hormone-secreting or not? *Ann Nucl Med* 2014;28:145–53.

101. Tessonnier L, Sebag F, Palazzo F et al. Does ^{18}F-FDG PET/CT add diagnostic accuracy in incidentally identified non-secreting adrenal tumours? *Eur J Nucl Mol Imaging* 2008;35:2018–25.

102. Williams A, Hammer GD, Else T. Transcutaneous biopsy of adrenocortical carcinoma is rarely helpful in diagnosis, potentially harmful, but does not affect patient outcome. *Eur J Endocrinol* 2014;170:829–35.

103. Hariskov S, Schumann R. Intraoperative management of patients with incidental catecholamine producing tumors: A literature review and analysis. *J Anaesthesiol Clin Pharmacol* 2013;29:41–6.

104. Grumbach M, Biller BMK, Braunstein G et al. Management of the clinically inapparent adrenal mass ("incidentaloma"). *Ann Int Med* 2003;138:424–9.

105. Paulker S, Kopelman R. Interpreting hoofbeats: Can Bayes help clear the haze? *N Engl J Med* 1992;327:1009–13.

106. Copeland P. The incidentally discovered adrenal mass. *Ann Intern Med* 1983;98:940–5.

107. Mansmann G, Lau J, Balk E, Rothberg M, Miyachi Y, Bornstein S. The clinically inapparent adrenal mass: Update in diagnosis and management. *Endocr Rev* 2004;25:309–40.

108. Terzolo M, Stigliano A, Chiodini I et al. AME position statement on adrenal incidentaloma. *Eur J Endocrinol* 2011;164:851–70.

109. Young WJ, Kaplan N, Kebebew E. The adrenal incidentaloma. Amsterdam: UpToDate, 2014. http://www.uptodate.com/contents/the-adrenal-incidentaloma/contributors?utdPopup = true

110. Shen J, Sun M, Zhou B, Yan J. Nonconformity in the clinical practice guidelines for subclinical Cushing's syndrome: Which guidelines are trustworthy? *Eur J Endocrinol* 2014;171:421–31.

111. Mazzaglia P, Monchik J. Limited value of adrenal biopsy in the evaluation of adrenal neoplasm: A decade of experience. *Arch Surg* 2009;144:465–70.

112. Barzon L, Fall F, Sonino N, Boscaro M. Development of overt Cushing's syndrome in patients with adrenal incidentaloma. *Eur J Endocrinol* 2002;146:61–6.

113. Barzon L, Scaroni C, Sonino N, Fallo F, Paoletta A, Boscaro M. Risk factors and long-term follow-up of adrenal incidentalomas. *J Clin Endocrinol Metab* 1999;84:520–6.

114. Siren J, Valimaki M, Huikuri K, Sivula A, Voutilainen P, Haapiainen R. Adrenalectomy for primary aldosteronism: Long-term follow-up study in 29 patients. *World J Surg* 1998;22:418–21.

115. Bülow B, Jansson S, Juhlin C et al. Adrenal incidentaloma—Follow-up results from a Swedish prospective study. *Eur J Endocrinol* 2006;154:419–23.

116. Vassilatou E, Vryonidou A, Michalopoulou S et al. Hormonal activity of adrenal incidentalomas: Results from a long-term follow-up study. *Clin Endocrinol* 2009;70:674–9.

117. Toniato A, Merante-Boschin I, Opocher G, Pelizzo M, Schiavi F, Ballotta E. Surgical versus conservative management for subclinical Cushing syndrome in adrenal incidentalomas: A prospective randomized study. *Ann Surg* 2009;249:388–91.

118. Hauch A, Al-Qurayshi Z, Kandil E. Factors associated with higher risk of complications after adrenal surgery. *Ann Surg Oncol* 2015;22:103–10.

119. Oshmyansky AR, Mahammedi A, Dackiw A et al. Serendipity in the diagnosis of pheochromocytoma. *J Comput Assist Tomogr* 2013;37:820–3.

120. Weingarten TN, Cata JP, O'Hara JF et al. Comparison of two preoperative medical management strategies for laparoscopic resection of pheochromocytoma. *Urology* 2010;76:508–11.

121. Burpee S, Jossart G, Gagner M. Laparoscopic adrenalectomy. In: Holzheimer RG, Mannick JA, eds., *Surgical Treatment: Evidence-Based and Problem-Oriented.* Munich: Zuckschwerdt, 2001. https://www.ncbi.nlm.nih.gov/books/NBK6872/ (accessed 12/5/2016).

122. Bharwani N, Rockall AG, Sahdev, A et al. Adrenocortical carcinoma: The range of appearances on CT and MRI. *AJR Am J Roentgenol* 2011;196:W706–14.

123. Sturgeon C, Shen WT, Clark OH, Duh QY, Kebebew E. Risk assessment in 457 adrenal cortical carcinomas: How much does tumor size predict the likelihood of malignancy? *J Am Coll Surg* 2006;202:423–30.

124. Miller BS, Doherty GM. Surgical management of adrenocortical tumours. *Nat Rev Endocrinol* 2014;10:282–92.

125. Gagner M, Lacroix A, Bolte E. Laparoscopic adrenalectomy in Cushing's syndrome and pheochromocytoma. *N Engl J Med* 1992;327:1033.

126. Gagner M, Lacroix A, Prinz RA et al. Early experience with laparoscopic approach for adrenalectomy. *Surgery* 1993;114:1120–4.

127. Duh QY, Siperstein AE, Clark OH et al. Laparoscopic adrenalectomy. Comparison of the lateral and posterior approaches. *Arch Surg* 1996;131:870–5.

128. Gagner M, Pomp A, Heniford BT, Pharand D, Lacroix A. Laparoscopic adrenalectomy: Lessons learned from 100 consecutive procedures. *Ann Surg* 1997;226:238–46.

129. Siperstein AE, Berber E, Engle KL, Duh QY, Clark OH. Laparoscopic posterior adrenalectomy: Technical considerations. *Arch Surg* 2000;135:967–71.

130. Li QY, Li F. Laparoscopic adrenalectomy in pheochromocytoma: Retroperitoneal approach versus transperitoneal approach. *J Endourol* 2010;24:1441–5.

131. Tiberio GA, Baiocchi GL, Arru L et al. Prospective randomized comparison of laparoscopic versus open adrenalectomy for sporadic pheochromocytoma. *Surg Endosc* 2008;22:1435–9.

132. Williams DT, Dann S, Wheeler MH. Phaeochromocytoma—Views on current management. *Eur J Surg Oncol* 2003;29:483–90.

133. Vanderveen KA, Thompson SM, Callstrom MR et al. Biopsy of pheochromocytomas and paragangliomas: Potential for disaster. *Surgery* 2009;146:1158–66.

134. Imai T, Kikumori T, Ohiwa M, Mase T, Funahashi H. A case-controlled study of laparoscopic compared with open lateral adrenalectomy. *Am J Surg* 1999;178:50–3.

135. Jacobs JK, Goldstein RE, Geer RJ. Laparoscopic adrenalectomy. A new standard of care. *Ann Surg* 1997;225:495–501.

136. Agcaoglu O, Sahin DA, Siperstein A, Berber E. Selection algorithm for posterior versus lateral approach in laparoscopic adrenalectomy. *Surgery* 2012;151:731–5.

137. Giebler RM, Walz MK, Peitgen K, Scherer RU. Hemodynamic changes after retroperitoneal CO2 insufflation for posterior retroperitoneoscopic adrenalectomy. *Anesth Analg* 1996;82:827–31.

138. Howell GM, Carty SE, Armstrong MJ et al. Outcome and prognostic factors after adrenalectomy for patients with distant adrenal metastasis. *Ann Surg Oncol* 2013;20:3491–6.

139. Vazquez BJ, Richards ML, Lohse CM et al. Adrenalectomy improves outcomes of selected patients with metastatic carcinoma. *World J Surg* 2012;36:1400–5.

140. Raffaelli M, Brunaud L, De CC et al. Synchronous bilateral adrenalectomy for Cushing's syndrome: Laparoscopic versus posterior retroperitoneoscopic versus robotic approach. *World J Surg* 2014;38:709–15.

141. Aliyev S, Karabulut K, Agcaoglu O et al. Robotic versus laparoscopic adrenalectomy for pheochromocytoma. *Ann Surg Oncol* 2013;20:4190–4.

142. Berber E, Mitchell J, Milas M, Siperstein A. Robotic posterior retroperitoneal adrenalectomy: Operative technique. *Arch Surg* 2010;145:781–4.

143. Callender GG, Kennamer DL, Grubbs EG, Lee JE, Evans DB, Perrier ND. Posterior retroperitoneoscopic adrenalectomy. *Adv Surg* 2009;43:147–57.

144. Kline GA, Pasieka JL, Harvey A, So B, Dias VC. Medical or surgical therapy for primary aldosteronism: Post-treatment follow-up as a surrogate measure of comparative outcomes. *Ann Surg Oncol* 2013;20:2274–8.

145. Gockel I, Heintz A, Polta M, Junginger T. Long-term results of endoscopic adrenalectomy for Conn's syndrome. *Am Surg* 2007;73:174–80.

146. Meyer A, Brabant G, Behrend M. Long-term follow-up after adrenalectomy for primary aldosteronism. *World J Surg* 2005;29:155–9.

147. Pang TC, Bambach C, Monaghan JC et al. Outcomes of laparoscopic adrenalectomy for hyperaldosteronism. *ANZ J Surg* 2007;77:768–73.

148. Sywak M, Pasieka JL. Long-term follow-up and cost benefit of adrenalectomy in patients with primary hyperaldosteronism. *Br J Surg* 2002;89:1587–93.

149. Catena C, Colussi G, Nadalini E et al. Cardiovascular outcomes in patients with primary aldosteronism after treatment. *Arch Intern Med* 2008;168:80–5.

150. Rossi GP, Bolognesi M, Rizzoni D et al. Vascular remodeling and duration of hypertension predict outcome of adrenalectomy in primary aldosteronism patients. *Hypertension* 2008;51:1366–71.

151. Stowasser M. New perspectives on the role of aldosterone excess in cardiovascular disease. *Clin Exp Pharmacol Physiol* 2001;28:783–91.

152. Hennings J, Andreasson S, Botling J, Hagg A, Sundin A, Hellman P. Long-term effects of surgical correction of adrenal hyperplasia and adenoma causing primary aldosteronism. *Langenbecks Arch Surg* 2010;395:133–7.

153. Zarnegar R, Young WF Jr, Lee J et al. The aldosteronoma resolution score: Predicting complete resolution of hypertension after adrenalectomy for aldosteronoma. *Ann Surg* 2008;247:511–8.

154. Favia G, Lumachi F, Scarpa V, et al. Adrenalectomy in primary aldosteronism: A long-term follow-up study in 52 patients. *World J Surg* 1992;16:680–3.

155. Midorikawa S, Sanada H, Hashimoto S, Suzuki T, Watanabe T. The improvement of insulin resistance in patients with adrenal incidentaloma by surgical resection. *Clin Endocrinol (Oxf)* 2001;54:797–804.

156. Bernini G, Moretti A, Iacconi P, Nami R, Lucani B, Salvetti A. Anthropometric, haemodynamic, humoral and hormonal evaluation in patients with incidental adrenocortical adenomas before and after surgery. *Eur J Endocrinol* 2003;148:213–9.

157. Emral R, Uysal A, Asik M et al. Prevalence of subclinical Cushing's syndrome in 70 patients with adrenal incidentaloma: Clinical, biochemical and surgical outcomes. *Endocr J* 2003;50:399–408.

158. Mitchell IC, Auchus RJ, Juneja K et al. "Subclinical Cushing's syndrome" is not subclinical: Improvement after adrenalectomy in 9 patients. *Surgery* 2007;142:900–5.

159. Zografos GN, Perysinakis I, Vassilatou E. Subclinical Cushing's syndrome: Current concepts and trends. *Hormones (Athens)* 2014;13:323–37.

160. Bilimoria KY, Shen WT, Elaraj D et al. Adrenocortical carcinoma in the United States: Treatment utilization and prognostic factors. *Cancer* 2008;113:3130–6.

161. Kutikov A, Mallin K, Canter D, Wong YN, Uzzo RG. Effects of increased cross-sectional imaging on the diagnosis and prognosis of adrenocortical carcinoma: Analysis of the National Cancer Database. *J Urol* 2011;186:805–10.

162. Deckers S, Derdelinckx L, Col V, Hamels J, Maiter D. Peritoneal carcinomatosis following laparoscopic resection of an adrenocortical tumor causing primary hyperaldosteronism. *Horm Res* 1999;52:97–100.

163. Gonzalez RJ, Shapiro S, Sarlis N et al. Laparoscopic resection of adrenal cortical carcinoma: A cautionary note. *Surgery* 2005;138:1078–85.

164. Jurowich C, Fassnacht M, Kroiss M, Deutschbein T, Germer CT, Reibetanz J. Is there a role for laparoscopic adrenalectomy in patients with suspected adrenocortical carcinoma? A critical appraisal of the literature. *Horm Metab Res* 2013;45:130–6.

165. Porpiglia F, Miller BS, Manfredi M, Fiori C, Doherty GM. A debate on laparoscopic versus open adrenalectomy for adrenocortical carcinoma. *Horm Cancer* 2011;2:372–7.

166. Cooper AB, Habra MA, Grubbs EG, et al. Does laparoscopic adrenalectomy jeopardize oncologic outcomes for patients with adrenocortical carcinoma? *Surg Endosc* 2013;27:4026–32.

167. Walz MK. Extent of adrenalectomy for adrenal neoplasm: Cortical sparing (subtotal) versus total adrenalectomy. *Surg Clin North Am* 2004;84:743–53.

168. Grubbs EG, Rich TA, Ng C et al. Long-term outcomes of surgical treatment for hereditary pheochromocytoma. *J Am Coll Surg* 2013;216:280–9.

169. Smith-Bindman R, Lipson J, Marcus R et al. Radiation dose associated with common computed tomography examinations and the associated lifetime attributable risk of cancer. *Arch Intern Med* 2009;169:2078–86.

170. Aron D, Kievit J. Adrenal incidentalomas. In: Schwartz A, Linos D, Gagner M, eds., *Endocrine Surgery*. New York: Marcel Dekker, 2004;411–428.

171. Melck AL, Rosengart MR, Armstrong MJ, Stang MT, Carty SE, Yip L. Immediate laparoscopic adrenalectomy versus observation: Cost evaluation for incidental adrenal lesions with atypical imaging characteristics. *Am J Surg* 2012;204:462–7.

172. Wang TS, Cheung K, Roman SA, Sosa JA. A cost-effectiveness analysis of adrenalectomy for non-functional adrenal incidentalomas: Is there a size threshold for resection? *Surgery* 2012;152:1125–32.

173. Young W. The incidentally discovered adrenal mass. *N Engl J Med* 2007;356:601–10.

34

Laparoscopic adrenalectomy with the transabdominal lateral approach

MICHEL GAGNER

INTRODUCTION

Since its first description in 1992 [1], laparoscopic adrenalectomy has proved to be the procedure of choice for the surgical treatment of benign adrenal disease. Multiple reports have consistently demonstrated the benefits of this surgery, including decreased analgesic requirements, less blood loss, and shorter hospital stay, over the conventional approach [2–8]. These results were not surprising considering that the procedure avoids an upper abdominal incision, does not require any reconstruction, benefits from magnification and clarity of view, is commonly performed for benign disease, and mostly involves small, easily extractable specimens. Proper application of minimally invasive surgery to the adrenal gland must take into account expertise in both endocrine and laparoscopic surgery [9]. For successful adrenalectomy, one must have knowledge of the anatomy and disease process, maintain meticulous hemostasis, and delicately handle tissue [9]. The alternative open conventional adrenalectomy invariably requires large incisions, and sometimes rib resections with posterior approaches, resulting in significant postoperative morbidity, including chronic pain syndromes because of injury to intercostal and other nerves [10]. Although those conventional approaches will undoubtedly still be required for certain adrenal pathologies, laparoscopic adrenalectomy, eliminating many of the problems of open surgery, has become the gold standard for treatment of most adrenal diseases [11,12].

INDICATIONS

The indications for laparoscopic adrenalectomy are basically the same as those for open adrenalectomy (Table 34.1). Laparoscopic adrenalectomy has been reported in several other conditions [13–15], but is not currently considered standard. These include neuroblastoma and congenital adrenal hyperplasia (CAH) in children and isolated adrenals [16–18]. The procedure is being performed with higher frequency than before, mainly due to an increase in the proportion of adrenalectomies performed for benign tumors [19,20].

General relative contraindications for laparoscopy include uncorrectable or untreated coagulopathy and unacceptable cardiopulmonary risk, previous surgery or trauma in the direct vicinity of the adrenal gland, diaphragmatic hernia, and surgeon's inexperience [3]. Obesity and previous major intra-abdominal surgery are no longer contraindications for laparoscopic adrenalectomy [21]. However, large obesity is an independent risk factor for wound and septic complications [22]. Currently, in experienced hands, the only specific absolute contraindication is known large adrenocortical carcinoma with frank tumor invasion

Table 34.1 Indications for laparoscopic transabdominal lateral decubitus tehnique

1. Functional adrenal cortical masses
   a. Cushing syndrome caused by benign cortisol producing adenoma
   b. Cushing's disease after failed pituitary surgery, or after failure to control or to find an ectopic-ACTH producing tumor
   c. Aldosterone producing adenoma (Conn's syndrome)
   d. Rare virilizing/feminizing tumors
2. Functional medullary adrenal masses
   a. Benign adrenal pheochromocytoma
3. Nonfunctional adrenal tumors
   a. Benign looking Incidentalomas (nonfunctioning adenomas) confined to the adrenal glands and meeting accepted criteria for adrenalectomy (size > 4 cm at presentation or growth in follow up
   b. Benign symptomatic lesions
   c. Rare entities such as cyst and myelolipoma

to adjacent structures like the vena cava, kidney, or diaphragm. In these cases, an open procedure is preferred in order to allow an *en bloc* resection and node dissection to be performed [23,24]. Rare entities such as various cysts, pseudocyst, hydatid cysts, myelolipoma, and chronic infections like tuberculosis constitute other indications [25,26].

Although controversy exists over the maximum acceptable tumor size for laparoscopic adrenalectomy, laparoscopy may not be advisable for adrenal tumors larger than 12–14 cm because of the technical difficulties associated with such surgery and the malignant potential of these large tumors.

OPERATIVE TECHNIQUES

Detailed knowledge of adrenal anatomy and its common variations is a prerequisite to laparoscopic adrenal surgery. Several laparoscopic approaches to the adrenal glands are demonstrated:

1. Transabdominal lateral (with the patient in the lateral decubitus position)
2. Transabdominal anterior (with the patient in the supine position)
3. Retroperitoneal endoscopic adrenalectomy (with the patient in the lateral or mostly prone posterior)

Although some advocate the retroperitoneal approach, usually practicing urologists [27–30], the technique of choice by most endocrine and general surgeons performing laparoscopic adrenalectomy is the transabdominal lateral approach, originally described by Gagner in 1992 [1,31]. In this positioning, the force of gravity helps retract the surrounding organs (including the bowel), and effectively exposes either adrenal gland for laparoscopic intervention.

As a result, there is reduced dissection and minimal retraction of the vena cava and other adjacent structure. The patient is positioned on the table to maximize the distance between the costal margin and the iliac crest. This is achieved by adjusting the laparoscopic operating table in the jackknife position, with the patient placed in the lateral decubitus position with the operated side up. Sufficient padding is placed over pressure points, and the patient is strapped and taped in position, especially avoiding a brachial plexus injury or iliac compression. The sterilization of the skin should extend from the nipple to the anterior superior iliac spine, and from the midline anteriorly to the spine posteriorly. This allows for conversion to an open procedure should this be necessary. Walz et al. have reported more than 500 procedures with this approach with excellent results. Between July 1994 and March 2006, 560 adrenalectomies for 21 Cushing's disease, 157 Conn's adenomas, 120 pheochromocytomas, 110 Cushing's adenomas, and 112 other tumors were performed. Tumor sizes ranged from 0.5 to 10 cm, and the procedures were performed in prone position, usually with three trocars. Conversion was necessary in 1.7%, with a mean operating time of 67 minutes. This may not be completely reproducible in less experienced hands [32]. Zhang et al. have reported faster operating times [33]. Recent meta-analyses have not demonstrated any superiority over the lateral transabdominal approach [34,35].

Transabdominal laparoscopic left adrenalectomy

Patients are placed in the lateral decubitus position with the left side up (Figure 34.1). The surgeon and the assistant stand on the side opposite the diseased gland, facing the abdomen (Figure 34.2). A flank cushion is positioned under the patient's right side, and the table is flexed so that the left side is hyperextended (Figure 34.1). The left arm is extended and suspended. The surgical area is prepared as previously described. An open technique is used to access the abdominal cavity in the left subcostal area at the level of anterior axillary line, and carbon dioxide, up to 15 mm of pressure, is insufflated. One 10 mm trocar is then inserted in this site, and a 30°, 10 mm laparoscope is introduced, through which the abdominal cavity is explored, for possible liver metastases, adhesions, or contiguous organ involvement or displacement. If the inspection is satisfactory, two more 5 or 10 mm trocars are inserted under direct vision in the flank, depending on available instrumentation: one under the 11th rib and one slightly more anterior and medial to the first trocar (Figure 34.3). Often, a fourth trocar is needed for retraction and is inserted at the costovertebral junction dorsally, since most left adrenalectomies are now performed with three trocars only more than 80% of the time. All trocars should be at least 5 cm and, more optimally, 8–10 cm apart. The laparoscope is then inserted in the most anterior trocar, and the surgeon will work laterally with a two-hand technique through the other two trocars. Working with the laparoscopic scissors with cautery or the ultrasonic scalpel,

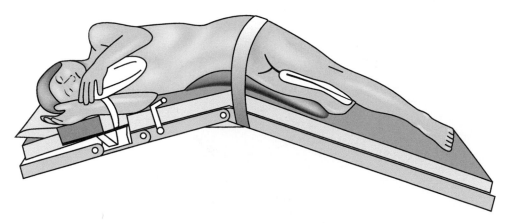

Figure 34.1 Patient positioning.

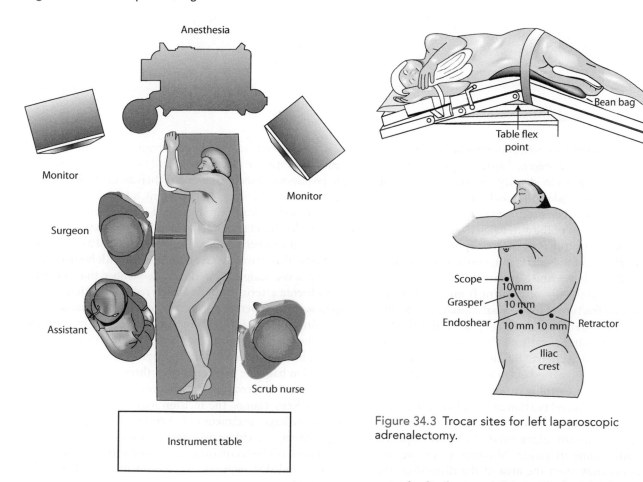

Figure 34.2 Laparoscopic left adrenalectomy: operating room layout.

Figure 34.3 Trocar sites for left laparoscopic adrenalectomy.

in the right hand, and a curved dissector in the left hand, the splenic flexure (or lienocolic ligament) is mobilized medially (Figure 34.4) to separate the colon from the inferior pole of the adrenal and expose the lineorenal ligament. Mobilization allows instruments to be inserted more easily and helps prevent inadvertent trauma to the colon or spleen during instrument insertion. Next, the lineorenal ligament is incised from inferior to superior approximately 1 cm from the spleen (Figures 34.5 and 34.6). The dissection is carried

up to the diaphragm and stopped when the short gastric vessels are encountered posteriorly behind the stomach. This maneuver allows the spleen to fall medially, thus exposing the retroperitoneal space. The lateral edge and anterior portion of the adrenal gland will become visible in the perinephric fat superiorly and medially. If necessary, a fourth 5 mm trocar is inserted dorsally at the costovertebral angle to gently retract large-size spleens, and open the space or push the left kidney or the surrounding fat downward to expose the inferior pole and lateral edge of the adrenal gland better. This trocar should always be inserted after the previous three because the splenorenal ligament must be divided first, so that the trocar will pass over the lateral and superior border

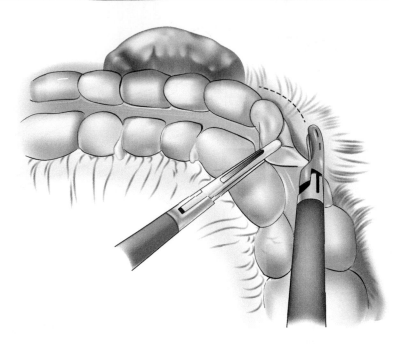

Figure 34.4 Dissection of splenic flexure.

of the kidney. This port, however, is usually not necessary in patients with normal-size spleen. Laparoscopic ultrasound may be used as an adjunct to identify the adrenal gland, the mass within the gland, and the adrenal vein [3]. Variants are common, and even so when dealing with pheochromocytomas [36]. The dissection of the adrenal gland can be easy or difficult, depending on the type of perinephric fat. Mainly two types may be encountered: (1) soft, nonadherent, areolar fat, which is easy to dissect, and (2) dense, adherent fat, which contains multiple small veins originating from the retroperitoneum. To avoid fracture of the adrenal capsule, it is helpful to leave a little periadrenal fat on the adrenal, so that this tissue, rather than the adrenal itself, can be retracted. Grasping the perinephric fat, dissection of the lateral and anterior part of the adrenal gland is carried out. Hook electrocautery or ultrasonic scalpels are useful instruments for this phase of dissection. Once the lateral portion of the adrenal gland has been exposed, the patient is moved to the Fowler position to permit further downward migration of the bowel loops and the spleen. Any saline irrigation, bleeding, or oozing will flow downward away from the area of the dissection. The dissection can either be continued inferiorly, so that the left adrenal vein can be clipped early in the dissection, or start superiorly and go down medially to clip the adrenal vein last. The dissection depends on the exposure gained after the spleen has been mobilized, the type of disease, and the size of the adrenal mass. In large adrenals (>5 cm), the left adrenal vein may be difficult to visualize. In such cases, dissecting the lateral and superior adrenal poles first will allow better mobilization and make clipping the adrenal vein easier later during the dissection (Figure 34.7). In smaller adrenals (angle dissector), the adrenal vein is dissected from its insertion into the left adrenal gland. It is not necessary to identify and dissect the origin of the vein from the left renal

vein. The adrenal vein is clipped about 1 cm from the renal vein: two clips are placed proximally to the gland and two are positioned distally. The vein is then divided with laparoscopic straight scissors. At this point, adrenal mobilization becomes easy because it is grasped on the perinephric fat with the left-hand grasper; the gland is then pushed upward and laterally to permit dissection of the medial and superior portions. This dissection is accomplished with hook cautery or ultrasonic scalpel. One should remember that the inferior phrenic arterial branches often require ligation as they approach the superior pole of the left adrenal gland. Once the adrenal gland is free, hemostasis is verified by repeated irrigation and aspiration. The gland is then extracted in total after it has been placed in an appropriately sized impermeable nylon bag. The bag is removed through the most anterior trocar by spreading the abdominal wall musculature using a Kelly clamp. The incision may have to be enlarged to remove large specimens (>4–5 cm) without rupturing the bag. Drainage is seldom necessary unless pancreatic injury is suspected. All fascia incisions are closed with 2-0 absorbable sutures, and skin incisions are closed with 4-0 subcuticular absorbable sutures.

Transabdominal laparoscopic right adrenalectomy

Patients are positioned in the lateral decubitus position with the right side up (Figure 34.8). Pneumoperitoneum is established in the same way as for left adrenalectomy. An open technique is used to access the abdominal cavity approximately 2 cm below and parallel to the costal margin. A 10 mm trocar is inserted at this site for the 30° angled laparoscope. Inspection of the abdominal cavity is carried out. Under direct vision, three additional 10 mm trocars are

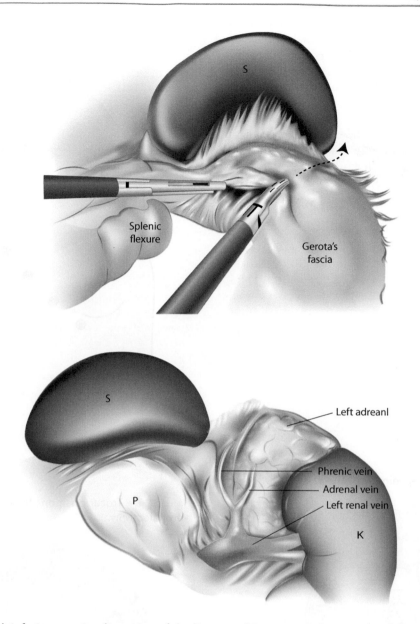

Figure 34.5 Left adrenal: inferio-superior dissection of the lienorenal ligament and exposure of the adrenal vessels.

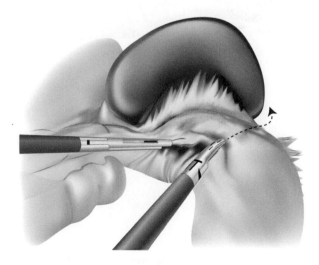

Figure 34.6 Use of a 5-mm ultrasonic endoscopic shear for division of the lienorenal ligament.

inserted 2 cm and parallel to the costal margin (Figure 34.9). The second trocar is positioned in the right flank, inferior and posterior to the tip of the 11th rib, just above the hepatic flexure of the colon, which seldom needs to be mobilized. The third trocar is then inserted in the most anterior position of the subcostal area between the epigastrium and the anterior axillary line. This most medial trocar should be lateral to the edge of the ipsilateral rectus muscle. The last trocar is introduced either at the tip of the 12th rib or sometimes at the costovertebral subcostal angle after the peritoneal reflection of the lateral edge of the right kidney has been dissected to avoid injury to the right kidney. Four trocars are necessary because the right lobe of the liver must be retracted to expose the most medial aspect of the right adrenal gland. It is therefore crucial that the liver retractor be inserted under direct vision, through the most anterior port, so that the right hepatic lobe can be lifted and pushed anteriomedially (Figure 34.10). The laparoscope is removed from the first

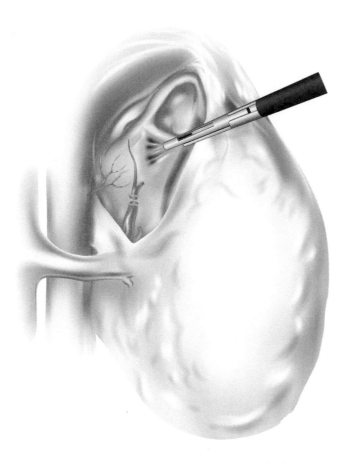

Figure 34.7 Left adrenal vein clipped and divided.

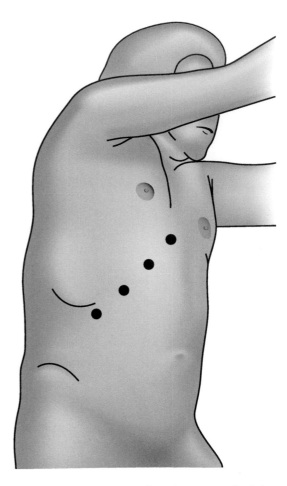

Figure 34.9 Trocar positions for a laparoscopic right adrenalectomy.

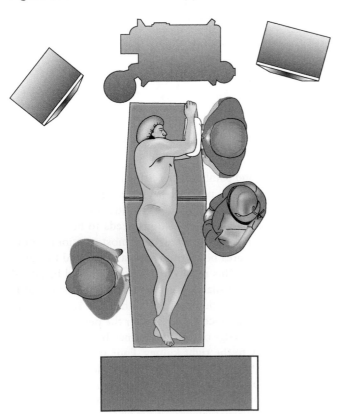

Figure 34.8 Operating room setup for a laparoscopic right adrenalectomy.

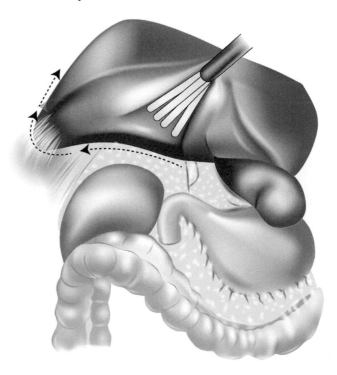

Figure 34.10 Retraction of the liver: the line of mobilization of the right lobe of the liver is demonstrated, including the right triangular ligament.

trocar and inserted in the second trocar, and the surgeon works with the two most lateral trocars. The camera can also be positioned dorsally, and the surgeon works with the two trocars in the middle to obtain another view of the dissection field. This is especially useful for dissecting the superior aspect of the adrenal gland. The liver often must be mobilized to obtain the best exposure of the junction between the adrenal gland and the inferior vena cava. The right lateral hepatic attachments and the triangular ligament are (Figure 34.10) therefore dissected from the diaphragm using laparoscopic scissors or ultrasonic scalpel. This dissection will permit more effective retraction to push the liver medially using a fan or some other atraumatic retractor. This is the key for providing adequate exposure of the right adrenal vein and its entry into the vena cava. We prefer to create a right-angle plane between the anterior aspect of the right kidney and the lateral portion of the liver. This plane will provide enough space to work and adequate exposure in case of bleeding. Laparoscopic ultrasound may be of assistance in identifying the anatomy. The right gland is dissected next. If the mass is smaller than 4 cm in diameter, gaining access to the right adrenal vein initially is possible, which permits easier dissection of the rest of the adrenal gland. The inferolateral edge is then mobilized (Figure 34.11), and dissection is continued afterwards medially (Figure 34.12) and upward (Figure 34.13), along the lateral edge of the vena cava (Figures 34.14 and 34.15). The adrenal vein should be visualized at this stage. This vein is often short and sometimes broad (Figures 34.16 and 34.17). Usually, the vein can be clipped with medium to large titanium clips, and at least two should be applied at the vena cava side. If there is not enough space for clips, then a vascular cartridge of a 30 or 35 mm laparoscopic stapler is used for secure division of the right adrenal vein (Figures 34.18 and 34.19). Smaller veins may be encountered superiorly; these should be clipped or cauterized to prevent bleeding (Figures 34.20 and 34.21). The superior pole of the gland is dissected next, and small branches from the inferior phrenic vessels can be clipped or cauterized with hook

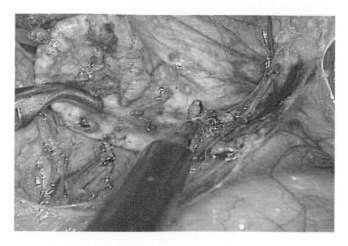

Figure 34.12 A similar dissection is achieved anteriorly.

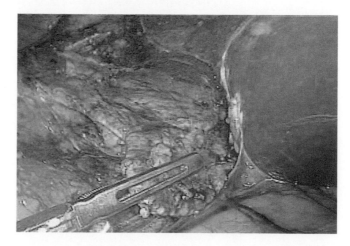

Figure 34.13 Demonstration of how a Dorsey bowel forcep (Karl Storz) can be used on the right adrenal gland to provide traction, between the gland and the vena cava.

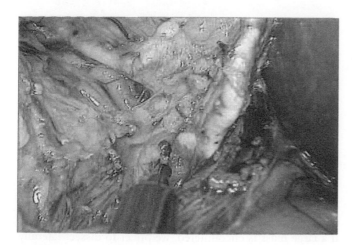

Figure 34.11 A 5-mm hook instrument (Karl Storz) is used to dissect the small vessels surrounding the inferior pole of the right adrenal gland.

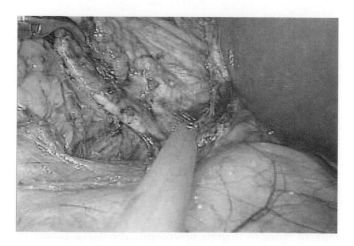

Figure 34.14 Blunt dissection between the vena cana (next to duodenum) and the right gland, using a 5-mm hydrodissection cannula.

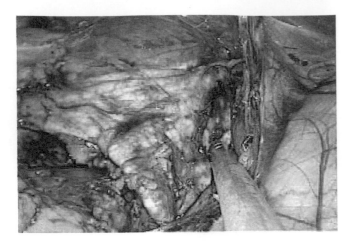

Figure 34.15 Inferior vena cava exposure.

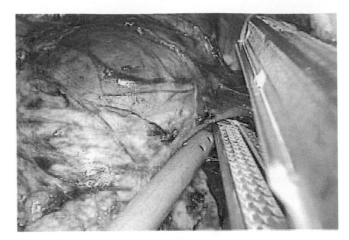

Figure 34.18 A cautious application of the endoscopic vascular stapler.

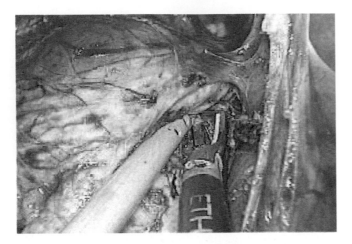

Figure 34.16 Posterior mobilization behind the right adrenal vein before clipping.

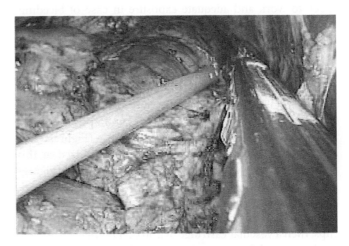

Figure 34.19 Vascular stapler applied to the right adrenal vein.

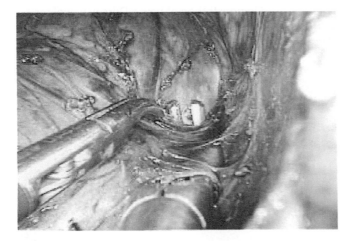

Figure 34.17 Right adrenal vein dissection using a 10-mm right angle dissector (Karl Storz).

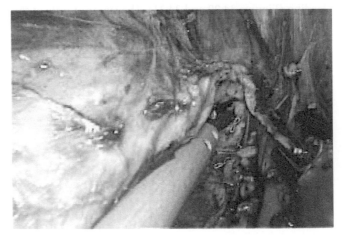

Figure 34.20 Clips applied to the right adrenal vein stump.

cautery or ultrasonic scalpel. Again, a Fowler position permits all fluids to migrate downward. The lateral border of the gland is then dissected from the perinephric fat using the same instruments (Figure 34.22). Meticulous dissection close to the gland will prevent tearing of the lateral branches

of the vena cava and other vessels from the retroperitoneum. If a large mass is encountered, we prefer to dissect laterally and superiorly first, and then move down along the vena cava to reach the adrenal vein. Once the mass has been dissected free, it is placed in an impermeable nylon bag (Figures 34.23

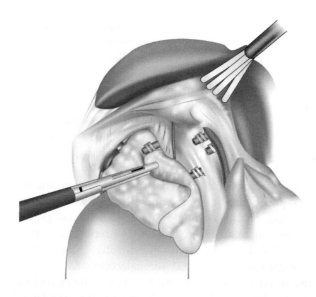

Figure 34.21 Right adrenal vessel dissection and control.

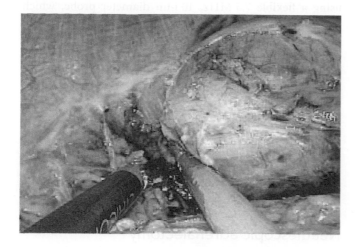

Figure 34.22 Lateral dissection of a large right pheochromocytoma.

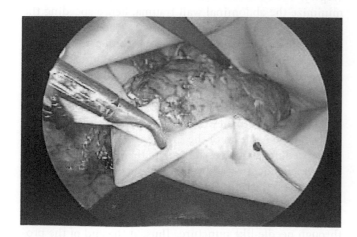

Figure 34.23 Gland extraction into an impermeable bag.

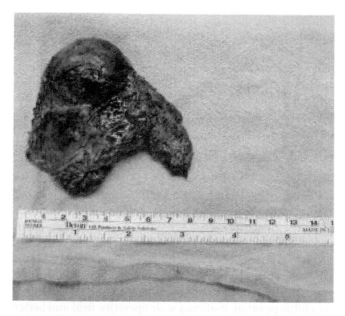

Figure 34.24 Macroscopic aspects of a resected right adrenal tumor after extraction.

and 34.24) and removed through the most anterior trocar site. All wounds are closed as described for the left side. The fascia of the fourth (dorsal) trocar site is not closed because of the depth of this wound.

Transabdominal anterior laparoscopic adrenalectomy

This approach can be a lengthy procedure due to the difficult dissection of the left colic flexure, spleen and pancreatic tail on the left side, and duodenum on the right. In addition, on the right side, the adrenal vein, found posterior to the vena cava, is very difficult to dissect and control. Although in bilateral adrenalectomy it is not necessary to change the position of the patient, the average operating time is similar to that for the lateral transabdominal approach. Nevertheless, because of its drawbacks, the majority of the teams have abandoned this approach. Lezoche et al. have reported a large series of >200 cases with excellent outcomes [37].

Bilateral laparoscopic adrenalectomy

The indications for bilateral laparoscopic adrenalectomy include the following [38]: (1) Cushing's disease refractory to transsphenoidal pituitary resection or irradiation, (2) Cushing's syndrome due to adrenocorticotropic hormone (ACTH)-independent macronodular or micronodular adrenal hyperplasia, (3) ectopic ACTH syndrome when the primary tumor cannot be resected or medical treatment has failed, (4) Conn's syndrome caused by bilateral adrenal adenomas, and (5) bilateral pheochromocytoma. Other less prevalent relative and possible indications include (1) unilateral pheochromocytoma in multiple endocrine neoplasia (MEN) type 2A, due to the fact that in 50% of cases a metachronous lesion will develop in the contralateral side within 10 years of resection of the affected side [39]; (2) idiopathic hyperaldosteronism (IHA) caused by bilateral symmetric adrenal hyperplasia refractory to medical treatment; and (3) congenital bilateral adrenal hyperplasia, which is difficult to manage medically [38]. There are several possible surgical approaches for bilateral laparoscopic adrenalectomy [40].

TRANSABDOMINAL LATERAL APPROACH

This is the preferred approach, in my opinion. The patient is placed in the lateral decubitus position; usually the left side is performed first because it is easier. After all trocar sites are closed, the patient is repositioned and redraped, to expose the right side. A 15- to 20-minute turnover time is necessary, not significantly adding to the operative length [2]. Nevertheless, we prefer this bilateral approach because gravity aids the dissection when the patient is in the lateral decubitus position; it offers a wide operative field and better control of blood vessels. Furthermore, it may be safer than the retroperitoneal approach for the right adrenal, where better control of a possible major vascular injury (i.e., vena cava) is needed. We have successfully performed bilateral laparoscopic adrenalectomy within a reasonable amount of time using a bilateral lateral technique [3]. Utilizing this approach, Chapuis et al. [41], with the largest published series on bilateral laparoscopic adrenalectomy in 24 patients with Cushing's syndrome, reported no major postoperative complications. The operative times have ranged from 243 to 386 minutes for the reported bilateral procedures using this approach. Steroid replacement may be necessary [42].

RETROPERITONEAL APPROACH

This can be accomplished using the lateral or posterior methods described earlier. It is worth mentioning that the few series with data on bilateral laparoscopic lateral and posterior retroperitoneal approaches have not shown greater elevations of carbon dioxide than with the lateral transabdominal approach [43–45].

ANTERIOR APPROACH

Despite its theoretical advantage in bilateral adrenalectomy, the drawbacks explained above regarding difficulty in exposure and dissection have led the majority of surgeons to abandon this approach. No randomized prospective studies have been conducted to compare laparoscopic bilateral adrenalectomy with open bilateral surgery, even though the available literature on bilateral laparoscopic adrenalectomy is encouraging, with low morbidity and mortality rates [1,3,41,43,46,47]. In the setting of Cushing's syndrome, the morbidity and mortality rates of the laparoscopic approach are noticeably lower than those for open surgery [1,3,41,43]. The typical operative length for bilateral laparoscopic adrenalectomy, including all approaches, is approximately 300 minutes [38]. There have been some reports of operative times longer than 300 minutes, with cases of hypercarbia requiring hyperventilation, but without significant sequelae

[43,45]. Fernandez-Cruz et al. [48,49] have recommended helium pneumoperitoneum for the bilateral laparoscopic procedure in order to prevent carbon dioxide retention and acidosis. The use of helium may be recommended in patients with pheochromocytoma with previous cardiovascular or respiratory disorders [49]. Gasless is another possibility, which is making a comeback from the early 1990s [50].

Laparoscopic partial adrenalectomy

Possible indications for adrenal-sparing surgery include bilateral pheochromocytoma and well-circumscribed bilateral cortisol or aldosterone-producing adenomas [51,52]. The purpose is to avoid lifelong cortisol replacement therapy [53]. The operative technique involves basically the same initial steps as for total adrenalectomy. After exposing the adrenal glands, dissection is first performed at the inferior borders and then carried upward along the lateral aspect using hook cautery or ultrasonic scalpel and gentle grasping forceps. One has to preserve as much blood supply as possible. An ultrasound of the gland is then performed using a flexible 7.5 MHz, 10 mm diameter probe, which demonstrates the location of the adrenal vein and arterial supply and confirms the location and borders of the adrenal lesion. It also should be possible to exclude the presence of other nodules or hyperplasia in the adrenal remnant. At this stage, the adrenal lesion can be easily dissected free and elevated. While concomitantly displaying the margins of the tumor with the ultrasound, the harmonic shears are used to bloodlessly transect the adrenal gland away from the lesion. The excised specimen is then placed in a bag, retrieved, and sent for immediate histopathologic examination to confirm histology and assess the margins. At least a 5 mm rim of normal adrenal tissue is preferred.

Needlescopic adrenalectomy

Initially described for diagnostic purposes or cholecystectomy, the availability of 2 mm instrumentation and camera technology has triggered the emergence of needlescopic surgery. The rationale behind this technique is to further minimize the abdominal wall trauma, hence speeding the convalescence and improving cosmesis. The positioning of the patient and number of trocars are similar to the traditional laparoscopic adrenalectomy. A 10–12 mm trocar is inserted in the superior aspect of the umbilicus to accommodate the 10 mm angled scope under which most of the procedure is conducted. It also enables the use of bigger instruments should they be required (e.g., vascular endostapler) and the retrieval of the specimen. During these steps, the procedure is monitored through the 2 mm needlescope. On the left side, two additional trocars of 2 and 5 mm are used, and on the right side, a fourth 2 mm trocar is utilized for liver retraction. Placement of the 2 mm ports does not require skin incisions. These ports can be readily inserted through needle-like puncture. Thus, at the end of the procedure, these miniature puncture sites require no skin closure, except for Steri-Strips. The 5 mm port is used by the surgeon's dominant hand in order to accommodate larger instruments, such as scissors, electrocautery, suction–irrigation devices, and clip appliers. Dissection is carried out using 2 mm graspers, scissors, and hook electrocautery, and vascular control is achieved with electrocautery (uni- or bipolar) and a 5 mm clip applier [54,55].

Single-port adrenalectomy

Hirano et al. had thought of a small incision (4.5 cm) and, using a resectoscope of 4 cm, performed retroperitoneoscopic adrenalectomy in 53 patients with an average procedure duration of 203 minutes. Still, the mean estimated blood loss was 252 mL and 7.4% required blood transfusion, perhaps related to the lack of triangulation [56]. Castellucci et al. had described a single-port access (SPA) adrenalectomy through a 2 cm supraumbilical incision [57]. This is in fact similar to needlescopic surgery performed a decade before, where a smaller umbilical port (10–12 mm) was used with smaller 1–2 mm instruments in the subcostal areas. The advantage of needlescopic surgery is the triangulation it confers, as opposed to "fencing", with all instruments being in the umbilical areas. Because of the nature of this surgery, with bleeding potentially involved, I prefer the needlescopic approach, even 20 years later. Walz et al. have recently analyzed the experience of single-access retroperitoneal adrenalectomy (SARA) vs. multiport surgery for retroperitoneoscopic adrenalectomy [58]. There were no major complications, and SARA was completed in 86% of cases attempted. Operative time was significantly longer for SARA (56 minutes) than for multiport surgery (40 minutes) ($p < 0.05$) by 40%, increasing costs. Postoperatively, less pain medication was administered to SARA patients [58]. Others have reported similar findings, with longer operative times, without increasing complications [59–69].

Robotic-assisted adrenalectomy

At first, this started with an assisted robotic arm to hold the camera (making it almost solo-surgeon surgery), and eventually moved to laparoscopic-assisted instruments in the late 1990s [70]. Initially reported by using the "Zeus" robot from Computer Motion and "Da Vinci" from Intuitive, both California companies, with almost 20 years of experience, they have failed to become mainstream [71–73]. The real benefits of robotic-assisted surgery compared with "standard" laparoscopic surgery are still evolving, and it is possible that with existing technology, there are no real advantages for both patients and surgeons. The first randomized trial on this question, from the University of Turin, showed clearly no advantages [74]. Conversion to standard laparoscopic surgery was necessary in 40% of robotic patients; morbidity was higher and total cost significantly higher ($p < 0.01$) [74]. Others reported no cost increases; however, they did not include the cost of the robot itself and its maintenance over time [75–80]. Partial

adrenalectomy can be safely done using an assisted robotic approach [81]. Obesity was thought to be a potential advantage of robotic techniques, but was recently studied and not confirmed [82]. The use of iodocyanin green helps in delineating the tumor from the normal parenchyma (as well as laparoscopic ultrasonography, but the latter necessitates an additional port) [83].

Perhaps robotic surgery will make single-port surgery easier and bring triangulation. The Mayo Clinic experience with single-site robotic-assisted adrenalectomy shows safety [76]. They have successfully operated on 33 patients with a mean age of 54 years and mean body mass index (BMI) of 32.7 kg/m². There were 18 left, 10 right, and 5 bilateral procedures for a total of 38 adrenal glands removed, but 7 were converted (about 20%). The main advantage was a short hospital stay (74% of patients were discharged on postoperative day 1 and 96% were discharged by postoperative day 2). A longer operating time and higher costs remained [84]. In a recent Korean series of 171 patients, 98 underwent conventional laparoendoscopic single-site surgery and 73 underwent robotic laparoendoscopic single-site surgery. The mean operative time was long at 190 minutes, and the mean estimated blood loss was 204 mL [85].

NOTES adrenalectomy

I was successful using a transgastric route, endoscopically in a human, to extract a left adrenal tumor, in Porto Alegre in Brazil, during the III Simposio Internacional de Videocirugia Avancada on May 8–10, 2008 [86]. This was a hybrid procedure in which microlaparoscopic surgery was entirely done with 3–5 mm laparoscopic guidance, and extraction of the tumor was done after a gastrotomy, for transoral extraction. This evolved from an earlier experience in transvaginal cholecystectomy at the same site [87]. An attempt was made by a team from the Department of Gastroenterology, Homerton University Hospital in London, for endoscopic transgastric removal of adrenal glands in pigs [88]. Adrenal gland removal failed in all procedures in which it was attempted. It appears that successful procedures were done via a transvaginal route in pigs [89]. A hybrid with transabdominal and transvaginal trocars for extraction has been used in female patients [90]. Eyraud reports on a transrectal route in cadavers, especially robotic, where transrectal hybrid natural orifice translumenal endoscopic surgery (NOTES) adrenalectomy was completed successfully. The total operative time was 145 minutes; right adrenalectomy, specimen extraction, and rectal closure were completed in 15, 30, and 20 minutes, respectively [91]. Instrumentation is not adequately made for NOTES, but no doubt this will be the future in one or two decades.

POSTOPERATIVE CARE

Oral fluids are started on the day of surgery and oral analgesics are provided to help patients tolerate the postoperative pain. However, during the first 12 hours, some patients require parenteral analgesia. The postoperative course is similar to that for laparoscopic cholecystectomy, except that some endocrine disorders will necessitate hormonal support and additional clinical laboratory data. It should be noticed that unexplained hypotension, fever, and confusion might be due to acute adrenocortical insufficiency. These patients should have blood drawn for determination of plasma cortisol levels and be immediately treated with 100 mg of hydrocortisone intravenously. Most patients will be ambulatory by the evening of the procedure, and the majority will be allowed to leave by the third postoperative day. However, discharge may be delayed in patients who require substantial hormonal support or adjustments of antihypertensive medications.

RESULTS

Since 1992, laparoscopic adrenalectomy has gained worldwide popularity, and in a search of Medline, we were able to retrieve more than 1500 articles dealing with laparoscopic adrenalectomy. Table 34.2 summarizes the reported results of selected large series of laparoscopic adrenalectomies performed with different laparoscopic techniques. Although no prospective randomized series exist, numerous studies have compared laparoscopic with open adrenalectomy (either retrospectively or nonrandomized prospectively), documenting the safety, decreased analgesic postoperative requirements, enhanced recovery, shorter hospital stay, and cost-effectiveness of the laparoscopic approach [4–8,45,92–101]. No differences in patient population, indications for surgery, or mean size of lesions were noticed. Our own experience, presented herein, with 100 procedures in 88 patients [3], further supports the superiority of this procedure. Table 34.3 lists the indications and pathology for our procedures. The overall mean age was 46 years (range 17–84 years), and the ratio of

female to male was >2:1. Fifty-two of the adrenalectomies were performed in the left and ten were performed bilaterally. The mean operating time was 132 minutes (range 80–360 minutes). In our initial experience, a right-sided procedure required an average of 138 minutes compared with 102 minutes for a left-sided procedure. However, review of the last 30 cases showed the time required for either side is essentially equal. The time required for bilateral adrenalectomy averaged approximately 45 minutes longer than the combined averages for the unilateral procedure alone. The indications for bilateral adrenalectomy are listed in Table 34.4. The average length of stay was 2.4 days (range 1–6 days), and the average size of the lesions was 4.95 cm (range 0.7–12 cm). The estimated intraoperative blood loss was approximately 70 mL, and the mean number of postoperative narcotic injections was 5.5. Conversion to open surgery was necessary in three patients (3%). These conversions occurred in our first attempt at laparoscopic adrenalectomy in a patient with a 15 cm right adrenal angiomyelolipoma, in a second patient with a locally invasive retroperitoneal sarcoma, and in a third patient with adrenal adenocarcinoma invading the inferior vena cava. More than half of our patient's population (55%) had had previous abdominal surgery. We have not viewed this as a contraindication for the laparoscopic approach, and no conversions occurred because of adhesions. We actually performed one procedure 6 weeks after a laparotomy failed to find the adenoma. In addition, 20 of the 88 patients underwent other associated laparoscopic procedures at the time of their adrenalectomy. These are listed in Table 34.5. Of the 100 procedures, 12% had postoperative complications, which are listed in Table 34.6. Reoperation within 30 days of surgery was required on two occasions (2%) for evacuation of a retroperitoneal hematoma in a patient who had been anticoagulated for mitral valve prosthesis, and for postoperative acute cholecystitis in the second case. These procedures were

Table 34.2 Summary of outcome of selected series with laparoscopic adrenalectomy

Study	No. of procedures	Operative time (min.)[a]	Blood loss (mL)	Conversion rate (%)	Complication rate (%)	Length of stay (days)	Mortality (%)
Gagner [3], 1997	100	123	70	3	12	2.4	0
Gill [151], 1999	110	188	125	NR[b]	16	1.9	0
Guazzoni [156], 2001	161	160	NR	2.5	5.1	2.8	0
Salomon [155], 2001	115	118	77	0.8	15.5	4	0
Terachi [180], 1997	100	240	77	3	12	NR	0
Mancini [181], 1999	172	132	NR	7	8.7	5.8	1.2
Thompson [6], 1997	50	167	NR	4.5	6	3.1	0
Suzuki [29], 2001	118	166	92	5	12.7	4.6	0
Lezoche [30], 2002	216	100	NR	1.9	2.3	3	0.05
Bonjer [153], 2000	111	114	65	4.5	11	2	0.9
Henry [106], 2000	169	129	NR	5	7.5	5.4	0
Brunt [118], 2001	72	176	107	2.8	19	3	0
Kebebew [182], 2001	176	168	NR	0	5.1	1.7	0
Miccoli [173], 2002	137	111	NR	4.3	3.9	3.8	0

[a] Of unilateral procedures.

[b] NR, not recorded.

Table 34.3 Indications for 100 laparoscopic adrenal procedures

Indication	N
Pheochromocytoma	25
Conn's syndrome	21
Nonfunctional adenoma	20
Cushing's adenoma	13
Cushing's disease	8
Carcinoma	3
Angiomyelolipoma	2
Paraneoplastic hypercortisolism	2
Macronodular hyperplasia	2
Androgen-producing adenoma	2
Others	2

Table 34.4 Indications for bilateral laparoscopic adrenalectomy in 88 patients undergoing adrenalectomy

Indication	Patients (n)
Malignant pheochromocytoma	3
Benign pheochromocytoma	2
Cushing's disease	3
Bilateral adenoma	1
Bilateral macronodular hyperplasia	1

Table 34.5 Additional laparoscopic procedures performed during adrenalectomy in 88 patients

Procedure	Patients (n)
Liver biopsy	8
Cholecystectomy	6
Peri-aortic node dissection	2
Ventral hernia repair	1
CBD exploration	1
Colorectal re-anastomosis	1
Left ovarian cystectomy	1

CBD = common bile duct.

Table 34.6 Complications occurring in 100 laparoscopic adrenalectomy/biopsies

Type of complication	N
Postoperative	
Deep venous thrombosis	3
Hematomas	2
Anemia	2
Subdural hematoma	1
Urinary tract infection	1
Colonic pseudo–obstruction	1
Pulmonary edema	1
Acute cholecystitis	1

accomplished laparoscopically with uneventful recovery thereafter. There have been no wound complications. There was no mortality. Injury to structures in the area of dissection is possible (transabdominally or retroperitoneally), adjacent to the adrenals, including the kidney, colon, tail of the pancreas, and stomach on the left side. On the right side, the liver and duodenum are at risk. Because both adrenals are located in close proximity to major blood vessels (the hilum of kidneys and the vena cava), massive bleeding is a potentially disastrous complication. Furthermore, dissection high in the abdomen could result in diaphragmatic injury, leading to potential tension pneumothorax. Conversion to hand-assisted or open adrenalectomy has been published by the San Francisco group to be around 3%. In three cases, the tumor was too adherent to surrounding structures to be resected laparoscopically; in another three cases, the tumor was found to have malignant features during laparoscopy, and the operation was converted to achieve proper resection margins. In two patients, the tumors were too large (15 and 16 cm, respectively) to be safely removed laparoscopically. There were no cases in which conversion was required emergently for bleeding [102]. National trends in the last decade seem to orient toward higher complication rates, perhaps due to inexperienced surgeons doing laparoscopic adrenalectomies [103]. A multi-institutional study by Terachi et al. from Japan has evaluated 370 patients who underwent laparoscopic adrenalectomy [104]. There was no mortality. Overall complications developed in 57 patients (15%), including intraoperative in 33 patients (9%) and postoperative in 24 patients (6%). Conversion to open surgery was necessary in 13 cases (3.5%). The 33 intraoperative complications involved vascular injury in 22 patients (5.9%) and visceral injury in 11 patients (3%). The 22 vascular injuries involved the vena cava in 2 patients, renal vein in 2 patients, adrenal vein in 4 patients, other adrenal vessels in 11 patients, and other vessels in 3 additional patients. The 11 visceral injuries included the liver in 4 patients, spleen in 3, pancreas in 2, gallbladder in 1, and adrenal gland in 1. The 24 postoperative complications involved bleeding in 6 patients, wound infection in 4, atelectasis in 3, ileus in 2, pneumothorax in 1, and other in 8. Most complications were minor and treated laparoscopically. Age, open surgery, preoperative anemia, American Society of Anesthesiologists score, and prolonged operative time are associated with an increased need for blood transfusions in laparoscopic and open adrenalectomy. Intraoperative transfusion was independently and incrementally associated with significant morbidity and mortality after laparoscopic and open adrenalectomy [105].

Henry et al. reported the complications of laparoscopic adrenalectomy in 169 consecutive procedures [106]. There was no mortality. Twelve patients (7.5%) had significant complications: three peritoneal hematomas requiring (in two cases) laparotomy and (in one case) transfusion, one parietal hematoma, three intraoperative bleeding episodes without need for transfusion, one partial infarction of the spleen, one pneumothorax, one tumor extraction, and two venous thrombosis. Another large multi-institutional study from France [107] reported a similar complication rate of 7.7% occurring in 10 patients out of 130 cases of laparoscopic adrenalectomy. Interestingly, neither this study nor others [104,108–111] have found significant differences between transperitoneal and retroperitoneal approaches, except for the risk of the intraperitoneal visceral injury.

Interestingly, 25% of the pathologies in our series were pheochromocytomas. These tumors were larger than in patients with other diseases: 6.3 cm versus 3.9 cm ($p < 0.05$). In addition, operative time was longer: 2.5 hours versus 1.8 hours ($p < 0.05$). During the removal of these tumors, hypertension occurred in 56% of patients and hypotension in 52%. Moreover, almost 60% (7/12) of our postoperative complications were observed in this subset. Associated MEN-2A syndrome was identified in six patients, and MEN-2B in two patients. Several studies have addressed the issue of hemodynamic changes during laparoscopic adrenalectomy for pheochromocytoma compared with open surgery [112–114]. The laparoscopic approach has resulted in less [114] or comparable [112,113] hemodynamic changes compared to traditional open surgery, although patients who underwent laparoscopy had a more rapid postoperative recovery. The retroperitoneal approach seems to offer no advantage over the intraperitoneal approach [115], and carbon dioxide pneumoperitoneum is well tolerated in this subset of patients [113]. In a literature review of large series on more than 300 laparoscopic adrenalectomies exclusively for pheochromocytoma, no mortality has been reported to date [49,114,116–127]. These cases included familial multiple endocrine hyperplasia syndromes, bilateral pheochromocytoma, and extra-adrenal pheochromocytoma. Both transperitoneal and extraperitoneal approaches were used. Although earlier experience was associated with more blood loss, longer operative time, and higher complication rate compared with other pathologies [116,117], the more recent large series demonstrated no significant difference. The occurrence of hypertension postoperatively is rare, and in fact, cure of hypertension was achieved in almost all patients. With regard to the functional outcome in other hormonally active tumors, during our follow-up period (range 1–44 months), patients appear to have responded well to laparoscopic adrenalectomy. Two have been found to have renovascular hypertension, and none have had hormonal recurrence. The renal arteriograms showed no stenosis and, in addition, excluded the possibility of superior arteriolar renal occlusions by metal clips. One patient operated upon for Cushing's disease who had a partial response to ACTH stimulation, however, was still having serum cortisone levels below the normal range by the end of the follow-up period. Other authors [118,128–131] have uniformly reported excellent results comparable to those of open surgery. The Mayo Clinic group reported bilateral laparoscopic adrenalectomy in 19 patients with ACTH-dependent Cushing's syndrome in whom the ACTH-secreting neoplasm could not be removed [128]. All patients experienced resolution of the signs and symptoms of Cushing's syndrome, as well as weight loss, improved glucose tolerance, and improved

control of blood pressure. No residual cortisol secretion was detected. Others reported similar success rates in more than 100 cases with Cushing's disease and syndrome [41,43,46]. Rossi et al. [129] reported the effectiveness of laparoscopic adrenalectomy in 30 patients with primary hyperaldosteronism. Twenty-nine of 30 (95%) patients were rendered normokalemic, and persisting hypertension was present in 10 of 30 (33%) patients. In these patients, the hypertension was easily controlled medically. Duration of the hypertension before surgery was a significant risk factor for persistent hypertension. Several other articles specifically focusing on laparoscopic adrenalectomy for aldosteronoma revealed that hypertension was cured or significantly improved in greater than 90% of patients [130,132,133]. In a recent study by Brunt et al. [118], involving 72 patients with hormonally active adrenal tumors, laparoscopic adrenalectomy resulted in an excellent clinical outcome. Resolution of clinical and biochemical signs was accomplished in 34 of 34 patients with pheochromocytoma, 25 of 26 patients with aldosteronomas, 5 of 5 patients with cortisol-producing adenomas, and 3 of 3 patients with ACTH-dependent Cushing's syndrome. Two patients with MEN-2 had contralateral pheochromocytomas removed 4 and 5 years after the initial surgery. Surprisingly, persistent hypertension necessitating medications was present in 72% of patients with aldosteronomas, although 92% of these patients had significantly improved blood pressure control after surgery. Recurrent hypokalemia developed in one patient (4%) with a cortical nodule in the contralateral adrenal. The authors concluded that the clinical and biochemical cure rates are comparable to those of open adrenalectomy during long-term follow-up. Since more complications are encountered with pheochromocytoma removal, it makes sense for the novice laparoscopic surgeon to start with small aldorestrone-producing tumors [134].

MALIGNANCY CONTROVERSY

During laparoscopic adrenalectomy, we have encountered in eight patients who were treated for malignant diseases, six primaries (three pheochromocytomas and three non-functioning tumors that showed microscopic features of carcinoma) and two secondaries, that had no evidence of local recurrence during our time period of follow-up (1–44 months). Laparoscopic adrenalectomy for solitary adrenal metastasis or cancer has also been investigated at a few centers, and to date, very few references are available in the literature. The experience from the Cleveland Clinic in 11 patients was reported by Heniford et al., essentially the series of my own patients that I personally did at the Cleveland Clinic between 1995 and 1998 (without including me as a coauthor) [135]. All of the tumors, except one, were due to metastatic cancer. The metastatic sources included renal cell cancer, lung cancer, colon cancer, and melanoma. The mean size of the tumors was 5.9 cm (range 1.9–12). One patient required conversion to open surgery due to local invasion of the tumor into the vena cava. At a mean follow-up of 8.3

months, there have been no port site or local recurrences. One patient has developed a new hepatic nodule, 10 of the 11 patients were alive at the time of the report, and 1 has died of extensive brain metastasis from melanoma. Valeri et al. [15], addressing the same issue in a series of eight neoplastic patients with adrenal masses, showed a 3-year survival rate of 63% (an adenoma was proved in two cases). Two other reports on laparoscopic adrenalectomy for large (>6 cm) and potentially malignant tumors were recently published and documented favorable outcome [136,137]. In the study by Henry et al. [136], out of six patients with adrenocortical carcinoma, only one patient developed liver metastasis 6 months after surgery and died. The five other patients were disease-free, with follow-up ranging from 8 to 83 months. The largest series with the longest follow-up to date was recently published by Kebebew et al. [138]. It included 23 patients who had a laparoscopic approach for suspected and unsuspected malignant adrenal tumors. Six of the patients showed primary adrenal cancers, 13 adrenal metastasis, and 2 lymphomas, and 2 cases showed no evidence of cancer. The tumor resection margin was negative on all adrenalectomies. There were three locoregional recurrences in the 6 patients with primary adrenal cancer, no port recurrences, and four distant recurrences in 13 patients with metastatic adrenal tumors. The disease-free survival was 65% at a mean follow-up time of 3.3 years (range 1–7 years). Interestingly, these results were comparable to the known results for conventional surgery [139]. It is worth mentioning that in all of these studies, no major complications occurred, conversions were required only in patients with intraoperative evidence of tumor invasion, the laparoscopic removal achieved free resection margins in all patients, and rare port site metastases were reported [140–142]. More recently, Gryn et al. [143] reported on 43 patients who underwent a total of 45 laparoscopic adrenalectomies. Positive surgical margins were found in 12 specimens (26.7%). After a median follow-up of 37 months, estimated overall survival rates were 89.5% and 51.5% at 1 and 5 years, respectively. In multivariable analysis, the only predictor of unfavorable surgical outcomes was a tumor size of >5 cm or pulmonary origin. Adrenalectomy provided better oncological outcomes in metastases from renal cell carcinoma. Most advanced laparoscopic surgeons can tackle tumors larger than 5 cm, and even 8 cm and above, without more morbidity. This may not be the case for all endocrine surgeons, but it may be for laparoscopic urologist and general surgeons [144–146]. A new meta-analysis comparing laparoscopic and open adrenalectomy for metastasis has reiterated the higher risk of peritoneal carcinomatosis with laparoscopic approaches; however, recurrences and cancer-specific mortality were not different [147].

ROLE OF LAPAROSCOPIC ULTRASONOGRAPHY

Laparoscopic ultrasonography has been used in 15 selected cases. It showed the location of the adrenal gland after an open surgery failed to find the organ; the presence of a 0.7 cm aldosteronoma, which was disputed before surgery; that no adenoma was present in two cases, necessitating only biopsy and closure rather than adrenalectomy; no vascular, extra-adrenal, or lymph node involvement in two large lesions (10 and 12 cm), which then were removed laparoscopically and found to be benign; vascular invasion in one patient with adrenal adenocarcinoma leading to conversion to open successful removal; the invasion of the periadrenal fat by one metastatic cancer that then was removed with negative margins; the right adrenal vein, which facilitated dissection and control in two operations; and bilateral hyperplasia requiring bilateral adrenalectomy. Other groups have reported similar results with the use of laparoscopic ultrasonography in adrenalectomy [148,149].

Brunt et al. [149] have utilized this modality during laparoscopic adrenalectomy in 27 patients. They concluded that laparoscopic ultrasound provided useful information to the surgeon in 11 of 28 procedures (39%) by (1) localizing the adrenal gland and tumor or guiding the dissection, (2) demonstrating that tumors of >4 cm were confined to the gland, and (3) investigating suspected pathology in other organs. The mean time for ultrasound was 10.9 minutes, and calculated hospital charges were $602. There were no intraoperative complications. Siperstein et al. [150] found that it was of extreme value in identification of small tumors in obese patients operated on with the posterior technique. Especially in patients with nodular hyperplasia, laparoscopic ultrasound enabled the complete excision of all lesions by demonstrating the absence or presence of residual tumor tissue in the adrenal bed after resection [150]. Thus, the information obtained from ultrasonography in many instances can affect the progression of the operation. It involves a simple technique, which can be easily mastered.

DISCUSSION

More than two decades after the advent of laparoscopic adrenalectomy, the worldwide accumulated experience indicates that the procedure is safe, successful, and in fact now considered a well-established and preferred treatment modality for the majority of endocrine and neoplastic disorders affecting the adrenal gland. The results of laparoscopic adrenalectomy must be compared with those of conventional open surgery. To the best of our knowledge, there are no prospective randomized studies comparing open with laparoscopic adrenalectomy, and the excellent results reported in the available retrospective comparative reports make such a study unnecessary, and possibly unethical. In our own retrospective comparative analysis [3], we have found no difference in operating time or adrenal dimensions. The estimated blood loss was 70 mL for the laparoscopic adrenalectomy versus approximately 200 mL for the open procedure. The mean hospital stay for the conventional surgery was 9 days versus less than 3 days in the laparoscopic group. The analgesia requirements and the mean time for ambulation were also significantly lower in the laparoscopic group. Other studies have reported similar outcomes [4–8,45,92–101].

The Cleveland Clinic retrospective comparison of 110 laparoscopic adrenalectomies and 100 open cases shows the superior results of the minimally invasive approach [151]. Open adrenalectomy was performed by various standard approaches. The laparoscopic group was superior in regard to mean surgical time, mean blood loss, mean narcotic analgesic requirements, mean intensive care unit admissions, mean resumption of oral fluid intake, and mean hospital stay. While intraoperative complication rates were similar, there were fewer postoperative complications in the laparoscopic group. Of special interest is the study by Thompson et al. from the Mayo Clinic [6], who compared the laparoscopic transabdominal laparoscopic approach in 50 patients and open posterior approach in 50 well-matched patients. In addition to the known reported advantages of laparoscopy, late incisional neuromuscular complications developed in 54% of the open group, including oblique muscles in 30%, chronic pain syndrome in 14%, and flank numbness in 10%. A recent meta-analysis of the English literature by Brunt [152] has compared the complications of laparoscopic with open adrenalectomy. Complications were tabulated from 50 studies of laparoscopic adrenalectomy involving 1522 patients and 48 studies of open adrenalectomy comprising 2273 patients. Among the reports, 22 compared laparoscopic and open adrenalectomy within a single institution. It was concluded that laparoscopic adrenalectomy has resulted in fewer adrenalectomy-related complications than seen historically with open adrenalectomy. Fewer wound and pulmonary complications and the reduced occurrence of incidental splenectomy are primarily responsible for this improved outcome. Finally, another variable of concern, addressed by several authors, is the cost of the procedure compared with the conventional surgery [5,6,8,93,100]. Although Thompson and coworkers [6] have demonstrated higher costs with the laparoscopic procedure, most other reports, in fact, have found no significant difference in overall cost between the two approaches. However, it should be noted that the impact of earlier return to work in patients undergoing the laparoscopic procedure has not been assessed yet, and future data will, most probably, show lower costs when this is taken into consideration. As described earlier, the technique of choice by most surgeons performing laparoscopic adrenalectomy is the transabdominal lateral approach. Several authors have successfully documented the feasibility, safety, and effectiveness of endoscopic adrenalectomy via the retroperitoneal approach in tumors smaller than 5–6 cm [27,28,30,153,154]. Since no peritoneum violation or bowel mobilization is required with this approach, it was postulated that this method would be less invasive and, consequently, be associated with better results, especially in small lesions and in obese patients [30,45].

Siperstein et al. [28], in a series of 31 patients, concluded that although more demanding, the retroperitoneal approach should be considered in patients with tumors smaller than 6 cm, bilateral tumors, or extensive previous abdominal surgery. In another large series from the Netherlands, the procedure was described in 111 consecutive cases and showed comparable results with the transabdominal approach [153].

These authors recommended the procedure for benign adrenal tumors smaller than 6 cm. Nevertheless, case history analysis has revealed no apparent difference in patient outcome, morbidity, or operative time for the two approaches to the adrenal gland [27,28,109,110,155]. Moreover, in our experience and the experience of others [156], no bowel injury or complications developed when using the transperitoneal approach. Comparison between the two techniques has, in fact, indicated no real difference for small masses, although for lesions more than 5–6 cm, the transabdominal route is considered preferable [29]. Disadvantages of the retroperitoneal approach include a lack of anatomic landmarks and a restricted working space. This combination of technical difficulties renders the retroperitoneal approach unsuitable for tumors larger than 6 cm. On the other hand, a major advantage of the transperitoneal approach is that the abdominal cavity, and particularly the liver, can be explored. In patients with pheochromocytoma, the liver can be examined by inspection and ultrasound, and suspicious lesions may be biopsied. Moreover, in our personal experience with the retroperitoneal approach, the exposure was inferior to that which an experienced surgeon can readily obtain via the transperitoneal approach to the adrenal gland. A randomized study from the Cleveland Clinic showed no differences [111]. The available data suggests that there are very few absolute contraindications for laparoscopic adrenalectomy. At the present time, we consider invasive adrenal carcinoma to be the only absolute contraindication for the laparoscopic approach, due to the possible extent and complexity of the operation required. An open technique also may be more desirable for patients with malignant pheochromocytoma when metastatic nodes are present in the periaortic chain or close to the bladder. Several authors differentiate between the biologic behavior of adrenal metastasis and primary adrenal cancer as to their suitability for the laparoscopic procedure [117,138]. Because solitary adrenal metastasis from an extra-adrenal primary is usually small and confined within the adrenal, the laparoscopic approach has considerable appeal for this specific indication [117]. Conversely, adrenal cancer is usually larger and often locally invasive. An important limitation in this regard is that adrenal imaging and even fine-needle aspiration are often insufficiently accurate to diagnose or exclude adrenal malignancy [138]. Given that no reliable and accurate preoperative diagnostic test to diagnose adrenal malignancy exists, it is difficult to determine when an open approach should be used. An initial laparoscopic approach can be used to establish the diagnosis with low morbidity, and allows curative resection in most instances [138]. Laparoscopic ultrasound is a simple and effective intraoperative technical adjunct that may be used to evaluate the nature and invasiveness of the suspected adrenal mass. Obviously, in patients who prove to have local invasion during surgery, the laparoscopic approach should be converted to an open procedure in order to allow curative wide radical resection.

Interestingly, the limited experience to date with laparoscopic adrenalectomy in malignant disease is promising, with short-term results comparable to those of conventional surgery [136,138]. Thus, it appears that a laparoscopic approach is reasonable for metastatic adrenal disease, provided the primary cancer is controlled and there is no evidence of extra-adrenal disease. Similarly, for primary neoplasms, if complete resection is technically feasible, and there is no evidence of local invasion, an initial laparoscopic approach is an acceptable option in experienced hands at selected centers [117,136,138]. The maximal acceptable size of lesion appropriate for laparoscopic adrenalectomy is another unsettled issue. Although size *per se* is not a definite contraindication, laparoscopy is not advisable in masses larger than 12–14 cm, because of the increased incidence of malignancy and the technical difficulties associated with their removal. The largest lesion that we have resected was 14 cm, but such a mass makes the dissection difficult and is time-consuming. The exposure also is problematic because of the limited space available in this area. Frequently, large masses have unusual and numerous retroperitoneal feeding vessels that require tedious and lengthy dissection. Only those surgeons with extensive laparoscopic experience should attempt resection of larger adrenal masses. Generally, the indications and contraindications for laparoscopic adrenalectomy, including the maximal size limit and other issues, are currently dictated largely by the experience of the individual laparoscopic surgeon. Management recommendations regarding an incidental adrenal mass are still a matter of controversy. Although generally adrenocortical carcinomas are seen in masses larger than 6 cm, reports are available of incidentally detected cancer in masses of 3–5 cm and even smaller [117,157]. Another confounding factor is the fact that computed tomography might be associated with 20%–40% underestimation of adrenal tumor size compared with the actual size on histopathology [157]. Definite indications for adrenalectomy include sizes larger than 4 cm, hormonally active lesions, suspicious mass characteristics based on imaging studies, and a documented increase in size. In light of the above-mentioned facts and the excellent results of the laparoscopic procedure, we and others [117] propose that laparoscopic adrenalectomy is the preferred management for young and low-operative-risk patients with 3–5 cm adrenal masses. Another argument against the watchful conservative policy in such cases is the observation that most adrenal nodules increase in size with age [117], and the annual need for imaging and biochemical testing throughout the patient's life. Moreover, the patient will be spared the anxiety, expense, and time lost from repeated follow-up appointments and the associated studies needed. At present, we believe it is beyond debate that this minimally invasive technique has become the procedure of choice for hyperaldosteronism [99,129,130], Cushing's syndrome and disease [3,41,43,46,47,128,133], and pheochromocytoma [39,49,114,116,119,120,124]. Bilateral laparoscopic adrenalectomy appears to be safe and effective in patients with pituitary-dependent Cushing's syndrome after failed transsphenoidal surgery and in cases with ectopic ACTH syndrome when the primary tumor cannot be identified or removed [128]. It is now obvious that laparoscopic

resection of pheochromocytomas can be accomplished safely despite frequent episodes of hemodynamic variability equal to those of historical open control subjects. The expedient recovery, fewer postoperative complications, and lack of endocrinopathy recurrence make this approach the procedure of choice for the management of pheochromocytoma [119,123]. In addition, a recent publication by Brunt et al. [118] has reported favorable results in cases of unilateral and bilateral familial pheochromocytoma (patients with MEN-2A, MEN-2B, Von Hippel–Lindau, and neurofibromatosis type 1). Another large series from Germany [121] has documented the successful outcome of the endoscopic approach in 61 chromaffin neoplasms (118 pheochromocytomas and 9 paragangliomas). The patient population included a wide spectrum of this disease: unilateral, hereditary, bilateral, recurrent, and multiple tumors. Interestingly, in patients with bilateral disease, partial bilateral adrenalectomy was performed and achieved preservation of the adrenocortical function in 86% of cases, without evidence of recurrence after 3 years of follow-up. Thus, in patients with hormonally active tumors of the adrenal, the procedure has proved feasible and safe and offers all the advantages of minimally invasive surgery. Additionally, it resulted in an excellent functional outcome and was associated with clinical and biochemical cure rates comparable to those of open surgery during long-term follow-up [3,118,119,121,123,128–130,158].

Recently, newer advances and innovations in the field of laparoscopic adrenalectomy have been introduced. Outpatient laparoscopic adrenalectomy has been performed in selected low-risk patients with small adrenal tumors (mainly hyperaldosteronism and excluding pheochromocytoma), with satisfactory results [131,159,160]. To further minimize the morbidity of conventional laparoscopic procedures, the needlescopic technique, utilizing smaller ports, was reported by several groups [159,161,162]. The limited experience to date with a small number of patients showed that the procedure is feasible; it resulted in improved wound cosmesis, and a trend toward decreased postoperative pain and hospital stay was observed, without prolonging operative time [159]. The continued technological advances, offering more effective 2 mm instruments, have the potential to convince more reluctant surgeons to embark on this new technique. Nevertheless, randomized prospective trials comparing needlescopic with conventional laparoscopy are still needed to validate these favorable initial results. Laparoscopic adrenal-sparing surgery in selected patients with bilateral pheochromocytoma and well-circumscribed bilateral cortisol or aldosterone-producing adenomas [53,125,163–167] was reported. This adrenal-sparing approach may be valuable in those who would otherwise require lifelong adrenal replacement therapy after complete adrenal gland extirpation. It was also reported in cases of unilateral aldosterone-producing adenomas [167]. Our limited experience [53] and that of others [163–168] confirm the technical feasibility and safety of laparoscopic partial adrenalectomy. It should be noted that recurrence rates in patients with bilateral pheochromocytomas in MEN syndromes approached 20% [53,166]. For this reason, it is recommended to avoid adrenal-saving surgery in these instances. Intraoperative ultrasound should be available if adrenal-sparing surgery is planned since it is not possible to rely solely on the direct laparoscopic view. Whenever a clear differentiation between tumor and normal parenchyma is impossible intraoperatively, total adrenalectomy becomes unavoidable. Total adrenalectomy is also undisputed in cases of suspected malignancy. There have been no studies in which failure to preserve adrenal function was clearly associated with main vein ligation; however, every attempt should be made to maintain the main vein during adrenal-sparing surgery. In the case of severe hypertension during surgery for pheochromocytoma, it has been suggested to temporarily occlude the vein with a laparoscopic bulldog clamp [125]. Due to the possibility of preserving a better cortical physiologic response to stress stimulation, even in cases of unilateral partial resections, adrenal-sparing surgery may represent a valuable alternative to total adrenalectomy for selected indications. However, more data from large prospective series with long-term follow-up is required before drawing definite conclusions. Another technical advance, further extending the scope of minimally invasive adrenal surgery, is the recent investigation of the thoracoscopic transdiaphragmatic approach to the adrenal gland [169]. Additional novel approaches under investigation are adrenal cryoablation [170] and robotic laparoscopic adrenalectomy [171,172]. Finally, two recent publications have addressed another interesting issue: whether the widespread introduction of laparoscopic adrenalectomy has broadened the indications of the surgical approach to adrenal lesions and changed the pattern of referral [173,174]. It has been found that the introduction of laparoscopic adrenalectomy has resulted in an increase in the number of patients referred, and consequently, more adrenalectomies are performed. While one study showed that the criteria for patient selection did not change, but more patients with adrenal metastasis and incidentalomas were operated on laparoscopically [173], the other study indicated that this was due to an increased number of cases with hyperaldosteronism and pheochromocytoma [174]. In this study, however, there was no change in the number of operations for incidentalomas and metastasis [174].

CONCLUSION

After two decades of worldwide experience, laparoscopic adrenalectomy has successfully achieved maturity [175]. Based on our experience [175], and that of others [176,177], laparoscopic adrenalectomy is a well-established technique and is currently the treatment of choice for benign functioning and nonfunctioning neoplasms of the adrenal gland. Although other laparoscopic approaches are feasible, they have their limitations and offer no clear advantage over the lateral transabdominal approach, the preferred technique practiced by most surgeons performing laparoscopic

adrenalectomy [178–187]. The limited experience with the procedure in malignancy shows some promise. It should be emphasized, however, that its definite role in this regard has yet to be clarified [188]. At the present time, invasive adrenocortical carcinoma and metastatic pheochromocytoma to periaortic nodes are the only absolute contraindications [189,190]. Needless to say, only experienced laparoscopic surgeons should attempt laparoscopic resection of large masses, and generally, the minimally invasive technique is not advisable for lesions greater than 12–14 cm.

REFERENCES

1. Gagner M, Lacroix A, Bolte E. Laparoscopic adrenalectomy in Cushing's syndrome and pheochromocytoma. N Engl J Med 1992;327:1003.
2. Gagner M, Lacroix A, Prinz RA et al. Early experience with laparoscopic approach for adrenalectomy. Surgery 1993;114:1120–5.
3. Gagner M, Pomp A, Heniford BT et al. Laparoscopic adrenalectomy. Lessons learned from 100 consecutive procedures. Ann Surg 1997;226:238–47.
4. Prinz RA. A comparison of laparoscopic and open adrenalectomies. Arch Surg 1995;130:489–94.
5. Brunt LM, Doherty GM, Norton JA et al. Laparoscopic adrenalectomy compared to open adrenalectomy for benign adrenal neoplasms. J Am Coll Surg 1996;183:1–10.
6. Thompson GB, Grant CS, van Heerden JA et al. Laparoscopic versus open posterior adrenalectomy: A case-control study of 100 patients. Surgery 1997;122:1132–6.
7. Dudley NE, Harrison BJ. Comparison of open posterior versus transperitoneal laparoscopic adrenalectomy. Br J Surg 1999;86:656–60.
8. Imai T, Kikumori T, Ohiwa M. A case-controlled study of laparoscopic compared with open lateral adrenalectomy. Am J Surg 1999;178:50–4.
9. Park HS, Roman SA, Sosa JA. Outcomes from 3144 adrenalectomies in the United States: Which matters more, surgeon volume or specialty? Arch Surg 2009;144(11):1060–7.
10. Mcleod MK. Complications following adrenal surgery. J Natl Med Assoc 1991;83:161.
11. Lee J, El-Tamer M, Schifftner T et al. Open and laparoscopic adrenalectomy: Analysis of the National Surgical Quality Improvement Program. J Am Coll Surg 2008;206(5):953–9.
12. Eichhorn-Wharry LI, Talpos GB, Rubinfeld I. Laparoscopic versus open adrenalectomy: Another look at outcome using the Clavien classification system. Surgery 2012;152(6):1090–5.
13. Wanaka T, Arai M, Ito M et al. Surgical treatment for abdominal neuroblastoma in the laparoscopic era. Surg Endosc 2001;15:751–4.
14. Castilho LN, Castillo OA, Denes FT et al. Laparoscopic adrenal surgery in children. J Urol 2002;168:221–4.

15. Valeri A, Borrelli A, Presenti L et al. Adrenal masses in neoplastic patients: The role of laparoscopic procedure. *Surg Endosc* 2001;15:90–3.

16. Skarsgard ED, Albanese CT. The safety and efficacy of laparoscopic adrenalectomy in children. *Arch Surg* 2005;140(9):905–8; discussion 909.

17. Pampaloni E, Valeri A, Mattei R et al. Initial experience with laparoscopic adrenal surgery in children: Is endoscopic surgery recommended and safe for the treatment of adrenocortical neoplasms? *Pediatr Med Chir* 2004;26(6):450–9.

18. Strong VE, D'Angelica M, Tang L et al. Laparoscopic adrenalectomy for isolated adrenal metastasis. *Ann Surg Oncol* 2007;14(12):3392–400.

19. Saunders BD, Wainess RM, Dimick JB, Upchurch GR, Doherty GM, Gauger PG. Trends in utilization of adrenalectomy in the United States: Have indications changed? *World J Surg* 2004;28(11):1169–75.

20. Gallagher SF, Wahi M, Haines KL et al. Trends in adrenalectomy rates, indications, and physician volume: A statewide analysis of 1816 adrenalectomies. *Surgery* 2007;142(6):1011–21.

21. Mazeh H, Froyshteter AB, Wang TS et al. Is previous same quadrant surgery a contraindication to laparoscopic adrenalectomy? *Surgery* 2012;152(6):1211–7.

22. Kazaure HS, Roman SA, Sosa JA. Obesity is a predictor of morbidity in 1,629 patients who underwent adrenalectomy. *World J Surg* 2011;35(6):1287–95.

23. Brix D, Allolio B, Fenske W et al. German Adrenocortical Carcinoma Registry Group. Laparoscopic versus open adrenalectomy for adrenocortical carcinoma: Surgical and oncologic outcome in 152 patients. *Eur Urol* 2010;58(4):609–15.

24. Constantinides VA, Christakis I, Touska P, Palazzo FF. Systematic review and meta-analysis of retroperitoneoscopic versus laparoscopic adrenalectomy. *Br J Surg* 2012;99(12):1639–48.

25. Kiriakopoulos A, Tsakayannis D, Linos D. Surgical management of adrenal myelolipoma: A series of 10 patients and review of the literature. *Minerva Chir* 2006;61(3):241–6.

26. Horchani A, Nouira Y, Nouira K, Bedioui H, Menif E, Safta ZB. Hydatid cyst of the adrenal gland: A clinical study of six cases. *Sci World J* 2006;6:2420–5.

27. Fernandez-Cruz L, Saenz A, Taura P et al. Retroperitoneal approach in laparoscopic adrenalectomy: Is it advantageous? *Surg Endosc* 1999;13:86–90.

28. Siperstein AE, Berber E, Engle KL et al. Laparoscopic posterior adrenalectomy. Technical considerations. *Arch Surg* 2000;135:967–71.

29. Suzuki K, Kageyama S, Hirano Y et al. Comparison of 3 surgical approaches to laparoscopic adrenalectomy: A randomized, background matched analysis. *J Urol* 2001;166:437–43.

30. Lezoche E, Guerrieri M, Feliciotti F et al. Anterior, lateral and posterior approaches in endoscopic adrenalectomy. *Surg Endosc* 2002;16:96–9.

31. Gagner M, Lacroix A, Bolte E et al. Laparoscopic adrenalectomy. The importance of a flank approach in the lateral decubitus position. *Surg Endosc* 1994;8:135–8.

32. Walz MK, Alesina PF, Wenger FA et al. Posterior retroperitoneoscopic adrenalectomy—Results of 560 procedures in 520 patients. *Surgery* 2006;140(6):943–8; discussion 948–50.

33. Zhang X, Fu B, Lang B et al. Technique of anatomical retroperitoneoscopic adrenalectomy with report of 800 cases. *J Urol* 2007;177(4):1254–7.

34. Nigri G, Rosman AS, Petrucciani N et al. Meta-analysis of trials comparing laparoscopic transperitoneal and retroperitoneal adrenalectomy. *Surgery* 2013;153(1):111–9.

35. Lombardi CP, Raffaelli M, De Crea C et al. Open versus endoscopic adrenalectomy in the treatment of localized (stage I/II) adrenocortical carcinoma: Results of a multiinstitutional Italian survey. *Surgery* 2012;152(6):1158–64.

36. Scholten A, Cisco RM, Vriens MR, Shen WT, Duh QY. Variant adrenal venous anatomy in 546 laparoscopic adrenalectomies. *JAMA Surg* 2013;148(4):378–83.

37. Lezoche E, Guerrieri M, Crosta F et al. Perioperative results of 214 laparoscopic adrenalectomies by anterior transperitoneal approach. *Surg Endosc* 2008;22(2):522–6.

38. Marescaux J, Mutter D, Forbes L et al. Bilateral laparoscopic adrenalectomy. In: Gagner M, Inabnet B, eds., *Minimally Invasive Endocrine Surgery*. Philadelphia: Lippincott Williams & Wilkins, 2002:205–16.

39. Lee JE, Curley SA, Gagel RF et al. Cortical sparing adrenalectomy for patients with bilateral pheochromocytoma. *Surgery* 1996;120:1064–71.

40. Chow JT, Thompson GB, Grant CS, Farley DR, Richards ML, Young WF Jr. Bilateral laparoscopic adrenalectomy for corticotrophin-dependent Cushing's syndrome: A review of the Mayo Clinic experience. *Clin Endocrinol (Oxf)* 2008;68(4):513–9.

41. Chapuis Y, Inabnet B, Abboud B et al. Bilateral laparoscopic adrenalectomy in Cushing's syndrome. Experience in 24 patients [in French]. *Ann Chir* 1998;52:35–56.

42. Shen WT, Lee J, Kebebew E, Clark OH, Duh QY. Selective use of steroid replacement after adrenalectomy: Lessons from 331 consecutive cases. *Arch Surg* 2006;141(8):771–4.

43. Fernandez-Cruz L, Saenz A, Benarroch G. Laparoscopic unilateral and bilateral adrenalectomy for Cushing's syndrome. *Ann Surg* 1996;224:727–36.

44. Walz MK, Pietgen K, Hoermann R et al. Posterior retroperitoneoscopy as a new minimally invasive approach for adrenalectomy: Results of 30 adrenalectomies in 27 patients. *World J Surg* 1996;20:769–74.

45. Bonjer HJ, Lange JF, Kazemier G et al. Comparison of three techniques for adrenalectomy. *Br J Surg* 1997;84:679–82.

46. Lanzi R, Montorsi F, Losa M et al. Laparoscopic bilateral adrenalectomy for persistent Cushing's disease after transsphenoidal surgery. *Surgery* 1998;123:144–50.

47. Ferrer FA, MacGillivray DC, Mlachoff DC et al. Bilateral laparoscopic adrenalectomy for adrenocorticotropic dependent Cushing's syndrome. *J Urol* 1997;157:16–8.

48. Fernandez-Cruz L, Saenz A, Taura P et al. Pheochromocytoma: Laparoscopic approach with CO2 and helium pneumoperitoneum. *Endosc Surg Allied Technol* 1994;2:300–4.

49. Fernandez-Cruz L, Saenz A, Pantoja JP. Laparoscopic adrenalectomy for pheochromocytoma. In: Gagner M, Inabnet B, eds., *Minimally Invasive Endocrine Surgery*. Philadelphia: Lippincott Williams & Wilkins, 2002:235–41.

50. Giraudo G, Pantuso G, Festa F, Farinella E, Morino M. Clinical role of gasless laparoscopic adrenalectomy. *Surg Laparosc Endosc Percutan Tech* 2009;19(4):329–32.

51. Diner EK, Franks ME, Behari A, Linehan WM, Walther MM. Partial adrenalectomy: The National Cancer Institute experience. *Urology* 2005;66(1):19–23.

52. Ishidoya S, Ito A, Sakai K et al. Laparoscopic partial versus total adrenalectomy for aldosterone producing adenoma. *J Urol* 2005;174(1):40–3.

53. Rubino F, Bellantone R, Gagner M. Laparoscopic adrenal-sparing surgery. In: Gagner M, Inabnet B, eds., *Minimally Invasive Endocrine Surgery*. Philadelphia: Lippincott Williams & Wilkinson, 2002:217–25.

54. Liao CH, Chueh SC, Wu KD, Hsieh MH, Chen J. Laparoscopic partial adrenalectomy for aldosterone-producing adenomas with needlescopic instruments. *Urology* 2006;68(3):663–7.

55. Liao CH, Lai MK, Li HY, Chen SC, Chueh SC. Laparoscopic adrenalectomy using needlescopic instruments for adrenal tumors less than 5 cm in 112 cases. *Eur Urol* 2008;54(3):640–6.

56. Hirano D, Minei S, Yamaguchi K et al. Retroperitoneoscopic adrenalectomy for adrenal tumors via a single large port. *J Endourol* 2005;19(7):788–92.

57. Castellucci SA, Curcillo PG, Ginsberg PC, Saba SC, Jaffe JS, Harmon JD. Single port access adrenalectomy. *J Endourol* 2008;22(8):1573–6.

58. Walz MK, Groeben H, Alesina PF. Single-access retroperitoneoscopic adrenalectomy (SARA) versus conventional retroperitoneoscopic adrenalectomy (CORA): A case-control study. *World J Surg* 2010;34(6):1386–90.

59. Colon MJ, Lemasters P, Newell P, Divino C, Weber KJ, Chin EH. Laparoscopic single site adrenalectomy using a conventional laparoscope and instrumentation. *JSLS* 2011;15(2):236–8.

60. Miyajima A, Maeda T, Hasegawa M et al. Transumbilical laparo-endoscopic single site surgery for adrenal cortical adenoma inducing primary aldosteronism: Initial experience. *BMC Res Notes* 2011;4:364.

61. Goo TT, Agarwal A, Goel R, Tan CT, Lomanto D, Cheah WK. Single-port access adrenalectomy: Our initial experience. *J Laparoendosc Adv Surg Tech A* 2011;21(9):815–9.

62. Kwak HN, Kim JH, Yun JS et al. Conventional laparoscopic adrenalectomy versus laparoscopic adrenalectomy through mono port. *Surg Laparosc Endosc Percutan Tech* 2011;21(6):439–42.

63. Vidal Ó, Astudillo E, Valentini M, Ginestà C, García-Valdecasas JC, Fernandez-Cruz L. Single-incision transperitoneal laparoscopic left adrenalectomy. *World J Surg* 2012;36(6):1395–9.

64. Sasaki A, Nitta H, Otsuka K et al. Laparoendoscopic single site adrenalectomy: Initial results of cosmetic satisfaction and the potential for postoperative pain reduction. *BMC Urol* 2013;13:21.

65. Wang L, Wu Z, Li M et al. Laparoendoscopic single-site adrenalectomy versus conventional laparoscopic surgery: A systematic review and meta-analysis of observational studies. *J Endourol* 2013;27(6):743–50.

66. Wang Y, He Y, Li BS et al. Laparoendoscopic single-site retroperitoneoscopic adrenalectomy versus conventional retroperitoneoscopic adrenalectomy in obese patients. *J Endourol* 2016;30(3):306–11.

67. Hora M, Ürge T, Stránský P et al. Laparoendoscopic single-site surgery adrenalectomy—Own experience and matched case-control study with standard laparoscopic adrenalectomy. *Wideochir Inne Tech Maloinwazyjne* 2014;9(4):596–602.

68. Vidal O, Astudillo E, Valentini M et al. Single-port laparoscopic left adrenalectomy (SILS): 3 years' experience of a single institution. *Surg Laparosc Endosc Percutan Tech* 2014;24(5):440–3.

69. Hu Q, Gou Y, Sun C, Xu K, Xia G, Ding Q. A systematic review and meta-analysis of current evidence comparing laparoendoscopic single-site adrenalectomy and conventional laparoscopic adrenalectomy. *J Endourol* 2013;27(6):676–83.

70. Hubens G, Ysebaert D, Vaneerdeweg W, Chapelle T, Eyskens E. Laparoscopic adrenalectomy with the aid of the AESOP 2000 robot. *Acta Chir Belg* 1999;99(3):125–7.

71. Sung GT, Gill IS. Robotic laparoscopic surgery: A comparison of the DA Vinci and Zeus systems. *Urology* 2001;58(6):893–8.

72. Del Pizzo JJ. Transabdominal laparoscopic adrenalectomy. *Curr Urol Rep* 2003;4(1):81–6.

73. Jacob BP, Gagner M. Robotics and general surgery. *Surg Clin North Am* 2003;83(6):1405–19.

74. Morino M, Benincà G, Giraudo G, Del Genio GM, Rebecchi F, Garrone C: Robot-assisted vs laparoscopic adrenalectomy: A prospective randomized controlled trial. *Surg Endosc* 2004;18(12):1742–6.

75. Winter JM, Talamini MA, Stanfield CL et al. Thirty robotic adrenalectomies: A single institution's experience. *Surg Endosc* 2006;20(1):119–24.

76. Wu JC, Wu HS, Lin MS, Chou DA, Huang MH. Comparison of robot-assisted laparoscopic adrenalectomy with traditional laparoscopic adrenalectomy–1 year follow-up. *Surg Endosc* 2008;22(2):463–6.

77. Brunaud L, Bresler L, Ayav A et al. Robotic-assisted adrenalectomy: What advantages compared to lateral transperitoneal laparoscopic adrenalectomy? *Am J Surg* 2008;195(4):433–8.

78. Brunaud L, Ayav A, Zarnegar R et al. Prospective evaluation of 100 robotic-assisted unilateral adrenalectomies. *Surgery* 2008;144(6):995–1001.

79. Karabulut K, Agcaoglu O, Aliyev S, Siperstein A, Berber E. Comparison of intraoperative time use and perioperative outcomes for robotic versus laparoscopic adrenalectomy. *Surgery* 2012;151(4):537–42.

80. Chai YJ, Kwon H, Yu HW et al. Systematic review of surgical approaches for adrenal tumors: Lateral transperitoneal versus posterior retroperitoneal and laparoscopic versus robotic adrenalectomy. *Int J Endocrinol* 2014;2014:918346.

81. Boris RS, Gupta G, Linehan WM, Pinto PA, Bratslavsky G. Robot-assisted laparoscopic partial adrenalectomy: Initial experience. *Urology* 2011;77(4):775–80.

82. Aksoy E, Taskin HE, Aliyev S, Mitchell J, Siperstein A, Berber E. Robotic versus laparoscopic adrenalectomy in obese patients. *Surg Endosc* 2013;27(4):1233–6.

83. Manny TB, Pompeo AS, Hemal AK. Robotic partial adrenalectomy using indocyanine green dye with near-infrared imaging: The initial clinical experience. *Urology* 2013;82(3):738–42.

84. Lee GS, Arghami A, Dy BM, McKenzie TJ, Thompson GB, Richards ML. Robotic single-site adrenalectomy. *Surg Endosc* 2016;30(8):3351–6.

85. Choi KH, Ham WS, Rha KH et al. Laparoendoscopic single-site surgeries: A single-center experience of 171 consecutive cases. *Korean J Urol* 2011;52(1):31–8.

86. Proceedings of the III Simposio Internacional de Videocirurgia Avancada, Porto Alegre, Brazil, May 8–10, 2008.

87. Decarli L, Zorron R, Branco A et al. Natural orifice translumenal endoscopic surgery (NOTES) transvaginal cholecystectomy in a morbidly obese patient. *Obes Surg* 2008;18(7):886–9.

88. Fritscher-Ravens A, Ghanbari A, Cuming T et al. Comparative study of NOTES alone vs. EUS-guided NOTES procedures. *Endoscopy* 2008;40(11):925–30.

89. Perretta S, Allemann P, Asakuma M, Dallemagne B, Marescaux J. Adrenalectomy using natural orifice translumenal endoscopic surgery (NOTES): A transvaginal retroperitoneal approach. *Surg Endosc* 2009;23(6):1390.

90. Zou X, Zhang G, Xiao R et al. Transvaginal natural orifice transluminal endoscopic surgery (NOTES)-assisted laparoscopic adrenalectomy: First clinical experience. *Surg Endosc* 2011;25(12):3767–72.

91. Eyraud R, Laydner H, Autorino R et al. Robot-assisted transrectal hybrid natural orifice translumenal endoscopic surgery nephrectomy and adrenalectomy: Initial investigation in a cadaver model. *Urology* 2013;81(5):1090–4.

92. Ishikawa T, Sowa M, Nagayama M, Nishiguchi Y, Yoshikawa K. Laparoscopic adrenalectomy: Comparison with the conventional approach. *Surg Lap Endosc* 1997;7:275–80.

93. Jacobs JK, Goldstein RE, Geer RJ. Laparoscopic adrenalectomy: A new standard of care. *Ann Surg* 1997;225:495–502.

94. Linos DA, Stylopoulos N, Boukis M et al. Anterior, posterior or laparoscopic approach for the management of adrenal disease? *Am J Surg* 1997;173:120–5.

95. MacGillivray DC, Shichman SJ, Ferrer FA et al. A comparison of open vs laparoscopic adrenalectomy. *Surg Endosc* 1996;10:987–90.

96. Nash PA, Leibovitch I, Donohue JP. Adrenalectomy via the dorsal approach: A benchmark for laparoscopic adrenalectomy. *J Urol* 1995;154:1652–4.

97. Staren ED, Prinz RA. Adrenalectomy in the era of laparoscopy. *Surgery* 1996;120:706–9.

98. Vargas HI, Kavoussi LR, Bartlett DL et al. Laparoscopic adrenalectomy: A new standard of care. *Urology* 1997;49:673–8.

99. Shen WT, Lim RC, Siperstein AE et al. Laparoscopic vs open adrenalectomy for the treatment of primary hyperaldosteronism. *Arch Surg* 1999;134:628–32.

100. Ortega J, Sala C, Garcia S et al. Cost-effectiveness of laparoscopic vs open adrenalectomy: Small savings in an expensive process. *J Laparoendosc Adv Surg Tech* 2002;12:1–5.

101. Ichikawa T, Mikami K, Komiya K et al. Laparoscopic adrenalectomy for functioning adrenal tumors: Clinical experience with 38 cases and comparison with open adrenalectomy. *Biomed Pharmacother* 2000;54(Suppl):178–82.

102. Shen WT, Kebebew E, Clark OH, Duh QY. Reasons for conversion from laparoscopic to open or hand-assisted adrenalectomy: Review of 261 laparoscopic adrenalectomies from 1993 to 2003. *World J Surg* 2004;28(11):1176–9.

103. Murphy MM, Witkowski ER, Ng SC et al. Trends in adrenalectomy: A recent national review. *Surg Endosc* 2010;24(10):2518–26.

104. Terachi T, Yoshida O, Matsuda T et al. Complications of laparoscopic and retroperitoneoscopic adrenalectomies in 370 cases in Japan: A multi-institutional study. *Bimed Phamacother* 2000;54(Suppl 1):211–4.

105. Venkat R, Guerrero MA. Risk factors and outcomes of blood transfusions in adrenalectomy. *J Surg Res* 2015;199(2):505–11.

106. Henry JF, Defechereux T, Raffaelli M et al. Complications of laparoscopic adrenalectomy: Results of 169 consecutive procedures. *World J Surg* 2000;24:1342–6.

107. Soulie M, Salomon L, Seguin P et al. Multi-institutional study of complications in 1085 laparoscopic urologic procedures. *Urology* 2001;58:899–903.

108. Suzuki K, Ushiyama T, Ihara H et al. Complications of laparoscopic adrenalectomy in 75 patients treated by the same surgeon. *Eur Urol* 1999;36:40–7.

109. Yoneda K, Shiba E, Watanabi T et al. Laparoscopic adrenalectomy: Lateral transabdominal approach vs. posterior retroperitoneal approach. *Biomed Pharmacother* 2000;54(Suppl 1):215–9.

110. Takeda M. Laparoscopic adrenalectomy: Transperitoneal vs. retroperitoneal approaches. *Biomed Pharmacother* 2000;54(Suppl 1):207–10.

111. Rubinstein M, Gill IS, Aron M et al. Prospective, randomized comparison of transperitoneal versus retroperitoneal laparoscopic adrenalectomy. *J Urol* 2005;174(2):442–5; discussion 445.

112. Sprung J, O'hara JF, Gill IS et al. Anesthetic aspects of laparoscopic and open adrenalectomy for pheochromocytoma. *Urology* 2000;55:339–43.

113. Inabnet B, Pitre J, Bernard D et al. Comparison of the hemodynamic parameters of open and laparoscopic adrenalectomy for pheochromocytoma. *World J Surg* 2000;24:574–8.

114. Fernandez-Cruz L, Taura P, Saenz A. Laparoscopic approach to pheochromocytoma: Hemodynamic changes and catecholamine secretion. *World J Surg* 1996;20:762–8.

115. Fernandez-Cruz L, Saenz A, Taura P et al. Retroperitoneal approach in laparoscopic adrenalectomy. *Surg Endosc* 1999;13:86–90.

116. Gagner M, Breton G, Pharand D et al. Is laparoscopic adrenalectomy indicated for pheochromocytomas? *Surgery* 1996;120:1076–80.

117. Gill IS. The case for laparoscopic adrenalectomy. *J Urol* 2001;166:429–36.

118. Brunt LM, Moley JF, Doherty GM et al. Outcome analysis in patients undergoing laparoscopic adrenalectomy for hormonally active tumors. *Surgery* 2001;130:629–34.

119. Kercher KW, Park A, Matthews BD et al. Laparoscopic adrenalectomy for pheochromocytoma. *Surg Endosc* 2002;16:100–2.

120. Brunt LM, Lairmore TC, Doherty GM et al. Adrenalectomy for familial pheochromocytoma in the laparoscopic era. *Ann Surg* 2002;235:713–20.

121. Walz MK, Peitgen K, Neumann H et al. Endoscopic treatment of solitary, bilateral, multiple and recurrent pheochromocytomas and paragangliomas. *World J Surg* 2002;26:1005–12.

122. Tanaka M, Tokuda N, Koga H et al. Laparoscopic adrenalectomy for pheochromocytoma: Comparison with open adrenalectomy and comparison of laparoscopic surgery for pheohromocytoma versus other adrenal tumors. *J Endourol* 2000;14:427–31.

123. Cheah WK, Clark OH, Horn JK et al. Laparoscopic adrenalectomy for pheochromocytoma. *World J Surg* 2002;26:1048–51.

124. Salomon L, Rabii R, Soulie M et al. Experience with retroperitoneal laparoscopic adrenalectomy for pheochromocytoma. *J Urol* 2001;165:1882–4.

125. Janetschek G, Finkenstedt G, Gasser R et al. Laparoscopic surgery for pheochromocytoma: Adrenalectomy, partial resection, excision of paragangliomas. *J Urol* 1998;160:330–4.

126. Mobius E, Nies C, Ruthmond M. Surgical treatment of pheochromocytomas. Laparoscopic or conventional? *Surg Endosc* 1999;13:35–9.

127. Col V, de Canniere L, Collard E et al. Laparoscopic adrenalectomy for pheochromocytoma: Endocrinological and surgical aspects of a new therapeutic approach. *Clin Endocrinol* 1999;50:121–5.

128. Vella A, Thompson GB, Grant CS et al. Laparoscopic adrenalectomy for adrenocorticotropin-dependent Cushing's syndrome. *J Clin Endocrinol Metab* 2001;86:1596–99.

129. Rossi H, Kim A, Prinz RA. Primary hyperaldosteronism in the era of laparoscopic adrenalectomy. *Am Surg* 2002;68:253–6.

130. Miyaki, Okuyama A. Surgical management of primary aldosteronism. *Biomed Pharmacother* 2000;54(Suppl 1):146–9.

131. Edwin B, Reader I, Trondsen E et al. Outpatient laparoscopic adrenalectomy in patients with Conn's syndrome. *Surg Endosc* 2001;15:589–91.

132. Siren J, Haglund C, Huikuri K et al. Laparoscopic adrenalectomy for primary aldosteronism: Clinical experience with 12 patients. *Surg Laparosc Endosc* 1999;9:9–13.

133. Go H, Takeda M, Imai T et al. Laparoscopic surgery for Cushing's syndrome: Comparison with primary aldosteronism. *Surgery* 1995;117:11–7.

134. Kim AW, Quiros RM, Maxhimer JB, El-Ganzouri AR, Prinz RA. Outcome of laparoscopic adrenalectomy for pheochromocytomas vs aldosteronomas. *Arch Surg* 2004;139(5):526–9.

135. Heniford BT, Arca MJ, Walsh RM et al. Laparoscopic adrenalectomy for cancer. *Semin Surg Oncol* 1999;16:293–306.

136. Henry JF, Sebag F, Iacobone M et al. Results of laparoscopic adrenalectomy for large and potentially malignant tumors. *World J Surg* 2002;26:1043–7.

137. MacGillivray DC, Whalen GF, Malchoff CD et al. Laparoscopic resection of large adrenal tumors. *Ann Surg Oncol* 2002;9:480–5.

138. Kebebew E, Siperstein AE, Clark OH et al. Results of laparoscopic adrenalectomy for suspected and unsuspected malignant adrenal neoplasms. *Arch Surg* 2002;137:948–53.

139. Vasilopoulou-Sellin R, Schultz PN. Adrenocortical carcinoma: Clinical outcome at the end of the twentieth century. *Cancer* 2001;92:1113–21.

140. Saraiva P, Rodrigues H, Rodrigues P. Port site recurrence after laparoscopic adrenalectomy for metastatic melanoma. *Int Braz J Urol* 2003;29(6):520–1.

141. Weyhe D, Belyaev O, Skawran S, Müller C, Bauer KH. A case of port-site recurrence after laparoscopic adrenalectomy for solitary adrenal metastasis. *Surg Laparosc Endosc Percutan Tech* 2007;17(3):218–20.

142. Marangos IP, Kazaryan AM, Rosseland AR et al. Should we use laparoscopic adrenalectomy for metastases? Scandinavian multicenter study. *J Surg Oncol* 2009;100(1):43–7.

143. Gryn A, Peyronnet B, Manunta A et al. Patient selection for laparoscopic excision of adrenal metastases: A multicenter cohort study. *Int J Surg* 2015;24(Pt A):75–80.

144. Feo CV, Portinari M, Maestroni U et al. Applicability of laparoscopic approach to the resection of large adrenal tumours: A retrospective cohort study on 200 patients. *Surg Endosc* 2016;30(8):3532–40.

145. Aksakal N, Agcaoglu O, Barbaros U et al. Safety and feasibility of laparoscopic adrenalectomy: What is the role of tumour size? A single institution experience. *J Minim Access Surg* 2015;11(3):184–6.

146. Palazzo FF, Sebag F, Sierra M, Ippolito G, Souteyrand P, Henry JF. Long-term outcome following laparoscopic adrenalectomy for large solid adrenal cortex tumors. *World J Surg* 2006;30(5):893–8.

147. Autorino R, Bove P, De Sio M et al. Open versus laparoscopic adrenalectomy for adrenocortical carcinoma: A meta-analysis of surgical and oncological outcomes. *Ann Surg Oncol* 2016;23(4):195–202.

148. Heniford BT, Iannitti DA, Hale J et al. The role of intraoperative ultrasonography during laparoscopic adrenalectomy. *Surgery* 1997;122:1068–73.

149. Brunt LM, Bennett HF, Teefey SA et al. Laparoscopic ultrasound imaging of adrenal tumors during laparoscopic adrenalectomy. *Am J Surg* 1999;178:490–5.

150. Siperstein AE, Berber E. Laparoscopic ultrasonography of the adrenal glands. In: Gagner M, Inabnet B, eds., *Minimally Invasive Endocrine Surgery*. Philadelphia: Lippincott Williams & Wilkinson, 2002:175–183.

151. Gill IS, Schweizer D, Nelson D. Laparoscopic versus open adrenalectomy in 210 patients: Cleveland Clinic experience with 210 cases. *J Urol Suppl* 1999;161:21.

152. Brunt LM. The positive impact of laparoscopic adrenalectomy on complications of adrenal surgery. *Endosc Surg* 2002;16:252–7.

153. Bonjer HJ, Sorm V, Berends FJ et al. Endoscopic retroperitoneal adrenalectomy: Lessons learned from 111 consecutive cases. *Ann Surg* 2000;232:796–803.

154. Ting AC, Lo CY, Lo CM. Posterior or laparoscopic approach for adrenalectomy. *Am J Surg* 1998;175:488–90.

155. Salomon L, Soulie M, Mouly F et al. Experience with retroperitoneal laparoscopic adrenalectomy in 115 procedures. *J Urol* 2001;166:38–41.

156. Guazzoni G, Cestari A, Montorsi F et al. Eight experiences with transperitoneal laparoscopic adrenal surgery. *J Urol* 2001;166:820–4.

157. Linos DA, Stylopoulos N. How accurate is computed tomography in predicting the real size of adrenal tumors? A retrospective study. *Arch Surg* 1997;132:740–3.

158. Goers TA, Abdo M, Moley JF, Matthews BD, Quasebarth M, Brunt LM. Outcomes of resection of extra-adrenal pheochromocytomas/paragangliomas in the laparoscopic era: A comparison with adrenal pheochromocytoma. *Surg Endosc* 2013;27(2):428–33.

159. Gill IS, Soble JJ, Sung GT et al. Needlescopic adrenalectomy: The initial series. Comparison with conventional laparoscopic adrenalectomy. *Urology* 1998;52:180–6.

160. Mohammad WM, Frost I, Moonje V. Outpatient laparoscopic adrenalectomy: A Canadian experience. *Surg Laparosc Endosc Percutan Tech* 2009;19(4):336–7.

161. Chueh SC, Chen J, Chen SC et al. Clipless laparoscopic adrenalectomy with needlescopic instruments. *J Urol* 2002;167:39–42.

162. Mamazza J, Schlachta CM, Seshadri PA et al. Needlescopic surgery. A logical evolution from conventional laparoscopic surgery. *Surg Endosc* 2001;15:1208–12.

163. Neumann HPH, Reincke M, Bender BU et al. Preserved adrenocortical function after laparoscopic bilateral adrenal sparing surgery for hereditary pheochromocytoma. *J Clin Endocrinol Metab* 1999;84:2608–10.

164. Walz MK, Peitgen K, Saller B et al. Subtotal adrenalectomy by the posterior retroperitoneoscopic approach. *World J Surg* 1998;22:621–7.

165. Imai T, Tanaka Y, Kikumori T et al. Laparoscopic partial adrenalectomy. *Surg Endosc* 1999;13:343–5.

166. Baghai M, Thompson GB, Young WF et al. Pheochromocytomas and paragangliomas in von Hippel–Lindau disease. *Arch Surg* 2002;137:682–9.

167. Al-Sobhi S, Peschel R, Bartsch G et al. Partial laparoscopic adrenalectomy for aldosterone-producing adenoma: Short and long-term results. *J Endourol* 2000;14:497–99.

168. Poulose BK, Holzman MD, Lao OB, Grogan EL, Goldstein RE. Laparoscopic adrenalectomy: 100 resections with clinical long-term follow-up. *Surg Endosc* 2005;19(3):379–85.

169. Gill IS, Meraney AM, Thomas JC et al. Thoracoscopic transdiaphragmatic adrenalectomy: The initial experience. *J Urol* 2001;165:1875–81.

170. Schulsinger DA, Sosa RE, Perlmutter AA et al. Acute and chronic interstitial cryotherapy of the adrenal gland as a treatment modality. *J Endourol* 1999;13:203–99.

171. Gill IS, Sung GT, Hsu TH et al. Robotic remote laparoscopic nephrectomy and adrenalectomy: The initial experience. *J Urol* 2000;164:2082–5.

172. Young JA, Chapman WHH, Kim VB et al. Robotic-assisted adrenalectomy for adrenal incidentaloma: Case and review of the literature. *Surg Laparosc Endosc Percutan Tech* 2002;12:126–30.

173. Miccoli P, Raffaelli M, Berti P et al. Adrenal surgery before and after the introduction of laparoscopic adrenalectomy. *Br J Surg* 2002;89:779–82.

174. Sidhu S, Bambach C, Pillinger S et al. Changing pattern of adrenalectomy at a tertiary referral center 1970–2000. *ANZ J Surg* 2002;72:463–6.

175. Gumbs AA, Gagner M. Laparoscopic adrenalectomy. *Best Pract Res Clin Endocrinol Metab* 2006;20(3):483–99.

176. Ramacciato G, Paolo M, Pietromaria A et al. Ten years of laparoscopic adrenalectomy: Lesson learned from 104 procedures. *Am Surg* 2005;71(4):321–5.

177. Emeriau D, Vallee V, Tauzin-Fin P, Ballanger P. Morbidity of unilateral and bilateral laparoscopic adrenalectomy according to the indication. Report of a series of 100 consecutive cases [in French]. *Prog Urol* 2005;15(4):626–31.

178. Barresi R, Prinz RA. Laparoscopic adrenalectomy. *Arch Surg* 1999;134:212–7.

179. Gill IS, Hobart M, Schweizer D et al. Outpatient adrenalectomy. *J Urol* 2000;163:717–20.

180. Terachi T, Matsuda T, Terai A et al. Transperitoneal laparoscopic adrenalectomy: Experience in 100 cases. *J Endourol* 1997;11:361–5.

181. Mancini F, Mutter D, Peix JL et al. Experiences with adrenalectomy in 1997. Apropos of 247 cases. A multicenter prospective study of the French-speaking Association of Endocrine Surgery [in French]. *Chirurgie* 1999;124:368–74.

182. Kebebew E, Siperstein AE, Duh QY et al. Laparoscopic adrenalectomy: The optimal surgical approach. *J Laparoendosc Adv Surg Tech* 2001;11:409–13.

183. Bittner JG 4th, Gershuni VM, Matthews BD, Moley JF, Brunt LM. Risk factors affecting operative approach, conversion, and morbidity for adrenalectomy: A single-institution series of 402 patients. *Surg Endosc* 2013;27(7):2342–50.

184. Elfenbein DM, Scarborough JE, Speicher PJ, Scheri RP. Comparison of laparoscopic versus open adrenalectomy: Results from American College of Surgeons-National Surgery Quality Improvement Project. *J Surg Res* 2013;184(1):216–20.

185. Porpiglia F, Fiori C, Bertolo R et al. Mini-retroperitoneoscopic adrenalectomy: Our experience after 50 procedures. *Urology* 2014;84(3):596–601.

186. Pędziwiatr M, Wierdak M, Ostachowski M et al. Single center outcomes of laparoscopic transperitoneal lateral adrenalectomy—Lessons learned after 500 cases: A retrospective cohort study. *Int J Surg* 2015;20:88–94.

187. DeLong JC, Chakedis JM, Hosseini A, Kelly KJ, Horgan S, Bouvet M. Indocyanine green (ICG) fluorescence-guided laparoscopic adrenalectomy. *J Surg Oncol* 2015;112(6):650–3.

188. Moreno P, de la Quintana Basarrate A, Musholt TJ et al. Adrenalectomy for solid tumor metastases: Results of a multicenter European study. *Surgery* 2013;154(6):1215–22.

189. Donatini G, Caiazzo R, Do Cao C et al. Long-term survival after adrenalectomy for stage I/II adrenocortical carcinoma (ACC): A retrospective comparative cohort study of laparoscopic versus open approach. *Ann Surg Oncol* 2014;21(1):284–91.

190. Inoue S, Ikeda K, Kobayashi K, Kajiwara M, Teishima J, Matsubara A. Patient-reported satisfaction and cosmesis outcomes following laparoscopic adrenalectomy: Laparoendoscopic single-site adrenalectomy vs. conventional laparoscopic adrenalectomy. *Can Urol Assoc J* 2014;8(1–2):E20–5.

35

Techniques of adrenalectomy

MINERVA ANGELICA ROMERO ARENAS, ASHLEY STEWART, AND NANCY D. PERRIER

INTRODUCTION

Adrenal pathologies have various patterns of presentation, depending on their endocrine functional hormone excess and oncologic potential. Evaluation of the patient with disease of the adrenal gland requires a thorough understanding of physiology and proper application of conventional and molecular (isotopic) imaging and biochemical testing to guide therapy. Selecting the best approach for surgical resection of an adrenal mass requires consideration of a multitude of factors, including the size of the tumor and degree of suspicion of malignancy. Tumors greater than 6 cm in size, because of the malignant potential, and those with features worrisome for adrenocortical carcinoma (ACC), should be resected by an open *en bloc* approach [1–3]. Other factors influencing the therapeutic approach include laterality of the disease, presence of multiple or extra-adrenal tumors, additional intra-abdominal disease, distant metastases, history of prior abdominal surgery, patient's body habitus, and the operating surgeon's experience.

ADRENAL GLAND PHYSIOLOGY

An adult adrenal gland weighs 4–5 g and is soft, yet rubbery in consistency. It is composed of two embryologically distinct structures: the outer cortex and inner medulla. The thin cortex, of mesodermal origin, synthesizes steroid hormones. Its bright yellow hue easily demarcates the adrenal gland from the surrounding retroperitoneal adipose tissue during surgery. The maroon inner medulla, formed by chromaffin cells from the neural crest, synthesizes neuroendocrine hormones involved with the sympathetic system.

The anatomic and physiologic differences in the adrenal structures result in distinct endocrinopathies and symptoms in the diseased state.

Three discrete functional layers comprise the adrenal cortex, each largely responsible for the production of a steroid hormone. The most superficial layer, the zona glomerulosa (ZG), produces mineralocorticoids; the zona fasciculata (ZF) produces glucocorticoids; and the zona reticularis (ZR) produces androgens. The hypersecreted hormone determines the clinical manifestations of functional adrenocortical lesions (Table 35.1).

However, not all tumors are functional. Nonfunctional tumors may also arise from the native tissue of the adrenal gland and other more rare tumors that are not composed of medullary or cortical tissues. These tumors can be found incidentally when a patient undergoes radiographic evaluation for an unrelated issue (commonly termed adrenal incidentaloma). Adrenal neoplasms, particularly those which are nonfunctional, can also grow to a size where the mass effect creates pain or adjacent organ dysfunction, such as ureteral or bowel obstruction. Identification of any adrenal lesion requires a thorough biochemical, radiographic, and, if indicated, genetic evaluation prior to any operative intervention.

RADIOGRAPHIC EVALUATION

Appropriate imaging is essential in the workup of adrenal lesions; it can both be diagnostic and provide critical anatomical detail necessary for surgical planning. Computed tomography (CT) is the mainstay of diagnostic imaging for adrenal tumors and provides a great deal

Table 35.1 Syndromes of hormone hypersecretion

	Cortisol	Androgen	Estrogen	Aldosterone
Manifestation[a]	• Truncal obesity • Buffalo hump • Moon facies • Abdominal purple striae • Easy bruising • Osteoporosis • Thin skin • Psychiatric changes • Glucose intolerance • Hypertension	• Hirsutism • Male pattern baldness • Voice changes • Breast atrophy • Libido change • Oligo- or amenorrhea • Increased muscle mass	• Gynecomastia • Mastodynia • Testicular atrophy • Decreased libido	• Hypertension • Hypokalemia • Polyuria • Weakness • Mild hypernatremia • Metabolic alkalosis

[a] Not all these signs and symptoms are present in all cases, and they may be absent or subtle in subclinical disease.

of information regarding the etiology of a given lesion, likelihood of malignancy, blood supply, and resectability. Characteristics such as size, homogenicity, density, presence of calcification or necrosis, and invasion into adjacent structures can be obtained from both the contrast and noncontrast phase of a CT. If the Hounsfield unit (HU) of a lesion in the noncontrast phase is greater than 10, the likelihood of a nonadenomatous lesion increases significantly. Delayed postcontrast images should be obtained to assess the relative and absolute percent washout of contrast of an adrenal lesion. Lesions with a relative percent washout (RPW) of >40% on delayed CT images are more likely to be benign adrenal adenomas [4]. Some series used a cutoff RPW of >50% but cite similar rates of sensitivity and specificity for adenoma vs. nonadenoma adrenal masses [5]. The absolute percent washout is also calculated, and values of >60% are consistent with adenomatous lesions. Calculation of washout is also particularly helpful when trying to distinguish lipid-poor adenomas from nonadenomas, which have very similar precontrast attenuation [6]. Employment of fine cuts, 1–2 mm, from the dome of the liver through the inferior pole of the kidneys is recommended through all phases, as lesions vary in size and can be poorly visualized or even missed with standard 5 mm cuts. Finer cuts also facilitate localization of the major adrenal vasculature. This is useful in planning the surgical approach and, in some cases, assessing the feasibility of a cortical-sparing procedure.

Magnetic resonance imaging (MRI) is currently not recommended as a first-line imaging modality in adrenal lesions, but it can be used in specific patient populations where CT is not feasible. It can have a role in the surveillance of patients who have a high likelihood of recurrent or metastatic disease, such as those with hereditary pheochromocytoma or paraganglioma.

Functional imaging is indicated in certain clinical scenarios. If a patient presents with clinical and biochemical confirmation of disease, yet none is identified on conventional cross-sectional imaging, functional imaging can be employed. Current guidelines for pheochromocytoma and paraganglioma recommend ^{123}I-metaiodobenzylguanidine

(MIBG) be reserved for lesions of >5 cm, as they have a higher likelihood of metastases [7]. Functional imaging also has a role in surveillance of patients who are at high risk for recurrent or metastatic pheochromocytoma or paraganglioma. When there is concern for metastatic disease, positron emission tomography (PET) imaging is recommended over MIBG and shows higher sensitivity for metastatic lesions [8]. This is felt to be secondary to tumor dedifferentiation within the metastatic tumor cells and loss of specific cell membrane transporters that show affinity for ^{123}I-MIBG. Antigens (chromogranin A, etc.) and receptors for catecholamines and somatostatin are present in functioning and silent neuroendocrine tumors. The common radiotracers ^{123}I, ^{111}In, ^{90}Y, and recently ^{68}Ga-labeled ligands (MIBG, somatostatin analogs, and gallium-DOTA compounds) are highly precise and cheaper.

Biopsy of adrenal lesions as part of a diagnostic workup is not recommended given their very vascular nature and high risk of bleeding. Even a small amount of hemorrhage within or around the gland increases the difficulty of resection secondary to scarring and inflammation within a small space. In the event of a percutaneous biopsy for pheochromocytoma, the presence of an anesthesiologist and intravenous alpha-blockade should be emphasized. Biopsy of the lesion can lead to a hypertensive crisis if it is producing catecholamines [9]. Seeding along the biopsy tract of malignant lesions has also been reported [10].

GENETIC EVALUATION

Approximately 40% of adrenal tumors are associated with a genetically inherited syndrome, although this percentage varies with the tumor type [11,12]. This includes multiple endocrine neoplasia (MEN) and Von Hippel–Landau, Li–Frameni, and Lynch syndromes. It is important that a clinician have an in-depth knowledge of the clinical manifestations of these various tumor syndromes. The family history of the patient and a careful physical examination are paramount, as they indicate whether a patient is at risk for an inherited adrenal lesion and therefore requires the appropriate genetic testing. This responsibility falls to the

Table 35.2 Genetic syndromes associated with adrenal neoplasms

ACC	Hyperaldosteronism	Cushing's syndrome	Pheochromocytoma
MEN1 (menin)	Familial hyperaldosteronism types 1 and 2	MEN1 (menin)	MEN2 (ret)
Li–Fraumeni (TP53)	Bilateral adrenal hyperplasia	Congenital adrenal hyperplasia	von Hippel–Lindau (VHL)
Adenomatous polyposis coli (APC)			Familial pheochromocystoma/paraganglioma syndrome (SDHB, SDHC, SDHD)
Beckewith–Wiedemann (IGF2)			Neurofibromatosis type 1

surgeon, as well as the referring provider. If the patient is believed to be at risk, genetic testing should ideally be obtained prior to surgical intervention.

Significant advancements have been made in the correlation of certain genetic mutations and the phenotypic expression of adrenal pathology. For example, in those patients with neurofibromatosis (NF1 tumor suppressor gene) who present with a pheochromocytoma later in life (average age 50), only about 10% are bilateral, and usually these tumors produce norepinephrine exclusively. A patient with pheochromocytoma in the context of known MEN2 disease has a high likelihood of bilateral disease but a lower likelihood of metastatic disease. This may prompt additional functional imaging to assess for bilateral disease and may alert the operating surgeon to plan for a cortical-sparing procedure at the time of the initial unilateral resection. It is also known that certain RET mutations within MEN2a are more strongly associated with the development of a pheochromocytoma. A genetic profile of a patient with adrenal disease can influence the timing of surgery, further workup necessary for safe surgical intervention, and the choice of surgical approach. A summary of hereditary genetic syndromes of interest and phenotypic expression in regards to adrenal disease is given in Table 35.2.

ANATOMIC CONSIDERATIONS

While the right and left adrenal glands have a similar gross location at the superior pole of each kidney, there are some important differences between the glands that impact the surgical approach and potential complications. They are both retroperitoneal, contained within the Gerota's fascia of the respective kidneys. The right adrenal gland is more triangular in shape and slightly smaller, whereas the left gland is flatter and slightly elongated, and rests more inferior than the right. The right adrenal gland is bordered on the medial side by the inferior vena cava (IVC), the liver along the anterior aspect, and superiorly by the diaphragm. The left adrenal is bordered medially by the aorta, the pancreas and stomach anteriorly, and the diaphragm superior and laterally.

The adrenal glands are highly vascularized (Figure 35.1); they receive small arterial blood from branches of the inferior phrenic arteries and renal artery and directly from the aorta. Nutrient arteries form a capsular arterial plexus that sends capillaries coursing through the cortex. These capillaries then form a venous portal system that drains into the adrenal medulla. There the vessels reach confluence with the central adrenal vein. The right adrenal vein is short and wide; it exits the gland and immediately enters the posterolateral aspect of the IVC. There can be smaller accessory veins that drain directly into the right renal vein inferiorly or into the inferior phrenic vein superiorly as well. The left adrenal vein exits anteriorly and usually drains into the left renal vein, although it occasionally enters the IVC directly.

PREOPERATIVE MANAGEMENT

Adequate preparation of a patient for adrenalectomy requires thorough attention to detail. It is the responsibility of the surgeon to ensure the workup is complete prior to operative intervention. Adequate multidisciplinary communication is a must, as there are often several specialties involved in the care of these patients. The biochemical preparation necessary depends on the etiology of the tumor. Excess hormone production should be managed medically and the effects mitigated as much as possible. In the case of some patients, such as those with irreversible Cushing's, surgery alone provides definitive hormonal control, and once a patient is optimized medically, surgical intervention should not be delayed in hopes of further correction. Communication with operating room personnel regarding equipment and the anesthesia team regarding positioning, venous access, potential need for blood products, and the plan for hemodynamic control should occur prior to the operative day. Available drugs should be clarified prior to procedure and available in all patient care areas, not just the operating room. Recommended drugs include nicardipine, esmolol, and levophed. Central venous access is recommended, as the response to medications is more rapid and vasopressors cannot be administered through peripheral intravenous lines. An immediate postoperative management plan in those patients with hormone-producing tumors should be discussed among the operative team in anticipation of the dynamic effects removal of these tumors can have.

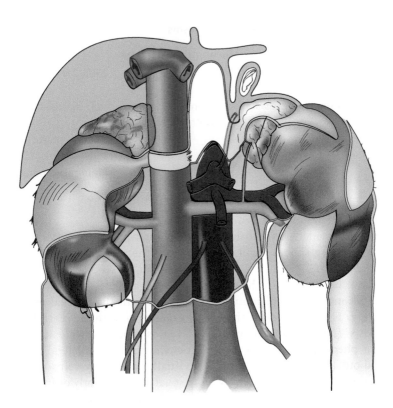

Figure 35.1 Adrenal gland and vascular supply. The adrenal glands are retroperitoneal structures with a rich vascular supply. Ligation of the adrenal vein is a critical step of the procedure.

OPEN ADRENALECTOMY

The traditional open approach to adrenalectomy can be divided into the anterior, lateral, and posterior approaches. Historically, the open approach has been the gold standard and remains such for tumors larger than 6–8 cm, for tumors that have a suspicion of malignancy, or when a minimally invasive technique is not feasible.

The anterior approach is the most common open approach and can be done via a variety of abdominal incisions. The preferred approach at our institution is the subcostal laparotomy, which can be extended to a chevron incision when greater exposure is needed or for bilateral disease. Another incision option for very bulky tumors extending into multiple surrounding organs or the diaphragm is the thoracoabdominal incision, also known as the Makuuchi incision. This incision begins just below the tip of the scapulae and is extended in an oblique fashion to the midline of the abdomen. This incision is utilized for many different procedures, as it provides extensive exposure of retroperitoneal organs and facilitates *en bloc* resection of tumors difficult to access through an abdominal incision [13–15]. There is debate, however, that this approach is associated with more morbidity postoperatively [14]. Patient positioning is of the utmost importance and facilitates an easier operation with better exposure. The patient is supine with arms extended on either side with arm boards. A bump is then placed under the side planned for resection, such that

the patient is extended maximally at the inferior costal margin. The bump, best made by rolled linens, should extend from the tip of the scapula to the top of the buttocks. The leg of the elevated side is flexed at the knee and rotated slightly over midline, while the opposite leg is straight and in anatomic position. Proper attention to pressure points in this position is always recommended. This patient positioning and abdominal incision provides excellent access to both adrenals and surrounding organs. Access to the right gland begins with mobilization of the hepatic flexure of the colon and partial "kocherization" of the curve of the duodenum to better visualize the IVC and take off of the right adrenal vein. For tumors that extend beyond Morrison's pouch and into the retrohepatic space, increased mobilization of the right lobe of the liver may be necessary for a safe *en bloc* resection of the tumor. This is achieved by division of the right triangular ligament of the liver, allowing for anteromedial retraction of the right lobe of the liver. Care should be taken to avoid injury to the right hepatic vein and any accessory inferior phrenic veins with this retraction on the liver. This maneuver can also cause compression of the IVC and decreased venous return; therefore, communication with the anesthesia team is imperative during this portion of the case. Incision into the parietal peritoneum and the lateral aspect of the hepatocolic ligament can then be made and the kidney retracted caudally, exposing the right adrenal.

Generally, with this exposure the right adrenal gland and its relationship to the IVC is clear, and the adrenal vein can readily be identified. The vein typically exits the gland from the superiomedial aspect and enters the IVC along its posterolateral aspect. Careful dissection along the medial aspect of the adrenal gland allows for circumferential isolation of the vein. Larger tumors that extend posterior to the cava require gentle retraction of the IVC to facilitate dissection of the gland from its posterior surface and identification of the adrenal vein. Variable anatomy with more than one adrenal vein can occur, draining into either the IVC or the right renal vein.

For large right adrenal tumors that show evidence of invasion into the right hepatic lobe or IVC with or without associated tumor thrombus, the "hanging technique" has been shown to be particularly useful. It is a technique described initially for hepatic resection, but its use has been extended to multiple types of large right upper quadrant tumors to facilitate necessary *en bloc* resection [16]. After the abdomen is opened via the incision of choice, the falciform ligament is divided and used as a guide to approach the hepatic hilum and prepare for Pringle's maneuver [17]. Segments II and III of the liver are retracted, and the lesser sac is entered, being mindful of a possible replaced left hepatic artery. A long fine clamp or pediatric suction tip is guided behind the caudate lobe and along the avascular plane between the anterior midline IVC and the posterior surface of the right lobe of the liver in the cranial direction. Some caudate branches to IVC may require careful ligation in order to access this plane. Ultrasound can be used to guide the passage of the clamp so as to avoid the right and middle hepatic veins. For right-sided tumor dissection, the clamp should be to the right of the middle hepatic vein. An umbilical tape or long slim Penrose drain is then placed in the clamp or sewn to the suction tip with silk suture and passed caudally back through the retrohepatic space. This then allows for control of the vasculature to the right liver without full mobilization of the liver, which is often not possible with large, bulky invasive tumors. Control of the right hepatic vein can also then be achieved from above the liver. Division of the liver parenchyma is then undertaken, separating involved liver tissue from healthy liver via a "two-surgeon technique," as described by Aloia et al. [18]. Once completely divided, the anterior surface of the IVC is exposed and can de dissected free of tumor. If there is known tumor thrombus extending from the adrenal vein, ultrasound can be used to assess the extent, proximal and distal control of the IVC can be secured, and excision with reconstruction can be performed via this exposure.

The left adrenal gland is exposed in a manner similar to that of the right, with mobilization of the splenic flexure of the colon and extension of this dissection inferiorly along the white line of Toldt and medially dividing the gastrocolic ligament to enter the lesser sac. The transverse and left colon can then be retracted inferiomedially, and the opening of the lesser sac widened to visualize the anterior surface of the pancreas. The retroperitoneum is then accessed by opening the peritoneum along the inferior border of the pancreas and dividing the splenocolic ligament. The spleen and pancreas can then be retracted superiomedially, allowing for exposure of the adrenal gland and hilum of the kidney. The

left adrenal vein typically exits the gland at the inferomedial aspect and drains directly into the left renal vein. It should be identified and ligated as previously described, taking care to preserve the renal hilum. Identification of renal hilar structures is recommended prior to ligation.

Risks of the open approach are inherent to the pathway taken. Iatrogenic injury to any of the surrounding organs is possible, resulting in hemorrhage, enteric fistulae, pancreatic leak, or splenic injury. It is known that in comparison to minimally invasive techniques, the open approach is associated with a longer operative time, longer convalescence, increased intraoperative blood loss, and more intraoperative complications [19,20]. This is nuanced by the fact that in the modern era, open surgery is primarily chosen for larger tumors, malignant tumors, and obviously invasive tumors. All of these factors increase the odds of complication regardless of surgical approach.

LAPAROSCOPIC ADRENALECTOMY

First described in 1992, laparoscopic adrenalectomy has become the procedure of choice for adrenalectomy for benign indications owing to its shorter convalescence period (the hospital stay is approximately 1 week for open adrenalectomy, but only 2–3 days following laparoscopic resection), reduced discomfort, and better cosmetic results. Patients with benign neoplasms and selected patients with adrenal metastasis may benefit from a laparoscopic approach. However, avoiding the minimally invasive approach is advised for any potentially malignant primary adrenal lesion, including radiographic evidence of invasion, suspicious finds of lobulation, tumors of >6 cm, and known tumor syndromes associated with ACC.

For anterior laparoscopic adrenalectomy, the patient is placed in the lateral decubitus position and the skin is prepared from the nipple to below the iliac crest, and from the umbilicus to the vertebral column. A port is placed below the costal margin approximately 10–15 cm anterior to the anterior axillary line for insufflation. Once pneumoperitoneum is established, three additional trocars (placed at the anterior axillary line, posterior axillary line, and 5 cm posterior to the posterior axillary port) are placed under direct visualization with the laparoscope. The adrenal gland is dissected from the retroperitoneal fat using a harmonic scalpel. The gland is mobilized entirely, and the adrenal vein is ligated just prior to specimen removal. The vein may be safely ligated using a vascular stapler or titanium clips placed on the proximal side of the vessel. The anterolateral approach makes bilateral adrenalectomy cumbersome, as the patient requires repositioning midway through the procedure.

The complications associated with the anterior laparoscopic approach are similar to those in open adrenalectomy. Injury to surrounding organs encountered in the exposure of the adrenal gland is an inherent risk. This is usually due to intraoperative detection of tumor invasion, uncontrolled bleeding from the adrenal vein, or known visceral injury requiring repair. Minimally invasive techniques inherently

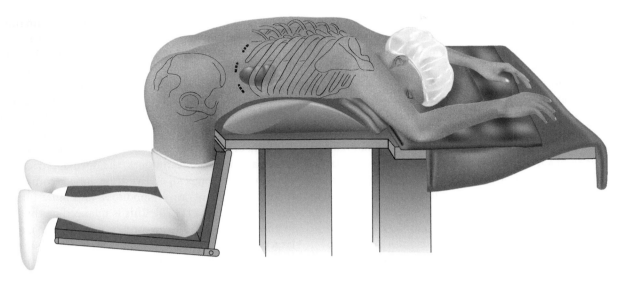

Figure 35.2 Patient in prone jackknife position on a Cloward surgical saddle. Appropriate padding at pressure points is necessary and the abdomen should be allowed to hang freely in the midline.

differ from open techniques in that they require mastery of techniques, as well as mastery of a different anatomical perspective. There is a learning curve for individual surgeons that must be overcome, but as laparoscopic training and tools have advanced, this learning curve is being shortened. More recent series, compared with those published 10–15 years ago, have a lower rate of complications and decreased operative time for minimally invasive techniques [21].

POSTERIOR RETROPERITONEOSCOPIC ADRENALECTOMY

The posterior retroperitoneoscopic adrenalectomy (PRA) is an excellent minimally invasive approach. It was first described by Mercan in 1995, and popularized by Walz [22]. It has the advantages of providing a direct approach to the adrenal glands without the need to enter the peritoneal cavity, mobilize adjacent organs, or navigate a potentially hostile abdomen if prior surgical intervention has occurred. Insufflation of the retroperitoneum does not alter cardiovascular and respiratory parameters as much as peritoneal insufflation and is generally better tolerated. This approach is also ideal for bilateral procedures because there is no need for patient repositioning. Patients who undergo PRA may be eligible for discharge as early as the first postoperative day.

Indications for PRA include a benign adrenal tumor (functional or nonfunctional), isolated metastases to the adrenal glands, and bilateral disease. Absolute contraindication is suspected or known primary adrenal malignancy. Relative contraindications are lesion size greater than 4–6 cm and limited distance between the ribs and iliac crest, both of which make the procedure more technically challenging.

The patient is placed in the prone jackknife position on a Cloward surgical table (Figure 35.2). The abdominal wall must be allowed to hang free from the hip support. The hips and knees are flexed at 90° angles, and all pressure points are appropriately padded. The anesthesia team needs to

be ready to manage adrenal-related pathologies with the patient in the prone position. Care must be taken to protect the endotracheal tube, eyes, and face.

The complications unique to the posterior approach are neuralgias caused by compression or damage to the intercostal neurovascular bundles. Given the location of the ports (Figure 35.3), the most common neurovascular bundle at risk of injury is beneath the 12th rib. Injury to these nerves can cause hypoesthesia and paresthesias in the area of associated intervention on the abdominal wall. A neuralgia associated with transversus abdominus laxity can result in an ipsilateral distention of the abdominal wall. These injuries can resolve over time, but if there is complete transection of

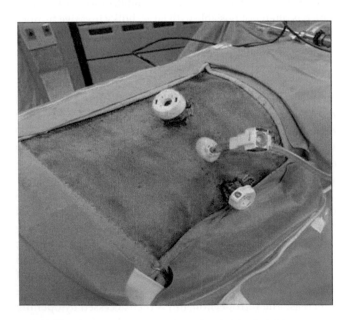

Figure 35.3 Photograph of port site placement for a posterior retroperitoneoscopic adrenalectomy. Critical landmarks for port positioning include the iliac crest, 12th rib, and the paraspinous muscles.

the nerve, they can be permanent. These injuries are rare, however, occurring in only 2.0%–3.4% of patients, depending on the series [21,23]. A challenge unique to the posterior approach is the novel anatomical perspective it creates. A thorough understanding of the anatomy on the part of the surgeon is paramount, particularly in right-sided operations, where the IVC is vulnerable to injury, as it is not readily seen.

ROBOT-ASSISTED ADRENALECTOMY

The approach for adrenalectomy using the surgical robot is similar to the laparoscopic transabdominal or retroperitoneal approach. The robotic system was designed to provide the potential advantages of enhanced three-dimensional visualization, improved ergonomics for the surgeon, and increased range of movement for laparoscopic instruments, which are designed with "wrists" that mimic the surgeon's hand. Disadvantages include increased cost, duration of anesthesia, and operative time to dock the robot. As surgeons become more familiar with the robotic system, the broader applicability in different fields may bring down the cost of robotic assistance.

As with laparoscopic surgery, port placement is essential to maximize the ease of operation. The surgeon or assistant must take care to place the ports approximately 8–10 cm apart to avoid collisions of the robotic arms. The patient's body habitus should be considered, as it may also require alteration of usual port placement to allow access to the adrenal glands. Robotic assistance during adrenalectomy is particularly useful when the adrenal gland is in an anatomically superior location that may limit access via conventional laparoscopy. It is also particularly helpful for dissection near the IVC on the right side. The improved visualization may also optimize exposure of the vasculature during cortical-sparing adrenalectomy for pheochromocytoma [24]. Otherwise, the operation proceeds in standard fashion with exposure of the gland, identification and control of the adrenal vein, dissection of the gland, and specimen removal.

Studies suggest the robotic-assisted approach can be performed safely. In a recent meta-analysis comparing laparoscopic and robotic adrenalectomy, primarily via the anterior approach, there were no complications unique to the robotic approach. Conversion of a robotic approach to open or laparoscopic adrenalectomy was most often due to bleeding in that meta-analysis (2.2%; 4/186 patients). A single surgeon demonstrated lower estimated blood loss in robotic-assisted cases than standard laparoscopy [25]. Recently, single-site robotic adrenalectomy has been described as a technically feasible alternative that led to a reduced need for narcotic pain medication with equivalency in costs when compared with standard laparoscopy [26].

CONTROVERSIES AND CHALLENGING ILLNESSES AND ISSUES

Cushing's disease has a widely variable treatment algorithm dependent largely upon the etiology of excess. It is a debilitating disease and gives rise to numerous complications. Patients with untreated disease have a mean survival of 5 years from presentation. Therefore, timely effective management and control of the cortisol production is critical. Eighty percent of Cushing's disease is adrenocorticotropic hormone (ACTH) dependent, meaning the cause is excess production of corticotropin (ACTH) from the pituitary or, less frequently, an ectopic source. Transsphenoidal surgery for resection of a pituitary adenoma results in substantial cure rates; however, persistent or recurrent disease occurs in 11.5%–25% of patients [27]. Another subset of patients has ectopic production of ACTH from an occult source or an unresectable tumor. There are pharmacologic agents aimed at inhibiting steroidogenesis, but these are successful in only about one-third to one-half of patients [28]. Recent data have suggested that patients with refractory Cushing's disease may benefit from a more timely surgical intervention, rather than surgery after failure of medical treatment [29]. The rapid progression of complications in this patient population, even while on medical therapy, can quickly render a patient inoperable because of such poor performance status. Ideally, decisions on timing of surgical intervention should be approached in a multidisciplinary fashion, such that consultation with a surgical endocrinologist occurs shortly after diagnosis, rather than in the later stages of disease, when a patient is in poorer health secondary to prolonged exposure to excess cortisol.

Cortical-sparing adrenalectomy is a technique that was initially described more than 30 years ago, but has only relatively recently gained acceptance as a preferred therapeutic option for certain adrenal pathologies. The goal of the procedure is to avoid steroid dependence resulting from bilateral adrenalectomy, and it is to be considered in patients with known or potential bilateral adrenal disease. Historically, total adrenalectomy has been the standard for any adrenal pathology for fear of recurrence, particularly in the setting of inherited adrenal disease, such as pheochromocytoma in VHL and MEN2a patients. There is significant variation in the data, but larger series show that recurrence rates are low in these syndromes and the time interval between these recurrences is quite long [30]. In the cases of recurrence, total adrenalectomy is often needed, but it is noteworthy that with cortical-sparing procedures, these patients have been afforded many years without steroid dependence and the risk of Addisonian crisis. It is suggested that at least one-third of one gland be spared, or 15% of both glands be preserved in order to maintain adequate function [30–32].

As previously mentioned, the standard surgical technique for ACC has been open surgical resection due to multiple series that demonstrate a higher rate of peritoneal recurrence and morbidity in those patients who undergo laparoscopic resection [2,3]. Other retrospective studies show no difference in long-term survival when tumors are at an earlier stage (stage I or II) [33]. Despite these previous results, ACCs are still removed laparoscopically because either the pathology is unknown prior to resection or they are of a small size and there are surgeons who believe oncologic outcome is not compromised by the laparoscopic approach when the lesion is small. Numerous series in the literature caution against this, however, as peritoneal carcinomatosis and local recurrence occur at unacceptably high rates regardless of size [1,2]. All agree, however, that for ACC, an appropriate oncologic resection is mandatory, including *en bloc* resection of all involved structures without invasion of the tumor capsule. There are few effective medical or adjuvant treatment options for ACC, and complete surgical resection remains the most important factor associated with improved survival. Therefore, superb exposure is of the utmost importance to remove these often friable tumors, and this is invariably best achieved with the open approach.

CONCLUSION

The last 20 years have brought new techniques that have significantly changed the landscape of adrenal surgery and, in many ways, improved the patient's experience. Experience and outcomes in this relatively short amount of time have also shown us, however, that each adrenal pathology and patient is unique, and the goals of the operations are far from generic. This serves as a reminder that innovation, while exciting and dynamic, should not replace validated methods, but rather be held to high standards of evaluation and trial.

REFERENCES

1. Gonzalez RJ, Shapiro S, Sarlis N et al. Laparoscopic resection of adrenal cortical carcinoma: A cautionary note. *Surgery* 2005;138:1078–85; discussion 1085–6.
2. Cooper AB, Habra MA, Grubbs EG et al. Does laparoscopic adrenalectomy jeopardize oncologic outcomes for patients with adrenocortical carcinoma? *Surg Endosc* 2013;27:4026–32.
3. Miller BS, Gauger PG, Hammer GD, Doherty GM. Resection of adrenocortical carcinoma is less complete and local recurrence occurs sooner and more often after laparoscopic adrenalectomy than after open adrenalectomy. *Surgery* 2012;152:1150–57.
4. Blake MA, Kalra MK, Sweeney AT et al. Distinguishing benign from malignant adrenal masses: Multi-detector row CT protocol with 10-minute delay. *Radiology* 2006;238:578–85.
5. Korobkin M, Brodeur FJ, Francis IR, Quint LE, Dunnick NR, Londy F. CT time-attenuation washout curves of adrenal adenomas and nonadenomas. *AJR Am J Roentgenol* 1998;170:747–52.
6. Caoili EM, Korobkin M, Francis IR, Cohan RH, Dunnick NR. Delayed enhanced CT of lipid-poor adrenal adenomas. *AJR Am J Roentgenol* 2000;175:1411–5.
7. Taieb D, Kebebew E, Castinetti F, Chen CC, Henry JF, Pacak K. Diagnosis and preoperative imaging of multiple endocrine neoplasia type 2: Current status and future directions. *Clin Endocrinol* 2014;81:317–328.
8. Timmers HJ, Chen CC, Carrasquillo JA et al. Comparison of 18F-fluoro-L-DOPA, 18F-fluorodeoxyglucose, and 18F-fluorodopamine PET and 123I-MIBG scintigraphy in the localization of pheochromocytoma and paraganglioma. *J Clin Endocrinol Metabol* 2009;94:4757–67.
9. Osman Y, El-Mekresh M, Gomha AM et al. Percutaneous adrenal biopsy for indeterminate adrenal lesion: Complications and diagnostic accuracy. *Urol Int* 2010;84:315–8.
10. Mody MK, Kazerooni EA, Korobkin M. Percutaneous CT-guided biopsy of adrenal masses: Immediate and delayed complications. *J Comput Assist Tomogr* 1995;19:434–9.
11. Dahia PL. Pheochromocytoma and paraganglioma pathogenesis: Learning from genetic heterogeneity. *Nat Rev Cancer* 2014;14:108–19.
12. Garber JE, Offit K. Hereditary cancer predisposition syndromes. *J Clin Oncol* 2005;23:276–92.
13. Chute R, Soutter L, Kerr WS Jr. The value of the thoracoabdominal incision in the removal of kidney tumors. *N Engl J Med* 1949;241:951–60.
14. Xia F, Poon RT, Fan ST, Wong J. Thoracoabdominal approach for right-sided hepatic resection for hepatocellular carcinoma. *J Am Coll Surg* 2003;196:418–27.
15. Kumar S, Duque JL, Guimaraes KC, Dicanzio J, Loughlin KR, Richie JP. Short and long-term morbidity of thoracoabdominal incision for nephrectomy: A comparison with the flank approach. *J Urol* 1999;162:1927–9.
16. Donadon M, Abdalla EK, Vauthey JN. Liver hanging maneuver for large or recurrent right upper quadrant tumors. *J Am Coll Surg* 2007;204:329–33.
17. Kim SH, Kim YK. Hanging manoeuver for a left hepatectomy using Glisson's approach with a focus on tape position in liver hilum. *HPB* 2013;15:681–6.
18. Aloia TA, Zorzi D, Abdalla EK, Vauthey JN. Two-surgeon technique for hepatic parenchymal transection of the noncirrhotic liver using saline-linked cautery and ultrasonic dissection. *Ann Surg* 2005;242:172–7.
19. Bittner JG 4th, Gershuni VM, Matthews BD, Moley JF, Brunt LM. Risk factors affecting operative approach, conversion, and morbidity for adrenalectomy: A single-institution series of 402 patients. *Surg Endosc* 2013;27:2342–50.
20. Guazzoni G, Montorsi F, Bocciardi A et al. Transperitoneal laparoscopic versus open adrenalectomy for benign hyperfunctioning adrenal tumors: A comparative study. *J Urol* 1995;153:1597–1600.
21. Chai YJ, Kwon H, Yu HW et al. Systematic review of surgical approaches for adrenal tumors: Lateral transperitoneal versus posterior retroperitoneal and laparoscopic versus robotic adrenalectomy. *Int J Endocrinol* 2014;2014:918346.
22. Mercan S, Seven R, Ozarmagan S, Tezelman S. Endoscopic retroperitoneal adrenalectomy. *Surgery* 1995;118:1071–5; discussion 1075–6.

23. Constantinides VA, Christakis I, Touska P, Palazzo FF. Systematic review and meta-analysis of retroperitoneoscopic versus laparoscopic adrenalectomy. *Br J Surg* 2012;99:1639–48.

24. Dickson PV, Alex GC, Grubbs EG et al. Posterior retroperitoneoscopic adrenalectomy is a safe and effective alternative to transabdominal laparoscopic adrenalectomy for pheochromocytoma. *Surgery* 2011;150:452–8.

25. Brandao LF, Autorino R, Zargar H et al. Robot-assisted laparoscopic adrenalectomy: Step-by-step technique and comparative outcomes. *Eur Urol* 2014;66:898–905.

26. Arghami A, Dy BM, Bingener J, Osborn J, Richards ML. Single-port robotic-assisted adrenalectomy: Feasibility, safety, and cost-effectiveness. *JSLS* 2015;19:e2014.00218.

27. Wong A, Eloy JA, Liu JK. The role of bilateral adrenalectomy in the treatment of refractory Cushing's disease. *Neurosurg Focus* 2015;38:E9.

28. Valassi E, Crespo I, Santos A, Webb SM. Clinical consequences of Cushing's syndrome. *Pituitary* 2012;15:319–29.

29. Morris LF, Harris RS, Milton DR et al. Impact and timing of bilateral adrenalectomy for refractory adrenocorticotropic hormone-dependent Cushing's syndrome. *Surgery* 2013;154:1174–83; discussion 1183–4.

30. Alesina PF, Hinrichs J, Meier B, Schmid KW, Neumann HP, Walz MK. Minimally invasive cortical-sparing surgery for bilateral pheochromocytomas. *Langenbecks Arch Surg* 2012;397:233–8.

31. Brauckhoff M, Thanh PN, Gimm O, Bar A, Brauckhoff K, Dralle H. Functional results after endoscopic subtotal cortical-sparing adrenalectomy. *Surg Today* 2003;33:342–8.

32. Walz MK, Peitgen K, Diesing D et al. Partial versus total adrenalectomy by the posterior retroperitoneoscopic approach: Early and long-term results of 325 consecutive procedures in primary adrenal neoplasias. *World J Surg* 2004;28:1323–29.

33. Donatini G, Caiazzo R, Do Cao C et al. Long-term survival after adrenalectomy for stage I/II adrenocortical carcinoma (ACC): A retrospective comparative cohort study of laparoscopic versus open approach. *Ann Surg Oncol* 2014;21:284–91.

PART 6

Pancreas

36

Pathology of the endocrine pancreas

HONGFA ZHU

DEFINITION AND TERMINOLOGY

Gastropancreatic neuroendocrine tumors (GEP-PanNETs) are epithelial neoplasms with predominant neuroendocrine differentiation that arise from the diffuse neuroendocrine cells in the gastrointestinal tract and the pancreas [1]. Although pancreatic neuroendocrine tumors (PanNETs) share similar histologic features with neuroendocrine tumors of the gastrointestinal tract (GEPs), it has become increasingly evident that they differ in molecular pathogenesis, clinical behavior, and responsiveness to certain therapies [2]. Since Oberndorfer first coined the term *carcinoid tumor* more than a century ago [3], a variety of nomenclatures have been proposed for this entity, such as "islet cell tumor," "endocrine tumor or neoplasm," "neuroendocrine tumor or neoplasm," and "endocrine or neuroendocrine carcinoma," which has caused great confusion clinically [4,5]. The term *islet cell tumors* has been disparaged because evidence suggests that PanNETs arise from the pluripotent cells among the acinar–ductal cells of the pancreas, and also, PanNETs produce hormones not normally found in normal islet cells [6]. In 2010, the World Health Organization (WHO), together with the European Neuroendocrine Tumor Society (ENETS), the American Joint Committee on Cancer (AJCC), and the North American Neuroendocrine Tumor Society (NANETS), made great efforts to standardize the nomenclature, developed guidelines for PanNETs, and recommended a minimal data set for pathologic reports [1,4,7]. It was also agreed by a panel of experts that the terms *endocrine* and *neuroendocrine* are essentially synonymous, and that *tumor* and *neoplasm* can be used interchangeably [4,8]. In the 2010 WHO classification system, PanNETs are separated into well-differentiated and poorly differentiated categories. The term *carcinoma* is reserved only for poorly differentiated pancreatic neuroendocrine carcinomas (PDPanNECs), consisting of small cell carcinoma and large cell neuroendocrine carcinoma.

EPIDEMIOLOGY

PanNETs are relatively rare tumors representing approximately 1%–2% of all pancreatic tumors and overall 7% of all neuroendocrine tumors [2]. According to the U.S. Surveillance, Epidemiology, and End Results (SEER) database, the incidence of neuroendocrine tumors in the United States increased nearly fivefold over the past three decades [9]. The annual incidence of PanNETs was 0.43 per 100,000 people in the United States, increasing greater than twofold since the 1980s [10]. However, data from an autopsy study indicated the prevalence of PanNETs varied between 0.8% and 3%, suggesting that the true occurrence of PanNETs may be underestimated [2,11]. Despite advanced detecting technology and improved modalities of clinical management, the overall prognosis of PanNETs has not changed significantly over the past few decades [7].

Most PanNETs are sporadic and occur in older patients, with a peak incidence between 30 and 60 years (mean age 50 years). There is a slight male predominance in the United States, with 55.2% men and 44.8% women. The vast majority of patients are Caucasian (84.3%), 9.4% African American, and 4.7% of Asian origin [12]. Patients with functional tumors tend to present at a younger age than those with nonfunctional tumors (55.2 years vs. 58.8 years) with improved survival (54 months vs. 26 months) [11].

Although PanNETs are indolent tumors with a favorable prognosis compared with pancreatic adenocarcinoma, they definitely have malignant potential. Most PanNET patients (60%–70%) present with metastatic disease [10,11]. Following surgical resection, the 5-year survival of PanNETs other than insulinoma is roughly 65%, with a 10-year survival of

45% [13]. The prognosis of high-grade PDNECs is dismal, where 5-year survival varies from 6% to 11% [14].

CLASSIFICATION

PanNETs can be classified as functional or nonfunctional tumors based on their hormone secretion and their corresponding clinical symptoms. Functional PanNETs are associated with syndromes caused by the hypersecretion of hormones, either appropriate (insulin, glucagon, and somatostatin) or inappropriate (e.g., gastrin, vasoactive intestinal peptide [VIP], growth hormone-releasing factor [GHRF], and adrenocorticotropic hormone [ACTH]), to the endocrine pancreas. Based on the types of biologically active peptides secreted, functional PanNETs can be classified as insulinomas, gastrinomas (Zollinger–Ellison syndrome), glucagonomas, VIPomas (Verner–Morrison syndrome), somatostatinomas, GRFomas, ACTHomas, PanNETs causing carcinoid syndrome, and PanNETs causing hypercalcemia [2,14].

Nonfunctional tumors do not produce any hormone, produce very small amounts that are insufficient to cause symptoms, or produce hormones that do not generate specific symptoms (such as pancreatic polypeptide). According to the SEER database, 90% of PanNETs diagnosed are nonfunctional tumors [7,11]. Most nonfunctional PanNETs present with symptoms of a mass effect that mimic carcinoma. It should be noted that functionality of PanNETs is defined by specific syndromes associated with secreted hormones, not by detection of hormones by immunohistochemical staining.

About 10% of PanNETs are associated with hereditary syndromes, including multiple endocrine neoplasia type 1 (MEN1), von Hippel–Lindau (VHL) disease, von Recklinghausen's diseases (neurofibromatosis 1), and tuberous sclerosis (TSC). Patients with hereditary syndromes generally have an earlier presentation, multiple synchronous tumors, and a positive family history of endocrine disorders.

GRADING

The previous 2004 WHO classification system attempted to subcategorize PanNETs as "benign or uncertain behavior"

versus frank "carcinoma," reserving the latter only for tumors that demonstrated unequivocal evidence of malignant behavior, such as gross local invasion or distant metastasis [15]. However, this system was based on the combined grading and staging parameters and lacked prognostic stratification. In addition, this system could cause great confusion in cases when the tumor initially presented as a well-differentiated neuroendocrine tumor (WDNET), but later would be redesignated as well-differentiated neuroendocrine carcinoma (WDNEC) because of subsequent liver or other organ metastasis. The 2010 WHO and ENETS adopted a risk stratification approach and classified PanNETs into a three-tiered grading system with great emphasis on the mitotic count and proliferation index Ki67 [1,8]. The 2010 WHO grading system has been repeatedly shown to provide prognostic significance for GEP-PanNETs [16–18]. By definition, the low-grade (G1) PanNETs have less than two mitoses per 10 high-power fields (hpf) and <3% Ki67 labeling; the intermediate-grade (G2) PanNETs have 2–20 mitoses per 10 hpf and a Ki67 labeling index of 3%–20%; and high-grade (G3) PanNETs are poorly differentiated carcinomas and have >20 mitoses per 10 hpf and >20% Ki67 labeling (Table 36.1).

The proliferation rate is generally assessed either by counting the mitotic figures (usually expressed as the number in 10 hpf or per 2 mm^2) or by calculating the percentage of cells labeled by immunohistochemistry for Ki67 [4]. It was recommended that at least 50 hpf should be examined for mitotic figures, and a minimum of 500 tumor cells should be counted for the Ki67 index [5]. Although the semiquantitative "eye balling" is a practically used and accepted methodology for evaluation of Ki67 labeling, the more accurate digital counting has been advocated [4,5,19]. The Ki67 index is particularly useful in small biopsies or on fine-needle aspiration cytology samples when the amount of tissue is very limited. It is important to realize that the proliferative activities are usually heterogeneous within tumors, and the tumor grade may be underestimated on small core biopsies [20,21].

Currently, there is no unified grading system for neuroendocrine tumors of different organ systems. The thoracic neuroendocrine tumors use different cutoff points and incorporate the presence or absence of necrosis for grading [22]. Even among the GEP-PanNETs, different cutoff values

Table 36.1 Comparison of the criteria for the tumor category in the ENETS and 7th edition AJCC TNM classification of PanNETs

ENETS TNM		AJCC/UICC TNM
Pancreatic neuroendocrine tumors		
T1	Confined to pancreas, <2 cm	Confined to pancreas, <2 cm
T2	Confined to pancreas, 2–4 cm	Confined to pancreas, >2 cm
T3	Confined to pancreas, >4 cm, or invasion of duodenum or bile duct	Peripancreatic spread, but without major vascular invasion (truncus coeliacus and a. mesent. sup.)
T4	Invasion of adjacent organs or major organs	Major vascular invasion

Source: Adapted from Klimstra DS. Semin Oncol 2013;40:23–36.

have been proposed [5]. Therefore, a multidisciplinary consensus group of experts has recommended a minimum pathology data set (checklists) to be included in a pathology report [4].

There are some controversies for PanNETs that are well differentiated based on histology and mitotic rate, but exhibit a high Ki67 labeling index (>20%) that would suggest PDPanNECs (G3) by definition [4,5,23]. True high-grade PDPanNECs, such as small cell carcinoma and large cell neuroendocrine carcinoma, commonly have 50–80 mitoses per 10 hpf and a Ki67 index usually above 75% [23]. One study indicated that only those neuroendocrine carcinomas with a Ki67 index greater than 55% responded to platinum-based chemotherapy, whereas the tumors with Ki67 between 20% and 55% did not respond [24]. Another study also suggested that the outcome of these WDPanNETs with an elevated Ki67 index was worse than that of G2 PanNETs, but not as bad as that of true PDPanNECs (5-year disease-specific survival rates of 22% vs. 66.5% vs. 17%, respectively) [23]. Therefore, it appears that G3 PanNETs comprise two distinct subgroups: one that is differentiated but more actively proliferating (Ki67 in the 20%–50% range) and the other comprising truly PDPanNECs, including small cell carcinoma and large cell neuroendocrine carcinoma [5,23].

STAGING

There were no formal tumor–node–metastasis (TNM)-based staging systems for neuroendocrine tumors until recently [8]. The SEER data categorized the extent of disease as "localized," "regional," or "distant" [10]. The 2000 and 2004 WHO combined grading parameters (such as proliferation index) and staging parameters (such as lymph node and distal metastasis) into a single prognostic system [25,26]. In 2006, ENETS published landmark papers proposing a separate stage system for PanNETs [8,27]. The AJCC, International Union Against Cancer (UICC), and College of American Pathologists (CAP) essentially adopted the staging system used for exocrine tumors of the pancreas [28–30]. The 2007 edition of the AJCC manual included staging parameters for neuroendocrine tumors of all anatomic sites [28]. Unfortunately, the staging systems of the ENETS and the WHO are not identical, although both systems attempt prognostic stratification well [31] (Table 36.2). Some studies suggested that the ENETS system may be superior to the AJCC/UICC system for stratifying by prognosis [31]. Therefore, it is important to document the critical basic information in the pathology report and the system used to reference particular staging.

HISTOPATHOLOGY

PanNETs can occur anywhere in the pancreas, but approximately two-thirds of the resected nonfunctional PanNETs arise in the head of the pancreas. Most PanNETs are well circumscribed, solitary, or cystic and tan–yellow in appearance (Figure 36.1). They are usually soft to firm. Areas of

Table 36.2 Grading systems for neuroendocrine tumors

Grade	Lung and thymus	Pancreas (ENETS and WHO)
Low grade	<2 mitoses/10 hpf and no necrosis	<2 mitoses/10 hpf and <3% Ki67 index
Intermediate grade	2–10 mitoses/10 hpf or foci of necrosis	2–20 mitoses/10 hpf or 3%–20% Ki67 index
High grade	>10 mitoses/10 hpf	>20 mitoses/10 hpf or >20% Ki67 index

Source: Adapted from Klimstra DS et al. *Pancreas* 2010;39: 707–12.

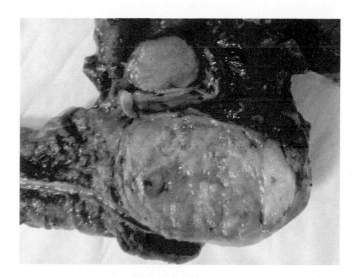

Figure 36.1 (Gross) The distal pancreatectomy specimen showing a 3 cm well-circumscribed, homogenous, tan–yellow tumor that is abutting the pancreatic duct. There is also one adjacent lymph node involved by the tumor.

hemorrhage or necrosis can occur, usually in larger tumors. Microscopically, WDPanNETs show classic "organoid" patterns with trabecular, nesting, glandular, gyriform, tubuloacinar, or pseudorosette arrangements that can be surrounded by eosinophilic, amyloid-like stroma, particularly in the case of insulinomas (Figure 36.2). Psammoma bodies are commonly observed in somatostatinomas, which more commonly occur in the duodenum. The neuroendocrine tumor cells are relatively uniform, with a fair amount of amphophilic to eosinophilic cytoplasm containing abundant neurosecretory granules that are immunohistochemically reactive to neuroendocrine markers such as chromogranin A and synaptophysin. The tumor cells have round to oval nucleus, indistinct nucleolus, and "salt and pepper" chromatin. Occasionally, clear cells, lipid-rich cells, oncocytes, and signet ring or "rhabdoid" histologic subtypes can be seen and present diagnostic challenges [5,9]. However, most of these histological patterns have no special

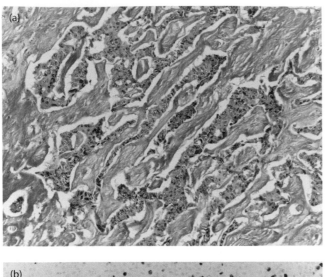

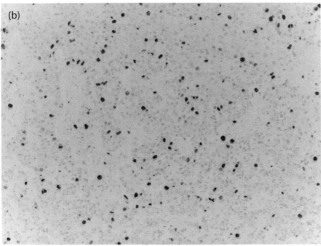

Figure 36.2 **(a)** Microscopic image of infiltrating neuroendocrine tumors composed of a monotonous cell population in trabecular and nesting patterns surrounded by eosinophilic fibrotic stroma. Mitotic figures are rare and tumor necrosis is absent. Original magnification, ×100. **(b)** Neuroendocrine tumor cells are stained with proliferation marker Ki67 immunohistochemically and show an approximate 10% proliferation rate (grade 2). Original magnification, ×100.

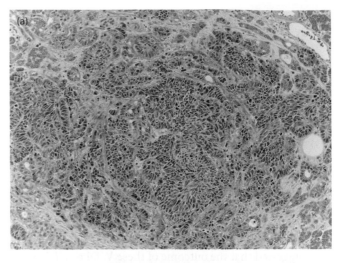

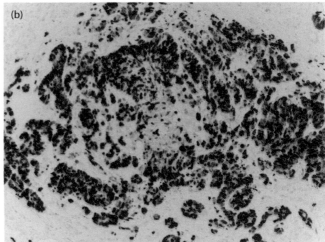

Figure 36.3 **(a)** Pancreas shows microscopic foci of small cell carcinoma. The tumor cells demonstrate histology resembling that of small cell carcinoma of the lung, comprising hyperchromatic tumor cells with nuclear molding, abundant individual tumor cell necrosis, and brisk mitosis. **(b)** The immunostains for proliferation index Ki67 are more than 90% (grade 3).

prognostic significance [9]. The PDPanNECs resemble small cell carcinoma or large cell neuroendocrine carcinoma from the lung with characteristic histology. Small cell carcinoma typically shows hyperchromasia, nuclear molding, and inconspicuous nucleoli with a brisk mitotic rate (50–80 per 10 hpf), high Ki67 index (above 75%), and abundant tumor necrosis (Figure 36.3).

In hereditary syndromes such as MEN1 and VHL, the tumors are frequently small and multifocal. Up to 80% of MEN1 patients develop multiple synchronous lesions (<0.5 cm) (microadenomatosis), as well as "dysplastic islets." Up to 17% of patients with VHL develop PanNETs. Most of these are nonfunctioning and may have a clear-cell morphology due to intracytoplasmic lipid [32,33]. The lipid-rich cells were once thought to be pathognomonic

of VLH-related WDNETs; however, similar cytological changes have been seen in other tumors [34].

MOLECULAR PATHOLOGY

The molecular alterations of PanNETs are very different from those of ductal or acinar tumors of the exocrine pancreas. The common genetic mutations identified in pancreatic ductal adenocarcinoma (e.g., TP53, KRAS, CDKN2A/p16, and SMAD4/DPC4) are infrequent in PanNETs [35,36]. A whole genome sequencing study showed that 44% of sporadic PanNETs harbored somatic inactivating mutations in MEN1, 25% a DAXX (death-domain-associated protein) mutation, 18% an ATRX (a thalassemia/mental retardation syndrome X-linked) mutation, and 14% mutations coding for members of the mammalian target of rapamycin (mTOR) signaling pathway [36]. Mutations in the ATRX and DAXX tumor suppressor genes appear to be mutually exclusive in PanNETs [36]. PanNET patients with mutations in MEN1, DAXX, or ATRX had better overall survival compared with those without mutation: 100% of PanNET patients who had these mutations survived at least 10 years, whereas more than 60% of the patients without these mutations died within 5 years of diagnosis [36].

Interestingly, the DAXX or ATRX mutation has been found only in WDPanNETs and not in PDPanNECs [36]. In contrast, p53 was positive in both small cell (100%) and large cell (90%) NECs, but was negative in WDPanNETs. Similarly, Rb protein was lost in 60%–90% of PDPanNECs. Among these tumors that retained Rb expression, there was usually concurrent loss of p16 staining, indicating that the two were mutually exclusive in PDPanNECs. Conversely, WDPanNETs retained both pRb and p16. Therefore, PDPanNECs are genetically related but are distinct from WDPanNETs [35].

WDPanNETs have been historically resistant to standard chemotherapy. The recent advance in our understanding of the molecular biology of PanNETs has opened the door for possible molecular-targeted therapy. Everolimus, an oral mTOR inhibitor, and sunitinib, an oral tyrosine kinase inhibitor, have been recently approved by the Food and Drug Administration (FDA) for advanced, nonresectable low- or intermediate-grade PanNETs [37,38]. Other potential molecular-targeted therapy, such as sorafenib (tyrosine kinase inhibitor) and bevacizumab (humanized monoclonal antibody against vascular endothelial growth factor), have been investigated in clinical trials. With further understanding of the genetics and molecular pathway of the PanNETs, additional medical and personalized therapies may become available in the future.

REFERENCES

1. Rindi G, Arnold R, Bosman FT et al. Nomenclature and classification of neuroendocrine neoplasms of the digestive system. In: Bosman FT, Carneiro F, Hruban RH et al., eds., *WHO Classification of Tumours of the Digestive System*. Lyon: IARC Press, 2010:13–4.
2. Metz DC, Jensen RT. Gastrointestinal neuroendocrine tumors: Pancreatic endocrine tumors. *Gastroenterology* 2008;135:1469–92.
3. Modlin IM, Shapiro MD, Kidd M et al. Siegfried Oberndorfer and the evolution of carcinoid disease. *Arch Surg* 2007;142:187–97.
4. Klimstra DS, Modlin IR, Coppola D et al. The pathologic classification of neuroendocrine tumors: A review of nomenclature, grading, and staging systems. *Pancreas* 2010;39:707–12.
5. Reid MD, Balci S, Saka B et al. Neuroendocrine tumors of the pancreas: Current concepts and controversies. *Endocr Pathol* 2014;25:65–79.
6. Vortmeyer AO, Huang S, Lubensky I et al. Non-islet origin of pancreatic islet cell tumors. *J Clin Endocrinol Metab* 2004;89:1934–8.
7. Rindi G, Kloppel G, Alhman H et al. TNM staging of foregut (neuro)endocrine tumors: A consensus proposal including a grading system. *Virchows Arch* 2006;449:395–401.
8. Klimstra DS. Pathology reporting of neuroendocrine tumors: Essential elements for accurate diagnosis, classification, and staging. *Semin Oncol* 2013;40:23–36.
9. Yao JC, Hassan M, Phan A et al. One hundred years after "carcinoid": Epidemiology of and prognostic factors for neuroendocrine tumors in 35,825 cases in the United States. *J Clin Oncol* 2008;26:3063–72.
10. Modlin IM, Oberg K, Chung DC et al. Gastroenteropancreatic neuroendocrine tumours. *Lancet Oncol* 2008;9:61–72.
11. Sadaria MR, Hruban RH, Edil BH. Advancements in pancreatic neuroendocrine tumors. *Expert Rev Gastroenterol Hepatol* 2013;7:477–90.
12. Halfdanarson TR, Rabe KG, Rubin J et al. Pancreatic neuroendocrine tumors (PNETs): Incidence, prognosis and recent trend toward improved survival. *Ann Oncol* 2008:19:1727–33.
13. de Wilde RF, Edil BH, Hruban RH et al. Well-differentiated pancreatic neuroendocrine tumors: From genetics to therapy. *Nat Rev Gastroenterol Hepatol* 2012;9:199–208.
14. Sorbye H, Strosberg J, Baudin E, Klimstra DS, Yao JC. Gastroenteropancreatic high-grade neuroendocrine carcinoma. *Cancer* 2014;120:2814–23.
15. Klimstra D, Perren A, Oberg K et al. Pancreatic endocrine tumours: Non-functioning tumours and microadenomas. In: DeLellis RA, Lloyd RV, Heitz PU, Eng C, eds., *Pathology and Genetics of Tumours of Endocrine Organs*. Lyon: IARC Press, 2004:201–4.
16. Jamali M, Chetty R. Predicting prognosis in gastro-tero-pancreatic neuroendocrine tumors: An overview and the value of ki-67 immunostaining. *Endocr Pathol* 2008;19:282–8.
17. Pape UF, Berndt U, Muller-Nordhorn J et al. Prognostic factors of long-term outcome in gastro-enteropancreatic neuroendocrine tumours. *Endocr Relat Cancer* 2008;15:1083–97.
18. Pelosi G, Bresaola E, Bogina G et al. Endocrine tumors of the pancreas: Ki-67 immunoreactivity on paraffin sections is an independent predictor for malignancy: A comparative study with proliferating-cell nuclear antigen and progesterone receptor protein immunostaining, mitotic index, and other clinicopathologic variables. *Hum Pathol* 1996;27:1124–34.
19. Tang LH, Gonen M, Hedvat C et al. Objective quantification of the Ki67 proliferative index in neuroendocrine tumors of the gastroenteropancreatic system: A comparison of digital image analysis with manual methods. *Am J Surg Pathol* 2012;36:1761–70.

20. Yang Z, Tang LH, Klimstra DS. Effect of tumor heterogeneity on the assessment of Ki67 labeling index in well-differentiated neuroendocrine tumors metastatic to the liver: Implications for prognostic stratification. *Am J Surg Pathol* 2011;35:853–60.

21. Yang Z, Tang LH, Klimstra DS. How many needle core biopsies are needed to comfortably predict the histologic grade of metastatic well differentiated neuroendocrine tumors to the liver? *Mod Pathol* 2012;25:426A.

22. Travis WD. The concept of pulmonary neuroendocrine tumours. In: Travis WD, Brambilia E, Muller-Hermelink HK, Harris CC, eds., *Pathology and Genetics of Tumours of the Lung, Pleura, Thymus and Heart.* Lyon: IARC Press, 2004:19–20.

23. Basturk O, Tang L, Hruban RH et al. Poorly differentiated neuroendocrine carcinomas of the pancreas: A clinicopathologic analysis of 44 cases. *Am J Surg Pathol* 2014;38:437–47.

24. Sorbye H, Welin S, Langer SW et al. Predictive and prognostic factors for treatment and survival in 305 patients with advanced gastrointestinal poorly differentiated neuroendocrine carcinoma: The NORDIC NEC study. *J Clin Oncol* 2012;30(Suppl; abstr 4015).

25. Capella C, Solcia E, Sobin LH et al. Endocrine tumours of the small intestine. In: Hamilton SR, Aaltonen LA, eds., *Pathology and Genetics of Tumours of the Digestive System.* Lyon: IARC Press, 2000:77–82.

26. Heitz PU, Komminoth P, Perren A et al. Pancreatic endocrine tumours: Introduction. In: DeLellis RA, Lloyd RV, Heitz PU, Eng C, eds., *Pathology and Genetics of Tumours of Endocrine Organs.* Lyon: IARC Press, 2004:177–82.

27. Rindi G, Kloppel G, Couvelard A et al. TNM staging of midgut and hindgut (neuro) endocrine tumors: A consensus proposal including a grading system. *Virchows Arch* 2007;451:757–62.

28. Edge SB, Byrd DR, Carducci MA et al. *AJCC Cancer Staging Manual.* 7th ed. New York: Springer, 2010.

29. Sobin L, Gospodarowicz M, Wittekind C. *UICC: TNM Classification of Malignant Tumors.* 7th ed. Oxford: Wiley-Blackwell, 2009.

30. College of American Pathologists. College of American Pathologists cancer protocols and checklists. Northfield, IL: College of American Pathologists, 2013. http://www.cap.org/.

31. Rindi G, Falconi M, Klersy C et al. TNM staging of neoplasms of the endocrine pancreas: Results from a large international cohort study. *J Natl Cancer Inst* 2012;104:764–77.

32. Lubensky IA, Pack S, Ault D et al. Multiple neuroendocrine tumors of the pancreas in von Hippel-Lindau disease patients: Histopathological and molecular genetic analysis. *Am J Pathol* 1998;153:223–31.

33. Hoang MP, Hruban RH, Albores-Saavedra J. Clear cell endocrine pancreatic tumor mimicking renal cell carcinoma: A distinctive neoplasm of von Hippel-Lindau disease. *Am J Surg Pathol* 2001;25:602–9.

34. Fryer E1, Serra S, Chetty R. Lipid-rich ("clear cell") neuroendocrine tumors of the pancreas in MEN I patients. *Endocr Pathol* 2012;23:243–6.

35. Yachida S, Vakiani E, White CM et al. Small cell and large cell neuroendocrine carcinomas of the pancreas are genetically similar and distinct from well-differentiated pancreatic neuroendocrine tumors. *Am J Surg Pathol* 2012;36:173–84.

36. Jiao Y, Shi C, Edil BH et al. DAXX/ATRX, MEN1, and mTOR pathway genes are frequently altered in pancreatic neuroendocrine tumors. *Science* 2011;331:1199–203.

37. Yao JC, Shah MH, Ito T et al. RAD001 in Advanced Neuroendocrine Tumors, Third Trial (RADIANT-3) Study Group. Everolimus for advanced pancreatic neuroendocrine tumors. *N Engl J Med* 2011;364:514–23.

38. Raymond E, Dahan L, Raoul JL et al. Sunitinib malate for the treatment of pancreatic neuroendocrine tumors. *N Engl J Med* 2011;364:501–13.

37

Imaging of the pancreas

WILLIAM L. SIMPSON JR.

ANATOMY OF THE PANCREAS

The pancreas is a tongue-shaped retroperitoneal organ (Figure 37.1). It is located within the anterior pararenal space, along with the ascending and descending colon, as well as the duodenum. The pancreas is divided into the uncinate process, head, neck, body, and tail. The long axis of the gland most commonly follows an oblique course, with the head at the eight o'clock position and the tail at two o'clock. The normal dimensions of the pancreas depend on many factors, the most important of which is age. It is normally 12–15 cm in length. The head should measure up to 3.0–3.5 cm, the body up to 2.5 cm, and the tail up to 2.0 cm. These sizes are variable, and there is a great deal of variation. Generally, the gland tapers in size from head to tail. Fatty infiltration of the gland lobules is common with age. This gives the gland a more lace-like or feathery appearance. The pancreatic duct runs through the entire length of the gland and may measure up to 3.0 mm in the head and body and gradually tapers in the tail. It is often partially visualized, more commonly on thin-section computed tomography (CT). The common bile duct (CBD) passes through the pancreatic head before it joins the pancreatic duct near the ampulla of Vater. The size of the CBD in the pancreatic head varies with age as well but should never exceed 10 mm, often attaining the larger diameters in patients postcholecystectomy.

Anatomically, the organ sits posterior to the stomach with the potential space of the lesser sac between them. The left lobe of the liver is anterior as well. The spine,

aorta, and inferior vena cava are posterior to the pancreas. The head of the organ sits within the duodenal sweep. The tail extends up into the splenic hilum. The transverse mesocolon attaches to the anterior aspect of the pancreatic head.

There are important vascular landmarks related to the pancreas. The splenic vein lies along the dorsal aspect. The splenic vein and superior mesenteric vein join at the portal confluence posterior to the pancreatic head and neck. The uncinate process extends between the superior mesenteric vein and the inferior vena cava. The splenic artery usually follows a tortuous, serpiginous course behind the organ. It can easily be mistaken for pancreatic cysts or a dilated pancreatic duct on a noncontrast scan by novice observers. Splenic artery calcifications can also be mistaken for pancreatic parenchymal or ductal calcifications. The superior mesenteric artery originates off of the aorta posterior to the body of the pancreas, with a fat plane separating the two. The gastroduodenal artery runs along the anterior surface of the pancreatic neck.

IMAGING MODALITIES

The pancreas can be imaged with several modern radiologic modalities, including ultrasound (US), CT, and magnetic resonance (MR) imaging. There are several goals for imaging a patient with a suspected tumor: (1) establish the diagnosis, (2) localize the mass, (3) evaluate the extent of disease, (4) assess vascular involvement, and (5) search for distant metastases.

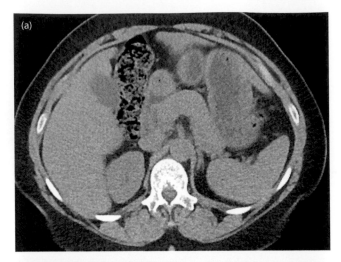

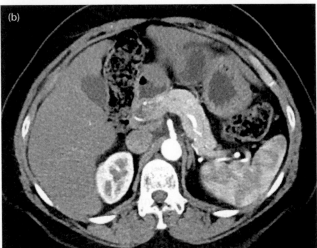

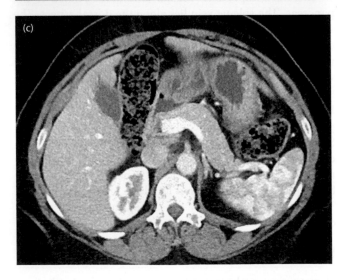

Figure 37.1 Normal CT appearance of the pancreas. The normal appearance of the pancreas on the non-contrast **(a)**, pancreatic **(b)** and portal venous **(c)** phases of a 3 phase pancreatic protocol scan. Due to the oblique positioning of the gland only portions of the neck and body are visualized on this axial slice. Notice the prominently enhanced splenic artery within the body on the pancreatic phase **(b)**. The portal confluence and part of the splenic vein are well seen on the portal phase **(c)**.

Ultrasound

In many patients, the pancreas can be visualized with transabdominal US. However, due to the deep retroperitoneal location of the organ and gas in the adjacent stomach, duodenum, and transverse colon, the evaluation is often limited. In addition, US is an operator-dependent modality that can also limit evaluation. Techniques such as fasting for 6–8 hours before the examination to limit bowel gas can be used to improve the study [1]. Conventional grayscale imaging is performed using 3–5 MHz multifrequency curved array transducers, with lower frequencies being used for better penetration. The pancreas should have a homogenous echotexture similar to that of the liver. However, with fatty infiltration the gland becomes echogenic. The use of tissue harmonic imaging has been shown to improve image quality and penetration when compared with grayscale US [2]. Color Doppler and power Doppler can be used to evaluate the vascular structures around the gland. Although not approved for use by the Food and Drug Administration in the United States, US contrast agents are used in many other countries for pancreatic assessment. Contrast-enhanced US can be used to identify lesions better than conventional grayscale US [3]. Similar to other cross section imaging modalities, contrast-enhanced sonography can be used to image the pancreas in various stages (pancreatic parenchymal, portal venous, and delayed) of enhancement.

Given the limitations listed above and the lack of availability of transabdominal US contrast agents in the United States, ultrasound is not a modality well suited for evaluation of pancreatic masses. However, many of these limitations are overcome by endoscopic US. With this form of US, the probe is inside the lumen of the stomach or duodenum, eliminating the issue of bowel gas. Given its proximity to the pancreas, a higher megahertz transducer can be used, resulting in higher-resolution images. The high resolution of these images permits identification of lesions as small as 2–3 mm and their relationship to adjacent blood vessels [4]. Endoscopic US is particularly useful in patients in whom a neuroendocrine tumor (NET) is suspected but not seen on other cross-sectional imaging modalities. In these patients, the sensitivity and specificity were found to be 82% and 92%, respectively [5].

Computed tomography

CT is the modality of choice for imaging the pancreas. Modern multidetector CT (MDCT) scanners permit rapid acquisition of thin-section data sets, high spatial resolution, multiphasic imaging, and multiplanar reconstruction. Although several different protocols can be used for pancreatic imaging, when a tumor is suspected, a three-phase protocol is utilized. It is important to acquire images of the pancreas and abdomen with thin sections of 3 mm or less. Current 64-channel scanners can image the entire abdomen with submillimeter sections within a single breath hold. A negative oral contrast medium such as water is used to evaluate for gastric or duodenal invasion by a pancreatic mass [6]. It is also helpful for evaluation of ampullary or periampullary tumors.

The three-phase pancreatic protocol consists of unenhanced, pancreatic parenchymal, and portal venous phases of the abdomen (Figure 37.1). Noncontrast images of the pancreas are useful for detecting parenchymal and ductal calcifications, as well as evaluating the size and contour of the gland. They also provide a baseline attenuation measurement for determination of enhancement of a mass after intravenous (IV) contrast administration. Since the pancreas is a very vascular gland, it enhances readily with contrast. The pancreatic parenchymal phase scan is obtained 35–40 seconds after intravenous contrast is injected. In this phase, there is maximal enhancement of the pancreatic parenchyma and also of the peripancreatic arteries. It allows easy differentiation of hypoattenuating masses such as adenocarcinoma and hyperattenuating masses such as NETs from the normal pancreatic parenchyma [7,8]. Since it is a late-arterial-phase scan, this phase can also be used to assess for hypervascular liver metastases. The portal venous phase is obtained 70 seconds after IV contrast is given. The portal, splenic, and superior mesenteric veins are well opacified in this phase. It can also be used to assess for hypodense liver metastases.

There are a few emerging CT techniques that hold promise for pancreas imaging. Dual-energy CT acquires data sets with at least two energy levels, commonly 140 and 80 kVp, although depending on the scanner configuration, additional energy levels are possible. Low-energy techniques have been shown to improve pancreatic enhancement after contrast administration and enhance the conspicuity of small pancreatic masses [9]. Dual-energy CT also allows for potential radiation dose reduction using a low tube voltage setting. In addition, with computer postprocessing, virtual unenhanced images can be produced from dual-energy data sets, saving radiation dose by eliminating the need for the unenhanced phase of the three-phase CT protocol [9]. Spectral CT is a form of dual-energy CT in which data sets are acquired using a single X-ray tube with rapid alternation between high-energy and low-energy settings. This allows (1) the data to be reconstructed along a spectrum of monochromatic energies and (2) the attenuation coefficients obtained at the two different energies to discriminate between different materials (such as fat, water, iodine, and calcium) to produce material density images [10]. CT perfusion refers to the transport of IV contrast material to a unit volume of tissue per unit of time. It involves the sequential CT scanning of the same volume over time, performed before, during, and after intravenous administration of contrast agents to trace the temporal changes in CT attenuation in the tissue volume of interest [11]. The CT perfusion technique has been used to evaluate and characterize pancreatic masses [12].

Magnetic resonance imaging

In the past, MR imaging of the pancreas was used mostly for problem solving when a diagnosis was unclear after CT. Today, with improvement in MR technology it is being used as a primary modality for evaluation (Figure 37.2). MR has several advantages over CT, including high soft tissue contrast, multiplanar imaging, and lack of ionizing radiation.

A typical MR pancreatic protocol includes a dual-echo T1-weighted sequence, a T2-weighted sequence, and a three-dimensional T1 sequence both before and after IV contrast administration. A magnetic resonance cholangiopancreatography (MRCP) sequence can also be added to the protocol. The pancreas has intrinsically high T1 signal. Therefore, it is well seen on a fat-suppressed T1 sequence. Moreover, with the India ink artifact seen at the interface of pancreatic tissue and the surrounding retroperitoneal fat on out-of-phase images, the pancreatic borders can be easily identified even in patients with a paucity of intra-abdominal fat. The pancreas has low to intermediate signal on a T2 sequence. T2-weighted images are helpful to show the pancreatic duct, the relationship of lesions to the duct, and the fluid content of pancreatic cystic lesions. A dynamic contrast-enhanced sequence includes precontrast, arterial, portal venous, and delay phase scans. These phases enable assessment of the briskly enhancing pancreatic parenchyma; the peripancreatic arteries, including the celiac axis, superior mesenteric, and splenic arteries; and the peripancreatic venous structures, including the splenic, superior mesenteric, and portal veins. The MRCP is a very heavily T2-weighted sequence that depicts the high signal within the biliary tree and pancreatic duct while suppressing signal from the surrounding organs. It is used to determine the relationship of a pancreatic mass to the pancreatic duct or CBD. A negative oral contrast can be used to null the high signal from fluid in the stomach and duodenum, which can obscure overlying ductal detail.

Similar to CT, there are emerging MR techniques that hold promise for pancreatic imaging. Perfusion imaging can be performed with MR similar to the CT technique to evaluate enhancement kinetics. Diffusion-weighted imaging (DWI) is an MR technique in which image contrast is due to differences in mobility of protons in water between different tissues [13]. Its application to oncologic imaging has shown that tumors generally restrict diffusion, leading to high signal on diffusion-weighted sequences. Thus, it can be used to detect pancreatic masses [14].

TUMORS

Adenocarcinoma

Most tumors of the pancreas arise from the ductal portion of the gland. These adenocarcinomas account for 85%–90% of all malignant pancreatic neoplasms, occur most commonly in the seventh and eighth decades of life, and have a 2:1 male-to-female prevalence [15]. Symptoms include abdominal pain, anorexia, weight loss, jaundice, and anemia, but they present late in the disease process. These tumors are most commonly located in the pancreatic head (70%–80%),

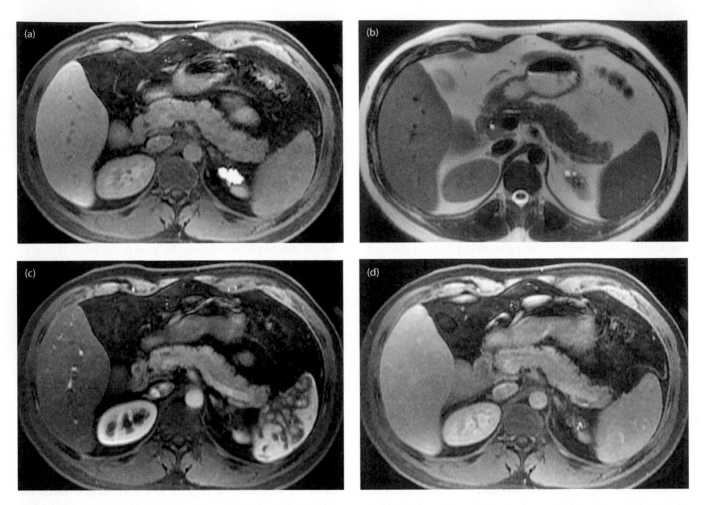

Figure 37.2 Normal MR appearance of the pancreas. The normal high signal intensity of the pancreas is seen on the fat saturated T1 sequence (a). On the T2 sequence the pancreatic parenchyma is low in signal and a portion of the high signal intensity pancreatic duct can be seen in the neck and body (b). Similar to the pancreatic phase on CT, the pancreas enhances briskly on the arterial phase after contrast administration (c). The pancreas homogenously enhances on the portal phase (d) with the pancreatic duct seen as a low signal structure.

with decreasing incidence in the body (10% to 20%) and tail (5% to 10%) [16]. Masses in the pancreatic head generally present earlier due to jaundice, whereas masses in the body and tail present later due to invasion of surrounding structures. The overall prognosis is poor, with a 1-year survival rate of <20% and a 5-year survival rate of <5% [17]. Surgery is the only potentially curative treatment, leading to a 20% 5-year survival rate when the tumor is small (<2 cm) without peripancreatic invasion [18]. However, only 10%–15% of tumors meet these criteria at diagnosis [19].

CT is the modality of choice for imaging pancreatic adenocarcinoma. The tumor is most commonly hypoattenuating on both the pancreatic and portal phases of scanning. The pancreatic phase shows optimal contrast between the tumor and the pancreatic parenchyma, as well as the peripancreatic arteries. The portal phase is best for evaluating metastatic disease to the liver and peritoneum and the peripancreatic veins. Approximately 10% of tumors are isoattenuating on all phases [17]. If the mass is not hypodense, then secondary signs such as a contour bulge, difference in parenchymal texture, duct obstruction, or distal glandular

atrophy can be sought. The classic double-duct sign is dilatation of both the CBD and the pancreatic duct due to an obstructing mass in the pancreatic head.

The main goals of imaging are to detect or localize the mass and determine resectability. CT is good for detecting tumors with a sensitivity of 89%–97% [20]. However, it does not fare as well when determining tumor resectability. For pancreatic carcinoma to be resectable, there must be no peripancreatic invasion and no metastatic disease. Criteria for unresectable tumors are listed in Table 37.1 [21]. CT has demonstrated a positive predictive value of 89%–100% for unresectability, but only a negative predictive value of 45%–79% for resectability [15]. Invasion of the peripancreatic vessels is one of the most common reasons for a pancreatic cancer not to be resectable. This includes not only occlusion of a vessel or complete encasement, but also if a mass is in contact with more than 180° of a vessel. Using these conditions, Vargas et al. showed an accuracy of 99% and negative predictive value of 100% in the detection of vascular invasion using MDCT and curved planar reconstructions [22].

Table 37.1 Criteria for unresectable pancreatic adenocarcinoma

1. Peri-pancreatic vascular invasion
   a. Vessel occlusion
   b. Complete vessel encasement
   c. Tumor touching >50% of the vessel circumference
2. Lymph node metastasis beyond the regional nodes
3. Liver metastasis
4. Peritoneal implants
5. Malignant ascites

On MR imaging, pancreatic adenocarcimoma is low signal on T1 images due to the high intrinsic signal in the normal pancreatic parenchyma. It is low signal on T2 images as well, likely due to a fibrotic component. After contrast administration, the tumor will enhance less than the normal pancreas, making it most conspicuous on the arterial phase images. The accuracy for the detection and staging of adenocarcinoma on MR is 90%–100% [23]. The use of DWI may allow earlier detection of pancreatic adenocarcinoma since these tumors demonstrate increased signal intensity [14].

Neuroendocrine tumors

NETs of the pancreas were formerly termed islet cell tumors, as they were believed to arise from the islet of Langerhans cells. However, new evidence suggests that these tumors may originate from pluripotential stem cells in ductal epithelium [24]. They are rare tumors with an incidence of 1.0–1.5 per 100,000 in the general population [25]. They account for 1%–5% of all pancreatic tumors, typically manifest in the fourth to sixth decades of life, and have equal gender distribution. Approximately half of these tumors are functional, meaning that they produce clinical symptoms from hormonal hypersecretion. The remainder are nonfunctional and come to medical attention due to symptoms from tumor size. The functional tumors include insulinoma, gastrinoma, glucagonoma, vasoactive intestinal peptide-oma (VIPoma), somatostatinoma, growth hormone–releasing factor-oma (GFRoma), adrenocorticotropic hormone-oma (ACTHoma), parathyroid hormone-like-oma (PTHoma), and neurotensinoma.

The majority of NETs occur sporadically, with 1%–2% associated with familial syndromes, including multiple endocrine neoplasia type 1 (MEN-1) and neurocutaneous syndromes, i.e., von Hippel–Lindau (VHL) syndrome, neurofibromatosis type 1 (NF-1), tuberous sclerosis, and Sturge–Weber syndrome. Tumors tend to be multiple when associated with syndromes. Tumor size and morphology are variable. In general, functioning tumors manifest early in the course of disease when they are small, due to the clinical manifestations of excessive hormone production. Nonfunctioning tumors manifest when they are large due to the lack of clinical symptoms.

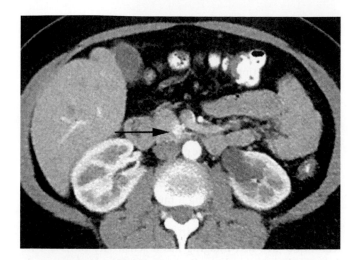

Figure 37.3 Functional NET. A small hypervascular insulinoma (arrow) is seen in the pancreatic head/uncinated process region on this pancreatic phase image.

Risk of malignancy increases with tumor size (especially in tumors of >5 cm), with 90% of nonfunctioning tumors being malignant at presentation. Small tumors are generally solid and homogeneous, whereas larger tumors are heterogeneous and may show cystic–necrotic degeneration and calcification [26].

The most common imaging feature of NETs is hypervasularity (Figure 37.3). These tumors are often more enhanced than the surrounding pancreatic parenchyma on arterial phase imaging due to a rich capillary network. Some remain enhanced compared with the pancreas on portal phase imaging, while many become isoattenuating. A sensitivity of 100% has been reported for the detection of NET on pancreatic phase CT scanning [27]. On MR imaging, these tumors are low signal on T1-weighted images and high signal on T2-weighted images. Similar to CT, they are hypervascular after contrast administration. DWI has not proven beneficial in the detection or evaluation of pancreatic NETs [14]. There are several imaging characteristics that can distinguish the more common adenocarcinoma from NET (Table 37.2).

Table 37.2 Differences between pancreatic adenocarcinoma and NETs

Characteristic	Adenocarcimona	Neuroendocrine Tumors
Enhancement	Hypovascular	Hypervascular
Vascular Involvement	Vessel encasement	Vessel infiltration
Calcification	Occurs in 2%	Occurs in 20%
Duct Involvement	Very common	Rare
Necrosis/cystic degeneration	Less common	More common especially in larger tumors

INSULINOMA

Insulinomas are the most common NET of the pancreas, accounting for about 40% of functioning NETs [28]. Due to the overproduction of insulin, they present with episodes of hypoglycemia that typically occur during fasting states or after exercise. They are predominantly benign (90%) and tend to be solitary and small (<2 cm) [29] (Figure 37.3). Moreover, 97% are located within the pancreas with an even distribution throughout the gland [28]. Due to the small size of these tumors, they are difficult to localize with CT preoperatively. Sensitivities ranging from 82% to 86% have been reported with MDCT using a multiphase protocol [29,30]. Since these tumors tend to be small, one study showed a sensitivity of 94.4% using thin sectioning with a dual-phase technique [31]. MR imaging has a sensitivity of 85%–94% for the detection of insulinomas [32,33]. Approximately 10%–30% of functioning NETs in patients with MEN-1 are insulinomas [28]. However, only 8% of patients with an insulinoma have MEN-1 syndrome [34]. MEN-associated insulinomas are more frequently multiple [16,21,28,34,35].

GASTRINOMA

Gastrinomas are the second most common NET [21,28,34,36]. The clinical manifestation of the tumor is due to the elevated levels of gastrin and is known as Zollinger–Ellison syndrome. The hypersecretion of gastrin stimulates the neuroendocrine cells to secrete histamine, which triggers the overproduction of gastric acid, resulting in peptic ulcer disease, often in unusual locations, as well as secretory diarrhea. As opposed to insulinomas, gastrinomas are predominantly malignant (60%–90%) [37]. These tumors tend to be small and preoperative localization is difficult; however, tumor size is a contributing factor, with the larger ones more easily identified. Up to 90% of gastrinomas are found in the gastrinoma triangle [38], a region bound by the junctions of the cystic duct and CBD superiorly, the second and third portions of the duodenum inferiorly, and the neck and body of the pancreas medially. CT can readily detect liver metastasis from malignant tumors. Approximately 20% of gastrinomas are associated with MEN-1 [28,36]. In fact, gastrinomas are the most common NET of the pancreas associated with MEN-1. As with insulinomas, MEN-associated gastrinomas are frequently multiple and malignant [25]. In addition, they are more commonly found located in the duodenum (~70%) than in the pancreas (~30%) [25,39].

GLUCAGONOMA

Glucagonoma is the third most common pancreatic NET. The clinical manifestation is known as the 4D syndrome: it consists of dermatitis, diabetes, deep venous thrombosis, and depression. The dermatitis refers to a specific rash termed necrolytic migratory erythema [28,34]. Glucagonomas most frequently occur between 40 and 60 years of age, and there is an equal gender distribution [40]. The majority of these tumors are single and originate in the pancreas, usually the body or tail [41]. They are usually larger than 4 cm at the time of imaging diagnosis. Tumor size is correlated with the malignancy risk. Up to 80% of glucagonomas larger than 5 cm demonstrate malignant behavior, and 50%–60% of patients have liver metastases at the time of diagnosis [42]. Glucagonomas are rarely associated with MEN-1 [28].

VASOACTIVE INTESTINAL PEPTIDE-OMA

VIP binds to receptors in the intestinal lumen to stimulate the secretion of sodium, chloride, potassium, and water into the bowel lumen, which results in secretory diarrhea, hypokalemia, and dehydration. Therefore, the clinical syndrome associated with VIPoma is often referred to as watery diarrhea, hypokalemia, and achlorhydria (WDHA) syndrome. The amount of diarrhea can be up to 6–8 L a day, leading to the other signs and severe dehydration. These tumors most frequently present in the fifth or sixth decade of life, have an equal gender distribution, and are rarely associated with MEN-1 [28]. At imaging, most VIPomas are solitary and larger than 5 cm and most commonly are located in the pancreatic tail [43]. At CT or MR imaging, smaller tumors may demonstrate homogeneous enhancement, while cystic change and calcification may be seen in larger ones [28]. The overwhelming majority of VIPomas are malignant, with metastases present in 60%–80% when they are initially diagnosed [44].

SOMATOSTATINOMA

Somatostatin functions to inhibit secretion of insulin, gastrin, glucagon, and cholecystokinin (CCK)-mediated pancreatic enzymes. The clinical presentation is nonspecific; however, the classic presentation of a somatostatinoma syndrome includes diabetes due to somatostatin's inhibitory effect on insulin secretion, cholelithiasis due to inhibition of CCK and gallbladder contractility, and steatorrhea due to inhibition of pancreatic enzyme and bicarbonate secretion [34]. The mean age at presentation is 50 years, and there is an equal gender distribution [42]. These tumors most frequently occur in the pancreatic head or periampullary region of the duodenum. Somatostatinomas demonstrate hypervascularity and can show cystic change and calcification when large. They are most commonly malignant often with metastases [42]. Duodenal somatostatinomas have a higher association with NF-1 than pancreatic tumors. In fact, one review showed that 43% of patients with a duodenal somatostatinoma have NF-1 compared with 1.2% of patients with a pancreatic somatostatinoma [45].

OTHER FUNCTIONAL NETs

The other functional NETs, including GFRoma, ACTHoma, PTHoma, and neurotensinoma, are extremely rare, similar to VIPoma and somatostatinoma. All these tumors have relatively nonspecific presentations. The tumors tend to be large at presentation and are frequently malignant [28,34].

NONFUNCTIONING NET

Nonfunctioning NET is somewhat of a misnomer. This term derives from the fact that these tumors do not have an associated syndrome related to hormone hypersecretion. In fact, these tumors may produce (1) high levels of a hormone that has no clinical symptoms, such as pancreatic polypeptide (PP); (2) small amounts of a functionally active hormone; (3) an inactive precursor hormone; or (4) an inactive form of a hormone [28,34]. The symptoms from non-functioning NET are most commonly due to mass effect. The most common symptom is abdominal pain, followed by weight loss. Jaundice can occur if the mass obstructs the CBD in the pancreatic head.

Without specific symptoms to prompt investigation, nonfunctioning NETs present later than functional NETs. They are increasingly found incidentally. In one study, 35% were incidentally discovered [46]. Nonfunctioning NETs are generally larger than functioning ones, with an average size of 5–6 cm, and can be located in any part of the pancreas [28]. Because of their large size, most demonstrate heterogeneity with areas of cystic degeneration and necrosis at

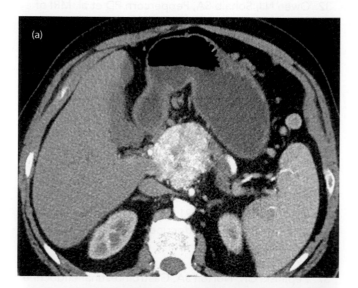

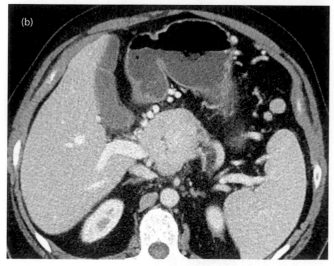

Figure 37.4 Nonfunctioning NET. A large hypervascular mass is seen in the pancreatic neck on the pancreatic phase **(a)** which become iso-attenuating to the pancreatic parenchyma on the portal phase **(b)**.

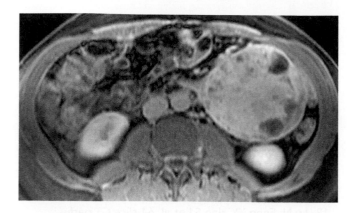

Figure 37.5 Metastatic disease to the liver from a malignant NET. A large prominently enhancing mesenteric lymph node is seen on the left side of the abdomen anterior to the lower pole of the left kidney on this MR image in a patient with a nonfunctioning pancreas NET. The mass demonstrates low signal areas around the periphery indicating areas of necrosis.

imaging (Figure 37.4). Calcification can commonly be seen [29]. These findings make them easily detected by CT or MR imaging. These tumors have a high incidence of malignancy with 60%–80% demonstrating metastatic disease at diagnosis [42,46] (Figure 37.5). The nonfunctioning NET is the most common NET in patients with MEN-1 or VHL syndrome [47]. Similar to other NETs, multiple tumors occur more commonly in familial syndromes.

REFERENCES

1. Zamboni GA, Ambrosetti MC, D'Onofrio M, Mucelli RP. Ultrasonogrphy of the pancreas. *Radiol Clin North Am* 2012;50:395–406.
2. Shapiro RS, Wagreich J, Parsons RB et al. Tissue harmonic imaging sonography: Evaluation of image quality compared with conventional sonography. *AJR Am J Roentgenol* 1998;171(5):1203–6.
3. D'Onofrio M, Zamboni G, Faccioli N et al. Ultrasonography of the pancreas. 4. Contrast-enhanced imaging. *Abdom Imaging* 2007;32(2):171–81.
4. Varadarajulu S, Eloubeidi MA. The role of endoscopic sonography in the evaluation of pancreaticobiliary cancer. *Surg Clin North Am* 2010;90:251–63.
5. Rosch T, Lightdale CJ, Botet JF et al. Localization of pancreatic endocrine tumors by endoscopic ultrasonography. *N Engl J Med* 1992;326:1721–6.
6. Bashir MR, Gupta RT. MDCT evaluation of the pancreas: Nuts and bolts. *Radiol Clin North Am* 2012;50:365–77.
7. Fletcher JG, Wiersema MJ, Farrell MA et al. Pancreatic malignancy: Value of arterial, pancreatic, and hepatic phase imaging with multi-detector row CT. *Radiology* 2003;229(1):81–90.
8. Balthhazar EJ. Staging of acute pancreatitis. *Radiol Clin North Am* 2002;40:1199–311.

9. Marin D, Nelson RC, Barnhart H et al. Detection of pancreatic tumors, image quality, and radiation dose during the pancreatic parenchymal phase: Effect of a low-tube-voltage, high-tube-current CT technique—Preliminary results. *Radiology* 2010;256(2):450–9.

10. Silva AC, Morse BG, Hara AK et al. Dual energy (spectral) CT: Applications in abdominal imaging. *Radiographics* 2011;31:1031–46.

11. Kim SH, Kamaya A, Willmann JK. CT perfusion of the liver: Principles and applications in oncology. *Radiology* 2014;272:322–44.

12. Lu N, Feng XY, Hao SJ et al. 64-slice CT perfusion imaging of pancreatic adenocarcinoma and mass-forming chronic pancreatitis. *Acad Radiol* 2011;18(1):81–8.

13. Taouli B, Koh DM. Diffusion weighted MR imaging of the liver. *Radiology* 2010;254:47–66.

14. Wang Y, Miller FH, Chen ZE et al. Diffusion weighted MR imaging of solid and cystic lesions of the pancreas. *Radiographics* 2011;31:E47–65.

15. Ros PR, Mortele KJ. Imaging features of pancreatic neoplasms. *JBR-BTR* 2001;84:239–49.

16. Low G, Panu A, Millo N, Leen E. Multimodality imaging of neoplastic and nonneoplastic solid lesions of the pancreas. *Radiographics* 2011;31:993–1015.

17. Brennan DD, Zamboni GA, Rastopoulos VD, Kruskal JB. Comprehensive preoperative assessment of pancreatic adenocarcinoma with 64 section volumetric CT. *Radiographics* 2007;27:1653–66.

18. Tsiotos GG, Farnell MB, Sarr MG. Are the results of pancreatectomy for pancreatic cancer improving? *World J Surg* 1999;23:913–9.

19. Beger HG, Rau B, Gansauge F et al. Treatment of pancreatic cancer: Challenge of the facts. *World J Surg* 2003;27:1075–84.

20. Freeny PC, Traverso LW, Ryan JA. Diagnosis and staging of pancreatic adenocarcinoma with dynamic computed tomography. *Am J Surg* 1993;165:600–6.

21. Paspulati RM. Multidetector CT of the pancreas. *Radiol Clin North Am* 2005;43:999–1020.

22. Vargas R, Nino-Murcia M, Trueblood W et al. MDCT in pancreatic adenocarcinoma: Prediction of vascular invasion and resectability using a multiphasic technique with curved planar reformations. *AJR Am J Roentgenol* 2004;182:419–25.

23. Hanbidge AE. Cancer of the pancreas: The best image for early detection—CT, MRI, PET or US? *Can J Gastroenterol* 2002;16(2):101–5.

24. Oberg K, Eriksson B. Endocrine tumours of the pancreas. *Best Pract Res Clin Gastroenterol* 2005;19(5):753–81.

25. Delcore R, Friesen SR. Gatrointestinal neuroendocrine tumors. *J Am Coll Surg* 1994;178:187–211.

26. Noone TC, Hosey J, Firat Z, Semelka RC. Imaging and localization of islet-cell tumours of the pancreas on CT and MRI. *Best Pract Res Clin Endocrinol Metab* 2005;19(2):195–211.

27. Fidler JL, Fletcher JG, Reading CC et al. Preoperative detection of pancreatic insulinomas on multiphasic helical CT. *AJR Am J Roentgenol* 2003;181(3):775–80.

28. Lewis RB, Lattin GE, Paal E. Pancreatic endocrine tumors: Radiologic-clinicopathologic correlation. *Radiographics* 2010;30:1445–64.

29. Van Hoe L, Gryspeerdt S, Marchal G et al. Helical CT for the preoperative localization of islet cell tumors of the pancreas. *AJR Am J Roentgenol* 1995;165:1437–9.

30. King AD, Ko GT, Yeung VT et al. Dual phase spiral CT in the detection of small insulinomas of the pancreas. *Br J Radiol* 1998;71:20–3.

31. Gouya H, Vignaux O, Augui J et al. CT, endoscopic sonography, and a combined protocol for preoperative evaluation of pancreatic insulinomas. *AJR Am J Roentgenol* 2003;181:987–92.

32. Owen NJ, Sohaib SA, Peppercorn PD et al. MRI of pancreatic neuroendocrine tumours. *Br J Radiol* 2001;74:968–73.

33. Thoeni RF, Mueller-Lisse UG, Chan R, Do NK, Shyn PB. Detection of small, functional islet cell tumors in the pancreas: Selection of MR imaging sequences for optimal sensitivity. *Radiology* 2000;214:483–90.

34. Heller MT, Shah AB. Imaging of neuroendocrine tumors. *Radiol Clin North Am* 2011;49:529–48.

35. Demeure MJ, Klonoff DC, Karam JH et al. Insulinomas associated with multiple endocrine neoplasia type 1: The need for a different surgical approach. *Surgery* 1991;110:998–1004.

36. Norton JA. Neuroendocrine tumors of the pancreas and duodenum. *Curr Probl Surg* 1994;31:77–164.

37. Peplinski GR, Norton JA. Gastrointestinal endocrine cancers and nodal metastases: Biological significance and therapeutic implications. *Surg Oncol Clin North Am* 1996;5:159–71.

38. Stabile BE, Morrow DJ, Passaro E Jr. The gastrinoma triangle: Operative implications. *Am J Surg* 1984;147(1):25–31.

39. Klöppel G, Anlauf M. Pancreatic endocrine tumors. *Pathol Case Rev* 2006;11:256–67.

40. Chastain MA. The glucagonoma syndrome: A review of its features and discussion of new perspectives. *Am J Med Sci* 2001;321:306–20.

41. Aldridge MC, Williamson RC. Surgery of endocrine tumors of the pancreas. In: Lynn JA, Bloom SR, eds., *Surgical Endocrinology*. New York: Butterworth, 1993:503.

42. Mansour JC, Chen H. Pancreatic endocrine tumors. *J Surg Res* 2004;120:139–61.

43. Ghaferi AA, Chojnacki KA, Long WD, Cameron JL, Yeo CJ. Pancreatic VIPomas: Subject review and one institutional experience. *J Gastrointest Surg* 2008;12:382–93.

44. Smith SL, Branton SA, Avino AJ et al. Vasoactive intestinal polypeptide secreting islet cell tumors: A 15-year experience and review of the literature. *Surgery* 1998;124:1050–5.

45. Soga J, Yakuwa Y. Somatostatinoma/inhibitory syndrome: A statistical evaluation of 173 reported cases as compared to other pancreatic endocrinomas. *J Exp Clin Cancer Res* 1999;18:13–22.

46. Gullo L, Migliori M, Falconi M et al. Nonfunctioning pancreatic endocrine tumors: A multicenter clinical study. *Am J Gastroenterol* 2003;98:2435–9.

47. Binkovitz LA, Johnson CD, Stephens DH. Islet cell tumors in von Hippel-Lindau disease: Increased prevalence and relationship to the multiple endocrine neoplasias. *AJR Am J Roentgenol* 1990;155:501–5.

38

Insulinoma

PER HELLMAN AND PETER STÅLBERG

INTRODUCTION

Insulinomas are rare tumors, with an approximated annual incidence of 1–4 per 1 million [1]. They may be sporadic or a part of an inherited syndrome, most often multiple endocrine neoplasia type 1 (MEN1). Similar symptoms exhibit in the even rarer condition of noninsulinoma pancreatogenous hypoglycemia syndrome (NIPHS). The key symptoms encompass neuroglycopenic and hypoglycemic ones, and diagnosis aims to verify this biochemically, while imaging is used to localize the tumor(s). For the surgeon, diagnosis and imaging are both extremely important before embarking on surgery; otherwise, unnecessary surgery may ensue. The main problems are the sometimes nonspecific symptoms not recognized as hypoglycemia, with potential devastating consequences, including permanent hypoglycemic brain damage; the sometimes difficult localization procedures; and the potential of malignancy, multiple tumors in MEN1, and, rarely, diffuse hyperplasia resembling nesidioblastosis.

HISTORY

The knowledge about insulin and insulin-producing tumors began in the 1920s, when Banting and Best discovered insulin [2]. Indeed, even earlier, Paul Langerhans had described the pancreatic islets [3,4]. The first attempt to surgically cure a patient with an unresectable insulin-producing tumor was performed in 1926 on an orthopedic surgeon, Dr. Dickinson, by William J. Mayo [5], followed by the first successful resection of a benign insulinoma by Dr. Graham in 1929 [6]. A couple of years later, Whipple discovered the triad of symptoms being so characteristic for hypoglycemia: hypoglycemia provoked by fasting, circulating glucose of less than 50 mg/dL at time of symptoms, and relief after administration of glucose. Since this discovery in the mid-1930s, development has until today been focused on more precise diagnostic methods, avoiding false-positive results, and more recently, highly sensitive imaging and minimally invasive and safe surgical methods to reduce complications.

DEMOGRAPHICS

Insulinoma is one of several causes for organic hyperinsulinism. The low annual incidence of approximately four per million seems to be constant over the years [7]. Epidemiological data of classical insulinoma patients describe a median age of approximately 48 years, but with a considerable range. In the literature, patients from 8 up to 88 years of age are reported. Slightly more than half are females (approximately 58%), about 7%–15% are ultimately found to suffer from MEN1, and approximately 8%–10% are found to be malignant [8–10].

A minority of patients suffer from NIPHS, also denoted as adult nesidioblastosis, associated with considerable difficulties in localization and surgical decision-making. Although extremely rare, there are studies indicating a higher incidence than anticipated [11].

PHYSIOLOGY AND PATHOPHYSIOLOGY

Glucose

Glucose is an obligatory and continuous supply from the circulation and is crucial for maintenance for brain function. Upon hypoglycemia, this is normally corrected by a decrease in insulin secretion, but also increased glucagon and eventually epinephrine release. Symptoms of hypoglycemia will usually develop below 55 mg/dL (3.0 mmol/L), and normally insulin secretion is reduced to below 3 µU/mL (18 pmol/L), with a concomitant fall in C-peptide levels (below 0.6 ng/mL; 0.2 nmol/L) [12]. In even lower glucose levels, insulin secretion is suppressed more or less totally [13]. The symptoms, and fall in hypoglycemia, occur when glucose utilization in muscles, kidney, and erythrocytes exceeds glucose production in the liver and kidney, together with carbohydrate ingestion. Thus, fasting and physical exercise are well-known triggers for hypoglycemia.

Insulin

Proinsulin is produced in the pancreatic beta-cell, and before secretion cleaved into insulin and the remaining C-peptide [12]. The secretory granules consist of equal molar amounts of insulin and C-peptide, which is important in the diagnostic assay (see below). In addition, exogenously administered insulin contains no C-peptide, which together with the longer half-life of C-peptide makes serum levels of this cleavage product an important marker to discover the occasional patients with factitious hypoglycemia due to self-administration of insulin or oral sulfonylurea preparations. Such individuals do occur, and are reported among patients who have undergone diagnostic and even operative procedures for supposed endogenous hyperinsulinism and hypoglycemia [14].

The unregulated autonomous secretion of insulin is characteristic of an insulin-producing tumor. Thus, even though serum glucose levels decline, and may worsen during fasting or physical exercise, the insulin level remains, although not necessary pathologically high.

Occasional ovarial carcinomas may rarely produce insulin. In addition, insulin growth factor (IGF) 1 or 2 may, if secreted in sufficient amounts, also cause hypoglycemia by binding to the insulin receptors. Such a mechanism may also be seen in hepatocellular or breast carcinomas [15,16].

GENETICS AND PATHOLOGY

Benign insulinomas

In a meta-analysis of 6222 cases, 87.1% of insulinomas were benign [17], and they have a good survival. Five-year survival rates are reported to be 60%–100%. The cause of insulinoma has for a long time been obscure. Studies in rats, however, have shown that the chemokine (C-X-C motif) ligand 12 (CXCL12) is a pre-beta-cell growth-stimulating factor [18,19], and overexpression of this gene leads to resistance to apoptosis, and consequently lack of diabetes [20]. Yin Yang 1 (YY1) is a ubiquitous zinc-finger transcription factor that regulates transcription [21], and studies have shown that YY1 strongly activates transcription of CXCL12 [22]. Mutations in YY1 are demonstrated at T372R in the third functional zinc-finger domain in YY1 responsible for transcriptional repression [23,24], implying an activation of the transcription of genes specific for leading to increased insulin secretion and beta-cell proliferation (ADCY1 and CACNAD2D2), and subsequently to insulinoma formation. The mutation was found in approximately 30% of investigated insulinomas. Other reports demonstrate a gain at chromosome locus 9q34 in insulinomas [25].

Histopathology of the usually benign tumor (World Health Organization [WHO] group 1) demonstrates a uniform tumor in 84% of cases smaller than 2 cm in size [17], while identification of tumors greater than 1 cm is rare (1.6% in Mehrabi et al. [17]). They are usually nonangioinvasive and have a <2% Ki-67 proliferation index, but they do not necessarily express insulin, possibly due to the enhanced release of peptides from active tumor cells. The tumor is generally yellow to reddish-brownish with a pseudocapsule, normally allowing extirpation without seriously affecting the surrounding normal pancreas. They may reside anywhere in the pancreas, and ectopic location is extremely rare.

Malignant insulinomas

Malignant insulinomas have a much worse clinical course and survival than the benign ones. Five-year survival rates range between 20% and 40% depending on extent of disease. Predictors for malignant disease are tumor size of ≥2 cm, Ki-67 of ≥2%, signs of angioinvasion and perineural space invasion, and findings of chromosomal lesions (loss at 3p or 6q and gain on 7q, 12q, or 14q) [26,27]. Also, mutations in YY1 were found in a subset of malignant insulinomas [23]. Some patients suffer from large pancreatic tumors classified as nonfunctioning but which may nevertheless secrete amounts of usually proinsulin (or IGF1 or IGF2) that may induce hypoglycemia. Malignant insulinomas may be discovered pre- or intraoperatively by the finding of metastases or tumor infiltration, or postoperatively by the pathologist who detects microscopic infiltration. The rate of malignancy is about 8%–10% in different series [17].

MEN1

It is of utmost importance to regularly exclude MEN1 in any patients who demonstrate an insulinoma, in particular multiple tumors, being present in 7%–15% [17]. MEN1 is an autosomal dominant disorder due to mutation in the *MEN1* gene on chromosome 11 encoding the nuclear protein menin [28,29], and characterized by primary hyperparathyroidism, anterior pituitary adenomas, and tumors of the endocrine pancreas and duodenum, and among the most common functional islet cell tumors are insulinomas and gastrinomas [30]. Today, genetic testing for mutations in the *MEN1* gene is possible and should be performed for all insulinoma patients. The protein product encoded for by the *MEN1* gene functions as a transcription factor, interacting with many proteins, such as histone–methylase transferase (HMT) complexes leading to epigenetic silencing due to hypermethylation [31], which seem to be important for especially the cell cycle regulators p18 (CDKN2C) and p27 (CDKN1β) [32].

Mutation in the *MEN1* gene is obviously present in MEN1 patients, but whether additional molecular derangements occur in those that develop specifically insulinomas is unknown. However, mutation in the *MEN1* gene seems to be absent, or very rare, in sporadic cases [23,24,33].

It should also be noted that the MEN1 patients usually demonstrate a number of pancreatic tumors, ranging in size from microscopically small over the whole pancreas to largely invasive and malignant tumors (Figure 38.1).

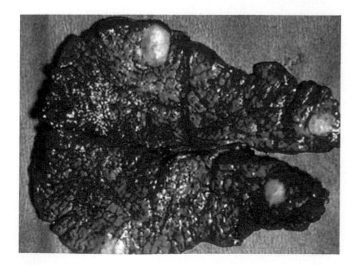

Figure 38.1 Multiple tumors in a resected pancreas from a patient with MEN1.

These tumors may produce a variety of hormones, and subsets of them may produce insulin, sometimes, due to the size of the tumor, in enough amounts to cause organic hyperinsulinism with the classical symptoms thereof [34].

The presence of MEN1 has great implications on treatment strategies, including the surgical procedure (see below).

NIPHS

NIPHS is rare and histopathologically characterizes the presence of enlarged islet cells—islet hypertrophy—and also an increased number of islets [35]. Also, some reports note budding of insulin-positive cells from the ducts of hormonally active cells budding off the ductular epithelium [36]. Genetically, not much is known in adult NIPHS, although an activating mutation in the *GCK* gene (glucokinase) has been reported [37]. Presumably, this occurs in families, but the penetrance is low and variable, clinically not detected in all mutated individuals.

CLINICAL FEATURES

The classical symptoms related to insulinoma described by Whipple [3] are (1) symptoms from hypoglycemia, such as the feeling of hunger, tremor, dizziness, etc.; (2) plasma glucose levels less than 50 mg/dL; and (3) relief of symptoms after glucose administration. These symptoms are typically aggravated after physical exercise.

One may be somewhat more specific regarding the symptoms and divide them into signs due to glycopenia, such as pure hunger, and neuroglycopenic symptoms, including tiredness, difficulties in awakening, confusion, seizures, abnormal behavior such as sudden aggressiveness, diplopia, blurred vision, paresthesias or even paralysis of a leg, lethargy, and even loss of consciousness and coma [38]. The neuroglycopenic symptoms, which may be vague and difficult to appreciate, are often the only signs of the underlying insulinoma, and should always suggest a diagnosis of hypoglycemia due to organic hyperinsulinism [38].

Psychological symptoms may be most apparent to the relatives of hypoglycemic patients. They often describe personality changes, various degrees of confusion, and aggressiveness or dementia-like behavior, which often occur fleetingly, and are sometimes difficult to recognize except by the closest relatives.

As a response, activation of the sympathetic system leads to palpitations, tremor, sweating, and anxiety. It is common that other diagnoses have been suggested before the glycopenia is discovered, mostly psychiatric or neurologic diagnoses.

As a usual consequence of this, weight gain over a defined period is commonly, but not always, seen. The reason is overconsumption of carbohydrates to relieve symptoms, but in physically active individuals, increased intake is consumed during exercise and no weight gain is seen.

Hypoglycemia, whether associated with coma or not, has the risk of causing permanent brain damage and persistent personality changes, even after a successful operation [8].

The symptoms may vary among the hypoglycemic individuals, although each patient seems to respond similarly during each attack [39]. The symptoms may lead to various incidents among the patients, including the relatively high frequency of patients involved in traffic accidents [40].

Although Whipple's symptomatic triad often is present, it is often not recognized immediately. The onset symptoms may precede the diagnosis by a considerably long interval: in one European study, an average of 3.1 years, and in a previous Mayo Clinic series, 46 months. Individual patients may have suffered several decades before diagnosis, as was the case of one patient in the Mayo series who had a 52-year-long history [40,41]. More recent reports have not demonstrated reduced time before diagnosis; in spite of that, imaging has improved dramatically in the last decade.

It is always important to suspect MEN1 in patients with organic hypoglycemia, especially if a lesion is diagnosed on imaging. Therefore, family history and associated measurements of serum calcium and serum parathyroid hormone should be performed routinely. In diagnosed individuals, genetic screening should be performed.

Not all patients with the above-mentioned symptoms have insulinoma, which should also be investigated (see below).

BIOCHEMICAL ASSAYS

Basal measurements

Neuroglycopenic symptoms associated with low blood glucose levels and concomitant inappropriately high serum insulin levels are the classical findings of organic hypoglycemia and insulinoma. To verify the diagnosis, a fasting test is mandatory (see below). Generally, a blood glucose of <55 mg/dL (3.0 mmol/L) is rarely seen, while levels of <40 mg/dL (<2 mmol/L) are never seen in healthy individuals, and symptoms associated with levels above 70 mg/dL (3.9 mmol/L) indicate that the symptoms are not due to hypoglycemia [42]. Also, in obese individuals with peripheral insulin resistance, as well as in patients who have undergone gastric bypass, similar symptoms and biochemical signs may appear [43]. Important to note is that a normal serum glucose level concomitant with developing symptoms excludes insulinoma as a diagnosis.

Serum insulin is nowadays measured by highly sensitive immunoradiometric or enzyme-linked immunological methods. The s-insulin level may, however, not be raised when measured during a hypoglycemic attack; in one series, only 10 out of 29 patients had elevated s-insulin [40]. However, lack of feedback regulation of insulin secretion in patients with hypoglycemia implies that a detectable s-insulin in patients with s-glucose of <40 mg/dL (2 mmol/L) supports a diagnosis of insulinoma [44]. However, insulin levels should be at least 3.0 μU/mL (18 pmol/L). Measurements of

the insulin/glucose ratio seem to be insensitive in several series, and should not be used [44].

Proinsulin may be selectively measured by specific assays, and is also reported to be pathologically high in insulinoma patients [45,46]. Ninety percent of insulinoma patients have increased basal proinsulin values (>0.2 ng/mL; 22 pmol/L). Remarkably, high proinsulin levels are indicative of malignant insulinoma.

Alternative diagnoses

Alternative diagnoses that cause hypoglycemia have to be ruled out, and most important is the factitious use of insulin or hypoglycemic drugs. Differentiation is done by measurements of C-peptide and proinsulin, which are normal in these cases. C-peptide is cleaved off from proinsulin, and is not present in commercial products. Therefore, a level of at least 0.6 ng/mL (0.2 nmol/L) indicates endogenous hyperinsulinism. A number of diagnoses other than pancreatogenous origin occur as noted (Table 38.1). After ruling out factitious insulin delivery, the increasing number of individuals who have undergone bariatric surgery may need specific attention. In a small subset of these, pancreatogenous nesidioblastosis may develop, especially after Roux-en-Y gastric bypass (RYGB), and in an initial Mayo series, they were treated with pancreatic resection [47]. The majority of patients with neuroglycopenic symptoms after RYGB respond to nutritional and medical treatment, and further investigations have focused on the importance of

Table 38.1 Differential diagnoses for hypoglycemia

Diabetes mellitus (approximately 2/3)[a]
Critical illness
Organ failure (liver, kidney, and cardiac)
Sepsis (approximately 1/4)
Tumors/organic lesions
Insulinoma
Noninsulinomic pancreategonous hypoglycemic syndrome
Post–gastric bypass hypoglycemia
IGF1 producing tumors (HCC)
IGF2 producing tumors (variety of tumors)
Autoimmune disorders
Insulin autoantibodies
Insulin receptor autoantibodies
Drugs
Insulin
Sulfonyl urea
Alcohol
Hormone deficiency
Cortisol (Addison's, postadrenalectomy, and adrenal insufficiency)
Glucagon

[a] From Fischer KF et al. N Engl J Med 1986;315:1245–50.

increased release of glucagon-like peptide 1 (GLP1). GLP1 is synthesized from the proximal jejunum, increases 10- to 15-fold after bariatric gastric bypass, and stimulates the receptors in beta-cells to produce excess insulin. A number of treatments are reported: low-carbohydrate diets, inhibition of glucose intestinal uptake, reduction of insulin secretion with calcium channel blockers, somatostatin analogs, diazoxide, a potassium ATP channel opener, and GLP1 analogs have been used [48]. In a review of the minority who apparently needed surgical correction for their symptoms, out of 75 patients, 51 had undergone pancreatic resection (of whom 34 [67%] were normalized), 17 RYGB reversal (76% normalized), and the remainder a number of other procedures to surgically cope with the problem [43].

Autoantibodies toward endogenous insulin may cause hypoglycemia; diagnostic testing is difficult, as the results may mimic insulinoma [49]. The condition is present at a higher frequency in persons of Japanese or Korean ethnicity [50]. The patients generally present with extreme levels of serum insulin, presumably due to cross-reaction with the antibodies, and the condition is usually treatable with lifestyle modifications. On the other hand, C-peptide levels may still be indicative of the diagnosis in these patients.

Fasting test

The most frequently used diagnostic test is a prolonged fast aimed at lasting originally 72 hours, but studies have shown that 48 hours is enough [45,46]. The fast must be supervised since the patient may develop symptoms, but also to hinder patients from taking food to reduce the developing symptoms. The latter is not unusual and must be clearly described to the patients. A patient with insulinoma extremely rarely stands a fast for more than 48 hours, and approximately 50% for only 12 hours [46]. The recent development of more sensitive assays for measurements of insulin and proinsulin, and thorough analyses of performed fasting tests have clarified cutoff values and increased the sensitivity of the test [45,46].

The appearance of neuroglycopenic symptoms and the presence of nonsuppressed serum insulin, which rarely falls below 10 µU/mL, and B-glucose lower than <55 mg/dL (<3.0 mmol/L) are highly suspicious for an insulinoma and the fast should be aborted. If levels of C-peptide are also >200 pmol/L (0.6 ng/mL) during a symptomatic episode, this strengthens the diagnosis. Serum measurements of proinsulin are nowadays also highly sensitive, and 80% of insulinoma patients have increased levels above 0.2 ng/mL (22 pmol/L) at the end of the fast [46]. In addition, samples for beta-hydroxybutyrate and sulfonylurea are drawn, to detect signs of exogenously administered drugs. The fasting test has a high positive predictive value, while a negative result is difficult to interpret, and does occur in patients who subsequently had successful resection of insulinoma.

If the diagnosis is still uncertain after the fasting test, the test should be repeated. Previously, provocative testing was common, which rarely is needed today, due to the increased sensitivity of imaging (see below).

Usually, in a patient with documented fasting endogenous hyperinsulinemic hypoglycemia, with negative screening for hypoglycemic agents, and without circulating insulin autoantibodies, the next step is localization.

LOCALIZATION

Surgery is the only method that may cure the patient, and therefore is the method of choice. The aim of the imaging is not only localization of the tumor, but also planning for type of surgery, to eventually avoid postoperative diabetes mellitus, as well as detect signs of eventual spread of disease. The preoperative workup has changed during the years, with most centers today applying two independent methods for localization, but also relying on intraoperative techniques. The success rate of localization procedures is slowly increasing [17,51].

Preoperative noninvasive methods

After the biochemical diagnosis is set or highly suspected, localization should be performed. Today, highly sensitive imaging is possible, and in up to 80%–90% of cases, insulinomas may be localized by endoscopic ultrasound (EUS), computed tomography (CT) with visualization in the arterial and venous contrast phases, or magnetic resonance tomography (MRT) using gadolinium enhancement and fat suppression (Figures 38.2 through 38.4) [44,52]. CT without dynamic contrast enhancement has an extremely low sensitivity, while triphasic CT may reach sensitivities up to 90% [53,54]. MRT has a slightly lower sensitivity and is usually not the first method of choice. Recent developments with diffusion-weighted MRT may enhance the sensitivity [55]. EUS has the highest sensitivity (70%–95%), which also allows clarification of eventual proximity to the pancreatic duct [56,57]. Two main instruments are available, one with

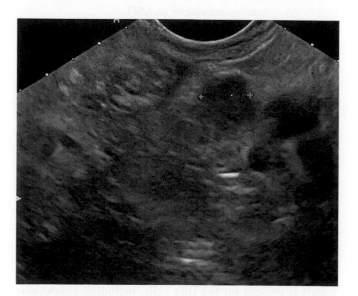

Figure 38.2 EUS image of an insulinoma in the body of the pancreas.

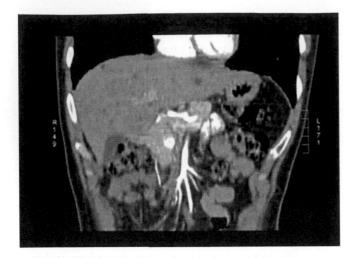

Figure 38.3 CT of a highly vascularized insulinoma in the head of the pancreas.

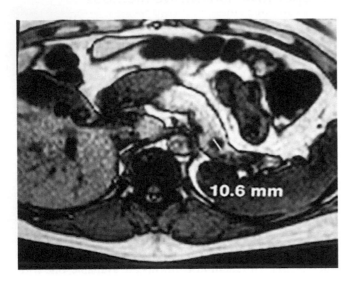

Figure 38.4 Insulinoma visible on MRT.

a rotating radial scanner allowing constant visualization of 360° and one with a sector scanner, in some cases noted to have difficulties in visualizing the leftmost part of the tail [58]. The resolution limit is about 4 mm.

If these methods fail to localize the insulinoma, somatostatin receptor–targeted imaging, such as scintigraphy with ^{111}In-labeled somatostatin analogs (Octreoscan®) or, better, ^{68}Ga-DOTATOC or ^{68}Ga-DOTATATE positron emission tomography (PET), may be used. However, the density of somatostatin receptors may be low in some insulinomas, leading to negative imaging, especially using the more insensitive scintigraphy [59,60]. In such cases, PET with ^{11}C-labeled 5-hydroxy-tryptophane (5-HTP) PET may also be used (Figure 38.5) [61]. In the future, the most promising tool seems to be using targets for the GLP1 receptor, which is present on the islet cells, including insulinoma cells. Initial studies are extremely promising [62–65].

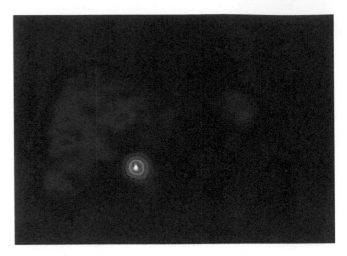

Figure 38.5 PET using ^{11}C-hydroxy-tryptophane as tracer for preoperative visualization of an otherwise unlocalized insulinoma.

Regular transabdominal US has a low sensitivity, in different series ranging from 8% to 66%, sometimes with a high false-positive rate. Contrast-enhanced transabdominal US has higher sensitivity (75%–85%) in some hands [66,67], but is highly dependent on the operator, as well as on the patient's body mass index (BMI) [68] and tumor size.

Invasive methods

Two invasive methods aimed at biochemical diagnosis have been used previously: transhepatic portal vein sampling and the arterial stimulation and venous sampling (ASVS) test (or selective arterial calcium stimulation [SACS]). The experience with portal venous sampling has more or less led to avoidance of this method today, leaving ASVS as the invasive method of choice in selected cases. It may be performed in conjunction with a conventional arteriography, which in some cases visualizes an insulinoma as a distinctive blush, due to the high vascularity of the tumor. However, ASVS/SACS seems to have high sensitivity, in some series close to 100% [69,70]. Calcium stimulates insulin secretion, and may be used to increase the insulin release from insulinomas [50]. In this method, a catheter is placed in the gastroduodenal, splenic, common hepatic, and superior mesenteric arteries, through which calcium gluconate is infused, leading to selective stimulation of different parts of the pancreas. A venous catheter is placed in a hepatic vein through which blood samples are drawn before injection, as well as after 30, 60, and 120 seconds (Figure 38.6). Regionalization of the insulinoma is possible after evaluation of the insulin concentrations in the samples collected after stimulation of different parts of the pancreas [51]. More than a two- to threefold increase in venous insulin concentration after calcium injection indicates excess insulin release in the region of the used artery.

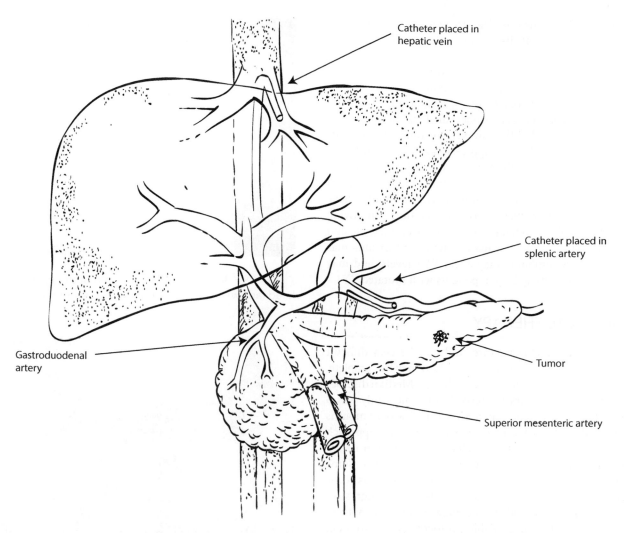

Figure 38.6 Schematic drawing of SACS with hepatic venous sampling. Through the catheter, which may be placed into the gastroduodenal, splenic (as in the drawing), superior mesenteric, and hepatic arteries, calcium is infused. Blood samples are drawn from the catheter placed at the final part of the hepatic veins.

Recommendation

Basal methods for localization are in most centers native CT scans, added by venous and arterial contrast enhancement phases, together with EUS. If no localization is demonstrated, review of the diagnosis should be done, and after confirming the likely pancreatogenous origin of the hypoglycemia, further imaging with MRT and somatostatin scintigraphy or preferably PET (using either ⁶⁸Ga-DOTATOC/DOTATATE or ¹¹C-5-HTP as tracer—or in the future, GLP1 receptor agonists as tracer) is recommended. If still no localization is seen, ASVS with concomitant arteriography should be performed. In most cases (80%–90%), the tumor is visualized after the initial CT and EUS, and surgery should follow.

In reoperative cases, CT and EUS are not enough as the only methods. PET scanning is highly recommended for thorough examination of spread disease, ASVS for further localization if not performed previously, and genetic screening should be performed to clarify eventual mutation in the MEN1 gene.

MEDICAL TREATMENT

The ultimate goal for the medical treatment is to avoid hypoglycemic episodes, and any patient scheduled for surgery needs to be preoperatively controlled to avoid these. Therefore, the patient should be told to have frequent meals and snacks, and to avoid prolonged intervals without intake of carbohydrates. This means that the patient has to wake up at night for a meal. Diazoxide is an antihypertensive and hyperglycemic drug that suppresses insulin secretion and enhances glycogenolysis, in doses between 50 and 300 (occasionally 600) mg/day [71]. However, diazoxide has a number of side effects, such as edema, renal impairment, and hirsutism. Usually, in a patient with a benign insulinoma, it is possible to avoid this drug. It is also important to await introduction of diazoxide until after the diagnosis of organic hyperinsulinism is clear, to avoid difficult workup. However, in malignant disease one often has to introduce the drug early.

Other possible drugs include calcium channel blockers, such as verapamil, and diphenylhydantoin or glucocorticoids may be used in refractory cases. In somatostatin receptor type 2-positive tumors, somatostatin analogs (octrotide and lanreotide) are useful [72]. However, in some patients, this treatment leads to efficient suppression of glucagon levels, leading to worsening of the hypoglycemia. Recently, mammalian target of rapamycin (mTOR) inhibitors (everolimus [Affinitor®] and sirolimus/rapamycin [Rapamune®]) have been successful in reducing insulin secretion, improving glycemic control, prolonging progression-free survival, and even reducing tumor size in mainly malignant insulinomas [73–75]. mTOR inhibitors may affect YY1 levels, and may therefore be a targeting drug in patients with mutated YY1.

ADDITIONAL THERAPY

Malignant insulinomas are rare, and may be very difficult to manage. In some patients, the resection may be complete, but the patient has to be under surveillance. Median disease-free survival after a curative resection in one study was 5 years, but after recurrence, median survival was 19 months [76]. Several studies have advocated an aggressive approach toward these tumors, with repeated resections and use of debulking or cytoreductive surgery [77]. However, some authors propose that at least 90% of the tumor has to be resected in order to achieve true palliation. The aggressive surgical approach should be accompanied by chemotherapy using the different available protocols (streptozotocin and 5-fluoro-uracil or Adriamycin, or temolozamide and capecitabine) [76]. Peptide receptor radiotherapy (PRRT) should be considered in somatostatin receptor-positive cases, and for massive liver metastases, embolization may be considered.

SURGICAL APPROACH

General considerations

All patients with pancreatogenous organic hypoglycemia should be considered for surgery. There is consensus that surgery should also be aimed for in metastatic disease. It is important to thoroughly question the diagnosis to avoid negative explorations and discover other reasons for the hypoglycemia preoperatively. It is also important to perform thorough localization procedures, and to verify or exclude hereditary syndromes, especially MEN1, which will affect the surgical procedure.

At surgery, regardless of whether performed by laparotomy or laparoscopy, a thorough exploration of the abdominal cavity should be performed in order to identify eventual metastases or, in rare cases, extrapancreatic tumors that

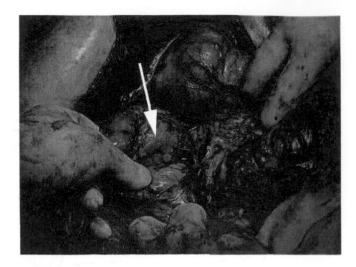

Figure 38.7 Intraoperative palpation of the pancreatic head (arrow) after a thorough Kocher's mobilization.

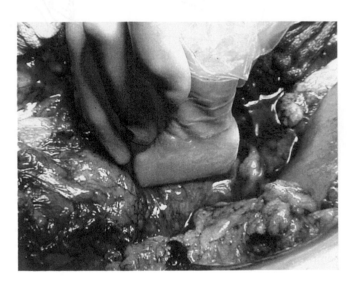

Figure 38.8 IOUS of the pancreas. The ultrasonic probe may be applied in direct contact with the pancreatic surface. Resolution may be enhanced by introduction of saline into the operative field.

may secrete IGFs, which may give rise to hypoglycemia (Figures 38.7 through 38.9).

Exploration, intraoperative palpation, and ultrasound

If the operation is done as an open laparotomy, palpation usually identifies the tumor (70% of cases), whereas adding intraoperative ultrasound (IOUS) of the entire pancreas will discover it in up to 100% of cases [44,78]. IOUS should always be performed to rule out multiple tumors and to clarify the relation to the pancreatic duct before the final decision of surgical method to remove the tumor. In some series, up to 8%–10% of cases are demonstrated with the

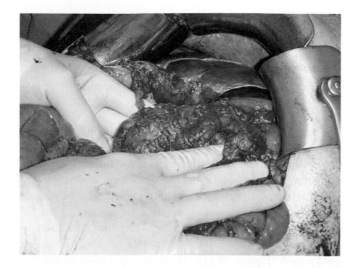

Figure 38.9 Bimanual palpation of the pancreas, allowing sensitive examination of the tissue.

tumor in another location than preoperatively estimated, or with multiple tumors [79].

In open surgery, a bilateral subcostal incision is made. A thorough examination of the peritoneal cavity is performed to rule out metastatic disease. The first aim is to perform a thorough visualization and exploration of the entire pancreas. A Kocher's maneuver is performed, after lowering of the hepatic colonic flexure, if necessary. The mobilization of the pancreatic head should be complete until the aorta can be palpated with the fingers. The mobilization of duodenum continues downward to include the third horizontal part. The mesentery of the transverse colon should be dissected away, and the superior mesenteric vein and its tributaries should be exposed. The lesser sac is now entered, either by lifting the major omentum from the transverse colon and retracting it upward, together with the stomach, or by dividing the gastrocolic ligament, distal to the gastroepiploic vessels, but well away from the colonic mesentery. The lower border of the pancreatic body and tail is now visualized. The adhesions between the posterior surface of the stomach and the anterior surface of the pancreas are divided. The peritoneum along the inferior border of the pancreas is incised, the transverse mesocolon separated, and the distal pancreas mobilized by using a blunt technique. The splenic artery should be identified along its entire course. The far end of the tail may be mobilized, together with the spleen, after dividing the splenocolic ligament. The tail can now be lifted up together with the spleen. After this thorough mobilization of the pancreas, bimanual palpation and IOUS are performed (Figures 38.8 and 38.9). Thus, even though an insulinoma is found early in the course, the whole pancreas should be examined, to avoid missing multiple tumors. The tumors are usually visible as reddish-brown on the surface, but occasionally are embedded within the parenchyma (Figure 38.10).

If laparoscopic surgery is performed similarly, thorough exploration may not be possible. An alternative is to use

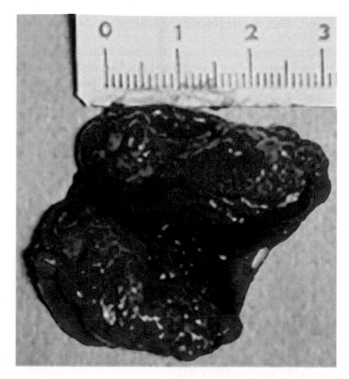

Figure 38.10 Typical insulinoma.

the hand port, allowing one hand to more easily perform a Kocher maneuver, as well as exploration of the body and tail of the pancreas. In laparoscopic surgery, relying on intraoperative laparoscopic US is important, possibly with contrast enhancement [66,67,80]. In most series, preoperatively localized insulinomas easily feasible for enucleation or a left-sided pancreatic resection are selected for laparoscopic surgery (Figure 38.11).

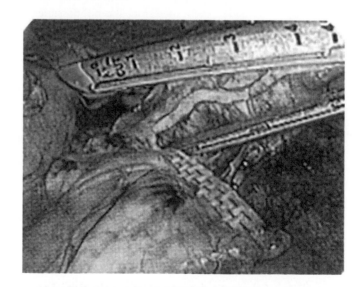

Figure 38.11 Left-sided laparoscopic resection is usually performed with a stapling device for dividing the pancreas.

Selecting resection procedure

Pancreatic surgery has been associated with a high complication rate, mostly from leakage of pancreatic fluid and development of fistulas and pseudocysts. These complications, as well as the history of high morbidity after pancreaticoduodenectomies, have had a hampering effect on the performance of pancreatic surgery, sometimes creating a conservative attitude. However, modern techniques, novel suture materials, and refinement of indications have reduced the rate of complications after pancreatic surgery.

Different authors reported an increased risk of leakage when handling insulinomas in the pancreatic head, whether by enucleation or resection. It is concluded that for pancreatic head tumors, it is important to define the relationship of the pancreatic and bile ducts and the vessels to the tumor. If the tumor is well away from these structures, enucleation is the method of choice (Figure 38.12). Even though rarely needed for insulinomas, a pylorus-preserving pancreaticoduodenectomy (PPPD) can be performed, even for benign disease. With thorough technique and postoperative care, PPPD may be performed with minimal morbidity and mortality [81].

Some authors have noticed a higher risk of fistula formation after enucleation in general [82]. This may, in the neck, be attributed to the oblique course of the pancreatic duct and the confluence with the accessory duct of Santorini in this part of the pancreas. Again, IOUS is helpful in clarifying the anatomical landmarks. The majority of the tumors in the uncinate process of the head, neck, and body of the pancreas may be enucleated. If the selection of the type of procedure is difficult, a resection should be performed. Alternatives that may be rarely used are duodenum-preserving resection of the pancreatic head and neck or central pancreatectomy [83,84].

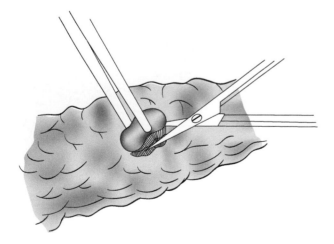

Figure 38.12 Schematic drawing of an enucleation of an insulinoma. Meticulous technique, fine instruments, and sutures should be used, after securing with IOUS that the pancreatic duct may not be injured due to a close location. This may also be done laparoscopically.

Tumors in the pancreatic tail may also be enucleated, especially the ones close to the body or protruding from the margin of the pancreas, but a liberal attitude toward a spleen-preserving left-sided pancreatic resection is suggested.

Enucleation

The insulinomas usually have a pseudocapsule, making it possible to enter a plane between the tumor and the surrounding normal pancreatic tissue. If the tumor is found to have unclear margins during the dissection and suspicions of malignancy appear, conversion to a resective procedure is proposed. By using a meticulous technique and fine instruments, applying small clips to any duct-like structures or using polypropylene 5-0 or 6-0, a safe enucleation can be performed (Figure 38.12). Thermocoagulation should be avoided. If there is suspicion of injury to the pancreatic duct, intravenous secretin will visualize extravasation of pancreatic fluid from the resected area. An injured duct may be closed using fine sutures, or alternatively and preferably, the operation is converted to a resection, segmental, distal spleen preserving, or PPPD. Helpful in the dissection is to lift the pancreas with one hand and, if possible, pull the tumor upward with a stitch placed through it. The defect should not be closed, since injury to the pancreatic tissue is likely to result in development of a pancreatic pseudocyst. It is wise to put some fibrin glue and possibly an omental flap to cover the defect. The area of enucleation should be carefully drained.

Left-sided and central pancreatic resections

A spleen-preserving left-sided pancreatic resection is a safe procedure [69,85], and has reduced morbidity compared with PPPD and enucleation [44,86]. The pancreatic tail is mobilized from the splenic vessels, often by dividing several smaller branches. A thorough search for the main pancreatic duct in the remaining pancreas is suggested, since ligation of this presumably reduces the risk of postoperative leakage. The pancreas may be cut with a scalpel according to the "fish mouth" technique. Smaller bleeders should be suture ligated with polypropylene 5-0 or 6-0. The cut edge is then carefully closed with sutures, avoiding large bites of pancreatic tissue in order to reduce the risk of devascularization. Fibrin glue is applied to the cut edge, and the area is carefully drained. However, recent developments with laparoscopic left-sided pancreatic resections using stapling devices to close the pancreas have been encouraging. Therefore, also in open surgery, this approach may be performed, and an Endo GIA Universal Green Reload (Covidien®) with 4.5 mm staples used in all patients (Figure 38.11) [87], and if reinforced with a running suture of polypropylene 5-0 around the stapled edge, as well as fibrin glue and Surgicel®, a very low incidence of postoperative fluid accumulation or fistulas occurs [77].

Central resections may be performed similarly, but leaving the tail of the pancreas *in situ*, to avoid diabetes mellitus.

The tail may be drained with a pancreaticojejunal anastomosis, or merely closed if considered to be small enough [53,84,88].

Pylorus-preserving pancreaticoduodenectomy

The PPPD is a development of the classical Whipple's procedure. In selected large and invasive cases, an extended operation, including resection of the mesenteric and portal veins or vascular bypass of the hepatic artery, may be needed [77]. In brief, after thorough examination of the entire pancreas, attention is drawn to the pancreatic head, and the common bile duct, common hepatic artery, and portal vein are exposed and isolated. The portal vein is freed and followed underneath the pancreatic neck. A similar dissection is performed from below, to isolate the mesenteric vein until the two veins are separated from the pancreatic neck using blunt dissection. The next step is ligation and division of the gastroduodenal artery, and the common hepatic artery is dissected away from the suprapancreatic area. To allow isolation of the uncinate process, the arterial branches and venous tributaries of the mesenteric vessels should be divided. Three structures now have to be divided: (1) the jejunum, approximately 20 cm inferior to the ligament of Treitz; (2) the duodenum; and (3) the common bile duct. The latter is usually divided immediately above the entrance of the cystic duct, making a cholecystectomy necessary. The jejunum and duodenum are divided with staplers. The pancreas is now divided over the portal vein, and the pancreatic duct identified in the remaining left part. The specimen is now free, and the reconstruction phase begins. An end-to-side pancreaticojejunostomy is performed using polydioxanone 4-0, and the classical invaginating technique with an inner row of sutures between the jejunal mucosa and the pancreatic rim, including the edges of the pancreatic duct, and an outer layer between jejunal serosa approximately 1 cm from the cut opening in the side of the gut and the pancreatic capsule. One may insert a small 3 cm piece of a pediatric feeding tube into the duct before closing the anastomosis. An end-to-side hepaticojejunostomy is constructed with polydioxanone 4-0 in a single layer. If the hepatic duct is narrow, one may consider using a stent to avoid stricture of the anastomosis. The catheter is passed down in the jejunal loop for about 10 cm before exiting through the intestinal and abdominal walls. The duodenojejunostomy is also constructed end-to-side with a single layer of running sutures of polydioxanone 4-0. A drain is used and positioned near the pancreatic and biliary anastomoses.

Minimally invasive techniques

The development of laparoscopic surgery has also made it possible to enucleate insulinomas and perform distal pancreatic resections (Figure 38.11) [53,66,89,90]. The postoperative recovery and hospital stay are shorter. The key to a technically successful laparoscopic operation of an insulinoma is a thorough exploration of the entire pancreas. As in open surgery, even though one tumor may be immediately seen, one has to examine the whole pancreas for the possibility of multiple tumors. Since bimanual palpation is impossible, one has to rely on laparoscopic US imaging [80]. The mobilization of the head of the pancreas, including the Kocher maneuver, entry into the lesser sac, and mobilization of the pancreatic tail demand high expertise in laparoscopic techniques. Nevertheless, selected cases with a surface-located insulinoma may be enucleated with laparoscopic techniques, and spleen-preserving pancreatic tail resection as well, using the stapling device described above for resection of the pancreas. An alternative is the hand-assisted laparoscopic technique that makes palpation of the pancreas possible, which presumably would increase the yield in comparison with conventional laparoscopic resection of insulinomas, but may increase postoperative recovery time [91].

Surgery in MEN1

All surgeons handling patients with endocrine pancreatic tumors have to consider the possibility of the patient having MEN1. If multiple tumors are found preoperatively, or other signs of hereditary disease, genetic screening has to be performed. If unanticipated multiple tumors are found intraoperatively, the surgical plan must be changed. Thus, measuring s-calcium and s-PTH (primary hyperparathyroidism) is easy and should be checked if not done preoperatively. There is a continuous debate about which pancreatic surgical procedure should be performed in MEN1 patients, and at which indication. However, most seem to stick with the advocated 1 cm rule, leading to resection of all tumors of at least 10 mm in size, usually by a subtotal pancreatic resection (tail and body), together with enucleation of tumors in the head. The reason for the 10 mm cutoff is the risk of malignancy, which becomes higher in larger tumors [92]. Others have suggested a more radical extended subtotal pancreatic resection, especially in families where malignant pancreatic tumors are known to occur [93]. However, if MEN1 is suspected intraoperatively, a left-sided resection, combined with enucleations from the head, is sufficient, followed by a thorough postoperative workup to confirm the diagnosis and proceed with eventual extended pancreatic reresection later.

The long-term results of pancreatic surgery in MEN1, as well as in conjunction with insulinomas and MEN1, are excellent [94,95], although some preliminary additional long-term follow-up reports state a high rate of diabetes mellitus.

Surgery in NIPHS

NIPHS is a rare disease, and is usually encountered after failure to localize an insulinoma in a patient with typical symptoms. Although some preoperative indications based on the response to ASVS, ^{68}Ga-DOTATOC/DOTATATE PET imaging [96], or a peroral glucose test exist, the diagnosis is still difficult [97,98]. GLP1 receptor–targeted PET may in the future facilitate the localization, including identifying individuals with NIPHS. However, series with successful surgery are documented, usually by a subtotal pancreatectomy, extending to the right of the superior mesenteric vessels, with preservation of the bile duct and the superior and inferior pancreaticoduodenal vessels [99]. Recurrences do occur, as well as induction of diabetes mellitus. Medical treatment of the disease may be an option, especially in recurrent situations.

Surgery in malignant insulinomas

Unless the tumor is widely spread, tumor resection is indicated, to reduce or avoid troublesome hypoglycemia. Since a number of tumors are found malignant only in the histopathological examination of the specimen, one may argue against enucleation as the procedure of choice, in order to comply with oncologic principles. However, these findings are extremely rare and do not justify pancreatic resections in all cases. Instead, one may consider resection in cases where the pseudocapsular margin is unclear, or the size is >2 cm. In the case of noncurative extended enucleation, a reoperative resection may have to be performed. In the case of liver metastases, these should be treated with any of the available methods (surgical resection, radiofrequency ablation, liver embolization, and chemotherapy). Some patients with malignant insulinomas, however, have a rapidly progressing disease and short survival prospects, and do not benefit from surgery.

Intraoperative biochemical monitoring

Approximately 30 minutes after tumor removal, a rebound increase in blood glucose occurs, raising the level by at least 30 mg/dL (1.5 mmol/L) [100], which may be used as an intraoperative indication of successful surgery.

Postoperative management

In the recovery room, immediately after surgery, blood glucose usually rises evidently to 120–140 mg/dL (6–7 mmol/L), and even higher if intravenous glucose administration is used. In fact, in some cases, insulin may have to be given, with frequent assays of serum glucose postoperatively. Drains may be removed if the output is less than 20 mL/day, or higher if the fluid contains low amylase concentrations.

Complications

Pancreatic surgery has been associated with a number of complications, mainly intraperitoneal leakage of pancreatic fluid or development of pancreatic fistula. Less frequently, a pseudocyst may develop. These complications previously had a hampering effect on pancreatic surgery. Serious attempts have been made to reduce morbidity and increase patient safety, and in a large meta-analysis, there are similar complication rates after open or laparoscopic surgery (35.4% or 32.8%) [17]. In the same review, pancreatic fistulas had rates of 14.6% (open) and 7.2% (laparoscopic), respectively. Indeed, different authors present varying results, and some reports fail to follow the criteria for definition of a fistula [101,102].

Different postoperative medical and surgical interventions for management of fistulas and pseudocysts have also been discussed. Most authors have reported that low-output fistulas noted as postoperative drainage containing high amylase concentrations in most cases resolve spontaneously within 6 weeks [82,103].

In some cases, one may leave the drain in place while the patient is fed. There seems to be no indication for somatostatin (or analog) treatment in these cases. This statement is supported by a prospective randomized trial using octreotide to prevent pancreatic fistulas after pancreaticoduodenectomy [104]. If the drainage does not resolve, various reoperative methods may be used to correct the leak, and in severe cases, endoscopic retrograde cholangiopancreatography with papillotomy or insertion of pancreatic stents may be necessary.

Overall postoperative mortality rate is 3.7% for an open procedure in the meta-analysis, including 6222 cases [17].

SURGICAL OUTCOMES REINFORCED BY EVIDENCE-BASED HIERARCHY

Extremely little has been performed to gain evidence higher than level II-2 (well-designed, cohort, or case-control analytic studies, preferably from more than one center or research group). The only randomized trial, leading to level I evidence, is the one considering use of somatostatin analogs to reduce the postoperative fistula rate, but after PPPD and in malignant disease [104].

Thus, the majority of the currently available data rely on studies of cohorts, either prospectively gathered without any control group, followed by a retrospective report, or pure retrospective data, and from single centers series (leading to not more than maximum level II-3 or level III evidence). On the other hand, this seems natural due to the scarcity of the disease. And even if including the experience of different neuroendocrine pancreatic tumors to increase the numbers, studies that increase the level of evidence are lacking. Nevertheless, the surgical results reported by several well-known large centers are acceptable, and development has occurred during the last decade to improve patient safety and outcome and reduce morbidity and mortality.

REFERENCES

1. Mathur A, Gorden P, Libutti SK. Insulinoma. *Surg Clin North Am* 2009;89(5):1105–21.
2. Banting F, Best C. Internal secretion of the pancreas. *J Lab Med* 1922;7:251.
3. Whipple AO, Frantz VK. Adenoma of islet cells with hyperinsulinism: A review. *Ann Surg* 1935;101(6):1299–335.

4. Langerhans P. *Beitrage zur mikroskopischen Anatomie der Bauchspeicheldrüse.* Berlin: Lange, 1869.

5. Wilder R, Allan F, Power M. Carcinoma of the islets of the pancreas: Hyperinsulinism and hypoglycemia. *JAMA* 1927;89:348–50.

6. Howland G, Campbell W, Maltby E. Dysinsulinism: Convuslions and coma due to islet cell tumor of the pancreas with operation and cure. *JAMA* 1929;93:674–7.

7. Service FJ, McMahon MM, O'Brien PC, Ballard DJ. Functioning insulinoma—Incidence, recurrence, and long-term survival of patients: A 60-year study. *Mayo Clin Proc* 1991;66(7):711–9.

8. Stefanini P, Carboni M, Patrassi N, Basoli A. Beta-islet cell tumors of the pancreas: Results of a study on 1,067 cases. *Surgery* 1974;75(4):597–609.

9. Jensen RT, Berna MJ, Bingham DB, Norton JA. Inherited pancreatic endocrine tumor syndromes: Advances in molecular pathogenesis, diagnosis, management, and controversies. *Cancer* 2008;113(7 Suppl):1807–43.

10. Vanderveen K, Grant C. Insulinoma. *Cancer Treat Res* 2010;153:235–52.

11. Soga J, Yakuwa Y, Osaka M. Insulinoma/hypoglycemic syndrome: A statistical evaluation of 1085 reported cases of a Japanese series. *J Exp Clin Cancer Res* 1998;17(4):379–88.

12. Cryer PE, Axelrod L, Grossman AB et al. Evaluation and management of adult hypoglycemic disorders: An Endocrine Society Clinical Practice Guideline. *J Clin Endocrinol Metab* 2009;94(3):709–28.

13. Heller SR, Cryer PE. Hypoinsulinemia is not critical to glucose recovery from hypoglycemia in humans. *Am J Physiol* 1991;261(1 Pt 1):E41–8.

14. Waickus CM, de Bustros A, Shakil A. Recognizing factitious hypoglycemia in the family practice setting. *J Am Board Fam Pract* 1999;12(2):133–6.

15. Bessell EM, Selby C, Ellis IO. Severe hypoglycaemia caused by raised insulin-like growth factor II in disseminated breast cancer. *J Clin Pathol* 1999;52(10):780–1.

16. Hizuka N, Fukuda I, Takano K, Okubo Y, Asakawa-Yasumoto K, Demura H. Serum insulin-like growth factor II in 44 patients with non-islet cell tumor hypoglycemia. *Endocr J* 1998;45(Suppl):S61–5.

17. Mehrabi A, Fischer L, Hafezi M et al. A systematic review of localization, surgical treatment options, and outcome of insulinoma. *Pancreas* 2014;43(5):675–86.

18. Rollins BJ. Chemokines. *Blood* 1997;90(3):909–28.

19. Nagasawa T, Kikutani H, Kishimoto T. Molecular cloning and structure of a pre-B-cell growth-stimulating factor. *Proc Natl Acad Sci USA* 1994;91(6):2305–9.

20. Yano T, Liu Z, Donovan J, Thomas MK, Habener JF. Stromal cell derived factor-1 (SDF-1)/CXCL12 attenuates diabetes in mice and promotes pancreatic beta-cell survival by activation of the prosurvival kinase Akt. *Diabetes* 2007;56(12):2946–57.

21. Shi Y, Lee JS, Galvin KM. Everything you have ever wanted to know about Yin Yang 1. *Biochim Biophys Acta* 1997;1332(2):F49–66.

22. Markovic J, Grdovic N, Dinic S et al. PARP-1 and YY1 are important novel regulators of CXCL12 gene transcription in rat pancreatic beta cells. *PloS One* 2013;8(3):e59679.

23. Cromer MK, Choi M, Nelson-Williams C et al. Recurrent somatic mutation altering DNA-binding motif of transcription factor YY1 explains pathogenesis of insulin-producing adenomas. Presented at 63rd Annual Meeting of the American Society of Human Genetics, Boston, 2013.

24. Cao Y, Gao Z, Li L et al. Whole exome sequencing of insulinoma reveals recurrent T372R mutations in YY1. *Nat Commun* 2013;4:2810.

25. Hessman O, Lindberg D, Einarsson A et al. Genetic alterations on 3p, 11q13, and 18q in nonfamilial and MEN 1-associated pancreatic endocrine tumors. *Genes Chromosomes Cancer* 1999;26(3):258–64.

26. Jonkers YM, Ramaekers FC, Speel EJ. Molecular alterations during insulinoma tumorigenesis. *Biochim Biophys Acta* 2007;1775(2):313–32.

27. Jonkers YM, Claessen SM, Perren A et al. DNA copy number status is a powerful predictor of poor survival in endocrine pancreatic tumor patients. *Endocr Relat Cancer* 2007;14(3):769–79.

28. Larsson C, Skogseid B, Oberg K, Nakamura Y, Nordenskjold M. Multiple endocrine neoplasia type 1 gene maps to chromosome 11 and is lost in insulinoma. *Nature* 1988;332(6159):85–7.

29. Chandrasekharappa SC, Guru SC, Manickam P et al. Positional cloning of the gene for multiple endocrine neoplasia-type 1. *Science* 1997;276(5311):404–7.

30. Thakker RV, Newey PJ, Walls GV et al. Clinical practice guidelines for multiple endocrine neoplasia type 1 (MEN1). *J Clin Endocrinol Metab* 2012;97(9):2990–3011.

31. Agarwal SK, Kennedy PA, Scacheri PC et al. Menin molecular interactions: Insights into normal functions and tumorigenesis. *Horm Metab Res* 2005;37(6):369–74.

32. Karnik SK, Hughes CM, Gu X et al. Menin regulates pancreatic islet growth by promoting histone methylation and expression of genes encoding p27Kip1 and p18INK4c. *Proc Natl Acad Sci USA* 2005;102(41):14659–64.

33. Cupisti K, Hoppner W, Dotzenrath C et al. Lack of MEN1 gene mutations in 27 sporadic insulinomas. *Eur J Clin Invest* 2000;30(4):325–9.

34. Akerstrom G, Stalberg P, Hellman P. Surgical management of pancreatico-duodenal tumors in multiple endocrine neoplasia syndrome type 1. *Clinics* 2012;67(Suppl 1):173–8.

35. Won JG, Tseng HS, Yang AH et al. Clinical features and morphological characterization of 10 patients with noninsulinoma pancreatogenous hypoglycaemia syndrome (NIPHS). *Clin Endocrinol* 2006;65(5):566–78.

36. Service FJ, Natt N, Thompson GB et al. Noninsulinoma pancreatogenous hypoglycemia: A novel syndrome of hyperinsulinemic hypoglycemia in adults independent of mutations in Kir6.2 and SUR1 genes. *J Clin Endocrinol Metab* 1999;84(5):1582–9.

37. Glaser B, Kesavan P, Heyman M et al. Familial hyperinsulinism caused by an activating glucokinase mutation. *N Engl J Med* 1998;338(4):226–30.

38. Dizon AM, Kowalyk S, Hoogwerf BJ. Neuroglycopenic and other symptoms in patients with insulinomas. *Am J Med* 1999;106(3):307–10.

39. Service FJ. Hypoglycemic disorders. *N Engl J Med* 1995;332(17):1144–52.

40. Hellman P, Goretzki P, Simon D, Dotzenrath C, Roher HD. Therapeutic experience of 65 cases with organic hyperinsulinism. *Langenbecks Arch Surg* 2000;385(5):329–36.

41. Service FJ, Dale AJ, Elveback LR, Jiang NS. Insulinoma: Clinical and diagnostic features of 60 consecutive cases. *Mayo Clin Proc* 1976;51(7):417–29.

42. Service FJ. Classification of hypoglycemic disorders. *Endocrinol Metab Clin North Am* 1999;28(3):501–17.

43. Mala T. Postprandial hyperinsulinemic hypoglycemia after gastric bypass surgical treatment. *Surg Obes Relat Dis* 2014;10(6):1220–5.

44. Grant CS. Insulinoma. *Best Pract Res Clin Gastroenterol* 2005;19(5):783–98.

45. Guettier JM, Lungu A, Goodling A, Cochran C, Gorden P. The role of proinsulin and insulin in the diagnosis of insulinoma: A critical evaluation of the Endocrine Society Clinical Practice Guideline. *J Clin Endocrinol Metab* 2013;98(12):4752–8.

46. Hirshberg B, Livi A, Bartlett DL et al. Forty-eight-hour fast: The diagnostic test for insulinoma. *J Clin Endocrinol Metab* 2000;85(9):3222–6.

47. Service GJ, Thompson GB, Service FJ, Andrews JC, Collazo-Clavell ML, Lloyd RV. Hyperinsulinemic hypoglycemia with nesidioblastosis after gastric-bypass surgery. *N Engl J Med* 2005;353(3):249–54.

48. Abrahamsson N, Engstrom BE, Sundbom M, Karlsson FA. GLP1 analogs as treatment of postprandial hypoglycemia following gastric bypass surgery: A potential new indication? *Eur J Endocrinol* 2013;169(6):885–9.

49. Lohmann T, Kratzsch J, Kellner K, Witzigmann H, Hauss J, Paschke R. Severe hypoglycemia due to insulin autoimmune syndrome with insulin autoantibodies crossreactive to proinsulin. *Exp Clin Endocrinol Diabetes* 2001;109(4):245–8.

50. Basu A, Service FJ, Yu L, Heser D, Ferries LM, Eisenbarth G. Insulin autoimmunity and hypoglycemia in seven white patients. *Endocr Pract* 2005;11(2):97–103.

51. Placzkowski KA, Vella A, Thompson GB et al. Secular trends in the presentation and management of functioning insulinoma at the Mayo Clinic, 1987–2007. *J Clin Endocrinol Metab* 2009;94(4):1069–73.

52. Fidler JL, Fletcher JG, Reading CC et al. Preoperative detection of pancreatic insulinomas on multiphasic helical CT. *AJR Am J Roentgenol* 2003;181(3):775–80.

53. Zhao YP, Zhan HX, Zhang TP et al. Surgical management of patients with insulinomas: Result of 292 cases in a single institution. *J Surg Oncol* 2011;103(2):169–74.

54. Gouya H, Vignaux O, Augui J et al. CT, endoscopic sonography, and a combined protocol for preoperative evaluation of pancreatic insulinomas. *AJR Am J Roentgenol* 2003;181(4):987–92.

55. Matsuki M, Inada Y, Nakai G et al. Diffusion-weighed MR imaging of pancreatic carcinoma. *Abdom Imaging* 2007;32(4):481–3.

56. Anderson MA, Carpenter S, Thompson NW, Nostrant TT, Elta GH, Scheiman JM. Endoscopic ultrasound is highly accurate and directs management in patients with neuroendocrine tumors of the pancreas. *Am J Gastroenterol* 2000;95(9):2271–7.

57. Patel KK, Kim MK. Neuroendocrine tumors of the pancreas: Endoscopic diagnosis. *Curr Opin Gastroenterol* 2008;24(5):638–42.

58. Sotoudehmanesh R, Hedayat A, Shirazian N et al. Endoscopic ultrasonography (EUS) in the localization of insulinoma. *Endocrine* 2007;31(3):238–41.

59. Kwekkeboom DJ, Krenning EP, Scheidhauer K et al. ENETS Consensus Guidelines for the standards of care in neuroendocrine tumors: Somatostatin receptor imaging with ^{111}In-pentetreotide. *Neuroendocrinology* 2009;90(2):184–9.

60. Bhate K, Mok WY, Tran K, Khan S, Al-Nahhas A. Functional assessment in the multimodality imaging of pancreatic neuro-endocrine tumours. *Minerva Endocrinol* 2010;35(1):17–25.

61. van Essen M, Sundin A, Krenning EP, Kwekkeboom DJ. Neuroendocrine tumours: The role of imaging for diagnosis and therapy. *Nat Rev Endocrinol* 2014;10(2):102–14.

62. Cases AI, Ohtsuka T, Fujino M et al. Expression of glucagon-like peptide 1 receptor and its effects on biologic behavior in pancreatic neuroendocrine tumors. *Pancreas* 2014;43(1):1–6.

63. Brand C, Abdel-Atti D, Zhang Y et al. In vivo imaging of GLP-1R with a targeted bimodal PET/fluorescence imaging agent. *Bioconjug Chem* 2014;25:1323–30.

64. Xu Y, Pan D, Xu Q et al. Insulinoma imaging with glucagon-like peptide-1 receptor targeting probe F-FBEM-Cys(39)-exendin-4. *J Cancer Res Clin Oncol* 2014;140(9):1479–88.

65. Eriksson O, Velikyan I, Selvaraju RK et al. Detection of metastatic insulinoma by positron emission tomography with [(68)ga]exendin-4—A case report. *J Clin Endocrinol Metab* 2014;99(5):1519–24.

66. Luo Y, Liu R, Hu MG, Mu YM, An LC, Huang ZQ. Laparoscopic surgery for pancreatic insulinomas: A single-institution experience of 29 cases. *J Gastrointest Surg* 2009;13(5):945–50.

67. Li W, An L, Liu R et al. Laparoscopic ultrasound enhances diagnosis and localization of insulinoma in pancreatic head and neck for laparoscopic surgery with satisfactory postsurgical outcomes. *Ultrasound Med Biol* 2011;37(7):1017–23.

68. Kuzin NM, Egorov AV, Kondrashin SA, Lotov AN, Kuznetzov NS, Majorova JB. Preoperative and intraoperative topographic diagnosis of insulinomas. *World J Surg* 1998;22(6):593–7; discussion 597–8.

69. Morganstein DL, Lewis DH, Jackson J et al. The role of arterial stimulation and simultaneous venous sampling in addition to cross-sectional imaging for localisation of biochemically proven insulinoma. *Eur Radiol* 2009;19(10):2467–73.

70. Guettier JM, Kam A, Chang R et al. Localization of insulinomas to regions of the pancreas by intraarterial calcium stimulation: The NIH experience. *J Clin Endocrinol Metab* 2009;94(4):1074–80.

71. Hirshberg B, Cochran C, Skarulis MC et al. Malignant insulinoma: Spectrum of unusual clinical features. *Cancer* 2005;104(2):264–72.

72. Vezzosi D, Bennet A, Rochaix P et al. Octreotide in insulinoma patients: Efficacy on hypoglycemia, relationships with Octreoscan scintigraphy and immunostaining with anti-sst2A and anti-sst5 antibodies. *Eur J Endocrinol* 2005;152(5):757–67.

73. Kulke MH, Bergsland EK, Yao JC. Glycemic control in patients with insulinoma treated with everolimus. *N Engl J Med* 2009;360(2):195–7.

74. Bourcier ME, Sherrod A, DiGuardo M, Vinik AI. Successful control of intractable hypoglycemia using rapamycin in an 86-year-old man with a pancreatic insulin-secreting islet cell tumor and metastases. *J Clin Endocrinol Metab* 2009;94(9):3157–62.

75. Yao JC, Shah MH, Ito T et al. Everolimus for advanced pancreatic neuroendocrine tumors. *N Engl J Med* 2011;364(6):514–23.

76. Jensen RT, Cadiot G, Brandi ML et al. ENETS Consensus Guidelines for the management of patients with digestive neuroendocrine neoplasms: Functional pancreatic endocrine tumor syndromes. *Neuroendocrinology* 2012;95(2):98–119.

77. Hellman P, Andersson M, Rastad J et al. Surgical strategy for large or malignant endocrine pancreatic tumors. *World J Surg* 2000;24(11):1353–60.

78. Lo CY, Lam KY, Kung AW, Lam KS, Tung PH, Fan ST. Pancreatic insulinomas. A 15-year experience. *Arch Surg* 1997;132(8):926–30.

79. Chung JC, Choi SH, Jo SH, Heo JS, Choi DW, Kim YI. Localization and surgical treatment of the pancreatic insulinomas. *ANZ J Surg* 2006;76(12):1051–5.

80. Grover AC, Skarulis M, Alexander HR et al. A prospective evaluation of laparoscopic exploration with intraoperative ultrasound as a technique for localizing sporadic insulinomas. *Surgery* 2005;138(6):1003–8; discussion 1008.

81. Yeo CJ, Cameron JL, Sohn TA et al. Six hundred fifty consecutive pancreaticoduodenectomies in the 1990s: Pathology, complications, and outcomes. *Ann Surg* 1997;226(3):248–57; discussion 257–60.

82. Nikfarjam M, Warshaw AL, Axelrod L et al. Improved contemporary surgical management of insulinomas: A 25-year experience at the Massachusetts General Hospital. *Ann Surg* 2008;247(1):165–72.

83. Beger HG, Schlosser W, Siech M, Poch B. The surgical management of chronic pancreatitis: Duodenum-preserving pancreatectomy. *Adv Surg* 1999;32:87–104.

84. Warshaw AL, Rattner DW, Fernandez-del Castillo C, Z'Graggen K. Middle segment pancreatectomy: A novel technique for conserving pancreatic tissue. *Arch Surg* 1998;133(3):327–31.

85. Lillemoe KD, Kaushal S, Cameron JL, Sohn TA, Pitt HA, Yeo CJ. Distal pancreatectomy: Indications and outcomes in 235 patients. *Ann Surg* 1999;229(5):693–8; discussion 698–700.

86. Hackert T, Hinz U, Fritz S et al. Enucleation in pancreatic surgery: Indications, technique, and outcome compared to standard pancreatic resections. *Langenbecks Arch Surg* 2011;396(8):1197–203.

87. Rosok BI, Marangos IP, Kazaryan AM et al. Single-centre experience of laparoscopic pancreatic surgery. *Br J Surg* 2010;97(6):902–9.

88. Sperti C, Pasquali C, Ferronato A, Pedrazzoli S. Median pancreatectomy for tumors of the neck and body of the pancreas. *J Am Coll Surg* 2000;190(6):711–6.

89. Vezakis A, Davides D, Larvin M, McMahon MJ. Laparoscopic surgery combined with preservation of the spleen for distal pancreatic tumors. *Surg Endosc* 1999;13(1):26–9.

90. Gagner M, Pomp A, Herrera MF. Early experience with laparoscopic resections of islet cell tumors. *Surgery* 1996;120(6):1051–4.

91. Kneuertz PJ, Patel SH, Chu CK et al. Laparoscopic distal pancreatectomy: Trends and lessons learned through an 11-year experience. *J Am Coll Surg* 2012;215(2):167–76.

92. Triponez F, Goudet P, Dosseh D et al. Is surgery beneficial for MEN1 patients with small (< or =2 cm), nonfunctioning pancreaticoduodenal endocrine tumor? An analysis of 65 patients from the GTE. *World J Surg* 2006;30(5):654–62; discussion 663–4.

93. Akerstrom G, Hessman O, Skogseid B. Timing and extent of surgery in symptomatic and asymptomatic neuroendocrine tumors of the pancreas in MEN 1. *Langenbecks Arch Surg* 2002;386(8):558–69.

94. Lopez CL, Waldmann J, Fendrich V, Langer P, Kann PH, Bartsch DK. Long-term results of surgery for pancreatic neuroendocrine neoplasms in patients with MEN1. *Langenbecks Arch Surg* 2011;396(8):1187–96.

95. Giudici F, Nesi G, Brandi ML, Tonelli F. Surgical management of insulinomas in multiple endocrine neoplasia type 1. *Pancreas* 2012;41(4):547–53.

96. Arun S, Rai Mittal B, Shukla J, Bhattacharya A, Kumar P. Diffuse nesidioblastosis diagnosed on a Ga-68 DOTATATE positron emission tomography/computerized tomography. *Indian J Nucl Med* 2013;28(3):163–4.

97. Starke A, Saddig C, Kirch B, Tschahargane C, Goretzki P. Islet hyperplasia in adults: Challenge to preoperatively diagnose non-insulinoma pancreatogenic hypoglycemia syndrome. *World J Surg* 2006;30(5):670–9.

98. Goretzki P, Starke A, Lammers B, Schwarz K, Roher HD. Pancreatic hyperinsulinism—Changes of the clinical picture and importance of differences in sporadic disease course (experience with 144 patients operated in the period 1986–2009) [in German]. *Zentralbl Chir* 2010;135(3):218–25.

99. Raffel A, Krausch MM, Anlauf M et al. Diffuse nesidioblastosis as a cause of hyperinsulinemic hypoglycemia in adults: A diagnostic and therapeutic challenge. *Surgery* 2007;141(2):179–84; discussion 185–6.

100. Gianello P, Gigot JF, Berthet F et al. Pre- and intraoperative localization of insulinomas: Report of 22 observations. *World J Surg* 1988;12(3):389–97.

101. Bassi C, Dervenis C, Butturini G et al. Postoperative pancreatic fistula: An international study group (ISGPF) definition. *Surgery* 2005;138(1):8–13.

102. Molinari E, Bassi C, Salvia R et al. Amylase value in drains after pancreatic resection as predictive factor of postoperative pancreatic fistula: Results of a prospective study in 137 patients. *Ann Surg* 2007;246(2):281–7.

103. Falconi M, Zerbi A, Crippa S et al. Parenchyma-preserving resections for small nonfunctioning pancreatic endocrine tumors. *Ann Surg Oncol* 2010;17(6):1621–7.

104. Lowy AM, Lee JE, Pisters PW et al. Prospective, randomized trial of octreotide to prevent pancreatic fistula after pancreaticoduodenectomy for malignant disease. *Ann Surg* 1997;226(5):632–41.

39

Congenital hyperinsulinism

CHRISTOPHER A. BEHR AND STEPHEN E. DOLGIN

INTRODUCTION

Hypoglycemia is especially dangerous to the developing brain of the newborn. While most causes of neonatal hypoglycemia are transient, those that persist can have devastating consequences. Therefore, it is of the utmost importance to identify, categorize, and appropriately treat these patients as promptly as possible. Most cases of persistent hypoglycemia seen in neonates are due to the overproduction of insulin. This condition was previously termed *nesidioblastosis*, and was thought to be due to diffuse hyperplasia of pancreatic islet cells. As we have learned more about the disease complex, this term is inaccurate. A more comprehensive and generally accepted term is *congenital hyperinsulinism* (CH). Insulinomas are a separate entity and are quite rare in childhood. They are not thought to be congenital and will not be addressed in this chapter [1]. Although CH may present throughout childhood and rarely even in adulthood, the most common age is within the neonatal period or infancy. The early-presenting cases invariably end up being more severe, more resistant to medical management, and more likely to require surgical intervention. Therefore, this chapter concentrates on CH specifically in the newborn patient, and highlights recent developments in genetics, diagnostic modalities, and surgical techniques that have improved the way clinicians manage this disease.

CLINICAL PRESENTATION

The clinical expression of hypoglycemia in neonates often includes nonspecific symptoms, such as lethargy, tachycardia, irritability, jitteriness, hypotonia, and poor feeding. It can lead to more specific symptoms, such as apnea, seizures, and coma. These neuroglycopenic symptoms are the most

dangerous to the development of the newborn because of a significant risk of irreversible neurological damage.

While transient hypoglycemia (blood glucose of <30 mg/dL) is common in healthy newborns 1–2 hours after birth, persistence of hypoglycemia is abnormal. It is difficult to define an exact plasma blood glucose value that denotes clinically significant hypoglycemia in neonates, but a 2011 report from the American Academy of Pediatrics states that the generally adopted cutoff value indicating significant hypoglycemia is <47 mg/dL (2.6 mmol/L) and proposed that the target glucose screen prior to routine feeds should be >45 mg/dL (2.5 mmol/L) [2].

Maternal diabetes is one of the most common reasons for neonatal hypoglycemia. This is attributed to intermittently high levels of blood glucose in the mother during pregnancy that cause beta cell hypertrophy in the fetus, resulting in a state of hyperinsulinemia in the fetus and, subsequently, the newborn. This typically resolves within 2–4 days of birth. The macrosomia that affects up to 40% of infants of diabetic mothers can be seen in cases of CH as well, and it is thought that the inappropriate fetal hyperinsulinism is the causative mechanism in both cases [3]. Perinatal insults resulting in poor oxygenation and hypoxia can cause hypoglycemia, but this too is transient. If hypoglycemia persists beyond this timeframe, it is most often due to hyperinsulinism, either as a result of a syndromic condition (Beckwith–Wiedemann, Costello, Perlman, Sotos, Kabuki, or congenital disorders of glycosylation) or as a result of CH [2]. It is the latter, CH, that is typically the most severe and refractory to medical management.

There are diagnostic criteria that help distinguish hyperinsulinism from other causes of hypoglycemia. The "critical blood sample," drawn while the patient is hypoglycemic, will most often show a number of abnormalities that indicate a hyperinsulinemic cause. These include an inappropriately high insulin level (>5 μU/mL), which should be generally undetectable during periods of hypoglycemia. Even a "normal" insulin value is abnormal in the face of a hypoglycemic episode. Similar to the insulin level, the level of C-peptide will be elevated. Intravenous or intramuscular administration of glucagon (0.5–1 mg or 0.3 mg/kg) will cause a marked increase in blood glucose (>30 mg/dL increase) within 30–40 minutes of administration. Ketone bodies in plasma and urine and free fatty acids in plasma will be low, as insulin inhibits lipolysis. There will likely be a decrease in the insulin-like growth factor binding protein 1 (IGFBP1) concentration, as production of IGFBP1 is inhibited by insulin. Finally, a specific, but insensitive, diagnostic indicator is the high rate of glucose infusion (>10 mg/kg/min) required to maintain a blood glucose value greater than 55 mg/dL (3 mmol/L) [3,4].

PATHOLOGICAL BASIS

The underlying pathological condition in a newborn whose hyperinsulinism persists is almost never a true insulinoma. Controversy has surrounded the actual underlying histopathology. The term *nesidioblastosis*, applied broadly to the congenitally abnormal pancreas producing excessive insulin and thought to be a diffuse abnormality in the pancreas, was introduced in 1939, curiously, in a paper actually about focal pancreatic lesions [5]. The author, Laidlaw, called the underlying causative lesions nesidioblastomas. Laidlaw speculated that if such lesions were multiple in a pancreas, the condition could be called nesidioblastosis. Laidlaw recognized islet cells budding from pancreatic ductal cells. The term *nesidioblastosis*, once thought to be the cause of CH, is no longer used because this histological finding described by Laidlaw has not consistently been associated with hyperinsulinism. Actually, the finding of beta cells budding from epithelium (ductuloinsular complexes) is characteristic of the fetal developmental process. It persists as a developmental stage postnatally [6]. It is reproduced in many states of injury, including pancreatic duct obstruction, and in recovery from these conditions. This histological condition has been recognized in the normal pancreas of newborns and infants. In the view of many pathologists, the finding of nesidioblastosis does not correlate with hypoglycemia [7–9].

Not only does this diffuse condition exist without hyperinsulinism, but it also has been shown that approximately 40% of cases of CH have unifocal lesions, as opposed to diffuse disease. Nesidioblastosis implies diffuse hyperplasia of beta cells throughout the pancreas. It has become an inappropriate term when applied broadly to patients with inborn pancreatogenous hyperinsulinism. The most current term for the condition is *congenital hyperinsulinism*, which includes diffuse and focal causes.

Histologically, the focal type of CH is defined as a focal adenomatous hyperplasia. The typical pathological picture is that of a small (2.5–7.5 mm) focus of hyperplastic islets. These are structurally normal, but the beta cells within the focus are hyperactive and abnormal. They show enlarged cellular components (cytoplasm, nucleus, and Golgi apparatus) with excessive proinsulin but a relative paucity of insulin granules and insulin staining. This is secondary to a scarcity of stored insulin due to its hypersecretion. Surrounding this focus of beta cells is a peripheral rim of nonbeta endocrine cells. Outside of the isolated focus, the other pancreatic islets are small, with reduced cytoplasm and tiny nuclei, and show a high amount of stored insulin. While these focal lesions are termed "adenomatous," they are not adenomas, as they show no dysplasia or neoplasia. In addition, adenomas are not composed of true islets [10,11].

In the diffuse type of CH, the entire pancreas is affected. While the focal form shows hyperactive beta cells in one distinct area, the diffuse form exhibits hyperactivity throughout. All of the islets show abnormally large beta cells, with enlarged nuclei (three to five times the size of nearby acinar nuclei) cytoplasm, and Golgi. They too stain very heavily for proinsulin and have scarce staining of insulin due to its excessive release [3,4,10].

GENETIC BASIS

There are both familial and sporadic forms of CH. The sporadic form has an incidence of approximately 1 in 50,000 live births, while the familial form can have an incidence of up to 1 in 2500 live births in some populations (most notably in Saudi Arabians and Ashkenazi Jews).

Some of the most important advances in the field of CH over the past 10 years have involved insights into the genetic basis of the disease. Researchers have been examining the genetics of CH since the 1990s, but until recently, the clinical application of these studies has been limited. A deeper understanding of the disease itself and the specific genetic disruptions, combined with the ability to clinically test for these mutations (and improved imaging studies), have revolutionized the treatment of CH.

Eight different genes have been identified as sites of mutations that can cause CH, all of which lead to dysregulated insulin secretion. However, mutations at these sites account for only 50%–55% of cases, with the remaining 45%–50% having no identifiable cause [12,13].

The most important mutations are those that affect the ATP-dependent potassium (K_{ATP}) channels in the pancreatic beta cells, resulting in the most severe form of CH. Two specific genes have been identified, *ABCC8* and *KCNJ11*, which together account for 80%–90% of the genetically identifiable forms of the disease (the other six genes make up the remaining 10%–20%) [4,14].

The K_{ATP} channel in the pancreatic beta cell plays an integral role in glucose-induced insulin release. It is composed of two subunits, the sulfonylurea receptor 1 and the inwardly rectifying potassium channel (Kir6.2) [15–17]. The K_{ATP} channels in the beta cell are normally in the open state. When the beta cell is stimulated by glucose, the resulting glycolysis increases the ratio of ATP/ADP within the cell. This increased ATP inhibits the activity of the K_{ATP}

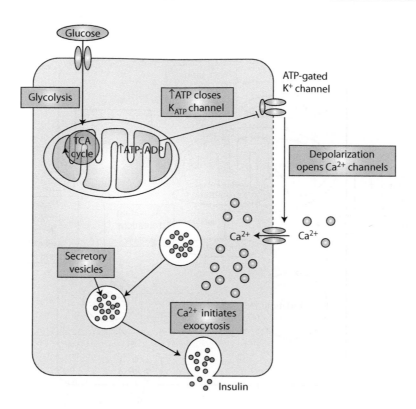

Figure 39.1 Outline of the molecular mechanisms that regulate insulin secretion in pancreatic beta cells. K_{ATP} channels of beta cells have a key role in transduction of the metabolic signals generated from glucose metabolism into changes in plasma membrane electrical activity and insulin secretion. Glucose metabolism in the pancreatic beta cell results in an increase in the intracellular ATP/ADP ratio, which leads to the closure of K_{ATP} channels and subsequent cell membrane depolarization. Depolarization results in increased Ca^{2+} influx via voltage-gated calcium channels, which leads to the exocytosis of insulin. TCA, tricarboxylic acid. (Reprinted by permission from Springer Nature. *Nat Clin Pract Endocrinol Metab*, Kapoor RR, James C, Hussain K. Advances in the diagnosis and management of hyperinsulinemic hypoglycemia. 2009;5(2):101–12, copyright 2009.)

channels, causing them to close. Once closed, the resultant change in ion flux across the membrane results in its depolarization. This in turn leads to the opening of voltage-gated Ca^{2+} channels, allowing for an influx of calcium into the cell. The increase in calcium is the final signal in the pathway that causes the release of insulin from secretory vesicles in the beta cell [12,18–20] (Figure 39.1).

The two subunits of the K_{ATP} channel, the sulfonylurea receptor 1 and the inwardly rectifying potassium channel (Kir6.2), are encoded by *ABCC8* and *KCNJ11*, respectively [15–17]. While an autosomal dominant mutation in one of these two genes causes a mild, medically responsive hyperinsulinism, the recessive inactivating mutations result in the more severe and often medically resistant form. Examining the mechanism of action of diazoxide, the principal medical treatment for CH, it becomes clear why this is the case. Diazoxide works as an agonist for the K_{ATP} channel in beta cells, specifically with the sulfonylurea receptor–potassium internal rectifier receptor complex (SUR-K_{ir}). In normal beta cells, it causes an opening of the K_{ATP} channel and halts the release of insulin. Not surprisingly, approximately 80% of the diazoxide treatment-unresponsive cases (the most severe form) are due to either *ABCC8* or *KCNJ11* inactivating mutations [4,14]. These recessive mutations most often

result in the diffuse form of CH. In contrast, the focal form of CH has been shown to be the result of a different genetic process, paternal uniparental disomy. Both the *ABCC8* gene and the *KCNJ11* gene are located on chromosome 11p15. The focal loss of the maternal allele with subsequent replacement by the paternal copy on the short arm of chromosome 11 at position 15.1 can lead to a clone of beta cells that develop into a focal lesion in the pancreas. If this paternal copy of the allele possesses a mutation in either the *ABCC8* or the *KCNJ11* gene, then the hemi- or homozygosity results in hyperinsulinemia of this focal lesion [3,4,21,22]. It is this paternal mutation and subsequent somatic loss of function of the maternal gene that is used clinically to differentiate between the diffuse and focal forms. Current genetic diagnostic testing allows the clinician to distinguish between a recessive homozygous mutation, and therefore diffuse disease, and a paternal mutation and subsequent loss of function of the maternal copy, indicating a focal disease. This, combined with recent advances in radiological imaging techniques, has made it possible to identify and localize these focal lesions, thus significantly changing the surgical management of CH.

While mutations in the genes affecting the K_{ATP} channel are implicated in 80%–90% of the identifiable causes of

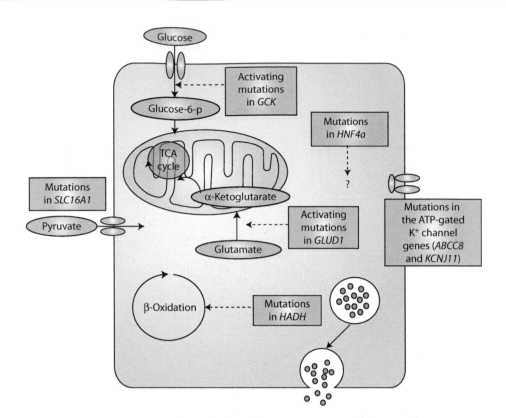

Figure 39.2 Summary of the molecular mechanisms that lead to congenital hyperinsulinemic hypoglycemia. Recessive inactivating mutations in *ABCC8* or *KCNJ11* cause continuous beta cell membrane depolarization and subsequent calcium influx, which result in unregulated insulin secretion. Activating mutations in *GLUD1* diminish the inhibitory effect of GTP on glutamate dehydrogenase and facilitate its activation by leucine. The activation of glutamate dehydrogenase causes increased oxidation of glutamate, thereby raising the ATP/ADP ratio in pancreatic beta cells, which leads to increased insulin secretion. Activating mutations in *GCK* lower the threshold for glucose-stimulated insulin secretion. The exact roles that HADH and HNF4A have in congenital HH are currently unclear, but HADH seems to be a negative regulator of insulin secretion. Dominant mutations in *SLC16A1* increase the expression of the MCT1R transporter, which allows pyruvate to act as an insulin secretagogue. GCK, glucokinase (hexokinase 4); glucose-6-P, glucose-6-phosphate; GTP, guanosine triphosphate. (Reprinted by permission from Springer Nature. *Nat Clin Pract Endocrinol Metab*, Kapoor RR, James C, Hussain K. Advances in the diagnosis and management of hyperinsulinemic hypoglycemia. 2009;5(2):101–12, copyright 2009.)

CH, the other 10%–20% of cases are caused by mutations in one of six different genes affecting other processes. The *GLUD1* (encoding glutamate dehydrogenase enzyme), *CGK* (encoding glucokinase), *HADH* (encoding short-chain L-3-hydroxyacyl-CoA dehydrogenase), *SLC16A1* (encoding a monocarboxylate transporter), and *UCP2* (encoding UCP2 protein) genes all affect the ATP/ADP ratio within the beta cells, which determines the status of the K_{ATP} channel [4, 23–26]. Likewise, a transcription factor defect in the *HNF4A* (hepatocyte nuclear factor 4 alpha) gene has been shown to cause neonatal hyperinsulinemia [27]. All of these mutations result in the diffuse, usually mild, form of CH, and all are diazoxide responsive (except *GCK*, which has variable diazoxide responsiveness) (Figure 39.2).

MEDICAL MANAGEMENT

When a newborn suffers hyperinsulinism, maximal steps are taken to correct the hypoglycemia in order to protect the developing brain. These steps include provision of glucose at rates greatly exceeding the normal demands. The normal newborn typically requires about 6 mg of glucose per kilogram of body weight per minute. The patient with hyperinsulinism frequently requires a central venous catheter to provide two to four times that amount of glucose. This supplements provision of enteral glucose often by nasogastric tube or gastrostomy. In addition, glucagon (intramuscular [IM] or intravenous [IV]) is useful for initial stabilization and as an adjunct on a short-term basis, but has little long-term usefulness.

After the initial emergency management has stabilized the patient, the standard first-choice treatment is administration of diazoxide. Diazoxide is an agonist of the SUR-K_{ir} complex in the K_{ATP} channel of pancreatic beta cells. It acts to open the K_{ATP} channel, inhibiting insulin secretion [28]. The typical dose of oral diazoxide is 5–15 mg/kg/day divided into two or three doses. Patients who are unresponsive to this dose rarely respond to increased dosing, which increases the potential for adverse effects of the medication. Diazoxide is not effective in all patients. Reviewing their results in a large number of children with hyperinsulinism, the group from Paris and Brussels showed that their success was largely limited to patients with onset of hypoglycemia at a somewhat later age [29]. They could effectively control the hypoglycemia with diazoxide in only 1 of 31 patients whose hypoglycemia began in the neonatal period. They were able to control the hypoglycemia in 12 of 39 children with early-infantile onset and all 7 of the uncommon late-infantile cases. These authors concluded that diazoxide is useful when hyperinsulinism occurs in infants and children, but not in newborns. We now know that these diazoxide-unresponsive newborns have mutations in *ABCC8* or *KCNJ11* in 80% of the cases. It seems evident that the patients presenting early in the newborn period (as opposed to later in infancy or childhood) are those with abnormalities in the sulfonylurea receptor complex. Patients with CH due to any of the other causes more often present later in life with more mild disease. When a neonate with hyperinsulinemia is unresponsive to diazoxide, genetic testing must be undertaken to identify the cause and guide treatment, specifically with respect to surgery. Rapid screening molecular genetic testing is used to screen for mutations in the *ABCC8* and *KCNJ11* genes [30]. Testing that shows homozygosity or compound heterozygosity for either of these genes indicates a diffuse disease. Alternatively, testing that shows a paternal *ABCC8* or *KCNJ11* mutation is highly indicative of focal disease [12,21]. If no mutation in either of these genes is identified, then the patient should undergo testing for *GCK*, as a select group of the patients with mutations in this gene can present early in life with severe disease [30]. Patients with diffuse disease most often undergo near-total pancreatectomy. Those with focal disease receive further radiological testing to localize the focus and subsequent surgical resection of the lesion (Figure 39.3).

Octreotide, a somatostatin analog, is frequently added in cases of diazoxide unresponsiveness. Octreotide has an inhibitory effect on the glucose-mediated release of insulin [31]. The typical dose is 5–20 µg/kg/day, either via constant infusion or divided into three daily doses, with the maximum dose range between 15 and 50 µg/kg/day [4]. The success of octreotide is variable. One study from a group in Israel noted that while octreotide was sometimes successful, 7 of 15 patients ultimately required pancreatic resection [29]. Even in patients who respond to octreotide, there are significant drawbacks to treatment. While some recent studies show potential for the use of long-acting-release octreotide, it generally has to be administered via either continuous subcutaneous infusion or four daily injections [32]. Tachyphylaxis develops quickly, and severe side effects, such as fatal necrotizing enterocolitis, have been observed [33].

Other medications have been used, including calcium channel blockers and steroids, but their efficacy has not been established, nor are they useful as stand-alone treatments.

RADIOLOGICAL IMAGING AND DIAGNOSTIC PROCEDURES

Advancements in diagnostic imaging in the last decade have changed the approach to patients with CH. Previously, there were no accurate imaging techniques to precisely identify the areas of hyperfunctioning beta cells within the pancreas, nor were there genetic tests to help distinguish between diffuse and focal lesions. The only method clinicians had at their disposal was highly selective arteriography and venography. These techniques do not image the lesions with the type of blush sometimes seen in insulinomas. Rather, they aid in localization through percutaneous transhepatic selective venous segmental sampling along the splenic and portal veins to measure the concentration of insulin. In addition, differential sequential arterial stimulation with tolbutamide was used along the arterial branches subserving different sites in the pancreas in order to detect the step-up of insulin concentration. These invasive techniques have been virtually abandoned.

The introduction of ^{18}F-L-3,4-dihydroxyphenylalanine positron emission tomography (^{18}F-L-DOPA-PET) scanning has revolutionized the preoperative assessment of these patients and has made the technique of venous and arterial sampling unnecessary. As noted earlier, we can now distinguish between the specific mutations causing the diffuse versus the focal forms of CH. When a patient has been found to have the mutation indicating a focal form, the next step in management is to obtain a ^{18}F-L-DOPA-PET scan. Pancreatic islet cells take up L-DOPA and convert it to dopamine via decarboxylases. The radiotracer labeled ^{18}F-L-DOPA is preferentially taken up by the hyperfunctioning beta cells that have an increased rate of insulin production compared with normal cells [12,34]. This technique can detect lesions as small a 10^5–10^6 cells, which is approximately 1 mm in diameter. Most focal lesions in CH measure 2.5–7.5 mm. The ability to localize these areas is even greater when paired with a computed tomography (CT) scan. The sensitivity for detecting focal lesions with ^{18}F-L-DOPA-PET-CT has been shown to be between 88% and 94%, with a specificity approaching 100% [35,36]. Recent meta-analyses have confirmed the superiority of ^{18}F-L-DOPA-PET-CT over other techniques in diagnosing and localizing the disease [37]. Most importantly, the focal form can be surgically cured by limited resection.

OPERATIVE APPROACH IN PAST DECADES

When medical therapy fails to control the symptoms of hyperinsulinemia, operative therapy is indicated. Until recently, clinicians have lacked the ability to adequately distinguish between focal and diffuse forms. Localizing the focal lesion was difficult and imperfect. Historically, surgeons have performed extensive pancreatic resections, believing the condition to be a diffuse hyperplasia of beta cells and generally considering lesser resections to yield unacceptable persistent hypoglycemia. While inadequate resection allows persistent hypoglycemia with the progression of neurological damage, excessive resection carries the increased risk of diabetes mellitus (DM) and glucose intolerance. A recent study of more than 50 patients who underwent a near-total pancreatectomy (>98% of the pancreas)

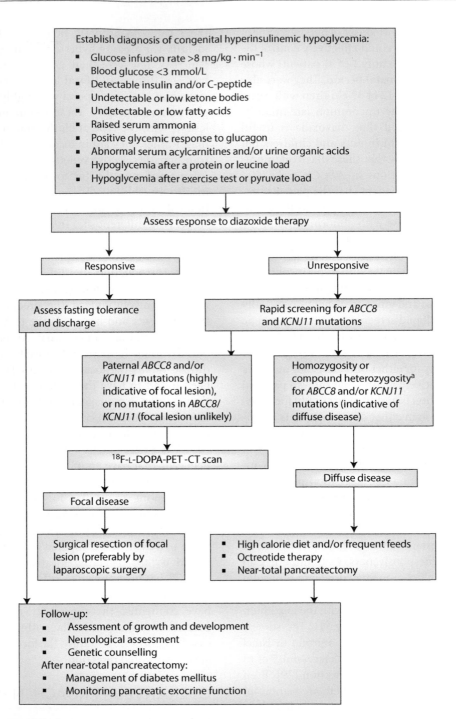

Establish diagnosis of congenital hyperinsulinemic hypoglycemia:

- Glucose infusion rate >8 mg/kg · min^{-1}
- Blood glucose <3 mmol/L
- Detectable insulin and/or C-peptide
- Undetectable or low ketone bodies
- Undetectable or low fatty acids
- Raised serum ammonia
- Positive glycemic response to glucagon
- Abnormal serum acylcarnitines and/or urine organic acids
- Hypoglycemia after a protein or leucine load
- Hypoglycemia after exercise test or pyruvate load

Assess response to diazoxide therapy

Responsive → Assess fasting tolerance and discharge

Unresponsive → Rapid screening for *ABCC8* and *KCNJ11* mutations

Paternal *ABCC8* and/or *KCNJ11* mutations (highly indicative of focal lesion), or no mutations in *ABCC8/KCNJ11* (focal lesion unlikely)

Homozygosity or compound heterozygosity^a for *ABCC8* and/or *KCNJ11* mutations (indicative of diffuse disease)

^{18}F-L-DOPA-PET-CT scan

Diffuse disease

Focal disease

Surgical resection of focal lesion (preferably by laparoscopic surgery)

- High calorie diet and/or frequent feeds
- Octreotide therapy
- Near-total pancreatectomy

Follow-up:
- Assessment of growth and development
- Neurological assessment
- Genetic counselling

After near-total pancreatectomy:
- Management of diabetes mellitus
- Monitoring pancreatic exocrine function

Figure 39.3 Outline of a diagnostic and management algorithm for patients with congenital hyperinsulinemic hypoglycemia. ^{18}F-L-DOPA-PET-CT examination is only indicated in patients who potentially have a focal lesion (i.e., those with a paternal *ABCC8* or *KCNJ11* gene mutation or those in whom the genetic basis of the disease is unknown). This imaging examination is not indicated in patients with genetically confirmed diffuse disease. In compound heterozygosity, the patient inherits two recessive alleles (in either *ABCC8* or *KCNJ11*) that can cause congenital hyperinsulinemic hypoglycemia in a heterozygous state. (Reprinted by permission from Springer Nature. *Nat Clin Pract Endocrinol Metab*, Kapoor RR, James C, Hussain K. Advances in the diagnosis and management of hyperinsulinemic hypoglycemia. 2009;5(2):101–12, copyright 2009.)

showed that by 13 years of age, 100% of patients had experienced episodes of hyperglycemia, and 91% required insulin therapy [38]. Another study of 27 infants found that 45% of children undergoing 95% pancreatectomy developed DM, as did 86% of those undergoing near-total pancreatectomy [39].

While excessive resection increases the risk of diabetes, inadequate resection allows for the persistence of hypoglycemia. The group at Children's Hospital of Philadelphia reviewed 35 years of surgical care for hyperinsulinism in 1999 [40]. The mean follow-up time was 9.8 ± 1.1 years. They found that what they refer to as "subtotal" (<95%)

(a)

(b)

(c)

(d)

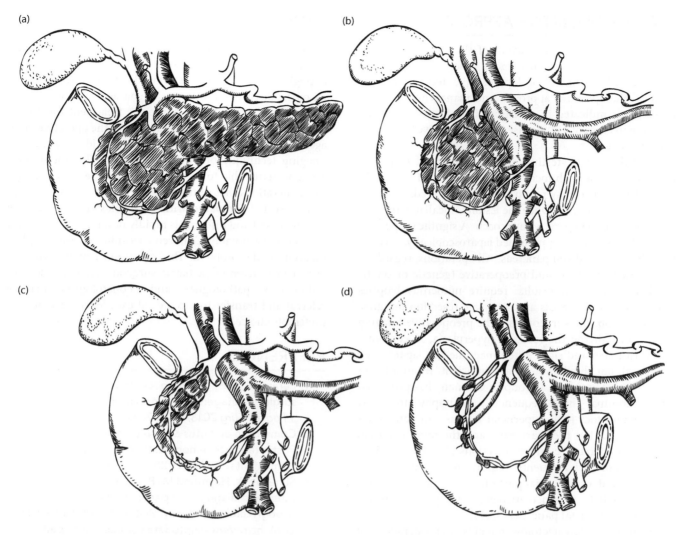

Figure 39.4 Pancreatic resections performed for glycemic control in diffuse forms of CH. **(a)** Normal pancreas. **(b)** 85% pancreatectomy. **(c)** 95% pancreatectomy. **(d)** 98% pancreatectomy. (Reprinted from *J Pediatr Surg*, 34, Lovvorn HN et al., Congenital hyperinsulinism and the surgeon: Lessons learned over 35 years, 786–93, Copyright 1999, with permission from Elsevier.)

pancreatectomy resulted in complete resolution of hyperinsulinism in only 19% of cases, compared with resolution in 50% of patients who received 95% or greater resection. Overall, complete resolution after surgery was seen in only 33% of diffuse lesions, but it was seen in 82% of focal lesions. The reresection rate was higher for the patients who underwent subtotal pancreatectomy, and the incidence of complications was not better than in those who underwent a >95% pancreatectomy [40].

The terminology surgeons have used in the past to describe the extent of resection has been murky. Sometimes, authors quantify the resection as between 70% and 98% pancreatectomy and often define these quantities poorly. Qualitative terms, also often poorly defined, include *leftsided pancreatectomy*, *subtotal pancreatectomy*, and *neartotal pancreatectomy*. Attempts have been made to define these assorted terms anatomically, although the inherent variability in gross morphology of the child's pancreas imposes inevitable inaccuracy. An autopsy study

of infants showed that anatomical landmarks often used to quantify a pancreatic resection are quite variable [41]. For instance, when all pancreatic tissue to the left of the superior mesenteric vessels was weighed and compared with the weight of the gland, this amount ranged from about 32% to about 67%. When all pancreatic tissue to the left of the pancreaticoduodenal vessels was assessed, that amount varied from 43% to 96%. The group at Children's Hospital of Philadelphia provided clear anatomical definitions for resections named by different numbered percentages. They defined a 95% pancreatectomy as a resection of the entire pancreas except for the tissue to the right of the common bile duct and a "thin rim along the second portion of the duodenum and pancreatico-duodenal arteries." A 98% pancreatectomy, in their words, "leaves only small islands of the pancreas along the pancreaticoduodenal arteries" [40] (Figure 39.4). These have become the generally accepted definitions used within the literature [42].

PRESENT OPERATIVE APPROACH

Over the last decade, the advent of ^{18}F-L-DOPA-PET-CT scan combined with sophisticated genetic testing, along with the advancement of laparoscopic techniques, has changed the operative approach and management of CH. Resection is indicated in all cases of confirmed focal disease, and in cases of diffuse disease unresponsive to medical management.

After the genetic testing distinguishes focal from diffuse forms, those with focal forms undergo a ^{18}F-L-DOPA-PET-CT scan. This may require transfer to a medical center with these capabilities. Once the lesion is localized, the surgeon can plan the operative approach. A significant percent of focal lesions can be approached laparoscopically, particularly those in the distal pancreas. All operations, regardless of the exact diagnosis and preoperative (genetic or scintigraphic) localization results, require numerous biopsies to confirm the diagnosis and adequate resection margins. At exploration, the surgeon uses the preoperative imaging to aid in localizing the focus of hyperplasia, in combination with touch and sight (often magnified by laparoscopy or loupes), but this is not always sufficient. In an attempt to rectify this problem, a group in Germany has promoted intra-abdominal high-frequency sonography to assist in localizing foci [43]. Superficial lesions can sometimes be enucleated, but these are rare, and the more common deeper lesions require larger resections [42]. Focal lesions in the head or neck frequently require an open approach to surgery and, if a substantial portion of the head is resected, often necessitate a pancreaticojejunostomy to allow for drainage of the distal pancreas [42,44].

Extensive pancreatectomy remains the operation of choice for diffuse disease. There is still no consensus regarding the optimal extent of resection. It is widely accepted that 98% resection results in very high rates of subsequent DM, and these operations are usually reserved for reresections rather than initial procedures. There is still some disagreement as to whether a 95% resection is actually superior to a subtotal (<95%) pancreatectomy. A group from Saudi Arabia (where CH is more prevalent due to consanguinity) has championed a laparoscopic approach that averages 90% resection [45]. In the largest reported series to date of laparoscopic resections for CH, 12 laparoscopic pancreatectomies were performed for diffuse disease. Two cases were converted to open, and one patient required reresection 3 months later due to persistent hypoglycemia. In total, four of the patients were euglycemic and showed complete resolution, while seven were controlled with medical management, and one progressed to DM. While these results are promising, average follow-up time was less than 2 years. More long-term data is needed to fully evaluate this approach. In addition, the group of patients treated laparoscopically were older (mean age = 14.5 months) than their cohort group who underwent open operations (mean age = 3.4 months) [45]. This group and a number of other case reports have provided evidence that laparoscopy can be a safe approach [46–48].

SUMMARY

CH is a rare and dangerous condition that requires prompt, often emergent medical efforts to control the significant hypoglycemia. Advances in our understanding of the genetics of the disease now allow us to characterize the disorder as either diffuse or focal. While the treatment for diffuse disease is still extensive pancreatectomy, the operative management of the focal form has evolved. Aided by the new imaging technique of ^{18}F-L-DOPA-PET-CT, practitioners are now better able to localize these focal lesions and perform operations that significantly limit the amount of pancreas resected compared with diffuse lesions. The field of CH treatment and research is rapidly developing, with a few centers, most notably Children's Hospital of Philadelphia, focused on the problem. This condition benefits from an experienced team of pediatric surgeons, endocrinologists, radiologists, pathologists, and neonatologists, making referral and transfer to a center of excellence a sound and preferable choice.

REFERENCES

1. Peranteau WH, Palladino AA, Bhatti TR et al. The surgical management of insulinomas in children. *J Pediatr Surg* 2013;48:2517–24.
2. Committee on Fetus and Newborn, Adamkin DH. Postnatal glucose homeostasis in late-preterm and term infants. *Pediatrics* 2011;127(3):575–9.
3. Sunehag A, Haymond M. Pathogenesis, clinical features, and diagnosis of persistent hyperinsulinemic hypoglycemia of infancy. Waltham, MA: UpToDate, 2014. http://www.uptodate.com/contents/pathogenesis-clinical-features-and-diagnosis-of-persistent-hyperinsulinemic-hypoglycemia-of-infancy/contributors.
4. Arnoux JB, Verkarre V, Saint-Martin C et al. Congenital hyperinsulinism: Current trends in diagnosis and therapy. *Orphanet J Rare Dis* 2011;6:63.
5. Laidlaw GF. Nesidioblastoma, the islet tumor of the pancreas. *Am J Pathol* 1938;14:125–34.
6. Jaffe R, Hashida Y, Yunis EJ. The endocrine pancreas of the neonate and infant. In: Rosenberg HS, Bernstein J, eds., *Perspectives in Pediatric Pathology*. Vol. 7. New York: Masson Publishing, 1982:137–65.
7. Jaffe R, Hashida Y, Yunis EJ. Pancreatic pathology in hyperinsulinemic hypoglycemia of infancy. *Lab Invest* 1980;42:356–65.
8. Witte DP, Greider MH, DeSchryver-Kecskemeti K, Kissane JM, White NH. The juvenile human endocrine pancreas: Normal v idiopathic hyperinsulinemic hypoglycemia. *Semin Diagn Pathol* 1984;1:30–42.
9. Rahier J, Guiot Y, Sempoux C. Persistent hyperinsulinaemic hypoglycaemia of infancy: A heterogeneous syndrome unrelated to nesidioblastosis. *Arch Dis Child Fetal Neonatal Ed* 2000;82:F108–12.

10. Rahier J, Guiot Y, Sempoux C. Morphological analysis of focal and diffuse forms of congenital hyperinsulinism. *Semin Pediatr Surg* 2011;20:3–12.

11. Capito C, de Lonlay P, Verkarre V et al. The surgical management of atypical forms of congenital hyperinsulinism. *Semin Pediatr Surg* 2011;20:54–5.

12. Kapoor RR, James C, Hussain K. Advances in the diagnosis and management of hyperinsulinemic hypoglycemia. *Nat Clin Pract Endocrinol Metab* 2009;5(2):101–12.

13. Glaser B, Thornton P, Otonkoski T, Junien C. Genetics of neonatal hyperinsulinism. *Arch Dis Child Fetal Neonal Ed* 2000;82:F79–86.

14. Bellanné-Chantelot C, Saint-Martin C, Ribeiro MJ et al. ABCC8 and KCNJ11 molecular spectrum of 109 patients with diazoxide-unresponsive congenital hyperinsulinism. *J Med Genet* 2010;47(11):752–9.

15. Palladino AA, Stanley CA. A specialized team approach to diagnosis and medical versus surgical treatment of infants with congenital hyperinsulinism. *Semin Pediatr Surg* 2011;20:32–7.

16. Thomas PM, Cote GJ, Wohllk N, Haddad B, Mathew PM, Rabl W. Mutations in the sulfonylurea receptor gene in familial persistent hyperinsulinemic hypoglycemia of infancy. *Science* 1995;268(5209):426–9.

17. Thomas PM, Ye Y, Lightner E. Mutation of the pancreatic islet inward rectifier Kir6.2 also leads to familial persistent hyperinsulinemic hypoglycemia of infancy. *Hum Mol Genet* 1996;5(11):1809–12.

18. Aguilar-Bryan L, Bryan J. Molecular biology of adenosine triphosphate-sensitive potassium channels. *Endocr Rev* 1999;20(2):101–35

19. Ashcroft SJ, Ashcroft FM. Properties and functions of ATP-sensitive K-channels. *Cell Signal* 1990;2(3):197–214.

20. Dukes ID, Philipson LH. K+ channels: Generating excitement in pancreatic beta-cells. *Diabetes* 1996;45(7):845–53.

21. de Lonlay P, Fournet JC, Rahier J et al. Somatic deletion of the imprinted 11p15 region in sporadic persistent hyperinsulinemic hypoglycemia of infancy is specific of focal adenomatous hyperplasia and endorses partial pancreatectomy. *J Clin Invest* 1997;100(4):802–7.

22. Verkarre V, Fournet JC, de Lonlay P et al. Paternal mutation of the sulfonylurea receptor (SUR1) gene and maternal loss of 11p15 imprinted genes lead to persistent hyperinsulinism in focal adenomatous hyperplasia. *J Clin Invest* 1998;102(7):1286–91.

23. Stanley CA, Lieu YK, Hsu BYL et al. Hyperinsulinism and hyperammonemia in infants with regulatory mutations of the glutamate dehydrogenase gene. *N Engl J Med* 1998;338(19):1352–7.

24. Clayton PT, Eaton S, Aynsley-Green A et al. Hyperinsulinism in short-chain L-3-hydroxyacyl-CoA dehydrogenase deficiency reveals the importance of beta-oxidation in insulin secretion. *J Clin Invest* 2001;108:457–65.

25. Otonkoski T, Jiao H, Kaminen-Ahola N et al. Physical exercise-induced hypoglycemia caused by failed silencing of monocarboxylate transporter 1 in pancreatic beta cells. *Am J Hum Genet* 2007;81(3):467–74.

26. Gonzalez-Barroso MM, Giurgea I, Bouillaud F et al. Mutations in UCP2 in congenital hyperinsulinism reveal a role for regulation of insulin secretion. *PLoS One* 2008;3(12):e3850.

27. Pearson ER, Boj SF, Steele AM et al. Macrosomia and hyperinsulinaemic hypoglycaemia in patients with heterozygous mutations in the HNF4A gene. *PLoS Med* 2007;4(4):e118.

28. Panten U, Burgfeld J, Goerke F et al. Control of insulin secretion by sulfonylureas, meglitinide and diazoxide in relation to their binding to the sulfonylurea receptor in pancreatic islets. *Biochem Pharmacol* 1989;38(8):1217–29.

29. Touati G, Poggi-Travert F, Ogier De Baulny H et al. Long-term treatment of persistent hyperinsulinaemic hypoglycaemia of infancy with diazoxide: A retrospective review of 77 cases and analysis of efficacy-predicting criteria. *Eur J Pediatr* 1998;157:628–33.

30. Glaser B. Familial hyperinsulinism. In: Pagon RA, Adam MP, Ardinger HH et al., eds., *GeneReviews®*. Seattle: University of Washington, 1993–2014. http://www.ncbi.nlm.nih.gov/books/NBK1375/.

31. Goel P, Choudhury SR. Persistent hyperinsulinemic hypoglycemia of infancy: An overview of current concepts. *J Indian Assoc Pediatr Surg* 2012;17(3):99–103.

32. Le Quan Sang KH, Arnoux JN, Mamoune A et al. Successful treatment of congenital hyperinsulinism with long-acting release octreotide. *Eur J Endocrinol* 2012;166(2):333–9.

33. Laje P, Halaby L, Adzick NS, Stanley CA. Necrotizing enterocolitis in neonates receiving octreotide for the management of congenital hyperinsulinism. *Pediatr Diabetes* 2010;11:142–7.

34. de Lonlay P, Simon-Carre A, Ribeiro MJ et al. Congenital hyperinsulinism: Pancreatic [18F]fluoro-L-dihyroxyphenylalanine (DOPA) positron emission tomography and immunohistochemistry study of DOPA decarboxylase and insulin secretion. *J Clin Endocrinol Metab* 2006;91(3):933–40.

35. Hardy OT, Hernandez-Pampaloni M, Saffer JR et al. Accuracy of [18F]fluorodopa positron emission tomography for diagnosing and localizing focal congenital hyperinsulinism. *J Clin Endocrinol Metab* 2007;92(12):4706–11.

36. Mohnike K, Blankenstein O, Minn H, Mohnike W, Fuchtner F, Otonkoski T. [18 F]-DOPA positron emission tomography for preoperative localization in congenital hyperinsulinism. *Horm Res* 2008;70(2):65–72.

37. Bloomberg BA, Moghbel MC, Saboury B, Stanley CA, Alavi A. The value of radiological interventions and 18F-DOPA PET in diagnosing and localizing focal congenital hyperinsulinism: Systematic review and meta-analysis. *Mol Imaging Biol* 2013;15:97–105.

38. Beltrand J, Caquard M, Arnoux JB et al. Glucose metabolism in 105 children and adolescents after pancreatectomy for congenital hyperinsulinism. *Diabetes Care* 2012;35(2):198–203.

39. Shilyansky J, Fisher S, Cutz E, Perlman K, Filler RM. Is 95% pancreatectomy the procedure of choice for treatment of persistent hyperinsulinemic hypoglycemia of the neonate? *J Pediatr Surg* 1997;32(2):342–6.

40. Lovvorn HN, Nance ML, Ferry RJ Jr et al. Congenital hyperinsulinism and the surgeon: Lessons learned over 35 years. *J Pediatr Surg* 1999;34:786–93.

41. Reyes GA, Fowler CL, Pokorny WJ. Pancreatic anatomy in children: Emphasis on its importance to pancreatectomy. *J Pediatr Surg* 1993;28:712–5.

42. Pierro A, Nah SA. Surgical management of congenital hyperinsulinism of infancy. *Semin Pediatr Surg* 2011;20:50–3.

43. von Rohden L, Mohnike K, Mau H et al. Visualization of the focus in congenital hyperinsulinism by intraoperative sonography. *Semin Pediatr Surg* 2011;20:28–31.

44. Laje P, Stanley CA, Palladino AA, Becker SA, Adzick NS. Pancreatic head resection and Roux-en-Y pancreaticojejunostomy for the treatment of the focal form of congenital hyperinsulinism. *J Pediatr Surg* 2012;47(1):130–5.

45. Al-Shanafey S, Habib Z, AlNassar S. Laparoscopic pancreatectomy for persistent hyperinsulinemic hypoglycemia of infancy. *J Pediatr Surg* 2009;44(1):134–8.

46. Al-Shanafey S. Laparoscopic vs open pancreatectomy for persistent hyperinsulinemic hypoglycemia of infancy. *J Pediatr Surg* 2009;44(5):957–61.

47. Liem NT, Son TN, Hoan NT. Laparoscopic near-total pancreatectomy for persistent hyperinsulinemic hypoglycemia of infancy: Report of two cases. *J Laparosc Adv Surg Tech* 2010;20(1):115–7.

48. Blakely ML, Lobe TE, Cohen J, Burghen GA. Laparoscopic pancreatectomy for persistent hyperinsulinemic hypoglycemia of infancy. *Surg Endosc* 2001;15(8):897–8.

40

Gastrinoma (Zollinger–Ellison syndrome) and rare neuroendocrine tumors

MARK SAWICKI

GASTRINOMA

Gastrinomas are uncommon neuroendocrine neoplasms (NENs) that secrete the hormone gastrin in excess, and result in the classic Zollinger–Ellison syndrome (ZES). First described in 1955, ZES includes the triad of diffuse gastroduodenal ulcerations, gastric acid hypersecretion, and pancreatic nonbeta islet tumors [1]. When Robert Zollinger and Edwin Ellison described their findings at the American Surgical Association meeting in 1955, they did not know gastrin was the culprit until Gregory and Tracy demonstrated that gastrinoma tumor extract increased acid secretion in dogs in a manner similar to that of antral gastrin extract [2]. Preoperative determination of gastrin was not feasible until gastrin was first measured by radioimmunoassay in 1968, which ushered in the "modern" era of ZES diagnosis [3].

Epidemiology

Gastrinomas, the second most common functional pancreatic neuroendocrine tumor (PanNET), have an annual incidence 0.4–4 cases per million population [4]. Most patients have sporadic gastrinomas, but as many as 30% are associated with multiple endocrine neoplasia type 1 (MEN1) syndrome [5].

Clinical presentation

The average ZES patient is 43 years old and presents with symptoms such as diarrhea, heartburn due to gastroesophageal reflux disease (GERD), and severe abdominal pain due to peptic ulcer disease (PUD) [6]. Patients with ZES have more severe acid secretion compared with patients with uncomplicated PUD, and historically, they present with increased severity of symptoms, such as an increased number of ulcers, ulcers at atypical locations (i.e., postbulbar duodenum or rarely jejunum), and increased abdominal pain. Currently, many patients with PUD or GERD are treated early with potent proton pump inhibitors (PPIs), such that the ravaging ulcer symptoms patients presented with in the early days of ZES are now often blunted by standard medical management and the diagnosis is often delayed 5 years or more. Even with potent PPI treatment shutting down acid secretion, patients with ZES develop prominent gastric folds due to gastrin-stimulated mucosal cell proliferation; this finding on endoscopy should prompt ZES diagnostic testing [6]. Failure to respond to conventional medical ulcer treatment, recurrence after adequate therapy, or PUD in the absence of *Helicobacter pylori* should also raise suspicion of ZES.

Anatomic location

Gastrinomas are anatomically and biologically different from other PanNETs. When ZES was first described, the gastrinoma was considered a pancreatic islet cell tumor, but it is now thought to also uniquely arise within extrapancreatic sites, most commonly the duodenum, but also within the peripancreatic soft tissues. This general area of the abdomen is referred to as the gastrinoma triangle (Figure 40.1) [7]. Rarely, they arise at other ectopic locations, including the liver, biliary tree, omentum, ovary, kidney, and heart [8–15].

Duodenal gastrinomas are small (<1 cm) and arise within the submucosa rather than the mucosa, and therefore are not readily identified by endoscopy [16,17]. Sporadic duodenal gastrinomas are usually solitary, whereas they are usually multiple in MEN1 patients with ZES [17]. In general, extrapancreatic gastrinomas such as those found in the duodenum have a better prognosis than pancreatic gastrinomas [18–20]. Although duodenal gastrinomas are often associated with lymph node metastases, they are less likely to go on to develop liver metastases. Perhaps they are biologically different from their pancreatic counterparts, as was proposed by Passaro [21]. Interestingly, molecular gene expression profiling suggests duodenal and pancreatic gastrinomas are different [22].

Primary lymph node gastrinomas are considered by some to be a true primary tumor rather than a metastasis

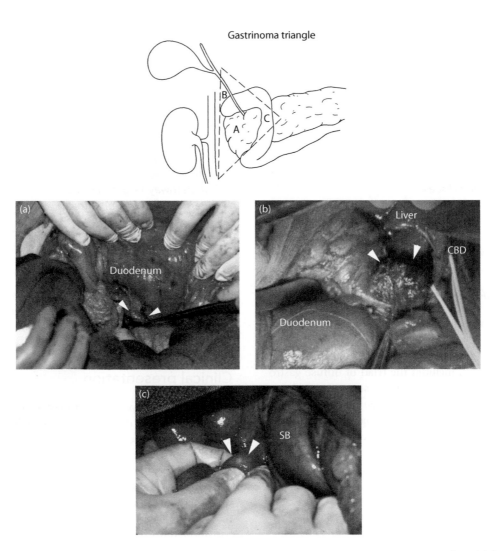

Figure 40.1 Gastrinoma triangle. The majority of gastrinomas (85%) occur in the gastrinoma triangle, which is an anatomic area bordered by imaginary lines connecting (1) the junction of cystic and common bile ducts, (2) the junction between the second and third portion of the duodenum, and (3) the junction between the neck and body of the pancreas. **(a)** Retropancreatic gastrinoma. **(b)** Hepatoduodenal ligament gastrinoma. **(c)** Duodenal gastrinoma. CBD, common bile duct; SB, small bowel. Arrowheads point to tumors.

because excision of some lymph node primary gastrinomas is curative [23,24]. It is hypothesized that such lymph node primary tumors arise from gastrinoma precursor cells scattered during embryonic development of the foregut [21,25]. Some have argued instead that these lymph node tumors are metastases from overlooked duodenal microgastrinomas that are slow to develop liver metastases [26].

Molecular biology

The molecular basis for PanNETs is incompletely understood. They are thought to arise through mutations in pancreatic islet cells or precursors [27]. This hypothesis fits well for the development of nonfunctional tumors and insulinomas, but is less clear for gastrinomas.

Menin, the protein product of the MEN1 gene, is a tumor suppressor protein commonly inactivated by mutation in sporadic and MEN1-associated PanNETs [28,29]. Menin is part of a large nuclear protein complex (histone methyltransferase) that activates gene transcription through histone (H3K4) methylation at target gene promoters [30]. This is a relatively common abnormality, but currently, there is no targeted therapy for menin inactivation in neuroendocrine tumors (NETs).

Genes in the mechanistic target of rapamycin (mTOR) signaling pathway are mutated in sporadic PanNETs. Members of this pathway mutated in PanNETs include PTEN, TSC2, and PIK3CA [31]. Reduced TSC2 (tuberin) and PTEN (phosphatase and tensin homolog deleted on chromosome 10) expression is also associated with worse prognosis, and Akt (serine/threonine kinase) activation is common in PanNETs [32,33]. mTOR is the catalytic subunit of two distinct serine/threonine kinase complexes: mTORC1 and mTORC2 [34]. Activated mTORC1 regulates protein synthesis and gene expression to regulate energy balance and metabolism, cell growth, and angiogenesis. mTORC1 in inhibited by the GTPase-activating protein activity of the TSC1 (hamartin)–TSC2 complex. Hence, mutation of TSC2 in PanNETs would be predicted to cause increased mTORC1 kinase activity. Insulin and insulin-like growth factor 1 (IGF-1) activate the mTOR pathway through PIK3CA and Akt. PIK3CA (phosphoinositide-3-kinase, catalytic, alpha-polypeptide) activity is inhibited by PTEN. Activating mutation of PIK3CA or inactivating mutation of PTEN would therefore lead to increased mTORC1 activity. mTORC1 is sensitive to inhibition by rapamycin [35]. Prior to the discovery of mTOR pathway mutations in PanNETs, studies showed promise of rapamycin-based mTOR inhibitors (rapalogs) in the treatment of these tumors.

Diagnosis

Serum gastrin measurement is the cornerstone for ZES diagnosis. Measurement of gastric acid pH is also very helpful to interpret the context of the fasting serum gastrin level.

Both of these tests should be performed in a controlled clinical setting after careful transition of PPI and H2-receptor antagonists [36]. This must be done carefully to avoid peptic ulcer complications. A fasting serum gastrin of >1000 pg/mL (475 pmol/L or >10 times the upper limit) and a gastric pH of ≤2 is virtually diagnostic for ZES. Unfortunately, more than half of ZES patients do not meet these criteria [5]. The secretin stimulation test can be helpful to confirm the diagnosis in patients with intermediate fasting serum gastrin elevations (200–1000 pg/mL).

PPIs can lead to loss of negative feedback on antral G-cells and result in significantly elevated serum gastrin levels in normal patients [37]. Therefore, patients will need to be briefly transitioned off of their antacid regimen to obtain an accurate measure of their fasting gastrin level and response to secretin injection. PPI therapy, however, should never be abruptly discontinued, as this can result in rebound acid secretion and devastating complications in ZES patients [38]. It is recommended that gastrin and gastric acid be measured after (1) patients transition from PPI to high-dose H2-receptor antagonist (ranitidine 450–600 mg every 4–6 hours), which can be stopped for 24 hours, or (2) progressive reduction of the PPI dose over 2–4 weeks [38,39]. With either approach, it is essential to ensure the patient's ulcer diathesis is controlled prior to testing and is not exacerbated during the weaning period. It is also important to remember that the duration of action of PPIs can be more than a week because the drug remains bound to the proton pump. One more challenge to measuring gastrin is that not all commercial kits are reliable, and care must be taken when evaluating gastrin measurements [40,41].

In order to interpret the hypergastrinemia, it is essential to know whether the elevated gastrin is due to a physiological response to decreased gastric acid secretion, as in pernicious anemia. Gastric acid production may be assessed by measurement of nasogastric (NG) tube aspirate pH or, less readily available, measurement of basal acid output (BAO) (mmol/h). Either a pH of ≤2 or a BAO of >15 mmol/h is suggestive of ZES if hypergastrinemia is also present [42]. Elevated gastrin may also be associated with gastric acid hypersecretion in other conditions, such as retained excluded antrum, or associated with achlorhydria or hypochlorhydria in patients with atrophic gastritis or pernicious anemia. The patient history, gastric pH, and secretin stimulation test will aid in making the correct diagnosis.

In patients with indeterminate fasting serum gastrin measurements (200–1000 pmol/L), a secretin stimulation test may be helpful to confirm ZES (Figure 40.2). Patients with gastrinoma typically have an increase in gastrin release shortly after intravenous recombinant secretin injection, whereas normal patients do not have a rise in gastrin. A positive response is a rise in gastrin of >120 pmol/L above baseline during the course of the test. False negatives are not common, but false positives can occur in atrophic gastritis and patients on PPI therapy [43].

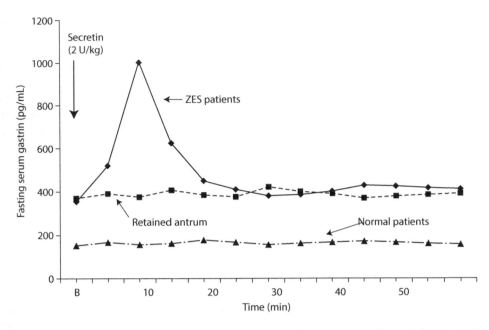

Figure 40.2 Secretin provocative test. Secretin (Kabi) was given at 2 U/kg intravenously, and the level of serum gastrin is measured over time. A rise in serum gastrin level within 15 minutes is diagnostic of ZES. This test is sensitive and specific, as other causes of hypergastrinemia do not respond to secretin with the paradoxical rise in gastrin level. B, baseline.

Imaging

Imaging of gastrinomas is essential for surgical planning, but challenging because the tumors are small, multiple, and frequently extrapancreatic. Conventional imaging (computed tomography [CT] or MRI) is usually obtained first, followed by somatostatin receptor scintigraphy (SRS). Gastrinomas are different from other PanNETs in that they are frequently extrapancreatic, so that imaging all tumor locations with a single modality can be very difficult. Even after extensive imaging, some gastrinomas are imaging negative.

CT scan has a sensitivity of approximately 50% for identifying gastrinomas [44,45]. In general, PanNETs are frequently isodense to pancreatic tissue, so they are not usually seen without contrast unless they are very large. Since they are quite vascular, gastrinomas frequently enhance with intravenous contrast. Multiplanar (coronal, sagittal, and axial) reconstruction is helpful to distinguish small tumors from blood vessels. Thin-slice (1 mm) biphasic studies have the highest sensitivity, with some tumors identified in the early arterial phase and others in the portal venous phase. In contrast to the modest sensitivity for pancreatic gastrinomas, CT scanning will identify <10% of duodenal tumors. Drinking a large amount of water (1.5 L) prior to the study, rather than standard oral contrast, provides the optimal negative contrast to visualize the ampulla and duodenal wall.

MRI has a sensitivity of 57% for identifying gastrinomas [44]. Gastrinomas have a lower concentration of aqueous protein and hydrogen protons than the surrounding normal pancreatic tissue. Therefore, islet cell tumors tend to be low signal intensity on T1-weighted fat-suppressed imaging and high signal intensity on T2-weighted fat-suppressed imaging. As in CT scanning, contrast enhancement is demonstrated due to their vascularity relative to the adjacent pancreas. MRI is better than CT for identifying duodenal tumors but inferior to SRS.

SRS should be obtained in every ZES patient (Figure 40.3). SRS takes advantage of the expression of somatostatin receptors on gastrinomas and other PanNETs (lower in insulinomas) [46]. SRS is more sensitive (87%) than other imaging modalities, although it does not provide the same anatomic detail obtained by CT or MRI. It is particularly helpful to identify bone and liver metastases [47,48]. While it is better than CT for duodenal gastrinomas, it still misses ~50% of duodenal gastrinomas [44,49]. As in all imaging modalities, smaller tumors (<1 cm) are more difficult to identify.

Although not yet Food and Drug Administration (FDA) approved ^{68}Ga-DOTA–positron emission tomography (PET)–CT will eventually become the gold standard for PanNET imaging (Figure 40.4). ^{68}Ga-labeled somatostatin analogs (SSTAs) bind to the cell surface SST receptors with preferential binding to somatostatin receptor subtypes 2 and 5, similar to SRS. ^{68}Ga-DOTA-PET-CT evaluation of a mixed population of neuroendocrine subtypes (i.e., not specific to PanNETs) has been shown to be superior to ^{111}In-DTPA-phenyloctreotide SRS chiefly because of better spatial resolution, as well as higher sensitivity [50,51]. Sensitivity and specificity are more than 90% in aggregate analysis. There is also the added benefit of faster study time (2 hours vs. 2 days) due to the shorter half-life of the tracer, less radiation, and no need for patient bowel prep. The imaging challenges

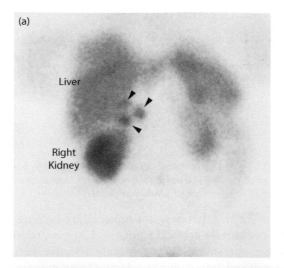

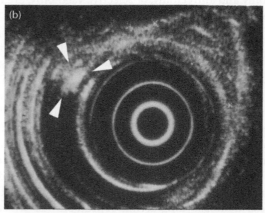

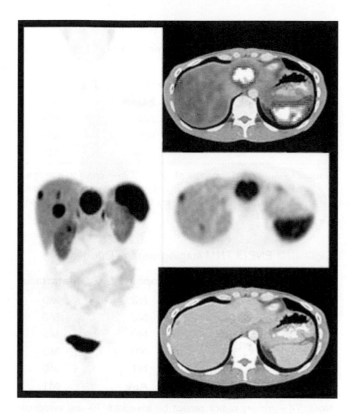

Figure 40.4 ^{68}Ga-DOTATATE-PET-CT showing multiple liver metastases from a PanNET occurring after Whipple resection. (Courtesy of Dr Martin Auerbach, University of California, Los Angeles.)

Figure 40.3 **(a)** SRS imaging showing multiple gastrinomas. **(b)** EUS of duodenum revealing occult gastrinoma within the bowel wall. Arrows point to tumor.

for gastrinomas may be helped with the introduction of ^{68}Ga-DOTA-PET-CT, but more gastrinoma-specific studies are needed, particularly comparing with SRS [52]. One unique problem for PanNETs is the physiological concentration of ^{68}Ga-DOTA-tracer in the uncinate process of the pancreas that can increase background [53].

Endoscopic ultrasound (EUS) is helpful to identify pancreatic and peripancreatic gastrinomas, but surprisingly not very sensitive for duodenal gastrinomas (Figure 40.3) [16,54,55]. Fine-needle aspiration (FNA) during EUS may be helpful but not necessary since the diagnosis is made by measuring fasting serum gastrin levels.

Staging

Recently, two staging and grading systems for NENs have been developed. In 2006, Rindi proposed a four-stage tumor–node–metastasis (TNM) staging system (Tables 40.1 and 40.2) and three-tier grading system (Table 40.3) that was adopted by the European Neuroendocrine Tumor Society (ENETS) [56,57]. In this scheme, NENs encompass lower-grade (G1 and G2) NETs and higher-grade (G3)

neuroendocrine cancers (NECs). This staging system has site-specific staging for duodenal and pancreatic tumors. Retrospective and prospective studies have validated this system for a variety of NENs, including PanNETs [58,59]. The World Health Organization (WHO) 2010 classification stratifies tumors based upon their Ki-67 index and their proliferative rate [56]. The American Joint Cancer Committee in 2010 published a second staging system (Table 40.4) adapted from the staging for pancreatic ductal adenocarcinomas that has also been validated for PanNETs [60,61]. Certainly, additional prospective studies need to be performed to further validate the utility of these new systems.

Treatment

Treatment of gastrinomas should follow published guidelines as recommended by the National Comprehensive Cancer Network (NCCN), ENETS, and current clinical trials (ClinicalTrials.gov). After controlling the PUD with medical management, patients with limited disease should undergo surgery for cure.

Medical management

Initial management of gastrinomas is to control acid secretion. Patients with inoperable, persistent or recurrent disease

Table 40.1 ENETS TNM staging system: Pancreas

Stage	Primary	Lymph node	Metastasis
I	T1	N0	M0
IIa	T2	N0	M0
IIb	T3	N0	M0
IIIa	T4	N0	M0
IIIb	Any	N1	M0
IV	Any	Any	M1

Note: T1—limited to pancreas of <2 cm; T2—limited to pancreas of 2–4 cm; T3— >4 cm or invading bile duct or duodenum; T4—invading adjacent organs (stomach, spleen, or colon) or vessels.

Table 40.2 ENETS TNM staging system: Duodenum

Stage	Primary	Lymph node	Metastasis
I	T1	N0	M0
IIa	T2	N0	M0
IIb	T3	N0	M0
IIIa	T4	N0	M0
IIIb	Any	N1	M0
IV	Any	Any	M1

Note: TX—primary tumor cannot be assessed; T0—no evidence of primary tumor; T1—tumor invades lamina propria or submucosa and size of ≤1 cm; T2—tumor invades muscularis propria or size of >1 cm; T3—tumor invades pancreas or retroperitoneum; T4—tumor invades peritoneum or other organs.

Table 40.4 AJCC TNM staging system

Stage	Primary	Lymph node	Metastasis
IA	T1	N0	M0
IB	T2	N0	M0
IIA	T3	N0	M0
IIB	T1-T3	N1	M0
III	T4	Any	M0
IV	Any	Any	M1

Note: T1—limited to pancreas of ≤2 cm; T2—limited to pancreas of >2 cm; T3—beyond pancreas but no SMA involvement; T4—involvement of SMA or celiac axis.

of these patients, but now it is unnecessary because of the efficacy of current antiacid regimens. Likewise, other acid-reducing operations, such as highly selective vagotomy, vagotomy and antrectomy, or selective vagotomy, are rarely necessary.

SSTAs (octreotide, lanreotide, and pasireotide) are useful to decrease hormone secretion-related symptoms and decrease tumor size (see below) [67–69]. Somatostatin binds to five different receptors, SSTR1–5, but the analogs have widely varying affinity [46]. Gastrinomas predominantly express SSTR2. Octreotide has high affinity for receptor subtypes SSTR2 and SSTR5. Pasireotide has a broader SSTR binding profile than octreotide and may be more effective [70]. Octreotide, with a longer half-life than somatostatin (2 hours vs. 2 minutes), is dosed two or three times daily subcutaneously. Long-acting forms of these analogs—long-acting repeatable (LAR)—allow monthly dosing, which improves patient compliance. Patients are initially treated with the short-acting analogs to determine tolerance to the medication. The dose can be escalated to control symptoms. Octreotide LAR may then be added to the regimen, and the shortened form transitioned off after 2 weeks of treatment with the short-acting analog. Side effects of SSTAs include nausea, abdominal pain, diarrhea, steatorrhea, hyperglycemia, and cholelithiasis. Approximately 1% of patients require cholecystectomy [71].

after surgery, or MEN1-ZES will require lifelong therapy. This is almost always successful with PPIs such as omeprazole, esomeprazole, pantoprazole, rabeprazole, or lansoprazole [62–64]. PPIs are used at higher than conventional doses administered once or twice a day. A starting dose is omeprazole at 60 mg/day. H2-receptor antagonists (cimetidine, ranitidine, and famotidine) can also be used, but at much higher than conventional dosing and inconveniently frequent dosing (every 4–6 hours) [65,66]. The high doses are well tolerated, with the notable exception that cimetidine is associated with antiandrogen effects with gynecomastia and impotence in men. Moreover, patients receiving H2-receptor antagonists require annual dose adjustments, whereas PPIs do not exhibit tachyphylaxis. For these reasons, PPIs are the optimum treatment for most patients. Total gastrectomy was at one time central to management

Surgery

After initiating medical management and completing preoperative localization studies, early surgical exploration for curative intent should be performed in every patient with limited disease, except for MEN1 patients, as described

Table 40.3 WHO 2010 grading classification

	Grade	Mitoses/10 hpf	Ki-67 index	
G1	Low	<2	<2%	Neuroendocrine tumor
G2	Intermediate	2–20	3%–20%	Neuroendocrine tumor
G3	High	>20	>20%	Neuroendocrine cancer

Note: 50 hpf is assessed if possible.
Ki-67 is assessed in area of highest labeling (hot spot).
Ki-67 values between 2 and 3 should be rounded to the nearest integer.

below. At initial presentation, approximately 15%–25% of gastrinoma patients will have liver metastases and cannot be operated on with curative intent [6,19]. Operative exploration by an experienced surgeon will identify the gastrinoma in most patients, but biochemical cure is difficult to achieve [72].

Patients with localized sporadic gastrinoma identified by preoperative imaging should undergo surgical resection for cure. Approximately 25% of patients will have localized disease at presentation [19]. Suspected lymph node spread is not a contraindication. Approximately 10% of patients will have "primary nodal" gastrinoma and benefit from excision. Negative imaging should not dogmatically deter surgical exploration either. Such patients will have small tumors, usually in the duodenum, and may be resected with curative intent [73].

MEN1 patients have multiple gastrinomas predominantly within the duodenum [74]. Patients with MEN1 and ZES generally have a good prognosis compared with their sporadic counterparts. This may be explained by the favorable biology of duodenal gastrinomas, as well as lead-time bias for patients being screened [75]. Risk of hepatic metastases increases, however, as the tumors grow larger, so there may be a survival benefit to earlier intervention [76–78]. Although most MEN1-associated gastrinomas are localized with the duodenum, it is possible that the gastrinoma is within the pancreatic head or, less likely, pancreatic body or tail. Localization requires specialized techniques to distinguish gastrinomas from other functioning and nonfunctioning pancreatic neoplasms in MEN1 patients [79,80]. Even with the selective arterial secretin injection (SASI) studies, it may not be possible to know whether a specific pancreatic tumor at the time of surgery is a gastrinoma. Because of these factors, there are several different surgical approaches to these patients: (1) resection of all localizable MEN1 gastrinomas [75,80], (2) selective resection based upon tumor size (>2 cm) [81,82], and (3) nonoperative management [83]. ENETS guidelines recommend surgery for patients whose pancreatic tumors are larger than 2 cm to reduce the risk of developing liver metastases, rather than the goal of biochemical cure (normal serum gastrin) [84].

The extent of surgery depends upon the size and location of the primary tumor. Every tumor identified by imaging should be accounted for during the exploration. Small pancreatic tumors may be enucleated so long as the main pancreatic duct will not be disrupted. This practice, however, does not follow traditional surgical oncology principles, and at least one retrospective study suggests formal resection may result in a longer disease-free interval [85]. There has not been a randomized controlled trial to determine whether formal pancreas resection or enucleation results in similar local control. The Whipple procedure is necessary for tumors within the pancreatic head that cannot be enucleated. Likewise, distal pancreatectomy should be performed for tumors located within the body and tail that cannot be safely enucleated. Patients with multiple tumors should have all tumors excised by either enucleation or *en bloc* with formal pancreatic resection. All extrapancreatic tumors, including nodal metastases, should be excised. Duodenal endoscopic transillumination and duodenotomy with palpation are essential in every patient undergoing exploration [86,87].

While the majority of gastrinomas are found within the triangle described by Stabile and Passaro, the surgical exploration must be thorough and encompass structures outside that area. The liver should be palpated for metastases. Wedge resection of limited metastases at the time of the first exploration may be performed, or formal resection may be required at a second operation. Throughout the remainder of the abdominal exploration, it should be remembered that as many as 30% of patients will have multiple primary tumors. The next maneuver is to thoroughly explore and palpate the pancreas after mobilizing the hepatic flexure. The body and tail of the pancreas should be palpated after incising the peritoneum along the inferior border. The pancreas head is bimanually palpated after wide kocherization of the duodenum. Careful attention should be paid to the soft tissues behind the pancreatic head (Figure 40.1). Any suspicious nodules or lymph nodes should be sent for frozen section. Intraoperative ultrasound is helpful to evaluate the pancreas and determine the distance from the tumor to the pancreatic duct. Tumors less than 3 mm from the pancreatic duct are not suitable for enucleation [88]. The duodenum should be opened opposite the papilla using a longitudinal incision that is closed transversely. Most duodenal gastrinomas will be either visible by initial endoscopic transillumination or palpable through the duodenotomy [89]. Duodenal wall tumors should be excised full thickness with a small margin. The porta hepatis should be palpated and any suspicious masses sent for frozen section. The root of the mesentery, omentum, splenic hilum, and celiac access should be palpated.

After surgery, patients should remain on their preoperative regimen of antiacid medications until repeat fasting serum gastrin and secretin testing confirms a biochemical cure. Initial follow-up should be every 3–4 months for the first 2 years. Recurrences can occur after many years, so patients must be followed at least annually for life. Approximately 50% of patients can be biochemically cured immediately after surgery.

Treatment of advanced disease

Approximately 25% of patients will present with liver metastases. Medical management with PPIs should continue to prevent ravaging ulcers. SSTAs may help decrease tumor size, as well as control hormone levels. Patients should be closely followed every 3–4 months with serial imaging to determine the rate of disease progression. Chemotherapy and cytoreductive surgery should be considered when this occurs and is discussed in the next section with nonfunctional PanNETs.

Prognosis

At initial presentation, at least 60% of gastrinomas are malignant with either lymph node or distant metastases. After resection with biochemical cure, recurrence is unfortunately common, but 5-year survival is still relatively good at 76% [90]. Importantly, patients with lymph node metastases do not always progress to hepatic metastases [20,91]. Patients with duodenal gastrinomas generally have a high rate of lymph node metastases but excellent survival with surgical resection [92]. These patients tend not to develop hepatic metastases. Pancreatic gastrinomas, on the other hand, have a propensity to develop liver metastases compared with extrapancreatic gastrinomas and have a worse prognosis [90,91]. It has been argued that patients with lymph node metastases need to be followed much longer to develop hepatic metastases [93]. There are no randomized trials comparing watchful waiting with surgery, but non-randomized studies demonstrate a survival benefit from surgical resection [15].

NONFUNCTIONAL PANNETS

Epidemiology

Many PanNETs do not have an identifiable clinical syndrome, although the tumors may produce a variety of peptide hormones demonstrated by immunohistochemistry. These so-called nonfunctional PanNETs are more common than their functional counterparts [94]. Over time, they are increasingly diagnosed as asymptomatic incidental findings (1.4 to 3 per million) on imaging performed for unrelated disease [94–96]. In MEN1 patients, they are the most common PanNET. They are also the most common sporadic PanNET [94–96].

Clinical presentation

In many respects, nonfunctional PanNETs present with clinical findings similar to those of the more common pancreatic adenocarcinoma. When they are symptomatic, they present with weight loss or mass effect-related symptoms, such as pain, bowel obstruction, bleeding, and obstructive jaundice. Increasingly, nonfunctional PanNETs are found incidentally on abdominal imaging. Incidental tumors are typically smaller than symptomatic tumors.

Diagnosis

There is no specific diagnostic serum marker for these tumors like there is for gastrinoma and other functional tumors, but the diagnosis can be supported by measuring both serum chromogranin A (CgA) and pancreatic polypeptide (PP) levels as recommended by the most recent North American Neuroendocrine Tumor Society (NANETS) consensus guidelines [97,98]. PanNETs may secrete other hormones, albeit at levels too low to cause symptoms, or the secreted hormone may not produce a clinical syndrome (e.g., serum PP). CgA is a member of the glycoprotein granin family that is cosecreted with peptide hormones and neuropeptides [99]. It is secreted by a variety of endocrine tumors, including nonfunctional PanNETs [100–102]. However, nonendocrine tumors such as pancreatic adenocarcinoma may also secrete CgA, so the differential diagnosis of a pancreatic mass may not be clear even with modestly elevated CgA levels [103]. CgA levels correlate with tumor burden, and tumor response to therapy can be monitored with CgA levels. Care must be taken, however, interpreting tumor growth response with octreotide analogs since they may decrease CgA secretion. High-grade PanNETs (WHO G3) are more likely to be CgA negative.

Imaging

Nonfunctional PanNETs are usually solitary and may be found throughout the pancreas. Both conventional (CT, MRI, and EUS) and functional (SRS and PET) imaging are used in most patients with nonfunctional PanNETs.

EUS is very sensitive for identifying nonfunctional PanNETs [104]. EUS-FNA biopsy has a diagnostic accuracy as high as 92% when compared with surgical pathology [105]. Cell morphology and immunostaining for neuroendocrine markers (CgA and synaptophysin) and Ki-67 should be combined to make the diagnosis [106]. Cytology specimens are difficult to stain for immunohistochemistry, and therefore fine-needle tissue acquisition can be stained [106]. Small tumors can be marked with either fiducial markers (tiny metal coils) or tattooing to facilitate identification of the tumor during surgery [107–109].

A contrast CT scan of nonfunctional PanNETs usually shows an enhancing mass [110]. This enhancement, suggesting a hypervascular tumor, may help distinguish PanNET from adenocarcinoma. A CT scan is useful but not infallible to determine the extent of disease, with staging accuracy of 78% when compared with operative findings.

MRI images of nonfunctional PanNETs also show contrast enhancement in the arterial phase and high signal intensity on T2- and diffusion-weighted images. CT and MRI have a similar accuracy. Multiphase postcontrast studies are essential for discriminating tumor from normal tissue [110]. The arterial pancreatic phase is the most discriminating, but some tumors are better visualized during the portal venous phase or the late phase.

Most nonfunctional PanNETs are SRS positive, and this study should be obtained in all patients. SRS is usually performed with ^{111}In-pentetreotide (OctreoScan) with imaging obtained at 24 and 48 hours after injection of the radiopharmaceutical. Not only can OctreoScan localize the tumor, but it also can predict response to peptide receptor radionuclide therapy (PRRT) [111].

Hybrid modalities such as PET-CT provide both morphological and functional characterization of the PanNET. The most widely available PET radiopharmaceutical for cancer imaging is ^{18}F-fluorodeoxy-D-glucose (^{18}F-FDG).

^{18}F-FDG PET is a good choice for nonfunctional tumors, particularly poorly differentiated tumors, and may be useful for staging [112,113]. The sensitivity is 90% for nonfunctional tumors and is much better than for functional tumors. Improved PET imaging for PanNETs is obtained with the positron-emitting isotope ^{68}Ga of gallium bound to octreotide analogs, as described for gastrinomas above.

Staging

Staging for nonfunctional PanNETs is based upon 2010 American Joint Committee on Cancer (AJCC) and 2006 ENTS TNM staging (Tables 40.1, 40.2, and 40.4) and the WHO classification (Table 40.3), similar to gastrinomas.

Treatment

Treatment of nonfunctional PanNETs should follow published guidelines as recommended by NCCN, ENETS, and current clinical trials (ClinicalTrials.gov). Patients with limited disease should undergo surgery for cure. Optimal management of unresectable disease or widely metastatic disease, on the other hand, is unclear because of a lack of randomized clinical trials comparing contemporary treatment regimens, including the role of cytoreductive surgery.

Surgery

The only curative treatment for nonfunctional PanNETs is surgical resection. Many patients present with distant metastases at the time of diagnosis. The extent of surgery depends upon the location of the tumor and extent of metastases. These tumors should be formally resected similar to pancreatic adenocarcinoma, rather than enucleated, as is often performed for gastrinomas. Considerations for surgical resection include local invasion, nodal and distant metastases, and vascular invasion. Survival is better when patients present with an incidental (asymptomatic) nonfunctional PanNET and size of <3 cm [114]. Cytoreductive liver resection is appropriate for selected patients with limited disease that is amenable to either nonanatomic partial hepatectomy (wedge or segmentectomy) or formal lobectomy [115]. The goal should be to remove >90% of the gross disease burden. Diffuse liver metastases should be treated with systemic therapy.

Treatment of advanced disease

Whether patients with surgically incurable disease are treated with either observation or systemic chemotherapy varies by institution. Randomized controlled trial data is lacking, and clear evidence-based treatment guidelines have not been developed. Moreover, many studies combine pancreatic and extrapancreatic GI NETs in the same study. Since the PanNETs behave differently than other GI NETs, it is difficult to extrapolate the results of such studies to the treatment of PanNETs. Everyone agrees, however, that

symptomatic patients with surgically unresectable disease should receive systemic treatment. Initial treatment should include streptozocin (STZ)-based cytotoxic combination (doxorubicin or 5-fluorouracil [5-FU]) chemotherapy. Patients who progress on this regimen should be considered for targeted therapy with either sunitinib or everolimus. The best supportive care should be used for patients with poor performance status who have high-grade tumors and a dismal prognosis [116,117].

Somatostatin analogs

Patients with hormone-related symptoms with advanced disease should be treated with an SSTA either as primary therapy or as an adjunct to liver targeted therapy. SSTAs such as octreotide and lanreotide bind to PanNET cell surface receptors SSTR2 and SSTR5 and have an antiproliferative effect in addition to decreasing hormone production. This was proven in two recent randomized control trials. The PROMID study showed an antiproliferative effect of octreotide LAR on midgut carcinoids [118]. The CLARINET study, which was larger and included PanNETs, demonstrated that treatment with lanreotide was associated with improved progression-free survival (PFS) [119].

Liver-directed therapy

Patients who are not candidates for partial hepatectomy may be candidates for liver transplantation if they do not have extrahepatic disease and their PanNET is well differentiated [120,121]. Even carefully selected candidates, however, have a high likelihood of recurrence. Radiofrequency ablation (RFA) and transhepatic artery embolization or chemoembolization (TACE) can be used for nonsurgical candidates or as an adjunct to partial hepatectomy [122]. RFA was effective for achieving symptom control in small series of NET patients, including PanNETs [123]. Patients selected for RFA should have tumors of <3 cm and a limited number of metastases.

Peptide receptor radionuclide therapy

[90]Y- and ^{177}Lu-DOTA may deliver a tumoricidal radiation dose for patients with tumors that are SRS positive. Nephrotoxicty has been seen, and amino acid infusions may provide some protection from this adverse side effect. There are no randomized controlled trials because the treatment has not been standardized, but response rates have been in the range of 15%–35% [124].

Chemotherapy

Cytotoxic chemotherapy regimens are based upon the WHO PanNET grade classification. High-grade tumors (G3: mitoses >20 per 10 hpf, Ki-67 >20%) can be treated with platinum (cisplatin or carboplatin)-based regimens combined with either etoposide (VP-16) or irinotecan [125–128].

Table 40.5 Outcomes of chemotherapy trials for advanced PanNETs

Agents	Study design	Patients	Response	References
CTZ + 5-FU	Phase II	44	32% ORR 25-month OS	136
STZ + dox (vs. STZ + 5-FU vs. CTZ)	Phase III	105	69% ORR 20-month PFS 2.2-year OS	130
STZ + 5-FU vs. STZ	Phase III	84	63% ORR 26-month OS	129
STZ + dox	Retrospective	45	36% ORR 16-month PFS	132
STZ + dox	Retrospective	16	6% ORR 3.9-month PFS	133
STZ + dox + 5-FU	Retrospective	84	39% ORR 18-month PFS 37-month OS	134
STZ + dox (liposomal)	Phase II	30	40% ORR	137
DTIC	Phase II	50	34% ORR 19.3-month OS	138
STZ + 5-FU + bevacizumab (BETTER trial)	Phase I	34	23.7-month PFS	139
TMZ	Retrospective	12 (PanNETs)	8% ORR	140
TMZ + capecitabine	Retrospective	18	61% ORR 14-month PFS	141
TMZ + capecitabine	Retrospective	30	70% ORR 18-month PFS	142
TMZ + thalidomide	Phase II	11 (PanNETs)	45% ORR 24-month OS	143
TMZ + bevacizumab	Phase II	15 (PanNETs)	33% ORR 14.3-month PFS 41.7-month OS	144
TMZ + bevacizumab + sandostain LAR	Phase II	15 (carcinoid + PanNETs)	64% ORR 9-month PFS	145
^{177}Lu-octreotate + capecitabine + TMZ	Phase I–II	17 (PanNETs)	82% ORR 31-month PFS	146

Note: OS, overall survival.

This treatment strategy is based upon experience with small cell lung cancer, and no regimen appears superior in a retrospective study [117].

Low- and intermediate-grade tumors (G1–G2) are treated with combination STZ-based regimens (Table 40.5), but this approach may change in the near future to temozolomide (TMZ)-based regimens that have lower toxicity. STZ was FDA approved in 1982 and, combined with either doxorubicin or 5-FU, has been the mainstay of systemic chemotherapy based upon an encouraging reported response rate of up to 69% of tumors in Eastern Cooperative Oncology Group (ECOG) randomized trials [129,130]. Combination therapy with STZ and doxorubicin had the highest response rate, but the cardiotoxicity of doxorubicin limits dosing and patient selection. These two randomized trials included both functional and nonfunctional PanNETs. Response rates in these studies were measured by one or more parameters, including decreased serum hormones, reduced hepatomegaly by physical exam, or decrease in size of metastases by imaging. More recent retrospective case series implementing more stringent CT-based tumor size criteria (WHO or Response Evaluation Criteria in Solid Tumors [RECIST]) suggest that the STZ combination therapy response rate is substantially lower [131–134]. Adding to the confusion, some have argued that the RECIST criteria are not applicable to these patients due to the indolent and slow-growing nature of many, but not all, of these tumors. Tumor stabilization (PFS) may be the more appropriate criteria to follow, rather than overall survival [135]. Toxicity of STZ-based therapy prompted development of derivatives including chlorozotocin (CTZ), but it caused significant renal toxicity [136].

Dacarbazine (DTIC), like STZ, is an alkylating agent with some efficacy in treating PanNETs, but it is infrequently used due to side effects, primarily myelodepression and nausea [138]. TMZ is an oral derivative of DTIC that also alkylates and methylates DNA, but is it better tolerated than DTIC or STZ. Single-agent TMZ therapy has some efficacy, but combination therapy is better [140]. In patients who had failed other treatments, the combination of capecitabine (oral prodrug for 5-FU) and TMZ (CAPTEM) was well tolerated and had a response rate of 61% (5.5% complete response [CR], 55.5% partial response [PR]) by RECIST criteria [141]. Better response rates were obtained in treatment-naïve patients [142].

Other TMZ-based combination regimens have been studied in small cohorts in single-arm studies, but also look promising. TMZ with ^{177}Lu-octreotate and capecitabine resulted in an overall radiological response rate or objective response rate (ORR) of 82% [146]. In this regimen, the tumor response determined by RECIST was thought to be due to the ^{177}Lu-octreotate and the PFS due to the capecitabine and TMZ combination therapy. In addition, the chemotherapy acted as a radiosensitizer. TMZ combined with antiangiogenic compounds shows efficacy: TMZ with bevacizumab, TMZ with bevacizumab and long-acting octreotide, and TMZ with thalidomide [143–145].

DNA damage induced by TMZ is repaired by the O-6-methylguanine-DNA methyltransferase (MGMT) protein. Regimens that have prolonged TMZ administration (called metronomic) are generally more effective. This is hypothesized to result from depletion of MGMT activity with prolonged TMZ administration. This is also why carcinoids with higher average MGMT expression than PanNETs respond poorly to TMZ-based therapy [147]. Interestingly, capecitabine is thought to act synergistically with TMZ by depleting MGMT levels before TMZ treatment. Future studies will include assessment of MGMT activity compared with TMZ efficacy [147].

Targeted therapy

Two agents (everolimus and sunitinib) have been FDA approved for targeted therapy, and other agents are in trials (Table 40.6).

mTOR pathway-targeted drugs

Evidence suggests that the phosphatidylinositol 3-kinase (PI3K)/Akt/mTOR pathway is important for PanNET development. Rapamycin analogs (temsirolimus, everolimus, and ridaforolimus) bind FK506 binding protein (FKBP12), and this drug–protein complex inhibits mTOR activity [35]. After a large international prospective randomized trial (RADIANT3), everolimus was approved by the FDA in 2011 for the treatment of PanNETs [150]. In this phase III trial, everolimus significantly increased the median PFS from 4.6 months to 11 months compared with placebo. Patients in the RADIANT3 trial had low- to intermediate-grade PanNETs with advanced and progressive disease.

The effectiveness of mTOR inhibitors is thought to be reduced by multiple feedback loops (such as IGF-1 signaling) in mTOR signaling, thus allowing escape [153]. Targeting these feedback pathways may help improve mTOR inhibitor effectiveness, and this was the rationale for including octreotide and IGF-1-specific inhibitors (cixutumumab) in some regimens [154]. It is thought that octreotide inhibits IGF-1 signaling, which is one of the upstream effectors in mTOR signaling. An alternative strategy is to directly target the catalytic kinase site in mTOR [155]. Subgroups of PanNETs that demonstrate activation of mTOR signaling may be more responsive to rapalogs [148].

Multitargeted kinase inhibitors

PanNETs overexpress vascular endothelial growth factor (VEGF), platelet-derived growth factor receptor (PDGFR)-alpha, PDGF-beta, c-Kit, and epidermal growth factor receptor [156–159]. PanNET angiogenesis is promoted by VEGF, and blood vessel pericytes are supported by the PDGF pathway. Sunitinib, a multitargeted tyrosine kinase inhibitor (TKI), was FDA approved in 2011. Sunitinib inhibits angiogenesis by blocking multiple receptor tyrosine kinases, including VEGF receptors (VEGF-R1, -R2, and -R3), PDGFR-alpha/beta, FML (formyl-Met-Leu)-like tyrosine kinase 3 receptor (FLT3R), c-Kit-R, and RET-R. In a phase III trial, sunitinib showed a significantly prolonged PFS (11.4 months vs. 5.5 months), increased overall response rate, and stable disease rate [152]. Sunitinib is approved for the treatment of metastatic or unresectable PanNETs with disease progression.

Table 40.6 Outcomes of targeted therapy trials for advanced PanNETs

Agents	Study design	Patients	Response	Reference
Temsirolimus	Phase II	37 (advanced carcinoid and PanNETs)	6% ORR	148
Everolimus + octreotide vs. everolimus (RADIANT1)	Phase II	30 (PanNETs)	27% ORR 50-week PFS	149
Everolimus (RADIANT3) vs. placebo	Phase III	410	5% ORR 11-month PFS	150
Sunitinib	Phase II	66 (PanNETs)	16.7% ORR 7.7-month PFS	151
Sunitinib vs. placebo	Phase III	171	9.3% ORR 11.4-month PFS	152

GLUCAGONOMA

Glucagonomas are exceedingly rare, occurring in approximately 1 in 20 million person-years. They occur at a mean age of 55 years and are more common in men. Patients present with "glucagonoma syndrome" characterized by necrolytic migratory erythema (NME), diabetes, and a glucagon-secreting pancreatic tumor [160–162]. Additional symptoms in these patients may include stomatitis, anemia, weight loss, venous thromboembolism (blood hyperviscosity), neurological and psychiatric disturbances (depression, dementia, and ataxia), dilated cardiomyopathy, and diarrhea. A useful mnemonic is the 6Ds (diabetes, dermatitis, depression, diarrhea, deep vein thrombosis, and dilated cardiomyopathy).

The characteristic NME rash, present in the majority of patients, occurs in waves, typically beginning on the extremities and intertriginous areas and then progressing to involve the trunk. Itchy, painful erythematous skin lesions become more confluent, blister, crust over, and then eventually turn black in 2–3 days and heal, resulting in hyperpigmented skin. This cycle repeats itself every few weeks. Not uncommonly, patients are treated for various skin disorders for years before the diagnosis is made. Skin biopsy can occasionally be diagnostic for NME but is not reliable. Moreover, NME is not specific to glucagonoma and can occur in other more common diseases, such as cirrhosis [163]. Diabetes eventually develops in the majority of patients and is generally mild but may require insulin treatment.

Obtaining at least two markedly elevated glucagon levels (usually 500–1000 pg/mL) makes the diagnosis. A clear correlation between tumor burden and glucagon levels has not been established. There is no provocative test.

The majority of glucagonomas are large (T3), solitary, and located to the left of the superior mesenteric artery (SMA), similar to the distribution of alpha-cell mass within the pancreas [164]. CT scan and octreotide scan are useful for localization of the primary and metastatic disease [165]. MRI or angiography may be helpful in small elusive tumors. EUS with biopsy can confirm the diagnosis [54]. Future developments may include ^{68}Ga-DOTANOC (1,4,7,10-tetraazacyclo- dodecane-1,4,7,10-tetraacetic acid-1-Nal3-octreotide) PET-CT, which may be more sensitive than conventional imaging [166,167].

The only curative treatment is partial pancreatectomy. Standard pancreatectomy anatomic resections are used. Less than half of the patients can be resected with R0/R1 results. However, given the relatively slow progression of these tumors, cytoreductive surgery may help palliate the patient's symptoms.

Medical management may be useful in patients with unresectable tumors. Treatment of the malnutrition (catabolism due to glucagon and tumor paraneoplastic syndrome) with periodic amino acid infusions (not enteral therapy) and suppression of glucagon secretion with octreotide analogs (lanreotide autogel, octreotide LAR, and octreotide) improves both the cutaneous and neurologic symptoms [168–171].

Due to their rarity (less than 500 cases in the literature), randomized controlled trials with systemic treatment have not been performed, so most treatment recommendations are based upon case series or case reports [172–174]. PRRT with the radiolabeled SSTA (90Y-DOTATOC 200 mCi, two doses) has resulted in minimal to moderate response in reduction of tumor size based upon RECIST criteria. Targeted therapy with everolimus (mTOR inhibitor) has been successful in the treatment of PanNETs, including glucagonoma [150]. Other systemic treatments with conventional chemotherapy and liver targeted therapy with TACE, partial hepatectomy, and external beam radiotherapy have been tried.

Because a "rash" and diabetes are common clinical problems, the diagnosis is frequently late. While most tumors are advanced at presentation, the survival is surprisingly long (66% at 5 years).

REFERENCES

1. Zollinger RM, Ellison EH. Primary peptic ulcerations of the jejunum associated with islet cell tumors of the pancreas. *Ann Surg* 1955;142(4):709–23; discussion 724–8.
2. Gregory RA et al. Extraction of a gastrin-like substance from a pancreatic tumour in a case of Zollinger-Ellison syndrome. *Lancet* 1960;1(7133):1045–8.
3. McGuigan JE, Trudeau WL. Immunochemical measurement of elevated levels of gastrin in the serum of patients with pancreatic tumors of the Zollinger-Ellison variety. *N Engl J Med* 1968;278(24):1308–13.
4. Halfdanarson TR et al. Pancreatic endocrine neoplasms: Epidemiology and prognosis of pancreatic endocrine tumors. *Endocr Relat Cancer* 2008;15(2):409–27.
5. Berna MJ et al. Serum gastrin in Zollinger-Ellison syndrome. I. Prospective study of fasting serum gastrin in 309 patients from the National Institutes of Health and comparison with 2229 cases from the literature. *Medicine (Baltimore)* 2006;85(6): 295–330.
6. Roy PK et al. Zollinger-Ellison syndrome. Clinical presentation in 261 patients. *Medicine (Baltimore)* 2000;79(6):379–411.
7. Stabile BE, Morrow DJ, Passaro E Jr. The gastrinoma triangle: Operative implications. *Am J Surg* 1984;147(1):25–31.
8. Wolfe MM, Alexander RW, McGuigan JE. Extrapancreatic, extraintestinal gastrinoma: Effective treatment by surgery. *N Engl J Med* 1982;306(25):1533–6.
9. Ito T, Jensen RT. Primary hepatic gastrinoma: An unusual case of Zollinger-Ellison syndrome. *Gastroenterol Hepatol (NY)* 2010;6(1):57–9.
10. Martignoni ME et al. Study of a primary gastrinoma in the common hepatic duct—A case report. *Digestion* 1999;60(2):187–90.

11. Wu PC et al. A prospective analysis of the frequency, location, and curability of ectopic (nonpancreaticoduodenal, nonnodal) gastrinoma. *Surgery* 1997;122(6):1176–82.

12. Price TN et al. Zollinger-Ellison syndrome due to primary gastrinoma of the extrahepatic biliary tree: Three case reports and review of literature. *Endocr Pract* 2009;15(7):737–49.

13. Noda S et al. Surgical resection of intracardiac gastrinoma. *Ann Thorac Surg* 1999;67(2):532–3.

14. Katkoori D et al. A rare case of renal gastrinoma. *Sci World J* 2009;9:501–4.

15. Norton JA et al. Surgery increases survival in patients with gastrinoma. *Ann Surg* 2006;244(3):410–9.

16. Ruszniewski P et al. Localization of gastrinomas by endoscopic ultrasonography in patients with Zollinger-Ellison syndrome. *Surgery* 1995;117(6):629–35.

17. Donow C et al. Surgical pathology of gastrinoma. Site, size, multicentricity, association with multiple endocrine neoplasia type 1, and malignancy. *Cancer* 1991;68(6):1329–34.

18. Imamura M et al. Clinicopathological characteristics of duodenal microgastrinomas. *World J Surg* 1992;16(4):703–9; discussion 709–10.

19. Weber HC et al. Determinants of metastatic rate and survival in patients with Zollinger-Ellison syndrome: A prospective long-term study. *Gastroenterology* 1995;108(6):1637–49.

20. Stabile BE, Passaro E Jr. Benign and malignant gastrinoma. *Am J Surg* 1985;149(1):144–50.

21. Passaro E Jr et al. The origin of sporadic gastrinomas within the gastrinoma triangle: A theory. *Arch Surg* 1998;133(1):13–6; discussion 17.

22. Fendrich V et al. Sonic hedgehog and pancreatic-duodenal homebox 1 expression distinguish between duodenal and pancreatic gastrinomas. *Endocr Relat Cancer* 2009;16(2):613–22.

23. Norton JA et al. Possible primary lymph node gastrinoma: Occurrence, natural history, and predictive factors: A prospective study. *Ann Surg* 2003;237(5):650–7; discussion 657–9.

24. MacGillivray DC et al. The significance of gastrinomas found in peripancreatic lymph nodes. *Surgery* 1991;109(4):558–62.

25. Perrier ND et al. An immunohistochemical survey for neuroendocrine cells in regional pancreatic lymph nodes: A plausible explanation for primary nodal gastrinomas? Mayo Clinic Pancreatic Surgery Group. *Surgery* 1995;118(6):957–65; discussion 965–6.

26. Anlauf M et al. Primary lymph node gastrinoma or occult duodenal microgastrinoma with lymph node metastases in a MEN1 patient: The need for a systematic search for the primary tumor. *Am J Surg Pathol* 2008;32(7):1101–5.

27. Vortmeyer AO et al. Non-islet origin of pancreatic islet cell tumors. *J Clin Endocrinol Metab* 2004;89(4):1934–8.

28. Wang EH et al. Mutation of the MENIN gene in sporadic pancreatic endocrine tumors. *Cancer Res* 1998;58(19):4417–20.

29. Guo SS, Sawicki MP. Molecular and genetic mechanisms of tumorigenesis in multiple endocrine neoplasia type-1. *Mol Endocrinol* 2001;15(10):1653–64.

30. Matkar S, Thiel A, Hua X. Menin: A scaffold protein that controls gene expression and cell signaling. *Trends Biochem Sci* 2013;38(8):394–402.

31. Jiao Y et al. DAXX/ATRX, MEN1, and mTOR pathway genes are frequently altered in pancreatic neuroendocrine tumors. *Science* 2011;331(6021):1199–203.

32. Missiaglia E et al. Pancreatic endocrine tumors: Expression profiling evidences a role for AKT-mTOR pathway. *J Clin Oncol* 2010;28(2):245–55.

33. Guo SS et al. Frequent overexpression of cyclin D1 in sporadic pancreatic endocrine tumours. *J Endocrinol* 2003;179(1):73–9.

34. Haissaguerre M, Saucisse N, Cota D. Influence of mTOR in energy and metabolic homeostasis. *Mol Cell Endocrinol* 2014;397(1–2):67–77.

35. Laplante M, Sabatini DM. mTOR signaling in growth control and disease. *Cell* 2012;149(2):274–93.

36. Metz DC. Diagnosis of the Zollinger-Ellison syndrome. *Clin Gastroenterol Hepatol* 2012;10(2):126–30.

37. Dhillo WS et al. Plasma gastrin measurement cannot be used to diagnose a gastrinoma in patients on either proton pump inhibitors or histamine type-2 receptor antagonists. *Ann Clin Biochem* 2006;43(Pt 2):153–5.

38. Poitras P, Gingras MH, Rehfeld JF. The Zollinger-Ellison syndrome: Dangers and consequences of interrupting antisecretory treatment. *Clin Gastroenterol Hepatol* 2012;10(2):199–202.

39. Ito T, Cadiot G, Jensen RT. Diagnosis of Zollinger-Ellison syndrome: Increasingly difficult. *World J Gastroenterol* 2012;18(39):5495–503.

40. Rehfeld JF et al. The Zollinger-Ellison syndrome and mismeasurement of gastrin. *Gastroenterology* 2011;140(5):1444–53.

41. Rehfeld, JF et al. Pitfalls in diagnostic gastrin measurements. *Clin Chem* 2012;58(5):831–6.

42. Roy PK et al. Gastric secretion in Zollinger-Ellison syndrome. Correlation with clinical expression, tumor extent and role in diagnosis—A prospective NIH study of 235 patients and a review of 984 cases in the literature. *Medicine (Baltimore)* 2001;80(3):189–222.

43. Shah P et al. Hypochlorhydria and achlorhydria are associated with false-positive secretin stimulation testing for Zollinger-Ellison syndrome. *Pancreas* 2013;42(6):932–6.

44. Alexander HR et al. Prospective study of somatostatin receptor scintigraphy and its effect on operative outcome in patients with Zollinger-Ellison syndrome. *Ann Surg* 1998;228(2):228–38.

45. Schirmer WJ et al. Indium-111-pentetreotide scanning versus conventional imaging techniques for the localization of gastrinoma. *Surgery* 1995;118(6):1105–13; discussion 1113–4.

46. Jais P et al. Somatostatin receptor subtype gene expression in human endocrine gastroentero-pancreatic tumours. *Eur J Clin Invest* 1997;27(8):639–44.

47. Gibril F et al. Somatostatin receptor scintigraphy: Its sensitivity compared with that of other imaging methods in detecting primary and metastatic gastrinomas. A prospective study. *Ann Intern Med* 1996;125(1):26–34.

48. Gibril F et al. Bone metastases in patients with gastrinomas: A prospective study of bone scanning, somatostatin receptor scanning, and magnetic resonance image in their detection, frequency, location, and effect of their detection on management. *J Clin Oncol* 1998;16(3):1040–53.

49. Cadiot G et al. Preoperative detection of duodenal gastrinomas and peripancreatic lymph nodes by somatostatin receptor scintigraphy. Groupe D'etude Du Syndrome De Zollinger-Ellison. *Gastroenterology* 1996;111(4):845–54.

50. Gabriel M et al. 68Ga-DOTA-Tyr3-octreotide PET in neuroendocrine tumors: Comparison with somatostatin receptor scintigraphy and CT. *J Nucl Med* 2007;48(4):508–18.

51. Geijer H, Breimer LH. Somatostatin receptor PET/CT in neuroendocrine tumours: Update on systematic review and meta-analysis. *Eur J Nucl Med Mol Imaging* 2013;40(11):1770–80.

52. Sharma P et al. Evaluation of (68)Ga-DOTANOC PET/CT imaging in a large exclusive population of pancreatic neuroendocrine tumors. *Abdom Imaging* 2014;40(2):299–309.

53. Krausz Y et al. Ga-68 DOTA-NOC uptake in the pancreas: Pathological and physiological patterns. *Clin Nucl Med* 2012;37(1):57–62.

54. Anderson MA et al. Endoscopic ultrasound is highly accurate and directs management in patients with neuroendocrine tumors of the pancreas. *Am J Gastroenterol* 2000;95(9):2271–7.

55. Zimmer T et al. Endoscopic ultrasonography of neuroendocrine tumours. *Digestion* 2000;62(Suppl 1):45–50.

56. Rindi G, Petrone G, Inzani F. The 2010 WHO classification of digestive neuroendocrine neoplasms: A critical appraisal four years after its introduction. *Endocr Pathol* 2014;25(2):186–92.

57. Rindi G et al. TNM staging of foregut (neuro) endocrine tumors: A consensus proposal including a grading system. *Virchows Arch* 2006;449(4):395–401.

58. Pape UF et al. Prognostic relevance of a novel TNM classification system for upper gastroenteropancreatic neuroendocrine tumors. *Cancer* 2008;113(2):256–65.

59. Rindi G et al. TNM staging of neoplasms of the endocrine pancreas: Results from a large international cohort study. *J Natl Cancer Inst* 2012;104(10):764–77.

60. Edge SB, Byrd DR, Compton CC, Fritz AG, Greene FL, Trotti A. *AJCC Cancer Staging Manual.* 7th ed. New York: Springer, 2010.

61. Strosberg JR et al. Prognostic validity of a novel American Joint Committee on Cancer staging classification for pancreatic neuroendocrine tumors. *J Clin Oncol* 2011;29(22):3044–9.

62. Desir B, Poitras P. Oral pantoprazole for acid suppression in the treatment of patients with Zollinger-Ellison syndrome. *Can J Gastroenterol* 2001;15(12):795–8.

63. Termanini B et al. A prospective study of the effectiveness of low dose omeprazole as initial therapy in Zollinger-Ellison syndrome. *Aliment Pharmacol Ther* 1996;10(1):61–71.

64. Hirschowitz BI, Mohnen J, Shaw S. Long-term treatment with lansoprazole for patients with Zollinger-Ellison syndrome. *Aliment Pharmacol Ther* 1996;10(4):507–22.

65. Shamburek RD, Schubert ML. Control of gastric acid secretion. Histamine H2-receptor antagonists and H + K(+)-ATPase inhibitors. *Gastroenterol Clin North Am* 1992;21(3):527–50.

66. Shamburek RD, Schubert ML. Pharmacology of gastric acid inhibition. *Baillieres Clin Gastroenterol* 1993;7(1):23–54.

67. Gaztambide S, Vazquez JA. Short- and long-term effect of a long-acting somatostatin analogue, lanreotide (SR-L) on metastatic gastrinoma. *J Endocrinol Invest* 1999;22(2):144–6.

68. Cives M, Kunz PL, Morse B et al. Phase II clinical trial of pasireotide long-acting repeatable in patients with metastatic neuroendocrine tumors. *Endocr Relat Cancer* 2015;22(1):1–9.

69. Saijo F et al. Octreotide in control of multiple liver metastases from gastrinoma. *J Gastroenterol* 2003;38(9):905–8.

70. Feelders RA et al. Pasireotide, a multi-somatostatin receptor ligand with potential efficacy for treatment of pituitary and neuroendocrine tumors. *Drugs Today (Barc)* 2013;49(2):89–103.

71. Oberg K et al. Consensus report on the use of somatostatin analogs for the management of neuroendocrine tumors of the gastroenteropancreatic system. *Ann Oncol* 2004;15(6):966–73.

72. Norton JA et al. Surgery to cure the Zollinger-Ellison syndrome. *N Engl J Med* 1999;341(9):635–44.

73. Norton JA et al. Value of surgery in patients with negative imaging and sporadic Zollinger-Ellison syndrome. *Ann Surg* 2012;256(3):509–17.

74. Pipeleers-Marichal M et al. Pathologic aspects of gastrinomas in patients with Zollinger-Ellison syndrome with and without multiple endocrine neoplasia type I. *World J Surg* 1993;17(4):481–8.

75. Lopez CL et al. Long-term results of surgery for pancreatic neuroendocrine neoplasms in patients with MEN1. *Langenbecks Arch Surg* 2011;396(8):1187–96.

76. Gibril F et al. Prospective study of the natural history of gastrinoma in patients with MEN1: Definition of an aggressive and a nonaggressive form. *J Clin Endocrinol Metab* 2001;86(11):5282–93.

77. Ito T et al. Causes of death and prognostic factors in multiple endocrine neoplasia type 1: A prospective study: Comparison of 106 MEN1/Zollinger-Ellison syndrome patients with 1613 literature MEN1 patients with or without pancreatic endocrine tumors. *Medicine (Baltimore)* 2013;92(3):135–81.

78. Cadiot G et al. Prognostic factors in patients with Zollinger-Ellison syndrome and multiple endocrine neoplasia type 1. Groupe d'Etude des Neoplasies Endocriniennes Multiples (GENEM) and Groupe de Recherche et d'Etude du Syndrome de Zollinger-Ellison (GRESZE). *Gastroenterology* 1999;116(2):286–93.

79. Imamura M, Takahashi K. Use of selective arterial secretin injection test to guide surgery in patients with Zollinger-Ellison syndrome. *World J Surg* 1993;17(4):433–8.

80. Imamura M et al. Biochemically curative surgery for gastrinoma in multiple endocrine neoplasia type 1 patients. *World J Gastroenterol* 2011;17(10):1343–53.

81. Norton JA et al. Comparison of surgical results in patients with advanced and limited disease with multiple endocrine neoplasia type 1 and Zollinger-Ellison syndrome. *Ann Surg* 2001;234(4):495–505; discussion 505–6.

82. Norton JA, Fang TD, Jensen RT. Surgery for gastrinoma and insulinoma in multiple endocrine neoplasia type 1. *J Natl Compr Canc Netw* 2006;4(2):148–53.

83. Mignon M. Diagnostic and therapeutic strategies in Zollinger-Ellison syndrome associated with multiple endocrine neoplasia type I (MEN-I): Experience of the Zollinger-Ellison Syndrome Research Group: Bichat 1958–1999 [in French]. *Bull Acad Natl Med* 2003;187(7):1249–58; discussion 1259–60.

84. Jensen RT et al. ENETS Consensus Guidelines for the management of patients with digestive neuroendocrine neoplasms: Functional pancreatic endocrine tumor syndromes. *Neuroendocrinology* 2012;95(2):98–119.

85. Giovinazzo F et al. Lymph nodes metastasis and recurrences justify an aggressive treatment of gastrinoma. *Updates Surg* 2013;65(1):19–24.

86. Norton JA. Surgery and prognosis of duodenal gastrinoma as a duodenal neuroendocrine tumor. *Best Pract Res Clin Gastroenterol* 2005;19(5):699–704.

87. Thompson NW, Pasieka J, Fukuuchi, A. Duodenal gastrinomas, duodenotomy, and duodenal exploration in the surgical management of Zollinger-Ellison syndrome. *World J Surg* 1993;17(4):455–62.

88. Heeger K et al. Increased rate of clinically relevant pancreatic fistula after deep enucleation of small pancreatic tumors. *Langenbecks Arch Surg* 2014;399(3):315–21.

89. Sugg SL et al. A prospective study of intraoperative methods to diagnose and resect duodenal gastrinomas. *Ann Surg* 1993;218(2):138–44.

90. Maire F et al. Recurrence after surgical resection of gastrinoma: Who, when, where and why? *Eur J Gastroenterol Hepatol* 2012;24(4):368–74.

91. Howard TJ et al. Biologic behavior of sporadic gastrinoma located to the right and left of the superior mesenteric artery. *Am J Surg* 1993;165(1):101–5; discussion 105–6.

92. Delcore R Jr, Cheung LY, Friesen SR. Outcome of lymph node involvement in patients with the Zollinger-Ellison syndrome. *Ann Surg* 1988;208(3):291–8.

93. Krampitz GW, Norton JA. Current management of the Zollinger-Ellison syndrome. *Adv Surg* 2013;47:59–79.

94. Vagefi PA et al. Evolving patterns in the detection and outcomes of pancreatic neuroendocrine neoplasms: The Massachusetts General Hospital experience from 1977 to 2005. *Arch Surg* 2007;142(4):347–54.

95. Fitzgerald TL et al. Changing incidence of pancreatic neoplasms: A 16-year review of statewide tumor registry. *Pancreas* 2008;37(2):134–8.

96. Franko J et al. Non-functional neuroendocrine carcinoma of the pancreas: Incidence, tumor biology, and outcomes in 2,158 patients. *J Gastrointest Surg* 2010;14(3):541–8.

97. Modlin IM et al. Chromogranin A–Biological function and clinical utility in neuroendocrine tumor disease. *Ann Surg Oncol* 2010;17(9):2427–43.

98. Panzuto F et al. Utility of combined use of plasma levels of chromogranin A and pancreatic polypeptide in the diagnosis of gastrointestinal and pancreatic endocrine tumors. *J Endocrinol Invest* 2004;27(1):6–11.

99. Kanakis G, Kaltsas G. Biochemical markers for gastroenteropancreatic neuroendocrine tumours (GEP-NETs). *Best Pract Res Clin Gastroenterol* 2012;26(6):791–802.

100. Stivanello M et al. Circulating chromogranin A in the assessment of patients with neuroendocrine tumours. A single institution experience. *Ann Oncol* 2001;12(Suppl 2):S73–7.

101. Nobels FR et al. Chromogranin A: Its clinical value as marker of neuroendocrine tumours. *Eur J Clin Invest* 1998;28(6):431–40.

102. Qiao XW et al. Chromogranin A is a reliable serum diagnostic biomarker for pancreatic neuroendocrine tumors but not for insulinomas. *BMC Endocr Disord* 2014;14:64.

103. Malaguarnera M et al. Elevated chromogranin A (CgA) serum levels in the patients with advanced pancreatic cancer. *Arch Gerontol Geriatr* 2009;48(2):213–7.

104. Khashab MA et al. EUS is still superior to multidetector computerized tomography for detection of pancreatic neuroendocrine tumors. *Gastrointest Endosc* 2011;73(4):691–6.

105. Unno J, Kanno A, Masamune A et al. The usefulness of endoscopic ultrasound-guided fine-needle aspiration for the diagnosis of pancreatic neuroendocrine tumors based on the World Health Organization classification. *Scand J Gastroenterol* 2014;49(11):1367–74.

106. Larghi A et al. Ki-67 grading of nonfunctioning pancreatic neuroendocrine tumors on histologic samples obtained by EUS-guided fine-needle tissue acquisition: A prospective study. *Gastrointest Endosc* 2012;76(3):570–7.

107. Gress FG et al. Preoperative localization of a neuroendocrine tumor of the pancreas with EUS-guided fine needle tattooing. *Gastrointest Endosc* 2002;55(4):594–7.

108. Lennon AM et al. EUS-guided tattooing before laparoscopic distal pancreatic resection (with video). *Gastrointest Endosc* 2010;72(5):1089–94.

109. Law JK et al. Endoscopic ultrasound (EUS)-guided fiducial placement allows localization of small neuroendocrine tumors during parenchymal-sparing pancreatic surgery. *Surg Endosc* 2013;27(10):3921–6.

110. Foti G et al. Preoperative assessment of nonfunctioning pancreatic endocrine tumours: Role of MDCT and MRI. *Radiol Med* 2013;118(7):1082–101.

111. van Essen M et al. Neuroendocrine tumours: The role of imaging for diagnosis and therapy. *Nat Rev Endocrinol* 2014;10(2):102–14.

112. Wang SC et al. Identification of unknown primary tumors in patients with neuroendocrine liver metastases. *Arch Surg* 2010;145(3):276–80.

113. Pasquali C et al. Neuroendocrine tumor imaging: Can 18F-fluorodeoxyglucose positron emission tomography detect tumors with poor prognosis and aggressive behavior? *World J Surg* 1998;22(6):588–92.

114. Gullo L et al. Nonfunctioning pancreatic endocrine tumors: A multicenter clinical study. *Am J Gastroenterol* 2003;98(11):2435–9.

115. Norton JA et al. Aggressive surgery for metastatic liver neuroendocrine tumors. *Surgery* 2003;134(6):1057–63; discussion 1063–5.

116. Oken MM et al. Toxicity and response criteria of the Eastern Cooperative Oncology Group. *Am J Clin Oncol* 1982;5(6):649–55.

117. Sorbye H et al. Predictive and prognostic factors for treatment and survival in 305 patients with advanced gastrointestinal neuroendocrine carcinoma (WHO G3): The NORDIC NEC study. *Ann Oncol* 2013;24(1):152–60.

118. Rinke A et al. Placebo-controlled, double-blind, prospective, randomized study on the effect of octreotide LAR in the control of tumor growth in patients with metastatic neuroendocrine midgut tumors: A report from the PROMID Study Group. *J Clin Oncol* 2009;27(28):4656–63.

119. Caplin ME et al. Lanreotide in metastatic enteropancreatic neuroendocrine tumors. *N Engl J Med* 2014;371(3):224–33.

120. Rossi RE, Burroughs, AK, Caplin ME. Liver transplantation for unresectable neuroendocrine tumor liver metastases. *Ann Surg Oncol* 2014;21(7):2398–405.

121. Chung H, Chapman WC. Liver transplantation for metastatic neuroendocrine tumors. *Adv Surg* 2014;48:235–52.

122. Nazario J, Gupta S. Transarterial liver-directed therapies of neuroendocrine hepatic metastases. *Semin Oncol* 2010;37(2):118–26.

123. Eriksson J et al. Surgery and radiofrequency ablation for treatment of liver metastases from midgut and foregut carcinoids and endocrine pancreatic tumors. *World J Surg* 2008;32(5):930–8.

124. Bergsma H et al. Peptide receptor radionuclide therapy (PRRT) for GEP-NETs. *Best Pract Res Clin Gastroenterol* 2012;26(6):867–81.

125. Mitry E et al. Treatment of poorly differentiated neuroendocrine tumours with etoposide and cisplatin. *Br J Cancer* 1999;81(8):1351–5.

126. Ramella Munhoz R et al. Combination of irinotecan and a platinum agent for poorly differentiated neuroendocrine carcinomas. *Rare Tumors* 2013;5(3):e39.

127. Strosberg JR et al. The NANETS consensus guidelines for the diagnosis and management of poorly differentiated (high-grade) extrapulmonary neuroendocrine carcinomas. *Pancreas* 2010;39(6):799–800.

128. Moertel CG et al. Treatment of neuroendocrine carcinomas with combined etoposide and cisplatin. Evidence of major therapeutic activity in the anaplastic variants of these neoplasms. *Cancer* 1991;68(2):227–32.

129. Moertel CG, Hanley JA, Johnson LA. Streptozocin alone compared with streptozocin plus fluorouracil in the treatment of advanced islet-cell carcinoma. *N Engl J Med* 1980;303(21):1189–94.

130. Moertel CG et al. Streptozocin-doxorubicin, streptozocin-fluorouracil or chlorozotocin in the treatment of advanced islet-cell carcinoma. *N Engl J Med* 1992;326(8):519–23.

131. Cheng PN, Saltz LB. Failure to confirm major objective antitumor activity for streptozocin and doxorubicin in the treatment of patients with advanced islet cell carcinoma. *Cancer* 1999;86(6):944–8.

132. Delaunoit T et al. The doxorubicin-streptozotocin combination for the treatment of advanced well-differentiated pancreatic endocrine carcinoma; a judicious option? *Eur J Cancer* 2004;40(4):515–20.

133. McCollum AD et al. Lack of efficacy of streptozocin and doxorubicin in patients with advanced pancreatic endocrine tumors. *Am J Clin Oncol* 2004;27(5):485–8.

134. Kouvaraki MA et al. Fluorouracil, doxorubicin, and streptozocin in the treatment of patients with locally advanced and metastatic pancreatic endocrine carcinomas. *J Clin Oncol* 2004;22(23):4762–71.

135. Kulke MH et al. Future directions in the treatment of neuroendocrine tumors: Consensus report of the National Cancer Institute Neuroendocrine Tumor clinical trials planning meeting. *J Clin Oncol* 2011;29(7):934–43.

136. Bukowski RM et al. Phase II trial of chlorozotocin and fluorouracil in islet cell carcinoma: A Southwest Oncology Group study. *J Clin Oncol* 1992;10(12):1914–8.

137. Fjallskog ML et al. Treatment with combined streptozotocin and liposomal doxorubicin in metastatic endocrine pancreatic tumors. *Neuroendocrinology* 2008;88(1):53–8.

138. Ramanathan RK et al. Phase II trial of dacarbazine (DTIC) in advanced pancreatic islet cell carcinoma. Study of the Eastern Cooperative Oncology Group-E6282. *Ann Oncol* 2001;12(8):1139–43.

139. Ducreux M et al. Bevacizumab combined with 5-FU/streptozocin in patients with progressive metastatic well-differentiated pancreatic endocrine tumours (BETTER trial)—A phase II non-randomised trial. *Eur J Cancer* 2014;50(18):3098–106.

140. Ekeblad S et al. Temozolomide as monotherapy is effective in treatment of advanced malignant neuroendocrine tumors. *Clin Cancer Res* 2007;13(10):2986–91.

141. Fine RL et al. Capecitabine and temozolomide (CAPTEM) for metastatic, well-differentiated neuroendocrine cancers: The Pancreas Center at Columbia University experience. *Cancer Chemother Pharmacol* 2013;71(3):663–70.

142. Strosberg JR et al. First-line chemotherapy with capecitabine and temozolomide in patients with metastatic pancreatic endocrine carcinomas. *Cancer* 2011;117(2):268–75.

143. Kulke MH et al. Phase II study of temozolomide and thalidomide in patients with metastatic neuroendocrine tumors. *J Clin Oncol* 2006;24(3):401–6.

144. Chan JA et al. Prospective study of bevacizumab plus temozolomide in patients with advanced neuroendocrine tumors. *J Clin Oncol* 2012;30(24):2963–8.

145. Koumarianou A et al. Combination treatment with metronomic temozolomide, bevacizumab and long-acting octreotide for malignant neuroendocrine tumours. *Endocr Relat Cancer* 2012;19(1):L1–4.

146. Claringbold PG, Price RA, Turner JH. Phase I-II study of radiopeptide 177Lu-octreotate in combination with capecitabine and temozolomide in advanced low-grade neuroendocrine tumors. *Cancer Biother Radiopharm* 2012;27(9):561–9.

147. Kulke MH et al. O6-Methylguanine DNA methyltransferase deficiency and response to temozolomide-based therapy in patients with neuroendocrine tumors. *Clin Cancer Res* 2009;15(1):338–45.

148. Duran I et al. A phase II clinical and pharmacodynamic study of temsirolimus in advanced neuroendocrine carcinomas. *Br J Cancer* 2006;95(9):1148–54.

149. Yao JC et al. Efficacy of RAD001 (everolimus) and octreotide LAR in advanced low- to intermediate-grade neuroendocrine tumors: Results of a phase II study. *J Clin Oncol* 2008;26(26):4311–8.

150. Yao JC et al. Everolimus for advanced pancreatic neuroendocrine tumors. *N Engl J Med* 2011;364(6):514–23.

151. Kulke MH et al. Activity of sunitinib in patients with advanced neuroendocrine tumors. *J Clin Oncol* 2008;26(20):3403–10.

152. Raymond E et al. Sunitinib malate for the treatment of pancreatic neuroendocrine tumors. *N Engl J Med* 2011;364(6):501–13.

153. Wan X et al. Rapamycin induces feedback activation of Akt signaling through an IGF-1R-dependent mechanism. *Oncogene* 2007;26(13):1932–40.

154. Bajetta E et al. Everolimus in combination with octreotide long-acting repeatable in a first-line setting for patients with neuroendocrine tumors: An ITMO group study. *Cancer* 2014;120(16):2457–63.

155. Feldman ME, Shokat KM. New inhibitors of the PI3K-Akt-mTOR pathway: Insights into mTOR signaling from a new generation of Tor Kinase Domain Inhibitors (TORKinibs). *Curr Top Microbiol Immunol* 2010;347:241–62.

156. Fjallskog ML et al. Expression of molecular targets for tyrosine kinase receptor antagonists in malignant endocrine pancreatic tumors. *Clin Cancer Res* 2003;9(4):1469–73.

157. Chaudhry A, Funa K, Oberg K. Expression of growth factor peptides and their receptors in neuroendocrine tumors of the digestive system. *Acta Oncol* 1993;32(2):107–14.

158. Chaudhry A et al. Expression of platelet-derived growth factor and its receptors in neuroendocrine tumors of the digestive system. *Cancer Res* 1992;52(4):1006–12.

159. Terris B et al. Expression of vascular endothelial growth factor in digestive neuroendocrine tumours. *Histopathology* 1998;32(2):133–8.

160. Mallinson CN et al. A glucagonoma syndrome. *Lancet* 1974;2(7871):1–5.

161. Church RE, Crane WA. A cutaneous syndrome associated with islet-cell carcinoma of the pancreas. *Br J Dermatol* 1967;79(5):284–6.

162. Braverman IM. Cutaneous manifestations of internal malignant tumors by Becker, Kahn and Rothman, June 1942. Commentary: Migratory necrolytic erythema. *Arch Dermatol* 1982;118(10):784–98.

163. Mullans EA, Cohen PR. Iatrogenic necrolytic migratory erythema: A case report and review of nonglucagonoma-associated necrolytic migratory erythema. *J Am Acad Dermatol* 1998;38(5 Pt 2):866–73.

164. Howard TJ et al. Anatomic distribution of pancreatic endocrine tumors. *Am J Surg* 1990;159(2):258–64.

165. Krausz Y et al. Somatostatin-receptor scintigraphy in the management of gastroenteropancreatic tumors. *Am J Gastroenterol* 1998;93(1):66–70.

166. Ambrosini V et al. 68Ga-DOTANOC PET/CT clinical impact in patients with neuroendocrine tumors. *J Nucl Med* 2010;51(5):669–73.

167. Sahoo MK et al. Necrolytic migratory erythema associated with glucagonoma syndrome diagnosed by (6)(8)Ga-DOTANOC PET-CT. *Asia Pac J Clin Oncol* 2014;10(2):190–3.

168. Alexander EK et al. Peripheral amino acid and fatty acid infusion for the treatment of necrolytic migratory erythema in the glucagonoma syndrome. *Clin Endocrinol (Oxf)* 2002;57(6):827–31.

169. Boden G et al. Treatment of inoperable glucagonoma with the long-acting somatostatin analogue SMS 201-995. *N Engl J Med* 1986;314(26):1686–9.

170. Tomassetti P et al. Treatment of gastroenteropancreatic neuroendocrine tumours with octreotide LAR. *Aliment Pharmacol Ther* 2000;14(5):557–60.

171. Tomassetti P, Migliori M, Gullo L. Slow-release lanreotide treatment in endocrine gastrointestinal tumors. *Am J Gastroenterol* 1998;93(9):1468–71.

172. Wermers RA, Fatourechi V, Kvols LK. Clinical spectrum of hyperglucagonemia associated with malignant neuroendocrine tumors. *Mayo Clin Proc* 1996;71(11):1030–8.

173. Kindmark H et al. Endocrine pancreatic tumors with glucagon hypersecretion: A retrospective study of 23 cases during 20 years. *Med Oncol* 2007;24(3):330–7.

174. Wermers RA et al. The glucagonoma syndrome. Clinical and pathologic features in 21 patients. *Medicine (Baltimore)* 1996;75(2):53–63.

41

The pancreas, the neuroendocrine system, neoplasia, traditional open pancreatectomy

DEMETRIUS PERTSEMLIDIS AND DAVID S. PERTSEMLIDIS

INTRODUCTION

This chapter is dedicated mainly to pancreatic endocrine surgery, but such narrow text cannot offer comprehensive education. Overviews of embryology, anatomy, physiology, clinical and biochemical assays, conventional and molecular isotopic imaging, correlation of risks and benefits of surgery, and prognostic profile are indispensable in any textbook [1].

Furthermore, the pancreatic neuroendocrine system comprising all the islets of Langerhans contributes to the integral function of the exocrine pancreas through the insular–acinar portal system. Insulin, somatostatin, and pancreatic polypeptide (PP) affect exocrine secretion, and conversely, they are affected by cholecystokinin (CCK),

gastric inhibitory polypeptide, and other gastrointestinal peptides [2,3].

EMBRYOLOGY

The human pancreas appears during the fourth week of fetal life. It is derived from two to three outpockets of the primitive gut. The dorsal outpocket (anlage) gives rise to the body and tail and fuses with the ventral anlage, which gives rise to the inferior portion of the pancreatic head and the uncinate process. It undergoes morphologic and physiologic changes during normal development, but anatomic differentiation does not always correlate with functional maturity.

The dorsal pancreas derives its blood supply from the celiac trunk through the splenic and gastroduodenal arteries and from the central (transverse) pancreatic artery arising from the superior mesenteric. The ventral pancreas is supplied from the superior mesenteric artery through the inferior pancreaticoduodenal artery. The venous drainage combines the splenic, superior and inferior mesenteric, and portal veins.

The volumes of the acinar cells and islets of Langerhans vary with age because their growth is discordant. The islet cells are initially present as single cells in the exocrine parenchyma and later in clusters separated from the exocrine tissue by a capsule of collagen and fibroblasts. The islets make up 20% of the pancreatic mass in the newborn and only 1%–2% of the adult pancreas, because of the exuberant growth of the exocrine pancreas in neonatal life. Remarkably, the blood flow to the endocrine pancreas is 15%–20% of the total pancreatic blood flow.

Glucagon-secreting α cells and somatostatin-containing δ cells develop before β cell differentiation, although insulin can be recognized before apparent maturity of the β cells. Fetal insulin secretion is low and does not respond to *acute changes in glucose*, but it is responsive to amino acids and glucagon as early as 14 weeks. Unlike the lack of response to acute changes in glucose, *chronic exposure* to hyperglycemia in diabetic mothers leads to increased secretion of insulin. This effect is apparently the cause of high birth weights in children of diabetic mothers.

Knowledge is limited on the impact of intrauterine growth retardation, postnatal malnutrition, modified infant formulas, and parenteral nutrition. In the first few months of neonatal life, there is a deficiency of lipase and amylase, which dictates caution in the use of lipid-rich and complex carbohydrate-containing formulas.

CONGENITAL MALFORMATIONS

Annular pancreas

Annular pancreas is a rare anomaly when normal pancreatic tissue completely or partially encircles the second portion of the duodenum (Figure 41.1). It is thought to arise from failure of normal clockwise rotation of the ventral pancreatic primordium (anlage), possibly due to abnormal fixation at the free end (Figure 41.2). Varying degrees of duodenal obstructive symptoms may be observed. Serious congenital anomalies such as intracardiac defects, Down's syndrome, and intestinal malrotation are commonly associated with annular pancreas. It is technically difficult or impossible to resect the annular pancreas without injury to the duodenum. Duodenojejunostomy or gastrojejunostomy is used to bypass the obstruction.

Heterotopic pancreas

The development of pancreatic tissue outside the main gland is a congenital abnormality referred to as heterotopic pancreas. Most commonly, heterotopic pancreatic tissue is found in the stomach, duodenum, small bowel, or Meckel's

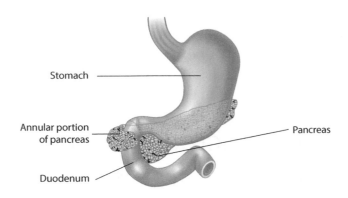

Figure 41.1 Annular pancreas. Failure of clockwise rotation of the ventral pancreatic anlage due to fixation of the free end (Figure 41.2), resulting in partial or complete encircling of the proximal duodenum. Association with serious congenital anomalies is common. Bypass with gastro- or jejunoduodenostomy is safer than surgical excision, which usually leads to destruction of the duodenum and pancreatic fistula. (From Mehrera, B.J., Marcel Dekker. Last modified by Demetrius Pertsemlidis.)

diverticulum. Rarely, such ectopic tissue may be found at the umbilicus, colon, appendix, gallbladder, or omentum. Heterotopic pancreas is usually an incidental finding at surgery or autopsy. Clinical small bowel obstruction may be caused by direct occlusion of the lumen or intussusception. Rarely, bleeding may occur.

Pancreas divisum

Pancreas divisum is the result of nonfusion of the dorsal and ventral pancreatic ducts (Figure 41.3). This anomaly has been recognized in about 10% of patients undergoing endoscopic retrograde cholangiopancreatography or magnetic resonance cholangiopancreatography (MRCP) for presumed pancreatic disease. In this anomaly, the major portion of the pancreas (superior head, neck, body, and tail) is drained by the duct of Santorini through the minor duodenal papilla. The major duodenal papilla usually communicates with a small duct of Wirsung, which drains the inferior head and uncinate process. The significance of the pancreas divisum remains controversial. In some series, endoscopic pancreatography for idiopathic pancreatitis revealed a high incidence of pancreas divisum approaching 25%, but it was not clear whether the ductal anomaly had any causal relationship to the pancreatitis. Speculation that functional stenosis of the minor duodenal papilla can cause pancreatitis has led to transduodenal sphincterplasty of the minor papilla, without success.

Nesidioblastosis

In this congenital anomaly, children are born with severe hypoglycemia from uncontrolled hypersecretion of insulin. The abnormal histology of the pancreas displays immature

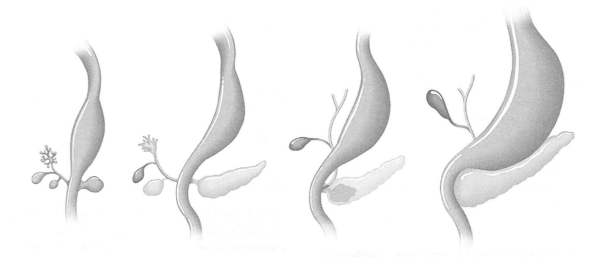

Figure 41.2 Development of the pancreas. The pancreas develops from two diverticula, one in the front and the other behind the duodenum. After complete clockwise rotation, the ventral anlage forms a portion of the head of the pancreas and the dorsal anlage forms the rest of the organ. Two types of cells create the mesentery of the duodenum, the ducts of the two anlagen anastomoses, thus creating the proximal part of the dorsal duct. In the adult, the main duct takes its origin from the ventral duct, and the ventral and dorsal ducts contribute to the formation of the ampulla.

Normal pancreatic duct

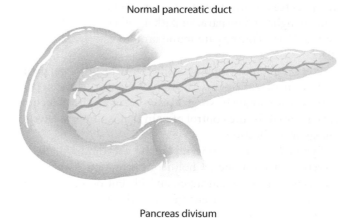

Pancreas divisum

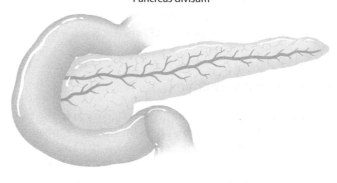

Figure 41.3 Pancreas divisum. Failure of fusion between the dorsal and ventral pancreatic ducts. The duct of Santorini drains most of the pancreatic fluid, and the narrowed duct of Wirsung, which normally drains the inferior head and uncinate process, may drain through the major papilla or not drain at all. The association with pancreatitis has been virtually dismissed, and surgical sphincterotomy or sphincteroplasty (personal experience) of the minor duodenal papilla failed to prevent pancreatitis.

β cells growing along the ducts. There is no formation of islets in this syndrome.

The disease is almost uniformly fatal in the neonatal period from severe hypoglycemia. Surgery in the form of subtotal or total pancreatectomy offers limited success.

In the multiple endocrine neoplasia (MEN) 1 syndrome, about 20% of patients have insulinomas, usually multicentric. A very small minority of these patients (children or adults) have diffuse or nodular hyperplasia resembling nesidioblastosis.

Noninsulinoma pancreatogenous hypoglycemia syndrome (NIPHS) was discovered in families with activated glucokinase mutations. Pathologically, the findings display hypertrophy and hyperplasia with insulin-containing cells budding from the ductal epithelium [4].

A similar syndrome resembling nesidioblastosis is the postprandial hyperinsulinemic hypoglycemia after gastric bypass surgery for obesity [5,6]. Surgical treatment with near-total (preserving the duodenum and the bile duct) or total pancreatectomy has been performed in small numbers.

Cystic fibrosis

Although not a primary pancreatic anomaly, cystic fibrosis is a recessive genetic disorder causing abnormalities of the pancreas and lungs beginning often in utero (Table 41.1) [7]. Two loss-of-function mutations in the cystic fibrosis transmembrane conductance regulator (CFTR) gene, mapped to chromosome 7, cause failure of chloride transport across epithelial cells in the exocrine pancreas, lungs, intestine, and sweat glands. The defective gene is present in 1 of 2000 Caucasian births. About 10% of affected newborns present with obstructive meconium ileus, and 40% of children older

Table 41.1 A defective gene of the transmembrane conductance regulation in chromosome 7 causes 10% of affected newborns to have meconium ileus and 40% of children older than 10 years to develop pancreatic endocrine insufficiency

Cystic fibrosis
• Autosomal recessive
• 1 in 2000 Caucasian births
• Mutations in CFTR gene
• Chromosome 7
• Chloride transport defect
• Pancreatic insufficiency (exocrine + endocrine)
• Chloride sweat test with pilocarpine

than 10 years develop pancreatic endocrine insufficiency. Decreased fluid secretion leads to mucus plugs in the lungs, exocrine pancreas, vas deferens, and sweat glands. Exocrine pancreatic insufficiency results in steatorrhea and growth retardation.

In patients with the nonclassic form of cystic fibrosis, one copy of the mutant gene confers partial function of the CFTR protein and some pancreatic function is preserved.

The chloride sweat test after pilocarpine administration offers a 99% diagnostic accuracy, if the chloride concentration is higher than 60 mmol/L. The test can be normal or borderline in the nonclassic form.

ANATOMY AND HISTOLOGY

The pancreas occupies a retroperitoneal position within the lesser peritoneal sac. It extends obliquely from the duodenal sweep to a more cephalad position in the hilum of the spleen. The normal adult pancreas weighs about 100 g and is 14–18 cm long, 2–9 cm wide, and 2–3 cm thick.

The gland is divided into four portions: the head, the neck, the body, and the tail. The uncinate process extends behind the superior mesenteric vein and ends at the right margin of the superior mesenteric artery. The neck and body of the pancreas lie anterior to the mesenteric and portal veins; the tail of the pancreas extends to the left and reaches the splenic hilum. The inferior vena cava and aorta lie posterior to the pancreatic head; the splenic artery runs along the superior border of the gland and divides into several branches along the 7 cm hilum of the spleen. The splenic vein runs along the posterior surface of the pancreas and joins the superior mesenteric vein near the neck and body.

Vascular anatomy

The head of the pancreas and the duodenum are supplied by two arterial arcades known as the anterior and posterior pancreaticoduodenal arteries, which originate from the gastroduodenal and superior mesenteric arteries, respectively (Figure 41.4a and b). The blood supply to the body and tail of the pancreas is more variable and is derived from the splenic and left gastroepeiploic arteries. The dorsal pancreatic artery from the splenic joins the central artery from the superior mesenteric to augment the blood supply to the distal pancreas. The venous drainage of the pancreas corresponds to the arterial anatomy. Veins draining the pancreatic parenchyma eventually terminate in the portal vein, which arises posterior to the neck of the pancreas by the union of the splenic and superior mesenteric veins.

Lymphatic system

Multiple lymph node groups drain the pancreas. From the head of the gland, nodes in the pancreaticoduodenal groove communicate with subpyloric, portal, mesocolic, mesenteric, and aortocaval nodes. Lymphatic vessels in the body and tail of the pancreas drain into retroperitoneal nodes, in the splenic hilum, or into celiac, aortocaval, mesocolic, or mesenteric nodes.

Autonomic innervation

The pancreas is innervated by sympathetic fibers from the celiac ganglia and by parasympathetic fibers from the vagus nerves. Nerve endings are found around vessels, acini, and islets.

Postganglionic sympathetic fibers are the principal pathways for pancreatic pain. Ablation of the splanchnic nerves or the celiac ganglia by surgical excision or alcohol injection is being used for the control of pain that is unresponsive to analgesic medications.

Sympathetic and parasympathetic nerves modulate the secretion of hormones. Cholinergic stimulation increases secretion of insulin, glucagon, and PP, but probably inhibits somatostatin. β-adrenergic stimulation increases the secretion of insulin, glucagon, PP, and somatostatin. α-adrenergic stimulation inhibits the release of insulin. Vasoactive intestinal peptide (VIP) and CCK also affect islet cell secretion.

Pancreatic parenchyma

Two distinct organs exist in the human pancreas, the exocrine and endocrine systems. The acini and ducts constitute the exocrine pancreas. The acinus (from the Latin berry) is the enzyme-secreting unit, and the ductules and ducts secrete water and electrolytes, aside from being the conduit for exocrine secretion. The acini and ducts resemble clusters of grapes on a stem (Figure 41.5).

Each acinus is composed of a single layer of cells (Figure 41.6) rich in endoplasmic reticulum, a large nucleus, a Golgi complex, and abundant symogen granules. Acinar cells make up 80% of the pancreatic parenchyma, and the remaining is made up by ducts, vessels, matrix, and islet cells.

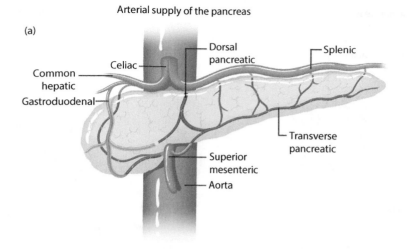

Arterial supply of the pancreas

(a)

Common hepatic
Celiac
Gastroduodenal
Dorsal pancreatic
Splenic
Transverse pancreatic
Superior mesenteric
Aorta

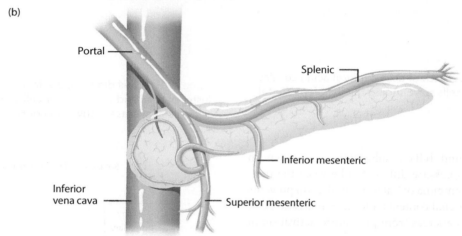

Venous drainage of the pancreas

(b)

Portal
Splenic
Inferior mesenteric
Inferior vena cava
Superior mesenteric

Figure 41.4a and b Pancreatic vasculature. Pancreatic and duodenal arteries originate from the gastroduodenal and superior mesenteric. The anterior and posterior pancreaticoduodenal arcades supply the pancreatic head and duodenum. The dorsal pancreatic from the splenic and the transverse pancreatic from the superior mesenteric arteries supply the body and tail. The splenic, superior, and inferior pancreatic veins join the portal vein to the portal venous system.

The pancreatic duct system originates in centroacinar cells, followed by formation of ductules and termination in the main excretory duct.

The endocrine pancreas is made up of about 1 million islets scattered throughout the exocrine tissue. The highly vascularized endocrine units contain several types of cells: β-producing insulin, α-secreting glucagon, δ-producing somatostatin, and PP cells secreting PP. Neuroendocrine cells, which are found infrequently, secrete VIP (δ1 cells), substance P, serotonin (enterochromaffin [EC] cells), and gastrin (G cells). β cells make up 60%–80% of the islets, α cells and PP cells 15%–20%, and δ cells 5%–10%.

Exocytosis

Zymogen granules release their enzymes into the acinar lumen by a complex mechanism called exocytosis. In the Golgi apparatus, they are packaged within a glycoprotein envelope and then migrate to the apex of the cell, where the zymogen envelope fuses with the acinar cell membrane (exocytosis), ultimately leading to extrusion into the centroacinar lumen (beginning of ductules).

The duct system

The duct system is the site of secretion of bicarbonate, ions, and water. It is subdivided into three parts. The *intralobular* ducts drain pancreatic juice from the acinar cells. The *interlobular* ducts run within connective tissue, together with vessels and nerves. The third part is the main pancreatic duct.

The final secretory product of the exocrine pancreas is a combined acinar and ductal fluid containing enzymes from the acinar cells and water, plus electrolytes from the ductal epithelium. The centroacinar cells comprising the beginning of pancreatic ductules contain high concentrations of the enzyme carbonic anhydrase, which catalyzes the reaction $H_2O + CO_2 = H^+ HCO_3^-$.

Histology of the exocrine pancreas

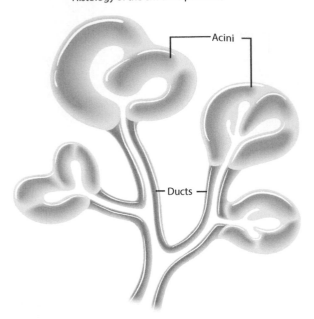

Figure 41.5 Artistic sketch of acinus (plural acini) consisting of two or three cells surrounding the incipient ductal system.

Histology of the exocrine pancreas

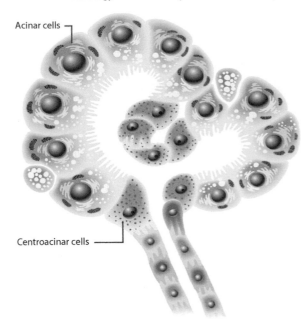

Figure 41.6 In this drawing, the focus is centered on a cluster of acini and centroacinar cells, the site of enzymatic (carbonic anhydrase) conversion of H_2O and CO_2 to H^+ and HCO_3^-.

The pancreatic and biliary sphincters are shown in Figure 41.7 [8]. The pressure differential between the pancreatic duct and the ampulla of Vater or duodenum prevents reflux of bile or duodenal contents into the pancreatic duct, thus protecting the pancreas from premature activation of the enzymes.

EXOCRINE PANCREATIC FUNCTION

Electrolyte and water secretion

The adult human pancreas secretes 800–1200 mL of pancreatic juice daily containing 60–120 mEq/L of bicarbonate, with a pH ranging from 7.6 to 8.2. The *basal* secretory rate is 0.2–0.3 mL/min, rising up to 5 mL/min after *maximal* stimulation with secretin. The other major anion is chloride.

The alkalinity of pancreatic juice is necessary for optimal function of the proteolytic, lipolytic, and amylolytic enzymes at a pH range of 7–9.

The secretion of electrolytes and water is regulated by humoral and vagal mechanisms. The concentrations of sodium and potassium are equal to those in the plasma, but the anion concentration depends on the secretory rate. At low secretory rates, the concentrations of chloride and bicarbonate are nearly equivalent to those of plasma, whereas with neurohumoral stimulation, bicarbonate increases and the chloride concentration is lowered. Secretion of bicarbonate into the duct lumen is an active transport mechanism, with bicarbonate ions leaving the cell by a chloride–bicarbonate exchanger, whose activity depends on

Sphincters of the pancreas and bile duct

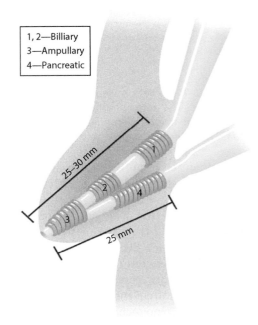

1, 2—Billiary
3—Ampullary
4—Pancreatic

Figure 41.7 The ductal system is composed of acinar and centroacinal cells, ductules, and ducts. The pressure differential of the three sphincters, pancreatic, biliary, and ampullary, protects the rise of pancreatic duct pressure and premature activation of enzymes. (The precise, artistic, highly educational periampullary sphincteric system is from Skandalakis, J.E. et al., *Contemp. Surg.*, 1979;15:17–40. With permission.)

the presence of chloride in the duct lumen. Secretin is the most potent endogenous stimulant of water and bicarbonate secretion. Secretin is synthesized in the proximal small intestine and is released into the bloodstream in the presence of luminal acid and bile. It binds to receptors on pancreatic ductal cells, effecting signal transduction through the intracellular adenylate cyclase system, to yield an increase in intracellular cyclic adenosine monophosphate. Several endogenous inhibitors of water and electrolyte secretion (somatostatin, PP, and glucagon) have been identified, but their inhibitory role has not been well defined.

Enzyme synthesis and secretion

1. *Synthesis.* The pancreas delivers 6–20 g of enzymes into the duodenum daily. An entirely distinct sequence of intracellular events mediates the synthesis and excretion of the digestive enzymes from acinar cells. The synthesis of all proteins occurs on ribosomes, where genetic information previously transferred to messenger RNA (mRNA) during nuclear transcription is translated into the appropriate amino acid sequence of the peptide chain. The synthesized preproenzymes, become free in the rough endoplasmic reticulum. During their transit through the rough endoplasic reticulum and the Golgi apparatus, the newly synthesized proteins undergo modification in a sequence of steps collectively referred to as post-translational processing.
2. *Secretion.* CCK, an integrin hormone produced in the proximal small bowel, and acetylcholine from parasympathetic (vagal) innervation are the most potent stimulants of enzyme secretion. The proenzymes subsequently pass to the Golgi apparatus through a vesicular shuttle system, where they are packaged within a glycoprotein vesicular membrane. The Golgi apparatus is responsible for sorting the proteins destined for either lysosomal pathways or zymogen granules. The packaged zymogen granules migrate to the acinar cell apex, where their membranes fuse with the acinar cell plasma membrane (exocytosis), leading to extrusion of the contents into the centroacinar lumen. Specific enzymes synthesized and released include endopeptidases (trypsin, chymotrypsin, elastase, and kallikrein) and exopeptidases (carboxypeptidases A and B). Other enzymes include phospholipase, lipase, colipase, nonspecific carboxylesterase, amylase, ribonuclease, and deoxyribonuclease. Most peptidases synthesized by acinar cells are released into the pancreatic ductal system in inactive forms. Peptide activation commences after the peptidases enter the duodenum, where mucosal enterokinase cleaves trypsinogen to trypsin and leaves trypsin to activate the other enzymes.

In contrast to other peptidases, ribonuclease, deoxyribonuclease, amylase, and lipase are released into the pancreatic ductal system in their active forms.

Proenzymes synthesized in the pancreatic acinar cell	
Proteolytic	**Lipolytic**
Trypsinogen	Lipase
Chymotrypsinogen	Prophospholipase A2
Proelastase	Carboxylesterase
Procarboxypeptidase A	**Nucleolytic**
Procarboxypeptidase B	Deoxyribonuclease (DNAse)
Amylolytic	Ribonuclease (RNAse)
Amylase	**Others**
	Procolipase
	Trypsin inhibitor

PHASES OF DIGESTION

1. *Cephalic phase.* Three classic phases of digestion occur in response of the pancreas to a meal. During the cephalic phase of digestion, stimuli such as the smell, sight, and taste of food activate vagal efferent signals, which stimulate pancreatic enzyme release. In addition, cephalic phase stimulation of gastric acid secretion causes duodenal acidification, which stimulates secretin release and subsequent pancreatic bicarbonate secretion. The net effect of cephalic phase stimulation is the secretion of an enzyme-rich, bicarbonate-poor fluid.
2. *Gastric phase.* During the gastric phase of digestion, gastric distention activates mechanoreceptors located in the body of the stomach. Antral distention and antral protein stimulate the release of gastrin, which promotes gastric acid secretion and also serves as a weak stimulator of pancreatic enzyme secretion. Gastrin-stimulated gastric acid secretion contributes to pancreatic bicarbonate secretion by duodenal acidification and subsequent secretin release. Stimulation of vagal afferents by antral distention also plays a role in the gastric phase of pancreatic exocrine secretion (antral distention-induced pancreatic exocrine secretion is reduced after truncal vagotomy).
3. *Intestinal phase.* During the intestinal (most important) phase of digestion, secretin and CCK serve a major function in mediating pancreatic exocrine secretion. Duodenal acid and bile stimulate secretin release, leading to bicarbonate and water secretion from duct cells. Duodenal fat and protein release CCK, with subsequent stimulation of pancreatic enzyme secretion from acinar cells. In addition to these humorally mediated events, bile salts, fatty acids, and amino acids in the duodenum can stimulate pancreatic exocrine secretion by neural pathways.

ENDOCRINE PHYSIOLOGY

The adult human pancreas has about 1 g of islet tissue comprising about 1 million islets, ranging in size from clusters of a few cells to more than 5000 cells [9–12].

Each islet is highly vascularized and contains four types of cells. Insulin-producing β cells make up 60%–80% of the islet cells, glucagon-secreting α cells and PP-secreting cells make up 15%–20% of the islet cells, and somatostatin-producing δ cells make up 5%–10% of the islet cells. Rarely, there are δ1: EC, and G cells producing vasoactive intestinal polypeptide, substance P, serotonin, and gastrin or adrenocorticotropic hormone (ACTH), respectively.

Initially (in fetal development), endocrine cells secrete more than one hormone, but ultimately secretion is restricted to one hormone.

Islet cell hormone secretion is modulated by autonomic nerves. Cholinergic stimulation increases insulin, glucagon, and PP secretion and probably inhibits somatostatin secretion.

β-adrenergic stimulation increases secretion of insulin, glucagon, PP, and somatostatin. Insulin secretion is inhibited by epinephrine and norepinephrine through α-adrenergic receptors. The hyperglycemia or frank diabetes seen in pheochromocytoma is due to inhibition of insulin secretion by excess catecholamines. This form of diabetes is cured after resection of the pheochromocytoma.

The influence of *peptidergic* nerves on islet cell secretion is unclear. They contain VIP, CCK, substance P, and enkephalin.

Islet cells are dispersed throughout the pancreas and may influence exocrine function and growth through an *insuloacinar* portal system. Insulin, somatostatin and PP can affect exocrine secretion, and conversely, they can be affected by CCK, gastric inhibitory polypeptide, and other gastrointestinal peptides.

1. *Insulin synthesis and secretion.* The human insulin gene is located in chromosome 11. In the endoplasmic reticulum, preproinsulin is converted to proinsulin, a single-peptide chain. Conversion to insulin in the secretory granules requires the action of two enzymes, a trypsin-like enzyme that removes the C-peptide, i.e., the segment connecting the two insulin chains, and a carboxypeptidase B-like enzyme.

   C-peptide is released into the circulation in the same amount as insulin. Proinsulin can be released into the circulation by exocytosis of granules when conversion to insulin is incomplete. In patients with insulinoma, the amount of circulating proinsulin is high, most likely because the normal orderly processing and secretion is disrupted, allowing excess secretion of insulin precursors.

2. *Insulin release.* Four mechanisms for acceleration or inhibition of the release of insulin by exocytosis are (a) metabolic (glucose), (b) hormonal (glucagon), neural (acetylcholine), and (c) neural (β-adrenergic).

   Glucose exerts its effect by entering the β cell by facilitated diffusion. The rate of insulin secretion is proportional to glucose metabolism, which is determined by glucokinase, the rate-limiting enzyme of glycolysis.

Aside from glucose, the release of insulin is accelerated by glucagon, amino acids, fatty acids, neural-mediated cholinergic and β-adrenergic stimulation, and a variety of gastrointestinal hormones, such as gastrin, CCK, gastric inhibitory peptide, secretin, and VIP.

Somatostatin and neural-mediated α-adrenergic stimulation inhibit the release of insulin.

3. *Insulin action and degradation.* Insulin is released directly into the portal vein and exerts its biologic effects by binding to specific membrane receptors on the target cells. Under physiologic conditions, 50% of insulin entering the liver is degraded in a single passage.

   The plasma concentration of insulin is 5–20 μU/mL in the fasting state and has a half-life of 5 minutes. C-peptide is secreted into the circulation in equimolar amounts but has a higher plasma concentration because of a longer half-life of 15 minutes. Proinsulin secretion is only 3% of that of insulin secretion but accounts for about 30% of the insulin immunoreactivity because of a long half-life of 17 minutes. C-peptide does not have significant biologic activity, and proinsulin has 10%–15% of the bioactivity of insulin.

   Insulin plays a key *anabolic* role by promoting the synthesis and storage of glycogen, fat, and protein.

   Degradation of insulin at the target organs is the result of insulin–receptor interaction. The insulin–receptor complex is internalized by the cells of target tissues and insulin is degraded.

   Under physiologic conditions, the kidney is another important site of degradation of insulin, proinsulin, and C-peptide.

4. *Glucagon, somatostatin, and PP.* The physiologic role of *glucagon* is to protect against hypoglycemia, but its loss (diabetes and pancreatectomy) does not have serious consequences, because catecholamines compensate for its absence. Patients with glucagon deficiency who have coexisting inadequate catecholamine response (dysautonomia) are vulnerable to hypoglycemia. Insulin-induced hypoglycemia increases plasma glucagon concentration in the nondiabetic patient.

   Glucose and somatostatin have an inhibitory effect on glucagon secretion. Most of the gut hormones, except secretin, accelerate the secretion of glucagon.

   The importance of pancreatic somatostatin has not been established. The most likely physiologic role is the inhibition of insulin and glucagon through paracrine mechanisms.

   The acceleration or inhibition of the release of somatostatin by the δ cells is similar to that by the β cells.

   The biologic significance of PP is unclear. Vagal stimulation and various gastrointestinal hormones stimulate secretion of PP.

   Serum PP is elevated in both functioning and nonfunctioning pancreatic and extrapancreatic neuroendocrine tumors. Together with chromogranin A and neuron-specific enolase, PP is a valuable serum and histochemical marker in all neuroendocrine tumors.

THE NEUROENDOCRINE SYSTEM

Historical perspectives

The neuroendocrine system was first described in 1914 by a French Canadian pathologist named Pierre Masson who called the chromoargentaffin cells of the intestine a diffuse endocrine gland [13–17]. In 1938, Friedrich Feyrter, an Austrian pathologist, expanded the definition of the neuroendocrine system beyond the intestine into a more disseminated or diffuse endocrine organ.

In 1966, Pearse, at the Hammersmith Hospital in London, defined the functional and cytochemical characteristics of the neuroendocrine system, especially the ability for uptake and decarboxylation of amine precursors (APUD cell system). Pollack and Bishop, students of Pearse, described the techniques for a cytochemical identification of the neuroendocrine tumors. Since then, more than 50 different cell types and more than 30 different peptide hormones, biogenic amines, neurotransmitters, and other markers have been identified. The most recently discovered neuropeptide was the atrial natriuretic hormone, which affects water and electrolyte regulation and the vascular system. The electron microscopic hallmark of neuroendocrine cells is the presence of cytoplasmic secretory granules (Figure 41.8).

The rapid advances of modern endocrinology were made possible in large measure by the radioimmunoassay of peptides, discovered by the late Solomon Berson, our former chairman of medicine, and his coworker Rosalyn Yalow, the recipient of the 1977 Nobel Prize for Medicine and emeritus professor of medicine in our medical school. She died on May 30, 2011.

Although the neuroendocrine cells cannot be fully integrated into a unified system, we have reasonably common morphologic and functional criteria, which permit recognition of these cells and of the neoplasms derived from them. The neuroendocrine system is distributed throughout the body, including the hypothalamic–pituitary unit, the thyroid and parathyroid, the heart, the bronchopulmonary system and thymus, the gastroenteropancreatic and sympathoadrenal system, and the skin and prostate (Table 41.2).

Table 41.2 Neural crest-derived neuroendocrine system is distributed from the brain to the pelvis, mostly in known hormonal organs

The neuroendocrine system embryology and anatomy

Embryological origin from the neural crest
Anatomic locations
  Hypothalamus and pituitary
  Thyroid and parathyroid
  Bronchopulmonary system and thymus
  Heart
  Pancreas and gastro-enteric system
  Adrenal medulla and sympathoneural paraganglia
  Prostate and skin

Table 41.3 Several abbreviated factors are released, including prolactin inhibitor, by the hypothalamus, and a variety of neuroendocrine hormones, including all islet cells of the pancreas, are located in mostly known endocrine organs

The neuroendocrine system

Hypothalamus (rel)	: ACTH Gn-Rh TRH releasing PIF
Anterior Pituitary	: ACTH prolactin GH TSH LH FSH
Thyroid + parathyroid	: Calcitonin, parathormone
Lungs and thymus	: Histamine
Heart	: Atrial natriuretic hormone
Pancreas, gut	: Glucagon insulin gastrin PP Somatostatin serotonin VIP
Adrenals/sympathetic paraganglia	: a) Catecholamines b) Ectopic amines + neuropeptide

Aside from listing the orthotopic hormones (Table 41.3), regulatory peptides, and amines, the neuroendocrine cells and their derivative neoplasms secrete a variety of silent cellular antigenic markers, such as chromogranin A, PP, neuron-specific enolase, and subunits α and β of the human chorionic gonadotropin, physostigmin, and pancreostatin (Table 41.4). The clinical significance of these silent markers is their presence in functioning and nonfunctioning neuroendocrine neoplasms and their utility as an index of therapeutic responses. Chromogranin A, isolated from the adrenal medulla, is a member of the granin family of proteins that is present in all neuroendocrine cells. Chromogranin A plasma levels reflect tumor load and may distinguish between benign and malignant tumors. *False elevations* of plasma chromogranin A are seen in end-stage renal disease, liver failure, and congestive heart failure. Neuroendocrine cells affect their secretory function by paracrine physiology.

Discovery of membrane receptors to somatostatin and catecholamines permitted both functional identification and anatomic localization of neuroendocrine tumors with ^{111}In-labeled somatostatin analogs (octreotide, pentetriotide,

Table 41.4 Antigens present in the serum and in the cytoplasmic neurosecretory granules of neuroendocrine cells and tumors

The neuroendocrine system common antigenic profile

Markers in serum, tissues (and tumors)
  Chromogranin A*
  Pancreatic polypeptide
  Neuron specific enolase
  α and β HCG subunits
  Pancreastatin
  Synaptophysine

Note: Their presence plays a key role in the diagnosis and detection of functioning and hormonally inactive tumors. Antigenicity also plays a role in the selection of ligands in isotopic imaging (low antigenicity is preferable).

* Chromogranin peptides antigens are multiple A, B, C, etc.

Table 41.5 Properties of affinity, antigenicity, and speed in the recognition, detection, and therapy of the commonly used tracers and ligands clinically

The neuroendocrine system common receptors			
Somatostatin (sst):	Affinity	Antigenicity	Half-life
	Low	High	Short
SST-analogs:	High	Low	Long
MIBG norepi-analog:	Mod	Mod	Mod
*Exendin-4, GLP-1: analog	High	Low	Long

* Receptors in beta islet cells.

and lanreotide) and ^{131}I-methyl-iodo-benzyl-guanidine, a norepinephrine analog (Table 41.5). Of the five somatostatin receptors (sstr), sstr-2 has the highest affinity to somatostatin or the long-acting analogs. Octreotide and lanreotide also exert effects on hormone secretion and antiproliferative activity by high-affinity binding to sstr-2 and, to a lesser degree, sstr-5. Hormonal hypersecretion is not a requisite for binding to somatostatin and its analogs, since nonfunctioning (silent) neuroendocrine tumors display similar receptor–ligand activity. Somatostatin receptor-based scintigraphy offers a high sensitivity and specificity (more than 90%), except for small tumors and insulinomas, where the diagnostic imaging accuracy drops to about 50%. Recent discovery of β cell receptors with high affinity to glucagon-like peptide (GLP-1) improved molecular imaging.

The common characteristics of neuroendocrine cells and neoplasm are displayed in Tables 41.4 through 41.8.

NEUROENDOCRINE ISLET CELL NEOPLASIA

Current nomenclature and abbreviations

Neuroendocrine neoplasia (NEN) includes benign hyperplasia and well-, intermediate-, and poorly-differentiated lesions [10–12].

Table 41.6 Majority, if not exclusive, etiology of secretory diarrhea from hypersecretion of neuroendocrine hormones

The neuroendocrine system secretory diarrhea	
Syndrome	***Hormone**
Carcinoid foregut	Histamine
Carcinoid midgut	Serotonin
Mastocytosis	Histamine
Gastrinoma	Gastrin
Medullary thyroid cancer	Calcitonin
VIP-oma	Vasoactive intestinal peptide
Cholera	Bacterial: *Vibrio cholerae*

Note: The similarity with cholera is purely a single enzymatic stimulation.
* ALL stimulate adenylate cyclase.

Table 41.7 Depicts close similarity in the high malignant potential

The neuroendocrine system malignant potential	
Tumor	**%**
• Gastrinoma	60–70
• Gucagonoma	60–70
• Vasoactive intestinal peptide	60–70
• Somatostatinoma	90
• Medullary thyroid cancer	90
• Carcinoid	Intermediate

Note: With the exception of somatostatinoma, all of the depicted neoplasms are small in size at the clinical expression.

Neuroendocrine tumor (NET) includes low- to intermediate-grade and well- to moderately-differentiated neoplastic lesions.

Neuroendocrine carcinoma (NEC) includes high-grade, moderately- to poorly-differentiated lesions [10].

Gastroenteropancreatic tumors

The islet cells are part of the neuroendocrine system, and the derivative neoplasms share numerous common characteristics in biologic behavior, hormonal functioning or nonfunctioning, potential for producing ectopic hormones, affinity to somatostatin and catecholamine receptors, antigenic profile to cytoplasmic secretory granules, and the enzymatic property of uptake and decarboxylation of amine precursors.

Neuroendocrine organs are derived embryologically from the neural crest. The neoplastic syndromes are inherited by autosomal dominance. The tumor cells have strong affinity to binding with silver and the ability for uptake and decarboxylation of amine precursors, display cytoplasmic secretory granules on electron microscopy, and have abundant membrane receptors to somatostatin and catecholamines.

Neuroendocrine functioning and nonfunctioning tumors secrete antigens (proteins and enzymes), which are measurable in serum and tissue markers, confirming the presence of such tumors and reflecting response to tumor load with treatment.

Table 41.8 The small size (subcentimeter to 2 cm) is common in their advanced stage at the time of clinical expression

The neuroendocrine system size and malignancy	
Medullary thyroid cancer > 1 cm	Nodal metastases
Carcinoid > 1 cm	Often metastatic
Gastrinoma < 1 cm	Often metastatic
VIPoma < 1 cm	Often metastatic

COMMON CHARACTERISTICS OF THE NEUROENDOCRINE CELLS AND NEOPLASMS

The commonality of features was recognized at the inception of the neuroendocrine system and ultimately the neuroendocrine neoplasms.

The enzymatic property, i.e., the uptake and decarboxylation of the amine precursors (APUD), the light and electron microscopy, and the recognition of cytoplasmic neurosecretory granules for hormone storage, as well as antigenic profile, are displayed in Tables 41.4 and 41.5 and Figure 41.8.

The common receptors to neuropeptides, mostly somatostatin and analogs, and amines (catecholamines, histamine, and serotonin and analogs), the secretory diarrhea, and aggressive neoplasia in spite of small size (mostly 1–2 cm) are shown in Tables 41.6 through 41.8.

The stem cell potential in all neuroendocrine tumors, mostly in advanced stage, have the capacity to produce ectopic hormones, i.e., ACTH, VIPoma, serotonin, calcitonin, etc.

In more than two decades, the radiotracers linked to somatostatin analogs (octreotide, pentetriotide, and lanreotide) or norepinephrine analog, methyl-iodo-benzylguanidine (MIBG), have been in clinical practice. There is recent introduction of ^{68}Ga-DOTA (tetra-aza-cyclo-dodecane-tetracetic acid), a chelator linked to stable complexes with six radiotracers.

^{68}Ga-DOTATOC (DOTA-Tyr^3-octreotide) offers better uptake of the isotope than ^{111}In-octreotide.

Neurosecretory granules
cytoplasmic feature in all NE cells

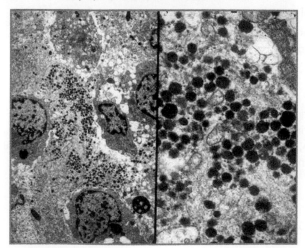

Figure 41.8 Under polarized microscopy, the cytoplasmic neurosecretory granules, a common neuroendocrine characteristic in normal and neoplastic cells, are the reservoir for neurohormones and antigens, and thus a histologic landmark. The presence of antigens and common receptors in functioning and nonfunctioning neuroendocrine tumors promotes completeness of diagnostic recognition in serum, tissue, and isotopic detection.

Table 41.9 Most common clinical use of radiotracers and ligands with high sensitivity and specificity, combined with high affinity, low antigenicity, and short half-life, and rapid completion of diagnostic imaging (1-hour ^{68}Ga-DOTA or DOTATOC/PET)

Receptor-based diagnostic imaging

^{111}In-octo, pente, lan-reotide SST analogs radio-tracers
^{123}I-MIBG, norepinephrine analog
^{111}In- or ^{68}Ga-exendin-4, GLP-1 analog (for insulinoma)
^{111}In-DOTA-lanreotide
^{68}Ga- DOTATOC or DOTANOC/PET
^{18}F- dopa or dopamine/PET
^{11}C- 5-htp/PET

^{68}Ga-DOTANOC (DOTA-1-NaI-octreotide) is the newest compound with high affinity to sstr-2, sstr-3, and sstr-5 ^{111}In or ^{68}Ga-exendin-4, a glucagon-like peptide 1 (GLP-1) analog for insulinoma (Table 41.9).

Scintigraphies are time-consuming (48 hours) compared with positron emission tomography (PET) imaging (about 1 hour).

Multiple neuroendocrine neoplasia

MENs are commonly inherited by autosomal dominance and classified according to clinical (phenotypic) expressions known as MEN 1 and MEN 2 (Tables 41.10 through 41.12, Figure 41.9) (2A, 2B, and familial medullary thyroid carcinoma only) [11–19]. This is to emphasize the unique presence of single medullary thyroid cancer (see Figure 41.10), unlike all the other MEN's. The striking characteristics of these syndromes are the plurality of involved endocrine organs, the centricity of neoplasms within the same gland,

Table 41.10 An overview—introduction to MEN 1 and 2

What are MEN 1 and MEN 2 Syndromes?

- * Multi-organ multicentric tumors
- Autosomal dominant inheritance
- Clinical Dx: 2/3 components + 1/3 first-degree relative
- Synchronous expression of all components only 20%
- Biochemical & receptor-based localization for Dx + therapy
- Surgery: total or subtotal resection
- Resistant to chemotherapy and external radiation
- 10-year survival with surgery 50%–70%

Note: The multiplicity of organs and multicentricity within each organ are highly frequent. The clinical definition, biochemical and receptor-based isotopic detection, and recognition of hormonal function or nonfunction offer unique achievement. The surgical difficulty is the need for total resection of the organ or bilateral removal with or without autotransplantation in benign neoplasms.

* Exception: familial medullary thyroid cancer only.

Table 41.11 Condensed information of MEN 1

	MEN-1 Components			
Component	**Clinical**	**Biochemical**	**Anatomy**	**Surgery**
Hyperparathyroidism Primary 95%	Kidney stones Peptic ulcer Bone disease Pancreatitis	Hypercalcemia High parathormone Hypercalcuria Hypophosphatemia	Hyperplasia All glands Benign!	Parathyroidectomy Autograft 90% 60% frozen tissue
Gastrinoma 50%	Peptic ulcer Secretory diarrhea Malabsorption	Hypergastrinemia Secretin Stimulation	Duodenal wall Multiple Malignant!	Transduodenal resection
Insulinoma 20%	Glucopenic encephalopathy and hyperadrenergic state	High C-peptide proinsulin, insulin Tolbutamid stimulation	Multiple Nesidioblastosis Benign!	Pancreatectomy: Enuclation Partial Subtotal, total
Carcinoid-foregut 40%	Secretory diarrhea "Asthma" Pulmonary fibrosis Valvular disease	High serum histamine Urine CH3- imidazole acetic acid Calcium stimulation	Bronchus, thymus stomach, pancreas Malignancy intermediate	Resection: Thoracoscopic Laparoscopic Open
Pituitary 30%	Amenorrhea Galactorrhea Cushing's	High prolactin High ACTH Other hormones	Anterior pituitary Microadenoma Benign!	Transsphenoidal adenomectomy

Note: The distribution of percentage of each component, symptomatology, biochemistry, anatomy, and surgical strategy are well defined. Analysis of each component is detailed, except for pituitary diseases managed by neurosurgery.

Table 41.12 MEN 2 components are analyzed as in MEN 1

	MEN-2 Components			
Component	**Clinical**	**Biochemical**	**Anatomy**	**Surgery**
Medullary thyroid cancer or C-cell hyperplasia >95%	Secretory diarrhea Neck mass in advanced disease	High serum calcitonin Gastrin stimulation	Multicentric tumors Malignant C-cell hyperplasia Benign	Thyroidectomy + lymphadenectomy Prophylactic in children
Pheochromocytoma 40%	Paroxysmal symptom Hypertention Diabates mellitus Diabates insipidus Cardiomyopathy	High metanephrines, plasma and urine Urine VMA, HVA, Avoid stimulation!	Adrenals bilateral Multicentric Benign	Adrenalectomy Bilateral Autotransplant of adrenal cortex?
Hyperparathyroidism MEN 2A 30% 2B absent	Kidney stones Bone disease Peptic ulcer Pancreatitis	Hypercalcemia Low phosphate High parathormone Hypercalcuria	Hyperplasia All glands Benign	Parathyroidectomy Autotransplant
Mucosal neuromas (MEN 2B only)	Facial disfiguring Abdominal pain from intestinal neuromas	NA	Conjuctiva Oral cavity Intestine	Removal for functional or esthetic reasons

Note: The vast majority are children and adolescents with medullary thyroid cancer managed by pediatric surgeons. Pheochromocytomas, almost always bilateral adrenal (synchronous or metachronous) and multicentric, are the most challenging for the surgeon. We have been able to perform 250 operations (85 laparoscopic) without mortality. We also achieved separation of pure adrenocortical tissue and implanted the cortex in heterotopic muscles. The results yielded limited success.

and the potential of hypersecretion of more than one hormone by a single organ. Common embryologic origin from the neural crest, serum markers, membrane receptors, and morphologic and histochemical features (secretory granules) are the ingredients of the neoplasms arising from the neuroendocrine cells.

The clinical manifestations and assays of hormones and their metabolites in the plasma and urine in the basal and provocative states permit diagnostic assessment with high accuracy. Molecular isotopic imaging augments the biochemical diagnosis, permits localization, and offers functional specificity in secretory tumors. In equivocal imaging results, selective venous sampling offers another method of localization by demonstrating unilateral or segmental step-up of the hormone concentration in comparison with that of the contralateral gland or the inferior vena cava.

Genetic studies revealed that the genes for MEN 1 and MEN 2 reside in chromosomes 11 and 10, respectively, and permit identification of affected family members before clinical expression of the syndrome and early treatment.

Hyperparathyroidism, usually from hyperplasia, is the earliest and universal component of MEN 1, whereas thyroid C-cell hyperplasia or medullary carcinoma is the earliest and universal key component in MEN 2. Hyperparathyroidism is less frequent in MEN 2A patients (about 30%) and absent in MEN 2B (Figure 41.9). Only a minority of affected patients (about 20%) display simultaneous phenotype of all main features of the MEN syndromes. Sequential phenotypic expression of the key components is the rule, with long intervals of many years or decades.

Familial medullary thyroid carcinoma is characterized by the presence of only one component. A minimum of 10 index cases in a family is necessary to distinguish it from MEN 2A because of overlap of genetic mutations. This definition of familial medullary thyroid carcinoma was chosen by the International RET Mutation Consortium in 2002.

Multiple neuroendocrine neoplasia type 1 (Wermer's syndrome)

The main components of MEN 1 are hyperparathyroidism, usually from hyperplasia, pituitary, or hypothalamic lesions, and gastroenteropancreatic tumors. Satellite neoplasms include adrenocortical tumors, foregut carcinoids, angiofibroma, lipoma, and ependymoma. Two of the three main components and a relative with one of the three key features are needed for clinical definition of the syndrome.

The autosomal dominant syndrome is caused by germline and somatic mutations of the gene encoding the protein menin, which is present in 80%–90% of the patients. The precise function of this protein is unknown. The gene is located in the long arm of chromosome 11q13. As mentioned before, complete simultaneous expression of the phenotype is seen in only 20% of the patients, and the remaining 80% display sequential development of the key clinical features, with intervals ranging from many years to decades.

GASTRINOMA

MEN 1-associated gastrinomas make up 25%–50% of all gastrinomas, and 50% have metastases at presentation [16,19] (Table 41.13). MEN 1 gastrinomas are multiple and located in the duodenal wall in 90% of cases (Figures 41.10 and 41.11). Pancreatic gastrinomas are less common and more malignant than those in the duodenum.

Peptic ulcer disease and secretory diarrhea are the dominant clinical features. Hypersecretion of gastrin results in a profound increase in the output of acid, pepsin, and gastric juice (3–5 L of output in 24 hours), as well as acceleration of ductal bile flow. The net effect is severe, intractable peptic ulcer disease (often multiple and ectopic ulcers). Diarrhea is in part the result of hypersecretion of gastric acid and volume and increase in bile flow, whereas steatorrhea is due to lack of activation of pancreatic enzymes due to low pH. Secretory diarrhea can be caused independently by gastrin-induced stimulation of adenylate cyclase (Table 41.6).

The biochemical diagnosis is based on high basal acid output, exceeding 15 mEq/h, and a gastrin serum basal concentration of more than 150 pg/mL. Following secretin stimulation, a rise of more than 200 pg over the basal gastrin concentration is diagnostic. The ratio of basal to stimulated gastric output is approaching 1 because of constant maximal stimulation of parietal cells in the basal state due to autonomous hypersecretion.

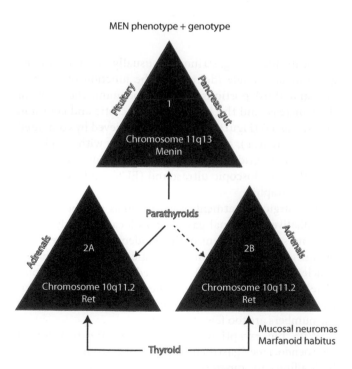

MEN phenotype + genotype

Figure 41.9 This triple triangle to display the multiple endocrine neoplasms can be classified as simplicity. The triple organ or system is limited to the major components of affected organs and systems. It ignores the "accessory" components, that is, the foregut carcinoids in MEN 1 and MEN 2, monocomponent familial medullary thyroid cancer, and Hirschsprung syndrome. The virtual absence of parathyroid hyperplasia in MEN 2B is unexplained.

Table 41.13 Clinical to molecular recognition

Sporadic	Solitary, in pancreas
Inherited	Multiple, in duodenal wall (MEN-1)
Symptoms	Flushing
	Hypotension
	Peptic ulcer, atypical
	Diarrhea, secretory
	Malabsorption
Biochemistry	High serum histamine
	High urinary methylimmidazole acetic acid
	Gastric acid >15 mEg/h
	Serum gastrin >150 pg/mL
	Secretin stimulation >200 pg over basal
Selective venous sampling	Percutaneous transhepatic catheterization to the hilus of the spleen. The segmental vein sampling is done sequentially every 3–4 cm until the hilus of the liver.
Anatomic localization	Helical computed tomography, magnetic resonant imaging, preoperative endoscopic and intraoperative ultrasound, are standard approaches
Molecular receptor based imaging	[111]Indium, [68]Gallium, and [99]Technicium radiotracers are coupled through chemical ligands, (tetra-aza-cyclo-dodecane tetra-acetic acid (DOTA), or diethylenetriamine penta-acetic acid (DTPA) to a somatostatin analogue. Scintigraphic detection is used for [111]Indium and [99]Technicium and PET detection for [68]Gallium. The current nuclear medicine has reached diagnostic accuracy up to 97% of neuroendocrine tumors.
Malignancy	About 60% of gastrinomas have metastases at presentation, in spite of small size of 1–2 cm

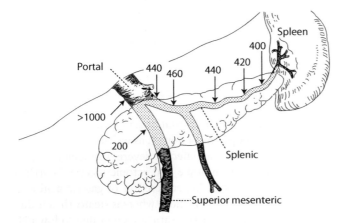

Gastrinoma: selective sampling of portal venous blood

Figure 41.10 Portal vein selective sampling. The percutaneous transhepatic access to the portal vein starts at the hilum of the spleen and ends at the liver hilum. The concentration of gastrin suddenly rises to more than threefold in comparison with the distant or peripheral vein. In the current era of noninvasive, highly sensitive and specific computed and magnetic tomography and resonance imaging, augmented by isotopic detection of subcentimeter neoplasms and recognition of function, portal vein sampling and segmental pancreatic arterial stimulation are approaching historical values.

Localization of gastrinomas, usually confined to the gastrinoma triangle (defined by the junction of the second and third portions of the duodenum, the body of the pancreas, and the junction of the cystic and common hepatic ducts) (Figure 41.11), can be achieved by computed tomography (CT), MRI, and scintigraphy with [111]indium-labeled octreotide scan, pentetriotide or lanreotide, ^{123}I-MIBG, endoscopic ultrasound (EUS), and intraoperative sonography.

The surgical treatment of gastrinomas may be curative or palliative. Duodenal gastrinomas located mostly in the first and second portions of the duodenum can be resected by transduodenal excision. Pancreatic tumors can be either enucleated (if <2 cm size) or treated with partial or complete resection of the pancreatic head and body. The experience with liver transplantation appears to be promising, but the numbers are too few at present.

With the exception of insulinomas, the majority of neuroendocrine gastroenteropancreatic tumors express high affinity to somatostatin receptors (subtypes 2 and 5). Therapeutic somatostatin receptor-based radiotherapy with indium-labeled octreotide analogs ^{68}Ga-DOTATOC and [90]yttrium has been disappointing. Complete remissions are rare (2%), and partial remission is 20%.

The 5-year survival is 20% with liver metastases, 30%–80% after liver resection, and 80% after liver transplantation.

Gastrinoma triangle

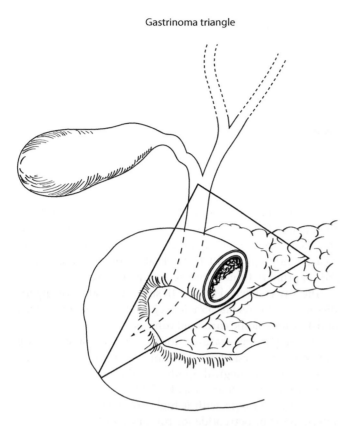

Figure 41.11 Anatomic predilection of gastrinoma. The predilection of gastrinoma to the head of the pancreas, distal duodenum, and mid-bile duct region was described by Passaro in 1991. In MEN 1, up to 50% of the affected have 90% of gastrinomas localized to the intramural wall of the duodenum and can be resected through the transduodenal approach.

INSULINOMA

About 20% of MEN 1 patients develop insulinoma, which is always located in the pancreas and is the second most common functioning tumor. Insulinomas may be single, multiple without predilection, or in the form of diffuse hyperplasia resembling nesidioblastosis [20,21]. Association with other functioning islet cell tumors, especially gastrinoma, is not infrequent. About 10% of insulinomas are malignant.

The autosomal dominant syndrome is caused by germline and somatic mutations of the gene encoding the protein menin, which is present in 80%–90% of the patients. The precise function of this protein is unknown. The gene is located in the long arm of chromosome 11q13. As mentioned before, complete simultaneous expression of the phenotype is seen in only 20% of the patients, and the remaining 80% display sequential development of the key clinical features, with intervals ranging from many years to decades.

Nesidioblastosis, unrelated to MEN 1, is seen mostly in the neonatal period and is associated with high mortality. The histologic features of nesidioblastosis in non-MEN premature infants are the absence of formed pancreatic islets and distribution of undifferentiated β cells in sheets along the ductules and ducts.

The symptoms are either from the effect of hypoglycemia on the brain (bizarre behavior to seizures) or due to release of catecholamines from the sympathoadrenal system, causing excess sweating and apprehension.

The biochemical diagnosis can be made by demonstrating hyperinsulinemia (>14 μU/mL) during fasting hypoglycemia (serum glucose of <50 mg). The ratio of fasting insulin to glucose must be in excess of 0.3. Elevated serum C-peptide (>1.9 ng/mL) and proinsulin in the hypoglycemic state permit differentiation from factitious hyperinsulinemia. Stimulation with intravenous tolbutamide induces the release of insulin by the tumor. Nonsuppression by exogenous insulin infusion implies autonomous hypersecretion.

Anatomic localization can be achieved by CT, MRI, preoperative endoscopic, and intraoperative US imaging. [111]Indium-labeled oct-reotide, or lanreotide, scan offers only a 50% diagnostic accuracy, but if positive, it verifies anatomic localization and function.

Exendin-4, an analog of GLP-1 that has abundant receptors in insulin-producing β cells, when linked to ^{111}In or ^{68}Ga increases enormously the diagnostic accuracy to more than 90%–97%.

More than 90% of insulinomas can be localized by noninvasive preoperative and intraoperative US imaging. The latter is essential to define the proximity anatomic relationship of the insulinoma to the pancreatic and biliary ducts, if the preoperative MRCP or EUS fail to provide this information.

Surgical treatment includes enucleation for peripheral small insulinomas, partial distal pancreatectomy, or pancreaticoduodenectomy. Subtotal pancreatectomy is used for multiple tumors or nesidioblastosis, usually in patients with MEN 1 syndrome. Liver resection or transplantation is justified for metastatic disease, if there are no extrahepatic metastases.

Palliative surgical cytoreduction (debulking) is justified. Octreotide, a powerful inhibitor of insulin secretion, is useful if the receptor-based isotopic imaging is positive. Receptor-based radiotherapy for unresectable or metastatic tumors has yielded very limited success.

CARCINOIDS

MEN 1-associated carcinoids are usually confined to the foregut and include bronchopulmonary, thymic, gastric, proximal duodenal, and pancreatic tumors. Hypersecretion of vasoactive amines and neuropeptides includes histamine, ACTH, substance P, neurotensin, prostaglandins, and kallikrein. The output of serotonin is low compared with that of midgut carcinoids, and elevated chromogranin A is found in 90%–100% of the patients. The incidence of malignancy is low (3%) with tumors smaller than 2 cm, and more than 30% in patients with tumors larger than 2 cm. Somatostatin receptors are present in more than 90% of the tumors.

Carcinoid tumors arise from gastroenteropancreatic and bronchopulmonary neuroendocrine cells. The hypersecretory states and histochemical characteristics vary according to anatomic location. Foregut carcinoids secrete mainly histamine and kallikrein, midgut tumors produce mainly serotonin, and hindgut carcinoids are usually hormonally inactive. Foregut carcinoids are commonly argyrophilic, whereas midgut carcinoids display mostly argentaffin staining and, less frequently, argyrophilic properties. The majority of bombesin-producing carcinoid tumors and those with "ectopic" secretion of neuropeptides like ACTH, parathormone, and VIP arise predominantly from the bronchopulmonary system.

About 70% of carcinoids originate in the gastrointestinal tract, and the remaining from the bronchopulmonary system, the thymus, and the ovary. Multiplicity is common in gastric, duodenal, and jejunoileal carcinoids. MEN 1 patients, not infrequently, have carcinoids coexisting with gastrinoma. Noncarcinoid neoplasms, mostly colon carcinoma, coexist with a frequency of 8%–17%.

Tryptamines from midgut carcinoids are normally cleared with one passage through the liver, by enzymatic degradation by monoamine oxidase. The *syndrome* is caused by functioning liver metastases or the release of amines and neuropeptides directly into the systemic circulation by bronchopulonary, thymic, or ovarian carcinoids.

Most carcinoids are discovered incidentally because of obstruction, bleeding, or routine physical examination and imaging for unrelated problems. Patients with bronchial carcinoids may present with coughing, hemoptysis, or infection. Gastrointestinal carcinoids may present with obstruction, bleeding, or intussusception. Other gastrointestinal tumors are discovered incidentally during endoscopy or other imaging for unrelated tumors.

Carcinoid syndrome occurs in about 10% of patients, mainly with jejunoileal carcinoids and liver metastases. The syndrome can be triggered by alcohol, aged cheese, coffee, and exercise and is manifested with flushing, hypotension, painful diarrhea, lacrimation, bronchial wheezing, and skin pigmentation.

The syndrome caused by bronchial and gastric carcinoids is characterized by severe atypical generalized flushing, bronchoconstriction, hypotension, lacrimation, and edema, mainly from release of histamine.

Pentagastrin stimulation results in release of serotonin and histamine not directly from the tumor, but through a flux of endogenous catecholamines. Pentagastrin is also used to test the adequacy of somatostatin receptor blockade when surgery or angioembolization is planned.

Adrenergic drugs to treat hypotension must never be used because carcinoid cells express receptors to catecholamines and cause excessive release of serotonin, histamine, and tachykinins.

The biochemical diagnosis can be made with assays of plasma serotonin and urinary 5-hydroxy-indolacetic acid (5-HIAA). Urinary excretion greater than 30 mg in 24 hours in the presence of malabsorbtion or higher than 15 mg in 24 hours in the absence of malabsorbtion establishes the diagnosis. Atypical carcinoid syndrome caused by excess histamine from bronchial and gastric carcinoids can be diagnosed by assays of serum histamine and urinary excretion of methyl-immidazole acetic acid (MeIm AA).

Classification of gastric carcinoids	
Type I	Small, multiple, located in the corpus and fundus
	Hypergastrinemia from chronic atrophic gastritis or pernicious anemia
	Hyperplasia of the EC-like cells
Type II	In MEN 1 patients often coexisting with gastrinoma
Type III	Sporadic tumor
	No hypergastrinemia

Carcinoid tumors can be localized with CT, MRI, EUS, PET, and octreotide scans with remarkable sensitivity and specificity. The combined use of conventional and receptor-based scintigraphy or PET scan leads to the identification of 95% of primary tumors and hepatic metastases.

The 5-year survival rates with surgery are 86% for appendiceal, 72% for rectal, 55% for jejunoileal, 49% for gastric, and 42% for colonic carcinoid tumors.

The important features for predicting outcome are tumor location and size, angiolymphatic invasion, hormone production, histological grade, and proliferative index. Streptozotocin, 5-fluorouracil (5-FU), and doxorubicin are used for tumors with a high proliferative index, and interferon-α or octreotide for tumors a with low proliferative index.

RARE NEUROENDOCRINE PANCREATIC NEOPLASMS

Glucagonoma

- A third common secretory neuroendocrine tumor.
- A large pancreatic tumor, highly (60%) malignant and 3% of pancreatic neuroendocrine tumors.
- There is a predilection to the distal pancreas. The signature symptom is the necrolytic erythema of the skin
- Cachexia, diabetes mellitus (>75%), and thromboembolism (30%). Other paraneoplastic symptoms are anorexia, anemia, ataxia, and dementia.
- The plasma glucagon is higher than 1000 pg/mL (normal is <150 pg/mL).

Somatostatinoma

- One-half of all functioning somatostatinomas are derived from the pancreas with predilection to the head; solitary and most are malignant (metastatic in 75%).
- Nonfunctioning somatostatinomas are found in the duodenum. Psammoma bodies are calcium deposits seen mostly in the papillary thyroid carcinoma.
- The majority of somatostatinomas present with mass effects like biliary obstruction and abdominal pain.
- The pancreatic secreting somatostatinoma causes 60% diabetes mellitus (suppressed insulin), 70%

cholelithiasis (CCK suppression), gall bladder stasis, 70% steatorrhea, and hypochlorhydria; malignant surgery, partial pancreatectomy, if resectable.

Glucagon-like peptide 1

- An incretin hormone produced in the proximal jejunum and increased 10- to 15-fold after gastric bypass for obesity or subtotal gastrectomy for ulcer or carcinoma (dumping syndrome).
- The hypersecretion of GLP-1 causes the syndrome of NIPHS through hyperstimulation of receptors in β cells.
- There is a similar mechanism in the dumping syndrome following subtotal gastrectomy and Billroth II gastrojejunostomy. The symptoms resemble the hypoglycemia following bariatric gastric bypass.

Pancreatic polypeptide tumors (PPomas)

PP tumors (PPomas) are generally silent, except for diarrhea in 1.3% of such patients with high levels of plasma PP. More common presentation when large enough to cause compression of adjacent organs. Anorexia and weight loss occur in 50%, but metastatic malignancy is exceedingly small.

Vasoactive intestinal peptide tumor (VIPoma)

(Verner–Morrison syndrome)

- One percent of pancreatic neuroendocrine tumors. Predilection to distal pancreas. Frequently malignant, large tumor.
- The signature of symptomatology is a constellation of secretory (watery) diarrhea, hypokalemia, and achlorhydria.
- The secretory diarrhea produces 3–5 L/day. The plasma VIP is very high, up to 1850 pg/mL (normal is <200 pg/mL).
- CT, MRI, scintigraphy with [111]Indium-labeled somatostatin analogs (octreotide, pentetriotide, or lanreotide) or [68]gallium-TOTATOC or TOTATATE/PET.
- Surgery is mostly distal pancreatectomy, if resectable. Octreotide for palliative treatment.
- *Nonfunctioning.* More common than functioning, multiple macro- and microadenomas, and malignant if larger than 3 cm. Elevated chromogranin A, PP, neuron-specific enolase, physostigmin, pancreastatin, and human chorionic gonadotropin α and β subunits.
- Localization with CT, MRI, [111]Indium-labeled scintigraphy with octreotide, pentetriotide, or lanreotide; ^{68}Ga-DOTATOC/DOTATE/PET has the highest sensitivity and specificity of 97%.

NONSURGICAL TREATMENT FOR ADVANCED OR METASTATIC NEUROENDOCRINE TUMORS

In the past, chemotherapy with streptozocin alone or in combination with doxorubicin was the only method approved for treatment of advanced disease. The benefit was very limited [22,23].

Recent discoveries of widespread expression of growth factor receptors (platelet-derived α and β stem cell, VEGEF-2, and VEGEF-3) in malignant pancreatic neuroendocrine tumors led to treatment with sunitinib malate. This agent inhibits these tyrosine kinases and delays tumor growth in animal models of pancreatic islet cell tumors and in phase 1, 2, and 3 clinical trials.

In a recent phase 3 trial, sunitinib improved progression-free survival, overall survival, and objective response in comparison with placebo among patients with advanced well-differentiated pancreatic neuroendocrine tumors. In a total of 171 patients, randomly assigned to treatment or placebo groups, the median progression-free survival was 11.4 months in the sunitinib group and 5.5 months in the placebo group (HR 0.42, $p < 0.001$). The objective response rate was 9.3% and 0% in the sunitinib and placebo groups, respectively. The death rate was 9 (10%) in the sunitinib group and 21 (25%) in the placebo group (HR 0.41, $p < 0.02$). The most frequent side effects of sunitinib were diarrhea, nausea, vomiting, weakness, and fatigue.

TRADITIONAL OPEN PANCREATECTOMY

1. Whipple pancreaticoduodenectomy
   Diagnostic laparoscopy is a routine precursor to pancreaticoduodenectomy to rule out metastases.
   The lower extremities should be included in the sterilization and draping for access of the deep femoral vein, if needed for an interposition to restore the portal venous flow.

Technical sequence

1. Whipple pancreaticoduodenectomy
   a. Bilateral subcostal or vertical incision.
   b. Mobilization of colonic hepatic flexure until the right kidney is exposed.
   c. Opening of the lesser peritoneal sac by dividing the gastrocolic omentum.
   d. Detachment of the transverse mesocolon from the anterior surface of the pancreas; ligation and division of the epiploic vessels near the origin from the right gastroepiploic artery.
   e. Mobilization of the duodenum (from the hepatoduodenal ligament containing the bile duct, hepatic artery, and portal vein) and the posterior surface of the pancreatic head until the vena cava, aorta, and superior mesenteric vessels crossing the third duodenal portion are exposed (Figure 41.12).

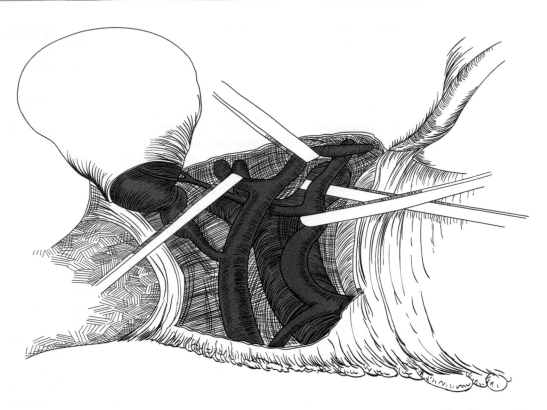

Figure 41.12 Mobilization and exposure of the pancreas surrounding organs and major vessels. The gastric branch of the gastroepiploic and right gastric arteries should be preserved, if pylorus preservation is planned. The hepatoduodenal ligament harboring the bile duct, hepatic artery, and portal vein is opened to expose and isolate each of the three structures. The gastroduodenal, a branch of the common hepatic artery, is seen in the lower part of the picture. The duodenal mobilization (Kocher maneuver) begins at the hepatoduodenal ligament until the superior mesenteric vessels are reached. The transverse mesocolon and splenic flexure are separated to expose the pancreas.

f. Separation of the transverse mesocolon from the inferior pancreatic margin using sharp dissection in this avascular plane.

g. Division of the lienocolic ligament. Avoid too much traction on the spleen.

h. The inferior mesenteric vein entering the splenic vein may have to be divided.

i. Creation of a plane between the pancreatic neck and the superior mesenteric and portal veins using a blunt gentle maneuver (even the fingernail must be manicured), pulling the pancreas upward to minimize the pressure on the vein (Figures 41.13 and 41.14). Never use sharp instruments.

j. Resection of one-third of the distal stomach, exposure of the common hepatic and hepatic artery proper, isolation, ligation, and division of the gastroduodenal artery. If aberrant right hepatic artery is known preoperatively, it usually originates from the superior mesenteric artery and runs behind the pancreatic head, posterior and right-lateral to the bile duct within the hepatoduodenal ligament.

k. Isolation and transection of the bile duct above the cystic–common hepatic duct junction. Separation of the gall bladder from the liver bed and inclusion into the resected specimen.

l. Transection of the proximal jejunum about 15 cm distal to the ligament of Treitz. The Treitz ligament and jejunal mesentery are divided close to the bowel to avoid injury to the superior mesenteric artery.

m. Transpose the proximal divided jejunum to the right behind the mesenteric vessels. The dissection between the uncinate process and the adjacent superior mesenteric and portal veins is the Achilles' heel. The venous tributaries and arterial branches from and to the pancreas are short and fragile, especially if surrounded by fibrosis.

2. Restoration of pancreaticobiliary and gastric continuity (Figure 41.14): Pancreaticojejunostomy end to side

a. The transected proximal jejunum is positioned into the supracolic, subhepatic space through the mesocolon.

b. The pancreatic stump is implanted into the side of the proximal jejunum, with or without duct-to-mucosa anastomosis, about 10–15 cm from the blind end.

c. The duct-to-mucosa anastomosis requires a greater than 5 mm calibre.

d. The entire pancreatic stump surface can be implanted into the seromuscular space and anchored with interrupted 2-0 silk or 2-0 polydioxanone suture (PDS).

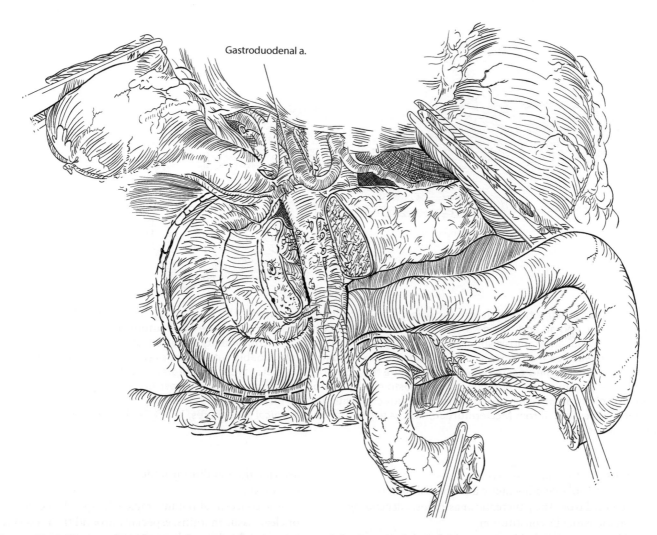

Gastroduodenal a.

Figure 41.13 Transection of stomach, gastroduodenal artery, bile duct, pancreatic neck, and proximal jejunum. The distal third of the stomach, the gastroduodenal artery, the bile duct above the junction of the cystic and hepatic ducts, and the proximal jejunum are transected. The gall bladder is included in the resected specimen. The transected jejunum and mesentery are transposed to the right behind the superior mesenteric vessels. The separation of the central pancreas from the superior mesenteric vessels, shown in the picture, is the last phase of decision making to proceed with curative operation. There are numerous small arteries from the superior mesenteric and tributaries to the mesenteric and portal veins. The uncinate process hidden behind the superior mesenteric vein and closely adjacent to the synonymous artery makes this difficult anatomy the Achilles' heel. (From McDermott Jr., W.V., *Atlas of Standard Surgical Procedures*, Lea & Febiger, Philadelphia, 1983. With permission.)

e. Without duct-to-mucosa anastomosis, the invagination of the pancreatic stump is also anchored with similar anchoring.

f. Expansion of the seromuscular plane created with injection of isotonic saline into the seromuscular space, cutting the serosa only and separating the muscle fibers for a distance of 5–6 cm.

g. The seromuscular plane can be expanded by injecting 3–4 mL of isotonic saline into the subserosal space until the tissue becomes visually edematous over a segment of 5–6 cm long at the antimesenteric side.

The expansion of the seromuscular plane facilitates cutting the serosa only and separating the muscle fibers until the submucosal layer is exposed.

The posterior suture line approximating the posterior pancreatic capsule to jejunal seromuscular should be done first, followed by duct-to-mucosa anastomosis, then the anterior suture line. The duct-to-mucosa anastomosis should be protected with an 8 mm polyethelene tube.

h. The opening of the submucosa–mucosa layer should be conforming to the caliber of the pancreatic duct.

i. Interrupted 5-0 Vicryl or Prolene is used to anastomose the duct to submucosa–mucosa of the jejunum. An 8 mm catheter is used to protect the anastomosis.

j. The anterior approximation of the pancreatic-to-jejunal seromuscular layer is similar to the posterior suture line.

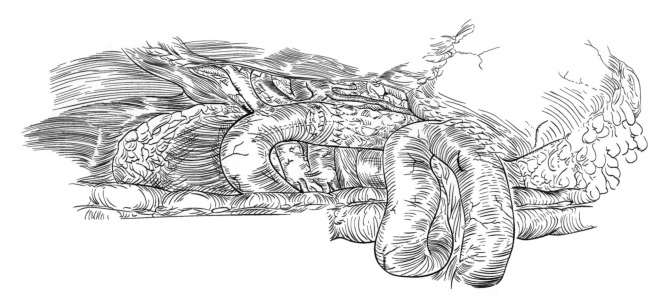

Figure 41.14 Reconstruction of pancreatic biliary and gastrojejunal continuity. The jejunum is placed retrocolic through the mesocolon, and an end-to-side anastomosis is performed with an interrupted one-layer suture line. The sutures for the pancreaticojejunal anastomosis should not be less than 0-2 silk or PDS, incorporating more capsule than parenchyma and more braided sutures than monolayer. For bilioenteric anastomosis, absorbable sutures are preferable. The antecolic end-to-side two-layer running gastrojejunostomy can be the Polya or Hofmeister type, with preferential hand-sewn technique. The pylorus-sparing end-to-side duodenojejunostomy requires preservation of the right gastroepiploic and right gastric arteries. The duodenojejunal anastomosis is constructed with a single interrupted 2-0 or 3-0 silk or PDS absorbable or unabsorbable suture. (From McDermott Jr., W.V., *Atlas of Standard Surgical Procedures*, Lea & Febiger, Philadelphia, 1983. With permission.)

3. Hepaticojejunostomy end to side
   a. The end-to-side bilioenteric anastomosis is constructed from the pancreatic anastomosis depending on the patient's constitution.
   b. Always use absorbable suture of 3-0 or 2-0 size depending on caliber and wall thickness of the bile duct.
   c. Use of a transanastomotic stent is personal or institutional idiosyncracy.
4. Gastrojejunostomy
   An end-to-side gastroenterostomy can be either a Polya or Hofmeister type, with either hand-sewn or stapling techniques. The gastroenterostomy should be placed in the antecolic position.
5. Pylorus-sparing pancreaticoduodenectomy
   The pylorus-saving modified Whipple procedure provides sparing of the entire stomach, but the slow gastric emptying in the early postoperative phase can be a problem.

   A segment of proximal duodenum, not less than 2 cm from the pylorus, and preservation of right gastroepiploic and right gastric arteries must exist to provide functional integrity.

   A single layer of interrupted nonabsorbable or PDS sutures are better to avoid a short and/or narrow duodenum.

   The prolonged gastroparesis in the early postoperative phase, and the small risk of instrumental arterial thrombosis of the right gastric or right gastroepiploic

arteries, did not diminish the acceptance by the surgical community.

   The concerns about incomplete lymphadenectomy or clear tissue margins, especially around the preserved proximal duodenum, have not influenced the long-term results of survival.
6. Central pancreatectomy and reconstruction (Figure 41.15a–c)
   The center of the pancreas is defined anatomically by the pancreatic neck (the thinnest portion) and the beginning of the pancreatic body, and on top of the superior mesenteric vessels. The central pancreatic segment can be easily separated from the superior mesenteric vessels by blunt finger dissection (Figure 41.13).

   Curative resection of the pancreatic centrum occupied by a tumor can be performed with at least 3 cm margins on each side and free of histologic involvement at the two transection surfaces.

   The reconstruction includes ligation of the transected duct at the pancreatic head and closure of the capsule with intermittent 2-0 silk or PDS. Creating a "fish mouth" during transection facilitates the approximation of the anterior and posterior capsular closure.

   The pancreaticoenteric continuity is achieved by end-to-side pancreaticojejunal anastomosis Roux-Y using interrupted 2-0 silk or PDS (braided, thick suture conforms to the soft consistency of the pancreatic parenchyma).

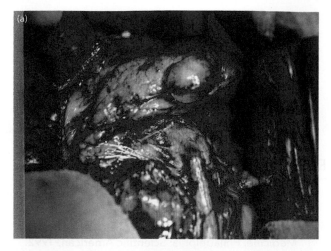

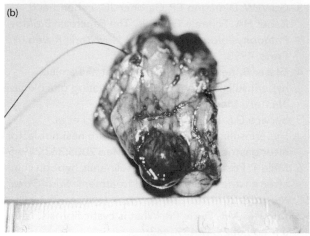

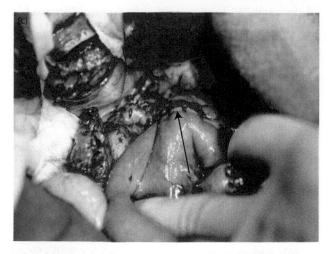

The duct-to-mucosa anastomosis is preferable if the diameter of the duct is suitable.

The central pancreatectomy offers the following advantages:

a. Preservation of 80%–90% of the pancreas and spleen
b. The Roux-Y reconstruction minimizes complications in comparison with pancreaticogastrostomy
c. In leaking of the Roux-Y pancreaticojejunal anastomosis, there is no activation of the proteolytic enzymes, since there is no presence of enterokinase, unless there is obstruction below the jejuno-jejunal anastomosis. Lipolytic enzymes are activated without enterokinase (Figures 41.14, 41.15a, b, c were used in the first edition of Endocrine Surgery).

7. Distal pancreatectomy—without splenectomy
Removal of a small benign tumor from the tail of the pancreas near the spleen can be performed with preservation of the splenic artery and vein.

The drawing should display the splenic artery and splenic vein with branches supplying and draining the tumor.

After ligation and division of the tumor vessels, the pancreatic stump is closed with interrupted sutures.

8. Distal pancreatectomy and splenectomy
Figure 41.16 shows a subtotal (85%) pancreatectomy and splenectomy after stenting the bile duct for protection and removal of the stent before closure.

The gastrocolic ligament (omentum) is divided to expose the lesser sac. The gastrosplenic ligament is divided up to the gastroesophageal junction. The short gastric vessels are ligated and cut. The splenic artery is isolated, ligated, and divided.

Figure 41.15 (a) Central pancreatectomy and reconstruction display a cystic neoplasm in the neck–body of the pancreas. **(b)** The resected specimen shows the adequacy of 3–4 cm margins on the proximal and distal transection with short and long suture markers for pathological orientation. **(c)** Closure of the pancreatic duct on the head side. End-to-side Roux-Y jejunostomy is constructed with or without duct-to-mucosa anastomosis. The posterior pancreatic capsule and full-thickness jejunum are reapproximated using interrupted 2-0 silk. A similar technic is used for the reapproximation of the anterior capsule to full-thickness jejunum. The distal pancreas and spleen are preserved.

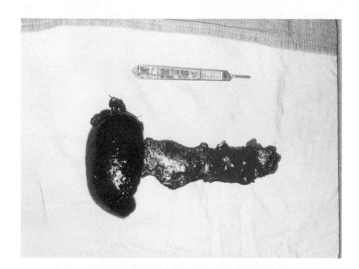

Figure 41.16 Distal pancreatectomy with splenectomy. Distal subtotal (85%) pancreatectomy and splenectomy after protection of the intrapancreatic bile duct with a stent, which is removed before closure. The entry for insertion of the stent through the distal bile duct is closed with a single suture.

The inferior margin of the pancreas is separated from the transverse mesocolon.

The lienocolic ligament is divided.

The spleen is lifted and retracted medially to expose the lienorenal ligament, which is divided with scissors.

The spleen is now suspended by the lienophrenic ligament, which is divided.

The distal pancreas is separated from the left kidney and adrenal until the transection site is placed between the right superior mesenteric vessels and the intrapancreatic bile duct. The splenic vein is ligated and divided.

9. Enucleation (Figure 41.17a and b)

Enucleation in any part of the pancreas, as long as it avoids the pancreatic or bile ducts, is feasible. A tumor size of less than 2 cm can be enucleated, especially located in the subcapsular space.

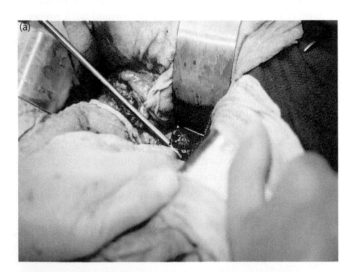

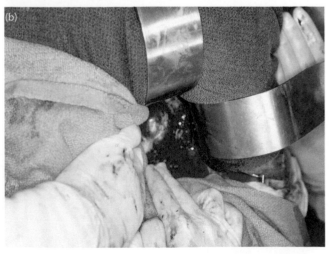

Figure 41.17 Enucleation. (a) and (b) display enucleation of small (<2 cm) gastrinoma and insulinoma near the pancreatic body. The desmoplastic reaction by the tumor facilitates the separation of the tumor from the pancreatic parenchyma. A drain is indispensable. Enucleating a tumor from the pancreatic head preserves the anatomic and functional integrity, and the morbidity of pancreaticoduodenectomy.

The neoplastic desmoplastic reaction facilitates enucleation with minimal bleeding.

Enucleation in the head of the pancreas requires greater attention to enucleation because of the morbidity of Whipple pancreaticoduodenectomy and the likely proximity to the pancreatic or bile ducts.

Drainage of the area of enucleation is mandatory to avoid leaking pancreatic enzymes causing fat necrosis.

REFERENCES

1. Simmons RL, Steed DL, eds. *Basic Science Review for Surgeons*. Philadelphia: WB Saunders, 1992.
2. Leder P, Clayton DA, Rubenstein E, eds. *Molecular Medicine*. Philadelphia: Scientific American, 1992.
3. Go VLW, Dimagno EP, Gardner JD, Lebenthal E, Reber HA, Scheele GA, eds. *The Pancreas: Biology, Pathophysiology and Disease*. New York: Raven Press, 1993.
4. Glaser B, Kesavan P, Heyman M et al. Familial hyperinsulinism caused by an activating glucokinase. *N Engl J Med* 1998;338:226–36.
5. Service GJ, Thompson GB, Service FJ et al. Hyperinsulinemic hypoglycemia with nesidioblastosis after gastric bypass. *N Engl J Med* 2005;353:249–54.
6. Mala T. Postprandial hyperinsulinemic hypoglycemia after gastric bypass surgical treatment. *Surg Obes Relat Dis* 2014;10:1220–5.
7. Knowles MR, Durie PR. What is cystic fibrosis. *N Engl J Med* 2002;347:439–442.
8. Braasch JW, Tompkins RK, eds. *Surgical Disease of the Biliary Tract and Pancreas*. St. Louis, MO: Mosby, 1994.
9. Weber BD, ed. *Molecular Endocrinology*. New York: Raven Press, 1995.
10. Solcia E, Rindi G, Capella C. In: Felpe M, Lake BD, eds., *Histochemistry in Pathology*. 2nd ed. Edinburgh: Churchill-Livingstone, 1990;397–409.
11. Schonhoff SE, Giel-Maloney M, Leiter AB. Minireview: Development and differentiation of gut endocrine cells. *Endocrinology* 2004;145:2639–44.
12. Lejonklu MH, Edfeldt K, Johansson TA, Stalberg P, Skogsteid B. Neurogenin 3 and neurogenic differentiation 1 are retained in the cytoplasm of multiple endocrine neoplasia type 1 islet and pancreatic endocrine tumor cells. *Pancreas* 2009;38:259–66.
13. Proye CAG, Farrell SG. Multiple endocrine neoplasia and other familial endocrine tumor syndromes. In: Schwartz AE, Pertsemlidis D, Gagner M, eds., *Endocrine Surgery*. New York: Marcel Decker, 1993:583–612.
14. Shepherd JJ. The natural history of multiple endocrine neoplasia type 1. Highly uncommon or highly unrecognized. *Arch Surg* 1991;126:935–52.
15. Burgess JR, Greenway TM, Shepherd JJ. Expression of the MEN-1 gene in a large kindred with multiple endocrine neoplasia type 1. *J Int Med* 1998;243:465–70.

16. Sizemore GW. Multiple endocrine neoplasia In: *Principles and Practice of Endocrinology and Metabolism*. Philadelphia: Lippincott Williams & Wilkins, 2001:1696–706.

17. Gagel RF, Tashjian AH Jr, Cummings T et al. The clinical outcome of prospective screening for multiple endocrine neoplasia type 2A. An 18-year experience. *N Engl J Med* 1988;318:478–84.

18. Kimura W, Tezuka K, Hizai I. Surgical management of pancreatic neuroendocrine tumors. *Surg Today* 2011;41:1332–43.

19. Norton JA, Frakel DL, Alexander HR et al. Surgery to cure the Zollinger-Ellison syndrome. *N Engl J Med* 1999;341:635–44.

20. Cases AI, Ohtsuka T, Fujino M et al. Expression of glucagon-like peptide 1 receptor and its effects on biologic behavior in pancreatic tumors. *Pancreas* 2014;43:1–6.

21. Eriksson D, Velikyan I, Selvaraju RK et al. Detection of metastatic insulinoma by positron emission tomography with ^{68}Ga-exendin-4: A case report. *J Clin Endocrinol Metab* 2014;99:1519–24.

22. Oeberg K. Chemotherapy and biotherapy in the treatment of neuroendocrine tumors. *Ann Oncol* 2001;12(Suppl 2):s111–4.

23. Raymond E, Dahan L, Raoul JL et al. Sunitinib malate for the treatment of pancreatic neuroendocrine tumors. *N Engl J Med* 2011;364:501–13.

42

Laparoscopic management of pancreatic islet cell tumors

MICHEL GAGNER

INTRODUCTION

Laparoscopy was first used for visual examination of the pancreas in 1911; this was revisited in 1972 where again examination of the pancreas using laparoscopy was suggested [1,2]. The advents of laparoscopic ultrasonography [3–5], along with improvement of surgeons' technical capabilities, have established a new chapter in the diagnosis, staging, and management of unresectable pancreatic carcinoma [6–8]. This approach was, however, slow to gain acceptance for resection of malignant pancreatic lesions due to the high morbidity and mortality in operating on this retroperitoneal structure. I set a new milestone in pancreatic surgery in 1992 for laparoscopic distal pancreatectomy [73], and a year later, in 1993, for laparoscopic Whipple [9], when the surgical field was challenged and led to explore unbroken territories. I performed, more specifically, a complete laparoscopic pylorus-preserving pancreatoduodenectomy for a patient with chronic pancreatitis localized in the head of the pancreas with pancreas divisum. Although technically feasible, the laparoscopic Whipple procedure did not improve the postoperative outcome or shorten the postoperative recovery period at that time, with limited staplers, early hand-sewn techniques, and limited energy sources. It appears that instrumentation improvements of the last decade have permitted us to see

a gain in laparoscopic pancreatiduodenectomy, provided that no complications occur. Attention was then drawn to more benign lesions, including laparoscopic distal pancreatectomy with splenectomy for chronic pancreatitis [10], and laparoscopic resections of islet cell tumors by enucleation or spleen-preserving distal pancreatectomy [11]. Laparoscopic pancreatic surgery began to gain acceptance and popularity [12] in the mid-1990s. It has been proved to lessen the stress response of individuals needing pancreatic resection [69]. Laparoscopic distal pancreatectomy or enucleation was felt to be technically feasible and safe, and seemed to benefit patients by shortening their hospital stay with no recurrence of disease [11,13–15,70,71,81,82,95]. Hand-assisted techniques and robotic assistance in small numbers were also attempted with success [16,17,81]. There is growing worldwide interest in performing laparoscopic enucleation or distal pancreatectomy for islet cell tumors [18–34,71].

INDICATIONS FOR ISLET CELL TUMOR REMOVAL

Insulinoma is by far the most common islet cell tumor. More than 90% of these are benign, often solitary, and distributed about a third each in the head, body, and tail of the pancreas. They measure <1 cm in about 40% and

<2 cm in 90% of cases. *In situ*, the lesion usually appears darker in color than the surrounding pancreas and is frequently found to have a network of small vessels around it. Patients can present with a spectrum of neurological, cardiovascular, and gastrointestinal symptoms due to hypoglycemia and catecholamine release. The classic finding is the Whipple triad, whereby the patient experiences (1) hypoglycemia during fasting or exertion, (2) blood sugar of <45 mg/dL at the time of symptoms, and (3) symptoms ameliorated by oral or intravenous glucose. Diagnostic studies include an elevated serum insulin level (normal is <10 μU/mL or more), an insulin-to-glucose ratio of >1.0, and a C-peptide suppression test. Provocative tests may be necessary in equivocal studies with high clinical suspicion. These include the intravenous tolbutamide test (80% sensitivity), intramuscular glucagon test (70% sensitive), oral glucose tolerance test (60% sensitive), and intravenous calcium infusion test. Preoperative localization studies remain controversial, as intraoperative ultrasound (US) has 75%–90% sensitivity. Depending on localization, surgical management should be enucleation or distal pancreatectomy with or without splenectomy [35].

Glucagonoma derives from alpha-cells and is usually found in patients over 50 years of age. Patients may present with the classic necrolytic migratory erythema whereby there is migratory scaling rash with intense puritus, usually in the groin and lower extremities. The plasma glucagon level can exceed 1000 pg/mL. The lesion tends to be large (>4 cm), malignant, and found within the body and tail of the pancreas. About 70% of patients are found to have liver metastasis at the time of diagnosis [36]. Other pancreatic endocrine lesions are rare, tend to be large, and have a higher malignant potential, i.e., gastrinomas. These lesions may be better approached via a standard laparotomy.

PREOPERATIVE CONSIDERATIONS

Patients undergo standard preoperative workup, including conventional blood tests, chest radiograph, electrocardiogram, and computed tomography (CT) scan. Preoperative endoscopic ultrasound (EUS) is performed in most cases. In anticipation of possible splenectomy, triple vaccination against *Streptococcus pneumonia*, *Haemophilus influenzae*, and *Neisseria meningitidis* is routinely administered. A modern state-of-the art operating room is equally important and must be equipped with high-flow insufflators, xenon light sources, and a digital mixer that permits switching from the laparoscopic view to laparoscopic ultrasonography, or has them on the same screen in a split mode (Figure 42.1).

SURGICAL TECHNIQUE

The patient is under general anaesthesia and should have large intravenous access for aggressive resuscitation; an arterial line may also facilitate hormone monitoring during the procedure. The patient is positioned in a supine, split-leg fashion with anchoring supports at both feet. Foam wedges should be placed under the left flank to elevate the retroperitoneal structures. In some cases, a steeper right-sided decubitus with the left side up about 45° is necessary. In fact, the degree of patient rotation is variable and primarily determined by surgeon preference, similar to the variation of patient position for laparoscopic splenectomy. However, patients are generally positioned with more rotation of the left side upwards for a distal pancreatectomy compared with an enucleation procedure. A Foley catheter, bilateral venous compressions, and an orogastric tube should be in place prior to final positioning. The surgeon stands between the patient's legs, with the scrub nurse to the patient's left side and the first assistant to the patient's right. Two video monitors, placed above each of the patient's shoulders, are usually used (Figure 42.1). The initial 10 mm port should be placed at supraumbilicus and pneumoperitoneum established to 15 mmHg. A state-of-the-art three-chip or digital camera coupled with a 30° angle scope is used (Figures 42.2 and 42.3); a general inspection of the abdomen should be performed to eliminate metastasis, especially on the liver surface. A total of five trocars are generally required, although the precise number and size of trocars may vary depending on the patient's body habitus, the surgeon's comfort, and the size of the available instruments. In order to use an endoscopic linear stapler and perform laparoscopic ultrasonography, a 12 mm port is necessary. This port should be placed on the left side at the midclavicular line, just below the level of the umbilicus, to facilitate smooth insertion of the stapler across the pancreas and thorough scanning with the ultrasonographic probe. The remaining cannulas are usually 5 mm ports for Maryland dissector (Figure 42.4), curved scissors (Figure 42.5), and retracting instruments.

Exposure and mobilization of the pancreas

With the patient in slight reverse Trendelenburg, the stomach is grasped and the gastrocolic ligament and distal inferior short gastric vessels lateral to the gastroepiploic artery are divided (Figure 42.6). The splenic flexure of the colon is also mobilized. These can be performed using the ultrasonic dissector, bipolar cautery (Ligasure, Valleylab, Boulder, Colorado), or simple diathermy and clips. Once access to the lesser sac is achieved, the posterior peritoneum is then incised along the inferior and superior borders of the body and tail of the pancreas using both sharp and blunt techniques. A high-definition linear array laparoscopic US probe is then inserted via the 12 mm port (Figure 42.7). A systematic approach in localizing the lesion is essential. Most surgeons prefer a 6.5–7.5 MHz frequency to scan the ventral and dorsal surfaces of the head, body, and tail of the pancreas, searching for the lesion, which should appear hypoechoic (Figure 42.8). Its spatial relationship to surrounding structures, such as pancreatic duct, splenic vessels, portal vein, superior mesenteric vessels, and spleen, should be noted.

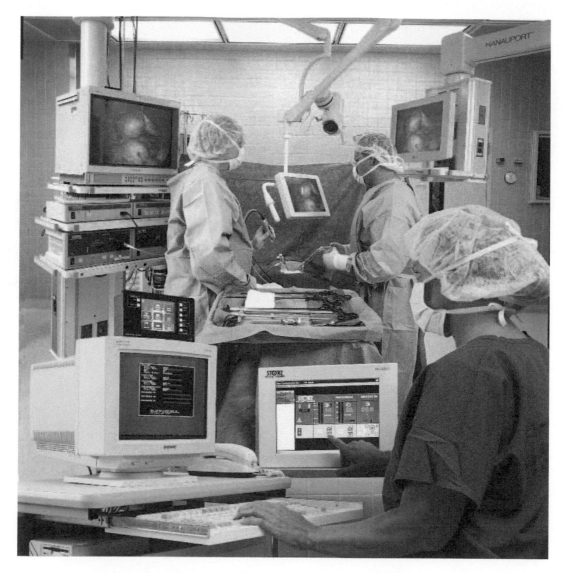

Figure 42.1 Minimally invasive surgery operating room. Suspended flat screens and booms for insufflators, light sources, and digital video systems are part of the new ergonomic environment. (Courtesy of Karl Storz Endoscopy.)

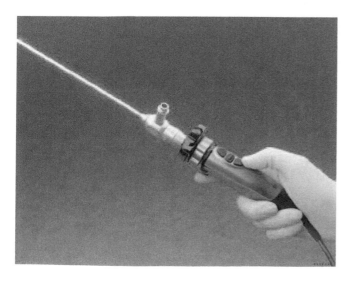

Figure 42.2 Digital camera mounted with a 5 mm laparoscope. (Courtesy of Karl Storz Endoscopy.)

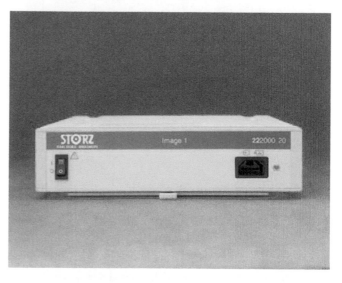

Figure 42.3 Digital camera ampificator. (Courtesy of Karl Storz Endoscopy.)

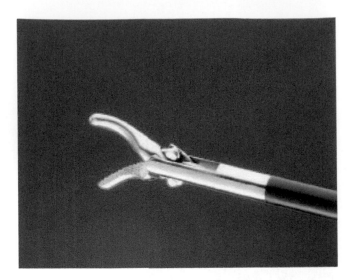

Figure 42.4 A laparoscopic curve dissector. (Courtesy of Karl Storz Endoscopy.)

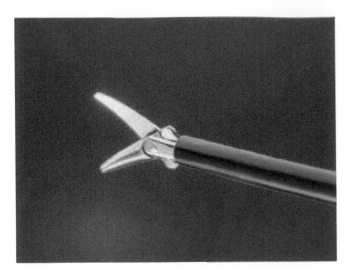

Figure 42.5 A laparoscopic curved scissor. (Courtesy of Karl Storz Endoscopy.)

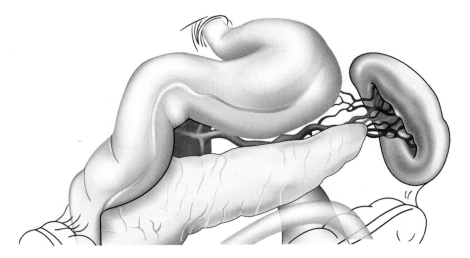

Figure 42.6 Exposure of the lesser sac content by opening the gastrocolic ligament.

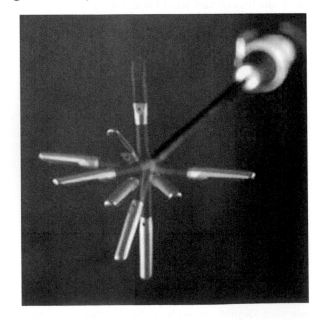

Figure 42.7 Laparoscopic probe.

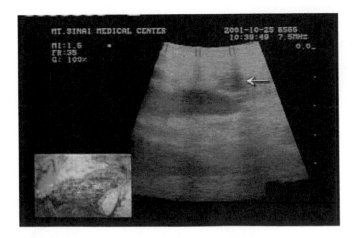

Figure 42.8 Laparoscopic ultrasonography on the anterior body of the pancreas, looking for an islet cell tumor. Note the split image of the laparoscope and of the laparoscopic ultrasonography.

Laparoscopic distal pancreatectomy with splenectomy

The splenic vessels are divided at the planned line of pancreatic transection, using either clips or endoscopic staplers (2.0 or 2.5 mm in height and 45 mm in length; Medtronic, Norwalk, Connecticut). The pancreas and splenic vein are usually divided as a single unit with an endoscopic stapler, and the vein stump doubly secured with clips, if possible. The pancreas is then mobilized from the body to the tail, in retrograde fashion (Figure 42.9). For resection of lesions in the tail of the pancreas, an alternative approach is sometimes taken, in which the spleen and pancreas are mobilized prior to division of the splenic vessels and the pancreas. Attachments of the spleen are divided, and the posterior spleen and tail of the pancreas are mobilized from the retroperitoneum, dissecting from lateral to medial, in an antegrade direction along the pancreas (Figure 42.10). After transecting the pancreas, the proximal stump is inspected for hemostasis and to ensure closure of the main pancreatic duct. If a patent duct is visualized, it is suture ligated intracorporeally, using a fine, nonabsorbable monofilament suture. Oversewing the proximal stump with a fine, nonabsorbable monofilament running suture may improve hemostasis and decrease leakage. The technique of buttressing an endoscopic mechanical stapler with strips of bovine pericardium has been shown to have preliminary success in resection of pulmonary bullous areas [37,38]. Applying a similar technique to pancreatic transection may decrease postoperative leak. Specimens are removed from the abdomen using sturdy, nonporous laparoscopic retrieval bags to prevent tissue spillage. When the opening of the retrieval bag is pulled out above the abdominal wall, ring forceps are used to morcellate the spleen while preventing intra-abdominal spillage. The umbilical trocar site is enlarged to 2.0–2.5 cm for removal of the pancreatic specimen. The abdomen is reinsufflated to check for hemostasis and a closed suction drain placed near the pancreas. Trocar sites greater than 5 mm diameter are closed. Splenectomy may be indicated when the lesion is at the very tip of the pancreas or when preservation of splenic vessels is not feasible. At times when the vein is densely adhered to the dorsal surface of the pancreas, it may be more feasible to divide it as a single unit with an endoscopic vascular stapler.

Laparoscopic distal pancreatectomy with splenic preservation

Following the laparoscopic exposure of the pancreas described above, the inferior border of the pancreas is dissected from the retroperitoneal fat until the splenic vein is reached posteriorly and superiorly. The tail of the pancreas is then gently grasped with 5 mm atraumatic forceps and retracted anteriorly and inferiorly to expose the transverse branches of the splenic artery and vein. These vessels are divided with the ultrasonic shears or 5 mm titanium clips until the desired length of pancreas is achieved. The entire pancreatic tail and body are mobilized, up to the portal vein, if necessary. The pancreas is transected with an endoscopic linear stapler (Figure 42.11). Occasionally, it is transected with ultrasonic shears (Ethicon EndoSurgery, Cincinnati, Ohio) or a bipolar device (Ligasure) to decrease blood loss.

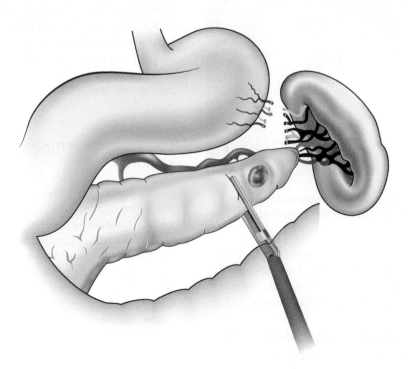

Figure 42.9 Laparoscopic distal pancreatectomy; the linear stapler divides and closes the pancreatic parenchyma.

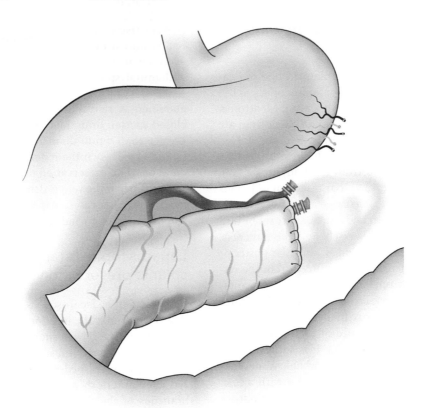

Figure 42.10 Laparoscopic distal pancreatectomy with en bloc splenectomy.

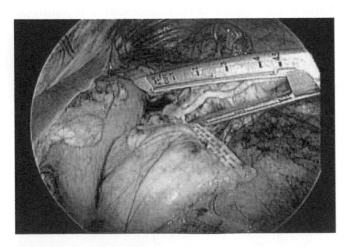

Figure 42.11 Laparoscopic distal pancreatectomy with splenic preservation; stapler across the pancreas.

The specimen is extracted in a rigid plastic bag through a minimally enlarged umbilical incision. Laparoscopic distal pancreatectomy with or without splenectomy should be performed when enucleation is not feasible or indicated.

Laparoscopic distal pancreatectomy with splenic vessels and spleen preservation

The spleen-preserving techniques are particularly indicated for patients with benign diseases, since lymphadenectomy

is expected to be insufficient for curative intent in malignancies [39]. Dissecting and clipping the superior edge of the pancreas from the vessels emerging from the splenic vein and artery is the most commonly performed splenic preservation technique (Figures 42.12 through 42.15). This technique requires a longer operative time and laparoscopic surgical expertise, and unfortunately, vascular damage when performing this procedure might occur due to the delicate maneuvers necessary in the upper margin of the pancreas.

Laparoscopic enucleation of islet cell tumors

Laparoscopic enucleation should be performed on lesions felt to be benign and technically extirpable due to their surface location or their physical distance away from vital (Figure 42.10). Laparoscopic intraoperative ultrasonography (LIOUS) is routinely used to confirm the location and relationship to the pancreatic duct and peripancreatic vessels. Once the islet cell tumor is localized, the dissection is carried out between the tumor and the normal parenchyma using an electrocautery hook or ultrasonic coagulating shears (Figures 42.16 and 42.17). Since insulinomas tend to have a vascular network, it is useful to dissect them with an electrocautery hook or ultrasonic device in one hand, while retracting and exposing with a suction tip in the other. A margin of normal parenchymal tissue should be included.

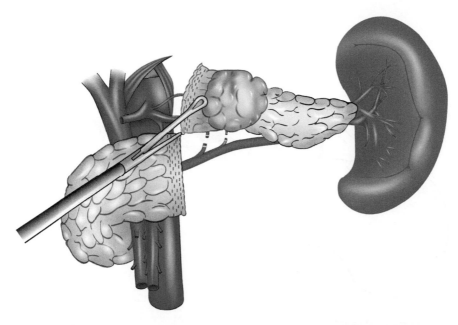

Figure 42.12 Laparoscopic distal pancreatectomy with spleen and splenic vessels preservation.

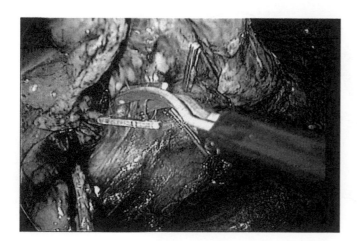

Figure 42.13 Endoshears dividing small pancreatic vessel branches.

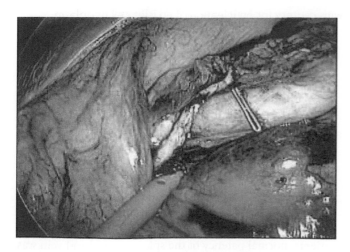

Figure 42.14 Titanium clips on arterial branch.

The pancreatic vessels feeding the tumor are ligated with medium to large titanium clips. Once the tumor is completely enucleated, it is extracted in a small sterile bag through the 12 mm port (Figure 42.18). A closed suction drain is placed in the lesser sac at the enucleation site. Depending on the depth of the defect and general appearance of the surrounding tissue, the enucleated crater may be filled with fibrin glue, although its efficacy in decreasing postoperative leak has not been determined (Figure 42.19) [40,41]. Preoperative imaging studies are required for localization, and the combined use of biphasic helical CT and EUS seems to be cost-effective. The use of laparoscopic US is an integral part of the laparoscopic procedure, and the information achieved is valuable for both confirming localization and making decisions concerning the most appropriate surgical procedure. If enucleation is not possible, for distal lesions, in cases of distal pancreatectomy, splenic salvage, preferably with preservation of splenic vessels, is feasible, albeit more demanding, and can be achieved in most cases [74].

Hand-assisted laparoscopic pancreatectomy

Conventional laparoscopy has been proved to be difficult in cases involving large tumors, massive intraoperative bleeding, dense adhesions, malignant diseases [43], and obesity [42]. Hand-assisted laparoscopic surgery may have an advantage in these groups of patients [43]. This technique basically involves the assistance of the surgeon's nondominant hand while still performing a laparoscopic procedure. It can be used either as the initial or as an intermediary step in cases in which the surgeon faces technical difficulties [34]. Although only a few such cases have been reported, the advantages described include the possibility of using the

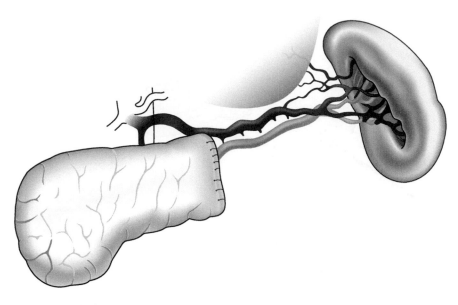

Figure 42.15 Splenic vessel branch dissection.

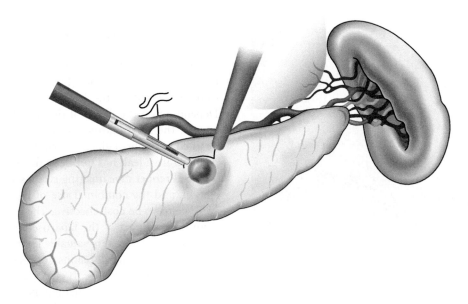

Figure 42.16 Demonstration on the use of a laparoscopic hook with cautery for enucleation of an islet cell neoplasm.

assistance of the hand for dissection (to palpate and identify tissues) [42,44], mobilizing large organs [44], having access to the instruments [42], protecting the wound during the extraction of malignant specimens [42], shortening the operative time required, and utilizing the fingers to rapidly stop unexpected bleeding.

Splenic Warshaw-preserving techniques

According to Fernandez-Cruz et al. from Barcelona [72], the intent-to-treat basis splenic vein preservation was achieved in only 54.5% of patients. In the remainder, conversion to the Warshaw technique (where the spleen is no longer irrigated by the main splenic vessels) was required for intraoperative

bleeding. Evaluation of intraoperative factors showed that the mean operative time was significantly shorter (165 vs. 222 minutes) and the mean blood loss significantly lower (225 vs. 495 mL) in the group with the Warshaw technique. But in my honest opinion, this may result in localized perisplenic vessel hypertension, with splenic complications, like infarct, abscesses, or localized infection [72]. What about the patency of the vein over time? A study to evaluate the short- and long-term patency of preserved splenic vessels after laparoscopic spleen-preserving distal pancreatectomy was undertaken, assessed by abdominal CT, and classified into three grades according to the degree of stenosis. Of 22 patients, normal patency of the splenic artery and vein was observed in 16 and 5 patients, respectively, within 1 month

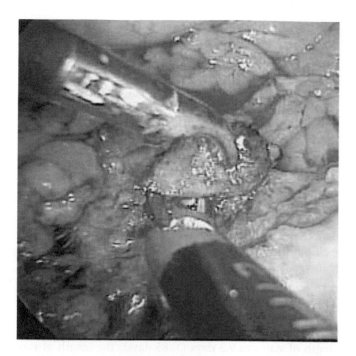

Figure 42.17 Enucleation using ultrasonic shears.

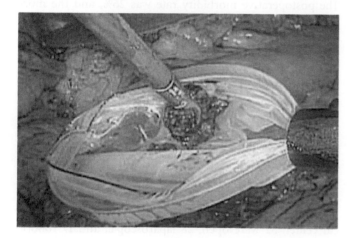

Figure 42.18 Extraction using an impermeable bag.

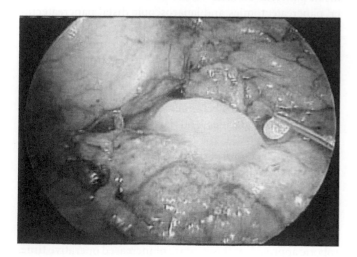

Figure 42.19 Application of fibrin glue to the enucleation site—a preventive method to avoid a pancreatic fistula.

of surgery, and in 19 and 9 patients 6 months or more after operation. Nine of 10 patients with complete splenic vein occlusion developed a collateral circulation in the late postoperative phase. Splenic perfusion was well preserved in all patients. Therefore, in the long term, there is a risk of left-sided portal hypertension if the splenic vein becomes occluded after surgery [83].

Laparoscopic pancreatoduodenectomy

The laparoscopic technique for a Whipple procedure is a modification of Longmire–Traverso pylorus-preserving pancreatoduodenectomy. The patient is placed in a supine position with the legs abducted. With an umbilical trocar, a 30 degrees scope is inserted to examine the peritoneal cavity, liver, stomach, and mesentery vessels. Then four to six more trocars are inserted under direct vision in the epigastrium and upper quadrants. The peritoneum covering the common bile duct (CBD) is opened anteriorly and laterally, and is then dissected free posteromedially from the portal vein and the right hepatic artery. The CBD is then transected at least 2 cm above the cystic duct junction using a stapler. The first portion of the duodenum is then divided 2 cm distal to the pylorus. After dissection of the gastrocolic ligament is completed, gastroepiploic vessels are double-clipped with titanium clips or suture ligated with intracorporeal techniques. Using a right-angled dissector under the pylorus, a window is created that allows passage of a stapler. Similarly, the duodenojejunal junction is transected as close to the proximal jejunum as possible, with the sample stapler to the right of the mesenteric vessels. The proximal jejunum retracts in the retroperitoneum and is freed at the ligament of Treitz. After transection, the gastroduodenal artery is exposed as the antrum of the stomach is pushed toward the left upper quadrant. The artery is dissected from the pancreatic neck and more so superiorly near its origin. The pancreas above the mesenteric vein and the portal vein is then transected using harmonic shears. The uncinate process is resected from the mesenteric vessels by using the ultrasonic dissector. The resected specimen is then inserted into a bag and left in the lower quadrant of the abdomen for later extraction. At this time, three anastomoses need to be created, and a good two-handed technique with fast intracorporeal knot tying is necessary. The proximal jejunal loop is prepared for this task by further mobilizing the Treitz ligament. The loop is passed and advanced behind the mesenteric vessels through the ligament of Treitz. The pancreas to jejunum anastomosis is created first because of its need for precision and delicate sutures, and it is easier to perform with the free jejunal loop. The anastomosis is created in two layers: an outer layer with interrupted 3-0 silk and an inner layer with 4-0 absorbable monofilament sutures placed with an small half curved needle, taking the duct to the antimesenteric side of the jejunum through the whole wall. Then four to six interrupted sutures are positioned beginning posteriorly. The hepaticojejunostomy is created in a similar fashion with intracorporeal sutures starting posteriorly, using 6–10 sutures. The distance between each anastomosis is 10 cm. The pylorojejunostomy is created using a 3-0 absorbable monofilament suture. The gall bladder can be removed after the sutures are placed. The specimen is extracted through the umbilical trocar. Drains are positioned below and above the anastomosis and passed through the trocar sites in the right subcostal and right paramedian areas.

In earlier Dulucq series, the hospital stay was 13.6 days after the Whipple procedure, and he believed that pancreatoduodenectomy should be performed only in selected cases and by a highly skilled laparoscopic surgeon. If there is any doubt, an open resection should be performed [75].

Laparoscopic central pancreatectomy

Once a decision is made to do a central pancreatectomy, as opposed to a distal pancreatectomy, the central segment is resected in a splenic vessel-preserving technique. The proximal pancreatic duct is ligated with added sutures on the staple line, or direct sutures if a harmonic scalpel was used in thick pancreas, for transection. The distal part is drained to the jejunum or posterior stomach. The pancreas-to-jejunum anastomosis is created with a Roux or in continuity using a free jejunal loop. The anastomosis is created in two layers: an outer layer with interrupted 3-0 silk and an inner layer with 4-0 absorbable monofilament sutures placed with an SH curved needle, taking the duct to the antimesenteric side of the jejunum through the whole wall. Then, four to six interrupted sutures are positioned beginning posteriorly. A similar technique is used with the posterior gastric wall. Drains are positioned posteriorly.

DiNorcia et al. report 11 laparoscopic central pancreatectomies from a large series of >100 cases. They note that there has been a significant increase in minimally invasive and parenchyma-sparing techniques for pancreatic neuroendocrine tumors. This shift did not increase morbidity or compromise survival. In addition, minimally invasive and parenchyma-sparing operations yielded shorter hospital stays [87]. Out of 200 cases, 4 were central pancreatectomies, performed laparoscopically with a robotically assisted approach using a camera holder [99]. This year, the largest series of such cases studied 14 patients who underwent laparoscopic central pancreatectomy over a 10-year period. The mean age of patients was 49 years. The mean operative time was 239.7 minutes, and the mean blood loss was 153.2 mL. It appears feasible and safe [101].

Preoperative tattooing of lesions may facilitate localization during the surgery and expedite intraoperative localization, which sometimes can be difficult and time-consuming. In a recent study, of 36 consecutive patients who had a laparoscopic distal pancreatectomy, 10 underwent preoperative tattooing via an endoscopic transgastric technique using US guidance, using 2–4 cc of sterile purified carbon particles injected immediately proximal and anterior to the pancreatic lesion. These tattoos were easily visible upon entering the lesser sac in all patients at laparoscopy. Patients with a tattoo had a shorter operative time (median 128.5 minutes, range 53–180) than patients without a tattoo (median 180 minutes, range 120–240, $p < 0.01$). None of the tattoo group required repeat surgery, whereas one patient who was not tattooed required reresection for a lesion missed in the initial specimen. There were no complications associated with the EUS-guided tattoo [86].

Robotic-assisted surgery

There have been many enthusiastic centers using robotic surgery, especially for reconstruction after pancreatoduodenectomy. The Department of Surgery from the University of Illinois in Chicago has been particularly vocal. During a 10-year period, 134 patients underwent robotic-assisted surgery for different pancreatic pathologies using the da Vinci robotic system (Intuitive, Sunnyvale, California). The mean operating room time was 331 minutes (75–660 minutes). There were 14 conversions to open surgery. The mean length of stay was 9.3 days (3–85 days). The length of stay for patients with no complications was 7.9 days (3–15 days). The postoperative morbidity rate was 26%, and the mortality rate was 2.23% (three patients). Among the procedures performed were 60 pancreaticoduodenectomies, 23 spleen-preserving distal pancreatectomies, 23 splenopancreatectomies, 3 middle pancreatectomies, 1 total pancreatectomy, and 3 enucleations. This largest series of robotic pancreatic surgery concludes that it enables difficult technical maneuvers during pancreatic minimally invasive surgery. Although the results demonstrate that it is feasible, its safety remains to be shown, as specific complications may be due to the robot itself, like infections due to a prolonged operating time and break in sterility [84]. Cost-effectiveness is the number one problem of this technology. Of 77 distal pancreatectomies performed at a single academic medical center, 32 were open, 28 laparoscopic, and 17 robotic assisted. Spleen preservation occurred in 65% of robotic distal pancreatectomies versus 12% and 29% in open distal pancreatectomies and laparoscopic distal pancreatectomies ($p < 0.05$). The operative time averaged 298 minutes in robotic distal pancreatectomies versus 245 and 222 minutes in open distal pancreatectomies and laparoscopic distal pancreatectomies ($p < 0.05$). Blood loss and morbidity were similar with no mortality. The length of stay was 4 days in robotic distal pancreatectomies versus 8 and 6 days in open distal pancreatectomies and laparoscopic distal pancreatectomies ($p < 0.05$). The total cost was $10,588 in robotic distal pancreatectomies versus $16,059 and $12,986 in open distal pancreatectomies and laparoscopic distal pancreatectomies. These data suggest direct hospital costs are comparable among all groups. They suggest a shorter length of stay in robotic versus laparoscopic or open approaches. Finally, spleen and vessel preservation rates may improve with a robotic approach at the expense of increased operative time. However, it did not include the cost and maintenance of the robot, which is quite substantial, and I do not agree with the authors that it is cost-effective [88]. In a recent systematic review, a total of 251 patients undergoing robot-assisted pancreatic surgery were analyzed. The weighted mean operation time was 404 ± 102 minutes (510 ± 107 minutes for pancreatoduodenectomy only). The rate of conversion was 11.0% (16.4% for pancreatoduodenectomy only). Overall morbidity was 30.7% ($n = 77$), most frequently involving pancreatic fistulas ($n = 46$). Mortality was 1.6%. Negative surgical margins were obtained in 92.9% of patients. The rate of spleen preservation in distal pancreatectomy was 87.1%. It seemed to be safe and feasible in selected patients and, in left-sided resections, may increase the rate of spleen preservation, but randomized studies should be done in order to conclude on the benefits for those patients, including costs [97].

Single-port and NOTES techniques

As far as single-port surgery, it has been described for pancreatectomy. Isolated reports and small series are starting to appear in the literature; however, due to the complexity, and need for localization with ultrasonography, it may not be suitable for many cases. A small transumbilical incision can be made for small benign lesions such as cysts [94]. Perhaps transvaginal extractions of specimens could be added in hybrid procedures. However, in seven cases subjected to this extraction, only two were possible [98]. Further, the robot and natural orifice translumenal endoscopic surgery (NOTES) technique could be combined, as experimented with in the use of a minimally invasive cardiac surgery (MICS) robot for transrectal distal pancreas exploration and resection in two nonsurvival porcine models. Future indications may include transgastric NOTES approaches, endoluminal procedures, and single-port applications [100].

Postoperative care

Nasogastric tubes are removed intraoperatively in all patients. Clear fluids are routinely begun on the evening of surgery. Patients are advanced to a regular diet after they pass flatus. Fluid from the closed suction drain is routinely sent for amylase-level determination, and is removed when it contains only serous fluid and the amylase level is approximately equal to the serum level. Drains can be managed as an outpatient and should not preclude discharge from the hospital. Antibiotics are not necessary in the postoperative period, and transfusions are usually avoided unless an extreme anemia is seen (in favor of iron treatment). With enhanced recovery protocols, antiemetics are used in the first 24 hours, and narcotics are changed to nonsteroidal anti-inflammatory medications. When thromboprophylaxis is administered, its duration is unknown; however, due to a higher rate of splenic vein thrombosis, a minimum of 7 days of low-molecular-weight heparin is usually administered, once the risk of bleeding is nil.

Complications

The incidence of bleeding in pancreatic open resections reported by Halloran et al. in 2002 was found to be 4.8% [45]. Factors like dense adhesions between the pancreas and the vessels (e.g., chronic pancreatitis) [46,11] increase the incidence of intraoperative hemorrhage. To prevent bleeding, ligature of the splenic artery as close as possible to its origin might reduce the risk of major bleeding and could also be used as an attempt to reduce the size of the spleen [47], facilitating the subsequent steps of the operation. Hemorrhage is a threatening complication that can also occur postoperatively and manifest itself as a serosanguineous fluid coming out from the drain or, if severe, with hemodynamic instability. Reoperation is the rule for the latter group of patients, while conservative management can be achieved for the former one. Pancreatic fistula is a notorious complication of distal pancreatectomies and enucleations, showing a higher incidence among the latter group of patients. Fistulization is the most common complication reported in laparoscopic series (17.9%) and seems to be higher than those reported in open series (10.4% [45] and 5% [48]). More specifically, we have seen them more often after enucleation, but the clinical course is benign in most instances [74]. The symptoms of this complication will primarily depend on the fistula output, varying from small peripancreatic collections up to high-output fistulas, requiring total parenteral nutrition (TPN), somatostatin analogs, or even reoperation. Distal pancreatectomies for chronic pancreatitis usually carry a lower incidence of pancreatic fistula or leak due to the firm consistency of the gland [34], as opposed to a normal, soft pancreas. There is consensus about leaving a drain near the pancreatic stump, which helps manage a pancreatic fistula and prevents pancreatic ascites. The utilization of somatostatin analogs (Sandostatin, Novartis AG, Basel, Switzerland) has been proposed to prevent fistulas or accelerate their closure. This proposed attempt to reduce the complication has not been confirmed to be effective; multiple trials had different outcomes [45]. If a fistula happens to occur, its management does not differ from the standard treatments. In general, external pancreatic fistulas are managed conservatively with continuous aspiration from the drain, clinical surveillance, octreotide, and enteral or even TPN, as most (>80%) fistulas have a successful outcome and close nonoperatively [49]. Reoperation might be required in those cases that do not respond to conservative medical management [49]. Fortunately, based on the literature, these kinds of fistulas rarely occur after a laparoscopic resection. Occasionally, a fistula will manifest itself as a fluid collection near the pancreatic stump or enucleated area. These collections are best treated percutaneously due to lowered morbidity and mortality rates [50], instead of by reoperation. The success rate for percutaneous drainage in postoperative pancreatic infected collections was reported by Cinat et al. to be 75% [51]. Abdominal pain, fever, and leukocytosis are the most common presenting symptoms. In these cases, surgery must be strongly considered when a second percutaneous attempt has failed [51]. Splenic abscesses often follow splenic-preserving procedures for spleen salvage. In his original description, Warshaw had one splenic abscess out of 22 patients, which occurred after 8 weeks. Splenomegaly might be a contraindication for this procedure, since these kinds of spleens require a greater vascular supply and short gastric vessels alone might be insufficient. Splenic abscesses will present with abdominal pain and fever, Tc99 sulfur colloid spleen scan will show abnormal uptakes, and CT scan will reveal sufficient or insufficient blood flow [52]. Depending on each particular case, either drainage [53] or splenectomy [54] might be performed to treat these patients. Infarction of the spleen can follow a pancreatic resection and happens only after splenic-preserving procedures, but could also appear after conventional spleen-sparing distal pancreatectomy. We recommend looking at the spleen before finishing the procedure and evaluating the need for splenectomy if major ischemia exists, since it can lead to abscess formation or severe postoperative pain. In Gagner's series, one patient presented with ischemic spleen after a spleen-sparing distal pancreatectomy, which necessitated removal [34]. In the Mount Sinai Series, indications for laparoscopic pancreatic resection included cystic lesions (10 patients), neuroendocrine tumors (7), chronic pancreatitis (1), and schwannoma (1). Pathological diagnoses of the cystic lesions are cystadenocarcinoma (1 patient), serous cystadenoma (2), mucinous cystadenoma (5), ductal papillary hyperplasia (1), lymphoid cyst (1), and congenital cyst (1]. An unsuspected small pancreatic adenocarcinoma was discovered in the distal pancreatectomy specimen for chronic pancreatitis. Of the neuroendocrine tumors, four were insulinomas and three were nonfunctioning islet cell tumors [34] (Table 42.1). The median operating time was

Table 42.1 Types of tumor removed by laparoscopic distal pancreatectomy, Mount Sinai series

Tumor type	No.
Chronic pancreatitis	8
Pancreatic adenocarcinoma	3 (1)
Neuroendocrine tumors	59
Insulinoma	49 (6)
Nonfunctioning tumor	6 (3)
Gastrinoma	2
VIPoma	1
Functioning tumor in MEN-1	1
Cystic pancreatic lesion	58
Mucinous cystadenoma	34 (5)
Serous cystadenoma	18 (2)
Cystadenocarcinoma	2 (1)
Ductal papillary hyperplasia	2 (1)
Lymphoid cyst	1 (1)
Congenital cyst	1 (1)
Schwannoma	1
Nesidioblastoma	1

Table 42.2 Intraoperative data and types of technique

Variables	Literature	Mount Sinai experience
Mean operative time[a]	3.7 h	4.1 h
Range	1.7–6.6 h	1.6–6.6 h
Median blood loss	300 mL	200 mL
Range[b]	100–733 mL	20–4000 mL
Type of resection[c]		
Distal pancreatectomy with splenectomy	57 (43.8%)	13 (59%)
Distal pancreatectomy with spleen preservation	46 (35.4%)	4 (18%)
Enucleation	27 (20.8%)	5 (18%)
Technique[d]		
Completed laparoscopically	123 (86.6%)	20 (90.9%)[e]
Converted to laparotomy	19 (13.3%)	2 (9%)

[a] Literature total 137 patients.
[b] Literature range is the mean range of series.
[c] Literature total 125 patients.
[d] Literature total 128 patients.
[e] One patient converted to hand-assisted.

4.4 hours (range 1.6–6.6). Median blood loss was 200 mL (range 20–4000). Four patients (21%) received blood transfusions during the hospital stay. Distal pancreatectomy with splenectomy was performed in 12 patients (63%). Spleen-preserving procedures were planned preoperatively in 4 of 15 patients (27%) undergoing distal pancreatectomy. Three of four spleens (75%) were successfully preserved, and one was removed because it appeared ischemic following completion of the pancreatic resection. Five patients (18%) underwent laparoscopic enucleation of islet cell tumors (Table 42.2). Sixteen of 19 (84%) pancreatic resections were completed laparoscopically. One distal pancreatectomy adhered to the splenic vein and artery. Two patients (11%) were converted from a laparoscopic (5%) to a hand-assisted technique, because in the first a densely adherent cystic mass precluded safe mobilization without bleeding, and in the second for suspicion of malignancy in a patient with a 6 cm solid tumor on CT scan in which splenic hilar invasion was discovered at laparoscopy. Cystadenocarcinoma of the pancreatic tail was confirmed pathologically. The major morbidity rate was 16%, and the minor morbidity rate was 10%, for a total morbidity of 26%. There were two minor postoperative complications: superficial phlebitis and prolonged ileus. Pancreatic fistulas developed postoperatively in three patients (16%): one patient who had an enucleation (25%), one patient who underwent distal pancreatectomy with splenectomy (8%), and one patient after spleen-preserving distal pancreatectomy (33%). Two of the patients with fistulas had the longest hospital stays of 18 and 26 days, respectively. The third patient had an initial hospital stay of 5 days and was readmitted to hospital several days later. All three patients were treated with CT-guided percutaneous drainage of a peripancreatic collection and TPN. They were discharged home on TPN until the fistula closed. There were no late postoperative complications and no deaths within 30 days of surgery. The median length of postoperative hospital stay was 6 days (range 1–26 days). In patients who had an uncomplicated course, the mean length of stay was 5 days, whereas patients with complications had a mean length of stay of 12 days, although this difference was not statistically significant.

Discussion and review of the literature

Since pancreatectomy is similar to adrenalectomy in that a relatively large incision is required to remove a small lesion, the potential benefits of the minimal access approach are substantial. The operative and postoperative results of laparoscopic pancreatic resection appear to be acceptable. Operative times of just more than 4 hours are identical to those of open pancreatectomy series [48]. Patients generally have minimal postoperative pain, a very short-lasting ileus, and a quick return to normal activity. An average of 7 days' postoperative hospital stay compares favorably with the 10–15 days reported in open series [48,55]. The total morbidity of 26% may appear high, but it is actually at the low end of the range of morbidities reported in other open and laparoscopic series (20%–60%) (Tables 42.3 and 42.4) [15,48,55,56]. The 16%–18% pancreatic fistula rate in the Mount Sinai series may also seem high, but the denominator is small. Broughan et al. reported a low fistula rate (6%) in a relatively large series of 84 patients with an open resection (Table 42.5) [57]. The laparoscopic procedures may have a complication rate of 31%, similar to recent series of open pancreatic procedures (33%) [48,55,57]. Only 29 patients (20%) had a major complication following the

laparoscopic procedures, and these complications were mostly due to a pancreatic leak (86%) (Table 42.6). The leak rate (mean 17.9%, range 0%–33%) seems higher when compared with the same open series (mean 7.2%, range 5%–23%). An appropriate control of fistulas and peripancreatic collections was always possible with CT-guided percutaneous drainage. Only in two cases did the pancreatic leak lead to reoperation. In addition, the pancreatic leak rate was higher in the enucleation patients than in the distal pancreatectomy patients. In addition, there were nine patients (11%) with intra-abdominal infections in that series, which are usually associated with pancreatic leaks; therefore, the true pancreatic leak rate is probably underestimated. Thus, the rate of postoperative pancreatic fistula formation in the Mount Sinai series is comparable to that in the open series. It is interesting that all three of the pancreatic leaks presented as peripancreatic collections, despite the presence of a functioning closed-suction drain in each patient. One could speculate that this phenomenon is due to decreased adhesion formation after laparoscopic versus open surgery, and therefore an increased risk of fluid collection formation if a pancreatic leak occurs. The consistency of the pancreatic parenchyma has previously been shown to correlate with the pancreatic fistula rate after distal pancreatectomy [58,59]. The firm pancreas, as seen in chronic pancreatitis, is associated with a lower fistula or leak rate than the normal, soft pancreas. The large open series reported by Lillemoe et al. had only a 5% incidence of fistula formation, but 24% of their patients were in the low-risk group with chronic pancreatitis. In the Mount Sinai series, only 1 of 19 patients (5%) had chronic pancreatitis, and thus our fistula rate is expected to be higher than the 5% incidence

Table 42.3 Laparoscopic pancreatic series: Postoperative results

First author, year	No.	Morbidity (%)	Minor complication (%)	Major complication (%)	Leak (%)	Mortality after 30 days (%)	Hospital stay (days)	References
Gagner, 2003	22	31.5	13.5	18	18	0	7	[34]
Fernandez-Cruz, 2002	18	27.7	0	27.7	27.7	0	5	[61]
Melotti, 2000	25	32.4	13.6	18.8	18.1	0	9	[62]
Fabre, 2002	13	38	23	15	15	0	7	[63]
Ferraina, 2002	5	20	0	20	20	0	5.3	[64]
Shinchi, 2001	2	0	0	0	0	0	7	[43]
Lo, 2000	3	33	0	33	33	0	NR	[27]
Mahon, 2002	3	0	0	0	0	0	4.7	[65]
Berends, 2000	10	50	20	30	20	0	7	[26]
Salky, 1996	7	28	28	0	0	0	4	[13]
Vezakis, 1999	6	33	0	33	33	0	34.5	[25]
Park, 1999	5	20	0	20	20	NR	5	[22]
Chapuis, 1998	5	20	8	31	8	0	4.7	[66]
Cuschieri, 1996	5	40	20	20	20	0	12	[12]
Total	142	31.6	10.8	20	17.9	0 (n = 137)	7.4 (n = 139)	

Table 42.4 Laparoscopic distal pancreatectomy and enucleation series: Peri-operative data

First author, year	No.	Operation time (h)	Enucleation	Distal pancreatectomy	Pancreatectomy "spleen preserving"	Conversion (%)	References
Gagner, 2003	22	4.1	5	17	4	13.5	[34]
Fernandez-Cruz, 2002	18	4.5	4	14	10	11.1	[61]
Melotti, 2000	25	2.8	3	22	17	0	[62]
Fabre, 2002	13	4.7	0	11	10	15.4	[63]
Ferraina, 2002	5	3.2	2	3	3	0	[64]
Shinchi, 2001	2	6.6	0	2	0	NR	[43]
Lo, 2000	3	NR	1	1	1	33	[27]
Mahon, 2002	3	1.7	0	3	2	0	[65]
Berends, 2000	10	3	5	1	NR	40	[26]
Salky, 1996	7	3.7	—	—	—	—	[13]
Vezakis, 1999	6	5.0	0	6	5	33	[25]
Park, 1999	5	5,0	0	5	NR	NR	[22]
Chapuis, 1998	5	2.4	3	2	—	20	[66]
Gagner, 1997	13	4	4	9	—	30.7	[15]
Cuschieri, 1996	5	4.5	0	5	5	0	[12]
Total	142	1.7–6.6 (range)	27	103	57	14.8[a] (n = 128)	

[a] The conversion rate of 142 patients is 13.3.

Table 42.5 Open distal pancreatectomy series: Postoperative results

First author, year	No.	Operation time (h)	Morbidity (%)	Minor complication (%)	Major complication (%)	Leak (%)	Mortality after 30 days (%)	Hospital stay (days)	References
Lillemoe, 1999	235	4.3	31	NR	31	5	0,9	10	[48]
Benoist, 1999	40	NR	63	5	58	23	0	15	[55]
Broughan, 1986	84	—	24	—	24	6	3.6	—	[57]
Total	359	4.3 (n = 235)	32.9 (n = 359)	5 (n = 40)	32.3 (n = 359)	7.2 (n = 359)	1.4 (n = 359)	10.7 (n = 275)	

in Lillemoe et al.'s study [48]. Pancreatic lesions requiring resection should be carefully evaluated and selected for a laparoscopic approach. Laparoscopic distal pancreatectomy for adenocarcinoma of the pancreatic tail is controversial. Unfortunately, patients with these lesions rarely present with curable disease. Laparoscopic resection for islet cell neoplasms and cystic lesions is feasible, but it is not widely performed. Insulinomas are ideal lesions for laparoscopic resection, as they are usually single and benign. Proven principles of open pancreatic surgery must be adhered to in laparoscopic resection, and insulinomas close to the pancreatic duct should be resected rather than enucleated. In retrospect, this was probably the case in our patient who developed a pancreatic fistula after enucleation of a 1.5 cm insulinoma from the neck of the pancreas. Laparoscopic pancreaticoduodenal resection (palliative) was successfully attempted for a malignant islet cell tumor invading the duodenal lumen and causing bleeding by Gagner in 1997, while he was at the Cleveland Clinic, during a live surgery for the American Hepato-Pancreato-Biliary Association (AHPBA). First performed in 1993 [9], laparoscopic pancreaticoduodenectomy remains in question because of the technical difficulty and the prolonged operating time, which may outweigh the potential benefits of the minimal access approach [60]. In the series of 10 patients, the operative time required to perform a laparoscopic Whipple procedure averaged 8.5 hours, the rate of conversion to laparotomy was 40%, and the mean hospital stay was 22.3 days [15]. Huscher from San Giovanni Hospital in Rome has recently revisited this procedure and may have better results due to improved instrumentation than was available 10 years ago. This will need to be confirmed by multiple teams and compared with open surgery.

The first multi-institutional series published concerned 25 European centers with 127 cases. Final diagnoses included benign pancreatic diseases in 111 patients (with 22 benign insulinomas) and malignant pancreatic diseases (of which three were insulinomas and five neuroendocrine

Table 42.6 Reported complications following a laparoscopic distal pancreatectomy

First author (Ref.)	No. cases	Surgery	Complication	Treatment
Cuschieri [10]	5	5 DP + S	1 pancreatic fistula	Resolved spontaneously
Gagner [11]	7	3 E	1 major bleeding (splenic vein)[a]	Multiple titanium clips
		4 DP	Small infected collection[a]	Percutaneous drainage
Vezakis [25]	4	4 DP	2 pancreatic fistula	Percutaneous drainage and PN
Ueno [67]	1	1 DP	Small splenic infarct (1 month)	Resolved spontaneously
Cuschieri [42]	4	2 HADP + S	1 intraop. bleeding	Conversion
		1 HACG	—	—
		1 HACJ	—	—
Patterson [34]	17	10 DP + S	1 intra-op bleeding	Conversion
			1 pancreatic fistula	CT-guided percutaneous drainage and PN
		3 DP	1 pancreatic fistula	
		4 E	1 pancreatic fistula	
Fabre [63]	13	13 DP	2 intraop bleeding from splenic vein	Conversion (1 splenectomy)
			1 pancreatic fistula	Conservative
			2 liquid cysts	
			1 bleeding from trocar	Reoperation
Fernandez-Cruz [54]	11	5 DP	Perforated duodenal ulcer	Reoperation
		2 LIGD	—	—
		4 TCG	—	—
Park [22]	28	9 CGLSA	1 myocardial infarction	Death
			1 necrotizing pancreatitis	Multiple (open) debridement
		5 MLIGCG	—	—
		11 TCG	2 postop bleeding	Transfusion
		3 LCJ	—	—
	23	21 DP	2 intraop bleeding	Transfusion
			1 pancreatic fistula	Percutaneous drainage
		2 HADP	1 wound infection	NR
Gramatica [68]	9	4 E	1 pancreatic fistula	Resolved spontaneously
		4 DP	1 pleural effusion	
		1 DP + S	1 fluid collection	
Mahon [65]	3	2 DP	Urinary retention	Catheterization
		1 DP + S		
Fernandez-Cruz [61]	16	4 E	2 pancreatic fistula	Drainage
		12 DP	3 pancreatic fistula	Drainage
			1 splenic abscess	Splenectomy
			1 intraop bleeding	Controlled w/stapler

Note: DP: Distal pancreatectomy; S: splenectomy; CGLSA: cyst gastrostomy by the lesser sac approach; MLIGCG: mini-laparoscopic intragastric cyst gastrostomy; TCG: transgastric cyst gastrostomy; LCJ: laparoscopic cyst jejunostomy; HADP: hand-assisted distal pancreatectomy; HACG: hand-assisted cyst gastrostomy; HACJ: hand-assisted cyst jejunostomy; E: enucleation; NR: nonreferred; PN: parenteral nutrition; LIGD: lsaparoscopic intragastric drainage.

[a] Surgery not specified.

neoplasms) in 16 patients (13%). Five patients with presumed benign pancreatic disease had malignancy at final pathology. The median tumor size was 30 mm (range 5–120 mm); 89% of tumors were located in the left pancreas. Laparoscopically successful procedures included 21 enucleations, 24 distal splenopancreatectomies, 58 distal pancreatectomies with splenic preservation, and 3 pancreatoduodenal resections. The overall conversion rate was 14%. There were no postoperative deaths. The rate of overall postoperative pancreatic-related complications was 31%, including a 17% rate of clinical pancreatic fistula. In laparoscopically successful operations, the median postoperative hospital stay was 7 days (range 3–67 days). During a median follow-up of 15 months (range 3–47 months), 23% of the patients with pancreatic malignancies had tumor recurrence [76]. A similar experience was recorded from the Spanish registry, where a total of 132 patients with lesions in the left pancreas were included, of which 42 neuroendocrine tumors were operated on laparoscopically. The conversion rate was 9.7%, and enucleation was performed only in patients with insulinoma. The most frequent technique was spleen-preserving distal pancreatectomy. There were no postoperative deaths. The overall rate of postoperative pancreatic-related complications was 16% [77].

Comparison between laparoscopic and open distal pancreatectomy started to appear in the mid-2000s, including in South Korea. Over a decade, 31 patients underwent laparoscopic distal pancreatectomy and 167 patients underwent open distal pancreatectomy at Seoul National University Hospital and Bundang Seoul National University Hospital. A case-control design was used with 2:1 matching to compare laparoscopic surgery with open surgery. There were no significant differences in operation time, rate of intraoperative transfusions, complications, recurrence, or mortality between the two groups. Laparoscopic distal pancreatectomy was associated with a statistically significant shorter hospital stay (11.5 days vs. 13.5 days, $p = 0.049$), but with more expensive hospital charges, than open distal pancreatectomy ($p < 0.01$) [78]. The Americans did a similar review from eight centers encompassing cases between 2002 and 2006. Of 667 pancreatectomies, 159 (24%) were attempted laparoscopically and 46% were for solid lesions. Positive margins occurred in 8% cases, and overall, 50% had complications, with significant leaks in 16%. Conversion to open pancreatectomy occurred in 20 (13%) of the laparoscopic group. In the matched comparison, there were no differences in positive margin rates (8% vs. 7%, $p = 0.8$), operative times (216 vs. 230 minutes, $p = 0.3$), or leak rates (18% vs. 11%, $p = 0.1$). But patients who had a laparoscopic resection had lower average blood loss (357 vs. 588 mL, $p < 0.01$), fewer complications (40% vs. 57%, $p < 0.01$), and shorter hospital stays (5.9 vs. 9.0 days, $p < 0.01$) [80]. Although not randomized, this confirms the superiority of the laparoscopic approach. In another series with a total of 360 patients, 95 laparoscopic were attempted and 71 were completed laparoscopically, with a 25.3% conversion rate. Compared to open surgery, the laparoscopic approach to distal pancreatectomy had similar rates of splenic preservation, pancreatic fistula, and mortality. Laparoscopy had lower blood loss (150 vs. 900 mL, $p < 0.01$), smaller tumor size (2.5 vs. 3.6 cm, $p < 0.01$), shorter length of resected pancreas (7.7 vs. 10.0 cm, $p < 0.01$), and fewer complications (28.2% vs. 43.8%, $p = 0.02$), as well as shorter hospital stays (5 vs. 6 days, $p < 0.01$) [85]. The Mayo Clinic experience of patients undergoing laparoscopic distal pancreatectomy ($n = 100$) matched them by age, pathologic diagnosis, and pancreatic specimen length to a cohort undergoing open pancreatectomy ($n = 100$). Tumor size was greater in the open group (mean 4.0 vs. 3.3 cm, $p = 0.02$). The laparoscopic group demonstrated decreased blood loss (mean 171 vs. 519 mL, $p < 0.001$) and shorter duration of hospital stay (mean 6.1 vs. 8.6 days, $p < 0.001$). There were no differences in operative time (mean 214 vs. 208 minutes, $p = 0.50$), pancreatic leak rate (17% vs. 17%, $p > 0.99$), overall 30-day morbidity (34% vs. 29%, $p = 0.45$), and 30-day

mortality (3% vs. 1%, $p = 0.62$) [89]. Finally, a recent meta-analysis on the subject encompassing 10 studies with 349 patients undergoing minimally invasive pancreatectomy and 380 patients undergoing open resection was considered suitable. The patients in the two groups were similar with respect to age, body mass index (BMI), American Society of Anesthesiology (ASA) classification, and indication for surgery. The rate of conversion from full laparoscopy to hand-assisted procedure was 37%, and that from minimally invasive to open procedure was 11%. Patients undergoing laparoscopic surgery had less blood loss, a shorter time to oral intake, and a shorter postoperative hospital stay. The mortality and reoperative rates did not differ between minimally invasive distal pancreatectomy (MIDP) and open distal pancreatectomy (ODP). The laparoscopic approach had fewer overall complications (odds ratio [OR] 0.49, 95% confidence interval [CI] 0.27–0.89), major complications (OR 0.57, 95% CI 0.34–0.96), surgical site infections (OR 0.32, 95% CI 0.19–0.53), and pancreatic fistulas (OR 0.68, 95% CI 0.47–0.98) [90]. In a longer follow-up study (53 months), the incidence of exocrine insufficiency and incisional hernias was significantly higher after open resections (both $p = 0.05$). After hospital discharge, median time to resume full-time work was 6 weeks in the open group and 3 weeks after laparoscopic resections ($p < 0.0001$). Laparoscopy also resulted as an independent factor for an early return to full-time activities in the multivariate analysis ($p < 0.0001$) [92]. It appears that some preoperative factors may favor one approach over the other. Patients with a BMI of ≤27, without adenocarcinoma, and with a pancreatic specimen length of ≤8.5 cm had significantly higher rates of significant fistulas after open than after laparoscopic pancreatic resection [93]. The largest analysis to date is from *HPB (Oxford)*, with 15 comparative studies that recruited 1456 patients. Again, it has confirmed that patients undergoing laparoscopic resection had less intraoperative blood loss, fewer blood transfusions, a shorter hospital stay, a higher rate of splenic preservation, an earlier oral intake, and fewer surgical site infections. However, there were no differences between the two approaches with regard to operation time, time to first flatus, and the occurrence of pancreatic fistula and other postoperative complications [96].

In 2008, Fernandez-Cruz updated their experience on 49 consecutive patients (43 women, with a mean age of 58 years) who underwent laparoscopic pancreatic surgery over a decade [79]. Other than nine pancreatic neuroendocrine tumors (PNTs) localized in the head of the pancreas, all tumors were located in the left pancreas. There were 33 patients with functioning tumors: 4 with gastrinomas (mean size 1.2 cm), 1 with a glucagonoma (4 cm), 3 with VIPomas (3.2 cm), 2 with carcinoids (5.2 cm), 20 with sporadic insulinomas (1.4 cm), 2 with insulinoma/multiple endocrine neoplasia type 1 (MEN-1) (4.4 cm), and 1 with a malignant insulinoma (13 cm). Sixteen patients had a nonfunctioning tumor (mean size 5 cm). Four cases (8.2%) were converted. Postoperative complications were significantly higher in the laparoscopic enucleations (42.8%) than in the laparoscopic distal pancreatectomies (mainly pancreatic fistula). Pathology examination of the specimen showed R0 resection in all patients with malignant PNT. The mean time to resumption of previous activities for patients was 3 weeks [79]. From South Korea, the very active group from Asian Medical Center in Seoul reported on 359 patients; 323 (90%) had benign or low-grade malignant neoplasms and 36 (10%) had malignancies. They performed spleen-preserving laparoscopic distal pancreatectomy on 178 patients (49.6%): 150 (84.3%) by main splenic vessel preservation and 28 (15.7%) supported by short gastric and gastroepiploic vessels (Warshaw technique). Postoperative complications occurred in 43 (12%) patients, including 25 (7%) with pancreatic fistula. The proportion of patients with pancreatic lesions who underwent laparoscopic distal pancreatectomy increased from 8.6% in 2005 to 66.9% in 2010. They concluded that laparoscopic distal pancreatectomy is feasible, safe, and effective for the treatment of benign and low-grade malignant lesions of the pancreas, and that the increased use of laparoscopic distal pancreatectomy for left-sided pancreatic lesions, including malignant lesions, represented a paradigm shift from open distal pancreatectomy [91].

CONCLUSION

One decade after the first laparoscopic pancreatic resection, the literature continues to show encouraging outcomes for laparoscopic distal pancreatectomies and enucleations. These procedures are technically feasible and result in acceptable complication and mortality rates. As with other laparoscopic procedures, the benefits include reduced postoperative pain, better cosmetic results, shorter hospitalization, and lower rate of major complications. Laparoscopic enucleation or distal pancreatectomy with or without splenectomy is technically feasible and safe and benefits patients. The ability to avoid a large incision and perform resection of an islet cell tumor that is predominantly small and benign is a meaningful advantage of laparoscopic surgery. Localization of these lesions by intraoperative inspection of the pancreas and contact ultrasonography has added significant merit to this approach. At the current time, given the small number of patients included in the series, the relatively short follow-up, and the possible increased risk of pancreatic leak, the laparoscopic approach needs further study.

REFERENCES

1. Bernheim B. Organoscopy. Cystoscopy of the abdominal cavity. *Ann Surg* 1911;53:764–7.
2. Meyer-Burg J. Laparoscopic examination of the pancreas [in Spanish]. *Rev Esp Enferm Apar Dig* 1972;38:697–704.
3. Hirata K, Mima S, Fukuda M. High-resolution ultrasonography in cancer diagnosis—Advances and indication of intraluminal sonography [in Japanese]. *Gan To Kagaku Ryoho* 1986;13:1661–7.
4. Cuesta MA, Meijer S, Borgstein PJ, Sibinga Mulder L, Sikkenk AC. Laparoscopic ultrasonography for hepatobiliay and pancreatic malignancy. *Br J Surg* 1993;80:1571–4.
5. Murugiah M, Paterson-Brown S, Windsor JA, Miles WF, Garden OJ. Early experience of laparoscopic ultrasonography in the management of pancreatic carcinoma. *Surg Endosc* 1993;7:177–81.
6. Cuschieri A. Laparoscopic surgery of the pancreas. *J R Coll Surg Edinb* 1994;39:178–84.
7. Gouma DJ, de Wit LT, Nieveen van Dijkum E et al. Laparoscopic ultrasonography for staging of gastrointestinal malignancy. *Scand J Gastroenterol Suppl* 1996;218:43–49.
8. Pietrabissa A, Di Candio G, Giulianotti PC, Mosca F. Laparoscopic exposure of the pancreas and staging of pancreatic cancer. *Semin Laparosc Surg* 1996;3:3–9.
9. Gagner M, Pomp A. Laparoscopic pylorus-preserving pancreatoduodenectomy. *Surg Endosc* 1994;8:408–410.
10. Cuschieri A, Jakimowicz JJ, van Spreeuwel J. Laparoscopic distal 70% pancreatectomy and splenectomy for chronic pancreatitis. *Ann Surg* 1996;223:280–5.
11. Gagner M, Pomp A, Herrera MF. Early experience with laparoscopic resections of islet cell tumors. *Surgery* 1996;120:1051–4.
12. Cuschieri A. Laparoscopic pancreatic resections. *Semin Laparosc Surg* 1996;3:15–20.
13. Salky BA, Edye M. Laparoscopic pancreatectomy. *Surg Clin North Am* 1996;76:539–45.
14. Sussman LA, Christie R, Whittle DE. Laparoscopic excision of distal pancreas including insulinoma. *Aust NZ J Surg* 1996;66:414–6.
15. Gagner M, Pomp A. Laparoscopic pancreatic resection: Is it worthwhile? *J Gastrointest Surg* 1997;1:20–6.
16. Klingler PJ, Hinder RA, Menke DM, Smith SL. Hand-assisted laparoscopic distal pancreatectomy for pancreatic cystadenoma. *Surg Laparosc Endosc* 1998;8:180–4.
17. Gagner M, Gentileschi P. Hand-assisted laparoscopic pancreatic resection. *Semin Laparosc Surg* 2001;8:114–25.
18. Yoshida T, Bandoh T, Ninomiya K, Matsumoto T, Baatar D, Kitano S. Laparoscopic enucleation of a pancreatic insulinoma: Report of a case. *Surg Today* 1998;28:1188–91.
19. Collins R, Schlinkert RT, Roust L. Laparoscopic resection of an insulinoma. *J Laparoendosc Adv Surg Tech A* 1999;9:429–31.
20. Dexter SP, Martin IG, Leindler L, Fowler R, McMahon MJ. Laparoscopic enucleation of a solitary pancreatic insulinoma. *Surg Endosc* 1999;13:406–8.
21. Marescaux J, Mutter D, Vix M, Leroy J. Endoscopic surgery: Ideal for endocrine surgery? *World J Surg* 1999;23:825–34.

22. Park A, Schwartz R, Tandan V, Anvari M. Laparoscopic pancreatic surgery. *Am J Surg* 1999;177:158–63.

23. Underwood RA, Soper NJ. Current status of laparoscopic surgery of the pancreas. *J Hepatobiliary Pancreat Surg* 1999;6:154–64.

24. Van Nieuwenhove Y, Delvaux G. Laparoscopic management of neuroendocrine tumours of the pancreas. *Acta Chir Belg* 1999;99:249–52.

25. Vezakis A, Davides D, Larvin M, McMahon MJ. Laparoscopic surgery combined with preservation of the spleen for distal pancreatic tumors. *Surg Endosc* 1999;13:26–9.

26. Berends FJ, Cuesta MA, Kazemier G et al. Laparoscopic detection and resection of insulinomas. *Surgery* 2000;128:386–91.

27. Lo CY, Lo CM, Fan ST. Role of laparoscopic ultrasonography in intraoperative localization of pancreatic insulinoma. *Surg Endosc* 2000;14:1131–5.

28. Raeburn CD, McIntyre RC Jr. Laparoscopic approach to adrenal and endocrine pancreatic tumors. *Surg Clin North Am* 2000;80:1427–41.

29. Spitz JD, Lilly MC, Tetik C, Arregui ME. Ultrasound-guided laparoscopic resection of pancreatic islet cell tumors. *Surg Laparosc Endosc Percutan Tech* 2000;10:168–73.

30. Cogliandolo A, Pidoto RR, Causse X, Kerdraon R, Saint Marc O. Minimally invasive management of insulinomas. A case report. *Surg Endosc* 2001;15:1042.

31. Furihata M, Tagaya N, Kubota K. Laparoscopic enucleation of insulinoma in the pancreas: Case report and review of the literature. *Surg Laparosc Endosc Percutan Tech* 2001;11:279–83.

32. Gentileschi P, Gagner M. Laparoscopic pancreatic resection. *Chir Ital* 2001;53:279–89.

33. Iihara M, Kanbe M, Okamoto T, Ito Y, Obara T. Laparoscopic ultrasonography for resection of insulinomas. *Surgery* 2001;130:1086–91.

34. Patterson EJ, Gagner M, Salky B et al. Laparoscopic pancreatic resection: Single-institution experience of 19 patients. *J Am Coll Surg* 2001;193:281–7.

35. Falconi M, Molinari E, Carbognin G, Zamboni G, Bassi C, Pederzoli P. What preoperative assessment is necessary for insulinomas? Calculating the degree of waste: An analysis of 29 cases. *Chir Ital* 2002;54(5):597–604.

36. Chu QD, Al-Kasspooles MF, Smith JL et al. Is glucagonoma of the pancreas a curable disease? *Int J Pancreatol* 2001;29(3):155–62.

37. Santambrogio L, Nosotti M, Baisi A, Bellaviti N, Pavoni G, Rosso L. Buttressing staple lines with bovine pericardium in lung resection for bullous emphysema. *Scand Cardiovasc J* 1998;32:297–9.

38. Olmos-Zuniga JR, Jasso-Victoria R, Sotres-Vega A et al. Suture-line reinforcement with glutaraldehyde-preserved bovine pericardium for nonanatomic resection of lung tissue. *J Invest Surg* 2001;14:161–8.

39. Warshaw A. Conservation of the spleen with distal pancreatectomy. *Arch Surg* 1988;123:550–3.

40. Tashiro S, Murata E, Hiraoka T, Nakakuma K, Watanabe E, Miyauchi Y. New technique for pancreaticojejunostomy using a biological adhesive. *Br J Surg* 1987;74:392–4.

41. Hiraoka T, Kanemitsu K, Tsuji T et al. A method for safe pancreaticojejunostomy. *Am J Surg* 1993;165:270–2.

42. Cuschieri A. Laparoscopic hand-assisted surgery for hepatic and pancreatic disease. *Surg Endosc* 2000;14:991–6.

43. Shinchi H, Takao S, Noma H et al. Hand-assisted laparoscopic distal pancreatectomy with mini-laparotomy for distal pancreatic cystadenoma. *Sugr Laparosc Endosc Percut Tech* 2001;11(2):139–43.

44. Klinger P, Hinder R, Menke DM et al. Hand-assisted laparoscopic distal pancreatectomy for pancreatic cystadenoma. *Surg Laparosc Endosc* 1998;3:180–4.

45. Halloran CM, Ghanch P, Bosennet L, Hartley MN, Sutton R, Neoptolemos JP. Complications of pancreatic cancer resection. *Dig Surg* 2002; 19(2):138–46.

46. Aldridge M, Williamson R. Distal pancreatectomy with and without splenectomy. *Br J Surg* 1991;78:976–979.

47. Cuschieri A, Jackimowicz J, van Spreeuwel J. Laparoscopic distal 70% pancreatectomy and splenectomy for chronic pancreatitis. *Ann Surg* 1996;3:280–285.

48. Lillemoe KD, Kaushal S, Cameron JL, Sohn TA, Pitt HA, Yeo CJ. Distal pancreatectomy: Indications and outcomes in 235 patients. *Ann Surg* 1999;229(5):693–700.

49. Ridgeway MG, Stabile BE. Surgical management and treatment of pancreatic fistulas. *Surg Clin North Am* 1996;76(5):1159–73.

50. McLean TR, Simmons K, Svensson LG. Management of postoperative intra-abdominal abscesses by routine percutaneous drainage. *Surg Gynecol Obstet* 1993;176(2):167–71.

51. Cinat M, Wilson S, Din A. Determinants for successful percutaneous image-guided drainage of intra-abdominal abscess. *Arch Surg* 2002;137(7):845–9.

52. Watanabe Y, Motomichi S, Kikkawa H et al. Spleen-preserving laparoscopic distal pancreatectomy for cystic adenoma. *Hepatogastroenterology* 2002;49:148–52.

53. Warshaw A. Conservation of the spleen with distal pancreatectomy. *Arch Surg* 1988;123:550–3.

54. Fernandez-Cruz L, Saenz A, Astudillo E et al. Laparoscopic pancreatic surgery in patients with chronic pancreatitis. *Surg Endosc* 2002;16:996–1003.

55. Benoist S, Dugue L, Sauvanet A et al. Is there a role of preservation of the spleen in distal pancreatectomy? *J Am Coll Surg* 1999;188:255–60.

56. Cuschieri A. Laparoscopic pancreatic resections. *Semin Laparosc Surg* 1996;3(1):15–20.

57. Broughan TA, Leslie JD, Soto JM, Hermann RE. Pancreatic islet cell tumors. *Surgery* 1986;99(6):671–8.

58. Buchler M, Friess H, Klempa I et al. Role of octreotide in the prevention of postoperative complications following pancreatic resection. *Am J Surg* 1992;163(1):125–30.

59. Montorsi M, Zago M, Mosca F et al. Efficacy of octreotide in the prevention of pancreatic fistula after elective pancreatic resections: A prospective, controlled, randomized clinical trial. *Surgery* 1995;117(1):26–31.

60. Cuschieri A. Whither minimal access surgery: Tribulations and expectations. *Am J Surg* 1995;169:9–19.

61. Fernandez-Cruz L, Saenz A, Astrdillo E et al. Outcome of laparoscopic pancreatic surgery: Endocrine and nonendocrine tumors. *World J Surg* 2002;26(8):1057–65.

62. Melotti G, Piccoli M, Bassi C et al. L'approccio laparoscopico ai tumori cistici del corpo-coda del pancreas: Indicazioni e tecnica. *Osp Ital Chir* 2000;6:411–5.

63. Fabre JM, Dulucq JL, Vacher C et al. Is laparoscopic left pancreatic resection justified? *Surg Endosc* 2002;16(9):1358–61.

64. Ferraina P, Ferraro A, Merello Lardies J, Cuenca Abente F. Academia Argentina de Cirugia, *Rev. Argent. Cirug.*, 2002.

65. Mahon D, Allen E, Rhodes M. Laparoscopic distal pancreatectomy. Three cases of insulinomas. *Surg Endosc* 2002;16:700–702.

66. Chapuis Y, Bigourdan JM, Massault PP, Pitre J, Palazzo L. Exérèse d'un insulinome pancreatique sous coelioscopie. *Chirugie* 1998;123(5):461–7.

67. Ueno T, Oka M, Nishihara K et al. Laparoscopic distal pancreatectomy with preservation of the spleen. *Surg Laparosc Endosc Percut Tech* 1999;4:290–3.

68. Gramatica L, Herrera M, Mercado-Luna A et al. Video-laparoscopic resection of insulinomas: Experience in two institutions. *World J Surg* 2002;26:1297–300.

69. Naitoh T, Garcia-Ruiz A, Vladisavljevic A, Matsuno S, Gagner M. Gastrointestinal transit and stress response after laparoscopic vs conventional distal pancreatectomy in the canine model. *Surg Endosc* 2002;16(11):1627–30.

70. Patterson EJ, Gagner M, Salky B et al. Laparoscopic pancreatic resection: Single-institution experience of 19 patients. *J Am Coll Surg* 2001;193(3):281–7.

71. Fernández-Cruz L, Herrera M, Sáenz A, Pantoja JP, Astudillo E, Sierra M. Laparoscopic pancreatic surgery in patients with neuroendocrine tumours: Indications and limits [review]. *Best Pract Res Clin Endocrinol Metab* 2001;15(2):161–75.

72. Fernández-Cruz L, Martínez I, Gilabert R, Cesar-Borges G, Astudillo E, Navarro S. Laparoscopic distal pancreatectomy combined with preservation of the spleen for cystic neoplasms of the pancreas. *J Gastrointest Surg.* 2004;8(4):493–501.

73. Gagner M. Pioneers in laparoscopic solid organ surgery. *Surg Endosc.* 2003;17(11):1853–4.

74. Assalia A, Gagner M. Laparoscopic pancreatic surgery for islet cell tumors of the pancreas. *World J Surg* 2004;28(12):1239–47.

75. Dulucq JL, Wintringer P, Stabilini C, Feryn T, Perissat J, Mahajna A. Are major laparoscopic pancreatic resections worthwhile? A prospective study of 32 patients in a single institution. *Surg Endosc* 2005;19(8):1028–34.

76. Mabrut JY, Fernandez-Cruz L, Azagra JS et al. Laparoscopic pancreatic resection: Results of a multicenter European study of 127 patients. *Surgery* 2005;137(6):597–605.

77. Fernández-Cruz L, Pardo F, Cugat E et al. Analysis of the Spanish National Registry of Laparoscopic Pancreatic Surgery [in Spanish]. *Cir Esp* 2006;79(5):293–8.

78. Eom BW, Jang JY, Lee SE, Han HS, Yoon YS, Kim SW. Clinical outcomes compared between laparoscopic and open distal pancreatectomy. *Surg Endosc* 2008;22(5):1334–8.

79. Fernández-Cruz L, Blanco L, Cosa R, Rendón H. Is laparoscopic resection adequate in patients with neuroendocrine pancreatic tumors? *World J Surg* 2008;32(5):904–17.

80. Kooby DA, Gillespie T, Bentrem D et al. Left-sided pancreatectomy: A multicenter comparison of laparoscopic and open approaches. *Ann Surg* 2008;248(3):438–46.

81. Luo Y, Liu R, Hu MG, Mu YM, An LC, Huang ZQ. Laparoscopic surgery for pancreatic insulinomas: A single-institution experience of 29 cases. *J Gastrointest Surg* 2009;13(5):945–50.

82. Isla A, Arbuckle JD, Kekis PB et al. Laparoscopic management of insulinomas. *Br J Surg* 2009;96(2):185–90.

83. Yoon YS, Lee KH, Han HS, Cho JY, Ahn KS. Patency of splenic vessels after laparoscopic spleen and splenic vessel-preserving distal pancreatectomy. *Br J Surg* 2009;96(6):633–40.

84. Giulianotti PC, Sbrana F, Bianco FM et al. Robot-assisted laparoscopic pancreatic surgery: Single-surgeon experience. *Surg Endosc* 2010;24(7):1646–57.

85. DiNorcia J, Schrope BA, Lee MK et al. Laparoscopic distal pancreatectomy offers shorter hospital stays with fewer complications. *J Gastrointest Surg* 2010;14(11):1804–12.

86. Newman NA, Lennon AM, Edil BH et al. Preoperative endoscopic tattooing of pancreatic body and tail lesions decreases operative time for laparoscopic distal pancreatectomy. *Surgery* 2010;148(2):371–7.

87. DiNorcia J, Lee MK, Reavey PL et al. One hundred thirty resections for pancreatic neuroendocrine tumor: Evaluating the impact of minimally invasive and parenchyma-sparing techniques. *J Gastrointest Surg* 2010;14(10):1536–46.

88. Waters JA, Canal DF, Wiebke EA et al. Robotic distal pancreatectomy: Cost effective? *Surgery* 2010;148(4):814–23.

89. Vijan SS, Ahmed KA, Harmsen WS et al. Laparoscopic vs open distal pancreatectomy: A single-institution comparative study. *Arch Surg* 2010;145(7):616–21.

90. Nigri GR, Rosman AS, Petrucciani N et al. Metaanalysis of trials comparing minimally invasive and open distal pancreatectomies. *Surg Endosc* 2011;25(5):1642–51.

91. Song KB, Kim SC, Park JB et al. Single-center experience of laparoscopic left pancreatic resection in 359 consecutive patients: Changing the surgical paradigm of left pancreatic resection. *Surg Endosc* 2011;25(10):3364–72.

92. Butturini G, Partelli S, Crippa S et al. Perioperative and long-term results after left pancreatectomy: A single-institution, non-randomized, comparative study between open and laparoscopic approach. *Surg Endosc* 2011;25(9):2871–8.

93. Cho CS, Kooby DA, Schmidt CM et al. Laparoscopic versus open left pancreatectomy: Can preoperative factors indicate the safer technique? *Ann Surg* 2011;253(5):975–80.

94. Chang SK, Lomanto D, Mayasari M. Single-port laparoscopic spleen preserving distal pancreatectomy. *Minim Invasive Surg* 2012;2012:197429.

95. Fernández-Cruz L, Molina V, Vallejos R, Jiménez Chavarria E, López-Boado MA, Ferrer J. Outcome after laparoscopic enucleation for non-functional neuroendocrine pancreatic tumours. *HPB (Oxford)* 2012;14(3):171–6.

96. In T, Altaf K, Xiong JJ et al. A systematic review and meta-analysis of studies comparing laparoscopic and open distal pancreatectomy. *HPB (Oxford)* 2012;14(11):711–24.

97. Strijker M, van Santvoort HC, Besselink MG et al. Robot-assisted pancreatic surgery: A systematic review of the literature. *HPB (Oxford)* 2013;15(1):1–10.

98. Mofid H, Emmermann A, Alm M, Zornig C. Transvaginal specimen removal after laparoscopic distal pancreatic resection. *Langenbecks Arch Surg* 2013;398(7):1001–5.

99. Gumbs AA, Croner R, Rodriguez A, Zuker N, Perrakis A, Gayet B. 200 consecutive laparoscopic pancreatic resections performed with a robotically controlled laparoscope holder. *Surg Endosc* 2013;27(10):3781–91.

100. Thakkar S, Awad M, Gurram KC et al. A novel, new robotic platform for natural orifice distal pancreatectomy. *Surg Innov* 2015;22(3):274–82.

101. Senthilnathan P, Gul SI, Gurumurthy SS et al. Laparoscopic central pancreatectomy: Our technique and long-term results in 14 patients. *J Minim Access Surg* 2015;11(3):167–71.

PART 7

Inherited Syndromes

43

Multiple endocrine neoplasia*

STEPHEN FARRELL

INTRODUCTION

Endocrine tumor syndromes are individually uncommon or rare. For most medical practitioners, these are unknown or barely known entities and are completely "out of mind."

Collectively, however, patients with these syndromes make up a significant portion of specialist endocrine surgery practice. One of the great rewards of such a practice comes when diligent inquiry into family history and specific investigation for related tumors reveals a patient to be an index

* This chapter is dedicated to the memory of Charles Proye.

case with an endocrine tumor syndrome. The consequences for the patient and family are profound, arising from the opportunity to prevent or minimize tumor-related illness.

Over the last 60 years, various endocrine tumor syndromes, beginning with multiple endocrine neoplasia type 1 (MEN1), have been described and subsequently genetically mapped. New mutations and syndromes continue to be identified. There is still much to discover. We still have patients who, based on the pattern of disease, must harbor a mutation yet have tested negative for all currently known gene mutations.

Around the world and even within countries or between institutions, there remain significant differences in management philosophies and strategies. The rarity of these disorders leaves us only with observational studies, pooled international experience, and expert opinion. Together, this has given rise to some guidelines for investigation and management [1–5]. Locally, the establishment of a "team" of persons with expertise is invaluable in making often complex and difficult decisions. The organs principally affected by endocrine tumors in MEN1 are easily remembered, the 3Ps: pituitary, pancreas, and parathyroid. MEN2 is dominated by medullary thyroid cancer (MTC) and, to a lesser extent, pheochromocytoma (PCC). Hyperparathyroidism (HPT) is a feature only in some patients with MEN2A and does not occur in MEN2B. Individuals with MEN2B have MTC, PCC, and a marfanoid habitus and pathognomonic facies. Familial medullary thyroid cancer (FMTC) is a variant of MEN2 without associated features.

MEN1 results from a germline mutation of the *MEN1* gene. Subsequent somatic mutation of the wild-type allele causes loss of function of this suppressor gene. In contrast, in MEN2, a germline mutation confers gain of function in the *RET* proto-oncogene. In both MEN1 and MEN2, penetrance is almost complete in carriers of a mutant gene, but the disease expression is remarkably varied. Interestingly, in MEN2, a strong genotype–phenotype correlation is found, while in MEN1 no such correlation is found. MEN1, MEN2, and other syndromes may arise as *de novo* mutations, which are then heritable.

Historically, complications due to hormone secretion were the major causes of morbidity and mortality in MEN1: in particular, renal complications of HPT, peptic ulcer due to gastrinoma, and hypoglycemia due to insulinoma. In MEN2, hypertensive stroke and cardiac disease due to PCC were frequent causes of death, but medullary carcinoma was also a major cause of death. Modern medical and surgical treatment has altered the natural history of both syndromes, and now malignant transformation is the most significant clinical problem: pancreaticoduodenal malignancy and thymic carcinoma in MEN1 and MTC in MEN2.

Patients with an inherited endocrine tumor syndrome fall into two very different groups: the first group present as an index case, often with advanced symptoms, from a tumor mass or from a hormone-mediated illness. The second group, now the larger group, are those identified to be gene carriers prior to development of any detectable disease.

The management of index patients with a new diagnosis and of those who are identified as gene carriers is fundamentally different. In the case of MEN2 gene carriers, timely prophylactic thyroidectomy affords nearly 100% protection against MTC. Uniquely, knowledge of the particular codon mutation is used to determine management. MEN2 is perhaps the best example in all of medicine of the way in which genetic diagnosis provides the opportunity to perform a surgical intervention (thyroidectomy) to prevent tumor (MTC).

In the case of MEN2 PCC, and in most other syndrome-associated tumors, screening is carried out with a view to timely intervention after a tumor has developed but before metastases or hormonal consequences arise. In principle, these tumors could be prevented by prophylactic organ extirpation, but the risks of surgery and the hormonal consequences do not justify such an approach. Examples might include prophylactic total pancreaticoduodenectomy in MEN1 and bilateral adrenalectomy in MEN2.

The timing, extent of surgery, and likely need for reoperation for new tumors are key discussions with patients. Decisions are based upon our knowledge of the natural history of all the different aspects of the patient's syndrome, as well as local expertise and opinion. Individual patient decisions will be strongly influenced by familial experience of outcomes, whether from the natural course of disease or surgical intervention. However, it cannot be assumed that children will follow the pattern of their parents in any of the syndromes. We can see, for example, a young adult presenting as the index case of MEN2A (V804M) with metastatic MTC while the 74-year old mother who carries the same gene has normal calcitonin and no tumor.

Controversies in the management of these syndromes remain. Perhaps the most difficult area of all is MEN1 pancreatic disease. How early and how radical should pancreatic surgery be for nonfunctioning tumors? Is Zollinger–Ellison syndrome (ZES) in MEN1 a surgical disease? If so, what is the best operation?

MEN1 (WERMER'S SYNDROME) (OMIM #131100)

MEN1 is the most well-known endocrine tumor syndrome. The defining three features, anterior pituitary adenoma, pancreaticoduodenal neuroendocrine tumors, and multigland parathyroid disease, occur in 40%, 70%, and almost 100% of patients, respectively. In MEN1 patients with ZES, multiple submucosal, duodenal, gastrin-secreting tumors are usually found and gastric carcinoids (enterochromaffin-like [ECL] type II) may be present. Additional features of MEN1 are bronchial, thymic, and gastric carcinoids; adrenocortical hyperplasia; adrenal adenoma and carcinoma; cutaneous and visceral lipomas; ependymoma; meningioma; facial angiofibromas; and truncal collagenomas (Table 43.1).

In 1954, Wermer [6] described the syndrome of familial pituitary, parathyroid, and pancreatic islet cell neoplasia and coined the term *adenomatosis* of the endocrine glands.

Table 43.1 Clinical characteristics of MEN1 syndrome

Key features

Parathyroid: Multigland primary HPT >95%

Pancreatic/duodenal endocrine tumor: 30%–75%

Pituitary tumor: 20%–40%

Other features

Adrenocortical hyperplasia, adenoma, and carcinoma

Bronchial, thymic, and gastric carcinoids

Lipomas

Facial angiofibromas and truncal collagenomas

Ependymomas

Clinical diagnosis

Two or more key features in index case

One or more key features in relative

The incidence of MEN1 is difficult to know. Shepherd [7] has emphasized the existence of unrecognized MEN1. In 1982, only three patients with MEN1 were known in Tasmania, an Australian island with a population then of 450,000. Thorough investigation of relatives led to the discovery of about 250 cases—a prevalence of 1 in 1800. Modern autopsy data or large population studies are lacking.

MEN1 is likely to remain significantly unrecognized. Each of the key MEN1 component tumors (apart from gastrinoma) is much more common as a sporadic tumor than in association with MEN1. Between 16% and 40% of gastrinomas, 2%–10% of HPT, and 5%–15% of insulinomas occur in the setting of MEN1 [8,9–14].

MEN1 tumors may not be recognized to be present even when symptomatic. Peptic ulcer, for example, is (or was) a very common disease, usually treated adequately by modern medications, and unless it presents in an unusual fashion, it may not evoke MEN1. Many cases of endocrine tumor are either asymptomatic or minimally symptomatic and may go entirely unrecognized during the life of the patient. In only 4 of 130 patients in one series [7] did the presentation evoke MEN1 as a diagnosis. The associated tumors often present metachronously, and may be separated by many years.

Management of MEN1 continues to be controversial, and every patient presents unique and challenging dilemmas. The approach to screening for tumors and the timing and extent of surgery are vexed issues. The lack of correlation between genotype and clinical evolution of disease even within families makes management difficult. Pancreaticoduodenal operations have a significant morbidity and a small risk of mortality. Screen-detected, likely premalignant pancreatic tumors in young, otherwise healthy people pose a difficult therapeutic conundrum.

MEN1 genetics

MEN1 is inherited as an autosomal dominant syndrome. The *MEN1* tumor suppressor gene was cloned in 1997. It is situated at 11q13, contains 10 exons, and encodes a 610-amino acid protein, menin. Menin is involved in regulation of transcription, genome stability, cell division, and proliferation. The interactions of menin are extremely complicated—more than 40 potential protein partners for menin have been examined [15]. In MEN1, menin interacts with JUND and represses JUND-activated transcription.

MEN1 mutations are enormously diverse, with a different mutation found in most families. More than 1000 different germline mutations have been identified, scattered throughout the entire coding region of the gene. The majority of these are inactivating, causing truncation [15]. When subsequent somatic mutation or loss of the second *MEN1* allele (Loss Of Heterozygosity, LOH) occurs in a cell, neoplastic clonal expansion may occur—in accordance with the Knudson two-hit hypothesis for tumor suppressor gene.

Germline mutations at the *MEN1* locus are only identified in <95% of families with clinical MEN1. Failure to find a genetic mutation in a proband does not exclude MEN1. Newer techniques. such as multiplex ligation-dependent probe amplification (MLPA) may detect whole or partial gene deletions. Mutations in the promoter or untranslated regions currently may not be detected. Mutations in cyclin-dependent kinase inhibitors *p15*, *p18*, and *p21* cause perhaps 2% of MEN1 [16]. Polymorphisms in the *MEN1* gene, which are not causative of MEN1, have also been reported.

Approximately 10% of MEN1 germline mutations arise *de novo* and can then be transmitted. Loss of function of both alleles is also evident in about a quarter of sporadic endocrine tumors. Somatic MEN1 gene mutations have been found in parathyroid adenoma (18%), gastrinoma (38%), insulinoma (14%), vasoactive intestinal peptide-oma (VIPoma) (57%), nonfunctioning PNET (16%), glucagonoma (60%), bronchial carcinoid (35%), and lipoma (28%) [8].

MEN1 PHENOCOPIES AND VARIANTS

Within known MEN1 families, sporadic development of a MEN1-related tumor (most likely HPT) in an unaffected relative is not rare [17] and was a cause of phenocopy and false diagnosis of MEN1 prior to genetic testing. Phenocopies may arise in patients with two sporadic endocrine tumors, but also occasionally in patients with mutations in other genes, such as *HRPT2*, which is responsible for HPT-jaw tumor syndrome, and *CDKN1B*, which causes MEN4.

A very small proportion of MEN1 families express variants of, or limited features of, the syndrome, such as familial isolated hyperparathyroidism (FIHP).

MEN1 clinical features

MEN1 has a high penetrance: more than 90% of individuals develop biochemical evidence of HPT by the age of 35, 30%–55% develop clinically significant pancreaticoduodenal neuroendocrine tumors (while more than 80% have demonstrable lesions at necropsy), and 15%–40% develop clinically significant pituitary tumors [7,17–21]. Approximately 80% of individuals express some clinical elements of the syndrome, and >95% biochemical markers by the age of 50 [19].

Occasionally, no clinical expression occurs despite being a gene carrier [17].

The first clinical manifestation of the syndrome in index cases is HPT in approximately 50% of patients, pancreaticoduodenal tumor in 30%, and pituitary tumor in 20% [7,19,21]. In 15 patients where the interval between first and second tumors was recorded, this ranged from 6 to 24 years [19]. In the study by Shepherd [7], younger patients presented more commonly with non-HPT symptoms. In patients under 25 years of age, 34 patients had MEN1 tumors: 25 were symptomatic and cause for presentation. Nine presented with symptomatic pituitary tumors (prolactinoma), 10 with symptomatic pancreatic tumors (5 insulinoma and 3 gastrinoma), and 6 with symptomatic HPT (altogether, 21/32 had HPT when tested).

MEN1 patients have a decreased life expectancy [20,22]. Untreated patients have a 50% chance of death by the age of 50. Seventy percent of patients die of MEN1-related illness [23]. In current patient cohorts, death is largely due to metastatic PNETs and thymic carcinoma. Males have a worse prognosis than females.

HYPERPARATHYROIDISM IN MEN1

While HPT is the feature most often leading to diagnosis of MEN1, in general, only patients with another MEN1 tumor, with a suggestive family history, younger than 40 years of age, and with multigland disease should be considered for further clinical or genetic investigation.

The age of onset and clinical severity of HPT are markedly varied, but HPT usually emerges around 20–25 years [17]. Even young women with MEN1 HPT have significant osteoporosis [24]. Significant and symptomatic hypercalcemia is common and may even lead to hypercalcemic crisis. In historical cohorts, death from hypercalcemia-related illness, including renal disease from stones, was a common outcome [17].

The pathological nature of HPT in MEN1 is not entirely clear. The distinction between adenoma and hyperplasia is not straightforward, and no universal or reliable tools for the pathologist exist. Mutation in a tumor suppressor gene might be expected to cause multiple tumors every time a second hit occurs in a cell, rather than hyperplasia. Single or double adenoma has been reported in some cases of MEN1 [25,26] (Figure 43.1a). The number of affected glands increases with time [27], and most parathyroid lesions in MEN1 are monoclonal [28], suggesting multiple metachronous adenomas. However, many other patients have apparent hyperplasia without a dominant nodular gland (Figure 43.1b). In a series from Proye of 307 glands seen at exploration for MEN1 HPT, 285 glands were examined histologically: 34 were normal (11.9%), 220 hyperplastic (77.1%), and 31 adenomas (10.9%). Adenomas were defined by the presence of a rim of normal parathyroid, and hyperplasia by the absence of this rim [29].

SURGERY FOR HYPERPARATHYROIDISM IN MEN1

The indication for surgery is clear when HPT is symptomatic or biochemically severe. Also, patients with ZES should

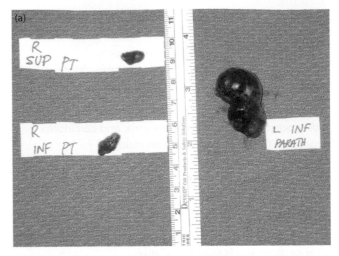

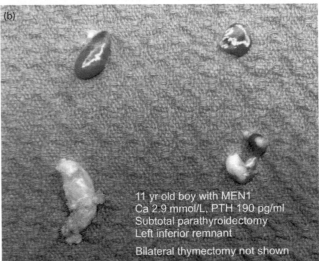

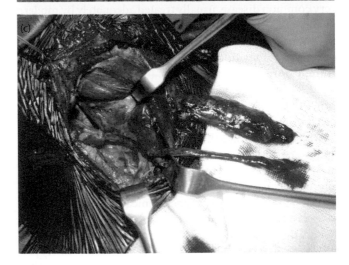

Figure 43.1 (a) Subtotal parathyroidectomy showing marked asymmetry of parathyroid glands (thymus not shown). (b) Subtotal parathyroidectomy in 11-year-old with nearly symmetrical enlargement of parathyroid glands (thymus not shown). (c) Dissection for subtotal parathyroidectomy in MEN1 showing the thymic horns and the superior and inferior parathyroid glands (blue arrows). The recurrent nerve, yellow arrow, is just visible. Note the lateral approach (strap muscles lie medially).

have their hypercalcemia corrected as the first therapeutic action because this leads to significant decrease in gastrin levels and symptoms. The timing and indication for surgery in mild, asymptomatic HPT is more contentious. Many surgeons would recommend surgery when the biochemical diagnosis is clear, just as they would for sporadic HPT. "Asymptomatic" sporadic HPT patients have subtle symptoms that improve with surgery [30]; this is likely true of MEN1 patients also. Untreated asymptomatic HPT in MEN1 has been shown to result in loss of bone density [24].

The aim of parathyroid surgery in MEN1 is to do more good than harm. The surgeon must strike the right balance between the consequences of hypercalcemia in patients either untreated or with persistent or recurrent HPT and operative complications, such as recurrent nerve palsy and permanent hypoparathyroidism. At the end of the procedure, there should ideally be a small but adequate amount of parathyroid tissue in a known location, such that a reoperation, if needed, is facilitated. Rather than aiming to "cure" patients, the aim is to achieve normocalcemia for as long as possible, with minimized risk of hypocalcemia. Reoperation is then expected to be required in some patients with recurrent hypercalcemia and is an integral part of the initial strategy [31].

There are two established surgical strategies. The first is subtotal parathyroidectomy [29,32], and the second is total parathyroidectomy with autograft [33,34]. Rates of hypoparathyroidism and persistent or recurrent hypercalcemia with each procedure vary widely from one institution to another, suggesting institutional experience and preference play a role in the outcome. It is clear that selective excision of large glands results in a high rate of persistence and recurrence and is not generally recommended [29,35].

The thymic horns should be resected as completely as possible using the transcervical route. In MEN1, supernumerary parathyroids or rests are found in the thymus in about 30% of cases and are a frequent cause of persistent or recurrent HPT [29]. Normally, 6–10 cm of right and left thymus can be extracted without difficulty via the neck. There is also a theoretical reduction in risk of thymic carcinoid, which occurs almost exclusively in males, and may be lethal. However, there is a significant portion of the thymus left behind requiring surveillance. There are few, if any, examples of thymic carcinoid found by cervical thymectomy during parathyroidectomy, and many cases of tumor developing afterward in the remnant [36,37].

Because all four glands are inevitably involved during a patient's lifetime, and recurrence in remnants, grafts, and supernumerary glands is common, it follows that reoperations are commonly needed. The first operation must be conducted with the utmost care. A bloodless field and meticulous, orderly, gentle dissection is key. The lateral approach facilitates visualization of the posterior aspect of the thyroid from the ipsilateral side.

If exploration fails to find one of the glands, it is preferable to have available intraoperative PTH assay to confirm biological cure and decide upon autotransplantation.

In multigland disease including MEN1, a drop in PTH by 50% at 10 minutes is not evidence of adequate surgery. A fall of PTH to subnormal levels is required to be confident of long-term cure [29]. Failure to fall by 50% predicts a supernumerary or unidentified gland and is perhaps the greatest use of the test.

Preoperative localization prior to initial parathyroid surgery has been considered to have little place in MEN1 because of the need for thorough exploration and thymectomy. Localizing studies, including sestamibi scintigraphy, are less informative in multigland disease than in the typical uniglandular disease of sporadic HPT. Nevertheless, sestamibi scan may be useful if it identifies an ectopic gland that might otherwise have been missed, particularly in a supernumerary gland.

A recent report [38] describes a thought-provoking contrary strategy if localization suggests a single large gland. Minimally invasive unilateral clearance and acceptance of likely reoperation was proposed. The rationale is that hypoparathyroidism is avoided at the first procedure, and the second can be done safely after a structured first operation. A prolonged period of normocalcemia is likely. Reflecting upon this approach, it may be more logical to be even more targeted, and find and remove only the enlarged gland, as the ipsilateral "normal" gland may be, in the long term, the one least affected and needed for preservation of function.

Reoperative surgery is potentially very difficult after a bilateral exploration that results in more than one residual parathyroid, especially if glands are present on both sides of the neck or are superior glands, or worse, if the number and site of residual glands is unknown.

SUBTOTAL PARATHYROIDECTOMY

The surgical strategy should be to identify all four parathyroid glands and any supernumerary glands. The thymus and all parathyroid glands should be resected, leaving only a well-vascularized remnant of one gland (Figure 43.1c).

The first step is to identify the preferred remnant before any resections take place. The ideal candidate should have a polar blood supply and be soft and hyperplastic without obvious nodularity. It is not necessarily the smallest. Preferably, the remnant should be an inferior parathyroid because of its more superficial location in the neck and greater distance from the recurrent laryngeal nerve, which reduces difficulty and risk in case of reoperation or alcohol ablation.

Before resection of the other glands, the remnant should be dissected and mobilized only sufficient to assess it fully and identify and clearly preserve its pedicle and therefore blood supply. The gland is then transected, removing the free end. The viability of the remnant can be confirmed by the presence of brisk bleeding. In principle, it should be possible to leave a well-positioned and viable remnant in most cases. In case of doubt, it may be better to prepare an alternate remnant or use an autograft in addition to [39] or in place of a remnant.

The remnant should be the size of a normal gland (30–60 mg). Larger remnants lead to persistent or recurrent disease. A 2–3 cm length of blue prolene suture knotted adjacent provides a "Hansel and Gretel" trail for reoperation. A metal clip adjacent may be useful to guide future ultrasound assessment. Patients with mild disease and a functioning remnant will require little or no calcium supplementation to avoid paraesthesia and cramps postoperatively. However, if the patient does not become transiently hypocalcemic and hypoparathyroid immediately after the surgery, the likelihood of persistence or recurrence is great.

Cryopreservation of parathyroid tissue is considered ideal because of the risk of hypoparathyroidism after initial or reoperative surgery. However, the cost of such a facility, the rarity with which patients in fact are transplanted with their own preserved tissue, and the high failure rate of grafts after cryopreservation have led most units to abandon storage of tissue for this purpose [40,41]. The onus is on the surgeon to be meticulous and experienced.

It is important to note that many early descriptions of subtotal parathyroidectomy are not the equivalent of the above definition of the operation. Some authors have not excised the thymus, and others have included in their category of subtotal parathyroidectomy resections of only one or two glands.

TOTAL PARATHYROIDECTOMY AND AUTOGRAFT

All four glands should be identified and excised. Supernumerary glands should also be removed and a cervical thymectomy carried out. The autograft is prepared from fresh parathyroid by dicing about 30 mg of the most normal parathyroid tissue into multiple morsels about 1 × 1 mm in size. These are implanted into pockets in muscle. Each pocket is marked with a blue prolene suture. The field may also be marked with metal clips to guide future ultrasound.

It is widely held that the transplant should be into the brachioradialis muscle of the nondominant forearm and not into the sternomastoid muscle because of the difficulty in determining the exact source of recurrent HPT by ultrasound, sestamibi scan, or venous sampling in this situation. By contrast, the function of a forearm graft can be reliably assessed by the Casanova test [42]. Tonelli et al. [43] have reported equal success with subcutaneous transplant in the arm, and others have used a subcutaneous cervical implantation site or the sternomastoid muscle. Resection of hyperfunctioning graft can be an awkward procedure (Figure 43.2a and b). There is great variation in the size and number of nodules of grafted tissue, which can be difficult to identify and selectively resect. Even with the aid of intraoperative isotope or ultrasound detection to try to ensure completeness of excision, generally a small "fillet" of muscle needs to be removed for adequate local control.

REOPERATION FOR PERSISTENT OR RECURRENT HPT IN MEN1

Persistent HPT, recurrent HPT, and hypocalcemia are more frequently observed in MEN1 than in sporadic HPT. The recurrence rate is affected by (1) no preoperative diagnosis of MEN1, (2) the surgeon's experience, (3) the timing of surgery, (4) the availability of intraoperative histologic

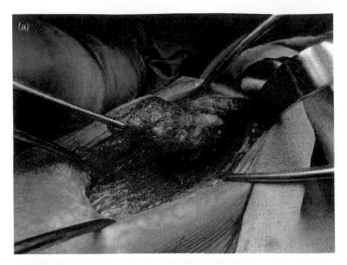

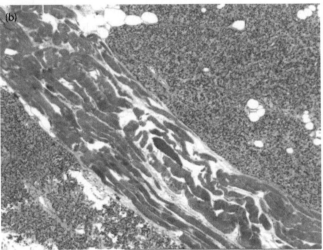

Figure 43.2 **(a)** Resection of forearm parathyroid graft as a fillet. **(b)** Histology of parathyroid graft. Nests of parathyroid cells within the striated muscle.

examination or rapid parathyroid hormone assay, and (5) the surgical strategy [43].

The first step is to review the original operation notes and pathology reports (which it should be remembered can be very misleading), along with all previous localization studies. The surgeon must keep in mind the possibility of multiple sites of recurrence. New localization studies are essential, regardless of the deductions made from original notes. The first investigations are sestamibi scan and ultrasonography and sometimes fine-needle aspiration (FNA) of suspected neck lesions for PTH assay [44]. MRI and computed tomography (CT) are both useful for cross-sectional localization. When localization by these methods is unconvincing, selective venous sampling is used to regionalize the lesion(s) or corroborate other results.

In the case of reoperation in the neck, the preference is to complete the resection to the equivalent of a total parathyroidectomy and thymectomy ± autograft, but to avoid unnecessary dissection of previously explored territory. It is better to limit the risk of complications and run the risk of needing further surgery than to blindly re-explore a scarred neck in the pursuit of an absent parathyroid gland. It is a matter of local preference and experience whether to autotransplant at this time, cryopreserve for later transplantation, or aim for a true total parathyroidectomy. There is a high risk of persistent functioning tissue even after reoperation.

If previous surgery was selective removal of only one or two glands, there is a choice of approaches: (1) to remove only lesions seen on localization in a targeted procedure or (2) to look for the remaining glands (hopefully marked) and remove the thymus. It may unfortunately become necessary to explore more widely if there is poor preoperative localization, and previous operative and pathology reports prove unhelpful. A low threshold for thyroidectomy, particularly in the presence of goiter, facilitates clearance of the central neck in difficult cases.

If previous surgery was subtotal and the remnant has hypertrophied, a targeted approach is advisable. Similarly, if previous subtotal or total parathyroidectomy was performed and there is a supernumerary gland recurrence, a targeted approach is advised. Ethanol ablation is an alternative to reoperation.

If no significant neck disease is found and the PTH does not fall, there may be a need to explore the mediastinum. In general, this should only be contemplated during the same procedure if hypercalcemia is a major clinical problem, this eventuality was planned from the outset, and ideally, it was indicated by imaging or venous sampling, or both. A targeted approach via the neck is preferred for inferior parathyroid glands in the anterior superior mediastinum and descended superior parathyroid glands in the posterior mediastinum, and via thoracoscopy for most other locations. If imaging is negative, then a full mediastinal exploration by thoracoscopy or sternotomy may be necessary. In the search for a middle mediastinal lesion, the aortopulmonary window should be examined [45].

If there is hyperfunctioning tissue in the forearm, this should be totally excised (± cryopreserved). There is usually an impressive initial response, but this is often followed by evidence of persistent disease either in the forearm or in the neck. Subsequent, painstaking reoperation on the forearm or the neck is often required.

The calcimimetic agent cinacalcet has become readily available and, in selected cases, is used to alter or delay the indications for primary or reoperative surgery by lowering serum calcium through stimulation of calcium receptors. However, it is expensive and the long-term efficacy and safety are still being evaluated. It may be strongly considered for use in patients with unlocalized recurrence, rare parathyroid cancer, or significant other medical illness, including widely metastatic neuroendocrine tumors.

Pancreatic and duodenal neuroendocrine tumors in MEN1

Endocrine pancreatic and duodenal lesions affect 30%–75% of individuals in clinical series [46–48]. In autopsy series,

these tumors are found in more than 80% of patients. They are nearly always multiple, and most of the lesions in a given patient remain asymptomatic (Figure 43.3). Twenty to forty percent of patients develop a clinical syndrome from excess pancreatic hormone. Clinical syndromes, most commonly ZES, are found more commonly from the age of 40, but in MEN1, insulinoma has a tendency to present early.

The earliest biochemical evidence of pancreaticoduodenal endocrine tumors precedes the clinical occurrence of disease by, on average, about 20 years [48]. Malignant disease occurs in approximately 40% of patients and is the leading cause of death in MEN1 today, often in middle age [20,22,49,50]. At the time of onset of symptoms related to functioning PNET, approximately 50% of patients will have malignant disease [51]. However, malignant disease most commonly runs an indolent clinical course over many years. A dramatically more aggressive clinical course is sometimes seen, but it is difficult to predict.

Thompson et al. [52] have shown that there is, early in the course of the disease and spread throughout the gland, a range of lesions, from nesidioblastosis and hyperplasia through micro- and macroadenomas to carcinoma. In their experience of patients with functioning tumors, there are always discrete tumors that stain for the symptomatic

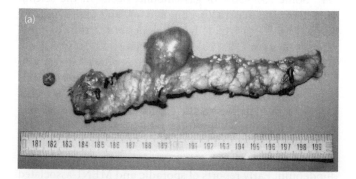

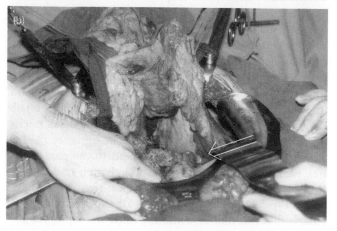

Figure 43.3 **(a)** Specimen of spleen-preserving subtotal pancreatectomy and enucleation of tumor of the head of pancreas. The large lesion was a functioning insulinoma. Multiple microadenomas were seen on histopathology. **(b)** Surgical exposure for the Thompson operation. Bilateral subcostal incision. Stomach and omentum elevated. A large tumor of the body of the pancreas is visible.

hormone, and in contrast, the hyperplastic tissue does not stain for this hormone. Islet cell hyperplasia is not responsible for clinical syndromes. In each patient, there are multiple tumors that display a variety of dominant cell and hormone types [53]. In MEN1, much more than in sporadic disease, a single tumor may elaborate (stain for) a multitude of hormones. Clinical evidence of this is usually a sign of malignancy.

Cystic or predominantly cystic endocrine pancreatic tumors are more common in MEN1 than sporadic disease and are equally as malignant as solid tumors. Therefore, diagnosis of cystadenoma of the pancreas in MEN1 on the basis of imaging studies should be regarded with skepticism.

The clinical syndromes, diagnosis, and differential diagnosis of gastrinoma and insulinoma and other islet cell tumors are covered in detail elsewhere. In cases where MEN1 can be confirmed, the management of these patients is quite different from the management of sporadic disease. When a genetic diagnosis of MEN1 precedes clinical disease, patients are entered into a screening protocol.

GASTRINOMAS IN MEN1

Of the functioning lesions, gastrinoma is the most common, occurring in up to 40%–60% of patients with MEN1 [54]. Some 25%–50% of gastrinomas occur in the setting of MEN1. The majority are malignant, and approximately half have metastasized to lymph nodes at the time of clinical presentation [55]. Peak age of onset is 40–50 years [18]. The syndrome of gastrin excess, ZES, is now relatively well controlled by parathyroidectomy to normalize serum calcium and proton pump inhibitors. Thus, in patients with a diagnosis of gastrinoma, the clinical consequence of concern has shifted from peptic ulcer to metastasis.

The vast majority of gastrinomas are situated in the gastrinoma triangle. In MEN1, 90% of gastrinomas are in the duodenum. Early reports of sporadic and MEN1-associated gastrinomas underestimate significantly the frequency of duodenal lesions because they were not systematically sought by duodenotomy. In MEN1, there are usually multiple duodenal, submucosal tumors, mostly <5 mm in size, predominantly in the first and second parts of the duodenum, but ranging through to the first part of the jejunum. They are frequently only possible to feel with a finger on the mucosal surface of the duodenum. These duodenal microadenomas have a high propensity to malignancy (>50%), which is characterized by early spread to the paraduodenal, peripancreatic, and gastrohepatic lymph nodes. Local invasion of the duodenum occurs in less than 50% of cases and is typically limited, with 16% extending into the muscularis mucosae and 27% into the muscularis propria [56]. Metastasis to lymph nodes confers a poorer prognosis but is still consistent with long-term survival. Distant metastasis to the liver occurs late in the course of disease in about 10% of cases and is a marker of poorer prognosis than lymph node metastasis.

True pancreatic gastrinomas are uncommon and are, in a sense, ectopic since the normal adult pancreas does not produce gastrin (gastrin may be found in fetal islet cells). They have a tendency to grow larger than the duodenal lesions, and at sizes greater than 1 cm, they are increasingly likely to metastasize to the liver [57]. Given most ZES patients have small duodenal tumors and islet cell staining is not particularly reliable, some cases of gastrinoma of the pancreas may be spurious. When a pancreatic tumor is the sole lesion removed and the gastrin normalizes, we can be confident of this entity. The gastric antrum is a rare location for gastrinoma. The features of gastrinoma conferring a poorer prognosis are pancreatic (rather than duodenal) tumor, metastases, ectopic Cushing's syndrome, and high gastrin level.

INSULINOMA IN MEN1

Insulinoma is the second most common functioning tumor of the pancreas in the setting of MEN1, occurring in 10%–20% of patients [58]. Twenty-five percent present before the age of 20 years, and uncommonly after the age of 40 years [14]. The hypoglycemic effects of proinsulin and insulin in these patients can be life threatening. Diazoxide and careful dietary manipulation are only partially successful in controlling symptoms. The syndrome may be due to one or more functioning lesions, as determined by intense insulin immunostaining, but many other nonfunctioning or minimally secreting lesions may be present [52,54]. Only 20% of patients had a single macroscopic tumor in the Japanese experience [14]. Insulinomas occur throughout the pancreas with equal distribution. Lesions typically begin to be symptomatic at small size, often less than 1 cm. About one-third are associated with another functioning islet cell tumor, usually gastrinoma. They are malignant in less than 20% of cases in MEN1 [58]. Metastatic spread is to regional lymph nodes and, more commonly, the liver.

Four to ten percent of insulinomas are found in association with MEN1 [5,14]. When insulinoma arises in a young patient, and especially if multiple neuroendocrine tumors are found, the diagnosis of MEN1 should be considered. Shepherd [7] has stressed that insulinoma may present in children and teenagers, and Sakurai et al. reported 20% present before the age of 20 years [14]. In 58% of cases with insulinoma in MEN1, insulinoma was the first presenting MEN1 lesion [59]. The earliest reported in association with MEN1 is 5 years of age [59].

GLUCAGONOMA, VASOACTIVE INTESTINAL PEPTIDE-OMA, AND OTHER FUNCTIONING TUMORS IN MEN1

Symptomatic glucagonoma and VIPoma are rare, 10% of them occurring in the setting of MEN1 and each occurring only in 2% of MEN1 patients. These tumors are frequently larger than 4 cm. About 60% are malignant, and they occur most often in the body and tail of the pancreas. The full clinical syndrome is only seen in index cases. There may be cosecretion of other pancreatic hormones and multiple other MEN1-related tumors. These patients are generally treated by curative or palliative debulking surgery to alleviate life-threatening symptoms. Other clinically significant hormones rarely produced by PNETs in MEN1 include somatostatin, adrenocorticotropic hormone (ACTH), growth hormone-releasing hormone (GHRH), and calcitonin.

NONFUNCTIONING TUMORS

Nonfunctioning tumors are the most common of all islet cell tumors in MEN1. Larger tumors (>3 cm) are more likely to be malignant and may sometimes be aggressive. Burgess reported a 30% rate of metastasis in lesions smaller than 2 cm in size [50]. In index cases, these tumors are likely to be large at presentation because it is not until they cause symptoms from mass effect that they are discovered. However, in a screened population, either elevation of chromogranin A and human pancreatic polypeptide (HPP) or a small mass lesion should be identified early in the course of the tumor.

PREOPERATIVE LOCALIZATION OF PNETS IN MEN1

Despite the fact that the usual surgical strategy for pancreaticoduodenal disease in MEN1 involves full exploration of the pancreas (and duodenum in ZES), with the aid of intraoperative ultrasound, there is vital information to be gained preoperatively. Careful preoperative assessment with CT, somatostatin receptor scintigraphy (SRS), or 5-hydroxytryptophane (5HTP) positron emission tomography (PET), gastroscopy, duodenoscopy, and EUS has several benefits: (1) identification of liver metastases, the single most important reason for imaging, as it may preclude surgery or lead to a different strategy; (2) mapping of the size and location of all visualized tumors; and (3) provision of advanced warning of findings, such as close relationship of a tumor to the pancreatic duct, a large tumor in the head of the pancreas, or major vascular involvement that would require resection and reconstruction.

The addition of calcium stimulation testing for insulinoma and gastrinoma may "regionalize" the source of excess hormone and help to avoid a surgical failure. However, there is no preoperative assessment as accurate as careful intraoperative assessment with intraoperative ultrasound.

SURGERY FOR MEN1 PANCREATICODUODENAL TUMORS

Pancreatic and duodenal disease in MEN1 is multifocal, with multiple synchronous and metachronous lesions being the norm. Nothing short of total pancreaticoduodenectomy could be hoped to be curative in the long term. The morbidity and potential mortality of this surgical strategy prohibit it as a prophylactic measure. Neither persistence nor recurrence of disease necessarily implies a poor prognosis. Even malignant disease frequently has a protracted course [60]. On the other hand, pancreatic endocrine cancer is the leading cause of death in MEN1 today [17,49], and progression is sometimes very rapid. Doherty et al. [22] reported that 46% of patients in 34 kindred died as a result of malignant endocrine tumors at a mean age of 47 years, and that islet cell tumors were the main cause of death. The French national series showed that after 1990, 71% of deaths were

MEN1 related, and of those, 65% were due to metastasis, principally from PNETs [23]. Resection of tumors prior to metastasis could in theory alter long-term survival.

There is general consensus with respect to the need for and type of surgical management of insulinoma, VIPoma, and glucagonoma in MEN1 because unresected, they pose significant clinical problems and risk of malignancy. Management of gastrinomas is, however, most controversial because the syndrome can be medically managed and historically most surgical procedures have resulted in high recurrence rates or significant morbidity. In part, poor surgical results stemmed from lack of awareness of the submucosal duodenal tumors. More recently, there is a growing enthusiasm for a variety of duodenal resection procedures. The timing of surgery for nonfunctioning PNET is also controversial.

In general, the principal aims of surgery are to (1) treat syndromes of hormone excess, (2) treat or prevent cancer, (3) preserve pancreatic function, and (4) do more good than harm. Secondary considerations include (1) facilitation of reoperations for recurrence, (2) cholecystectomy to prevent cholecystitis caused by future somatostatin therapy or liver embolization, and (3) being aware that choledochojejunostomy is a portal for ascending infection if liver therapy such as embolization is needed.

SURGERY FOR INSULINOMA, GLUCAGONOMA, AND VIPOMA IN MEN1

Insulinoma, glucagonoma, and VIPoma, in particular, share some common features. They are usually located in the pancreas. They produce a florid and life-threatening clinical syndrome from hormone excess. Medical treatment becomes increasingly unsatisfactory if the tumor is allowed to grow unchecked. Symptomatic glucagonoma and VIPoma are highly likely to be malignant, while insulinoma may be malignant in up to 20% of cases in MEN1. They should therefore always be resected unless there is significant, untreatable liver metastasis.

It might be possible to cure insulinoma in MEN1 by enucleation of a single tumor, but this is not often a wise practice. In the setting of multiple pancreatic lesions, it is difficult to determine accurately the source of the excess hormone: the functional lesion may remain. Enucleation is suboptimal treatment for larger, potentially malignant lesions, and furthermore, the remaining pancreatic pathology is ignored by such management.

A surgical approach popularized by Thompson [61] and used by others [3,58,62,63] aims to cure insulinoma, remove multiple other tumors, and decrease the likelihood of recurrent PNET. The procedure comprises subtotal pancreatectomy, and depending on the size of tumors and presence of lymph node metastases, the spleen may be resected or preserved. Tumors in the remaining pancreas are enucleated. Intraoperative ultrasound is used to aid identification of all lesions larger than 5 mm, the pancreatic and biliary ductal system, and the portal vein. Prophylactic pancreaticoduodenal lymph node dissection, either in principle [54] or in the case of a pancreatic head lesion greater than 2–3 cm [61], may be added. In the original series [61], all six patients with MEN1-associated insulinoma achieved prolonged cure from hypoglycemia. This operation in the setting of ZES is described in more detail below.

Because VIPoma and glucagonoma are generally large at presentation, concomitant small tumors deep in the residual pancreas may be left without jeopardizing functional cure. On the other hand, for insulinomas, in the absence of very clear regionalization by calcium stimulation to the body or tail, all lesions above 5mm ideally should be resected from the remnant pancreas.

Metachronous lesions can be managed on their merits, by re-enucleation or by completion pancreaticoduodenectomy when the need arises [64].

For large and malignant lesions of the head of the pancreas, either pancreaticoduodenectomy (Whipple) or, sometimes in the presence of widespread PNETs, total pancreaticoduodenectomy is indicated. In the absence of metastatic disease, life expectancy is good [65]. Resection and reconstruction of involved vascular structures (e.g., superior mesenteric artery or vein) is sometimes indicated [65,66].

SURGERY FOR GASTRINOMAS IN MEN1

The indications for surgery and surgical strategy for MEN1 gastrinoma continue to be a most contentious subject of debate. There are three points of general agreement. (1) ZES must first be well controlled with proton pump inhibitors. (2) Correct the hyperparthyroidism. Normalizing serum calcium removes the stimulatory effect of calcium on gastrin secretion. (In one patient [7], parathyroidectomy reduced serum gastrin from 21,000 ng/L to 150 ng/L.) (3) Do not operate if metastatic disease in the liver is extensive and not amenable to excision or ablative therapy.

There are two divergent, broad groups of management strategies. (1) Observe these patients, treat them with proton pump inhibitors, and do not operate unless there is another indication for pancreatic surgery. (2) Operate in cases with clinical ZES regardless of findings of imaging studies, provided there is no evidence of distant metastasis.

The first approach, somewhat nihilistic, is founded on the fact that the pathology is widespread and recurring and the prospect of long-lasting cure by conservative surgery is remote, while extended surgery may produce significant complications. This is the approach of many physicians and perhaps half of the surgeons with expertise in this field [3,55,60,67–69].

But this approach has its disadvantages. By the time operation is undertaken, metastases are frequently present. Imaging is positive due to pancreatic primary or metastatic disease, but rarely due to the small duodenal tumors, which are the usual cause of ZES. It seems rather paradoxical to wait for a tumor to become likely incurable before operating. On the other hand, survival after surgical resection, in patients with advanced disease, may be the same as in patients with limited disease [60].

The second attitude, adopted by many surgeons, may produce long-term remissions from ZES [51,61,70]. In Thompson's series of 43 patients with neuroendocrine pancreaticoduodenal tumors, 37 of whom had gastrinomas, only one patient (with ZES) developed metastasis to the liver after operation [71]; 22/34 (68%) had a normal serum gastrin level at follow-up of up to 19 years, and 9/27 (33%) had a negative secretin test [61]. The 5-, 10-, and 15-year survival in this series was 97%, 94%, and 94%, respectively. In an update from the same center, 8 out of 49 of these patients have been reoperated upon by completion pancreaticoduodenectomy. Seven of these eight had another interim procedure: five had pancreatic enucleation and two had duodenotomy for enucleation [64]. There is a good argument in favor of this approach. Most, if not all, patients with ZES have duodenal microadenomas that are the cause of hypergastrinemia. Half of the patients with duodenal microadenomas will have lymph node metastases. Thorough exploration of the duodenum and resection of potentially involved lymph nodes will result in clinical remission of hypergastrinemia in a majority of patients, and only 10% or fewer of these patients will develop liver metastases. The steps of Thompson's operation [72] (Figure 43.4a and b) are subtotal pancreatectomy, with the line of section to the right of the portal vein, in order to remove all distal tumors; enucleation of all tumors of the head of the pancreas, whether palpable or detected by intraoperative ultrasound; lymph node dissection of the gastrinoma triangle and frozen section examination; routine D1–D3 duodenotomy and excision of all gastrinomas found by endoscopic transillumination and bimanual palpation (submucosal resection is usually adequate, but full-thickness local excision may be required for lesions greater than 5 mm; if duodenotomy is negative, the first jejunal loop should be opened); cholecystectomy; secretin testing [73] to verify the completeness of resection; and excision of adrenal tumors, certainly those greater than 3–4 cm.

OTHER SURGICAL STRATEGIES FOR MEN1 ZES: EXTENDED RESECTIONS

Indications for pancreaticoduodenectomy in MEN1 are arguable, but include periampullary tumors, large or invasive tumors of the head, extensive nodal involvement, numerous duodenal tumors, or a positive intraoperative secretin test. In addition, tumors in the remainder of the pancreas will need to be treated on their merits, if possible leaving adequate pancreas for function. Thus, a Whipple procedure, for example, may be combined with distal pancreatectomy and enucleations, or extended to include the neck and part of the body.

There are a number of surgical groups favoring total duodenectomy and lymph node clearance for MEN1 ZES as the only hope for prolonged surgical control of ZES. Arguably, this is the most logical approach given the distribution of duodenal tumors, the frequency of nodal metastases, and the increasing difficulty of reoperations for recurrence. Surgical procedures to achieve this include Whipple, pylorus-preserving pancreaticoduodenectomy (PPPD), and

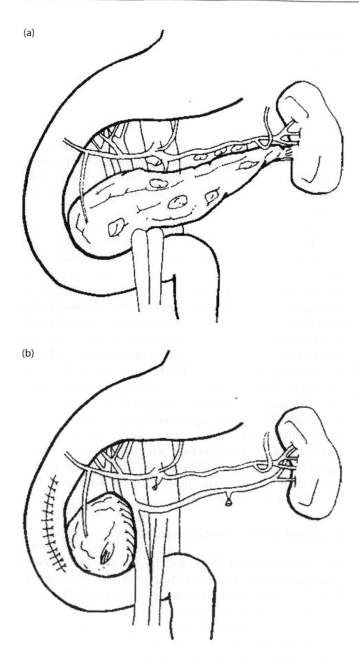

(a)

(b)

Figure 43.4 (a) Diagrammatic representation of the Thompson operation for ZES: preoperation, demonstrating multiple pancreatic tumors and lymph nodes. **(b)** After resection of the distal pancreas, cephalic tumors, lymph nodes, and duodenal lesions.

pancreas-preserving total duodenectomy (PPTD) [74–76]. Each of these can be combined with enucleations or limited distal resections.

As surgical technique evolves and perioperative care of complications improves, these more radical operations have become relatively safe with low mortality, perhaps around 1%, but data from large numbers of patients is lacking. In MEN1 patients, the greatest technical difficulty is the usually soft pancreas with nondilated bile duct.

Bartsch and colleagues [75] have recently reported favorable results from pancreaticoduodenectomy. Thirteen

patients with duodenal gastrinomas underwent pancreaticoduodenectomy resections (group 1, partial pancreaticoduodenectomy [n = 11], total pancreaticoduodenectomy [n = 2]), whereas nine patients had no-pancreaticoduodenectomy resections (group 2) as the initial operative procedure. Perioperative morbidity and mortality, including postoperative diabetes, was similar for groups 1 and 2. After a median follow-up of 136 [3–276] months, 12 (92%) patients of group 1 were eugastrinemic compared with only 3 of 9 (33%) patients of group 2 (p = 0.023). Three (33%) patients of group 2 underwent reoperations for recurrent disease compared with none of group 1.

In uncommon cases with extensive involvement of the entire pancreas, or if there have been prior resections, complications, or pancreatitis, a total pancreaticoduodenectomy may be the best surgical option.

SELECTIVE ENUCLEATION AND NODE RESECTION FOR MEN1 ZES

In the case of ZES, there has been recent increased success with careful assessment and enucleation of duodenal tumors combined with node resection. The advantage of this approach is the lesser procedure, which in the future can be repeated or upgraded to a more extended resection. The disadvantage is a higher rate of persistent or recurrent ZES and perhaps loss of the chance of true cure [75].

SURGERY FOR NONFUNCTIONING PANCREATIC NEUROENDOCRINE TUMORS IN MEN1

The aim of prophylactic surgery for nonfunctioning lesions is prevention of metastasis. Surgical strategy should facilitate future reoperation. Broadly, the strategies are to (1) operate for tumors larger than 1 cm [62,71] or (2) wait until they are >2 cm [46]. The first approach, initially recommended by the Uppsala group [77], is radical in its timing. Can early resection prevent the occurrence of cancer? And is the apparent benefit seen in the early studies more than just a lead-time bias? If reresection is performed for recurrent tumors found by imaging, perhaps one can keep a step ahead of the development of cancer. The concern many surgeons have is that pancreatic surgery is accompanied by a significant morbidity and occasional mortality. Exposure of patients to these risks perhaps 20 years before otherwise necessary is a bold step. Only long-term comparative studies could answer the questions.

The second approach aims for an optimal timing of surgery: to avoid premature surgery and risk of complications in the majority of patients and allowing for a calculated, approximately 10%, risk of metastasis developing prior to surgery [46].

MANAGEMENT OF HEPATIC METASTASES OF PANCREATICODUODENAL DISEASE IN MEN1

Surgery for metastases may be considered if they are favorably located for resection. It is rare to find suitable cases in MEN1. Newer techniques utilizing staged resections may extend the option of surgery to more patients. Literature regarding benefit of surgical treatment over other treatments is lacking. A recent analysis found surgery to be the preferred management only for symptomatic tumors with <25% liver involvement [78]. Ablative therapy has been available in many forms for a long time. Recently, radiofrequency ablation of hepatic lesions has shown promising results. It is suitable for multiple lesions, but not more than about ten. It may be combined with resection and can be repeated.

Medical therapy may be required for symptomatic control of hormone excess: diazoxide for insulinoma, proton pump inhibitors for gastrinoma, and somatostatin for VIPoma. Long-acting somatostin analogs have become a major component of palliation of neuroendocrine tumors. Other therapeutic options include chemotherapy, chemoembolization, radioisotope-labeled somatostatin analogs, and, more recently, tyrosine kinase inhibitors (TKIs) and mammalian target of rapamycin (mTOR) inhibitors.

Pituitary lesions in MEN1

Anterior pituitary lesions are one of the three defining features of MEN1 syndrome. The prevalence in MEN1 varies widely from 30% to 76% in various series. About two-thirds are microadenomas. Prolactinoma is by far the most common lesion, followed by growth hormone-secreting tumor, ACTH secreting, and nonfunctioning (or α subunit secreting). Nearly all types of anterior pituitary tumor have been reported in MEN1. Some large families have a high penetrance of pituitary tumors or predominance of prolactinoma. In 1980, MEN1-Burin, a syndrome of prolactinoma, carcinoid, and HPT in four large families from the Burin Peninsula, Newfoundland, was described [79]. Among 1500 pituitary adenomas surgically resected at the Mayo Clinic, 41 (2.7%) occurred in the setting of MEN1 [80].

Treatment is similar to that of sporadic tumors. Most prolactinomas respond well to medical therapy with cabergoline, although MEN1 prolactinoma may have a more aggressive and therapy-resistant course than sporadic tumors [81].

Foregut-derived carcinoids in MEN1

Thymic carcinoid occurs in less than 5% of MEN1 patients, predominantly in males, with a male-to-female ratio of 20:1 and often with familial clustering [37,82]. It may be aggressively malignant, apparently more so in MEN1 than sporadic tumors. Death from thymic carcinoid is now recognized to be a significant component of the overall death risk from MEN1 [83]. Vigilant screening, especially in males, by CT or MRI at least every 2 years is recommended, and total thymectomy as soon as a lesion is discovered. Radical thymectomy, including, if necessary, pleura, pericardium, vessel wall, or nerve, is the best hope for cure of malignant and locally invasive tumor. Currently, the frequency of thymic carcinoid does not seem to justify routine prophylactic thoracoscopic thymectomy. Note that cervical thymectomy performed during parathyroidectomy only removes the thymic horns and does not preclude the development of thymic carcinoid. It presumably does slightly reduce the risk [84]. Six of 21 patients in the study by Goudet et al. developed thymic carcinoma after cervical thymectomy [37].

Bronchial carcinoid occurs in about 5% of patients, and is seen mostly in females with a ratio of 15:4. Seventy-four percent are benign in behavior with indolent growth. In MEN1, they may be more prone to carcinoid syndrome. Smaller, slow-growing carcinoids of the lung may be managed by observation. There is an association between bronchial carcinoid and pituitary tumor [82].

Type II gastric ECL cell carcinoids are mainly found in MEN1 patients with ZES during endoscopy. They are common (30%–50%), multiple (90%), and small (usually < 1.5 cm) and are associated with a proliferation of extratumoral ECL cells from which the tumor is thought to originate [85,86]. In 90% of cases, invasion is limited to the submucosa, but metastases to lymph nodes occur in 30% and to the liver in 10%. It is proposed that they arise as a result of gastrin and acid stimulation of increased histamine production in MEN1 ZES. These lesions rarely secrete hormones. They are apparently, in part, genetically determined by mutation of *MEN1*, because they are rarely seen in sporadic ZES [86]. Gauger and Thompson reported two cases, which spontaneously regressed after resection of the gastrinoma [71]. They have been reported to be occasionally aggressive malignancies [87]. It is not clear whether proton pump inhibitors have any direct effect on the natural history of these tumors [88].

Adrenal cortical lesions in MEN1

These occur in about 40% of patients and are often bilateral hyperplasia and nonsecreting. Adenomas (10%–20%) mostly have an indolent clinical course; approximately 10% secrete excess aldosterone or corticosteroid [89]. Adrenocortical carcinomas (2%) may also occur [89,90]. Adrenal lesions are usually seen only in patients who also have pancreatic lesions. Previously, most groups have had a conservative approach to adrenal lesions. There are now multiple reports of unexpected cases of rapid growth while under surveillance, and death from malignant transformation of adrenal disease in MEN1 [89]. Regular screening and resection of lesions with reduced or heterogenous lipid content, growth, size of >3 cm, or excess function is now recommended. Resection of any adrenal lesions during pancreatic surgery should be considered.

Cutaneous manifestations of MEN1

In one study [91], a consecutive sample of 32 individuals with previously diagnosed MEN1 who were not preselected for the presence of skin lesions were examined for cutaneous abnormalities. Multiple facial angiofibromas were observed in 28 (88%) of the patients, with 16 patients (50%) having five or more. Angiofibromas were clinically and histologically identical to those in individuals with tuberous sclerosis. Truncal collagenomas were observed in 23 patients (72%). Also observed were café au lait macules in 12 patients (38%) and lipomas in 11 patients (34%). These are encapsulated and typically do not recur after surgery.

Other lesions

Ependymoma, meningioma, fibrosarcoma, phaeochromocytoma, visceral lipomas, and other lesions have been reported more commonly in MEN1 than in control populations, but remain uncommon in MEN1.

Screening for MEN1

The aims and elements of different screening protocols reflect the resources and management philosophies of the groups involved. For example, the Uppsala group, which has a policy of early surgical intervention for pancreatic disease, has an extensive screening protocol [51]. The most effective initial step is to determine gene carriers by genetic testing. Hormone assays and imaging studies can be rationalized according to the clinical impact of the screened for tumor and the cost-effectiveness of the tests. The range of tests is age dependent, just as the various tumors have characteristic age-related probabilities of onset (Table 43.2). Potential consequences of false-positive results, radiation exposure, and complications of surgical treatment need to be considered.

Table 43.2 Suggested screening protocol for MEN1

Essential biochemical screening: Annual from age 5 years

Serum calcium (prefer ionized) and PTH

Glucose with simultaneous insulin

Gastrin (from age 15 years)

Prolactin and IGF-1

Comprehensive biochemical screening: 2-yearly from age 10 years

Pancreatic polypeptide

Chromogranin A

VIP

Glucagon

Calcitonin, GHRH, ACTH, and somatostatin

Essential imaging: 2-yearly from age 15 years

High-quality contrast-enhanced spiral CT of chest and abdomen

(Abdominal CT may be replaced by MRI)

MRI of pituitary

Imaging: Optional

Upper gastrointestinal endoscopy/endoscopic ultrasound of the pancreas

Octreotide or PET scan

HPT is easily screened with annual ionized calcium or corrected calcium and PTH. Screening should certainly begin by 10 years of age and be continued for life—even after surgery [3,5]. Imaging is not indicated for screening.

Screening for pituitary disease is also relatively straightforward; a typical program might be annual prolactin and insulin-like growth factor 1 (IGF-1), with 2- to 3-yearly MRI for nonfunctioning tumors. Screening should begin at around 5 years of age, as the earliest reported morbid lesion was an aggressive pituitary macroadenoma at the age of 5 years [92].

With respect to pancreaticoduodenal disease, the most common functioning lesions, insulinoma and gastrinoma, and any pancreatic lesions greater than 2 cm have the most impact on patients. Thus, screening should at least aim to detect subclinical insulinoma and gastrinoma and tumors of this size. A minimal program would include annual fasting glucose with simultaneous insulin and proinsulin (from age 5 to 40 years), gastrin (age 15+), and high-quality imaging every 2–3 years (CT, MRI, or EUS) [3,5]. Glucagon, chromogranin A, HPP, and VIP should be monitored at least every 2–3 years. More rigorous biochemical screening may include somatostatin and other rarer hormones.

A 72-hour supervised fast may be indicated to confirm the diagnosis of insulinoma. A secretin stimulation test may be used to confirm gastrinoma. Endoscopic ultrasound is the most sensitive imaging study for pancreatic tumors [93], being able to detect lesions of around 3 mm in size in favorable patients, and should be considered along with CT. MRI may be used to spare radiation exposure. A variety of PET tracers, including 5HTP, L-DOPA, and Ga-octreotate, can be used for PNETs and have the highest sensitivity of all radiological imaging modalities. Duodenal microadenomas will not usually be detected by any scan, and EUS has only been able to detect perhaps half to two-thirds of lesions.

MEN2

MEN2 encompasses MEN2A, MEN2B, and FMTC. MEN2A comprises MTC, PCC, and HPT. MEN2B is a syndrome of precocious MTC, PCC, characteristic facies, marfanoid habitus, and intestinal ganglioneuromatosis. FMTC is a subset of MEN2A, formally defined by expression only of MTC in a family with more than 10 kindred members over multiple generations.

Sipple [94] first described the association of thyroid carcinoma and PCC in 1961, and the MEN2A syndrome is sometimes referred to as Sipple's syndrome. In 1966, Williams and Pollock described a family with the features of MEN2B [95]. Subsequently, in 1968 Gorlin et al. [96] and Steiner et al. [97] described the MEN2B syndrome. A recent study in Germany estimated the incidence is 1 in 100,000 and prevalence is 1 in 80,000 [98].

MEN2A is dominated by the development of MTC, with almost 100% penetrance. Multifocal C-cell hyperplasia (CCH) is the universal precursor to MTC. PCC occurs in 50% and is bilateral in most patients with MEN2B and patients with a codon 634 mutation in MEN2A, but is an uncommon feature of most other MEN2A mutations. HPT is most common in patients with a codon 634 mutation (reaching 80% penetrance after 70 years of age [99]) and is uncommon in most other MEN2A mutations. HPT is clinically relatively insignificant in MEN2 and does not occur in MEN2B.

Two other MEN2 phenotypic variants have been described: MEN2 with cutaneous lichen amyloidosis (CLA) and MEN2 with Hirschsprung's disease (HSCR) (Table 43.3).

MEN2 syndromes result in disease-related death in perhaps 50% of index cases and obligate carriers because of sudden death from PCC, or because MTC or PCC is metastatic at the time of clinical recognition. The outlook for known gene carriers is vastly different. It is now routine to perform prophylactic thyroidectomy to prevent MTC and to screen for and excise PCC before morbidity arises.

Up to 20% of newly diagnosed MTC and less than 5% of new PCC may prove to be associated with MEN2. MEN2 rarely presents as HPT. One of the fundamental tenets of endocrine surgery is that one must always think of and rule out the presence of PCC when assessing a patient with MTC, and certainly before proceeding to an anesthetic to remove the thyroid.

Table 43.3 Clinical characteristics of MEN2 syndromes

Syndrome	Characteristics
MEN2A: Codon 634	MTC: Childhood onset usually 95% penetrance by age 60
	PCC: 70% penetrance by age 60 >80% bilateral
	HPT: 33% penetrance by age 60
MEN2A: Other codons	MTC: 50%–95% penetrance by age 60
	PCC: 0%–20%; codon-specific penetrance
	HPT: 0%–4%; codon-specific penetrance
MEN2B	MTC: <1 year age; lymph node metastases at not of <5 years age
	PCC: >50%; >50% bilateral
	Intestinal and submucosal ganglioneuromas
	Characteristic facies and marfanoid habitus
	Mucosal ganglioneuromas: Tongue, lips, and eyelids
FMTC	MTC: Least aggressive variant
	By definition: No PCC or HPT in kindred
MEN2A and CLA	MEN2A: Almost exclusively codon 634
	Pruritic, lichenoid lesions of the interscapular region
MEN2A or FMTC and HSCR	MEN2A or FMTC: Exon 10; majority codon 620 and Hirschsprung's disease

MEN2 genetics

The *RET* proto-oncogene was identified as the locus of mutations causing MEN2 in 1993. The following year, evidence of a correlation between specific mutations and phenotypes was noted [100] (Table 43.4). The *RET* (rearranged during transfection) gene is located near the centromere of chromosome 10 at 10q11.2. *RET* contains 21 exons and encodes ret, a membrane-bound tyrosine kinase enzyme with an extracellular cadherin-like ligand binding site, cysteine-rich extracellular domains, a transmembrane domain, two intracellular tyrosine kinase domains, and an intracellular catalytic core (Figure 43.5).

RET is expressed mainly in cells of neural crest origin, but particularly the thyroid C-cells, adrenal medullary chromaffin cells, and to a lesser extent, parathyroid cells. Ret is involved in cell growth, differentiation, and survival.

MEN2 results from activating germline mutations in *RET*. In most cases, there is a change of a single amino acid. Mutations may occur in both the extracellular and intracellular domain sites of the gene. The result is activation of ret by different means:

1. Directly activating the enzyme's intracellular catalytic core, rendering the receptor activated in the monomeric state. This is the mechanism for MEN2B and has the highest transforming activity.
2. Homodimerization of the extracellular component (this normally occurs only as a result of ligand binding), which leads to autophosphorylation of the intracellular tyrosine kinase residues and activation of downstream pathways. This is the mechanism involved in MEN2A and some FMTCs, and it has variable transforming activity.
3. Interference with ATP binding at the intracellular tyrosine kinase domains. This mechanism causes principally FMTC and has the lowest transforming activity.

The oncogenic activation of the RET receptor as an inherited "first hit" is believed to cause CCH. Progression to MTC is thought to depend on secondary somatic hits' in activated C-cells [101] occurring by "the play of chance" or, more technically, in a stochastic manner. The factors behind this are still a matter of investigation.

Genetic testing in MEN2 is far simpler than for MEN1 and is extremely reliable. The false-positive and false-negative rates are very low. A mutation can be identified in the *RET* gene in 98% of index cases. A limited number of common mutations have been identified, principally involving exons 10, 11, 13, 14, 15, and 16. MEN2A patients have mutations in the extracellular, cysteine-rich residues. Forty to seventy-five percent of MEN2A patients have a mutation in codon 634 of exon 11; others principally in exon 10 (codons 609, 610, 611, 618, and 620). FMTC patients have mutations in the extracellular, cysteine-rich residues, spread over exons 10, 11, 13, and 14 and some in the intracellular tyrosine kinase domain in exon 15. There is overlapping of the

Table 43.4 Genotype–phenotype correlation in MEN2*

Syndrome	Mutation					
	Exon 10	Exon 11	Exon 13	Exon 14	Exon 15	Exon 16
MEN2A	609, 611, 618, 620	630, **634**, 635, 637	790		891	
MEN2A and CLA		**634**				
MEN2A and HSCR	609, 611, 618, **620**					
MEN2B				804a	883	**918**
FMTC	609, 611, 618, 620	630	768, **790, 791**	**804**		

* In conjunction with second mutation on the same allele.

mutations found in FMTC with those in MEN2A. Ninety-five percent of MEN2B patients have a mutation in codon 918 of exon 16, occasionally in codon 883 of exon 15, and rarely tandem mutations (V804M is one of the two mutations in each of these). In recent years, many new pathogenic mutations have been identified, including some arising in exons 5 and 8, and other mutations of uncertain significance in exons 9 and 18. An online repository for sharing of information on RET mutations was created in 2009 [102] (Table 43.4) has a more detailed analysis of the location of mutations and genotype–phenotype relations.

Currently, genetic testing in possible index cases is directed to sequencing of particular exons in an order based on phenotype and frequency of mutations. Typically, testing for the MEN2A phenotype would start with exon 11 and then exon 10: 95% of mutations will be found here. Subsequent testing would be of exons 13–15. When the clinical diagnosis is clear but no mutation has been found after testing exons 10–15, the next step is sequencing of the entire coding region [103]. New techniques of next-generation and whole exome sequencing are likely to revolutionize testing.

MEN2A (Sipple's syndrome) (OMIM #171400)

MEN2A is a clinical syndrome of MTC in 90%–100% of cases, PCC in 50%, and multigland parathyroid disease (HPT) in 30%–50% (Table 43.3) [99,103,104]. Prior to recognition of the syndrome, and screening of family members, death from MTC occurred in about 20% of cases. Sudden death from PCC was equally as frequent. New index cases arising from *de novo* germline mutations in 5% of MEN2A [105], and previously unrecognized kindred still result in late presentations and death from MTC and PCC. The most frequent mutation is codon 634, although throughout the world, the percentage of MEN2A due to 634 mutation is widely variable, ranging from 40% [106,107] up to 100% reported in mainland China [108]. The codon 634 mutation in MEN2A is also the most penetrant and aggressive, and frequently associated with PCC and HPT. As more investigation is carried out, the proportion of 634 cases is falling as cases of apparently sporadic MTC are discovered to be milder variants, and families thought to have been FMTC

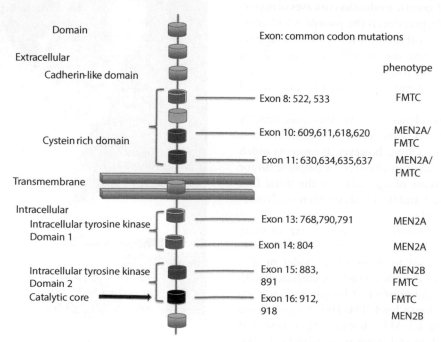

Figure 43.5 Schematic representation of the RET receptor protein and relationship between *RET* mutations and phenotype.

are reclassified as MEN2A [109]. Outside of the 634 muta-tion, PCC and HPT are less common. Frank-Raue et al. reported genotype–phenotype correlations in 340 patients with exon 10 mutations: PCC was seen in 26% of 609, 10% of 611, 23% of 618, and 13% of 620 mutations, and PCC was bilateral in 28% of cases [110]. For exon 10 overall, the penetrance of PCC by age 60 was 33% compared with 70% in the 634 mutation. The penetrance of HPT at age 60 was 3.7% compared with 33.8% for the 634 mutation. Exon 13 and 14 mutations are even less often associated with PCC and HPT.

C-CELL HYPERPLASIA

CCH is defined as more than six C-cells per follicle, clus-ters of C-cells, or more than 50 C-cells per low-power field. Outside of the setting of MEN2, CCH (secondary CCH) has been described in men, smokers, aging individuals, and patients with thyroiditis, renal impairment, HPT, hyper-gastrinemia, and near follicular derived tumors, usually malignancies.

CCH in MEN2 has a penetrance of nearly 100%, is mul-ticentric, and mirrors the normal distribution of C-cells: primarily in the upper half of each lobe.

MTC may be diagnosed when there is focal loss, redupli-cation, or disruption of the basement membrane, but usu-ally it is more obvious: characterized by follicles infiltrated, filled, or replaced by C-cells.

MEDULLARY THYROID CANCER IN MEN2A

Medullary cancer of the thyroid is genetically linked in 12%–25% of cases [1] almost exclusively to MEN2. Of these, 95% have MEN2A/FMTC and 5% have MEN2B. MTC is a nearly constant finding in MEN2A [104,111].

What is the value of genetic evaluation in cases of appar-ently sporadic MTC? In practice, if the patient is >40 years of age and there is a unifocal tumor, the likelihood of appar-ently sporadic MTC being due to MEN2 is around 2% [112,113]. Nevertheless, the importance of a positive genetic test for MEN2 means that most patients with MTC should be tested.

In MEN2A, the prevalence of MTC increases steadily with age. By the age of 60 years, about 90% of individuals will have clinical MTC. Often, however, it presents much earlier and may be detected in children. A palpable tumor is unusual before 10 years of age. MTC is the usual first manifestation of MEN2A and the most common syndrome-related cause of death today.

When the tumor is greater than 2 cm in size, or there are >10 neck nodes involved, it is usually incurable because of unresectable metastases to mediastinal nodes or dis-tant organs. The risk of distant metastasis correlates with the number of nodes, the number of lymph node regions involved, and the calcitonin level [114–116]. Surgery is the sole effective treatment for MTC because MTC does not take up radioactive iodine and is not responsive to chemo-therapy, radiotherapy, or hormonal treatment.

HISTOPATHOLOGY AND BIOCHEMISTRY OF MTC IN MEN2

MTC in MEN2 variants is characteristically multifocal and arises in a background of CCH (Figure 43.6).

There is otherwise no distinction between sporadic and hereditary MTC histologically. The progression from CCH to MTC is very variable and may be precocious, as in MEN2B, or never clinically evident in some low-risk gene carriers with FMTC. The aggressiveness of the disease depends upon the transforming potential of the specific genetic mutation.

CCH and MTC almost always are accompanied by secretion of calcitonin, but also a number of other peptide hormones, particularly CEA and chromogranin A. The stimulated calcitonin level may be elevated in the presence of CCH, and the basal or stimulated level may be elevated in MTC [117]. A tumor greater than 5 mm in size can always be biochemically detected [118]. In general, tumor burden is well correlated with calcitonin level. However, occasional patients with negative stimulated calcitonin and small lymph node metastases are reported [114,119]. Elevated cal-citonin is a useful marker of persistent disease after surgery for MTC.

Palpable MTC is associated with high rates of nodal invasion: 80% to the central compartment (level VI), 75% to the ipsilateral and 50% to the contralateral neck (levels II–V), and 30% to the upper mediastinum (level VII) [120]. Distant metastasis is primarily to the liver, central medias-tinal lymph nodes, and lungs.

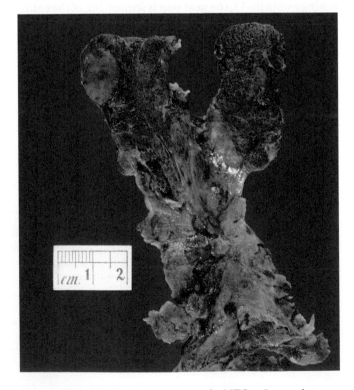

Figure 43.6 "Owl's-eye" upper-pole MTCs: Coronal sec-tion of thyroid in a 16-year-old girl with 634 mutation.

SURGERY FOR CLINICAL MTC IN MEN2

Total thyroidectomy plus central lymph node dissection (CLND) is required in all cases of clinical MTC in MEN2 (Figure 43.7a and b). Management of the parathyroid glands is discussed below. The indications for ipsilateral and contralateral neck and mediastinal lymph node dissections have been debated. Previously, there was a near consensus toward extensive surgery, including bilateral neck dissections, as a routine for MTC [114,117,120–122]. There is an emerging preference to tailor the extent of surgery according to factors, including specific mutated codon; level of basal or stimulated calcitonin; ultrasound and CT examination of nodes, size, and bilaterality of the primary; and operative finding of central lymphadenopathy [1,123,124]. Tumor biology is variable between patients. For example, some patients with larger primary tumors and FMTC have no nodal involvement, while some patients with microscopic MTC and the 634 mutation have extensive node involvement.

While single-stage surgery is ideal, lateral neck or mediastinal node dissection has potential morbidity and may

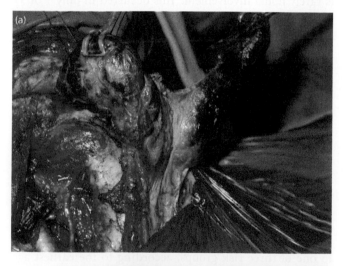

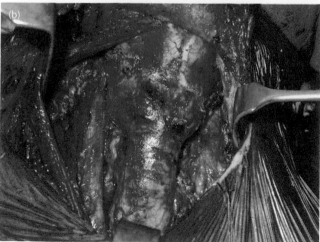

Figure 43.7 **(a and b)** Bilateral central and lateral neck dissections for MEN2A with nodal disease.

yield no pathological nodes. The smaller the tumor and lower the calcitonin, the more unlikely that N1b nodes will be involved. Furthermore, unlike central node dissections, lateral node dissections can be readily performed as a second procedure if disease persistence is confirmed and localized.

It is doubtful whether delayed removal of lateral nodes, until the time they are first identified by ultrasound, has any survival disadvantage compared with removal at the time of thyroidectomy, although this has been reported [121].

The presence of ipsilateral, lateral neck nodes reduces the biochemical cure rate from >90% to <40% [126]. The presence of contralateral, lateral neck nodes is, of itself, an indication of likely metastatic disease with little hope of biochemical cure [115,116,126].

When serum calcitonin is high (>5000 pg/mL), the likelihood of distant metastatic disease is great. In these cases, staging of the disease by CT scan of the chest and abdomen is indicated. If CT staging is negative, laparoscopy to identify liver metastasis may be considered prior to radical thyroid surgery.

The finding of metastatic disease changes the goal of surgery from possible cure to local control of disease. Distant metastasis is not, however, incompatible with long-term survival, as many cases of MTC are relatively indolent despite their tendency to metastasize early. Total thyroidectomy and central node clearance may prevent death and morbidity from local tumor growth in the neck.

PROPHYLACTIC THYROID SURGERY FOR GENE CARRIERS IN MEN2

In principle, all gene carriers might be prevented from developing MTC by timely prophylactic thyroidectomy. However, the details of how this is best achieved, optimizing the timing and extent of surgery, are debated. When surgery is performed early enough, central node dissection, with its small incremental risks of injury to the recurrent laryngeal nerve and hypoparathyroidism, is not necessary. However, the risks of surgery in very young children are greater. There are risks associated with persistence and recurrence when surgery is delayed too long for cure at the initial operation.

Prior to the genetic revolution, all first-degree relatives had to be screened. The pentagastrin stimulation test was not sufficiently reliable because of false positives and the inability to differentiate CCH from MTC [114,119]. Kindred members without MEN2 have undergone surgery on the basis of elevated calcitonin [119]. Eighty percent of patients with a stimulated calcitonin test of >100 but less than 560 pg/mL have CCH and not MTC [117]. Conversely, by the time stimulated calcitonin testing becomes positive, rare patients with normal basal calcitonin will have nodal metastasis [114]. Today, 50% of first-degree relatives can be confirmed not to have the mutation and therefore set free from surveillance. The 50% who are gene carriers have a near 100% lifetime risk of developing a potentially lethal tumor and have a strong indication for prophylactic thyroid surgery.

There is evidence that prophylactic thyroidectomy can remove the risk of MTC for life. Prophylactic total thyroidectomy and central node dissection in teenagers, on the basis of positive calcitonin testing, have shown evidence of cure, in most cases, at long-term follow-up [114,127]. There is also evidence that the risk of recurrence, morbidity, and death is greatly reduced, even when "prophylactic" surgery is undertaken after malignant transformation has occurred [123,128,129].

Wells and colleagues [128] in 1994 were the first to report prophylactic thyroidectomy on the basis of positive genetic testing in children. These patients had an average age of 13 years. The absence of nodal involvement in the 13 patients in this series gave hope for cure in these patients. However, in 10 of the patients, macroscopic or microscopic MTC was found; thus, the operation was effectively therapeutic or secondary prophylactic, rather than primary prophylactic. In three out of six of these patients, who had negative pentagastrin tests, microscopic MTC was already present.

There was no persistent or recurrent MTC in a series of 50 children when they underwent prophylactic thyroidectomy *and* central neck dissection before age 8 years [130]. By contrast, six children who had undergone surgery at ages 8, 10, 11, 14, 16, and 19 years with RET mutations in codons 634, 620, 618, 620, 634, and 618, respectively, had persistent or recurrent disease postoperatively. Two had major postoperative elevations of basal calcitonin. In four, the stimulated levels were only 6, 7, 20, and 22 pg/mL. The long-term clinical significance of such minimal biochemical recurrences is yet to be seen. Interestingly, of these six children, four had no evidence of lymph node metastases on histopathology, and of the three patients with lymph node metastases at surgery, only one remained biochemically free of disease.

In another series of 46 MEN2A or FMTC children who underwent prophylactic thyroidectomy between age 4 years and 21 years, no patient was found to have involved nodes, but 5 (11%) experienced biochemical persistence (2 patients) or recurrence (3 patients) after more than 10 years' follow-up, all of whom were operated on at age 13 years or later, and all of whom had central node dissection [131]. Thus, histopathologic node-negative status does not equate to cure. The obvious conclusion must be drawn that surgery was too late in many of these children.

At the other end of the age scale, three MEN2A (634 mutation) children under 12 months of age were operated upon on the basis of elevated calcitonin [132]. In the second and third patients, central node dissection was performed. Micro-MTC was found in all three, but no nodes were involved. Some have argued from such cases that prophylactic surgery needs to be performed at this young age in some patients with 634 (and other) mutations when calcitonin is elevated.

The time from development of MTC to node development seems to be significant and somewhat predictable. Machens et al. [133] reported that for codon 634 mutations, the mean age of the patients at progression to various stages was 6.9 years for CCH, 10.1 years for node-negative medullary thyroid carcinoma, and 16.7 years for node-positive medullary thyroid carcinoma: a 6.6-year mean interval from intrathyroidal cancer to nodal spread. Based on this information, it seems that curative surgery can be achieved, without central node dissection, even in the presence of microscopic MTC at histopathology.

The risk of nodal disease as determined by genotype, the age of the child at the time of surgery, and the calcitonin level may be used to decide the need for node dissection in individual cases [1,114,134]. Up to the age of 5 and with only very rare exceptions, nodal metastasis does not occur in MEN2A, but only in MEN2B [115].

Pentagastrin stimulation has a low sensitivity for small tumors. In one study of patients with stimulated calcitonin below the upper reference range for normal (on various assays), 6 of 27 cases had pathologically proven micro-MTC, and in 1 of 27 cases, a lymph node metastasis was present [114]. However, in another study totaling 170 patients, no case with positive nodes in patients with a basal calcitonin of <30 ng/L has been reported [129]. In patients with a positive provocation test but normal baseline calcitonin, there is rarely nodal involvement. This occurred in only 1 of 34 patients in one series [125]. Similarly, when the stimulation test was positive but the level was less than 130 pg/mL, none of 20 patients had nodal involvement [119].

The reference values for basal serum calcitonin levels are <12 pg/mL for males and <5 pg/mL for females. They vary in children, especially in neonates (<40 pg/mL in children under 6 months of age, <15 pg/mL in children between 6 months and 3 years of age). Beyond the age of 3 years, the values are indistinguishable from those observed in adults [135].

GUIDELINES FOR PROPHYLACTIC SURGERY ACCORDING TO RISK STRATIFICATION IN MEN2

Pooled international experience of MEN2 syndromes led to the first guidelines, known as the Gubbio consensus [3]. Each of the known *RET* mutations was allocated to one of three risk groups, according to the earliest age at which MTC is likely to develop. The American Thyroid Association (ATA) 2009 guidelines for MTC [1] provided more detailed codon-by-codon analysis and, rightly, separated the 634 mutation into a risk group of its own. See Table 43.5 for more detail.

As defined in the ATA 2009 guidelines, the four risk groups and surgical strategies are as follows:

Risk group D. The highest-risk group is that of children with MEN2B associated with *RET* mutations of codon 918. MTC develops in the first year of life. Surgery for these children should be in infancy.

Risk group C. The very high-risk group, a subset of MEN2A, comprising *RET* mutations of codon 634. Surgery is recommended before 5 years of age. In rare patients with codon 634 mutations, involved lymph nodes have been found at the age of 5 [136], while in others, microscopic MTC has been found at the ages of 1 [132] and of 2 [133,137].

Table 43.5 Correlation of RET codon mutation, risk of MTC, and recommended age for prophylactic thyroidectomy or calcitonin screening (for more common mutations)

Risk group	Mutations	Recommended age for surgery / Role for calcitonin screening
Extreme	918	1–6 months / No role for calcitonin screening?
Very high	883, 634, 804 tandem, 630	2–5 years / Calcitonin screening from 2 years
High	609, 611, 618, 620	5–10 years / Determined by calcitonin from 2 years
Least high	768, 790, 791, 804, 891	>10 years / Determined by calcitonin from 5 years

Risk group B. The high-risk group comprising exon 10 and codon 609, 611, 618, and 620 mutations. Group B mutations present slightly later and more variably than group C mutations. Prophylactic thyroidectomy is recommended at <5 years of age to ensure cure. Surgery may be delayed if the parents wish, if ultrasound and stimulated calcitonin are normal, and if family history is less aggressive.

Risk group A. The least high-risk group comprising children with *RET* mutations in exons 13, 14, and 15 and codons 768, 790, 791, 804, and 891. The natural history of MTC in carriers of these mutations is variable, but generally, MTC develops at a later age, occasionally not at all, and grows more slowly. Lymph node metastasis or death is uncommon in patients with these mutations [114,138]. They should be recommended to undergo total thyroidectomy. However, in risk group A, this can be delayed beyond 5 years of age. Some recommend 10 years of age, when the child is larger and more mature, and others wait for provocation testing to become positive.

Publication of the ATA 2009 guidelines stimulated a new round of international discussion. Most recently, the ATA 2015 guidelines were released [2]. The main change was a merging of risk groups A and B, recognizing the highly variable age of onset of MTC within these groups and increasing reliance upon calcitonin testing rather than age alone to dictate timing of surgery for these groups. MEN2B 883 and tandem mutations involving V804M are no longer treated as aggressively as 918, and given their rarity, care should be individualized.

Within risk group B, the 620 mutation has a much earlier age of onset of MTC (median 9 years) and a much greater penetrance of 85%–95% by 50 years than other mutations [110,139]. Within the group of exon 10 mutations, there is a trend to earlier presentation and more aggressive disease from codon 609, in numerical order, to codon 620; however, one patient with 609 had MTC at age 4, and another nodal metastasis at age 9 [110].

RET mutation-based risk stratification is considered by some authors a crude tool that does not match clinical experience [123]. In a cohort of 84 patients, 53 were operated upon but 30 are still under surveillance. Intrathyroidal tumors were found when basal CT was below 60 pg/mL, whereas either node metastases or larger tumors were observed when CT was above 60 pg/mL. No correlation between serum CT, age, and type of *RET* mutation was observed [123]. The authors recommended stimulated calcitonin to define the timing of surgery.

In a multicenter study of 170 patients [129], cure was observed in all patients with a preoperative basal CT level below 30 ng/L regardless of the genotype, suggesting a simple definition of timely surgery. It should be noted that many patients in this retrospective study had central and lateral neck dissections because they already had tumors and elevated calcitonin. For less aggressive FMTC classes A or B, a higher basal threshold of 100 pg/mL was recommended as timely; in their study, only one of 56 patients had MTC below this cutoff, and all were N0.

Machens and Dralle [140] proposed, "The mutation's risk profile determines the frame within which screening for the tumor marker calcitonin is employed to refine the accuracy of the prediction." The 2012 European Thyroid Association Guidelines for Genetic Testing and Its Clinical Consequences in Medullary Thyroid Cancer placed more reliance upon calcitonin testing than genetic, risk-based stratification [4] (Figure 43.8).

The European Society of Endocrine Surgeons (ESES) consensus describes the genotype–age–calcitonin (GAC) concept [142]: "Although no data are as yet available, calcitonin measurements are recommended every 6 months in 'C,' annually in 'B' and every 2 years in 'A,' respectively. The moment of transition from C-cell hyperplasia to MTC seems to occur when calcitonin levels rise upon stimulation" [140,141].

These calcitonin-based approaches have the advantage that surgical complications are delayed until "necessary." This is perhaps particularly relevant when discussing surgery in children prior to 5 years of age. The concern remains that the opportunity to cure may be missed and the patient will have a lifetime of anxiety and unpleasant annual stimulation test.

Is it necessary to perform CLND for prophylactic surgery in MEN2A? The answer is that it should not be; i.e.,

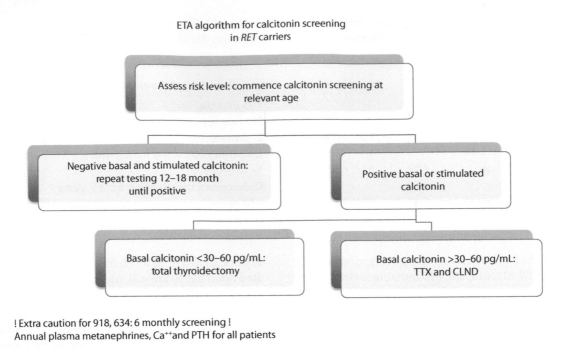

ETA algorithm for calcitonin screening
in *RET* carriers

Assess risk level: commence calcitonin screening at relevant age

Negative basal and stimulated calcitonin: repeat testing 12–18 month until positive

Positive basal or stimulated calcitonin

Basal calcitonin <30–60 pg/mL: total thyroidectomy

Basal calcitonin >30–60 pg/mL: TTX and CLND

! Extra caution for 918, 634: 6 monthly screening !
Annual plasma metanephrines, Ca⁺⁺and PTH for all patients

Figure 43.8 Algorithm for calcitonin-directed prophylactic thyroid surgery in MEN2A/FMTC. (Modified from Elisei R et al. *Eur Thyroid J* 2013;1:216–31.)

surgery should be performed before node resection is indicated. Up to the age of 5 years, CLND should rarely be necessary. For level B and A mutations, early prophylactic surgery before 10 years of age or before basal calcitonin reaches 30–60 pg/mL should not be required [4,123,129]. German guidelines recommend CLND if the basal CT is elevated but do not consider groups A and B separately [124]. The ATA's 2009 Guideline Recommendation 42 is that in MEN2A and FMTC, when all lesions are <5 mm and if basal CT is less than 40 pg/mL, CLND may be omitted. The ATA's 2015 Guideline Recommendation 35 for the 634 mutation is for CLND for basal CT greater than 40 or evidence of nodal metastases. Notably, for all other MEN2A and FMTC mutations, CLND is not mentioned with prophylactic surgery: timely surgery is prior to the need for CLND.

If prophylactic total thyroidectomy with or without central node clearance is to be performed in children, it is important that the complications of surgery do not outweigh the benefit of prophylaxis.

PHEOCHROMOCYTOMA IN MEN2

PCC in MEN2 once carried a significant morbidity and a mortality rate of around 20%. Only index cases should now be at risk. Never should medullary carcinoma of the thyroid be tackled before exclusion of PCC.

PCC occurs in 30%–50% of patients with MEN2, with a wide family variation, between 0% and 100% [103,104,110,137,142,143]. The penetrance and the age at diagnosis of PCC among different MEN2 kindred varies by *RET* mutation with a 50%–92% occurrence in codon 634, 22%–42% in codon 618, 9%–23% in codon 620, and 4%–47% in

codon 609, rarely in patients with exon 14 and 15 mutations, but in 40%–50% of MEN2B patients with codon 918 mutation [110,129,139,142] (the highest figure given for each codon in exon 10 represents the prevalence at age 60 years [110]).

In approximately 60% of patients with PCC (>80% in 634 mutation) there is a synchronous or metachronous contralateral PCC (Figure 43.9). In 10%–27% of cases, they are the presenting lesion, occurring 10 years prior to MTC in 8.5% of cases [144,145]. In 15 cases when PCC was the first presentation, only 5 had MTC at that time [144]. They are ectopic in 4% and malignant in 3% of cases. They preferentially secrete adrenaline rather than noradrenaline [143].

Codon 634 mutation carriers have a 92% likelihood of developing PCC by 70 years of age [143], and PCC has been reported as early as 12 years of age. Screening for PCC can be stratified by risk according to mutation, just as for MTC [3,98].

Screening for early evidence of PCC in MEN2 should begin at 10 years for 634 and 918 mutations and by 20 years of age in all others with at-risk codon mutations. The diagnosis, imaging, and preparation for surgery of patients with PCC are covered elsewhere in this book.

Adrenal medullary hyperplasia is a feature of MEN2, preceding tumor development. In approximately 50% of cases of unilateral PCC, a lesion develops in the contralateral gland after an average interval of 7 years [146]. Some groups in the past therefore advocated systematic bilateral adrenalectomy in MEN2 [147]. The main objection to this strategy is that the patient risks Addisonian crisis in up to 25% of cases [146,148]. Perhaps 50% of patients will not develop a contralateral tumor and have no clinical need for bilateral surgery. Screening for development of another

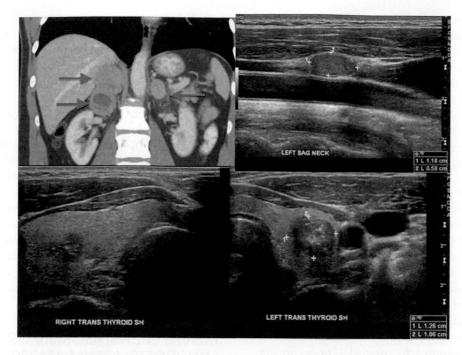

Figure 43.9 Thirty-eight-year-old male, index case of MEN2A, 634 mutation, presented with typical adrenergic symptoms and calcitonin-induced diarrhea. Three adrenal PCCs, bilateral MTC with lateral nodes, no HPT present.

PCC is simple and has shown no increase in morbidity due to delayed diagnosis. More recently, partial or subtotal adrenalectomy has increasingly been performed for PCC [149–151]. In one series, there was only a 3% recurrence after subtotal compared with 2% after total adrenalectomy [150]. In another series [149], metachronous tumors in the remnant occurred in 21% of patients, with a follow-up of 11 years, but this may result in no survival disadvantage to the patient and the risk of Addisonian crisis is delayed. Despite the presence of medullary hyperplasia, there does not seem to be a concern regarding fracturing of the medulla and seeding the abdomen. Some surgeons would preserve adrenal tissue even at the first side to be addressed; others would do so only for the second side.

PHEOCHROMOCYTOMA IN MEN2: SURGICAL APPROACH

The traditional approach to PCC in the setting of MEN2 was a large midline or bisubcostal incision allowing bilateral adrenal examination and exploration of all sites of possible paragangliomas and nodal and liver metastasis prior to resection of the tumor. Now that laparoscopic surgery is the optimal approach and preoperative localization is undertaken, routine exploration of the entire abdomen is no longer necessary. Modern imaging with CT, MRI, metaiodobenzylguanidine (MIBG), or Ga-DOTATATE has virtually eliminated the unexpected finding of multifocal, malignant, or metastatic disease [152].

Open adrenal resection for PCC requires gentle handling to avoid hypertensive crises. Early control of venous drainage is usually recommended, but in practice, even right-sided tumors have multiple significant veins and catechols

may freely enter the circulation until resection is near complete. For larger tumors, a total adrenalectomy including the periadrenal fat is recommended to minimize the risk of capsular rupture and ensure complete resection of the tumor. Rare malignant lesions may require open, *en bloc* resection of adjacent organs and lymph nodes.

There is evidence that patients are more stable during laparoscopy than in open surgery [153–155]. Most authors would now perform bilateral adrenalectomy or subtotal adrenalectomy, when indicated and technically possible, laparoscopically.

HYPERPARATHYROIDISM IN MEN2

HPT is reported in only 17%–30% of cases of MEN2A [104,156]. It often has a late presentation, after 40 years of age, and uncommonly reveals the syndrome. Frequently, patients with HPT are normocalcemic or asymptomatic. But 23% of patients had stones, and the mean calcium was 2.8 mmol/L, with a calcium of up to 3.7 mmol/L, in the French GETC report [156]. HPT in MEN2 is genetically determined, is not a secondary response to calcitonin, and is highly associated with a mutation of codon 634. Its overall prevalence in patients with codon 634 mutation is 19%, but it rises to 82% at 70 years [99]. The natural history of HPT in MEN2A is nowadays routinely altered by thyroid surgery with frequent removal of parathyroid glands. Mutations in codons 609, 611, 618, 620, 790, and 791 are less frequently associated with HPT. Those with codon 768, 804, and 891 mutations rarely develop HPT.

In the GETC series, apparently single-gland disease was observed at initial operation in 24 of 44 (54%) cases. Of the remaining patients, two had no glands removed, five had two removed, and the remainder had either subtotal parathyroidectomy or total parathyroidectomy with autograft. The cure rate was 89%, including 22% who were hypoparathyroid, and there were eight reoperations [156].

With respect to the parathyroid glands, the primary surgical concern in MEN2A is to avoid hypocalcemia after thyroid surgery for MTC or its prophylaxis. A secondary consideration is the future risk of HPT—primarily in 634 mutations. There are three different strategies for three different surgical groups:

1. In normocalcemic patients, who have mutations associated with low penetrance of HPT, it is suggested to preserve all parathyroid tissue if possible, either *in situ* or transplanted to the sternomastoid muscle.
2. By contrast, in hyperparathyroid patients, subtotal parathyroidectomy or total parathyroidectomy with autograft is indicated, based on high lifetime risk of multigland disease.
3. For patients without evidence of HPT at the time of thyroid surgery, but with increased risk for development of HPT, a considered approach is needed. If nodes are not resected, it may be wise to leave a limited number (one or two) of residual, vascularized, and marked parathyroid glands. Where two glands are preserved, reoperation will be easier after preservation of either both inferior or both ipsilateral glands. If nodes are resected, it may still be possible to leave a vascularized superior gland or an intrathymic inferior gland; otherwise, an autograft is needed. In the setting of clinical MTC, another strategy is routine total parathyroidectomy and autograft regardless of the presence or risk of HPT, to facilitate a radical central neck dissection.

MEN2A with Hirschsprung's disease

Inactivating mutations of the *RET* proto-oncogene are known to cause HSCR. In contrast, MEN2A is caused by activating mutations. It is at first, therefore, difficult to conceptualize the coexistence of these two disorders in the same patient or within the same family, but there are many clearly reported familial studies showing this does indeed occur [157–159].

MEN2A with HSCR is associated with mutations in the cysteine-rich area of RET—principally codon 620—although others (e.g., 609, 611, and 618) have been reported. These RET mutations approximate the transmembrane domain of the gene. Codon 620 has been described as the "Janus gene," which, like the Roman god of doorways, can face in both directions (i.e., activation in MEN and inactivation in HSCR) [160]. A unique mutation can be activating or inactivating depending on the tissue in which RET is expressed [161].

Genetic testing of neonates presenting with HSCR is recommended, and when mutations consistent with MEN2A are found, screening of relatives should follow. The index child should be monitored or considered for a subsequent prophylactic thyroidectomy. In one family, an infant boy and his sister were diagnosed with HSCR as neonates. Genetic testing demonstrated a C620R gene mutation consistent with MEN2A. Total thyroidectomies revealed metastatic MTC in the father and CCH in both children [159].

MEN2A with cutaneous lichen amyloidosis

This is a variant of MEN2A with the addition of pruritic, macular, cutaneous lesions of the interscapular region of the upper back [162]. CLA is associated almost exclusively with mutation of codon 634. In one study, 9 of 25 patients (36%) with codon 634 mutations presented CLA, although 2 of them did not show CLA skin lesions but the typical neurological pruritus in the upper back. In all patients, neurological pruritus was present since infancy as a precocious marker of the disorder. Pruritus has a pivotal role in the development of CLA, the amyloid deposition being the consequence of repeated scratching [163].

MEN2B (MEN3) (GORLIN OR STEINER'S SYNDROME) (OMIM #162300)

MEN2B is characterized by MTC, PCC, characteristic facies, and marfanoid habitus. MEN2B is much less common than MEN2A, accounting for 5% of MEN2 cases. The clinical presentation is dominated by that of the associated MTC, which is more precocious and aggressive in MEN2B than in any other clinical setting.

PCC is observed in about one-half of patients and is usually bilateral, often synchronous, and occurs at a later age of onset than MTC, typically in the teenage years or early adulthood. It may not have time to manifest in many cases because of premature death from MTC. HPT is not a feature of MEN2B.

MEN2B has pathognomonic facies and marfanoid habitus that allow instant diagnosis if recognized but are usually only subtly present in infancy (Figure 43.10a and b). The most striking features are thickened, nodular, and everted lips, eyelids, and nares as a result of submucosal neuromas. The tongue is nodular and dentition usually deranged with gaps. Neural hypertrophy is most evident in the retina, as seen by slit lamp examination. Medulated corneal fibers are present. Orthopedic problems, including pes cavus, talipes, hypotonia, proximal weakness, kyphosis, scoliosis, joint laxity, and pectus excavatum, may be the initial presentation. During infancy and childhood, constipation is a major clinical problem. Megacolon development due to intestinal ganglioneuromatosis may necessitate surgery in 50% or more of patients [164].

In index cases, the appearance of a lump in the neck, which gives rise to the diagnosis of metastatic MTC, is commonly the trigger to the diagnosis of MEN2B.

The condition is sufficiently rare that in sporadic cases, the diagnosis is usually delayed despite multiple presentations to a variety of healthcare professionals during infancy and childhood. A subset of patients with constipation who

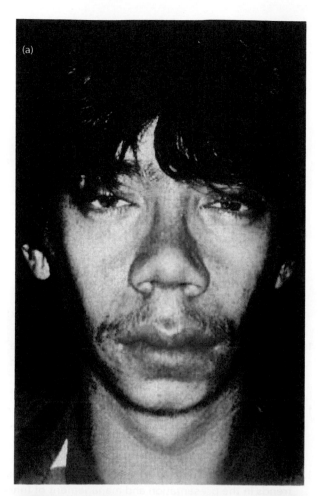

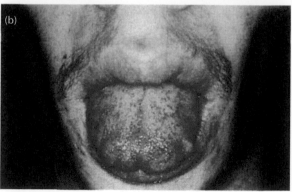

Figure 43.10 (a) MEN2B. Thickened lips and characteristic facies. (b) MEN2B. Submucosal neuromas of the tongue.

have a rectal biopsy may fortuitously be diagnosed early with intestinal ganglioneuromatosis. Gene analysis in these patients allows prophylactic thyroidectomy for cure at an early age. Tearless crying beyond 1 year is characteristic, and when associated with constipation, it could be used to identify these patients [165,166].

MTC in MEN2B typically presents in childhood with advanced disease and nodal and distant metastases. Locoregional disease may be unresectable at presentation even as a child. It is well recognized that in MEN2B, MTC may develop in infancy, suggesting the possibility of malignant change in utero. Despite metastatic disease, patients may live for many years with minimal morbidity due to indolent behavior of metastases. Diarrhea from calcitonin secretion by metastatic MTC can be troublesome despite octreotide therapy. New vascular endothelial growth factor and epidermal growth factor (EGF) inhibitors such as vandetanib are of benefit for progressive disease.

PCC may occasionally be diagnosed before any other feature of the syndrome is recognized, but MTC and the other features are always evident at that time.

MEN2B is associated almost exclusively with a mutation of codon 918 of the *RET* proto-oncogene resulting in activation of the intracellular catalytic core. Other rarer mutations causing MEN2B are codon 883 and the V804M mutation with a tandem *RET* mutation (805, 806, or 904) [167,168]. The transforming potential of the 883 mutation is slightly less than that of 918, and in the tandem mutations, it is about 50% less. There appears to be an equal sex distribution. Sporadic germline mutation is the cause of the syndrome in about 50% of cases. Kindreds may be short-lived (particularly in the past) due to the lethality of the mutation.

The surgical strategy for MTC in MEN2B is similar to that for MEN2A. In sporadic cases, surgery is carried out at diagnosis. The presence of PCC must be sought and treated before thyroid surgery. Assessment for distant metastases by imaging and level of calcitonin may influence the aim and extent of surgery. In cases with clear evidence of metastatic disease to the chest or liver, or markedly elevated calcitonin, the aim is palliative, with the hope to prevent locoregional complications. Typically, in advanced disease, surgery is total thyroidectomy with CLND, transcervical mediastinal node clearance, and bilateral neck dissection. However, every effort should be made to avoid morbidity—particularly bilateral nerve palsy, tracheostomy, radical neck dissection, and sternotomy when cure is not possible. With the availability of systemic therapeutic options such as vandetanib, radical, exenterating neck surgery should be a last resort.

Prophylactic total thyroidectomy should be performed before the age of 1 year, perhaps in the first few months, to avoid the need for concomitant central node dissection. Microscopic MTC is commonly found within the first year of life, and lymph node metastasis in infants has also been described [127]. Calcitonin testing in this age group is difficult to manage and interpret. The use of calcitonin screening to guide the timing of surgery in MEN2B is therefore questionable.

Familial medullary thyroid cancer (OMIM# 155240)

In this variant of MEN2, only MTC is expressed. Recently, consensus opinion is that FMTC is not a distinct entity from MEN2A. FMTC simply represents a phenotype with much less frequent penetrance of PCC or HPT. In general, onset of MTC is at a later age and the clinical course is more indolent than in MEN2A. Mutations of many codons in both the extracellular and intracellular domains of the *RET* proto-oncogene have been associated with FMTC (Table 43.4). There is overlap of the genetic mutations giving rise to MEN2A and FMTC, and thus the two phenotypes often cannot be differentiated by the genotype. FMTC patients should still have intermittent investigation for PCC: plasma metanephrines, perhaps every 3–5 years, because it is impossible to be sure PCC will not arise. There are strict inclusion criteria that can be applied before assuming a diagnosis of FMTC [3]. There should be more than 10 carriers in the kindred and multiple carriers or affected members over the age of 50 who have been thoroughly investigated.

Prophylactic thyroid surgery should be undertaken in FMTC at the appropriate age as determined by mutation analysis or in conjunction with calcitonin level, just as in MEN2A.

MEN4 (OMIM# 610755)

Studies initially in a rat model with spontaneous MEN-like syndrome led to the recent discovery of a new gene responsible for some cases of MEN syndrome primarily causing pituitary and parathyroid tumors now called MEN4. The gene *CDKN1B* encodes pKIP1, a tumor suppressor that binds to and inhibits cyclin/cyclin-dependent kinase complexes, preventing cell cycle progression [169,170].

In the small number of patients so far described, HPT was due usually to one tumor, but in some cases, there was multigland disease. Pituitary tumors of various kinds occurred in about half of the patients, and a variety of other endocrine lesions were also found: ZES, bronchial carcinoid, gastric carcinoid, and bilateral adrenal masses [171].

MIXED MEN1 AND MEN2?

There have in the past been rare observations of apparent mixed syndromes, such as ZES and PCC. Now that the distinct genetic basis of each condition has been clearly determined, they will most likely be classified as MEN1 or MEN2, with an additional uncharacteristic endocrine tumor. Very rarely, MEN1 and MEN2 gene mutations may occur in the same patient [172]. There remains the possibility of other very rare syndromes yet to be recognized.

REFERENCES

1. Kloos RT, Eng C, Evans DB et al. Medullary thyroid cancer: Management guidelines of the American Thyroid Association. *Thyroid* 2009;19:565–12.
2. Wells SA, Asa SL, Dralle H et al. Revised American Thyroid Association guidelines for the management of medullary thyroid carcinoma. *Thyroid* 2015;25:567–610.
3. Brandi ML, Gagel RF, Angeli A et al. Guidelines for diagnosis and therapy of MEN type 1 and type 2. *J Clin Endocrinol Metab* 2001;86:5658–71.
4. Elisei R, Alevizaki M, Conte-Devolx B et al. 2012 European Thyroid Association guidelines for genetic testing and its clinical consequences in medullary thyroid cancer. *Eur Thyroid J* 2013;1:216–31.
5. Thakker RV, Newey PJ, Walls GV et al. Clinical practice guidelines for multiple endocrine neoplasia type 1 (MEN1). *J Clin Endocrinol Metab* 2012;97:2990–3011.
6. Wermer P. Genetic aspects of adenomatosis of endocrine glands. *Am J Med* 1954;16:363–71.
7. Shepherd JJ. The natural history of multiple endocrine neoplasia type 1. Highly uncommon or highly unrecognized? *Arch Surg* 1991;126:935–52.
8. Thakker RV. Multiple endocrine neoplasia type 1 (MEN1). *Best Pract Res Clin Endocrinol Metab* 2010;24:355–70.
9. Marx SJ. Multiple endocrine neoplasia type 1. In: Scriver CR, Sly WS, Childs B, eds., *The Metabolic and Molecular Basis of Inherited Disease*. New York: McGraw-Hill, 2001:943–66.
10. Uchino S, Noguchi S, Sato M et al. Screening of the Men1 gene and discovery of germ-line and somatic mutations in apparently sporadic parathyroid tumors. *Cancer Res* 2000;60:5553–7.
11. Sakurai A, Yamazaki M, Shinichi S. Clinical features of insulinoma in patients with multiple endocrine neoplasia type 1: Analysis of the database of the MEN Consortium of Japan. *Endocrine J* 2012;59:859–66.
12. Placzkowski KA, Vella A, Thompson GB et al. Secular trends in the presentation and management of functioning insulinoma at the Mayo Clinic, 1987–2007. *J Clin Endocrinol Metab* 2009;94:1069–73.
13. Roy PK, Venzon DJ, Shojamanesh H et al. Zollinger-Ellison syndrome. Clinical presentation in 261 patients. *Medicine* 2000;79:379–411.
14. Sakurai A, Yamazaki M, Suzuki S et al. Clinical features of insulinoma in patients with multiple endocrine neoplasia type 1: Analysis of the database of the MEN Consortium of Japan. *Endocr J* 2012;59:859–66.
15. Agarwal SK. Multiple endocrine neoplasia type 1. *Front Horm Res* 2013;41:1–15.
16. Agarwal SK, Mateo CM, Marx SJ. Rare germline mutations in cyclin-dependent kinase inhibitor genes in multiple endocrine neoplasia type 1 and related states. *J Clin Endocrinol Metab* 2009;94:1826–34.
17. Burgess JR, Greenaway TM, Shepherd JJ. Expression of the MEN-1 gene in a large kindred with multiple endocrine neoplasia type 1. *J Intern Med* 1998;243:465–70.
18. Machens A, Schaaf L, Karges W et al. Age-related penetrance of endocrine tumours in multiple endocrine neoplasia type 1 (MEN1): A multicentre study of 258 gene carriers. *Clin Endocrinol* 2007;67:613–22.
19. Trump D, Farren B, Wooding C et al. Clinical studies of multiple endocrine neoplasia type 1 (MEN1). *QJM* 1996;89:653–69.

20. Ito T, Igarashi H, Uehara H et al. Causes of death and prognostic factors in multiple endocrine neoplasia type 1: A prospective study: Comparison of 106 MEN1/Zollinger-Ellison syndrome patients with 1613 literature MEN1 patients with or without pancreatic endocrine tumors. *Medicine* 2013;92:135–81.

21. Calender A, Giraud S, Porchet N et al. Clinicogenetic study of MEN1: Recent physiopathological data and clinical applications. Study Group of Multiple Endocrine Neoplasia (GENEM) [in French]. *Ann Endocrinol (Paris)* 1998;59:444–51.

22. Doherty GM, Olson JA, Frisella MM et al. Lethality of multiple endocrine neoplasia type I. *World J Surg* 1998;22:581–6; discussion 586–7.

23. Goudet P, Murat A, Binquet C et al. Risk factors and causes of death in MEN1 disease. A GTE (Groupe d'Etude des Tumeurs Endocrines) cohort study among 758 patients. *World J Surg* 2010;34:249–55.

24. Burgess JR, David R, Greenaway TM et al. Osteoporosis in multiple endocrine neoplasia type 1: Severity, clinical significance, relationship to primary hyperparathyroidism, and response to parathyroidectomy. *Arch Surg* 1999;134:1119–23.

25. van Heerden JA, Kent RB, Sizemore GW et al. Primary hyperparathyroidism in patients with multiple endocrine neoplasia syndromes. Surgical experience. *Arch Surg* 1983;118:533–6.

26. Kraimps JL, Duh QY, Demeure M, Clark OH. Hyperparathyroidism in multiple endocrine neoplasia syndrome. *Surgery* 1992;112:1080–6; discussion 1086–8.

27. Doherty GM, Lairmore TC, DeBenedetti MK. Multiple endocrine neoplasia type 1 parathyroid adenoma development over time. *World J Surg* 2004;28:1139–42.

28. Friedman E, Sakaguchi K, Bale AE et al. Clonality of parathyroid tumors in familial multiple endocrine neoplasia type 1. *N Engl J Med* 1989;321:213–8.

29. Arnalsteen LC, Alesina PF, Quiereux JL et al. Long-term results of less than total parathyroidectomy for hyperparathyroidism in multiple endocrine neoplasia type 1. *Surgery* 2002;132:1119–24; discussion 1124–5.

30. Pasieka JL, Parsons L, Jones J. The long-term benefit of parathyroidectomy in primary hyperparathyroidism: A 10-year prospective surgical outcome study. *Surgery* 2009;146:1006–13.

31. Elaraj DM, Skarulis MC, Libutti SK et al. Results of initial operation for hyperparathyroidism in patients with multiple endocrine neoplasia type 1. *Surgery* 2003;134:858–64; discussion 864–5.

32. O'Riordain DS, Obrien T, Grant CS et al. Surgical management of primary hyperparathyroidism in multiple endocrine neoplasia types 1 and 2. *Surgery* 1993;114:1031–7.

33. Wells SA, Farndon JR, Dale JK et al. Long-term evaluation of patients with primary parathyroid hyperplasia managed by total parathyroidectomy and heterotopic autotransplantation. *Ann Surg* 1980;192:451–8.

34. Waldmann J, López CL, Langer P. et al. Surgery for multiple endocrine neoplasia type 1-associated primary hyperparathyroidism. *Br J Surg* 2010;97:1528–34.

35. Goudet P, Cougard P, Vergès B et al. Hyperparathyroidism in multiple endocrine neoplasia type I: Surgical trends and results of a 256-patient series from Groupe d'Etude des Néoplasies Endocriniennes Multiples Study Group. *World J Surg* 2001;25:886–90.

36. Burgess JR, Giles N, Shepherd JJ. Malignant thymic carcinoid is not prevented by transcervical thymectomy in multiple endocrine neoplasia type 1. *Clin Endocrinol* 2001;55:689–93.

37. Goudet P, Murat A, Cardot-Bauters C et al. Thymic neuroendocrine tumors in multiple endocrine neoplasia type 1: A comparative study on 21 cases among a series of 761 MEN1 from the GTE (Groupe des Tumeurs Endocrines). *World J Surg* 2009;33:1197–207.

38. Versnick M, Popadich A, Sidhu S et al. Minimally invasive parathyroidectomy provides a conservative surgical option for multiple endocrine neoplasia type 1–primary hyperparathyroidism. *Surgery* 2013;154:101–5.

39. Burgess JR, David R, Parameswaran V et al. The outcome of subtotal parathyroidectomy for the treatment of hyperparathyroidism in multiple endocrine neoplasia type 1. *Arch Surg* 1998;133:126–9.

40. Borot S, Lapierre V, Carnaille B et al. Results of cryopreserved parathyroid autografts: A retrospective multicenter study. *Surgery* 2010;147:529–35.

41. Shepet K, Alhefdhi A, Usedom R et al. Parathyroid cryopreservation after parathyroidectomy: A worthwhile practice? *Ann Surg Oncol* 2013;20:2256–60.

42. Casanova D, Sarfati E, De Francisco A et al. Secondary hyperparathyroidism: Diagnosis of site of recurrence. *World J Surg* 1991;15:546–9.

43. Tonelli F, Giudici F, Cavalli T, Brandi ML. Surgical approach in patients with hyperparathyroidism in multiple endocrine neoplasia type 1: Total versus partial parathyroidectomy. *Clinics* 2011;67:155–60.

44. Kiblut NK, Cussac J-F, Soudan B et al. Fine needle aspiration and intraparathyroid intact parathyroid hormone measurement for reoperative parathyroid surgery. *World J Surg* 2004;28:1143–7.

45. Proye C, Lefebvre J, Bourdelle-Hego MF et al. Middle mediastinal parathyroid adenoma of the aorto-pulmonary window. 2 cases [in French]. *Chirurgie* 1988;114:166–73.

46. Triponez F, Goudet P, Dosseh D et al. Is surgery beneficial for MEN1 patients with small (≤2 cm), nonfunctioning pancreaticoduodenal endocrine tumor? An analysis of 65 patients from the GTE. *World J Surg* 2006;30:654–62.

47. Ito T, Sasano H, Tanaka M et al. Epidemiological study of gastroenteropancreatic neuroendocrine tumors in Japan. *J Gastroenterol* 2010;45:234–43.

48. Skogseid B, Eriksson B, Lundqvist G et al. Multiple endocrine neoplasia type 1: A 10-year prospective screening study in four kindreds. *J Clin Endocrinol Metab* 1991;73:281–7.

49. Dean PG, van Heerden JA, Farley DR et al. Are patients with multiple endocrine neoplasia type I prone to premature death? *World J Surg* 2000;24:1437–41.

50. Burgess JR, Greenaway TM, Parameswaran V et al. Enteropancreatic malignancy associated with multiple endocrine neoplasia type 1: Risk factors and pathogenesis. *Cancer* 1998;83:428–34.

51. Skogseid B, Oberg K, Eriksson B et al. Surgery for asymptomatic pancreatic lesion in multiple endocrine neoplasia type I. *World J Surg* 1996;20:872–7.

52. Thompson NW, Lloyd RV, Nishiyama RH et al. MEN I pancreas: A histological and immunohistochemical study. *World J Surg* 1984;8:561–72.

53. Le Bodic M-F, Heymann M-F, Lecomte M et al. Immunohistochemical study of 100 pancreatic tumors in 28 patients with multiple endocrine neoplasia, type I. *Am J Surg Pathol* 1996;20:1378.

54. Bartsch DK, Langer P, Wild A et al. Pancreaticoduodenal endocrine tumors in multiple endocrine neoplasia type 1: Surgery or surveillance? *Surgery* 2000;128:958–66.

55. Norton JA, Fraker DL, Alexander HR et al. Surgery to cure the Zollinger-Ellison syndrome. *N Engl J Med* 1999;341:635–44.

56. Thom AK, Norton JA, Axiotis CA, Jensen RT. Location, incidence, and malignant potential of duodenal gastrinomas. *Surgery* 1991;110:1086–91; discussion 1091–3.

57. Cadiot G, Vuagnat A, Doukhan I et al. Prognostic factors in patients with Zollinger-Ellison syndrome and multiple endocrine neoplasia type 1. Groupe d'Etude des Néoplasies Endocriniennes Multiples (GENEM) and Groupe de Recherche et d'Etude du Syndrome de Zollinger-Ellison (GRESZE). *Gastroenterology* 1999;116:286–93.

58. Cougard P, Goudet P, Peix JL et al. Les insulinomes dans les néoplasies endocriniennes multiples de type 1 (NEM1). À propos d'une série de 44 cas du groupe d'étude des néoplasies endocriniennes multiples (GENEM). *Ann Chir* 2000;125:118–23.

59. Borson-Chazot F, Cardot-Bauters C, Mirallie É et al. Insulinoma of genetic aetiology [in French]. *Ann Endocrinol (Paris)* 2013;74:200–2.

60. Norton JA, Alexander HR, Fraker DL et al. Comparison of surgical results in patients with advanced and limited disease with multiple endocrine neoplasia type 1 and Zollinger-Ellison syndrome. *Ann Surg* 2001;234:495–505; discussion 505–6.

61. Thompson NW. Current concepts in the surgical management of multiple endocrine neoplasia type 1 pancreatic-duodenal disease. Results in the treatment of 40 patients with Zollinger-Ellison syndrome, hypoglycaemia or both. *J Intern Med* 1998;243:495–500.

62. Akerstrom G, Stalberg P, Hellman P. Surgical management of pancreatico-duodenal tumors in multiple endocrine neoplasia syndrome type 1. *Clinics* 2012;67:173–8.

63. Proye CA. Endocrine tumours of the pancreas: An update. *Aust N Z J Surg* 1998;68:90–100.

64. Gauger PG, Doherty GM, Broome JT et al. Completion pancreatectomy and duodenectomy for recurrent MEN-1 pancreaticoduodenal endocrine neoplasms. *Surgery* 2009;146:801–8.

65. Hellman P, Andersson M, Rastad J et al. Surgical strategy for large or malignant endocrine pancreatic tumors. *World J Surg* 2000;24:1353–60.

66. Lairmore TC, Chen VY, DeBenedetti MK et al. Duodenopancreatic resections in patients with multiple endocrine neoplasia type 1. *Ann Surg* 2000;231:909–18.

67. Krampitz GW, Norton JA. Current management of the Zollinger-Ellison syndrome. *Adv Surg* 2013;47:59–79.

68. Mignon M, Ruszniewski P, Podevin P et al. Current approach to the management of gastrinoma and insulinoma in adults with multiple endocrine neoplasia type I. *World J Surg* 1993;17:489–97.

69. MacFarlane MP, Fraker DL, Alexander HR et al. Prospective study of surgical resection of duodenal and pancreatic gastrinomas in multiple endocrine neoplasia type 1. *Surgery* 1995;118:973–9.

70. Wiedenmann B, Jensen RT, Mignon M et al. Preoperative diagnosis and surgical management of neuroendocrine gastroenteropancreatic tumors: General recommendations by a consensus workshop. *World J Surg* 1998;22:309–18.

71. Gauger PG, Thompson NW. Early surgical intervention and strategy in patients with multiple endocrine neoplasia type 1. *Best Pract Res Clin Endocrinol Metab* 2001;15:213–23.

72. Thompson NW, Pasieka J, Fukuuchi A. Duodenal gastrinomas, duodenotomy, and duodenal exploration in the surgical management of Zollinger-Ellison syndrome. *World J Surg* 1993;17:455–62.

73. Imamura M, Takahashi K. Use of selective arterial secretin injection test to guide surgery in patients with Zollinger-Ellison syndrome. *World J Surg* 1993;17:433–8.

74. Tonelli F, Giudici F, Fratini G, Brandi ML. Pancreatic endocrine tumors in multiple endocrine neoplasia type 1 syndrome: Review of literature. *Endocr Pract* 2011;17(Suppl 3):33–40.

75. Lopez CL, Falconi M, Waldmann J et al. Partial pancreaticoduodenectomy can provide cure for duodenal gastrinoma associated with multiple endocrine neoplasia type 1. *Ann Surg* 2013;257:308–14.

76. Imamura M. Biochemically curative surgery for gastrinoma in multiple endocrine neoplasia type 1 patients. *World J Gastroenterol* 2011;17:1343–53.

77. Skogseid B, Oberg K, Benson L et al. A standardized meal stimulation test of the endocrine pancreas for early detection of pancreatic endocrine tumors in multiple endocrine neoplasia type 1 syndrome: Five years experience. *J Clin Endocrinol Metab* 1987;64:1233–40.

78. Mayo SC, de Jong MC, Bloomston M et al. Surgery versus intra-arterial therapy for neuroendocrine liver metastasis: A multicenter international analysis. *Ann Surg Oncol* 2011;18:3657–65.

79. Farid NR, Buehler S, Russell NA et al. Prolactinomas in familial multiple endocrine neoplasia syndrome type I. Relationship to HLA and carcinoid tumors. *Am J Med* 1980;69:874–80.

80. Scheithauer BW, Laws ER, Kovacs K et al. Pituitary adenomas of the multiple endocrine neoplasia type I syndrome. *Semin Diagn Pathol* 1987;4:205–11.

81. Burgess JR, Shepherd JJ, Parameswaran V et al. Spectrum of pituitary disease in multiple endocrine neoplasia type 1 (MEN 1): Clinical, biochemical, and radiological features of pituitary disease in a large MEN 1 kindred. *J Clin Endocrinol Metab* 1996;81(7):2642–46.

82. Duh Q-Y, Hybarger CP, Geist R et al. Carcinoids associated with multiple endocrine neoplasia syndromes. *Am J Surg* 1987;154:142–8.

83. Goudet P, Murat A, Binquet C et al. Risk factors and causes of death in MEN1 disease. A GTE (Groupe d'Etude des Tumeurs Endocrines) cohort study among 758 patients. *World J Surg* 2009;34:249–55.

84. Ferolla P, Falchetti A, Filosso P et al. Thymic neuroendocrine carcinoma (carcinoid) in multiple endocrine neoplasia type 1 syndrome: The Italian series. *J Clin Endocrinol Metab* 2013;90:2603–9.

85. Rindi G, Bordi C, Rappel S et al. Gastric carcinoids and neuroendocrine carcinomas: Pathogenesis, pathology, and behavior. *World J Surg* 1996;20:168–72.

86. Jensen RT. Management of the Zollinger-Ellison syndrome in patients with multiple endocrine neoplasia type 1. *J Intern Med* 1998;243:477–88.

87. Norton JA, Melcher ML, Gibril F, Jensen RT. Gastric carcinoid tumors in multiple endocrine neoplasia-1 patients with Zollinger-Ellison syndrome can be symptomatic, demonstrate aggressive growth, and require surgical treatment. *Surgery* 2004;136:1267–74.

88. Modlin IM, Lye KD, Kidd M. A 50-year analysis of 562 gastric carcinoids: Small tumor or larger problem? *Am J Gastroenterol* 2004;99:23–32.

89. Gatta-Cherifi B, Chabre O, Murat A et al. Adrenal involvement in MEN1. Analysis of 715 cases from the Groupe d'etude des Tumeurs Endocrines database. *Eur J Endocrinol* 2012;166:269–79.

90. Skogseid B, Rastad J, Gobl A et al. Adrenal lesion in multiple endocrine neoplasia type 1. *Surgery* 1995;118:1077–82.

91. Darling TN, Skarulis MC, Steinberg SM et al. Multiple facial angiofibromas and collagenomas in patients with multiple endocrine neoplasia type 1. *Arch Dermatol* 1997;133:853–7.

92. Stratakis CA, Schussheim DH, Freedman SM et al. Pituitary macroadenoma in a 5-year-old: An early expression of multiple endocrine neoplasia type 1. *J Clin Endocrinol Metab* 2000;85(12):4776–80.

93. Hellman P, Hennings J, Akerstrom G, Skogseid B. Endoscopic ultrasonography for evaluation of pancreatic tumours in multiple endocrine neoplasia type 1. *Br J Surg* 2005;92:1508–12.

94. Sipple JH. The association of pheochromocytoma with carcinoma of the thyroid gland. *Am J Med* 1961;31:163–6.

95. Williams ED, Pollock DJ. Multiple mucosal neuromata with endocrine tumours: A syndrome allied to von Recklinghausen's disease. *J Pathol Bacteriol* 1966;91:71–80.

96. Gorlin RJ, Sedano HO, Vickers RA, Červenka J. Multiple mucosal neuromas, pheochromocytoma and medullary carcinoma of the thyroid—A syndrome. *Cancer* 1968;22:293–9.

97. Steiner AL, Goodman AD, Powers SR. Study of a kindred with pheochromocytoma, medullary thyroid carcinoma, hyperparathyroidism and Cushing's disease: Multiple endocrine neoplasia, type 2. *Medicine* 1968;47:371–409.

98. Machens A, Lorenz K, Dralle H. Peak incidence of pheochromocytoma and primary hyperparathyroidism in multiple endocrine neoplasia 2: Need for age-adjusted biochemical screening. *J Clin Endocrinol Metab* 2013;98:E336–45.

99. Schuffenecker I, Virally-Monod M, Brohet R et al. Risk and penetrance of primary hyperparathyroidism in multiple endocrine neoplasia type 2A families with mutations at codon 634 of the RET proto-oncogene. Groupe D'etude des Tumeurs à Calcitonine. *J Clin Endocrinol Metab* 1998;83:487–91.

100. Mulligan LM, Eng C, Healey CS et al. Specific mutations of the RET proto-oncogene are related to disease phenotype in MEN 2A and FMTC. *Nat Genet* 1994;6:70–74.

101. Machens A, Dralle H. Genotype-phenotype based surgical concept of hereditary medullary thyroid carcinoma. *World J Surg* 2007;31:957–68.

102. Margraf RL, Crockett DK, Krautscheid PMF et al. Multiple endocrine neoplasia type 2 RET protooncogene database: Repository of MEN2-associated

RET sequence variation and reference for genotype/phenotype correlations. *Hum Mutat* 2009;30:548–56.

103. Moline J, Eng C. Multiple endocrine neoplasia type 2: An overview. *Genet Med* 2011;13:755–64.

104. Howe JR, Norton JA, Wells SA. Prevalence of pheochromocytoma and hyperparathyroidism in multiple endocrine neoplasia type 2A: Results of long-term follow-up. *Surgery* 1993;114:1070–7.

105. Schuffenecker I, Ginet N, Goldgar D et al. Prevalence and parental origin of *de novo* RET mutations in multiple endocrine neoplasia type 2A and familial medullary thyroid carcinoma. Le Groupe d'Etude des Tumeurs a Calcitonine. *Am J Hum Genet* 1997;60:233–7.

106. Romei C, Mariotti S, Fugazzola L et al. Multiple endocrine neoplasia type 2 syndromes (MEN 2): Results from the ItaMEN network analysis on the prevalence of different genotypes and phenotypes. *Eur J Endocrinol* 2010;163:301–8.

107. Machens A, Dralle H. Familial prevalence and age of RET germline mutations: Implications for screening. *Clin Endocrinol* 2008;69:81–87.

108. Zhou Y, Zhao Y, Cui B et al. RET proto-oncogene mutations are restricted to codons 634 and 918 in mainland Chinese families with MEN2A and MEN2B. *Clin Endocrinol* 2007;67:570–6.

109. Raue F, Frank-Raue K. Genotype-phenotype relationship in multiple endocrine neoplasia type 2. Implications for clinical management. *Hormones (Athens)* 2009;8:23–28.

110. Frank-Raue K, Rybicki LA, Erlic Z et al. Risk profiles and penetrance estimations in multiple endocrine neoplasia type 2A caused by germline RET mutations located in exon 10. *Hum Mutat* 2011;32:51–58.

111. Raue F, Frank-Raue K, Grauer A. Multiple endocrine neoplasia type 2. Clinical features and screening. *Endocrinol Metab Clin North Am* 1994;23:137–56.

112. Eng C, Mulligan LM, Smith DP et al. Low frequency of germline mutations in the RET proto-oncogene in patients with apparently sporadic medullary thyroid carcinoma. *Clin Endocrinol* 1995;43:123–7.

113. Erdogan MF, Gürsoy A, Ozgen G et al. Ret proto-oncogene mutations in apparently sporadic Turkish medullary thyroid carcinoma patients: Turkmen study. *J Endocrinol Invest* 2005;28:806–9.

114. Machens A, Ukkat J, Brauckhoff M et al. Advances in the management of hereditary medullary thyroid cancer. *J Intern Med* 2005;257:50–9.

115. Machens A, Holzhausen H-J, Dralle H. Contralateral cervical and mediastinal lymph node metastasis in medullary thyroid cancer: Systemic disease? *Surgery* 2006;139:28–32.

116. Machens A, Gimm O, Ukkat J et al. Improved prediction of calcitonin normalization in medullary thyroid carcinoma patients by quantitative lymph node analysis. *Cancer* 2000;88:1909–15.

117. Scheuba C, Kaserer K, Bieglmayer C et al. Medullary thyroid microcarcinoma recommendations for treatment—A single-center experience. *Surgery* 2007;142:1003–10.

118. Wells SA, Dilley WG, Farndon JA et al. Early diagnosis and treatment of medullary thyroid carcinoma. *Arch Intern Med* 1985;145:1248–52.

119. Murat A, Modigliani E, Conte-Devolx B et al. Early therapeutic management of patients genetically predisposed to medullary thyroid cancer [in French]. *Ann Chir* 1998;52:455–60.

120. Moley JF, DeBenedetti MK. Patterns of nodal metastases in palpable medullary thyroid carcinoma: Recommendations for extent of node dissection. *Ann Surg* 1999;229:880–7.

121. Fleming JB, Lee JE, Bouvet M et al. Surgical strategy for the treatment of medullary thyroid carcinoma. *Ann Surg* 1999;230:697–707.

122. Dralle H, Damm I, Scheumann GF et al. Compartment-oriented microdissection of regional lymph nodes in medullary thyroid carcinoma. *Surg Today* 1994;24:112–21.

123. Elisei R, Romei C, Renzini G et al. The timing of total thyroidectomy in RET gene mutation carriers could be personalized and safely planned on the basis of serum calcitonin: 18 years experience at one single center. *J Clin Endocrinol Metab* 2012;97:426–35.

124. Dralle H, Musholt TJ, Schabram J et al. German Association of Endocrine Surgeons practice guideline for the surgical management of malignant thyroid tumors. *Langenbecks Arch Surg* 2013;398:347–75.

125. Gimm O, Ukkat J, Dralle H. Determinative factors of biochemical cure after primary and reoperative surgery for sporadic medullary thyroid carcinoma. *World J Surg* 1998;22:562–7; discussion 567–8.

126. Machens A, Hinze R, Thomusch O, Dralle H. Pattern of nodal metastasis for primary and reoperative thyroid cancer. *World J Surg* 2002;26:22–28.

127. Skinner MA, DeBenedetti MK, Moley JF et al. Medullary thyroid carcinoma in children with multiple endocrine neoplasia types 2A and 2B. *J Pediatr Surg* 1996;31:177–81; discussion 181–2.

128. Wells SA Jr, Chi DD, Toshima K et al. Predictive DNA testing and prophylactic thyroidectomy in patients at risk for multiple endocrine neoplasia type 2A. *Ann Surg* 1994;220:237.

129. Rohmer V, Vidal-Trecan G, Bourdelot A et al. Prognostic factors of disease-free survival after thyroidectomy in 170 young patients with a RET germline mutation: A multicenter study of the Groupe Francais d'Etude des Tumeurs Endocrines. *J Clin Endocrinol Metab* 2011;96:E509–18.

130. Skinner MA, Moley JA, Dilley WG et al. Prophylactic thyroidectomy in multiple endocrine neoplasia type 2A. *N Engl J Med* 2005;353:1105–13.

131. Frank-Raue K, Buhr H, Dralle H et al. Long-term outcome in 46 gene carriers of hereditary medullary thyroid carcinoma after prophylactic thyroidectomy: Impact of individual RET genotype. *Eur J Endocrinol* 2006;155:229–36.

132. Zenaty D, Aigrain Y, Peuchmaur M et al. Medullary thyroid carcinoma identified within the first year of life in children with hereditary multiple endocrine neoplasia type 2A (codon 634) and 2B. *Eur J Endocrinol* 2009;160:807–13.

133. Machens A, Niccoli-Sire P, Hoegel J et al. Early malignant progression of hereditary medullary thyroid cancer. *N Engl J Med* 2003;349:1517–25.

134. Dralle H, Gimm O, Simon D et al. Prophylactic thyroidectomy in 75 children and adolescents with hereditary medullary thyroid carcinoma: German and Austrian experience. *World J Surg* 1998;22:744–50; discussion 750–1.

135. Basuyau J-P, Mallet E, Leroy M, Brunelle P. Reference intervals for serum calcitonin in men, women, and children. *Clin Chem* 2004;50:1828–30.

136. Gill JR, Reyes-Múgica M, Iyengar S et al. Early presentation of metastatic medullary carcinoma in multiple endocrine neoplasia, type IIA: Implications for therapy. *J Pediatr* 1996;129:459–64.

137. Leung K, Stamm M, Raja A, Low G. Pheochromocytoma: The range of appearances on ultrasound, CT, MRI, and functional imaging. *AJR Am J Roentgenol* 2013;200:370–8.

138. Gimm O, Niederle BE, Weber T et al. RET proto-oncogene mutations affecting codon 790/791: A mild form of multiple endocrine neoplasia type 2A syndrome? *Surgery* 2002;132:952–9; discussion 959.

139. Rich TA, Feng L, Busaidy N et al. Prevalence by age and predictors of medullary thyroid cancer in patients with lower risk germline RET proto-oncogene mutations. *Thyroid* 2014:24:1096–1106.

140. Machens A, Dralle H. Prophylactic thyroidectomy in RET carriers at risk for hereditary medullary thyroid cancer. *Thyroid* 2009;19:551–4.

141. Niederle B, Sebag F, Brauckhoff M. Timing and extent of thyroid surgery for gene carriers of hereditary C cell disease—A consensus statement of the European Society of Endocrine Surgeons (ESES). *Langenbecks Arch Surg* 2014;399:185–97.

142. Milos IN, Frank-Raue K, Wohllk N et al. Age-related neoplastic risk profiles and penetrance estimations in multiple endocrine neoplasia type 2A caused by germ line RET Cys634Trp (TGC > TGG) mutation. *Endocr Relat Cancer* 2008;15:1035–41.

143. Casanova S, Rosenberg Bourgin M et al. Phaeochromocytoma in multiple endocrine neoplasia type 2 A: Survey of 100 cases. *Clin Endocrinol* 1993;38:531–7.

144. Inabnet WB, Caragliano P, Pertsemlidis D. Pheochromocytoma: Inherited associations, bilaterality, and cortex preservation. *Surgery* 2000;128:1007–11; discussion 1011–2.

145. Modigliani E, Vasen HM, Raue K et al. Pheochromocytoma in multiple endocrine neoplasia type 2: European study. The Euromen Study Group. *J Intern Med* 1995;238:363–7.

146. Lairmore TC, Ball DW, Baylin SB et al. Management of pheochromocytomas in patients with multiple endocrine neoplasia type 2 syndromes. *Ann Surg* 1993;217:595.

147. van Heerden JA, Sizemore GW, Carney JA et al. Surgical management of the adrenal glands in the multiple endocrine neoplasia type II syndrome. *World J Surg* 1984;8:612–9.

148. de Graaf JS, Dullaart RP, Zwierstra RP. Complications after bilateral adrenalectomy for phaeochromocytoma in multiple endocrine neoplasia type 2—A plea to conserve adrenal function. *Eur J Surg* 1999;165:843–6.

149. Lee JE, Curley SA, Gagel RF et al. Cortical-sparing adrenalectomy for patients with bilateral pheochromocytoma. *Surgery* 1996;120:1064–70; discussion 1070–1.

150. Castinetti F, Qi X-P, Walz MK et al. Outcomes of adrenal-sparing surgery or total adrenalectomy in phaeochromocytoma associated with multiple endocrine neoplasia type 2: An international retrospective population-based study. *Lancet Oncol* 2014;15:648–55.

151. Brauckhoff M, Thanh PN, Gimm O et al. Functional results after endoscopic subtotal cortical-sparing adrenalectomy. *Surg Today* 2003;33:342–8.

152. Pattou FN, Combemale FP, Poirette JF et al. Questionability of the benefits of routine laparotomy as the surgical approach for pheochromocytomas and abdominal paragangliomas. *Surgery* 1996;120:1006–11; discussion 1012.

153. Fernández-Cruz L, Taurá P, Sáenz A et al. Laparoscopic approach to pheochromocytoma: Hemodynamic changes and catecholamine secretion. *World J Surg* 1996;20:762–8; discussion 768.

154. Cheah WK, Clark OH, Horn JK et al. Laparoscopic adrenalectomy for pheochromocytoma. *World J Surg* 2002;26:1048–51.

155. Tiberio GAM, Baiocchi GL, Arru L et al. Prospective randomized comparison of laparoscopic versus open adrenalectomy for sporadic pheochromocytoma. *Surg Endosc* 2008;22:1435–9.

156. Kraimps JL, Denizot A, Carnaille B et al. Primary hyperparathyroidism in multiple endocrine neoplasia type IIa: Retrospective French multicentric study. Groupe d'Etude des Tumeurs á Calcitonine (GETC,

French Calcitonin Tumors Study Group), French Association of Endocrine Surgeons. *World J Surg* 1996;20:808–12; discussion 812–3.

157. Caron P, Attié T, David D et al. C618R mutation in exon 10 of the RET proto-oncogene in a kindred with multiple endocrine neoplasia type 2A and Hirschsprung's disease. *J Clin Endocrinol Metab* 1996;81:2731–3.

158. Mulligan LM, Eng C, Attié T et al. Diverse phenotypes associated with exon 10 mutations of the RET proto-oncogene. *Hum Mol Genet* 1994;3:2163–7.

159. Fialkowski EA, DeBenedetti MK, Moley JF, Bachrach B. RET proto-oncogene testing in infants presenting with Hirschsprung disease identifies 2 new multiple endocrine neoplasia 2A kindreds. *J Pediatr Surg* 2008;43:188–90.

160. Moore SW, Zaahl M. The Hirschsprung's–multiple endocrine neoplasia connection. *Clinics* 2012;67:63–7.

161. Chappuis-Flament S, Pasini A, De Vita G et al. Dual effect on the RET receptor of MEN 2 mutations affecting specific extracytoplasmic cysteines. *Oncogene* 1998;17:2851–61.

162. Donovan DT, Levy ML, Furst EJ et al. Familial cutaneous lichen amyloidosis in association with multiple endocrine neoplasia type 2A: A new variant. *Henry Ford Hosp Med J* 1989;37:147–50.

163. Verga U, Fugazzola L, Cambiaghi S et al. Frequent association between MEN 2A and cutaneous lichen amyloidosis. *Clin Endocrinol* 2003;59:156–61.

164. Oriordain D, Obrien T, Crotty T et al. Multiple endocrine neoplasia type 2B: More than an endocrine disorder. *Surgery* 1995;118:936–42.

165. Brauckhoff M, Machens A, Lorenz K et al. Surgical curability of medullary thyroid cancer in multiple endocrine neoplasia 2B. *Ann Surg* 2014;259:800–6.

166. Brauckhoff M, Machens A, Hess S et al. Premonitory symptoms preceding metastatic medullary thyroid cancer in MEN 2B: An exploratory analysis. *Surgery* 2008;144:1044–50; discussion 1050–3.

167. Miyauchi A, Futami H, Hai N et al. Two germline missense mutations at codons 804 and 806 of the RET proto-oncogene in the same allele in a patient with multiple endocrine neoplasia type 2B without codon 918 mutation. *Jpn J Cancer Res* 1999;90:1–5.

168. Cranston AN, Carniti C, Oakhill K et al. RET is constitutively activated by novel tandem mutations that alter the active site resulting in multiple endocrine neoplasia type 2B. *Cancer Res* 2006;66:10179–87.

169. Pellegata NS, Quintanilla-Martinez L, Siggelkow H et al. Germ-line mutations in p27Kip1 cause a multiple endocrine neoplasia syndrome in rats and humans. *Proc Natl Acad Sci USA* 2006;103:15558–63.

170. Molatore S, Marinoni I, Lee M et al. A novel germline CDKN1B mutation causing multiple endocrine tumors: Clinical, genetic and functional characterization. *Hum Mutat* 2010;31:E1825–35.

171. Lee M, Pellegata NS. Multiple endocrine neoplasia type 4. *Front Horm Res* 2013;41:63–78.

172. Frank-Raue K, Rondot S, Hoeppner W et al. Coincidence of multiple endocrine neoplasia types 1 and 2: Mutations in the RET protooncogene and MEN1 tumor suppressor gene in a family presenting. *J Clin Endocrinol Metab* 2005;90:4063–7.

Gastro-Entero-Pancreatic System

44

Radionuclide imaging of carcinoid tumors, neurendocrine tumors of the pancreas and adrenals

LALE KOSTAKOGLU

INTRODUCTION

The heightened awareness of neuroendocrine tumors (NETs), coupled with the availability of advanced technology to measure secreted proteins, improved immunohistochemistry, and the parallel increase in the use of advanced imaging techniques, has significantly contributed to the increasing incidence of NETs [1–3]. However, early detection of NETs remains a clinical challenge, particularly in patients with no clinical symptoms. Additionally, sensitive detection of NETs is hindered by the small size and slow growth of these tumors, causing delays in the diagnosis, which is associated with the high incidence of metastatic disease at initial presentation. Surgical resection has been the established curative treatment in localized disease, to some extent in advanced stages. Preoperative imaging strongly contributes to patient care for determining the extent of disease, localization of unknown primaries, lesion characterization,

treatment planning, and subsequent follow-up. Because of diverse tumor properties and clinical behavior, the disease presentation is varied in individual patients. In this chapter, the different nuclear imaging techniques and tracers for the imaging of NETs are discussed.

CARCINOID TUMORS

Somatostatin receptor imaging

The expression of somatostatin receptors (SSTRs) by the vast majority of NETs constitutes the basis for both somatostatin receptor imaging (SRI) [4,5] and peptide receptor radionuclide therapy (PRRT) [6]. SRI has an important role for the localization of NETs as an important functional imaging test that is adjunct to morphologic diagnostic modalities, i.e., diagnostic computed tomography (CT) and magnetic resonance imaging (MRI). At staging, because of its ability to detect otherwise undetected NETs, SRI has a significant impact on patient management by providing critical information for either confirming resectability or avoiding unnecessary surgery, and evaluation of patients whose tumors have spread to distant sites that cannot be detected with conventional imaging alone.

There are five well-characterized SSTR subtypes expressed on the tumor cell surface: SSTR1 to SSTR5. The expression and the density of the SSTR subtypes vary among tumors [7], but SSTR2 is the predominantly expressed SSTR subtype on well-differentiated NETs, and it binds to various synthetic analogs of somatostatin (e.g., octreotide and lanreotide) with high affinity [8–10]. After a diagnosis of NET based on elevated biomarkers and clinical symptoms and confirmatory findings by CT or MRI, the goals for the initial SRI are the determination of disease extent and the identification of the primary tumor site to help formulate treatment planning. In the post-therapy setting, follow-up SRI studies are performed for surveillance, even without elevated biomarkers, to confirm the presence of recurrence. SRI can also be performed after surgery to ensure the completeness of resection and to confirm the presence or absence of recurrence after treatment.

Currently, SRI can be performed by either using gamma camera-based imaging with ^{111}In-DTPA^0-octreotide, commercially available as Octreoscan (Covidien, Hazelwood, Missouri), or using positron emission tomography (PET) technology with ^{68}Ga-labeled somatostatin analogs. Somatostatin receptor scintigraphy (SRS), i.e., Octreoscan, targets SSTR2 and, to a lesser extent, SSTR5 and has long been considered the gold standard in functional imaging in NETs [4,7–9,11]. However, the emergence of PET technology and its attendant advantage of higher sensitivity has shifted the paradigm toward ^{68}Ga-labeled somatostatin analog [12–15]. The most common of these labeled analogs are ^{68}Ga-DOTATOC, ^{68}Ga-DOTANOC, and ^{68}Ga-DOTATATE. Importantly, the slightly different affinities of these radiolabeled molecules for the SSTR subtypes have not resulted in variable diagnostic effectiveness [12]. Besides staging and restaging, the overexpression of SSTRs in NETs is currently being investigated as a molecular target for PRRT [16]. Both imaging techniques, SRS or PET-based SRI, can be clinically utilized to test *in vivo* for the presence of SSTR2 to determine the eligibility of a patient for PRRT because intense radiotracer accumulation at tumor sites is considered a good predictor of favorable response to PRRT [16].

SRI using either technique should be performed 3–6 weeks after the last dose of long-acting octreotide to minimize competition between cold octreotide and radiolabeled octreotide at the receptor site and avoid false-negative results. Short-acting octreotide or continuous octreotide infusion should be stopped for 48 hours before and during the 1- to 2-day period of imaging. Interferon (IFN-α) is known to upregulate SSTRs [17], and thus can lead to increased uptake and false-positive findings without disease progression. In cases of suspected gastrointestinal and pancreatic NETs, it may be beneficial to have the patient use a laxative the night before the imaging test to minimize the tracer accumulation in the bowel.

^{111}IN-DTPA^0-OCTREOTIDE SCINTIGRAPHY

SRS with ^{111}In-DTPA^0-octreotide is currently the most important tracer in the diagnosis, staging, and selection for PRRT. Although ^{111}In-DTPA^0-octreotide binds to both SSTR2 and SSTR5, the primary targeting is through SSTR2 for a positive imaging result [9,18,19].

An optimized protocol for ^{111}In-DTPA^0-octreotide will ensure superior image quality and diagnostic performance. The detailed recommended imaging protocols are provided by the current guidelines published by various international organizations [20–23]. Upon completion of whole body planar imaging, single-photon emission computed tomography (SPECT) with CT fusion (SPECT/CT) or at least SPECT imaging should be additionally obtained to provide three-dimensional images to minimize the interference of physiologic uptake with NET detection. This topic is further discussed later in this section.

Biodistribution

The visualized organs in normal distribution of ^{111}In-DTPA^0-octreotide include the thyroid, spleen, liver, kidneys, urinary bladder, and bowel. On SPECT imaging, the adrenals and the pituitary gland can be seen [24]. The pituitary, thyroid, adrenals, and spleen express SSTRs, but the uptake in the kidneys is mainly due to reabsorption of the radiolabeled somatostatin analog in the renal tubules after glomerular filtration. Clearance of the radiopharmaceutical is predominantly via the kidneys and, to some extent, via the hepatobiliary system; thus, the gall bladder can be visualized in 7%–10% of patients. The use of laxatives may be sometimes necessary to differentiate between nonspecific bowel uptake and NETs.

CLINICAL APPLICATIONS OF ^{111}IN-DTPA^0-OCTREOTIDE IN WELL-DIFFERENTIATED CARCINOIDS

The overall sensitivity of SRS with ^{111}In-DTPA^0-octreotide for detecting NETs is 60%–90%, for both functioning and nonfunctioning pancreatic NETs (PNETs), and 80% to more than 90% for carcinoids, depending on tumor anatomic site and size [8,11,26–31] (Figures 44.1 through 44.3). SRS combined with SPECT, particularly SPECT/CT, proved improved sensitivity compared with planar imaging for detection of both the primary NETs (except nonmetastatic insulinomas) and metastatic NETs [8,9]. Because the specificity of planar SRS is low at 50%–80% [11,27,29,30,32–34] a SPECT or preferably SPECT/CT of the abdomen and pelvis is beneficial to limit the interference from nearby structures with high physiological tracer activity [35–38]. The benefits of SPECT are discussed later in this chapter.

Pulmonary carcinoids

Pulmonary carcinoids (PCs) are well-differentiated NETs and are classified into low-grade malignant, i.e., typical

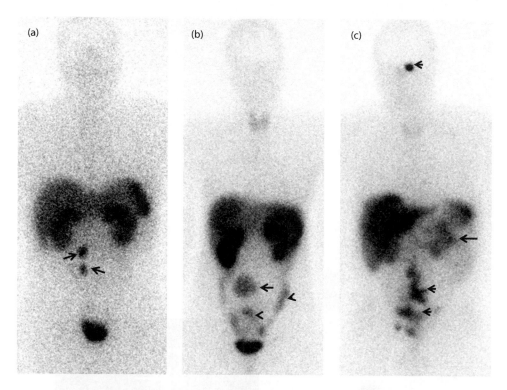

Figure 44.1 ^{111}In-DTPA^0-octreotide (Octreoscan) whole body images in anterior planes in three different carcinoid patients. **(a)** Patient with a carcinoid tumor metastasis from an unknown primary (CUPNET) who has been maintained on long-acting octreotide therapy, now referred for evaluation of disease status. Anterior whole body image shows radio-tracer uptake in multiple retroperitoneal lymph nodes (arrows) compatible with metastatic disease. There is otherwise no evidence for other sites of metastasis or the primary disease. **(b)** Patient with a recent diagnosis of metastatic carcinoid tumor on a liver biopsy. Anterior whole body image shows radiotracer uptake in the right mid-to-lower quadrant (arrow) corresponding to a large mesenteric mass involving the ileum consistent with the primary NET. There is also physiologic bowel uptake in the colon (arrowheads). Note that the hepatic metastasis is not well appreciated on the planar image but was clearly seen on SPECT images (not shown here). **(c)** Patient with a recent diagnosis of metastatic glucagonoma referred for evaluation of the extent of the disease. Anterior whole body image shows increased uptake in the pancreas (primary disease site) (arrow) and multiple metastatic disease sites involving the retroperitoneal lymph nodes and pelvic lymph nodes (small arrows), as well as the orbit (small arrow).

carcinoid (TC), and intermediate-grade malignant, i.e., atypical carcinoid (AC) subgroups. SRS may play a role in the diagnosis of PCs because of its higher specificity than conventional imaging for low-grade PCs, including TCs and lower-grade ACs. Nearly 80% of the primary tumors that are predominantly TCs may be visualized with this technique [39]. SPECT/CT usually reveals a corresponding peripheral lung nodule with smooth or lobular margins [40]. Central PCs may present with indirect signs of obstruction on CT. Diffuse idiopathic pulmonary neuroendocrine cell hyperplasia (DIPNECH) is characterized by proliferation of neuroendocrine cells within the lung. They are diagnosed on high-resolution CT, and there is no role for a nuclear medicine imaging technique.

Gastroenteropancreatic neuroendocrine tumors

The primary NETs are most commonly located in the gastrointestinal tract or the pancreas; hence, these tumors are collectively referred to as gastroenteropancreatic neuroendocrine tumors (GEPNETs). The majority of GEPNETs consists of small intestine carcinoid tumors (~55%) and pancreatic neuroendocrine tumors (PNETs) [21]. Tumors of PNET origin are known by the hormones they secrete, e.g., insulinoma, glucagonoma, and gastrinoma. SSTR2 is expressed in approximately 90% of gastrointestinal NETs and in almost 80% of PNETs with the exception of insulinomas, in which the SSTR2 expression is usually present in less than 50% of the tumors [5,7]. While modalities such as small bowel series and MR enterography have been described as potential options in the initial workup of small bowel NETs, the two most commonly used tests are SRS and contrast-enhanced CT. The overall sensitivity of SRS for GEPNETs is reported to be approximately 90% [41].

In jejunum, ileum, and cecum carcinoids, in cases where the primary site is not directly identified (e.g., a mesenteric mass), the overall sensitivity of SRS is 85%–95% [9,42]. The 48-hour imaging may be helpful better delineate abdominal lesions because of the decreased bowel uptake, which may potentially obscure lesions at earlier imaging periods. As discussed before, SPECT/CT imaging also benefits clinical management by minimizing indeterminate lesions

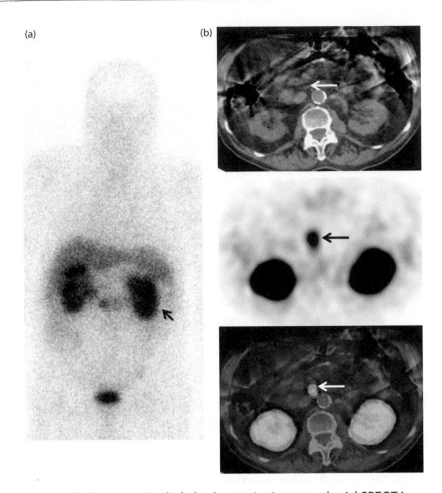

Figure 44.2 ^{111}In-DTPA^0-octreotide (Octreoscan) whole body anterior image and axial SPECT images in a patient with a diagnosis of ileum carcinoid who had undergone surgery in the past and now has been referred for evaluation for recurrent disease based on rising tumor markers but otherwise no evidence of disease on other cross-sectional imaging tests. **(a)** Anterior whole body image shows an area of increased uptake in the right of the midline in the upper abdomen; however, anatomic localization of this focus is not possible without a cross-sectional imaging technique. **(b)** Axial image of the SPECT/CT shows increased uptake in a small paracaval lymph node (arrow) consistent with metastatic disease. Note that the CT component of the SPECT study helps define the exact location of the metastasis.

(Figures 44.2 and 44.3). SRS is a good adjunct to CT or MRI to detect distant metastases at staging. The SRS sensitivity for detection of hepatic metastases ranges from 50% to 90% [27,43,44]. SRS is also used to localize primary GEPNETs when the primary tumor site is unknown. The identification of the primary tumor is crucial in treatment planning, as resection of the primary tumor may improve symptom-free survival, overall survival (OS), and quality of life [45].

In patients with distal colon and rectum carcinoids, staging SRS is not routinely recommended because they are localized to the mucosa or submucosa and associated with a low risk of metastatic spread. However, patients with known large (>2 cm) or invasive tumors should undergo SRS to rule out distant metastases. In patients with known metastases, SRS can help establish whether metastatic tumors express SSTRs, specifically SSTR2 for therapeutic implications.

PNETs

In patients with PNETs, SRS detects the primary disease site with a relatively high sensitivity (60%–90%), but it is less sensitive in nonmetastatic insulinomas and duodenal gastrinomas [8,11,27–31,46–49]. SRS has a high sensitivity of more than 90% in cases with metastatic disease [8–10,50] (Figure 44.2). Generally, the sensitivity of SRS is lower in small lesions measuring less than the resolution of gamma cameras (i.e., 1 cm for SPECT); in insulinomas (sensitivity of <50%), likely due to the low-density expression of SSTR2 [42]; in NETs with a high proliferation index (Ki-67) of >10%; and in poorly differentiated NETs [51]. The use of SRS has reportedly resulted in a change in clinical management in 25%–50% of PNET patients [8–10,50]. False-positive results can occur in 10%–15% of patients, but when the results are interpreted within the clinical context, the false-positive rate can be reduced by 75% [10,28].

In a multicenter trial, the sensitivities of histologically or biochemically proven PNETs or gastrointestinal carcinoids, in decreasing order, were 100% in glucagonomas, 88% in VIPomas, 87% in gastrointestinal carcinoids, 82% in nonfunctioning islet cell tumors, and 72% in gastrinomas [52]. These favorable imaging characteristics led

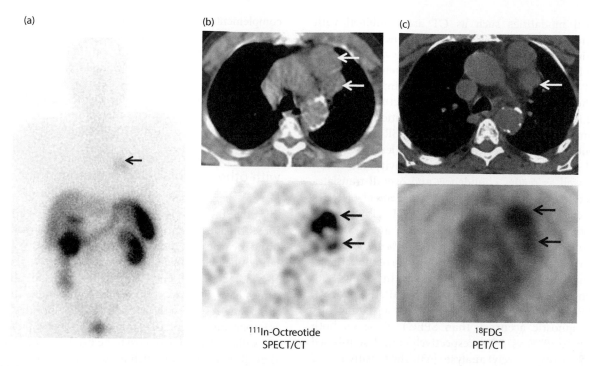

(a) (b) (c)

^{111}In-Octreotide
SPECT/CT

^{18}FDG
PET/CT

Figure 44.3 A patient with a diagnosis of well-differentiated (Ki-67 < 5) midgut NET on treatment with long-acting octreotide now presents with rising tumor markers and clinical symptoms of flushing and diarrhea. (a) ^{111}In-DTPA^{0}-octreotide (Octreoscan) anterior planar image shows vague radiotracer uptake in the chest left of the midline without a clear anatomic delineation. (b) SPECT/CT axial images show that the radiotracer uptake seen on the planar image corresponds to masses located in the prevascular region (small arrow on planar and large arrows on SPECT/CT), corresponding to several enlarged lymph nodes, probably representing carcinoid metastases. (c) FDG PET/CT axial images show increased glucose metabolism corresponding to the prevascular lymph nodes (arrows). Note the lesser degree of FDG uptake compared with the octreotide accumulation, which is in line with well-differentiated histology with adequate SSTR2 expression.

^{111}In-DTPA^{0}-octreotide SRS to be integrated into the clinical workup of GEPNETs as an essential test.

Insulinomas constitute a special subgroup of PNETs, in which SRS has a particularly low sensitivity at 20%–60%, although there is usually uptake in the metastatic lesions [11,53–55]. In addition to the low number of patients included in each study and varying scanning protocols, the small size of tumors, as well as the variability in the expression and density of SSRTs between benign and malignant insulinomas, is considered to account for the wide variability in SRS sensitivity [5,53–56]. In this regard, the most sensitive diagnostic procedure was reportedly endoscopic ultrasound (EUS), with a sensitivity of 93%, vs. 14% with SRS and 21% with CT [48]. One potential area of confusion relates to the association of carcinoids with multiple endocrine neoplasia (MEN) 1 syndrome. Because of the coexistance of multiple tumor sites, the imaging findings should not be confused with a metastatic site or a second cancer [57].

Recently, glucagon-like peptide 1 (GLP-1)-like radioligands retaining high binding affinity to GLP-1 receptor have been developed based on the overexpression of the GLP-1 receptor in insulinomas [58,59] and can be used as a potential target. Preliminary data using the ^{111}In-labeled specific ligand [Lys^{40}(Ahx-DOTA)NH$_2$]exendin-4 (^{111}In-DOTA-exendin-4) in humans indicate that GLP-1 imaging is capable of localizing insulinomas *in vivo* by displaying a high sensitivity for insulinomas [58,60]. Although the preliminary results are promising, the need for staging of benign insulinomas has yet to be justified, particularly in the face of a proven high sensitivity for EUS [61] in this category of tumors.

Because NETs are slow-growing tumors and metastatic spread may occur many years after the initial diagnosis and therapy, long-term surveillance beyond 5 years should be considered in the management algorithm. However, following the surgical resection, the impact of long-term surveillance on survival of NET patients is unknown. Especially for submucosal tumors measuring less than or equal to 2 cm (stage I), the low risk of recurrence does not support an imaging surveillance approach. For patients with tumors invading the muscularis propria or involving locoregional lymph nodes (stage II or III), annual surveillance imaging should be considered.

Addition of anatomical imaging: SPECT/CT with radiolabeled somatostatin analog

The spatial resolution of CT (1–2 mm) is significantly higher than that of SPECT (~10 mm); however, the detection sensitivity of SPECT is significantly higher than that of structural modalities through detection of tracer concentration in the picomolar or nanomolar range [62]. When anatomical modalities such as CT are combined with SPECT in one imaging session, the obtained synergistic information improves the diagnostic accuracy. This is especially useful for localizing abdominal and pelvic disease in GEPNET patients because of the close proximity of disease sites to the visceral organs and osseous structures.

There is sufficient evidence that the addition of SPECT/CT to conventional ^{111}In-DTPA^0-octreotide SRS provides an incremental and complementary value for lesion localization and characterization; increases sensitivity and specificity, as well as reader confidence; and overall translates to a positive clinical impact in the management of NETs (Figures 44.2 and 44.3). When SRS SPECT/CT was compared with planar scintigraphy and SPECT alone, SPECT/CT improved lesion localization for 50%–70% of the lesions, improved diagnostic confidence in 50%–65% of the patients, and provided incremental diagnostic value in 30%–40% of the patients [14,36,37,63–65]. In a cohort of 81 NET patients, ^{111}In-DTPA-octreotide SPECT/CT yielded a significantly higher diagnostic accuracy than SPECT alone on both patient-based (93% vs. 79%, respectively) and lesion-based (96% vs. 81%, respectively) analyses [63]. The sensitivity and specificity for SPECT/CT were 95% and 92%, respectively, with significantly lower equivocal findings on SPECT/CT than SPECT alone.

PRRT using the somatostatin analogs attached to a β-emitter, such as ^{90}Y-DOTA^{0}Tyr^3-octreotide and ^{177}Lu-DOTA^{0}Tyr^3-octreotate, is an effective targeted treatment modality [66,67]. SRS is useful for both prognostication and selection of NET patients. This information can be derived from greater radiotracer avidity in GEPNET lesions. Notably, the ^{111}In-DTPA-octreotide uptake in each NET focus can be scored visually on planar images according to Krenning's 4-point scale as follows: lower than (grade 1), equal to (grade 2), or greater than (grade 3) normal liver tissue, or higher than normal spleen or kidney uptake (grade 4) [67]. However, this strategy may change in time with the clinical implementation of PET imaging using ^{68}Ga-labeled somatostatin analogs.

As alluded to before, higher expression of SSTR positively correlates with higher radiotracer uptake and a more effective PRRT [16]. In this regard, in both the pretherapy and post-treatment settings, SPECT/CT is useful to better assess the extent of radionuclide uptake for predicting the efficacy of ^{177}Lu-labeled somatostatin analogs and, to some extent, ^{90}Y-labeled somatostatin analogs using bremsstrahlung imaging. The dose to critical organs following PRRT can also be calculated using post-therapeutic SPECT/CT.

In the published literature, SPECT/CT was consistently reported to lead to a management change in 15%–65% of the patients, and the treatment approach was influenced in 10%–15% of the patients through improving surgical planning or obviating unnecessary surgery by demonstrating otherwise undetected metastatic sites [35,38,64].

In summary, SPECT/CT is a preferred modality in imaging NET patients with SRS because of its incremental and complementary value for improved therapy planning and patient management. Following the international guidelines is essential both to ensure optimal acquisition protocols and accurate diagnostic evaluations and to yield data for generalizable comparative results across centers. It is recommended that all available European and U.S. guidelines be reviewed for better understanding and execution of diagnostic studies in NETs [20–23,49].

^{111}In-DTPA-octreotide SRS versus SRS with other radiolabeled somatostatin receptor analogs

The other investigational radiolabeled somatostatin analogs for SRS include, but are not limited to, ^{99m}Tc-6-hydrazinopyridine-3-carboxylic acid (HYNIC)-TOC [65], ^{111}In-DOTA-lanreotide [68], ^{111}In-DOTA-octreotide [26,69], ^{111}In-DOTA [1-NaI3]octreotide, and ^{111}In-DOTANOC [70]. These molecules have different affinities for SSTR and demonstrated promising results with favorable affinity profiles [39,40]. It is important to emphasize that DTPA-labeled molecules are not sufficiently stable *in vivo* to be used in a therapy setting; thus, β-emitting radionuclides used for PRRT, i.e., ^{90}Y and ^{177}Lu, are compounded with 1,4,7,10-tetraazacyclodecane-1,4,7,10-tetraacetic acid (DOTA)-conjugated somatostatin analogs to ensure stability [16]. It would be preferred to use the same conjugate (i.e., DOTA) for SRS if a subsequent PRRT is considered. Although these novel imaging compounds are promising, they are not readily available and not well studied in humans; therefore, clinical experiences are limited [71].

Technetium-labeled investigational somatostatin analogs have also been investigated with favorable results in GEPNETs, and these included ^{99m}Tc-depreotide, which binds with high affinity to SSTR2, SSTR3, and SSTR5; ^{99m}Tc-vapreotide, which binds with high affinity to SSTR2 and SSTR5 and, to a lesser extent, SSTR3 and SSTR4; ^{99m}Tc-HYNIC-TOC; and ^{99m}Tc-HYNIC-[Tyr^3,Thr^8]-octreotide (TATE) [29,65,72]. There are advantages of ^{99m}Tc-labeled somatostatin analogs over ^{111}In-DTPA-octreotide imparted by superior imaging capabilities of the extrahepatic metastases and better individual separation of lesions. However, these results should be analyzed with caution since most of these reported comparisons did not use the optimal imaging protocols for ^{111}In-DTPA-octreotide SRS defined by the European and U.S. guidelines [20–23].

Positron emission tomography radiotracers labeled with somatostatin analogs

Somatostatin analogs labeled with PET radiotracers are increasingly favored over SRS radiotracers because of their superior sensitivity and specificity [69,73,74]. The short half-life of PET radiotracers allows for imaging only 1 hour after injection, which makes the operations convenient for patients and clinicians alike. Moreoever, because of their short half-lives, the majority of PET radiotracers have a favorable dosimetry for the patient compared with the γ-emitting tracers, such as ^{111}In-DOTATOC, which results in approximately twice the radiation dose to the patients [75].

The introduction of DOTA as a chelator has improved peptide labeling by ensuring stability using the metal group radiotracers, including ^{111}In, ^{68}Ga, ^{90}Y, and ^{177}Lu, of which the latter two are the mainstay for radionuclide therapy [16,67,68]. The most commonly used PET tracer for labeling a somatostatin analog has been [68]gallium, which has the great advantage of being produced from a generator without a cyclotron investment.

[68]GA-LABELED SOMATOSTATIN ANALOGS

The radiolabeled PET molecule ^{68}Ga-DOTATOC ([68]Ga-[DOTA[0],Tyr[3]]octreotide) was the first ^{68}Ga-labeled somatostatin analog investigated in humans [69,75]. Subsequently, other clinically applicable ^{68}Ga-labeled somatostatin analogs were developed to increase the imaging sensitivity and expand their affinity profile. These later-generation molecules include ^{68}Ga-DOTANOC ([68]Ga-[DOTA]-1-Nal3-octreotide) [14,70,76,77] and ^{68}Ga-DOTATATE ([68]Ga-[DOTA0,Tyr[3]]octreotate) [78]. The intensity of radiotracer uptake with all of these compounds is directly related to the density of SSTR expressed on the cell membrane and the binding affinity of the peptides. The binding to the relevant SSTRs plays a significant factor for both imaging and therapy purposes. ^{68}Ga-DOTATATE, similar to In-DTPA-octreotide, binds to only SSTR2 with high affinity, while ^{68}Ga-DOTATOC binds to both SSTR2 and SSTR5, and ^{68}Ga-DOTANOC to SSTR2, SSTR3, and SSTR5 [79]. Reubi et al. demonstrated that the binding affinity of ^{68}Ga-DOTATATE toward SSTR2 is about 10-fold higher than that of ^{68}Ga-DOTATOC and ^{68}Ga-DOTANOC [80]. ^{68}Ga-DOTANOC had a 10-fold higher affinity than ^{68}Ga-DOTATOC [31,80] (Table 44.1).

[68]Ga-labeled somatostatin analogs significantly contribute to improved patient management owing to a higher spatial resolution than afforded by SRS-SPECT [46], and a higher affinity for GEPNETs compared with ^{111}In-DTPA-Octreotide, as well as providing easy access to all centers by being a generator-produced positron-emitting radiotracer. The radiation absorbed dose associated with radiotracers is a crucial factor in determining a preferable tracer, especially in NET patients based on

their relatively long survival, allowing for multiple scans during the follow-up period of disease. For ^{68}Ga-emitting SSTR tracers, the spleen receives the highest dose, followed by the bladder, kidneys, and liver. A wait period of 45–60 minutes is allowed after the injection of the radiotracer for ^{68}Ga-PET SRI.

Biodistribution

The biodistribution of ^{68}Ga-labeled somatostatin analogs is similar to that of ^{111}In-DTPA-Octreotide, with physiological uptake seen in the thyroid, adrenal, pituitary, and salivary glands; liver; spleen; pancreas; and kidneys. The uptake in the adrenal and pituitary glands is particularly high with ^{68}Ga-DOTATATE and ^{68}Ga-DOTATOC. The physiologic uptake in pituitary and salivary glands is higher for ^{68}Ga-DOTATATE than ^{68}Ga-DOTANOC [81]. The significant uptake in the accessory spleen should not be mistaken for a disease site. The most challenging interpretations involve the disease sites in the liver and the uncinate process of the pancreas because of the significant overlap with the physiologic uptake in these predominant localizations of both primary and metastatic sites of NETs. More recent standardized uptake value (SUV) cutoff definitions did not lead to a resolution of the challenge [13]; thus, cautious interpretation of the pancreatic uptake is recommended.

CLINICAL APPLICATIONS OF [68]GA-LABELED SOMATOSTATIN RECEPTOR PET IMAGING FOR NETS

The diagnostic performance of the three most commonly used SSTR PET tracers is shown in Table 44.2. In a meta-analysis of 16 studies and 567 cases, the pooled sensitivity and specificity of ^{68}Ga-DOTA PET, irrespective of tracer type, were 93% (91%–95%) and 91% (82%–97%), respectively [82]. On a patient-based evaluation, the sensitivity of ^{68}Ga-DOTATOC was 92%–100% and the specificity was 83%–100%. For ^{68}Ga-DOTATATE, the sensitivity was slightly lower (72%–96%), and the specificity could not be meaningfully reported because only a few studies reported on it. For ^{68}Ga-DOTANOC, the sensitivity was variable (68%–100%), but the specificity was high at 93%–100%. Collectively, all of these molecules seem to have comparative diagnostic utility. Compared with CT, ^{68}Ga-DOTANOC PET has demonstrated a higher sensitivity (80% vs. 100%,

Table 44.1 Binding profiles for commonly used somatostatin analogs

Somatostatin analog	Name	SSTR2	SSTR3	SSTR4	SSTR5
In-DTPA-octreotide	In-DTPA-OC	22 ± 3.6	182 ± 13	[a]	237 ± 52
Ga-DOTA-Tyr[3]-octreotide	Ga-DOTATOC	2.5 ± 0.5	613 ± 140	[a]	73 ± 21
Ga-DOTA-I-Nal[3]-octreotide	Ga-DOTANOC	1.9 ± 0.4	40 ± 5.8	260 ± 74	7.2 ± 1.6
Ga-DOTA-Tyr[3]-octreotate	Ga-DOTATATE	0.2 ± 0.04	>1000	300 ± 140	377 ± 18
DOTA-lanreotide	DOTALAN	26 ± 3.4	771 ± 229	[a]	73 ± 12

Source: Modified from Johnbeck CB, Knigge U, Kjær A. *Future Oncol* 2014;10:2259–77.
Note: SSTR1 affinity for all is >100,000.
[a] SSTR4 affinity is >1000.

Table 44.2 ^{68}Ga-labeled SSTR PET imaging data in NETs

Investigator	Year	Reference	Patients	NET subtype	Sensitivity %	Specificity %
DOTATOC						
Hofmann et al.	2001	75	8	Lung carcinoid and GEPNET	100	—
Buchmann et al.	2007	114	27	Mixed NETs (CUP, GEPNET, and lung carcinoid)	100	—
Gabriel et al.	2007	69	84	Mixed NETs (CUP, GEPNET, and lung carcinoid)	97	92
Putzer et al.	2009	160	51	Bone metastases of NETs	97	92
Versari et al.	2010	87	19	GEPNET	92	83
DOTATATE						
Kayani et al.	2008	161	38	Mixed NETs (CUP, GEPNET, and lung carcinoid)	82	—
Kayani et al.	2009	78	18	Lung carcinoid	72	—
Haug et al.	2009	113	51	Metastatic NET	96	—
Srirajaskanthan et al.	2010	74	25	GEPNET	87	—
Kabasakal et al.	2012	81	20	Mixed NETs (CUP, GEPNET, and lung carcinoid)	100	—
Wild et al.	2013	70	18	GEPNET	94	—
DOTANOC						
Ambrosini et al.	2008	76	13	GEPNET and lung carcinoid	100	—
Ambrosini et al.	2009	83	11	Lung carcinoid	100	—
Ambrosini et al.	2010	73	223	Metastatic GEPNET	100	—
Naswa et al.	2011	84	109	GEPNET	78 (P), 97 (M)	92.5 (P), 100 (M)
Krausz et al.	2011	14	19	Mixed NETs (CUP and GEPNET)	10	—
Naswa et al.	2013	88	25	Gastrinoma	68	—
Kabasakal et al.	2012	81	20	Mixed NETs (CUP, GEPNET, and lung carcinoid)	93	100
Ambrosini et al.	2012	12	1239	Mixed NETs (CUP, GEPNET, and lung carcinoid)	92	98
Wild et al.	2013	70	18	GEPNET	94	—

Note: P, primary; M, metastatic.

respectively) and specificity (98% vs. 100%) in the detection of NET bone metastases [73].

Pulmonary NETs

Seventy percent of bronchial carcinoids express SSTR1, SSTR2, and SSTR5, with SSTR2 being the predominantly expressed receptor subtype [5]. Kayani et al. examined 18 pulmonary NET patients with ^{68}Ga-DOTATATE and found that typical, well-differentiated bronchial NETs showed significantly higher uptake of ^{68}Ga-DOTATATE and significantly less uptake of ^{18}F-fluorodeoxyglucose (FDG) than did tumors of higher grade ($p = 0.002$ and 0.005) [78]. There was no instance of false-positive uptake of ^{68}Ga-DOTATATE, but there were three false positives with FDG PET secondary to inflammation. ^{68}Ga-DOTATATE was also superior to FDG in discriminating endobronchial tumor from distal collapsed lung ($p = 0.02$) [78]. A pilot study using ^{68}Ga-DOTATOC showed an equally high detection rate for the typical bronchial carcinoids, while high-grade tumors were not visualized

consistently, and high sensitivity and specificity for typical, well-differentiated pulmonary NETs [83].

GEPNETs

In 109 GEPNET patients, Naswa et al., found that ^{68}Ga-DOTANOC PET/CT had a sensitivity and specificity of 78% and 92.5%, respectively, for detecting the primary tumor, and 97% and 100% for identification of metastases, proving a superiority to conventional imaging modalities ($p < 0.001$) [84]. Other smaller studies reported sensitivities ranging between 94% and 100% for GEPNETs [70,76].

^{68}Ga-DOTATOC also shows high sensitivities exceeding 90% in GEPNET patients [69,85–87] (Figures 44.4 and 44.5). In 84 patients, Gabriel et al. showed a 45% higher detection rate for ^{68}Ga-DOTATOC than conventional SRS SPECT ($p < 0.001$) using ^{99m}Tc-HYNIC-TOC and ^{111}In-DOTATOC [69]. ^{68}Ga-DOTATOC PET had a sensitivity of 97% and a specificity of 92%, which was approximately 35% higher than that of CT.

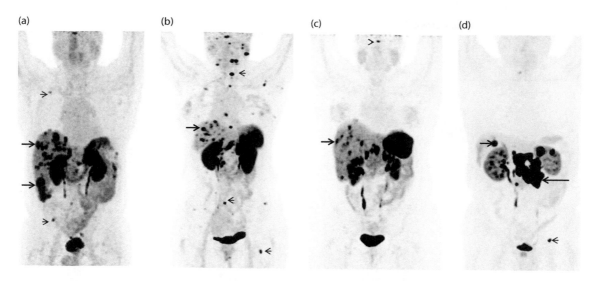

Figure 44.4 **(a–d)** ^{68}Ga-DOTATOC PET studies in four different patients with GEPNETs. On the volume-rendered whole body images, all patients demonstrate hepatic metastases (selective left arrows pointing to some of the lesions). In addition, patients a, b, and d are noted to have otherwise unknown bone metastases (selective short arrows). Note the ^{68}Ga-DOTATOC avid large conglomerate retroperitoneal mass in patient d (long right arrow). Note the physiologic uptake in the pituitary gland, most clearly seen in patient c (arrowhead).

Versari et al. found a comparable accuracy for EUS, ^{68}Ga-DOTATOC PET, and diagnostic CT in the diagnosis of duodenopancreatic NETs in 19 patients [87]. On a lesion basis, EUS, PET, and CT correctly identified NETs in 96%, 87%, and 72% of the lesions ($p = 0.08$ EUS vs. CT). Both on a patient and lesion basis, the specificities were 67%, 83%, and 80% for EUS, PET, and CT, respectively. It should be emphasized that the accuracy of interpretation was challenged by the significant physiologic uptake in the normal pancreatic tissue. These results suggest that a combination of these modalities may allow for an optimal preoperative diagnosis.

In 25 gastrinoma patients with clinical or biochemical diagnosis, diagnostic performance of ^{68}Ga-DOTANOC PET/CT was better than that of CT in cases with equivocal or negative CT findings. ^{68}Ga-DOTANOC PET/CT yielded an overall detection rate of 68% [88]. As expected, the pretest probability always affects the test results; of the patients who had a negative CT result, ^{68}Ga-DOTANOC PET/CT was positive in 36%, while it was abnormal in 93% of patients who had equivocal CT findings.

Carcinoma of unknown primary NET

Detection of the primary tumor site is important to optimize the treatment strategy. Although immunohistochemistry is quite helpful in characterizing tumors (e.g., serotonin expression consistent with a small bowel primary), the molecular imaging coupled with cross-sectional imaging may overcome tumor heterogeneity and sampling errors. The incidence and clinical course of carcinoma of unknown primary neuroendocrine tumors (CUP-NETs) is not well studied, but it is known that hepatic metastases of a NET primary can occur in the absence of any evidence for a primary tumor on conventional imaging. There is also a correlation between the size of the primary tumor

and the probability of metastases for small intestine carcinoids, which makes it clinically crucial to detect the primary tumor at an earlier stage for better management. In a study of 59 NET patients, Prasad et al. reported a 59% detection rate in CUP-NETs for ^{68}Ga-DOTANOC PET/CT in the localization of the primary site [15], while CT alone confirmed CUP-NETs in only 20% of patients. Interestingly, the SUVmax values of the unknown PNET and small intestine NETs were significantly lower ($p < 0.05$) than the ones with known primary tumor sites, and 81% of the patients had low-grade NETs. Corroborating results were also obtained by Naswa et al. with ^{68}Ga-DOTANOC PET, reporting a detection rate of 60% for the primary tumors in NET patients with unknown primary tumors [89]. These data indicate that ^{68}Ga-DOTA PET/CT is highly superior to ^{111}In-Octreoscan (~60% vs. ~40%) and can play a major role in the management of patients with a CUP-NET.

In the context of false-positive and negative findings, similar to SRS, the small lesions that fall below the PET resolution limits (<7 mm), and tumors with low SSTR expression, such as poorly differentiated neuroendocrine carcinoma and insulinomas, were the main reasons for false-negative PET imaging. The contributing conditions to false-positive results include inflammatory processes that can be associated with increased uptake, and physiologic uptake in the above-mentioned anatomic locations.

Comparison of the somatostatin receptor PET tracers

There are scarce data with respect to direct comparison of the performance of the available somatostatin analogs labeled with [68]Ga. Several studies reported direct comparisons of different PET tracers using the same patient cohort [81,90,91]. In 40 NET patients, Poeppel et al. reported 262

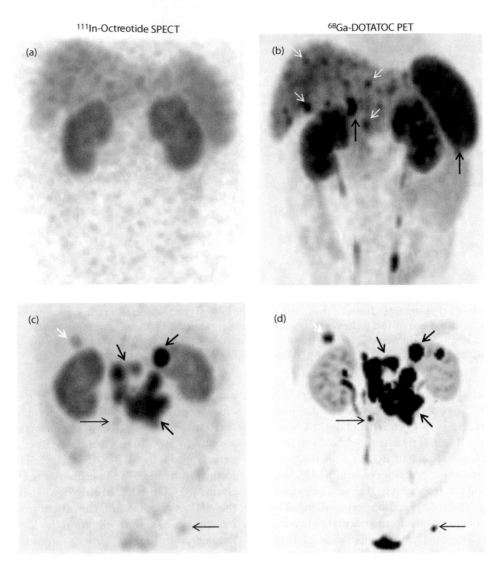

Figure 44.5 (a and b) A patient with an unknown primary NET diagnosed on biopsy of a hepatic lesion who has been maintained on long-acting octreotide. The patient is now referred for evaluation of disease status. **(a)** ^{111}In-DTPA^0-octreotide (Octreoscan) SPECT coronal image (left panel) shows no focally increased uptake in the liver. **(b)** ^{68}Ga-DOTATOC PET coronal image (right panel) of the same patient shows innumerable foci of increased radiotracer uptake consistent with extensive involvement of the liver by carcinoid metastases (selective white arrows). These findings emphasize the increased sensitivity provided by ^{68}Ga-DOTATOC PET, which guides management better than conventional diagnostic tests. Note the intense physiologic uptake in the spleen and adrenal (black vertical arrows) **(c and d)** A patient with a diagnosis of midgut carcinoid who has been maintained on long-acting octreotide. The patient is now referred for evaluation of disease status. **(c)** ^{111}In-DTPA^0-octreotide (Octreoscan) SPECT coronal image (left panel) shows multiple foci of increased uptake in coalescing retroperitoneal lymph nodes (known from CT) (small black arrows). These findings are consistent with SSTR2-positive metastatic carcinoid. There is also a faint focus of uptake in the liver (white arrow), in a separate para-aortic lymph node (known from CT) (right long arrow) and in the left iliac bone (mapped from CT) (left long arrow), suggesting additional carcinoid metastases. **(d)** ^{68}Ga-DOTATOC PET coronal image (right panel) of the same patient shows similar findings in the retroperitoneal lymph nodes (small black arrows). However, note that the uptake in the hepatic lesion (white arrow), additional para-aortic lymph node (right long arrow), and left iliac bone (left long arrow) is impressively higher than that seen on the SPECT study. These findings emphasize the superiority of ^{68}Ga-DOTATOC PET over ^{111}In-DTPA^0-octreotide (Octreoscan).

CT-verified lesions compared with 254 lesions detected by ^{68}Ga-DOTATATE PET [90]. The SUVmax was overall higher with ^{68}Ga-DOTATOC than with ^{68}Ga-DOTATATE. On a regional basis, there was no significant difference between ^{68}Ga-DOTATATE and ^{68}Ga-DOTATOC, making the differences less clinically relevant.

Kabasakal et al. found a similar diagnostic performance for ^{68}Ga-DOTATATE and ^{68}Ga-DOTANOC in 20 NET patients. ^{68}Ga-DOTATATE detected 12% more lesions than ^{68}Ga-DOTANOC [81], but this was not significantly different. Sensitivity on a patient level was calculated to be equally high at 93% for both scans, and the specificity was 100%.

The ^{68}Ga-DOTATATE accumulation in the lesions was significantly higher compared with that of ^{68}Ga-DOTANOC, a finding that is expected in light of the higher affinity of ^{68}Ga-DOTATATE for SSTR2. Interestingly, the additional affinities for SSTR3 or SSTR5 of ^{68}Ga-DOTANOC did not improve the tracer performance.

Putzer et al. evaluated the impact of ^{68}Ga-labeled DOTA[0]-lanreotide (^{68}Ga-DOTALAN) on the diagnostic assessment of NET patients with low to moderate uptake on planar SRS or ^{68}Ga-DOTATOC PET. ^{68}Ga-DOTATOC revealed twice as many tumor sites than ^{68}Ga-DOTALAN, with a significantly higher tumor-to-background ratio ($p < 0.02$) [91].

The extent of hepatic metastasis is a significant factor for management decisions. The choice of treatment decisions for surgical resection, embolization, PRRT, or hepatic transplantation heavily relies on the extent and localization of liver metastases. In this regard, the optimal somatostatin analog is expected to have the least physiologic hepatic uptake. Thus far, the data on both ^{68}Ga-DOTANOC [15] and ^{68}Ga-DOTATOC revealed a similar ratio between the tumor and normal tissue uptake, which was approximately 3 [13]. In a limited comparison study, with the use of ^{68}Ga-DOTANOC, Wild et al. reported that on a lesion-based analysis, ^{68}Ga-DOTANOC performed significantly better than ^{68}Ga-DOTATATE, with a sensitivity of 93.5%, compared with 85.5% ($p = 0.005$). The better performance of ^{68}Ga-DOTANOC PET was attributed to the significantly higher detection rate of liver metastases because of lower background liver uptake (tumor-to-background ratios were 2.7 and 2.0, respectively) [70]. However, based on these small series, it is fair to say that the superiority of one SSTR PET radiotracer over the other has not been proved with the currently available data.

The presence of bone metastases is associated with a poor prognosis [92]; thus, different treatment strategies may be preferred over surgical intervention. In 51 NET patients with no evidence of bone metastases on conventional bone scintigraphy, ^{18}F-Na-fluoride PET, or CT, ^{68}Ga-DOTATOC PET proved to be a superior modality in the detection of bone metastases, with a sensitivity of 97% and a specificity of 92% [91]. Moreover, ^{68}Ga-DOTATOC PET detected bone metastases at a significantly higher rate than did CT [69,91] ($p \leq 0.001$). These results lent further credence to the use of ^{68}Ga-DOTATOC PET as a reliable first-line imaging test at staging or restaging of NET patients. On a lesion-based analysis in 18 patients, Wild et al. reported a higher detection rate of bone lesions with ^{68}Ga-DOTATATE compared with ^{68}Ga-DOTANOC (89% vs. 82%) because of a lower bone marrow activity with ^{68}Ga-DOTATATE, resulting in a higher tumor-to-background activity and a high detection rate of bone metastases [70]. These results lent further credence to the use of ^{68}Ga-DOTATOC PET as a reliable first-line imaging test at staging or restaging of NET patients.

^{68}Ga-DOTATOC PET proved to be the most accurate test in 51 NET patients [85]. The sensitivity was 73% for PET compared with 77% for combined triple-phase CT, 66% for portal venous CT, 67% for venous CT, and 53% for arterial CT. The respective specificities were 97%, 85%, 92%, 90%, and 93%. The interobserver reproducibility was highest with PET and lowest for venous CT. Given these data, ^{68}Ga-DOTATOC PET/CT is strongly recommended and the triple-phase protocol continues to be strongly recommended for delivering synergistic information with an improved sensitivity [93]. With the superior soft tissue contrast contributed by MRI, the combination of PET and MRI is hypothesized to be superior to multiphase contrast-enhanced PET/CT using a somatostatin analog. In a study by Schreiter et al., Gd-EOB-DTPA-enhanced MRI increased the detection sensitivity of liver metastases from 74% to 91%, and specificity was raised from 88% to 96% compared with ^{68}Ga-DOTATOC PET/CT [94]. Therefore, Gd-EOB-DTPA-enhanced MRI seems to be the imaging modality of choice for combination with ^{68}Ga-DOTATOC to provide complementary tumor characterization in hepatic metastases of NETs. Nonetheless, the clinical value of ^{68}Ga-DOTATOC PET/MR with additional diagnostic MR sequences is yet to be evaluated against PET/CT with multiphase contrast-enhanced CT protocols in future studies to evaluate its full benefit.

In summary, the incremental role of morphologic imaging to PET/CT is irrefutable. The latest consensus guidelines state that imaging studies that are generally recommended for the initial diagnostic workup and staging of patients with a tissue diagnosis of a NET include CT of the soft tissues of the head and neck and the chest, a triple-phase CT protocol or MRI of the abdomen and pelvis, and ^{111}In-DTPA-octreotide scintigraphy [21,23]. In addition, because of the availability, PET/CT using a ^{68}Ga SSTR PET tracer should be performed in NET patients with unknown primary tumors. Furthermore, MRI proved to be superior to CT in the detection and follow-up of liver metastases, so if the CT scan of liver metastases is inconclusive, T2-weighted, dynamic, contrast-enhanced MRI should be considered [95].

Impact on clinical management

Overall, the clinical use of PET imaging to selectively visualize SSTRs as an adjunct to cross-sectional imaging by CT or MRI leads to management change in 20%–60% of cases [76,84,96,97], essentially in those patients being considered for PRRT [73]. In 59 NET patients, compared with conventional and ^{111}In-DTPA-octreotide imaging, additional information was provided by ^{68}Ga-DOTATATE in 83% of patients. Management impact was high (intermodality change) in 47% and moderate (intramodality change) in 10% of cases [97]. High management impact included directing patients to curative surgery by identifying a primary site and directing patients with multiple metastases to systemic therapy. In another study using ^{68}Ga-DOTANOC PET/CT in the detection of undiagnosed primary sites of NETs, PET/CT findings resulted in a management change in approximately 10% of patients with respect to surgical planning. In the remaining patients, because of the advanced stage, the primary tumors were not operated on [15]. There is still a need for larger prospective studies to determine the actual clinical impact of receptor peptide PET imaging with respect to change in quality of life, patient outcomes, survival, and cost–benefit ratio.

Although PET selective receptor imaging has great potential to change therapy choices, it is important to realize that there is no data showing that a significant survival gain can be obtained favoring any of these most used tracers—^{68}Ga-DOTATOC, ^{68}Ga-DOTATE, and ^{68}Ga-DOTANOC.

Other alternatives for radionuclide imaging of NETs

META-IODOBENZYLGUANIDINE

^{131}I-MIBG and, more recently, ^{123}I-MIBG imaging are also used as an alternative to SRS for imaging NETs [98]. Cellular uptake of meta-iodobenzylguanidine (MIBG) is mediated by the noradrenalin transporter, and intracellular uptake in secretory vesicles is mediated by the vesicular monoamine transporter (VMAT). Imaging of NETs with ^{123}I-MIBG is used but is not routinely recommended in the diagnostic workup of these patients because of its lower sensitivity (~50%) in GEPNETs and PNETs (~10%) compared

with the more frequently used ^{111}In-DTPA-octreotide SRS [99]. Nonetheless, in ^{111}In-DTPA-octreotide, negative NETs may be identified with ^{123}I-MIBG in some cases. Interestingly, despite the lower sensitivity of ^{123}I-MIBG in carcinoid tumors, a complementary role for it was noted with patterns of different intensities of ^{123}I-MIBG in non-octreotide-avid regions [99]. However, with the increasing use of ^{68}Ga-labeled PET radiotracers for SRI, false-negative results have significantly decreased in NETs, as previously discussed in this section. Further discussions on the role of MIBG in other NETs can be found in the next section.

^{18}F-FLUORODEOXYGLUCOSE PET/CT IMAGING

FDG PET/CT imaging is the first-line test of choice for many solid tumors; however, its role in well-differentiated NETs is limited because of their lower grade and rate of growth. The SUVs for FDG are generally higher in higher-grade NETs with a high proliferation index and those of a poorly differentiated histology [100] (Figures 44.3 and 44.6). Binderup et al. showed a sensitivity of 92% for FDG PET in the detection of NETs with a proliferation index

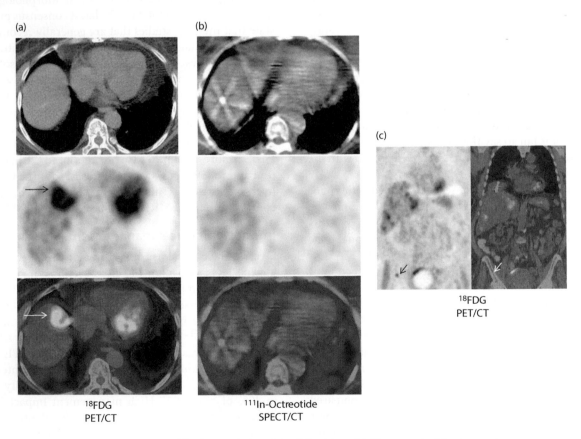

Figure 44.6 A patient with a diagnosis of high-grade (Ki-67 > 15) midgut NET treated with chemotherapy now presents with rising tumor markers and clinical symptoms of flushing and diarrhea. (a) FDG PET/CT axial images show increased glucose metabolism in a large hepatic dome lesion (arrows). (b) ^{111}In-DTPA^0-octreotide (Octreoscan) SPECT/CT axial images show no appreciable radiotracer uptake in the corresponding hepatic lesion seen on the FDG PET/CT study. (c) FDG PET/CT coronal images show additional hepatic lesions with increased FDG uptake, which were all negative on the Octreoscan (not shown here). Additionally, a right iliac bone metastasis is detected (diagonal arrows) that was otherwise not detected by CT and Octreoscan. These findings underscore the importance of FDG PET/CT imaging in the management of patients with high-grade NETs, especially when Octreoscan is negative. Note the lesser degree of FDG uptake compared with the octreotide accumulation, which is in line with well-differentiated histology with adequate SSTR2 expression.

exceeding 15%, compared with a sensitivity of 69% for conventional SRS [46]. In support of these findings, multiple other data have been published corroborating the correlation between tumor aggressive behavior and increased FDG uptake [51,78]. More recent published data are also in line with these earlier studies, confirming a role for FDG PET in characterizing NET aggressiveness to determine the clinical behavior and thereby prognosis [12,70,101–104]. Wild et al. reported that the tumor uptake of ^{68}Ga-DOTATATE and ^{68}Ga-DOTANOC was dependent on tumor grade; the median SUVmax decreased as the tumor grade increased. Multivariate analysis revealed a significantly higher SUVmax in low-grade (G1) than in-high grade (G3) tumors ($p = 0.009$) [70]. In another study by Ambrosini et al., ^{68}Ga-DOTATATE PET was also found superior to FDG PET imaging in the detection of lower-grade (G1 and G2) NETs (SUVmax 29 and 15.5, respectively), compared with values for FDG PET of 2.9 and 10.5 [12]. In contrast, FDG PET imaging was superior to ^{68}Ga-DOTATATE in high-grade (G3) NETs (SUVmax of 12 and 4.4, respectively). Has et al. found statistically significant differences between different grades of GEPNETs with respect to ^{68}Ga-DOTATATE and FDG PET/CT, with higher-grade tumors favoring the latter [102]. The impact of the combined FDG and ^{68}Ga-DOTATATE PET/CT on the therapeutic decision was about 60%. The results of a study by Pattenden et al. confirmed that well-differentiated NET metastases can be false negative on FDG PET in TC patients in a series of 207 pulmonaryl carcinoid patients [103]. Extrapolating from these findings that the aggressive NETs are often negative on SRI and will often be positive on FDG PET, there may be a role for the diagnostic use of FDG PET in SRI-negative cases.

FDG avidity also correlated with survival in NET patients with a strong prognostic value that exceeded that of traditional markers [46]. In a prospective study of 98 NET patients, the diagnostic sensitivity of FDG PET was 58% and a positive FDG PET result was associated with a significantly higher risk of death (hazard ratio [HR] = 10.3). In a multivariate analysis including SUVmax, Ki-67, and chromogranin A, an SUVmax of >3 was the only predictor of progression-free survival (PFS) (HR = 8.4, $p < 0.001$) [46]. In 38 GEPNETs, Bahri et al. reported that a positive FDG PET with an SUV ratio (tumor/normal tissue) of ≥2.5 was a poor prognostic factor, with a 4-year survival rate of 0% [104]. The median PFS and OS were significantly higher for patients with a negative FDG PET than for patients with a positive FDG PET ($p < 0.003$). FDG PET provided complemenary prognostic information regardless of SRS results; even for patients with a low-grade GEPNET and a positive SRS, PFS and OS were significantly shorter when the FDG PET was positive ($p < 0.003$). The tumor/normal tissue ratio was the only parameter associated with OS on multivariate analysis.

In summary, FDG PET imaging is usually clinically useful with favorable sensitivity in undifferentiated tumors when [^{111}In-DTPA^0]octreotide is negative or equivocal. In the context of the above discussions, a positive conventional SRS does not necessarily eliminate the need for performing FDG PET/CT, because it may add further prognostic value. Furthermore, combined radionuclide functional imaging of NETs using SRS and FDG PET imaging may allow *in vivo* determination of biological behavior in the entire tumor mass, which may not be possible with histopathological analysis because of biopsy sampling errors. Therefore, combined ^{68}Ga-DOTATATE and FDG PET/CT seems to be a reasonable approach for an individualized therapeutic strategy of GEPNETs; however, further validation studies are necessary to determine the clinical impact of this approach.

OTHER NOVEL MOLECULES FOR IMAGING NETS

β-^{11}C-5-hydroxy-L-tryptophan (^{11}C-5-HTP) and 6-^{18}F-L-3,4-dihydroxyphenylalanine (^{18}F-DOPA) were developed for the diagnosis of NETs. DOPA is a catecholamine precursor that accumulates in neuroendocrine cells [105], whereas 5-HTP is a direct precursor for the serotonin pathway, and therefore provides a potentially universal method for NET detection [106]. Published data have suggested ^{11}C-5-HTP PET to be a better imaging modality than SRS for identification of NET disease sites [106]. However, the necessity of an on-site cyclotron and the short half-life of ^{11}C ($t_{1/2} = 20$ min) impart an insurmountable disadvantage for the use of ^{11}C-labeled molecules in a routine clinical setting. ^{18}F is favored over other PET radiotracers based on its favorable chemical and nuclear properties, such as 110-minute half-life, which allows for time-consuming radiosynthesis and delivery; abundance of positron emission; low β+ energy of 0.63 MeV, which ensures a short positron range associated with a high spatial resolution; and lower radiation doses to patients [107].

A significant number of NETs accumulate and decarboxylate amino acid precursors, such as L-DOPA, a feature that is exploited for obtaining tumor NET functional information. In gastrointestinal carcinoids, early studies showed good results for ^{18}F-FDOPA PET, with better sensitivity than SRS (65% vs. 57%) [108]. These findings were replicated in later studies demonstrating a better performance by ^{18}F-FDOPA PET than the combination of SRS and CT, with a sensitivity of 95%–98% and 73–79%, respectively ($p < 0.001$) [109,110], while in noncarcinoid digestive NETs, SRS was better [111,112]. More recently, ^{18}F-FDOPA PET/CT has been reported to be a sensitive functional imaging tool for the detection of primary NETs occult on SRS, especially tumors with a well-differentiated pattern and serotonin secretion. In one comparative study of midgut carcinoids, ^{18}F-DOPA PET was found to be more sensitive than ^{11}C-5-HTP PET (98% vs. 89%), while the opposite was noted for PNETs (80% vs. 96%) [110]. In another study, a correlation between the ^{18}F-DOPA SUVmax and plasma serotonin in ^{18}F-DOPA-positive patients suggested a role for ^{18}F-DOPA imaging in serotonin-secreting tumors that are not visible on SRI by PET [113]. In recent years, comparisons between ^{68}Ga-labeled somatostatin analogs and ^{18}F-DOPA revealed a lower diagnostic value for ^{18}F-DOPA PET [69,74,76,91,106,113,114]. Moreover, one has to bear in mind that in the selection of patients for PRRT, it is imperative that the imaging radiotracer should be in a group similar to that used for PRRT; thus, SRI methods are superior to other molecules used in imaging NETs.

The majority of PNETs are well differentiated and thus have a slow growth pattern, but some may exhibit a locally invasive behavior and others may metastasize. ^{18}F-FDOPA PET/CT has a lower sensitivity in the identification and staging of PNETs when compared with carcinoid tumors of midgut origin. Therefore, FDOPA should be considered as a second-line imaging tool to SRI with SPECT/CT or PET/CT. In a meta-analysis performed by Ambrosini et al., ^{68}Ga-DOTANOC identified more lesions than ^{18}F-FDOPA on a lesion basis analysis [76].

When compared with FDG PET, ^{18}F-FDOPA offers an advantage for the detection of carcinoids, because many of these tumors are well differentiated and have an indolent disease course because of low proliferation activity [41,49]. ^{18}F-FDG PET/CT, on the other hand, detects high-grade lesions with aggressive histology and is associated with a negative SRS due to insufficient expression of SSTRs [115]. Hence, it has been suggested that a positive ^{18}F-FDG scan and negative SRS scan or F-DOPA scan may be a sign of poor prognosis.

Gastrin receptor scintigraphy (GRS) is a new imaging method primarily developed for the detection of medullary thyroid carcinoma, but it was also evaluated in a pilot study in NETs because gastrin binding CCK2 receptors are also expressed on a variety of other NETs [116]. GLP-1 receptors may also be targeted for imaging of other tumors, such as gastrinoma, pheochromocytoma (PHEO), and medullary thyroid cancer, which overexpress this receptor subtype. The results of preliminary studies suggest a role for GLP-1 receptor imaging, particularly in patients with benign insulinomas, gastrinoma, PHEO, or medullary thyroid cancer [117,118]. Wild et al. showed the superiority of GLP-1 receptor SPECT/CT using ^{111}In-labeled [Lys[40](Ahx-DTPA)NH$_2$]-exendin-4 as a radiopharmaceutical [117]. Recently, using [Lys[40](Ahx-HYNIC-^{99m}Tc/EDDA)NH$_2$]-exendin-4, Sowa-Staszczak et al. demonstrated 100% sensitivity and specificity in patients with benign insulinomas [118]. The authors emphasized that the GLP-1 receptor tracer labeled with ^{99m}Tc instead of ^{111}In is characterized by a lower radiation exposure to patients and staff, and potential usefulness for intraoperative localization of insulinoma foci using a gamma probe. However, these results require verification in a larger series of patients to prove the clinical usefulness of this indication.

SUMMARY

Currently, ^{111}In-DTPA[0]-octreotide remains the most widely used tracer in the management of carcinoid tumors and PNETs because of its availability with an established place in the clinical management algorithm. However, of ^{68}Ga-labeled peptides, ^{68}Ga-DOTATOC, ^{68}Ga-DOTATATE, and ^{68}Ga-DOTANOC have recently emerged as strong contenders to SRS, consistently demonstrating superior results to ^{111}In-DTPA-octreotide imaging in the diagnosis, staging, and restaging of NETs. ^{11}C-5-HTP PET, ^{18}F-fluorodopamine

(^{18}F-DA) PET, and ^{18}F-DOPA PET are also robust PET radiopharmaceuticals for imaging NETs. The availabilities of these novel molecules, however, are even more limited than that of ^{68}Ga-DOTA-labeled somatostatin analogs. Although large prospective data sets are not available, based on retrospective data, the sensitivities of these latter molecules seem to be inferior to that of ^{68}Ga-DOTA peptides. Thus, with the proven superiority, it is expected that over time, with the increasing availability, ^{68}Ga-DOTA peptide PET will replace SRS SPECT. The long-lived radionuclides, such as ^{18}F, may further improve clinical operations in NET patients. In this regard, however, the easy access to PET tracers is a crucial step to overcome limited use of this advanced technology. FDG PET is particularly helpful for visualizing more aggressive NETs, although there are limited data showing that FDG avidity confers a poor prognosis. A combined used of SRI and FDG PET may be a future consideration for better disease characterization. Furthermore, the more targeted radiopharmaceuticals, e.g., GLP-1 receptor imaging, are promising for localization of benign insulinomas with a greater sensitivity; however, the availability of these radiotracers is rather limited and costly. More research is warranted to prove their clinical value.

Finally, combining different radiotracers reflecting different tumor behaviors (e.g., FDG PET and ^{68}Ga-DOTA PET) exploits varying avidities and targets within the tumor for different mechanisms to pan out a genomic profile that may help better plan therapies.

PHEOCHROMOCYTOMA AND PARAGANGLIOMA

MIBG imaging

The tumor cells of chromaffin origin, such as PHEO, paraganglioma (PGL), and neuroblastomas, exclusively express a norepinephrine transporters, which function as a facilitator for the uptake of norepinephrine and epinephrine into the presynaptic sympathetic neurons. This system enables functional imaging with [131]I- or ^{123}I-MIBG, an analog of guanethidine, and is structurally similar to noradrenaline [98]. MIBG is avidly taken up by neuroendocrine cells originating from the sympathomedullary tissues through both diffusion and active transport by norepinephrine transporters. [123]I has replaced ^{131}I as a radiolabel for MIBG imaging because of its greater photon flux, with superior image quality and increased sensitivity, as well as shorter half-life and better radiation dosimetry [119,120]. Despite the high specificity (95%–100%) for detecting PHEO, and being superior to ^{131}I-MIBG, ^{123}I-MIBG scintigraphy has intrinsic disadvantages, such as suboptimal spatial resolution, which limits the detection sensitivity; the need for multiple imaging sessions; and the relatively high radiation exposure [119].

BIODISTRIBUTION

After intravenous administration, radiolabeled MIBG is taken up by adrenergic tissues without binding to postsynaptic adrenergic receptors. In normal subjects, MIBG accumulates in the myocardium, lungs, salivary glands, liver, spleen, large intestine, and urinary bladder. MIBG uptake can be observed in the cerebellum, basal nuclei, and thalamic regions. Bilateral symmetrical activity is sometimes seen in the supraclavicular region corresponding to the brown adipose tissue that has an abundant supply of sympathetic nerves [121]. The normal adrenal medulla may show physiological uptake, and this finding is more frequently seen when ^{123}I-MIBG is used (75% of patients versus 10% with ^{131}I-MIBG) [122]. The adrenal uptake exceeding that seen in the liver is usually considered outside the normal range [123].

Similar to SRS, the accuracy of ^{123}I-MIBG planar imaging is hampered by the overlapping of structures and the interference of adjacent high physiological tracer uptake. In these patients, SPECT/CT allows precise lesion localization, leading to an accurate demonstration of the site of tracer uptake despite the close proximity of structures such as the abdominal viscera, nodes, and bones.

DRUGS INTERFERING WITH MIBG UPTAKE

A complete list of interfering medications is available in review articles and procedure guidelines in the literature [22,124]. All medications should be discontinued for 1–3 days with the exception of labetalol (approximately 10-day withdrawal) and depot forms of antipsychotics (1-month withdrawal) to avoid false-negative results. The combination of alpha-receptor blockade and beta-receptor blockade may not significantly reduce MIBG uptake [125]. However, manipulation of medications should be discussed with the referring clinician.

Procedure guidelines on the use of MIBG scintigraphy in NETs have been published previously [22,124]. It is essential to protect thyroid blockade with potassium iodide, starting from the day before injection of the radiotracer and continuing during the duration of imaging: 2 days for ^{123}I-MIBG and 5 days for ^{131}I-MIBG. The standard time of imaging with ^{123}I-MIBG is at 20–24 hours after injection (with optional images at 48 hours), compared with 24 and 48 hours when ^{131}I-MIBG is used (with optional images at 72 hours).

CLINICAL APPLICATIONS OF MIBG IMAGING IN PHEO AND PGL

Surgery is the first line of treatment for resectable PHEOs and PGLs. Therefore, accurate staging is essential to determine the extent of disease and the feasibility of surgery. The overall sensitivity of ^{131}I-MIBG scintigraphy in PHEO and PGL ranges between 75% and 90%, and the specificity is usually above 95%, but the use of ^{123}I-MIBG with SPECT improved its sensitivity to greater than 85% (88–96%) with no change in specificity for detecting PHEO [122,124,126,127]. Hence, ^{123}I-MIBG scintigraphy has become the first choice for imaging functional PHEOs, PGLs, and neuroblastomas for assessing PHEOs and PGLs [22,124].

Because ^{123}I-MIBG uptake represents the presence of a functional norepinephrine transport system, both benign

and malignant PHEO and PGL can be imaged by this modality (Figure 44.7). Generally, foci of increased MIBG uptake in the adrenal gland or at a site compatible with the sympathetic paraganglia of the nervous system are consistent with a benign tumor, whereas multiple sites of uptake outside the adrenal and sympathetic ganglia are in line with malignant lesions. Positive MIBG imaging results have been obtained in oligosecretory or nonsecretory adrenal tumors [22,124]. MIBG scintigraphy can also identify PHEO associated with various familial syndromes and simple familial PHEO [31].

Current treatment for malignant inoperable PHEO/PGL and neuroblastomas also includes ^{131}I-MIBG-targeted internal radiotherapy. Similar to that discussed in the previous section for SRI and PRRT, the avidity of tracer uptake on ^{123}I-MIBG imaging is one of the important factors that determine the eligibility for ^{131}I-MIBG therapy. Recently, histone deacetylase (HDAC) inhibitors have been investigated to increase the expression of norepinephrine transporters and thereby increase the entry of ^{131}I-MIBG into PHEO cells in an attempt to enhance the therapeutic efficacy of ^{131}I-MIBG therapy in patients with advanced malignant PHEO/PGL [128]. However, this is an area of ongoing research and long-term results are yet to be published.

Not surprisingly, the rate of lesion detection with MIBG imaging further improves at post-therapy high-dose ^{131}I-MIBG [129] (Figure 44.8). A prospective multicenter study involving 81 primary or metastatic PHEO or PGL patients and 69 with suspected PHEO or PGL reported an overall sensitivity of 82%–88% and specificity of 82%–84% for ^{123}I-MIBG imaging with or without SPECT [130]. For patients evaluated for suspected disease, the sensitivity and specificity were 88% and 84%, respectively. In a subgroup analysis for adrenal (PHEO) and extra-adrenal (PGL) tumors, sensitivities were 88% and 67%, respectively. The addition of SPECT increased reader confidence with no significant effect on sensitivity or specificity. These favorable results are supported by a recent meta-analysis of 15 well-controlled clinical studies that yielded a calculated sensitivity of 94% and specificity of 92% for ^{123}I-MIBG scintigraphy in detecting PHEO [131]. In this analysis, the sensitivity of MIBG scans for detection of neuroblastomas was 97%.

SPECT or SPECT/CT improves diagnostic accuracy and confidence in interpretation with respect to lesion localization and characterization that usually leads to better management in patients with NETs. In multiple small studies in patients with PHEO or suspected PHEO or neuroblastoma who had equivocal diagnostic CTs, overall ^{123}I-MIBG SPECT/CT had a sensitivity of 100% and a specificity of 89%. ^{123}I-MIBG SPECT/CT provided additional information in more than half of the cases and increased the diagnostic certainty in 50%–90% of studies [132,133]. However, these are limited studies with a retrospective design; therefore, the results should be judiciously interpreted.

More recently published data indicate that the overall sensitivity of ^{123}I-MIBG imaging is considerably low at approximately 65%, which is below the historically

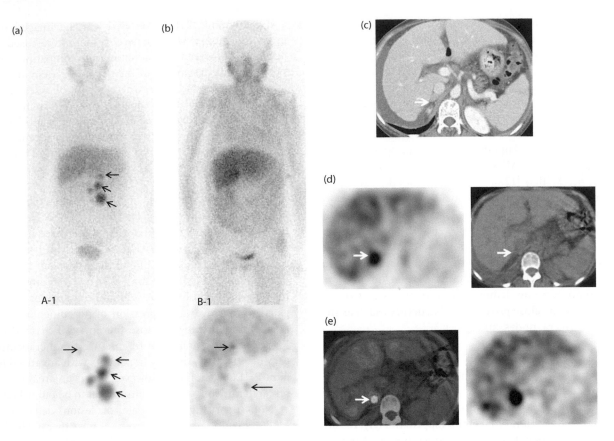

Figure 44.7 **(a)** A patient with a diagnosis of PHEO evaluated with [123]MIBG prior to surgery. The whole body planar image of the [123]MIBG study shows multiple foci of increased radiotracer uptake in the region of the left adrenal gland (arrow) and multiple retroperitoneal lymph nodes (diagonal arrows) consistent with malignant PHEO and regional nodal metastases, respectively. (A-1) Coronal image of the SPECT study performed subsequent to the whole body imaging shows similar findings (arrow and the diagonal arrows) consistent with the primary tumor and metastases. Note the faint uptake in the region of the right adrenal gland (left arrow) consistent with physiologic uptake. **(b)** The same patient is referred for follow-up study after 4 months to determine disease status after surgery, consistent with partial left adrenalectomy and retroperitoneal lymph node dissection. The whole body planar image shows no appreciable abnormal finding. (B-1) Coronal image of the SPECT study performed subsequent to the whole body imaging shows complete disappearance of the previously seen uptake in multiple retroperitoneal lymph nodes except for a faint focus of uptake in the midabdomen suggesting residual nodal metastasis (right arrow). Note the faint uptake in the region of the right adrenal gland (left arrow), which is again consistent with physiologic uptake. **(c)** A contrast CT study done in the postsurgical period shows an enhancing nodule in the adrenal gland that may represent another focus of PHEO. **(d)** Axial image of the SPECT/CT (same time period as B) shows uptake corresponding to the right adrenal that is more pronounced than seen in the planar image. This uptake was slightly higher than that seen on the preoperative study (axial SPECT image not shown here) and that seen on SPECT/CT. This finding was equivocal and may represent either uptake in the PHEO (may be benign) or normal physiologic uptake in the adrenal gland. **(e)** Further imaging with ^{18}F-DOPA PET/CT and ^{18}F-DA PET/CT was unrevealing with respect to the presence of an additional PHEO in the right adrenal gland due to intense physiologic uptake of ^{18}F-DOPA (^{18}F-DA PET not shown here) in the adrenal gland (arrow); the intense uptake might have obscured an underlying small adrenal tumor.

reported results, especially for the detection of extra-adrenal or metastatic disease [130,134–137]. In particular, a low MIBG sensitivity was obtained in PHEOs associated with von Hippel–Lindau (VHL) syndrome, probably due to the low expression of NET in VHL-related PHEO cells [138]. Particularly, lower MIBG sensitivity was associated with VHL syndrome, probably due to the low expression of transporters of norepinephrine (tNEs) in VHL-related PHEO cells. In support of these findings, Timmers et al. reported a sensitivity of only 65% for ^{123}I-MIBG in patients with mutations in succinate dehydrogenase subunit B

(SDHB) genes [137]. Therefore, patients with false-negative MIBG SPECT may be considered for further testing for SDHB mutations.

Several studies have shown lower sensitivities in the range of 60%–85%, particularly in patients with bilateral disease and hereditary syndromes [126,139]. A limitation of MIBG scintigraphy is the inability to differentiate between medullary hyperplasia and neoplasia in familial PHEOs, mainly because the size of familial tumors is usually smaller than that of sporadic PHEOs. De Graaf et al. reported a specificity of only 17% in patients with MEN2 syndrome,

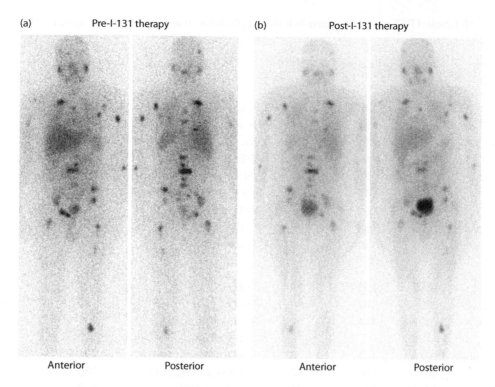

(a) Pre-I-131 therapy   **(b)** Post-I-131 therapy

Anterior   Posterior   Anterior   Posterior

Figure 44.8 A 22-year-old male with a diagnosis of metastatic PHEO who underwent high-dose ^{131}I-MIBG therapy. **(a)** ^{131}I-MIBG whole body imaging was performed 7 days after high-dose MIBG therapy. On anterior and posterior planar images, there are multiple foci of ^{131}I-MIBG accumulation involving multiple bones in the axial and appendicular skeleton, consistent with metastatic disease. **(b)** The patient underwent repeat high-dose ^{131}I-MIBG therapy after 3 months, and 7 days later, a whole body scan was obtained in the anaterior and posterior planes. Note the decrease in intensity of uptake in the lesions throughout the involved sites. These findings are consistent with favorable response to therapy. A whole body screening to reflect the tumor functional status provided by MIBG study would not be possible with morphologic (CT or MRI) imaging studies, and a whole body bone scan would not be as specific as the MIBG study.

while CT and MRI were clearly superior in this regard [140], although the sensitivity of MIBG was similar to or slightly higher than that of CT and MRI (92% vs. 87%). Based on these findings, MIBG scintigraphy can be restricted to those patients in whom MRI findings are negative despite a clinical suspicion of PHEO.

MIBG accumulation by sympathomedullary tissue is mediated by tNEs and the VMAT types 1 and 2 [135]. Therefore, false-negative MIBG findings can be a result of low affinity to NETs, the lack of storage granules, or the loss of NET or VMAT by dedifferentiation of tumor cells [127]. In a study by Fottner et al. for a positive ^{123}I-MIBG functional imaging, the expression of VMAT-1 was found to be essential because all VMAT-1-negative tumors on immunohistochemical analysis remained undetected on ^{123}I-MIBG scintigraphy [141]. In this study, clinical predictors for MIBG negativity also included a predominant norepinephrine/normetanephrine secretion, age of <45 years, and a hereditary cause.

In summary, ^{123}I-MIBG used to be considered the imaging test choice in the evaluation of PHEOs and PGLs; however, the sensitivity of these imaging tests has been scaled downwards because of the above-reviewed limitations related to both this agent's physical characteristics and pharmacokinetics. Therefore, evaluation of PHEOs and

PGLs with PET/CT is increasingly gaining importance with the availability of novel PET radiopharmaceuticals labeled with somatostatin peptide derivatives, as discussed in the following section.

Positron emission tomography of PHEO and PGL

Diagnostic performance from studies comparing PET tracers and MIBG in patients with PHEO/PGL is shown in Table 44.3. Overall, the higher spatial resolution of PET than of SPECT enables the acquisition of excellent-quality images of NET entities. In addition, fast scan completion and readout within hours, compared to days, with ^{123}I-MIBG SPECT/CT makes this imaging modality highly favorable. This advantage of PET/CT is especially beneficial for children, where the shorter scanning time improves compliance. Other advantages of PET radiotracers versus MIBG include less radiation exposure and no need for thyroid blockade. A wide range of PET tracers that are associated with catecholamine synthesis, transport, and storage pathways have been used for imaging PHEO/PGL. These include ^{11}C-hydroxyephedrine (^{11}C-HED) [139], ^{18}F-DA [138,142], and ^{18}F-DOPA [105,141,143,144]. All of these tracers allow imaging tumors of chromaffin cell origin based

Table 44.3 ^{18}F-labeled PET molecules used in imaging pheochromocytomas and paragangliomas

Investigator	Year	Reference	No. of patients	NET subtype	PET sensitivity %	MIBG sensitivity %
^{18}F-DA						
Ilias et al.	2003	122	16	Metastatic PHEO	100	56
Kaji et al.	2007	138	7	PHEO	100	57
Timmers et al.	2007	137	30	PGL	88	80
Ilias et al.	2008	142	53	PHEO	90	71
Zelinka et al.	2008	162	71	Metastatic PHEO/PGL	90	71
Timmers et al.	2009	144	52	Nonmetastatic PGL	78	78
				Metastatic PGL	76	57
Timmers et al.	2009	163	99	PGL	92	83
King et al.	2011	136	10	Head/neck PGL	46	31
^{18}F-DOPA						
Hoegerle et al.	2002	108	14	PHEO	100	71
Fiebrich et al.	2009	151	48	PHEO	90	65
Timmers et al.	2009	144	52	Nonmetastatic PGL	81	78
				Metastatic PGL	45	57
Fottner et al.	2010	141	30	PHEO/PGL	96	80
Rufini et al.	2011	164	12	Malignant PHEO/PGL	100	75
King et al.	2011	136	10	Head/neck PGL	100	31
^{18}F-FDG						
Mann et al.	2006	139	14	PHEO	100	50
Timmers et al.	2007	137	30	PGL	100	80
Zelinka et al.	2008	162	71	Metastatic PHEO/PGL	76	71
Timmers et al.	2009	144	52	Nonmetastatic	88	78
				Metastatic PHEO/PGL	74	57
King et al.	2011	136	10	Head/neck PGL	77	31
Timmers et al.	2012	155	216	Nonmetastatic PGL	77	75
				Metastatic PGL	82	50

on the increased activity of large amino acid transporter systems in NETs such as PHEOs and PGLs [134,144]. ^{18}F-FDG has also been implicated in imaging PHEO/PGL to evaluate glucose metabolism. Most relevant radiotracers are further discussed in the following section. In a systematic review of 28 studies comprising 852 PHEO/PGL patients who underwent both MIBG scintigraphy and PET or PET/CT with different radiopharmaceuticals, including ^{18}F-DA, ^{18}F-DOPA, ^{18}F-FDG, and ^{68}Ga-DOTA peptides, Rufini et al. showed a clear diagnostic superiority of PET over that of MIBG scintigraphy [145]. However, except for ^{18}F-FDG, these novel PET radiotracers may not be routinely available at most imaging centers worldwide because of limited infrastructure and cost.

^{18}F-DOPA PET

^{18}F-DOPA is a dopamine precursor that targets the catecholamine metabolic pathways and is taken up into the cells via the amino acid transporter (LAT1/4F2hc), which is also coupled to the mammalian target of rapamycin (mTOR) signaling pathway [146]. ^{18}F-DOPA PET/CT may be performed

for confirmation of diagnosis of PHEO or PGL, staging at initial presentation, restaging, and follow-up of such patients (Figure 44.9). The imaging protocol requires 4-hour fasting and has been published elsewhere [147]. Physiologic uptake of ^{18}F-DOPA is seen in the striatum, kidneys, pancreas, liver, gall bladder, biliary tract, esophagus, myocardium, and duodenum [147]. Adrenal glands may be faintly visible. The liver uptake is used as a reference for defining pathological uptake.

In an earlier study, Hoegerle et al. reported a much higher sensitivity for ^{18}F-DOPA than for ^{123}I-MIBG (100% vs. 71%), for the detection of PHEOs, and an even better performance than MRI in head and neck PGLs [108]. However, later studies have suggested an inferior performance for ^{18}F-DOPA, with a relatively low sensitivity for localizing malignant PHEOs. In a study of 52 PGL patients, Timmers et al. reported favorable detection rates for localizing nonmetastatic PGL, with ^{18}F-DOPA showing a similar sensitivity at 88% as that of the other radiopharmaceuticals, including ^{18}F-DA, ^{18}F-FDG, and ^{123}I-MIBG (78%) [144]. However, for metastatic tumors, ^{18}F-DA performed better than the other radiotracers, with a reported sensitivity of 76%. In a recent

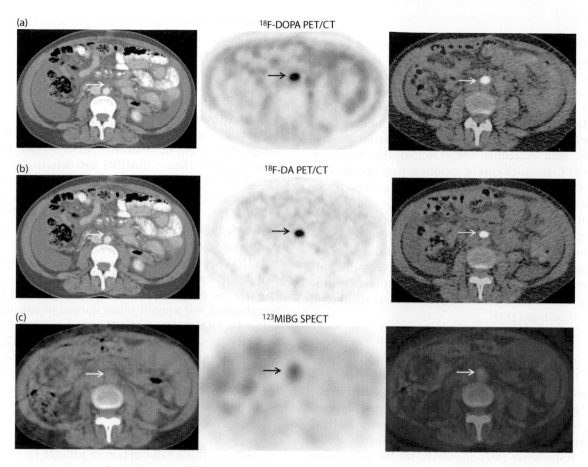

Figure 44.9 The same patient presented in Figure 44.7. Subsequent to MIBG imaging, the patient underwent ¹⁸F-DOPA PET/CT and ¹⁸F-DA PET/CT imaging to further evaluate the disease status. **(a)** Axial image of the ¹⁸F-DOPA PET/CT shows intense uptake in a small aortocaval lymph node (white and black arrows), consistent with residual lymph node metastasis. **(b)** Axial image of the ¹⁸F-DA PET/CT shows similar findings to those seen on ¹⁸F-DOPA PET/CT. **(c)** ¹²³MIBG SPECT/CT (lower abdominal images of the same study presented in Figure 44.7) axial images reveal a faint focus of uptake in the aortocaval region, consistent with the presence of residual lymph node metastasis. These studies confirm the superiority of both ¹⁸F-DOPA PET/CT and ¹⁸F-DA PET/CT over ¹²³MIBG SPECT/CT with respect to clear visualization of PHEOs because of increased sensitivity provided by both the radiotracer and PET technology.

meta-analysis, the pooled sensitivity of ¹⁸F-FDOPA PET for the detection of PGLs was 91% and 79% on a patient-based and lesion-based analysis, respectively [82]. For both analyses, the specificity was approximately 95%.

SDHB gene mutation is one of the causes of of hereditary PHEO/PGL syndrome, and it is associated with a high rate of malignancy. ¹⁸F-DOPA was found to have a low sensitivity for SDHB-related metastatic disease [144,148,149]. In SDHB-related metastatic forms of PHEO/PGL, ¹⁸F-FDG PET/CT was able to detect more lesions than ¹⁸F-FDOPA PET [149]. The inferior performance of ¹⁸F-DOPA in localizing metastatic disease may be on the grounds of the loss of tNEs in the setting of aggressive disease. However, in another study by Rischke et al., ¹⁸F-DOPA uptake ratios could not differentiate between various genotypes of VHL syndrome, which is associated with a low predisposition to malignancy, and SDHB-related disease, which is associated with a higher malignancy rate [150]. The available limited data suggest that ¹⁸F-DA PET is superior to ¹²³I-MIBG for VHL-related metastatic PHEO/PGL [143], while ¹⁸F-DOPA

PET and FDG PET are superior to ¹⁸F-DA PET and ¹²³I-MIBG for detecting metastatic SDH-related head and neck PGLs [136]. Overall, ¹⁸F-DA showed a high sensitivity for detecting both intra- and extra-adrenal, as well as metastatic PHEO [138,142] (Figure 44.8); however, the main disadvantage of imaging with ¹⁸F-DA is the limited access to it. It is fair to say that the definitive value of ¹⁸F-FDOPA PET in distinguishing between various genotypes of PHEO/PGL is not established, and this important area requires further investigations.

In an era of hybrid imaging, it is important to report results with the synergistic value of anatomic and functional imaging harnessed to the overall analysis. Fiebrich et al. showed that ¹⁸F-DOPA PET with CT/MRI was superior to ¹²³I-MIBG with CT/MRI (93% vs. 76%, $p < 0.001$), and there was good correlation between ¹⁸F-FDOPA PET/CT and plasma normetanephrine ($r = 0.82$) [151]. A more recent study also reported a high sensitivity and specificity ¹⁸F-DOPA PET/CT (93% and 88%, respectively) for detection of PHEOs and PGLs [150].

[11]C-HED

[11]C-HED is a catecholamine analog whose uptake reflects catecholamine transport, storage, and catecholamine recycling and accumulates in organs with rich sympathetic innervations, such as the heart and adrenal medulla [152]. Although ^{11}C-HED has been shown to be more useful than ^{123}I-MIBG SPECT/CT for the detection of tumors of the sympathetic nervous system with a high sensitivity and specificity, both exceeding 90% [126,153], the 20-minute half-life of ^{11}C and high cost of cyclotron-based production limit its widespread availability and application. Low tracer accumulation in soft tissue, muscle, gut, lungs, and bones is an advantage, but the relatively high physiologic liver and pancreatic uptake of ^{11}C-HED may impede the detection of small liver metastases and metastases around the pancreas. In addition, no clear advantage was observed with this tracer compared with ^{123}I-MIBG in the detection of neuroblastoma; however, the number of patients was small for a definitive conclusion [153].

^{18}F-FDG

Primary PHEOs and PGLs are equally well identified by ^{18}F-FDG PET/CT and ^{123}I-MIBG SPECT, which are currently the standard imaging modalities. According to the results of a large prospective study in 216 patients, Timmers et al. reported a superiority for FDG PET over ^{123}I-MIBG SPECT for metastatic PHEO/PGL, with sensitivities of 80% and 49%, respectively [137]. Moreover, for the localization of metastases of the bone, a frequent site of involvement in malignant PHEO/PGL, FDG PET was superior to CT and MRI (sensitivity 94% vs. 79%), whereas for soft tissue metastases, its accuracy was similar. Regarding the specificity of FDG PET, tracer uptake by non-PHEO/PGL lesions and by normal adrenal glands might be of concern. But, in most patients, FDG uptake by normal adrenal glands did not exceed that of the liver [154]. For differentiating benign from malignant PHEO/PGL, an SUVmax of >4.6 was suggested to be in line with malignant disease. For metastatic PCs and PGLs, especially those related to SDHB gene mutations, FDG/PET is the modality of choice regardless of tumor location, whereas the majority of MEN2-related PHEO/PGL are FDG PET negative [155]. In addition, there is evidence that FDG/PET SUV may distinguish PHEO/PGL related to different genetic defects [156]. Briefly, following the establishment of a biochemical diagnosis of PHEO/PGL, FDG PET appears superior to ^{123}I-MIBG and should be used as the first-line functional imaging modality to determine the extent of disease.

In conclusion, compared with ^{123}I-MIBG SPECT, FDG PET/CT allows better detection of metastases of PHEO/PGL with a high specificity. Although not validated in large data sets, the observations of a high FDG uptake in SDHB-related tumors and low uptake in MEN2-related tumors suggest a role for tumor functional characterization for a hereditary syndrome underlying PHEO/PGL. However, ^{123}I-MIBG imaging remains necessary to establish the eligibility of patients with metastatic PHEO/PGL for ^{131}I-MIBG treatment. FDG PET also appears useful in the identification of head and neck PGLs, but its comparative role with other imaging modalities remains to be investigated.

SOMATOSTATIN RECEPTOR IMAGING

Metastatic PHEOs and PGLs may also be evaluated with SRS. Nonetheless, generally, the sensitivity of ^{111}In-DTPA-octreotide is inferior to that of ^{123}I-MIBG for detecting benign PHEO, but in contrast, ^{111}In-octreotide is usually more sensitive than ^{123}I-MIBG for detecting malignant PHEO and metastatic lesions [126]. Similarly, although in limited series, ^{111}In-octreotide proved to be superior to ^{123}I-MIBG for diagnosing head and neck PGL with a sensitivity of 93% for ^{111}In-octreotide and CT/MRI, compared with 44% for ^{123}I-MIBG [110]. Recently, the ^{68}Ga-DOTA peptide PET has gained popularity with a well-documented role in NETs, as dicussed earlier in this chapter. The use of these peptides in PHEO and PGL has been limited, but a small series showed promising results with ^{68}Ga-DOTATOC [157]. There is some evidence that ^{68}Ga-DOTA peptide PET detects malignant PGL otherwise not identified on ^{123}I-MIBG, ^{111}In-octreotide scans, and cross-sectional imaging [96,158,159]. However, there is a need for a validation study to confirm the true role of ^{68}Ga-DOTA peptides in the management of PHEO/PGL.

SUMMARY

^{123}I-MIBG is still a valid option in patients with nonmetastatic PHEO/PGL due to its high sensitivity and wide availability; however, based on collective data, ^{123}I-MIBG has been removed from clinical use in the evaluation of metastatic tumors, except in situations where targeted radiotherapy can be planned using ^{131}I-MIBG. There is published evidence that ^{18}F-dopamine, ^{18}F-DOPA, and ^{18}F-FDG perform better than ^{123}I-MIBG to assess disease extent in malignant PHEO/PGL. The true clinical gain from PET radiotracers appears to be related to malignant and metastatic disease, but with the ability to target different mechanisms driving the biological behavior through various pathways, including gene mutations, multiple PET tracers may characterize tumors better. Preliminary data seem to indicate a primary role of ^{68}Ga-labeled somatostatin analogs not only in patients with head and neck PGL, but also in those at high risk of PGL and metastatic disease. Nonetheless, until larger prospective series confirm a definitive role for ^{68}Ga-DOTA peptides, routine investigation of PHEO and PGL should be performed using cross-sectional imaging and ^{123}I-MIBG. In cases with negative or equivocal results on MIBG and CT/MRI, other sensitive PET radiotracers can also be used (e.g., F-DOPA or F-DA) if feasible and accessible.

REFERENCES

1. Fraenkel M, Kim MK, Faggiano A, de Herder WW, Valk GD. Incidence of gastroenteropancreatic neuroendocrine tumours: A systematic review of the literature. *Endocr Relat Cancer* 2014;21:R152–63.

2. Yao JC, Hassan M, Phan A et al. One hundred years after 'carcinoid': Epidemiology of and prognostic factors for neuroendocrine tumors in 35,825 cases in the United States. *J Clin Oncol* 2008;26:3063–72.

3. Klöppel G. Classification and pathology of gastroenteropancreatic neuroendocrine neoplasms. *Endocr Relat Cancer* 2011;18(Suppl 1):S1–16.

4. Krenning EP, Kwekkebom DJ, Pauwels S, Kvols LK, Reubi JC. Somatostatin receptor scintigraphy. In: Freeman LM, ed., *Nuclear Medicine Annual*. New York: Raven Press, 1995:1–50.

5. Reubi JC, Waser B. Concomitant expression of several peptide receptors in neuroendocrine tumors as molecular basis for *in vivo* multireceptor tumor targeting. *Eur J Nucl Med* 2003;30:781–93.

6. Modlin IM, Oberg K, Chung DC et al. Gastroenteropancreatic neuroendocrine tumours. *Lancet Oncol* 2008;9:61–72.

7. Reubi JC. Somatostatin and other peptide receptors as tools for tumor diagnosis and treatment. *Neuroendocrinology* 2004;80(Suppl 1):51–6.

8. Virgolini I, Traub T, Decristoforo C. Nuclear medicine in the detection and management of pancreatic islet-cell tumours. *Best Pract Res Clin Endocrinol Metab* 2005;19:213–27.

9. Krenning EP, Kwekkeboom DJ, Oei HY et al. Somatostatin-receptor scintigraphy in gastroenteropancreatic tumors. An overview of European results. *Ann NY Acad Sci* 1994;733:416–24.

10. Metz DC, Jensen RT. Gastrointestinal neuroendocrine tumors: Pancreatic endocrine tumors. *Gastroenterology* 2008;135:1469–92.

11. Krenning EP, Kwekkeboom DJ, Bakker WH et al. Somatostatin receptor scintigraphy with [111In-DTPA-D-Phe1]- and [123I-Tyr3]-octreotide: The Rotterdam experience with more than 1000 patients. *Eur J Nucl Med* 1993;20:716–31.

12. Ambrosini V, Campana D, Tomassetti P et al. 68Ga-labelled peptides for diagnosis of gastroenteropancreatic NET. *Eur J Nucl Med Mol Imaging* 2012;39:s52–60.

13. Kroiss A, Putzer D, Decristoforo C et al. 68Ga-DOTA-TOC uptake in neuroendocrine tumour and healthy tissue: Differentiation of physiological uptake and pathological processes in PET/CT. *Eur J Nucl Med Mol Imaging* 2013;40:1800–8.

14. Krausz Y, Freedman N, Rubinstein R et al. 68Ga-DOTA-NOC PET/CT imaging of neuroendocrine tumors: Comparison with 111In-DTPA-octreotide (OctreoScan®). *Mol Imaging Biol* 2011;13:583–93.

15. Prasad V, Baum RP. Biodistribution of the Ga-68 labeled somatostatin analogue DOTA-NOC in patients with neuroendocrine tumors: Characterization of uptake in normal organs and tumor lesions. *Q J Nucl Med Mol Imaging* 2010;54:61–7.

16. Van Essen M, Krenning EP, De Jong M et al. Peptide receptor radionuclide therapy with radiolabelled somatostatin analogues in patients with somatostatin receptor positive tumours. *Acta Oncol* 2007;46:723–34.

17. Fjallskog ML, Sundin A, Westlin JE, Oberg K, Janson ET, Eriksson B. Treatment of malignant endocrine pancreatic tumors with a combination of alpha-interferon and somatostatin analogs. *Med Oncol* 2002;19(1):35–42.

18. John M, Meyerhof W, Richter D et al. Positive somatostatin receptor scintigraphy correlates with the presence of somatostatin receptor subtype 2. *Gut* 1996;38:33–9. Erratum: Positive somatostatin receptor scintigraphy correlates with the presence of somatostatin receptor subtype 2 and 5. *Gut* 1996;38:302.

19. Hofland LJ, Lamberts SWJ, van Hagen PM et al. Crucial role for somatostatin receptor subtype 2 in determining the uptake of [111In-DTPA-D-Phe1] octreotide in somatostatin receptor-positive organs. *J Nucl Med* 2003;44:1315–21.

20. Balon HR, Brown TLY, Goldsmith SJ et al. Procedure guideline for somatostatin receptor scintigraphy 2.0. *J Nucl Med* 2011;39:317–24.

21. Vinik, A, Woltering, E, Warner R et al. NANETS consensus guidelines for the diagnosis of neuroendocrine tumor. *Pancreas* 2010;39:713–34.

22. Bombardieri E, Coliva A, Maccauro M et al. Imaging of neuroendocrine tumours with gamma-emitting radiopharmaceuticals. *Q J Nucl Med Mol Imaging* 2010;54:3–15.

23. Klöppel G, Couvelard A, Perren A et al. ENETS Consensus Guidelines for the Standards of Care in Neuroendocrine Tumors: Towards a standardized approach to the diagnosis of gastroenteropancreatic neuroendocrine tumors and their prognostic stratification. *Neuroendocrinology* 2009;90:162–6.

24. Jacobson AF, Deng H, Lombard J, Lessig HJ, Black RR. 123I-meta-iodobenzylguanidine scintigraphy for the detection of neuroblastoma and pheochromocytoma: Results of a meta-analysis. *J Clin Endocrinol Metab* 2010;95:2596–606.

25. Westlin JE, Janson ET, Arnberg H, Ahlstrom H, Oberg K, Nilsson S. Somatostatin receptor scintigraphy of carcinoid tumours using the [111In-DTPA-D-Phe1]-octreotide. *Acta Oncology* 1993;32:783–6.

26. Kwekkeboom DJ, Kooij PP, Bakker WH, Mäcke HR, Krenning EP. Comparison of 111In-DOTA-Tyr3-octreotide and 111In-DTPA-octreotide in the same patients: Biodistribution, kinetics, organ and tumor uptake. *J Nucl Med* 1999;40:762–7.

27. Chiti A, Fanti S, Savelli G et al. Comparison of somatostatin receptor imaging, computed tomography and ultrasound in the clinical management of neuroendocrine gastro-enteropancreatic tumours. *Eur J Nucl Med* 1998;25:1396–403.

28. Gibril F, Reynolds JC, Chen CC et al. Specificity of somatostatin receptor scintigraphy: A prospective study and effects of false-positive localizations on management in patients with gastrinomas. *J Nucl Med* 1999;40:539–53.

29. Lebtahi R, Cadiot G, Sarda L et al. Clinical impact of somatostatin receptor scintigraphy in the management of patients with neuroendocrine gastroenteropancreatic tumors. *J Nucl Med* 1997;38:853–8.

30. Gibril F, Reynolds JC, Doppman JL et al. Somatostatin receptor scintigraphy: Its sensitivity compared with that of other imaging methods in detecting primary and metastatic gastrinomas. A prospective study. *Ann Intern Med* 1996;125:26–34.

31. Rufini V, Calcagni ML, Baum RP. Imaging of neuroendocrine tumors. *Semin Nucl Med* 2006;36:228–47.

32. Mariani G, Bruselli L, Kuwert T et al. A review on the clinical uses of SPECT/CT. *Eur J Nucl Med Mol Imaging* 2010;37:1959–85.

33. Ricke J, Klose KJ. Imaging procedures in neuroendocrine tumours. *Digestion* 2000;62(Suppl 1):39–44.

34. Krenning EP, Kwekkeboom DJ, Reubi JC. Peptide receptor scintigraphy in oncology. In: Murray IPC, Ell PJ, eds., *Nuclear Medicine in Clinical Diagnosis and Treatment*. Edinburgh: Churchill Livingstone, 1998:859–70.

35. Krausz Y, Keidar Z, Kogan I et al. SPECT/CT hybrid imaging with 111In-pentetreotide in assessment of neuroendocrine tumours. *Clin Endocrinol* 2003;59:565–73.

36. Hedlund E, Karlsson JE, Starck SA. Automatic and manual image fusion of In-pentetreotide SPECT and diagnostic CT in neuroendocrine tumor imaging— An evaluation. *J Med Phys* 2010;35:223–8.

37. Amthauer H, Denecke T, Rohlfing T et al. Value of image fusion using single photon emission computed tomography with integrated low dose computed tomography in comparison with a retrospective voxel-based method in neuroendocrine tumours. *Eur Radiol* 2005;15:1456–62.

38. Castaldi P, Rufini V, Treglia G et al. Impact of 111In-DTPA-octreotide SPECT/CT fusion images in the management of neuroendocrine tumours. *Radiol Med* 2008;113:1056–67.

39. Caplin ME, Baudin E, Ferolla P et al. Pulmonary neuroendocrine (carcinoid) tumors: European Neuroendocrine Tumor Society expert consensus and recommendations for best practice for typical and atypical pulmonary carcinoids. *Ann Oncol* 2015;26:1604–20.

40. Meisinger QC, Klein JS, Butnor KJ, Gentchos G, Leavitt BJ. CT features of peripheral pulmonary carcinoid tumors. *AJR Am J Roentgenol* 2011;197:1073–80.

41. Toumpanakis C, Kim MK, Rinke A et al. Combination of cross-sectional and molecular imaging studies in the localization of gastroenteropancreatic neuroendocrine tumours. *Neuroendocrinology* 2014;99:63–74.

42. Sundin A. Radiological and nuclear medicine imaging of gastroenteropancreatic neuroendocrine tumors. *Best Pract Res Clin Gastroenterol* 2012;26:803–18.

43. Dahdaleh FS, Lorenzen A, Rajput M et al. The value of preoperative imaging in small bowel neuroendocrine tumors. *Ann Surg Oncol* 2013;20:1912–7.

44. Kumbasar B, Kamel IR, Tekes A et al. Imaging of neuroendocrine tumors: Accuracy of helical CT versus SRS. *Abdom Imaging* 2004;29:696–702.

45. Rothenstein J, Cleary SP, Pond GR et al. Neuroendocrine tumours of the gastrointestinal tract: A decade of experience at the Princess Margaret Hospital. *Am J Clin Oncol* 2008;31:64–70.

46. Binderup T, Knigge U, Loft A, Federspiel B, Kjær A. 18F-fluorodeoxyglucose positron emission tomography predicts survival of patients with neuroendocrine tumors. *Clin Cancer Res* 2010;16:978–85.

47. Kwekkeboom D, van Urk H, Pauw KH et al. Octreotide scintigraphy for the detection of paraganglioma. *J Nucl Med* 1993;34:873–8.

48. Zimmer T, Stolzel U, Bader M et al. Endoscopic ultrasonography and somatostatin receptor scintigraphy in the preoperative localisation of insulinomas and gastrinomas. *Gut* 1996;39:562–8.

49. de Herder WW. GEP-NETS update: Functional localisation and scintigraphy in neuroendocrine tumours of the gastrointestinal tract and pancreas (GEP-NETs). *Eur J Endocrinol* 2014;170:R173–83.

50. Termanini B, Gibril F, Reynolds JC et al. Value of somatostatin receptor scintigraphy: A prospective study in gastrinoma of its effect on clinical management. *Gastroenterology* 1997;112:335–47.

51. Abgral R, Leboulleux S, Déandreis D et al. Performance of (18)fluorodeoxyglucose-positron emission tomography and somatostatin receptor scintigraphy for high Ki67 (≥10%) well-differentiated endocrine carcinoma staging. *J Clin Endocrinol Metab* 2011;96:665–71.

52. Krenning EP, Kwekkeboom DJ, Oei HY et al. Somatostatin-receptor scintigraphy in gastroenteropancreatic tumors. An overview of European results. *Ann NY Acad Sci* 1994;733:416–24.

53. Schillaci O, Massa R, Scopinaro F. 111In-pentetreotide scintigraphy in the detection of insulinomas: Importance of SPECT imaging. *J Nucl Med* 2000;41:459–62.

54. Vezzosi D, Bennet A, Rochaix P et al. Octreotide in insulinoma patients: Efficacy on hypoglycemia, relationships with OctreoScan scintigraphy and immunostaining with anti-sst2A and anti-sst5 antibodies. *Eur J Endocrinol* 2005;152:757–67.

55. de Herder WW, Niederle B, Scoazec JY et al. Well-differentiated pancreatic tumor/carcinoma: Insulinoma. *Neuroendocrinology* 2006;84:183–8.

56. Bertherat J, Tenenbaum F, Perlemoine K et al. Somatostatin receptors 2 and 5 are the major somatostatin receptors in insulinomas: An in vivo and in vitro study. *J Clin Endocrinol Metab* 2003;88:5353–60.

57. Thakker RV, Newey PJ, Walls GV et al. Clinical practice guidelines for multiple endocrine neoplasia type 1 (MEN1). *J Clin Endocrinol Metab* 2012;97:2990–3011.

58. Christ E, Wild D, Forrer F et al. Glucagon-like peptide-1 receptor imaging for localization of insulinomas. *J Clin Endocrinol Metab* 2009;94:4398–405.

59. Estall JL, Drucker DJ. Glucagon and glucagon-like peptide receptors as drug targets. *Curr Pharm Des* 2006;12:1731–50.

60. Wild D, Béhé M, Wicki A, Storch D et al. [Lys40(Ahx-DTPA-111In)NH2]exendin-4, a very promising ligand for glucagon-like peptide-1 (GLP-1) receptor targeting. *J Nucl Med* 2006;47:2025–33.

61. Nelsen EM, Buehler D, Soni AV, Gopal DV. Endoscopic ultrasound in the evaluation of pancreatic neoplasms—solid and cystic: A review. *World J Gastrointest Endosc* 2015;7:318–27.

62. Seo Y, Mari C, Hasegawa BH. Technological development and advances in single-photon emission computed tomography/computedtomography. *Semin Nucl Med* 2008;38:177–98.

63. Perri M, Erba P, Volterrani D et al. OctreoSPECT/CT imaging for accurate detection and localization of suspected neuroendocrine tumors. *Q J Nucl Med Mol Imaging* 2008;52:323–33.

64. Wong KK, Cahill JM, Frey KA, Avram AM. Incremental value of 111-In pentetreotide SPECT/CT fusion imaging of neuroendocrine tumors. *Acad Radiol* 2010;17:291–7.

65. Gabriel M, Hausler F, Bale R et al. Image fusion analysis of (99m)Tc-HYNIC-Tyr(3)-octreotide SPECT and diagnostic CT using an immobilisation device with external markers in patients with endocrine tumours. *Eur J Nucl Med Mol Imaging* 2005;32:1440–551.

66. Teunissen JJ, Kwekkeboom DJ, Valkema R, Krenning EP. Nuclear medicine techniques for the imaging and treatment of neuroendocrine tumors. *Endocr Relat Cancer* 2011;18(Suppl 1):S27–51.

67. Kwekkeboom DJ, Teunissen JJ, Bakker WH et al. Radiolabeled somatostatin analog [177Lu-DOTA0,Tyr3]octreotate in patients with endocrine gastroenteropancreatic tumors. *J Clin Oncol* 2005;23:2754–62.

68. Rodrigues M, Traub-Weidinger T, Li S, Ibi B, Virgolini I. Comparison of 111In-DOTA-DPhe1-Tyr3-octreotide and 111In-DOTA-lanreotide scintigraphy and dosimetry in patients with neuroendocrine tumours. *Eur J Nucl Med Mol Imaging* 2006;33:532–40.

69. Gabriel M, Decristoforo C, Kendler D et al. ^{68}Ga-DOTA-Tyr3-octreotide PET in neuroendocrine tumors: Comparison with somatostatin receptor scintigraphy and CT. *J Nucl Med* 2007;48:508–18.

70. Wild D, Bomanji JB, Benkert P et al. Comparison of 68Ga-DOTANOC and 68Ga-DOTATATE PET/CT within patients with gastroenteropancreatic neuroendocrine tumors. *J Nucl Med* 2013;54:364–72.

71. Bombardieri E, Seregni E, Villano C, Chiti A, Bajetta E. Position of nuclear medicine techniques in the diagnostic work-up of neuroendocrine tumors. *Q J Nucl Med Mol Imaging* 2004;48:150–63.

72. Graham MM, Menda Y. Radiopeptide imaging and therapy in the United States. *J Nucl Med* 2011;52(Suppl 2):56S–63S.

73. Ambrosini V, Nanni C, Zompatori M et al. (68)Ga-DOTA-NOC PET/CT in comparison with CT for the detection of bone metastasis in patients with neuroendocrine tumours. *Eur J Nucl Med Mol Imaging* 2010;37:722–7.

74. Srirajaskanthan R, Kayani I, Quigley AM et al. The role of 68Ga-DOTATATE PET in patients with neuroendocrine tumors and negative or equivocal findings on 111InDTPA-octreotide scintigraphy. *J Nucl Med* 2010;51:875–82.

75. Hofmann M, Maecke H, Börner R et al. Biokinetics and imaging with the somatostatin receptor PET radioligand 68Ga-DOTATOC: Preliminary data. *Eur J Nucl Med* 2001;28:1751–7.

76. Ambrosini V, Tomassetti P, Castellucci P et al. Comparison between 68Ga-DOTA-NOC and 18F-DOPA PET for the detection of gastro-enteropancreatic and lung neuro-endocrine tumours. *Eur J Nucl Med Mol Imaging* 2008;35:1431–8.

77. Fanti S, Ambrosini V, Tomassetti P et al. Evaluation of unusual neuroendocrine tumours by means of 68Ga-DOTA-NOC PET. *Biomed Pharmacother* 2008;62:667–71.

78. Kayani I, Conry BG, Groves AM et al. A comparison of 68Ga-DOTATATE and 18FFDG PET/CT in pulmonary neuroendocrine tumors. *J Nucl Med* 2009;50:1927–32.

79. Antunes P, Gin JM, Zhang H et al. Are radiogallium-labelled DOTA-conjugated somatostatin analogues superior to those labelled with other radiometals? *Eur J Nucl Med Mol Imaging* 2007;34:982–93.

80. Reubi JC, Schär JC, Waser B et al. Affinity profiles for human somatostatin receptor subtypes SST1–SST5 of somatostatin radiotracers selected for scintigraphic and radiotherapeutic use. *Eur J Nucl Med* 2000;27:273–82.

81. Kabasakal L, Demirci E, Ocak M et al. Comparison of 68Ga-DOTATATE and 68Ga-DOTANOC PET/CT imaging in the same patient group with neuroendocrine tumours. *Eur J Nucl Med Mol Imaging* 2012;39:1271–7.

82. Treglia G, Castaldi P, Rindi G, Giordano A, Rufini V. Diagnostic performance of gallium-68 somatostatin receptor PET and PET/CT in patients with thoracic and gastroenteropancreatic neuroendocrine tumours: A meta-analysis. *Endocrine* 2012;42:80–7.

83. Ambrosini V, Castellucci P, Rubello D et al. 68Ga-DOTA-NOC: A new PET tracer for evaluating patients with bronchial carcinoid. *Nucl Med Commun* 2009;30:281–6.

84. Naswa N, Sharma P, Kumar A et al. Gallium-68-DOTA-NOC PET/CT of patients with gastroenteropancreatic neuroendocrine tumors: A prospective single-center study. *AJR Am J Roentgenol* 2011;197:1221–8.

85. Ruf J, Schiefer J, Furth C et al. 68Ga-DOTATOC PET/CT of neuroendocrine tumors: Spotlight on the CT phases of a triple-phase protocol. *J Nucl Med* 2011;52:697–704.

86. Hofmann M, Maecke H, Börner R et al. Biokinetics and imaging with the somatostatin receptor PET radioligand 68Ga-DOTATOC: Preliminary data. *Eur J Nucl Med* 2001;28:1751–7.

87. Versari A, Camellini L, Carlinfante G et al. Ga-68 DOTATOC PET, endoscopic ultrasonography, and multidetector CT in the diagnosis of duodenopancreatic neuroendocrine tumors: A single-centre retrospective study. *Clin Nucl Med* 2010;35:321–8.

88. Naswa N, Sharma P, Soundararajan R et al. Diagnostic performance of somatostatin receptor PET/CT using 68Ga-DOTANOC in gastrinoma patients with negative or equivocal CT findings. *Abdom Imaging* 2013;38:552–60.

89. Naswa N, Sharma P, Kumar A et al. 68Ga-DOTANOC PET/CT in patients with carcinoma of unknown primary of neuroendocrine origin. *Clin Nucl Med* 2012;37:245–51.

90. Poeppel TD, Binse I, Petersenn S et al. 68Ga-DOTATOC versus 68Ga-DOTATATE PET/CT in functional imaging of neuroendocrine tumors. *J Nucl Med* 2011;52:1864–70.

91. Putzer D, Kroiss A, Waitz D et al. Somatostatin receptor PET in neuroendocrine tumours: 68Ga-DOTA (0), Tyr (3)-octeotide versus 68Ga-DOTA (0)-lanreotide. *Eur J Nucl Med Mol Imaging* 2013;40:364–71.

92. Panzuto F, Nasoni S, Falconi M et al. Prognostic factors and survival in endocrine tumor patients: Comparison between gastrointestinal and pancreatic localization. *Endocr Relat Cancer* 2005;12:1083–92.

93. Mayerhoefer ME, Schuetz M, Magnaldi S, Weber M, Trattnig S, Karanikas G. Are contrast media required for 68Ga-DOTATOC PET/CT in patients with neuroendocrine tumours of the abdomen? *Eur Radiol* 2012;22:938–46.

94. Schreiter NF, Nogami M, Steffen I et al. Evaluation of the potential of PET–MRI fusion for detection of liver metastases in patients with neuroendocrine tumours. *Eur Radiol* 2012;22:458–67.

95. Giesel FL, Kratochwil C, Mehndiratta A et al. Comparison of neuroendocrine tumor detection and characterization using DOTATOC-PET in correlation with contrast enhanced CT and delayed contrast enhanced MRI. *Eur J Radiol* 2012;81:2820–5.

96. Frilling A, Sotiropoulos GC, Radtke A et al. The impact of 68Ga-DOTATOC positron emission tomography/computed tomography on the multimodal management of patients with neuroendocrine tumors. *Ann Surg* 2010;252:850–6.

97. Hofman MS, Kong G, Neels OC, Eu P, Hong E, Hicks RJ. High management impact of Ga-68 DOTATATE (GaTate) PET/CT for imaging neuroendocrine and other somatostatin-expressing tumours. *J Med Imaging Radiat Oncol* 2012;56:40–7.

98. Vallabhajosula S, Nikolopoulou A. Radioiodinated metaiodobenzylguanidine (MIBG): Radiochemistry, biology, and pharmacology. *Semin Nucl Med* 2011;41:324–33.

99. Kaltsas G, Korbonits M, Heintz E et al. Comparison of somatostatin analog and meta-iodobenzylguanidine radionuclides in the diagnosis and localization of advanced neuroendocrine tumors. *J Clin Endocrinol Metab* 2001;86:895–902.

100. Daniels CE, Lowe VJ, Aubry MC, Allen MS, Jett JR. The utility of fluorodeoxyglucose positron emission tomography in the evaluation of carcinoid tumors presenting as pulmonary nodules. *Chest* 2007;131:255–60.

101. Oh S, Prasad V, Lee DS, Baum RP. Effect of peptide receptor radionuclide therapy on somatostatin receptor status and glucose metabolism in neuroendocrine tumors: Intraindividual comparison of Ga-68 DOTANOC PET/CT and F-18 FDG PET/CT. *Int J Mol Imaging* 2011;2011:524130.

102. Has Simsek D, Kuyumcu S, Turkmen C et al. Can complementary 68Ga-DOTATATE and 18F-FDG PET/CT establish the missing link between histopathology and therapeutic approach in gastroenteropancreatic neuroendocrine tumors? *J Nucl Med* 2014;55:1811–7.

103. Pattenden H, Leung M, Beddow E et al. Test performance of PET-CT for mediastinal lymph node staging of pulmonary carcinoid tumors. *Thorax* 2015;70:379–81.

104. Bahri H, Laurence L, Edeline J et al. High prognostic value of 18F-FDG PET for metastatic gastroenteropancreatic neuroendocrine tumors: A long-term evaluation. *J Nucl Med* 2014;55:1786–90.

105. Becherer A, Szabó M, Karanikas G et al. Imaging of advanced neuroendocrine tumors with F-18-FDOPA PET. *J Nucl Med* 2004;45:1161–7.

106. Orlefors H, Sundin A, Garske U et al. Whole-body (11)C-5-hydroxytryptophan positron emission tomography as a universal imaging technique for neuroendocrine tumors: Comparison with somatostatin receptor scintigraphy and computed tomography. *J Clin Endocrinol Metab* 2005;90:3392–400.

107. Chen K, Chen X. Positron emission tomography imaging of cancer biology: Current status and future prospects. *Semin Oncol* 2011;38:70–86.

108. Hoegerle S, Nitzsche E, Altehoefer C et al. Pheochromocytomas: Detection with 18F DOPA whole body PET—Initial results. *Radiology* 2002;222:507–12.

109. Koopmans KP, de Vries EG, Kema IP et al. Staging of carcinoid tumours with ^{18}F-DOPA PET: A prospective, diagnostic accuracy study. *Lancet Oncol* 2006;7:728–34.

110. Koopmans KP, Neels OC, Kema IP et al. Improved staging of patients with carcinoid and islet cell tumours with 18F-dihydroxy-phenyl-alanine and 11C-5-hydroxy-tryptophan positron emission tomography. *J Clin Oncol* 2008;26:1489–95.

111. Montravers F, Grahek D, Kerrou K et al. Can fluoro-dihydroxyphenylalanine PET replace somatostatin receptor scintigraphy in patients with digestive endocrine tumours? *J Nucl Med* 2006;47:1455–62.

112. Balogova S, Talbot JN, Nataf V et al. ^{18}F-fluorodihydroxyphenylalanine vs other radiopharmaceuticals for imaging neuroendocrine tumours according to their type. *Eur J Nuc Med Mol Imaging* 2013;40:943–66.

113. Haug A, Auernhammer CJ, Wängler B et al. Intraindividual comparison of 68Ga-DOTA-TATE and 18F-DOPA PET in patients with well-differentiated metastatic neuroendocrine tumours. *Eur J Nucl Med Mol Imaging* 2009;36:765–70.

114. Buchmann I, Henze M, Engelbrecht S et al. Comparison of 68Ga-DOTATOC PET and 111In-DTPAOC (Octreoscan) SPECT in patients with neuroendocrine tumours. *Eur J Nucl Med Mol Imaging* 2007;34:1617–26.

115. Adams S, Baum R, Rink T et al. Limited value of fluorine-18 fluorodeoxyglucose positron emission tomography for the imaging of neuroendocrine tumours. *Eur J Nucl Med* 1998;25:79–83.

116. Gotthardt M, Béhé MP, Grass J et al. Added value of gastrin receptor scintigraphy in comparison to somatostatin receptor scintigraphy in patients with carcinoids and other neuroendocrine tumours. *Endocr Relat Cancer* 2006;13:1203–11.

117. Wild D, Mäcke H, Christ E, Gloor B, Reubi JC. Glucagon-like peptide 1-receptor scans to localize occult insulinomas. *N Engl J Med* 2008;359:766–8.

118. Sowa-Staszczak A, Pach D, Mikołajczak R et al. Glucagon-like peptide-1 receptor imaging with [Lys40(Ahx-HYNIC-99mTc/EDDA)NH2]-exendin-4 for the detection of insulinoma. *Eur J Nucl Med Mol Imaging* 2013;40:524–31.

119. Shulkin BL, Ilias I, Sisson JC, Pacak K. Current trends in functional imaging of pheochromocytomas and paragangliomas. *Ann NY Acad Sci* 2006;1073:374–82.

120. Bhatia KS, Ismail MM, Sahdev A et al. 123I-metaiodobenzylguanidine (MIBG) scintigraphy for the detection of adrenal and extra-adrenal phaeochromocytomas: CT and MRI correlation. *Clin Endocrinol (Oxf)* 2008;69:181–8.

121. Hadi M, Chen CC, Whatley M, Pacak K, Carrasquillo JA. Brown fat imaging with (18)F-6-fluorodopamine PET/CT, (18)F-FDG PET/CT, and (123)I-MIBG SPECT: A study of patients being evaluated for pheochromocytoma. *J Nucl Med* 2007;48:1077–83.

122. Ilias I, Divgi C, Pacak H. Current role of metaiodobenzylguanidine in the diagnosis of pheochromocytoma and medullary thyroid cancer. *Semin Nucl Med* 2011;41:364–8.

123. Cecchin D, Lumachi F, Marzola MC et al. A meta-iodobenzylguanidine scintigraphic scoring system increases accuracy in the diagnostic management of pheochromocytoma. *Endocr Relat Cancer* 2006;13:525–33.

124. Taïeb D, Timmers HJ, Hindié E et al. EANM 2012 guidelines for radionuclide imaging of phaeochromocytoma and paraganglioma. *Eur J Nucl Med Mol Imaging* 2012;39:1977–95.

125. Rufini V, Treglia G, Perotti G, Giordano A. The evolution in the use of MIBG scintigraphy in pheochromocytomas and paragangliomas. *Hormones* 2013;12:58–68.

126. van der Harst E, de Herder WW, Bruining HA. [(123)I]metaiodobenzylguanidine and [(111)In]octreotide uptake in benign and malignant pheochromocytomas. *J Clin Endocrinol Metab* 2001;86:685–93.

127. Havekes B, Lai EW, Corssmit PM, Romijn JA, Timmers HJLM, Pacak K. Detection and treatment of pheochromocytomas and paragangliomas: Current standing of MIBG scintigraphy and future role of PET imaging. *Q J Nucl Med Mol Imaging* 2008;52:419–29.

128. Martiniova L, Perera SM, Brouwers FM et al. Increased uptake of [123I]meta-iodobenzylguanidine, [18F]fluorodopamine and [3H]norepinephrine in mouse pheochromocytoma cells and tumors after treatment with the histone deacetylase inhibitors. *Endocr Related Cancer* 2011;18:143–57.

129. Kayano D, Taki J, Fukuoka M et al. Low-dose (123)I-metaiodobenzylguanidine diagnostic scan is inferior to (131)I-metaiodobenzylguanidine post-treatment scan in detection of malignant pheochromocytoma and paraganglioma. *Nucl Med Commun* 2011;32:941–6.

130. Wiseman GA, Pacak K, O'Dorisio MS et al. Usefulness of 123I-MIBG scintigraphy in the evaluation of patients with known or suspected primary or metastatic pheochromocytoma or paraganglioma: Results from a prospective multicenter trial. *J Nucl Med* 2009;50:1448–54.

131. Jacobson AF, Deng H, Lombard J, Lessig HJ, Black RR. 123I-meta-iodobenzylguanidine scintigraphy for the detection of neuroblastoma and pheochromocytoma: Results of a meta-analysis. *J Clin Endocrinol Metab* 2010;95:2596–606.

132. Rozovsky K, Koplewitz BZ, Krausz Y et al. Added value of SPECT/CT for correlation of MIBG scintigraphy and diagnostic CT in neuroblastoma and pheochromocytoma. *AJR Am J Roentgenol* 2008;190:1085–90.

133. Meyer-Rochow GY, Schembri GP, Benn DE et al. The utility of metaiodobenzylguanidine single photon emission computed tomography/computed tomography (MIBG SPECT/CT) for the diagnosis of pheochromocytoma. *Ann Surg Oncol* 2010;17:392–400.

134. Havekes B, King K, Lai EW, Romijn JA, Corssmit EP, Pacak K. New imaging approaches to phaeochromocytomas and paragangliomas. *Clin Endocrinol* 2010;72:137–45.

135. Vaidyanathan G. Meta-iodobenzylguanidine and analogues: Chemistry and biology. *Q J Nucl Med Mol Imaging* 2008;52:351–68.

136. King KS, Chen CC, Alexopoulos DK et al. Functional imaging of SDHx-related head and neck paragangliomas: Comparison of 18F-fluorodihydroxyphenylalanine, 18F-fluorodopamine, 18F-fluoro-2-deoxy-D-glucose PET, 123I-metaiodobenzylguanidine scintigraphy, and 111In-pentetreotide scintigraphy. *J Clin Endocrinol Metab* 2011;96:2779–85.

137. Timmers HJ, Kozupa A, Chen CC et al. Superiority of fluorodeoxyglucose positron emission tomography to other functional imaging techniques in the evaluation of metastatic SDHB-associated pheochromocytoma and paraganglioma. *J Clin Oncol* 2007;25:2262–9.

138. Kaji P, Carrasquillo JA, Linehan WM et al. The role of 6-[18F]fluorodopamine positron emission tomography in the localization of adrenal pheochromocytoma associated with von Hippel-Lindau syndrome. *Eur J Endocrinol* 2007;156:483–7.

139. Mann GN, Link JM, Pham P et al. [11C]metahydroxyephedrine and [18F]fluorodeoxyglucose positron emission tomography improve clinical decision making in suspected pheochromocytoma. *Ann Surg Oncol* 2006;13:187–97.

140. De Graaf JS, Dullaart RP, Kok T, Piers DA, Zwierstra RP. Limited role of meta-iodobenzylguanidine scintigraphy in imaging phaeochromocytoma in patients with multiple endocrine neoplasia type II. *Eur J Surg* 2000;166:289–92.

141. Fottner C, Helisch A, Anlauf M et al. 6-18F-fluoro-L-dihydroxyphenylalanine positron emission tomography is superior to 123I-metaiodobenzyl-guanidine scintigraphy in the detection of extraadrenal and hereditary pheochromocytomas and paragangliomas: Correlation with vesicular monoamine transporter expression. *J Clin Endocrinol Metab* 2010;95:2800–10.

142. Ilias I, Chen CC, Carrasquillo JA et al. Comparison of 6-18F-fluorodopamine PET with I-123 metaiodobenzylguanidine and In-111 pentetreotide scintigraphy in localisation of nonmetastatic and metastatic phaeochromocytoma. *J Nucl Med* 2008;49:1613–9.

143. Charrier N, Deveze A, Fakhry N et al. Comparison of [111In]pentetreotide-SPECT and [18F]FDOPA-PET in the localization of extra-adrenal paragangliomas: The case for a patient-tailored use of nuclear imaging modalities. *Clin Endocrinol* 2011;74:21–9.

144. Timmers H, Chen C, Carrasquillo J et al. Comparison of 18F-fluoro-L-DOPA, 18Ffluoro-deoxyglucose, and 18F-fluorodopamine PET and 123IMIBG

145. Rufini V, Treglia G, Castaldi P, Perotti G, Giordano A. Comparison of metaiodobenzylguanidine scintigraphy with positron emission tomography in the diagnostic work-up of pheochromocytoma and paraganglioma: A systematic review. *Q J Nucl Med Mol Imaging* 2013;57:122–33.

146. Ganapathy V, Thangaraju M, Prasad PD. Nutrient transporters in cancer: Relevance to Warburg hypothesis and beyond. *Pharmacol Ther* 2009;121:29–40.

147. Santhanam P, Taïeb D. Role of (18) F-FDOPA PET/CT imaging in endocrinology. *Clin Endocrinol* 2014;81:789–98.

148. Gabriel S, Blanchet EM, Sebag F et al. Functional characterization of nonmetastatic paraganglioma and pheochromocytoma by (18)F-FDOPA PET: Focus on missed lesions. *Clin Endocrinol* 2013;79:170–7.

149. Taïeb D, Tessonnier L, Sebag F et al. The role of 18F-FDOPA and 18F-FDG-PET in the management of malignant and multifocal phaeochromocytomas. *Clin Endocrinol* 2008;69:580–6.

150. Rischke HC, Benz MR, Wild D et al. Correlation of the genotype of paragangliomas and pheochromocytomas with their metabolic phenotype on 3,4-dihydroxy-6-18F-fluoro-L-phenylalanin PET. *J Nucl Med* 2012;53:1352–8.

151. Fiebrich HB, Brouwers AH, Kerstens MN et al. 6-[F-18]Fluoro-L-dihydroxyphenylalanine positron emission tomography is superior to conventional imaging with (123)I-metaiodobenzylguanidine scintigraphy, computer tomography, and magnetic resonance imaging in localizing tumors causing catecholamine excess. *J Clin Endocrinol Metab* 2009;94:3922–30.

152. Shulkin BL, Wieland DM, Schwaiger M et al. PET scanning with hydroxyephedrine: An approach to the localization of phaeochromocytoma. *J Nucl Med* 1992;33:1125–31.

153. Franzius C, Hermann K, Weckesser M et al. Whole-body PET/CT with 11C-meta-hydroxyephedrine in tumors of the sympathetic nervous system: Feasibility study and comparison with 123I-MIBG SPECT/CT. *J Nucl Med* 2006;47:1635–42.

154. Bagheri B, Maurer AH, Cone L, Doss M, Adler L. Characterization of the normal adrenal gland with 18F-FDG PET/CT. *J Nucl Med* 2004;45:1340–3.

155. Timmers HJ, Chen CC, Carrasquillo JA et al., Staging and functional characterization of pheochromocytoma and paraganglioma by 18F-fluorodeoxyglucose (18F-FDG) positron emission tomography. *J Natl Cancer Inst* 2012;104:700–8.

156. Blanchet EM, Gabriel S, Martucci V et al. 18F-FDG PET/CT as a predictor of hereditary head and neck paragangliomas. *Eur J Clin Invest* 2014;44:325–32.

157. Kroiss A, Putzer D, Uprimny C et al. Functional imaging in phaeochromocytoma and neuroblastoma with 68Ga-DOTA-Tyr 3-octreotide positron emission tomography and 123I-metaiodobenzylguanidine. *Eur J Nucl Med Mol Imaging* 2011;38:865–73.

158. Naji M, Zhao C, Welsh SJ et al. 68Ga-DOTA-TATE PET vs. 123I-MIBG in identifying malignant neural crest tumours. *Mol Imaging Biol* 2011;13:769–75.

159. Johnbeck CB, Knigge U, Kjær A. PET tracers for somatostatin receptor imaging of neuroendocrine tumors: Current status and review of the literature. *Future Oncol* 2014;10:2259–77.

160. Putzer D, Gabriel M, Henninger B et al. Bone metastases in patients with neuroendocrine tumor: 68Ga-DOTA-Tyr3-octreotide PET in comparison to CT and bone scintigraphy. *J Nucl Med* 2009;50:1214–21.

161. Kayani I, Bomanji JB, Groves A et al. Functional imaging of neuroendocrine tumors with combined PET/CT using 68Ga-DOTATATE (DOTA-DPhe1,Tyr3-octreotate) and 18F-FDG. *Cancer* 2008;112:2447–55.

162. Zelinka T, Timmers HJ, Kozupa A et al. Role of positron emission tomography and bone scintigraphy in the evaluation of bone involvement in metastatic pheochromocytoma and paraganglioma: Specific implications for succinate dehydrogenase enzyme subunit B gene mutations. *Endocr Relat Cancer* 2008;15:311–23.

163. Timmers HJ, Eisenhofer G, Carrasquillo JA et al. Use of 6-[18F]-fluorodopamine positron emission tomography (PET) as first-line investigation for the diagnosis and localization of non-metastatic and metastatic phaeochromocytoma (PHEO). *Clin Endocrinol (Oxf)* 2009;71:11–7.

164. Rufini V, Treglia G, Castaldi P et al. Comparison of 123I-MIBG SPECT-CT and 18F-DOPA PET-CT in the evaluation of patients with known or suspected recurrent paraganglioma. *Nucl Med Commun* 2011;32:575–82.

References 387

45

Carcinoid tumors

DANI O. GONZALEZ, RICHARD R.P. WARNER, AND CELIA M. DIVINO

INTRODUCTION

Carcinoid tumors represent a type of neuroendocrine tumor (NET) of primarily enterochromaffin cells that can present in a number of ways. In 1907, these tumors were first termed *karzinoide*, or carcinoid, by the German pathologist Obendorfer. They were described as tumors of the ileum, with a more indolent presentation than one would expect from an adenocarcinoma [1]. Forty years earlier, in 1867, Langhans first described the histology of what is known as a carcinoid today [2]. In 1888, Lubarsch reported carcinoid tumors in the ileum of two patients discovered during autopsy [3]. Since the initial description, scientific and clinical research has elucidated many details about these tumors; however, much remains to be discovered.

These tumors represent the most common endocrine tumors of the gastrointestinal tract and behave quite differently from other tumors of the gastrointestinal tract. Familiarity with their biochemical and pathologic behaviors is important for planning the management of these malignancies. The optimal treatment team for one with a carcinoid tumor includes an interdisciplinary team comprised of gastroenterologists, radiologists, surgeons, and oncologists.

This chapter provides an updated review of several aspects of carcinoid tumors, including epidemiology, clinical features, site-specific disease, tumor localization, and management. As is true with many clinical entities, further research is necessary in order to discover additional therapeutic modalities, screening protocols, or even preventative strategies.

EPIDEMIOLOGY

True prevalence and incidence data are difficult to determine because many carcinoid tumors may go undiagnosed. Databases like the Surveillance, Epidemiology, and End Results (SEER) Program aid in obtaining epidemiologic data, but also have their limitations. Only malignant tumors are included in this registry, which may limit the completeness of the database and cause bias when assessing survival data.

Modlin et al. identified 13,715 carcinoid tumors over a 50-year period using a cancer database. Of those cases, nearly 67% occurred in the gastrointestinal tract and 24.5% in the tracheobronchopulmonary tree. Different subsets of this cancer registry revealed varying frequencies of tumor sites, but in the most recent subset of data, 41.8% of gastrointestinal carcinoids occurred in the small intestine, 27.4% in the rectum, and 8.7% in the stomach. Figure 45.1 demonstrates the distribution of digestive system carcinoid tumors in this registry. Of all small intestinal carcinoid tumors, 47.3% occurred in the ileum and 24.1% in the appendix (Figure 45.2) [4]. The most common site of carcinoid tumors may face an epidemiologic change in the next several years. With the use of screening colonoscopy, there may be an increase in the number of colorectal carcinoid tumors detected.

Distribution of digestive tract carcinoid tumors

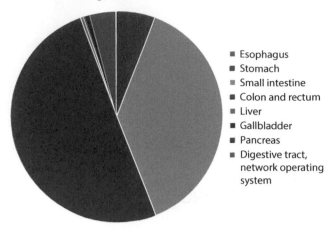

- ■ Esophagus
- ■ Stomach
- ■ Small intestine
- ■ Colon and rectum
- ■ Liver
- ■ Gallbladder
- ■ Pancreas
- ■ Digestive tract, network operating system

Figure 45.1 Distribution of digestive tract carcinoid tumors by site, according to a five-decade analysis of 13,715 carcinoid tumors. (Adapted from Modlin IM, Lye KD, Kidd M. *Cancer* 2003;97:934–59.)

Distribution of small intestine carcinoid tumors

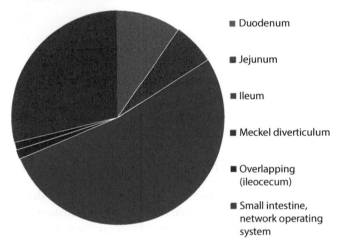

- ■ Duodenum
- ■ Jejunum
- ■ Ileum
- ■ Meckel diverticulum
- ■ Overlapping (ileocecum)
- ■ Small intestine, network operating system

Figure 45.2 Distribution of small intestine carcinoid tumors according to a five-decade analysis of 13,715 carcinoid tumors. (Adapted from Modlin IM, Lye KD, Kidd M. *Cancer* 2003;97:934–59.)

According to a large SEER study, the average age of patients diagnosed with carcinoid tumors is between 59 and 61, depending on the SEER subset that is analyzed [4]. For some carcinoid tumors, like appendiceal tumors, the average age of diagnosis is slightly younger than that for patients with noncarcinoid tumors at the same site.

When considering the effect of ethnicity on the incidence of carcinoid tumors, there may be higher incidence in some ethnic groups for certain tumor locations. Rectal carcinoids, for example, are more common among minorities, including Asian, black, and Hispanic patients, than in white patients [5].

In a large population-based study, the overall 5-year survival for carcinoid tumors at all sites was 69.7% [6]. This included patients with and without surgery. Rectal carcinoid

Table 45.1 Five-year survival of carcinoid tumors by site

Tumor site (n)	5-year survival (%)		
	Localized (%)	Distant (%)	Overall (%)
Stomach (n = 449)	90	18	75
Small intestine (n = 2778)	95	51	76
Appendix (n = 1040)	96	38	76
Colon (n = 661)	94	28	70
Rectum (n = 1217)	95	15	88

Source: Adapted from Maggard MA, O'Connell JB, Ko CY. *Ann Surg* 2004;240:117–22.

tumors had the highest 5-year survival (87.5%). If disease is localized, the 5-year survival was almost 95%, whereas in distant disease, the survival is 14.6%. Colonic carcinoid tumors have a 5-year survival of 69.5% for all stages, 94% for local stage, and 27.8% for those with distant disease. All-stage 5-year survival in gastric carcinoid tumors was 75%, with 90% and 18% 5-year survival for local and distant stage disease, respectively. Small bowel and appendiceal carcinoid tumors had similar all-stage 5-year survival, about 76%. Local stage 5-year survival was 94.5% for small bowel carcinoid tumors and 95.6% for appendiceal carcinoids. Finally, the 5-year survival for distant disease is 51% for small bowel carcinoid tumors and 37.5% for appendiceal carcinoid tumors. See Table 45.1 for the 5-year survival of carcinoid tumors across tumor locations.

CLINICAL FEATURES

These tumors can present in various ways. Their clinical manifestations range from an absence of symptoms to very aggressive clinical courses. The reason for the variety in presentation is due to the broad range of biochemical activity and localization of disease. All NETs, including carcinoids, have the stem cell potential to secrete ectopic hormones. Furthermore, the ectopic secretion is not limited to peptides, but extends to amines (histamines, catecholamines, and serotonin). These tumors can occur in many locations throughout the body, including the gastrointestinal tract and bronchopulmonary system, and are generally classified as occurring in the foregut, the midgut, or the hindgut. The thymus, part of the neuroendocrine system, can also be involved. In fact, prophylactic thymectomy during parathyroidectomy in multiple endocrine neoplasia (MEN) 1 and 2 patients yielded 13% of thymic carcinoids. The clinical presentation of carcinoid tumors depends on the primary site of the tumor and whether metastatic disease has reached the liver. Site-specific disease information will be presented later in the chapter.

The tumors secrete a number of biologically active mediators, which play a role in the presence and severity of symptoms. Some of the mediators released include serotonin, 5-hydroxytryptophan, histamine, pancreatic polypeptide, prostaglandins, kallikrein, and bradykinin.

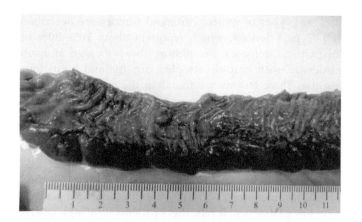

Figure 45.3 Gross specimen of a 7 mm solid, well-circumscribed polypoid lesion in the small intestine. Pathology was consistent with a carcinoid tumor.

On gross examination, these tumors may appear as polypoid lesions protruding through mucosa (Figure 45.3). The overlying mucosa may appear either intact or ulcerated. These tumors may appear bright yellow after formalin fixation. The surrounding tissue may be encased in a desmoplastic reaction. Histologically, these tumors are submucosal and may demonstrate patterns of insular, trabecular, or glandular collections of cells with peripheral palisading (Figure 45.4). The cytoplasm is finely granular with small nucleoli and a "salt and pepper" chromatin appearance. Mitotic figures are rarely seen.

Carcinoid syndrome refers to the symptoms occurring as a result of the biochemical mediators secreted by the carcinoid tumors. A variety of hormones are catabolized by one enzyme during passage through the liver. Once disease has metastasized to the liver, these mediators forgo liver metabolism and are secreted into the systemic circulation, thus causing the symptoms of carcinoid syndrome. It may

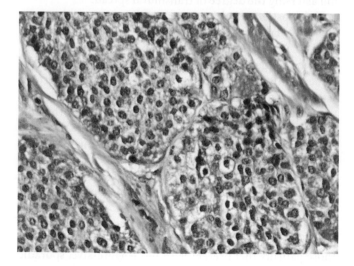

Figure 45.4 Histopathologic image of small intestinal carcinoid tumor stained by hematoxylin and eosin. The image shows a homogeneous population of tumor cells arranged in insular and trabecular patterns.

also occur in the absence of liver metastases if the venous drainage of the tumor bypasses the liver.

The most common feature of carcinoid syndrome is cutaneous flushing. It occurs in about 80% of patients with carcinoid syndrome. The flushing has a characteristic appearance, involving the face, neck, and trunk and ranging from a pink or red flush to a violaceous flush. In severe cases, the flush can even involve the entire body [7]. The episodes typically last less than 3 minutes. Carcinoid syndrome may also include telangectasia, chronic watery diarrhea, wheezing, and valvular heart disease.

A carcinoid crisis may also occur during induction of anesthesia, in which patients may demonstrate flushing, bronchospasm, or profound hypotension. The crisis may be reversed by the administration of a somatostatin analog [8]. Prior to resection, administration of octreotide (300–500 µg intravenously or subcutaneously) reduces the incidence of carcinoid crisis. Octreotide dosing should be repeated throughout the surgery as needed. If carcinoid crisis does occur, one can treat it with a continuous infusion of octreotide at a rate of 50–200 µg/h or an intravenous dose of 500–1000 µg.

SITE-SPECIFIC DISEASE

Overview

Derived from neural crest cells, carcinoid tumors can be broadly classified as occurring in the foregut, midgut, or hindgut. Those in the foregut occur in the respiratory tract, the stomach, the first portion of the duodenum, and the pancreas. Carcinoid tumors in the midgut occur throughout the small bowel, beginning at the second portion of the duodenum, through the ascending colon, and those in the hindgut affect the distal transverse and descending colon, as well as the rectum. Most carcinoids arise from the embryologic midgut.

The activity of the carcinoid tumors and their clinical presentation vary based on the location of their origin. The metabolic agents secreted from the tumors occurring at various cells of origin can drastically alter the clinical activity and behavior of the tumor. For example, foregut tumors secrete mostly histamine, and its urine metabolite is methyl-imidazole acetic acid. They may present early with localized symptoms within the bronchial tract. These patients may display coughing, wheezing, hemoptysis, etc. These tumors have a low serotonin content compared with mid- and hindgut carcinoids, and therefore may present with no systemic symptoms. Midgut carcinoids, which have higher levels of serotonin and tachykinins, produce the systemic systems, such as diarrhea, flushing, and wheezing, once they have metastasized to the liver. Watery diarrhea is almost exclusively caused by excess neurohormones (serotonin, histamine, gastrin, calcitonin, and vasoactive intestinal peptide) and cholera. Hindgut carcinoid tumors synthesize several agents, including somatostatin and tachykinins, which are not clearly proved to be secreted into the circulation. Serotonin is rarely produced by hindgut carcinoids, but chromogranin A (CgA) may be produced. CgA is only one of six antigens that are present in functioning and nonfunctioning NETs. It is safe to assume that they are in the hindgut tumors as well.

Esophagus

Esophageal carcinoid tumors are rare clinical entities. There appears to be a 6:1 male predominance. Largely, the data published are single-institution series with small numbers. To date, the largest series of carcinoid tumors included more than 13,000 carcinoid tumors, only six of which were reported as esophageal tumors [4].

Reflecting their embryologic origin, most esophageal carcinoids occur in the lower third of the esophagus and at the gastroesophageal junction because of the distribution of endocrine cells. The tumors arise in the submucosa. These tumors can present as polypoid lesions or as incidental findings associated with adenocarcinoma in patients with Barrett esophagus. An increased number of endocrine cells have been found in those with metaplasia [9], and may therefore lead to an increase in the incidence of esophageal carcinoid tumors.

While esophageal carcinoid tumors were previously thought to have a poor prognosis, one case series published four cases with favorable outcomes [10]. Prior reports of atypical esophageal carcinoid tumors with poor prognoses may have actually included cases that were small cell carcinomas. In this study, histological and immunohistochemical studies were performed to confirm the diagnosis. Their patients had a median age of 61, with a range from 48 to 72 years. The sizes of the tumors ranged from 0.3 to 3.5 cm, with the mean size of 1.5 cm. Two tumors involved the lamina propria, and two invaded the muscular wall. One patient underwent polypectomy, and two underwent esophagectomy. The fourth patient underwent esophagectomy 9 years later because of a recurrence of the tumor. One of the four patients died of a postoperative pneumonia, while the other three were alive and disease-free at 1, 6, and 23 years after surgery when the data were published.

The diagnostic approach in these patients should be similar to that of all esophageal lesions—including endoscopy for tissue diagnosis and full imaging to rule out distant metastases. While no randomized studies have been performed to determine the ideal treatment modality for these patients, based on case reports, it appears that subtotal esophagectomy with gastroesophageal anastomosis offers promising outcomes.

Stomach

Historically, it was believed that carcinoid tumors of the stomach were rare. Gastric carcinoids may actually represent about 4%–5% of all carcinoid tumors [4]. It is unknown whether the increased incidence is due to an epidemiologic trend or a difference in the reporting of disease.

Three types of gastric carcinoid tumors are described [11]. Type 1 lesions, which represent about 70%–80% of all gastric carcinoids, are almost always benign and are associated with chronic atrophic gastritis and pernicious anemia. These lesions are found in the fundus and body and are typically small tumors (<1 cm). Patients may have multiple lesions. Type 2 carcinoids represent 5%–10% of all gastric carcinoid tumors and are associated with MEN 1 and Zollinger–Ellison syndrome (ZES). These are also small tumors (<1 cm) located in the fundus and body, and sometimes in the antrum. These patients also have a good prognosis. In contrast with type 1 lesions, in which patients have low gastric acid levels, these patients have high gastric acid levels. Type 3 (sporadic) gastric carcinoid tumors represent 10%–15% of all gastric carcinoid lesions and have no well-defined associated disease processes. These patients have a poorer prognosis. The tumors are often solitary and larger lesions located in the antrum or fundus. These patients have normal gastric acid levels.

The clinical presentation for gastric carcinoid tumors is nonspecific. Patients may report pain, vomiting, upper gastrointestinal bleeding, and reflux. Rarely do these patients present with carcinoid syndrome. Typically, type 1 lesions are noted incidentally on endoscopy. Immunohistochemically, the majority of cases are positive for chromogranin, synaptophysin, and Leu-7, with serotonin and neuron-specific enolase (NSE) positivity less frequently. A variety of cell types are found histopathologically in gastric carcinoid tumors, including enterochromaffin cells, enterochromaffin-like cells, and x-cells.

When multiple lesions are present (as in types 1 and 2), they are typically small, yellow, and round, located in the submucosa. When larger, solitary lesions (type 3) are present, they are typically ulcerated, erythematous nodules. These lesions can be seen endoscopically and biopsied. Endoscopic ultrasound may play a role in identifying submucosal lesions and assessing the degree of transmural spread.

Those patients with multiple, small lesions can be managed with endoscopic resection and then surveillance. If these lesions recur, antrectomy may be considered to remove the source of gastrin. In those patients with large and more numerous carcinoid tumors, antrectomy can be performed with restoration of gastrointestinal continuity by either a Roux-en-Y or Billroth I or II reconstruction. The role of laparoscopic antrectomy has been established as a safe and minimally invasive approach in the treatment of nonmetastatic type 1 gastric carcinoid tumors [12]. Although antrectomy alone is not a definitive cure, it will remove the stimulus, with reported regression of disease. Whether treatment is pursued via endoscopic mucosal resection or surgical excision and antrectomy, these patients require surveillance with endoscopy and biopsies every 6 months. Those patients that present with more aggressive, sporadic disease demonstrating malignant potential require aggressive surgical management with either partial or total gastrectomy and regional lymph node dissection. All-stage 5-year survival in gastric carcinoid tumors was 75% in one large population-based study, with 90% and 18% 5-year survivals for local and distant stage disease, respectively [6].

Small intestine

The small intestine is the most common site of gastrointestinal carcinoid tumors, representing 25% of tumors in one study of 13,715 carcinoid tumors [4]. Carcinoid tumors of the small bowel, especially jejunoileal tumors, are thought to have a more aggressive course than appendiceal carcinoid tumors. This may be attributed, in part, to the fact that these tumors pose a challenge for diagnosis. They are not as readily identified as gastric and rectal carcinoid tumors, which can be detected early endoscopically. In fact, many of these tumors are diagnosed at the time of surgery for another reason—a bowel obstruction or bleeding.

The presenting symptoms can vary, depending on the part of the small bowel that is affected. For tumors in the duodenum, patients may present with dyspepsia, upper gastrointestinal bleed, abdominal pain, jaundice, nausea, and vomiting. Those patients with jejunoileal carcinoid tumors may go undiagnosed until exploration. At the time of diagnosis, these patients often have metastatic disease, either to regional lymph nodes or to the liver. For small duodenal lesions that are discovered on endoscopy, endoscopic excision may be sufficient treatment. Lesions that are larger may require more aggressive surgical resection. For periampullary carcinoid tumors, pancreaticoduodenectomy should be considered in those patients that are candidates. For jejunoileal tumors, resection with lymphadenectomy should be performed. One should be mindful that multiple lesions might be present throughout the length of the small bowel (Figure 45.5). In cases where there is extensive disease and mesenteric adenopathy, surgical management can be challenging. Oftentimes, these tumors cause shortening of the mesentery because of the desmoplastic reaction. Encasement of the vasculature may also occur, which can also complicate surgical planning. Figure 45.6 demonstrates one complicated case in which the patient

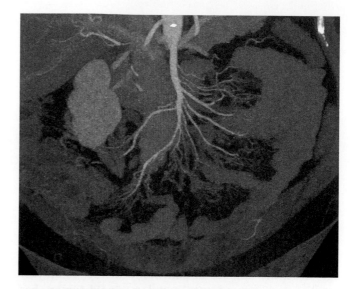

Figure 45.6 CT scan demonstrating metastatic carcinoid tumor encasing the superior mesenteric artery in a patient with primary tumor localized to the small intestine.

had encasement of the superior mesenteric artery by metastatic tumor. In those cases, it is of critical importance to implement a multidisciplinary approach to the treatment planning. The overall 5-year survival for carcinoid tumors of the small bowel is about 76%. For those tumors that are local stage, the 5-year survival is 94.5%, and for distant disease, the 5-year survival is 51% [6].

Appendix

Although historically reported as the most frequent site for carcinoid tumors, the relative frequency of appendiceal carcinoid tumors has decreased over time. Previously, it was believed that carcinoid tumors comprised the majority of appendiceal malignancies; it is now believed that they may only represent one-quarter of appendiceal malignancies [4].

Patients with appendiceal carcinoid tumors present earlier (mean age 49.3) than those with noncarcinoid appendiceal tumors (mean age 59.8) [4]. Patients with appendiceal carcinoid tumors often present with appendicitis. After appendectomy for suspected appendicitis, the diagnosis is often made histopathologically. Traditionally, when these tumors are detected pathologically, no additional treatment is necessary if the tumor is less than 1 cm and does not involve the base of the appendix. For tumors larger than 2 cm, or involving the base of the appendix, or those with goblet cell features, a right hemicolectomy is performed [13]. To date, there are no randomized studies that support this practice. For appendiceal carcinoid tumors, the all-stage 5-year survival is about 76%, and the local and distant stage 5-year survival is 95.6% and 37.5%, respectively [6].

Colorectal

The incidence of colonic carcinoid tumors is lower than that of rectal carcinoid tumors. In a large study of 13,715

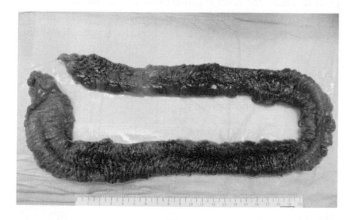

Figure 45.5 Segment of small bowel revealing multiple solid, polypoid lesions that were pathologically consistent with carcinoid tumors.

carcinoid tumors, 13.7% of patients had rectal carcinoid tumors and 7.8% had colonic carcinoid tumors [4]. With the use of screening colonoscopy, the early detection of colorectal carcinoid tumors is on the rise. The presentation of these tumors is variable. A large number are discovered incidentally. When patients develop symptoms as a result of a colonic carcinoid tumor, it is usually late in the course. These patients can present with abdominal pain, diarrhea, nausea, weakness, or bleeding. When these lesions are less than 1 cm in size and are histologically well differentiated, complete endoscopic removal may be sufficient. Large colonic carcinoid tumors should be treated as adenocarcinomas are—with a standard resection and locoregional lymphadenectomy.

Rectal carcinoid tumors are increasing in incidence. With the use of screening colonoscopy for patients at the age of 50, the number of patients in the 50- to 59-year age group diagnosed with rectal carcinoid tumors has increased. As mentioned previously in this chapter, rectal carcinoids are more common among minorities, including Asian, black, and Hispanic patients, than in white patients [5].

While rectal carcinoid tumors are thought to have an indolent course, there is risk for metastasis. Patients at risk for metastasis are those with tumors of >1 cm or with an atypical surface; age of >60; and muscular, perineural, or lymphovascular invasion. While there is no consensus on the optimal management of these tumors, those without the above-mentioned risk factors can be managed with endoscopic or local resection. Tumors more than 2 cm in size require surgical resection, whereas the treatment of those within the 1–2 cm range is still debated [14]. The all-stage 5-year survival for colonic and rectal carcinoid tumors is 69.7% and 87.5%, respectively. For colonic carcinoid tumors, the 5-year survival is 94% for local disease and 27.8% for distant disease. For rectal carcinoid tumors, the 5-year survival is 95% for local disease and 14.6% for distant disease [6].

Meckel's diverticulum

The majority of the data on carcinoid tumors of a Meckel's diverticulum are case reports and case series. Carcinoid tumors are the most common malignant tumors discovered in Meckel's diverticula [15]. While most patients with carcinoid tumors in a Meckel's diverticulum are identified incidentally on postmortem examination or laparotomy, they can present like other patients with Meckel's diverticula—with either small bowel obstruction or gastrointestinal bleeding. A Meckel's diverticulum can cause an intestinal obstruction through either a fibrotic reaction, producing adhesions and causing folds in the bowel, or intussusception. The management of patients with that presentation is more straightforward; it usually involves resection of the diverticulum and the adjacent segment of the small bowel. Without bleeding or obstruction, simple diverticulectomy can be performed.

The management of those patients that are identified incidentally on laparotomy or laparoscopy for another reason is not yet standardized. The majority of the literature on the subject is from case series and case reports. Because of the low incidence of tumors at this site, there are not large case series or randomized studies on the optimal treatment of these asymptomatic patients. Some authors propose resection of these lesions that are found incidentally.

Pancreas

Pancreatic carcinoid tumors are relatively rare clinical entities. They are often difficult to differentiate from other endocrine tumors of the pancreas. The most common clinical symptoms are abdominal pain and diarrhea. Flushing and pancreatitis have also been reported. These patients rarely present with jaundice. Most carcinoid tumors are slow growing and originate from the tail or body of the pancreas. At the time of diagnosis, most tumors are advanced and either have metastasized or are >2 cm in size. Tumor size correlates with malignancy potential.

The management of these lesions is generally the same as for adenocarcinoma of the pancreas—resection with regional lymphadenectomy. Endoscopic ultrasound and intraoperative ultrasound are especially useful for the diagnosis of pancreatic carcinoid tumors. Intraoperative ultrasound may be used to assist in cases where the tumor is small or nonpalpable.

DIAGNOSIS

Biochemical markers

Several biochemical markers are useful in aiding to diagnose carcinoid tumors. Refer to Table 45.2 for a list of biochemical markers that can be used for the detection of carcinoid tumors.

Urinary 5-hydroxyindole acetic acid (5-HIAA), a breakdown product of serotonin, can be collected over a 24-hour period. There are several limitations to the use of 5-HIAA. A 24-hour urine collection may prove cumbersome to patients. In addition, there are certain tryptophan- and

Table 45.2 Sensitivity and specificity of various biochemical markers in the detection of carcinoid and other neuroendocrine tumors

Marker	Sensitivity (%)	Specificity (%)
Chromogranin A	67–93	85–96
Serotonin	75	100
Urinary 5-HIAA	35	88
Plasma 5-HIAA	89	74
Neuron-specific enolase	33	100
Pancreastatin	64	100

serotonin-containing foods, like aged red wine, cheese, spinach, bananas, tomatoes, and eggplant, that can cause falsely elevated levels of excreted 5-HIAA. The sensitivity and specificity of its use as a biochemical marker in carcinoid tumors varies by laboratory and depending on the cutoff value that is set. One study reported the sensitivity and specificity of urinary 5-HIAA to be 77% and 88%, respectively. That same group assessed the sensitivity and specificity of plasma 5-HIAA levels and blood serotonin levels. The sensitivity and specificity of plasma 5-HIAA were 89% and 74%, respectively. The sensitivity and specificity for whole blood serotonin were 75% and 100%, respectively [16]. Those authors concluded that measuring a fasting plasma 5-HIAA level was more convenient for screening for carcinoid than a 24-hour urinary level of 5-HIAA, without compromising diagnostic precision. Urinary 5-HIAA is more commonly used, however.

Another marker that can be used is CgA, one of six antigens that are present in the cytoplasmic neurosecretory granules of all neuroendocrine cells and tumors. Levels of chromogranin correlate with the tumor burden. The sensitivity and specificity of these values vary by laboratory, as there are no international standards for CgA values in carcinoid tumors. One study compared three different commercial kits for CgA measurement and found that the sensitivity ranged from 67% to 93% and the specificity ranged from 85% to 96% [17].

CgA is less specific than 5-HIAA, as it may be elevated in other NETs. Levels of CgA may vary depending on the cutoff value set at the laboratory, as well as the location of the carcinoid tumor. False positives may occur in patients on proton pump inhibitors. Chromogranins B and C are also useful markers for the detection of carcinoid tumors, although less sensitive.

In addition to 5-HIAA and CgA, several other markers have been investigated and may play a role in the detection of carcinoid and other NETs. Serum pancreastatin holds promise as a marker for detecting NETs. In one group of patients with NETs, the sensitivity and specificity of pancreastatin were 64% and 100%, respectively, while the sensitivity and specificity of CgA in that same group were 43% and 64%, respectively [18].

NSE is another biochemical marker that has been investigated for its use in detecting NETs. While the specificity of NSE in one study was 100%, the sensitivity was quite low at 32.9% [19]. Foregut tumors are unique in that they secrete mostly histamine. The urine metabolite of histamine is methyl-imidazole acetic acid, which can be measured. Pancreatic polypeptide, produced primarily in the islet cells of the pancreas, can also be produced by pancreatic NETs and some gastrointestinal NETs. In one study, it was elevated in 13% of patients with carcinoid tumors. Additional research is necessary in order to establish the significance of this marker. In the same study, gastrin was only elevated in 3% of patients with carcinoid tumors. While it is useful in the detection of other NETs, its use in the detection of carcinoid tumors remains limited [20].

Localization

Several imaging modalities are available for tumor localization and staging. Computed tomography (CT) scans are noninvasive studies that can be performed quickly and can provide information about the location of tumors and sometimes evidence of metastatic disease. Like other studies, CT scans are not without limitation. Small tumors are often difficult to visualize unless surrounded by a desmoplastic reaction. In certain instances, it may be difficult to differentiate carcinoid tumors from other tumors based on CT findings. Nevertheless, CT scans are helpful and should be performed on most patients with suspected carcinoid tumors.

Somatostatin receptor scintigraphy (SSTRS), also known as OctreoScan, involves using a radiolabeled form of octreotide, 111-indium octreotide. A more recent development involving the use of radiolabeled 111-indium pentetreotide offers a higher affinity to receptors than octreotide. This study is limited by the poor anatomic delineation of tumor. Some centers have combined SSTRS with single-photon emission computed tomography (SPECT) because it can improve the accuracy of SSTRS. Although not necessary for the diagnosis of a carcinoid tumor, some advocate the use of SSTRS to detect extra-abdominal carcinoid tumors, like bone metastases. Foregut carcinoids secrete mostly histamine; therefore, the uptake of somatostatin analogs by the receptors should be unchanged.

Magnetic resonance imaging (MRI) is helpful with the detection of liver metastases. It has been noted to be more sensitive than CT scanning for the detection of metastatic NETs in the liver [21].

Another study that is useful for the imaging of carcinoid tumors is a positron emission tomography/computed tomography (PET/CT) using gallium-radiolabeled somatostatin analogs—Ga-68-Dota-Phe-Tyr-octreotide (Ga-68-DOTA-Phe-Tyr3). This imaging modality can be useful in detecting small lesions and liver metastases. Figure 45.7 demonstrates a Ga-68-DOTA-Phe-Tyr3 PET/CT, which reveals multiple liver metastases in a patient with carcinoid syndrome. In a large meta-analysis, the pooled sensitivity and specificity of somatostatin receptor PT or PET/CT were 93% and 91%, respectively [22].

Endoscopic studies, like upper endoscopy, capsule endoscopy, and colonoscopy, are useful in certain cases of carcinoid tumors. Upper endoscopy is a useful diagnostic, and even therapeutic, modality in patients with some gastric carcinoid tumors. Capsule endoscopy can be used to detect lesions in the small bowel that are not readily seen on other imaging studies. Colonoscopy, as mentioned in the chapter, has proved useful for the identification and diagnosis of colorectal carcinoid tumors. With guidelines for screening colonoscopy, there will be higher detection of rectal carcinoid tumors.

THERAPY

The goal of treatment for patients with carcinoid tumors should be curative whenever possible. Resection of the

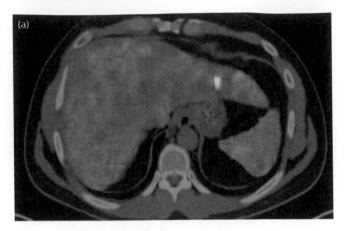

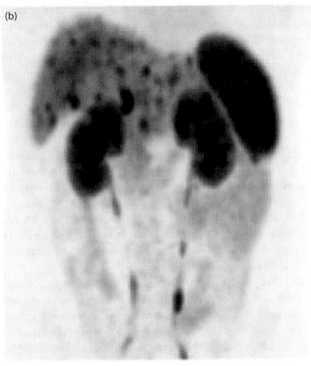

Figure 45.7 PET/CT images using Ga-68-DOTA-Phe-Tyr3 demonstrating multiple liver metastases. (a) Imaging of one organ with metastases; (b) isotopic (nuclear) imaging with uptake by the liver + metastases, the normal spleen, the kidneys, the ureters and sparse isotope in the gut.

debulking may play a role as a palliative therapy in these patients by decreasing the tumor burden, thus facilitating the control of symptoms [23] with pharmacologic therapy [24]. In addition, surgery may serve a role in preventing complications that result from extensive intra-abdominal metastases, including bleeding, bowel obstruction, and even perforation. Since there may be an improvement in quality of life and survival with debulking, metastatic disease should not preclude surgical intervention. Those patients with complex cases can be managed utilizing a multi-disciplinary approach. Gastroenterologists, radiologists, and surgeons should all partake in the treatment of these patients. Constructing individualized treatment plans for patients based on the extent and location of their tumors may prove beneficial. The management of these patients can include a combination of medical therapy, embolization and cytoreductive surgery, and heated infusion of peritoneal chemotherapy (HIPEC).

Long-term therapy of these patients primarily aims to control symptoms. Somatostatin analogs, such as octreotide, have aided in the management of symptoms in patients with carcinoid tumors. A majority of patients experience relief of diarrhea and flushing after treatment with octreotide. While useful, daily injections of octreotide may prove cumbersome for patients. Lanreotide, which is a long-acting somatostatin analog that has effects and efficacy similar to those of octreotide, can be injected every 10–14 days. In a randomized study, lanreotide use was associated with a prolonged progression-free survival among select patients with advanced NETs [25]. A depot formulation of a long-acting repeatable (LAR) octreotide and a slow-release preparation of lanreotide have also been created. Octreotide LAR significantly lengthened the time to tumor progression in patients with both functionally active and inactive midgut NETs in a randomized, placebo-controlled study [26]. The use of these agents is usually limited by the development of tachyphylaxis or progression of disease.

Another application of somatostatin analogs is during carcinoid crises. Although there are no randomized studies to corroborate this indication, there are case reports documenting the use of intravenous somatostatin analogs during carcinoid crises.

Interferons (IFNs) have also been used for the management of carcinoid tumors. Like somatostatin analogs, IFN-α has been reported to relieve diarrhea and flushing in a majority of patients. Unlike octreotide, however, IFN-α has also been demonstrated to play a role in tumor regression [24]. Some studies have combined the use of somatostatin analogs and IFNs in order to assess for a synergistic effect, but to date there are no data to support this.

Studies of the use of single agents in the management of these patients have shown little benefit. Studied agents include 5-fluorouracil (5-FU), doxorubicin, streptozocin, etoposide, and cisplatin, among others. The use of multiple agents in the management of these patients has also been extensively studied. There is no standard chemotherapeutic regimen for patients with carcinoid tumors.

primary tumor and local lymph nodes is the only potentially curative option for patients with carcinoid tumors. In addition to removing all gross disease, managing the patient's symptoms is another aim of therapy. The specific surgical treatment for carcinoid tumors varies by location. The details for the management of tumors at each location were described in detail in the "Site-Specific Disease" section of this chapter. Cholecystectomy is recommended at the time of surgical exploration in patients with carcinoid tumors because of the cholestasis occurring as a result of somatostatin analogs.

While the definitive role of surgery in metastatic disease has not been established in the literature, surgery may offer selected patients an improvement in quality of life. Tumor

In addition to the previously listed therapeutic options for patients with carcinoid tumors, supportive care may also help improve their quality of life. Patients can be advised to avoid certain factors that may cause symptoms, like alcohol, aged wine, and capsaicin-containing foods. Patients with diarrhea may be treated with antidiarrheal medications, like loperamide.

REFERENCES

1. Obendorfer S. Karzinoide tumoren des dunndarms. *Frankf Zschr Pathol* 1907;1:426–30.
2. Langhans T. Ueber einen Drüsenpolyp im Ileum. *Virchows Arch Pathol Anat* 1867;38:550–60.
3. Lubarsch O. Ueber dem primären Krebs des Ileum nebst Bemerkungen über das gleichzeitige Vorkommen von Krebs und Tuberculose. *Virchows Arch Pathol Anat* 1888;111:280–317.
4. Modlin IM, Lye KD, Kidd M. A 5-decade analysis of 13,715 carcinoid tumors. *Cancer* 2003;97:934–59.
5. Taghavi S, Jayarajan SN, Powers BD, Davey A, Willis AI. Examining rectal carcinoids in the era of screening colonoscopy: A Surveillance, Epidemiology, and End Results analysis. *Dis Colon Rectum* 2013;56:952–9.
6. Maggard MA, O'Connell JB, Ko CY. Updated population-based review of carcinoid tumors. *Ann Surg* 2004;240:117–22.
7. Grahame-Smith DG. What is the cause of the carcinoid flush? *Gut* 1987;28:1413–6.
8. Marsh HM, Martin JK, Kvols LK et al. Carcinoid crisis during anesthesia: Successful treatment with a somatostatin analogue. *Anesthesiology* 198;66:89–91.
9. Tateishi R, Taniguchi H, Wada A et al. Argyrophil cells and melanocytes in esophageal mucosa. *Arch Pathol Lab Med* 1974;98:87–9.
10. Hoang MP, Hobbs CM, Sobin LH, Albores-Saavedra J. Carcinoid tumor of the esophagus: A clinicopathologic study of four cases. *Am J Surg Pathol* 2002;26:517–22.
11. Zhang L, Ozao J, Warner R, Divino C. Review of the pathogenesis, diagnosis, and management of type I gastric carcinoid tumor. *World J Surg* 2011;35:1879–86.
12. Ozao-Choy J, Buch K, Strauchen JA, Warner RRP, Divino CM. Laparoscopic antrectomy for the treatment of type I gastric carcinoid tumors. *J Surg Res* 2010;162:22–5.
13. Byrn JC, Wang JL, Divino CM, Nguyen SQ, Warner RR. Management of goblet cell carcinoid. *J Surg Oncol* 2006;94:396–402.
14. McDermott FD, Heeney A, Courtney D, Mohan H, Winter D. Rectal carcinoids: A systematic review. *Surg Endosc* 2014;28:2020–6.
15. Thirunavukarasu P, Sathaiah M, Sukumar S et al. Meckel's diverticulum—A high-risk regional for malignancy in the ileum. Insights from a population-based epidemiologic study and implications in surgical management. *Ann Surg* 2011;253:223–30.
16. Carling RS, Degg TL, Allen KR, Bax NDS, Barth JH. Evaluation of whole blood serotonin and plasma 5-hydroxyindole acetic acid in diagnosis of carcinoid disease. *Ann Clin Biochem* 2002;39:577–82.
17. Stridsberg M, Eriksson B, Oberg K, Janson ET. A comparison between three commercial kits for chromogranin A measurements. *J Endocrinol* 2003;177:337–41.
18. Rustagi S, Warner RRP, Divino CM. Serum pancreastatin: The next predictive neuroendocrine tumor marker. *J Surg Oncol* 2013;108:126–8.
19. Bajetta E, Ferrari L, Matinetti A et al. Chromogranin A, neuron specific enolase, carcinoembryonic antigen, and hydroxyindole acetic acid evaluation in patients with neuroendocrine tumors. *Cancer* 1999;86:858–65.
20. Calhoun K, Toth-Fejel S, Cheek J, Pommier R. Serum peptide profiles in patients with carcinoid tumors. *Am J Surg* 2003;186:28–31.
21. Dromain C, de Baere T, Lumbroso J et al. Detection of liver metastases from endocrine tumors: A prospective comparison of somatostatin receptor scintigraphy, computed tomography, and magnetic resonance imaging. *J Clin Oncol* 2005;23:70–8.
22. Treglia G, Castaldi P, Rindi G, Giordano A, Rufini V. Diagnostic performance of gallium-68 somatostatin receptor PET and PET/CT in patients with thoracic and gastroenteropancreatic neuroendocrine tumours: A meta-analysis. *Endocrine* 2012;42:80–7.
23. Gulec SA, Mountcastle TS, Frey D et al. Cytoreductive surgery in patients with advanced-stage carcinoid tumors. *Am J Surg* 2002;68:667–71
24. Modlin IM, Latich I, Zlkusoka M et al. Gastrointestinal carcinoids: The evolution of diagnostic strategies. *J Clin Gastroenterol* 2006;40:572–82.
25. Caplin ME, Pavel M, Ćwikła JB et al. Lanreotide in metastatic enteropancreatic neuroendocrine tumors. *N Engl J Med* 2014;371:224–33.
26. Rinke A, Muller HH, Schade-Brittinger C et al. Placebo-controlled, double-blind, prospective, randomized study on the effect of octreotide LAR in the control of tumor growth in patients with metastatic neuroendocrine midgut tumors: A report from the PROMID study group. *J Clin Oncol* 2009;27:4656–63.

46

Serotonin receptors and valvular heart disease

JAVIER G. CASTILLO AND DAVID H. ADAMS

SEROTONIN PRODUCTION, ACTION AND METABOLISM

5-Hydroxytryptamine (5-HT) or serotonin is a vital cellular signaling molecule mostly present in the central and peripheral nervous systems (serotoninergic neurons), gastrointestinal tract (intestinal myenteric plexus and enterochromaffin cells), bronchopulmonary system (enterochromaffin cells) and cardiovascular system (blood platelets) [1]. While serotoninergic neurons and enterochromaffin cells can synthesize serotonin, platelets only rely on uptake mechanisms to proceed with serotonin storage [2]. The synthesis of serotonin is a complex biochemical pathway that initially involves the conversion of the essential amino acid L-tryptophan to 5-hydroxytryptophan (5-HTP) by the enzyme L-tryptophan hydroxylase (TPH) [3]. It is important to highlight that this reaction is a rate-limiting step for serotonin production in non-neuronal tissues. Subsequently, the aromatic L-amino acid decarboxylase (AADC) catalyzes the final production of 5-HT, and this is internalized by the vesicular monoamine transporter (VMAT) and released to induce both autocrine and paracrine actions [4] (Figure 46.1a).

Serotonin participates in a wide array of unrelated physiologic processes, including sleep–wake cycles, maintenance of mood [5], control of food intake, regulation of blood pressure, and platelet aggregation [6]. In this regard, with the exception of the 5-HT3 receptor subtype [7], which is a transmitter-gated sodium channel, signaling of 5-HT is

mediated by six (5-HT1, 2, 4, 5, 6, 7) transmembrane G protein-coupled receptors (GPCRs) located in the cell membrane of the targeted biological tissues [8]. Upon GPCR activation, G proteins release guanosine diphosphate, which in turn triggers a metabolic cascade that results in the production of secondary messengers such as cAMP, inositol 1,4,5-triphosphate (IP3), and diacylglycerol [9] (DAG).

After signal transduction, 5-HT is taken up by the serotonin reuptake transporter (SERT) and is either stored (blood platelets) or recycled in a sodium-dependent manner. Intracellular metabolism of 5-HT is primarily catalyzed by the outer mitochondrial membrane enzyme monoamine oxidase (MAO) [10]. The action of MAO converts 5-HT to its inactive form 5-hydroxyindole acetaldehyde (5-HIA) and then this is mostly degraded into 5-hydroxyindole acetic acid (5-HIAA) by an isoform of the enzyme aldehyde dehydrogenase (ALDH2) for final renal clearance [11].

5-HT RECEPTORS

The action mechanisms of 5-HT have been extensively studied by the pharmaceutical industry for the past decade [12]. Although most of the research has focused on the production of more efficient serotonin selective reuptake inhibitors (SSRIs), many other biological agents with serotonin-related mechanisms have been proposed [13]. These include anorexigens (fenfluramine and dexfenfluramine) [14], ergot derivatives for the treatment and prophylaxis of migraine (ergotamine and methysergide), certain

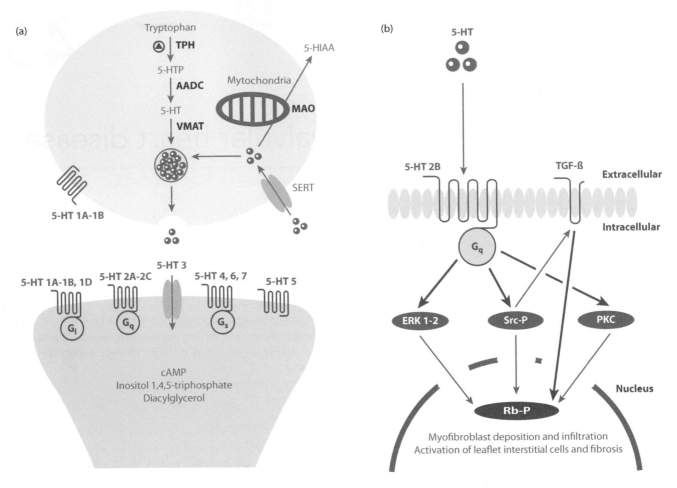

Figure 46.1 **(a)** Serotonin production, action mechanism, and metabolism. **(b)** Proposed pathway of 5-HT2B activation through the expression of Src and cross-activation of TGF-β1 signaling.

drugs for the treatment of Parkinson's disease (pergolide or cabergoline) [15] or hyperprolactinemia (bromocriptine), antidepressants, atypical antipsychotics, antiemetics, adjuvant therapies for dyslipemia (benfluorex) [16], and some drugs of abuse, such as 3,4-methylenedioxymethamphetamine (MDMA) (also known as ecstasy) [17]. However, both the direct action of abnormally elevated levels of 5-HT (i.e., carcinoid syndrome) and the indirect action of some of the aforementioned bioactive agents have been found to be related to a number of adverse cardiovascular effects, including alterations of the rhythm, pulmonary hypertension, and valve disease [18]. In this regard, research has provided initial insights, but the etiology remains incompletely understood, particularly when it comes to the occurrence of valvular heart disease.

Among the seven families of 5-HT receptors, the 5-HT2 family has been traditionally linked to secondary cardiovascular disease, especially 5-HT2A and 5-HT2B [19]. This family consists of three different GPCRs (5-HT2A, 5-HT2B, and 5-HT2C) that induce a sudden increase in the intracellular concentration of IP3, thus generating the production of DAG and calcium. Parallel to these reactions, 5-HT2 receptors also generate secondary organ-specific responses, among which the brain is the most prevalent

target [20]. In the brain, 5-HT2C receptors are uniformly distributed in all brain areas and represent an important target for psychoactive agents (i.e., atypical antipsychotics and anorectics), whereas the presence of 5-HT2A receptors is only important in cortical regions and the concentration of 5-HT2B receptors is very low (minor involvement) [21]. However, a very characteristic trait of 5-HT2 receptors is the lack of selectivity. This is due to an approximate 50% homology among receptors, and as a consequence, drugs intended to target 5-HT2A or 5-HT2C receptors located in the brain may interact with peripheral 5-HT2B receptors and vice versa [22].

Recent publications have suggested a more concrete and selective link between 5-HT2B receptors and heart valve disease secondary to a mitogenic and secretory response in ventricular and valvular fibroblasts [23]. Accordingly, several authors have reproduced animal models of long-term administration of 5-HT to elucidate the mechanism of serotonin-induced valvular alterations [24]. After analysis, the data has unanimously pointed toward a significant correlation between the expression of 5-HT2B receptors and the occurrence of histopathological cardiac valve changes. The activation of 5-HT2B receptors [25], already demonstrated to be present in aortic leaflet tissue, has been reported to directly promote the proliferation and fibrosis of the leaflets by accumulation of extracellular matrix secreted by the valvular interstitial cells [26]. In this context, the signal transduction has been shown to upregulate the cytokine transforming growth factor β1 (TGF-β1), which then acts as a key mediator in the appearance of leaflet changes due to myofibroblast deposition and increased production of collagen and glycosaminoglycans [27]. Evidence postulates that the signaling pathway from 5-HT2B receptors may be identical to the TGF-β1 signaling pathway [28] in that both are mediated by the tyrosine kinase Src [29] (Figure 46.1b).

DRUG-INDUCED HEART VALVE DISEASE

The pathologic features of drug-induced heart valve disease (DIHVD) are very similar to those occurring in patients with carcinoid heart disease (CHD) [30]. Elevated 5-HT levels in plasma are the well-known link between these two conditions. Patients with CHD characteristically present with excess 5-HT production after developing hepatic metastases and carcinoid syndrome (see below), whereas those patients who develop DIHVD suffer from an overt serotoninergic activity. Among these, the most classic example is the fenfluramine–phentermine (fen-phen) syndrome [31]. The use of fenfluramine (usually administered with phentermine for better tolerance) or dexfenfluramine promotes the release of 5-HT, also blocking its subsequent neuronal uptake. This triggers an increase in 5-HT levels and therefore in serotoninergic activity with a strong anorectic effect. However, up to 25% of patients on these regimens have been reported to have abnormal echocardiographic findings after 12 months [32]. In addition, it has been demonstrated that although phentermine alone does not cause any valve abnormality, the incidence of DIHVD is 7.1 per 10,000 in patients treated with fenfluramine for 4 months, and as high as 35 per 10,000 in patients treated for longer periods of time [33].

Ergot derivatives have been similarly linked to DIHVD [32]. Ergotamine and methysergide (classically prescribed for the treatment and prophylaxis of migraine), as well as nonspecific dopamine agonists such as pergolide and cabergoline (routinely recommended for the treatment of Parkinson's disease), share a similar chemical structure with 5-HT and therefore can interact with its receptors, particularly 5-HT2B receptors [34]. Accordingly, the incidence of valve disease (on echocardiography) in patients taking pergolide or cabergoline has been published to be 23% and 28%, respectively, versus none in those patients on nonergot dopamine agonists [35]. Interestingly, those ergot derivatives with more affinity for 5-HT2A receptors, such as lisuride, bromocriptine, and terguride, have not been associated with DIHVD. These findings lead to support for the specific implication of 5-HT2B receptors in the development of valvulopathies [36]. As a consequence, multiple drugs have been tested for agonist activity at the 5-HT2B receptor, including guanfacine, oxymetazoline, quinidine, xylometazoline, and fenoldopam. Among the latter, although still under investigation, guanfacine (antihypertensive agent in adults and recently indicated to treat attention deficit in infants) and quinidine (antiarrhythmic) are of special concern.

Diagnosis

Current guidelines from the American College of Cardiology, the American Heart Association, and the American Society of Echocardiography recommend baseline echocardiography in all patients with a history of use of any drug known to be associated with DIHVD (particularly anorectic drugs) and symptoms of valve disease or present auscultatory abnormalities [37]. The absence of murmurs has been correlated to the absence of echocardiographic findings in more than 90% of the patients [38]. A repeat physical examination every 6 months is advised if that is the case.

DIHVD may involve left- and right-sided valves, but there is a clear predilection for the left-sided valves (aortic valve > mitral valve > tricuspid valve). Characteristic echocardiographic features in the aortic position include decreased cusp mobility due to thickening and restriction, as well as various degrees of leaflet doming with rolling of the free edge, mainly leading to aortic regurgitation [39]. In atrioventricular positions, there is leaflet thickening and restriction of the subvalvular apparatus due to chordal shortening (chordal fusion has only been described in isolated cases of severe disease). Most patients present with regurgitation combined with varying degrees of stenosis (Table 46.1).

Surgical management

From a cardiac point of view, DIHVD shares numerous pathologic findings with rheumatic disease, CHD, radiation-induced valve disease, systemic lupus erythematosus, hypereosinophilic syndrome, and mucopolysaccharidosis in that all of these clinical entities present with type IIIA leaflet dysfunction. However, in terms of quantification, the severity of valvular regurgitation or stenosis is only mild to moderate in most cases. In addition, withdrawal of the drug has been associated with improvement or at least stabilization of the valvular function (only 4%–5% of patients have continuous disease progression). These two facts not only distinguish DIHVD from other forms with similar pathophysiology, but also change the potential surgical approach. In fact, some data in the literature suggests that when indicated, these patients may benefit from valve reconstruction (valves are more amenable to repair techniques) more than patients with, for example, CHD or radiation-induced valve disease.

Surgical technique

Surgical exploration of the valves reveals a glistening-white appearance of the leaflets with diffuse and irregular

Table 46.1 Characteristics of the main clinical entities causing changes in the leaflet architecture due to an inflammatory process or deposition/infiltration

Characteristics	RD	DIVHD	CHD
Etiology	Microorganisms	Drugs (5-HT2B)	Mainly serotonin (5-HT2B)
Valves	Left > right	Left > right	Right > left
Histopathology	Inflammatory reaction and neovascularization	Leaflet glistening with diffuse thickening	Deposition of pearly white plaques (smooth muscle, myofibroblasts, and collagen)
Leaflet thickening	Severe	Irregular	Severe
Leaflet architecture	Distorted	Preserved	Distorted
Calcification	Yes	No	No
Commissural fusion	Yes	No	No
Dysfunction	S > R	R > S	R and S
Quantification	Severe	Moderate	Severe
Disease progression	Continuous	Stable or reversible (if drug is withdrawn)	Continuous

Note: R, regurgitation; RD, rheumatic disease; S, stenosis.

thickening. Retraction of the subvalvular apparatus with occasional chordal fusion might also be seen. In the aortic position, valve replacement is frequently the procedure of choice. In the mitral and tricuspid positions, valve reconstruction might be considered using techniques such as chordal cutting and fenestration, chordal replacement (neochordoplasty with polytetrafluoroethylene sutures), leaflet enlargement with a pericardial patch in favorable cases (preserved leaflet mobility), and remodeling annuloplasty. It is important to emphasize that the surgical experience with this particular patient population is very limited, and currently there is scarce data regarding surgical outcomes.

CARCINOID SYNDROME AND CARCINOID HEART DISEASE

Carcinoid tumors are rare slow-growing neuroendocrine malignancies most commonly originating from enterochromaffin cells located in the gastrointestinal tract [40]. They are uncommon and only occur in between 2.5 and 5 cases per 100,000 of the population [41]. The most common primary site of carcinoid tumors is the gastrointestinal tract (60%), followed by the bronchopulmonary system (27%). More infrequent sites are the gonads, liver, biliary tree, and pancreas.

In subjects with local disease (absence of metastases), 5-HT is recaptured and undergoes hepatic conversion into urinary 5-HIAA for renal clearance [42]. In the presence of hepatic metastases, metastatic active foci of enterochromaffin cells secrete copious amounts of 5-HT that will exceed and bypass the degradation capacity of the liver [43]. As a result, a significant concentration of these substances (10%–15% of patients) might be integrally released into the systemic circulation, leading to a constellation of clinical symptoms known as carcinoid syndrome [44] (Figure 46.2). Exceptions to this are ovarian carcinoids, which drain directly into the systemic circulation, or very rare (<1%)

cases of extensive retroperitoneal lymph node metastases, with drainage to the thoracic duct [45,46]. The vasoactive amines eventually enter the inferior vena cava and then reach the right-sided chambers of the heart in up to 60% of patients. In the absence of a primary endobronchial carcinoid tumor (additional satellite production of serotonin or isolated left-sided CHD), the development of left-sided CHD implies the presence of a cardiac shunt or uncontrolled tumor burden that may overcome the pulmonary potential to inactivate 5-HT. Left-sided CHD occurs in approximately 20% of the patients with carcinoid syndrome. The prevalence of direct myocardial carcinoid metastasis is about 4%.

Clinical diagnosis

Clinical diagnosis mandates a high index of suspicion. Careful examination of the jugular venous pressure is essential, as an early prominent V wave of tricuspid regurgitation (TR) may be observed. A coincident V wave with carotid pulse is also characteristic of moderate to severe TR. TR usually yields a pansystolic murmur, which increases intensity during inspiration. Similarly, an early diastolic murmur or a systolic murmur can be heard in pulmonic position in the presence of pulmonic regurgitation or stenosis, respectively.

Biochemical markers

Measurement of 24-hour urinary 5-HIAA excretion is usually the initial diagnostic test, with a sensitivity of 75% and a specificity of up to 100% for the diagnosis of carcinoid syndrome [47]. In cases where the measurement of urinary 5-HIAA is inconclusive, determination of blood serotonin concentrations can be helpful as a first step. Although not useful in the diagnosis of CHD, peak urinary levels of 5-HIAA have been identified as a predictor of worse long-term survival in patients with cardiac involvement [48]. Plasma levels of chromogranin A (CgA)

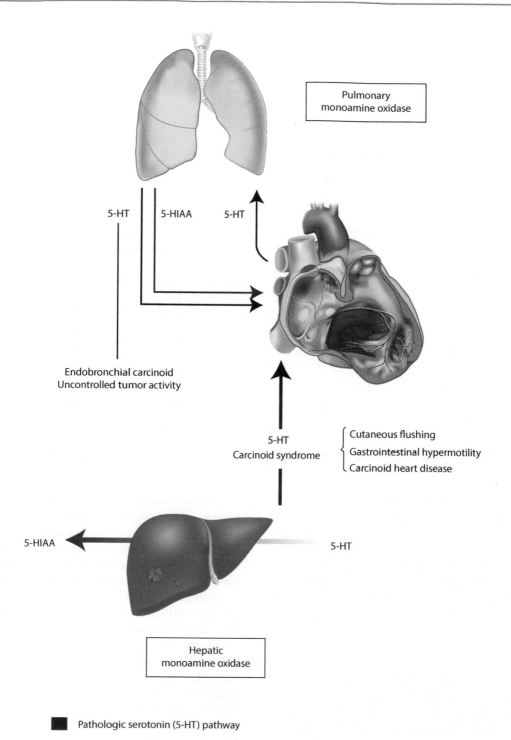

Figure 46.2 Pathophysiology of carcinoid syndrome and CHD. Although possible, the occurrence of carcinoid syndrome secondary to the presence of an endobronchial tumor is rare.

are elevated in more than 80% of patients with a carcinoid tumor and have been reported to correlate with tumor burden and disease activity (best marker for recurrence) [49]. This is particularly important during the perioperative period, when tumor stabilization before and after valve replacement might become crucial to avoid carcinoid crises and to choose an appropriate prosthesis type. Patients with suspected CHD should have a complete panel of biomarkers, including 5-HIAA, CgA, neurokinin A,

brain natriuretic peptide (BNP), gastrin, serum 5-HT, and pancreastatin [50].

Imaging techniques

Echocardiography is the primary imaging modality used for diagnosis and assessment of extent and severity of CHD [51] (Figure 46.3). Tricuspid (TV) and pulmonary (PV) valves are typically thickened and retracted (type IIIA

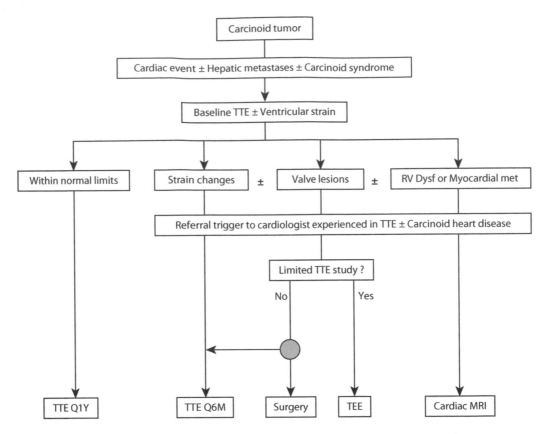

Figure 46.3 Imaging algorithm for patients with CHD. Dysf, dysfunction; Q, every; TTE, transthoracic echocardiography; TEE, transesophageal echocardiography.

valve dysfunction). In the early stages, there is insidious valve thickening (requires echocardiographic expertise) with changes in leaflet concavity [52]. Disease progression results in further thickening of the leaflet and the subvalvular apparatus, including the papillary muscles, which leads to additional leaflet retraction and restriction of motion. In the tricuspid position, chordae are commonly fused and very thickened. In advanced stages, the manifest deterioration of valvular architecture results in a fixed noncoaptation of the valve leaflets. Consequently, valve function is severely impaired [53] and a combination of regurgitation secondary to a semiopen noncoapting position and stenosis due to severe leaflet thickening is commonly found [54].

Severe TR is characterized by an early-peaking Doppler spectral profile, followed by a rapid decline. Peak regurgitant velocity may be increased due to coexistence of pulmonary stenosis. A color-flow Doppler examination of the hepatic veins may also show a systolic flow reversal, consistent with severe TR. The TV inflow pressure half-time may also be prolonged, indicative of associated tricuspid stenosis. An increase in peak jet velocity of >4 m/s (peak gradient of >64 mmHg) on continuous-wave Doppler examination is consistent with severe pulmonary stenosis [55], whereas a sharp deceleration slope is a typical finding for severe pulmonic regurgitation [56]. The severity of pulmonary stenosis may in some cases be underestimated due to a combination of low cardiac output (right ventricular [RV] dysfunction) and severe TR.

Chronic tricuspid and pulmonary dysfunction results in continuous right atrium and ventricle enlargement secondary to volume overload and, subsequently, RV dysfunction. In this setting, an accurate assessment of the RV function might be challenging due to severe elevation of the RV pressure, paradoxical motion of the interventricular septum, reopening of a patent foramen ovale, and potentially RV hypokinesis [57]. In this context, unpublished data from our institutional ongoing research has revealed a potential role of speckle tracking echocardiography and strain techniques in surgical referral. Classically, the evaluation of patients with CHD has been exclusively focused on estimations of functional valve disease. However, strain techniques have been recently proposed for the assessment of RV function as an indirect measure of endocardial fibrosis. Recent series have shown a significant reduction in RV function (assessed by strain) in those patients with CHD when compared with healthy controls [58]. Moreover, RV strain was reduced in patients with 5-HIAA levels above the normal range compared with those with normal levels. In our opinion, this is a seminal study that might open a novel application of strain measurement to assess RV function and fibrosis in patients with early-stage CHD. Early diagnosis might have a significant impact on prognosis by providing critical information to avoid late referral to surgical intervention.

Cardiac magnetic resonance imaging (CMRI) is an alternative imaging modality for the evaluation of CHD that can affect decision making and management since it provides several attractive advantages [59]. First, it provides reproducible and accurate assessment of the volume and function of the right heart. In fact, nowadays CMRI is considered the gold standard for the quantification of RV volumes and the ejection fraction. Furthermore, CMRI enables quantification of the size of possible myocardial metastases and offers information regarding extension into surrounding structures [60].

Future directions in the imaging field comprise the evaluation and quantification of inflammatory activity. The basis of molecular imaging is to target specific receptors or hormones with radiotracers that allow the visualization of high-activity processes using positron emission tomography (PET). Carcinoid tumors express different somatostatin receptors, particularly receptors 2 and 5, and it has been demonstrated that gallium-68 octreotide PET could be a specific ligand for these receptors. After the radiotracer injection, imaging with PET could be performed to specifically visualize the presence and extension of uptake if carcinoid tumor is present [61].

Surgical management: General considerations

The replacement of the right-sided valves, including the patch enlargement of the right ventricular outflow tract (RVOT), is currently the only definitive treatment to potentially improve quality of life and provide survival benefit. Although cardiac surgery has been traditionally reserved for patients with symptomatic RV failure, a current trend toward improved surgical outcomes has triggered a more liberal referral for valve replacement [62]. Poor functional class and ventricular failure are independently associated with adverse outcomes in this population, so much so that surgery is indicated unless imminent demise is anticipated.

Characteristic lesions of CHD involve the right-sided endocardium, valves, and subvalvular apparatus. The deposition of carcinoid plaques, a pearly white fibrotic conglomerate of smooth muscle cells, myofibroblasts, and collagen, leads to annular constriction, leaflet or cusp thickening and retraction, and subvalvular fusion and shortening [63] (Figure 46.4). Chordae are usually fused and present with different patterns of disease, from thick and focal to thin and diffuse [64].

Although left-sided pathology has not been as well characterized as right-sided lesions, several observations have been made describing a less aggressive and more diffuse pattern of lesions (more amenable to repair versus replacement) when present [65]. The aortic valve will show thickening of the valve cusps and loss of normal concavity during diastole. The mitral leaflets might

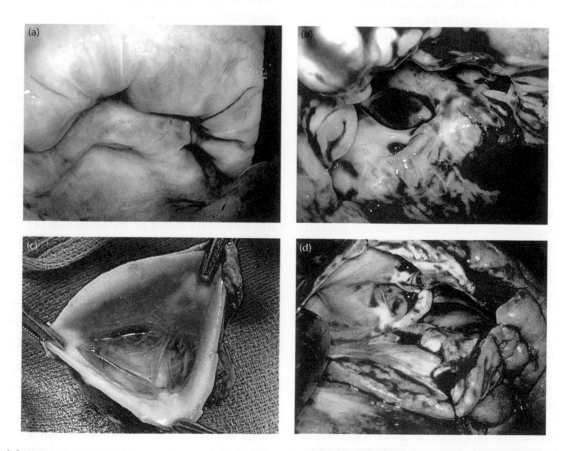

Figure 46.4 Intraoperative atrial views of a normal tricuspid valve (a) and a pathologic tricuspid valve with CHD (b). (c) Normal PV as an autograft during a Ross procedure. (d) Outflow view of a pathologic PV in a patient with CHD. Note the severe fibrotic reaction on the leaflets and subvalvular apparatus with chordal fusion, thickening, and retraction. (Courtesy of Paul Stelzer, MD.)

be thickened, and the subvalvular apparatus is most frequently affected, resulting in chordal thickening and fusion, leading to retraction and restricted leaflet motion. Left-sided involvement rarely results in stenosis, but rather regurgitation.

Surgical management: Anesthesia

Anesthetic management for any interventional procedure in patients with CHD may pose two distinct challenges: the occurrence of a "carcinoid crisis" and the identification and subsequent management of low cardiac output syndrome [66]. A carcinoid crisis (mainly characterized by hypotension, respiratory wheezing, and facial hyperemia) [67] may be precipitated by the administration of histamine-releasing neuromuscular relaxants (atracurium, mivacurium, and tubocurarine), inotropes or vasopressors (catecholamines), and long-acting opioids such as meperidine and morphine [68,69]. The administration of medications with histamine-releasing properties results in the release of bradykinin, which in turn triggers the release of catecholamines (especially in the setting of gastric carcinoid tumors). Additionally, carcinoid crises have been shown to be precipitated by emotional stress, hypercapnia, hypothermia, or tumor necrosis after chemoembolization. Therefore, the administration of anxiolytics might be useful during the preoperative period and induction. In our experience, anesthetic induction can be accomplished safely with etomidate and maintained with isoflurane, and muscle relaxation might be achieved with rorcuronium or vecuronium. Short-acting synthetic opioids such as fentanyl or sufentanil are also safe. Finally, antifibrinolytics such as epsilon-aminocaproic acid have been used to avoid facial edema [70]. In the event of hypotension secondary to carcinoid crisis, standard management with optimal volume replacement, correction of electrolyte abnormalities, and octreotide administration should be the first choice. If this is not effective, only certain vasopressors (they are generally contraindicated), like phenylephrine, calcium, or dopamine (rescue infusion), may be considered if administered in conjunction with octreotide [71].

Octreotide has been shown to prevent the release of serotonin and bradikinin in more than 70% of the patients [72,73]. Our institutional octreotide protocol starts with a pre-emptive infusion of octreotide at 50–100 µg/h the night before surgery (day admission surgery is preferably avoided) or in the holding area before the insertion of the arterial catheter. Then, the infusion is continued throughout the case and until up to 48 hours after surgery. During induction, an additional bolus of 50–100 µg is routinely given. Also, octreotide might be administered intermittently throughout the procedure as bolus injections of 20–100 µg to patients with carcinoid symptoms or unexplained decline in central venous pressures during cardiopulmonary bypass. The infusion of octreotide is increased to a maximum dose of 300 µg/h if necessary.

Surgical technique

Although TV replacement has been traditionally accepted by most authors, the need for PV replacement (versus isolated valvectomy) has been debatable. It is certainly true that some patients may tolerate pulmonary regurgitation; however, long-standing pulmonary regurgitation after valvectomy may have a negative impact on RV remodeling. Additionally, a more uneventful postoperative recovery has been described among those patients undergoing PV replacement and additional patch enlargement of the RVOT [74].

Surgical technique: Tricuspid valve replacement

Our current surgical strategy for replacement of the TV implies beating heart (without aortic cross-clamping) cardiopulmonary bypass provided there are no shunts (atrial septal defect or patent foramen ovale) that would increase the risk of left-sided air entry. In this context, it is crucial to look for shunts during anesthetic induction (transesophageal echocardiography). Standard central cannulation techniques are used, including aortic and bicaval cannulation. Vacuum assistance at 40 mmHg is routinely used with cardiopulmonary bypass, allowing the use of smaller cannulas and smaller incisions [75].

A generous right atriotomy extending from the base of the right atrial appendage toward the inferior vena cava allows ample exposure of the tricuspid valve. A weighted suction catheter is placed into the coronary sinus to aspirate venous return and obtain further visualization. Valve analysis is then made under direct vision. If possible (in the absence of significant stenosis due to severe leaflet thickening), the leaflets and their subvalvular attachments will be preserved to maintain ventricular geometry and function. Pledgeted 2-0 Ethibond sutures are then placed along the annulus and leaflet junction in an everting fashion. In the region of the septal leaflet, near the atrioventricular node, the sutures are placed on the leaflet side of the annulus to avoid postoperative conduction block. The valve is then seated into position such that a strut is not aligned over the RVOT, causing obstruction.

Surgical technique: Pulmonary valve replacement and patch enlargement of the right ventricular outflow tract

The main pulmonary artery is dissected away from the aorta and surrounding structures, allowing clear visualization of the RVOT and main pulmonary artery. This maneuver should be done with the cautery being as close to the aorta as possible. A longitudinal incision is then made in the main pulmonary artery and carried across the pulmonary annulus into the RVOT (Figure 46.5a). A pulmonary valvectomy is performed, and a valve sizer is brought to the field so that two-thirds of the posterior valve fits within

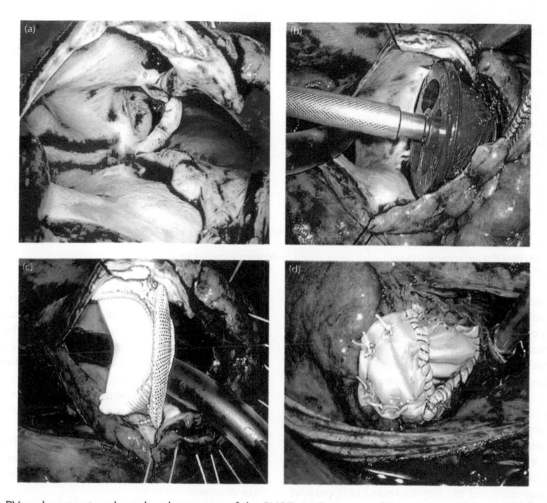

Figure 46.5 PV replacement and patch enlargement of the RVOT. **(a)** Exposure of the PV through a longitudinal incision in the main pulmonary artery carried across the pulmonary annulus into the RVOT. **(b)** Valve sizer brought to the field so that two-thirds of the posterior valve fits within the native annulus. **(c)** The struts of the prosthesis are placed at the two, six, and ten o'clock positions. **(d)** A patch is used to enlarge the infundibulum of the pulmonary artery and accommodate the prosthesis.

the native pulmonary annulus (Figure 46.5b). Interrupted pledgeted 2-0 Ethibond (Ethicon Inc., Somerville, New Jersey) sutures are placed along the posterior two-thirds of the pulmonary annulus, and the prosthesis is oriented in its intended position. Struts are placed at the two, six, and ten o'clock positions (avoiding the twelve o'clock position to prevent excessive tenting of the patch) (Figure 46.5c). After placing sutures through the sewing ring (spacing of the sutures should match the spacing in the annulus), the sutures are tightened to secure the prosthesis. Interrupted pledgeted (very important in infudibular sutures) 2-0 Ethibond sutures are then placed along the infundibular side of the incision, and a glutaraldehyde-fixed bovine pericardial patch (a Dacron graft [MediTech, Boston Scientific, Natick, Massachusetts] might also be a reasonable option) is used to enlarge the infundibulum and the pulmonary artery. The patch is then tailored so that its greatest width corresponds to the remaining circumference of the anterior portion of the prosthesis. The length of the patch is longer than the RVOT incision to avoid leaks and allow billowing and therefore tilting of the prosthesis, which

reduces turbulence. The patch is then anchored using a 4-0 Prolene (Ethicon) running suture, beginning at the apex of the pulmonary arteriotomy and working in each direction toward the prosthesis. Once the distal portion of the patch has covered the pulmonary artery, the patch is then folded back on itself over the prosthesis to mark the positioning of the remaining one-third of the sewing cuff. A 4-0 Prolene running suture is finally sewn across the anterior third of the prosthesis and through the patch (Figure 46.5d).

Surgical outcomes

The first surgical series on the management of CHD was published in the early 1990s [76]. In 1995, Robiolio and colleagues observed an operative mortality of 63% [77]. Subsequently, Connolly et al. reported the Mayo Clinic experience presenting a surgical series of 26 patients with a mortality of 35% [78]. Later on, Moller and colleagues updated the Mayo Clinic experience, analyzing 87 patients who underwent surgery over two decades and demonstrated a significant decrease in perioperative mortality to 16% [79].

Table 46.2 Surgical outcomes of patients with carcinoid heart disease

Author (reference)	Year	N	TVR (%)	PVR[a] (%)	RVOT (%)	AVI (%)	MVI (%)	Prostheses	Mortality (%)
Robiolio et al. [77]	1995	8	100	25	—	—	—	Biological	63
Connolly et al. [78]	1995	26	100	11	50	8	11	Both	35
Moller et al. [79]	2005	87	100	30	68	11	9	Both	16
Castillo et al. [83]	2008	10	100	90	90	10	30	Biological	20
Bhattacharyya et al. [80]	2011	22	100	86	—	9	18	Biological	18
Komoda et al. [81]	2011	12	75[a]	25	—	8	—	Biological	17
Mokhles et al. [82]	2012	19	100	21	10	5	—	Both	7[b]
Castillo et al. (unpublished data)	2014	30	100	96	96	12	18	Biological	10

Note: AVI, aortic valve involvement; MVI, mitral valve involvement; PVR, pulmonary valve replacement; TVR, tricuspid valve replacement.

[a] Patients who did not receive tricuspid valve replacement underwent tricuspid valve repair.

[b] Hospital mortality as opposed to 30-day mortality.

Very recent series from United Kingdom, Germany, and the Netherlands have shown mortality rates below 20% [80–82]. Our own surgical experience has shown a decrease in 30-day mortality from 20% to 11% over a 5-year period [83] (Table 46.2). Thus, it seems obvious that a clear trend toward improved surgical outcomes has been accomplished over time. In addition, better oncologic therapies have significantly contributed to achieving a threefold increase in median survival over the last two decades. On this basis, it may be prudent to consider an early surgical intervention in patients with mildly symptomatic CHD. This is crucial, since watchful waiting for severe symptoms due to RV failure has been observed to carry increased perioperative mortality [84].

Midterm survival among patients with cardiac manifestations has been demonstrated to be significantly reduced in comparison with those patients without echocardiographic evidence of carcinoid lesions (31% vs. 68% at 3 years). Although the assessment of patients with CHD has been traditionally limited to echocardiographic estimations [85], new prognostic values and techniques have contributed to empower the preoperative assessment of these patients [86]. Among these are the ratio of the early transmitral flow velocity (E) to the early diastolic mitral annulus velocity (e') (equal to or above 8 is a significant prognostic factor of mortality) [58] and novel techniques for the detection of regional myocardial contraction for the assessment of RV function as an indirect measure of endocardial fibrosis [87]. In addition, ongoing trials are trying to correlate levels of biomarkers in plasma and urine with subclinical myocardial fibrosis, hence potentially providing a threshold value to proceed with echocardiographic surveillance and maybe earlier referral.

Valve replacement in patients with CHD has been demonstrated to mitigate symptoms, provide survival benefit, and present outcomes similar to those of patients undergoing hepatic resection for carcinoid syndrome, but without CHD. While right-sided valve replacement has been well accepted, the choice of prosthesis remains debatable. Historical series have favored the use of mechanical

prostheses based on the potential structural valve deterioration due to high levels of vasoactive substances and the relatively young age of these patients [88]. Indeed, recent reports have emphasized the increasing use of mechanical prostheses even in the pulmonary position. However, limited available data suggests that bioprosthetic valve replacement might be preferable to mechanical valves in these patients, who often present with an abnormal liver profile and associated coagulopathies [89]. Additionally, mandatory anticoagulation represents an additional risk for bleeding during hepatic artery embolization or other surgical procedures focused on achieving hormonal control of the disease.

REFERENCES

1. Erspamer V, Asero B. Identification of enteramine, the specific hormone of the enterochromaffin cell system, as 5-hydroxytryptamine. *Nature* 1952;169:800–1.
2. Lesurtel M, Graf R, Aleil B et al. Platelet-derived serotonin mediates liver regeneration. *Science* 2006;312:104–7.
3. Rapport MM, Green AA, Page IH. Serum vasoconstrictor, serotonin; isolation and characterization. *J Biol Chem* 1948;176:1243–51.
4. Torres GE, Gainetdinov RR, Caron MG. Plasma membrane monoamine transporters: Structure, regulation and function. *Nat Rev Neurosci* 2003;4:13–25.
5. Lucki I. The spectrum of behaviors influenced by serotonin. *Biol Psychiatry* 1998;44:151–62.
6. Nichols DE, Nichols CD. Serotonin receptors. *Chem Rev* 2008;108:1614–41.
7. Maricq AV, Peterson AS, Brake AJ, Myers RM, Julius D. Primary structure and functional expression of the 5ht3 receptor, a serotonin-gated ion channel. *Science* 1991;254:432–7.
8. Hoyer D, Hannon JP, Martin GR. Molecular, pharmacological and functional diversity of 5-HT receptors. *Pharmacol Biochem Behav* 2002;71:533–54.

9. Idzko M, Panther E, Stratz C et al. The serotoninergic receptors of human dendritic cells: Identification and coupling to cytokine release. *J Immunol* 2004;172:6011–9.

10. Giannaccini G, Betti L, Palego L et al. The expression of platelet serotonin transporter (sert) in human obesity. *BMC Neurosci* 2013;14:128.

11. Rooke N, Li DJ, Li J, Keung WM. The mitochondrial monoamine oxidase-aldehyde dehydrogenase pathway: A potential site of action of daidzin. *J Med Chem* 2000;43:4169–79.

12. Cosyns B, Droogmans S, Rosenhek R, Lancellotti P. Drug-induced valvular heart disease. *Heart* 2013;99:7–12.

13. Huot P, Johnston TH, Lewis KD et al. Uwa-121, a mixed dopamine and serotonin re-uptake inhibitor, enhances L-DOPA anti-parkinsonian action without worsening dyskinesia or psychosis-like behaviours in the MPTP-lesioned common marmoset. *Neuropharmacology* 2014;82:76–87.

14. Connolly HM, Crary JL, McGoon MD et al. Valvular heart disease associated with fenfluramine-phentermine. *N Engl J Med* 1997;337:581–8.

15. Van Camp G, Flamez A, Cosyns B et al. Treatment of Parkinson's disease with pergolide and relation to restrictive valvular heart disease. *Lancet* 2004;363:1179–83.

16. Boudes A, Lavoute C, Avierinos JF et al. Valvular heart disease associated with benfluorex therapy: High prevalence in patients with unexplained restrictive valvular heart disease. *Eur J Echocardiogr* 2011;12:688–95.

17. Droogmans S, Cosyns B, D'Haenen H et al. Possible association between 3,4-methylenedioxymethamphetamine abuse and valvular heart disease. *Am J Cardiol* 2007;100:1442–5.

18. Mekontso-Dessap A, Brouri F, Pascal O et al. Deficiency of the 5-hydroxytryptamine transporter gene leads to cardiac fibrosis and valvulopathy in mice. *Circulation* 2006;113:81–9.

19. Hutcheson JD, Setola V, Roth BL, Merryman WD. Serotonin receptors and heart valve disease—It was meant 2b. *Pharmacol Ther* 2011;132:146–57.

20. Kozikowski AP, Cho SJ, Jensen NH, Allen JA, Svennebring AM, Roth BL. HTs and rational drug design to generate a class of 5-HT(2C)-selective ligands for possible use in schizophrenia. *ChemMedChem* 2010;5:1221–5.

21. Kursar JD, Nelson DL, Wainscott DB, Baez M. Molecular cloning, functional expression, and mRNA tissue distribution of the human 5-hydroxytryptamine2B receptor. *Mol Pharmacol* 1994;46:227–34.

22. Setola V, Dukat M, Glennon RA, Roth BL. Molecular determinants for the interaction of the valvulopathic anorexigen norfenfluramine with the 5-HT2B receptor. *Mol Pharmacol* 2005;68:20–33.

23. Yabanoglu S, Akkiki M, Seguelas MH, Mialet-Perez J, Parini A, Pizzinat N. Platelet derived serotonin drives the activation of rat cardiac fibroblasts by 5-HT2A receptors. *J Mol Cell Cardiol* 2009;46:518–25.

24. Gustafsson BI, Tommeras K, Nordrum I et al. Long-term serotonin administration induces heart valve disease in rats. *Circulation* 2005;111:1517–22.

25. Rothman RB, Baumann MH, Savage JE et al. Evidence for possible involvement of 5-HT(2B) receptors in the cardiac valvulopathy associated with fenfluramine and other serotonergic medications. *Circulation* 2000;102:2836–41.

26. Etienne N, Schaerlinger B, Jaffre F, Maroteaux L. The 5-HT2B receptor: A main cardio-pulmonary target of serotonin [in French]. *J Soc Biol* 2004;198:22–9.

27. Li B, Zhang S, Zhang H et al. Fluoxetine-mediated 5-HT2B receptor stimulation in astrocytes causes EGF receptor transactivation and ERK phosphorylation. *Psychopharmacology (Berl)* 2008;201:443–58.

28. Walker GA, Masters KS, Shah DN, Anseth KS, Leinwand LA. Valvular myofibroblast activation by transforming growth factor-beta: Implications for pathological extracellular matrix remodeling in heart valve disease. *Circ Res* 2004;95:253–60.

29. Merryman WD, Lukoff HD, Long RA, Engelmayr GC Jr, Hopkins RA, Sacks MS. Synergistic effects of cyclic tension and transforming growth factor-beta1 on the aortic valve myofibroblast. *Cardiovasc Pathol* 2007;16:268–76.

30. Roth BL. Drugs and valvular heart disease. *N Engl J Med* 2007;356:6–9.

31. Gardin JM, Schumacher D, Constantine G, Davis KD, Leung C, Reid CL. Valvular abnormalities and cardiovascular status following exposure to dexfenfluramine or phentermine/fenfluramine. *JAMA* 2000;283:1703–9.

32. Sachdev M, Miller WC, Ryan T, Jollis JG. Effect of fenfluramine-derivative diet pills on cardiac valves: A meta-analysis of observational studies. *Am Heart J* 2002;144:1065–73.

33. Dahl CF, Allen MR, Urie PM, Hopkins PN. Valvular regurgitation and surgery associated with fenfluramine use: An analysis of 5743 individuals. *BMC Med* 2008;6:34.

34. Rasmussen VG, Ostergaard K, Dupont E, Poulsen SH. The risk of valvular regurgitation in patients with Parkinson's disease treated with dopamine receptor agonists. *Mov Disord* 2011;26:801–6.

35. Corvol JC, Anzouan-Kacou JB, Fauveau E et al. Heart valve regurgitation, pergolide use, and Parkinson disease: An observational study and meta-analysis. *Arch Neurol* 2007;64:1721–6.

36. Huang XP, Setola V, Yadav PN et al. Parallel functional activity profiling reveals valvulopathogens are potent 5-hydroxytryptamine(2b) receptor agonists: Implications for drug safety assessment. *Mol Pharmacol* 2009;76:710–22.

37. Cheitlin MD, Armstrong WF, Aurigemma GP et al. ACC/AHA/ASE 2003 guideline update for the clinical application of echocardiography: Summary article. A report of the American College of Cardiology/American Heart Association Task Force on Practice Guidelines (ACC/AHA/ASE Committee to Update the 1997 Guidelines for the Clinical Application of Echocardiography). *J Am Soc Echocardiogr* 2003;16:1091–10.

38. Roldan CA, Gill EA, Shively BK. Prevalence and diagnostic value of precordial murmurs for valvular regurgitation in obese patients treated with dexfenfluramine. *Am J Cardiol* 2000;86:535–9.

39. Bhattacharyya S, Schapira AH, Mikhailidis DP, Davar J. Drug-induced fibrotic valvular heart disease. *Lancet* 2009;374:577–85.

40. Oberndorfer S. Karzinoide tumoren des dünndarms. *Frank Z Pathol* 1907;1:426–32.

41. Modlin IM, Lye KD, Kidd M. A 5-decade analysis of 13,715 carcinoid tumors. *Cancer* 2003;97:934–59.

42. Manolopoulos VG, Ragia G, Alevizopoulos G. Pharmacokinetic interactions of selective serotonin reuptake inhibitors with other commonly prescribed drugs in the era of pharmacogenomics. *Drug Metabol Drug Interact* 2012;27:19–31.

43. Lundin L, Norheim I, Landelius J, Oberg K, Theodorsson-Norheim E. Carcinoid heart disease: Relationship of circulating vasoactive substances to ultrasound-detectable cardiac abnormalities. *Circulation* 1988;77:264–9.

44. Druce M, Rockall A, Grossman AB. Fibrosis and carcinoid syndrome: From causation to future therapy. *Nat Rev Endocrinol* 2009;5:276–83.

45. Bernheim AM, Connolly HM, Pellikka PA. Carcinoid heart disease in patients without hepatic metastases. *Am J Cardiol* 2007;99:292–4.

46. Mordi IR, Bridges A. A rare case of ovarian carcinoid causing heart failure. *Scott Med J* 2011;56:181.

47. Aggarwal G, Obideen K, Wehbi M. Carcinoid tumors: What should increase our suspicion? *Cleve Clin J Med* 2008;75:849–55.

48. Westberg G, Wangberg B, Ahlman H, Bergh CH, Beckman-Suurkula M, Caidahl K. Prediction of prognosis by echocardiography in patients with midgut carcinoid syndrome. *Br J Surg* 2001;88:865–72.

49. d'Herbomez M, Do Cao C, Vezzosi D, Borzon-Chasot F, Baudin E, Groupe des Tumeurs Endocrines. Chromogranin A assay in clinical practice. *Ann Endocrinol* 2010;71:274–80.

50. Dobson R, Burgess MI, Banks M et al. The association of a panel of biomarkers with the presence and severity of carcinoid heart disease: A cross-sectional study. *PLoS One* 2013;8:e73679.

51. Zoghbi WA, Enriquez-Sarano M, Foster E et al. Recommendations for evaluation of the severity of native valvular regurgitation with two-dimensional and Doppler echocardiography. *J Am Soc Echocardiogr* 2003;16:777–802.

52. Bhattacharyya S, Toumpanakis C, Burke M, Taylor AM, Caplin ME, Davar J. Features of carcinoid heart disease identified by 2- and 3-dimensional echocardiography and cardiac MRI. *Circ Cardiovasc Imaging* 2010;3:103–11.

53. Castillo JG, Adams DH, Fischer GW. Absence of the tricuspid valve due to severe carcinoid heart disease. *Rev Esp Cardiol* 2010;63:96.

54. Pellikka PA, Tajik AJ, Khandheria BK et al. Carcinoid heart disease. Clinical and echocardiographic spectrum in 74 patients. *Circulation* 1993;87:1188–96.

55. Baumgartner H, Hung J, Bermejo J et al. Echocardiographic assessment of valve stenosis: EAE/ASE recommendations for clinical practice. *Eur J Echocardiogr* 2009;10:1–25.

56. Lancellotti P, Tribouilloy C, Hagendorff A et al. European Association of Echocardiography recommendations for the assessment of valvular regurgitation. Part 1. Aortic and pulmonary regurgitation (native valve disease). *Eur J Echocardiogr* 2010;11:223–44.

57. Ueti OM, Camargo EE, Ueti Ade A, de Lima-Filho EC, Nogueira EA. Assessment of right ventricular function with Doppler echocardiographic indices derived from tricuspid annular motion: Comparison with radionuclide angiography. *Heart* 2002;88:244–8.

58. Mansencal N, McKenna WJ, Mitry E et al. Comparison of prognostic value of tissue Doppler imaging in carcinoid heart disease versus the value in patients with the carcinoid syndrome but without carcinoid heart disease. *Am J Cardiol* 2010;105:527–31.

59. Champion HC, Michelakis ED, Hassoun PM. Comprehensive invasive and noninvasive approach to the right ventricle-pulmonary circulation unit: State of the art and clinical and research implications. *Circulation* 2009;120:992–1007.

60. Sandmann H, Pakkal M, Steeds R. Cardiovascular magnetic resonance imaging in the assessment of carcinoid heart disease. *Clin Radiol* 2009;64:761–6.

61. Gabriel M, Decristoforo C, Kendler D et al. 68Ga-DOTA-Tyr3-octreotide pet in neuroendocrine tumors: Comparison with somatostatin receptor scintigraphy and CT. *J Nucl Med* 2007;48:508–18.

62. Castillo JG, Silvay G, Solis J. Current concepts in diagnosis and perioperative management of carcinoid heart disease. *Semin Cardiothorac Vasc Anesth* 2013;17:212–23.

63. Rajamannan NM, Caplice N, Anthikad F et al. Cell proliferation in carcinoid valve disease: A mechanism for serotonin effects. *J Heart Valve Dis* 2001;10:827–31.

64. Bhattacharyya S, Davar J, Dreyfus G, Caplin ME. Carcinoid heart disease. *Circulation* 2007;116:2860–5.

65. Castillo JG, Filsoufi F, Rahmanian PB, Adams DH. Quadruple valve surgery in carcinoid heart disease. *J Card Surg* 2008;23:523–5.

66. Castillo JG, Filsoufi F, Adams DH, Raikhelkar J, Zaku B, Fischer GW. Management of patients undergoing multivalvular surgery for carcinoid heart disease: The role of the anaesthetist. *Br J Anaesth* 2008;101:618–26.

67. Thorson A, Biorck G, Bjorkman G, Waldenstrom J. Malignant carcinoid of the small intestine with metastases to the liver, valvular disease of the right side of the heart (pulmonary stenosis and tricuspid regurgitation without septal defects), peripheral vasomotor symptoms, bronchoconstriction, and an unusual type of cyanosis; a clinical and pathologic syndrome. *Am Heart J* 1954;47:795–817.

68. Gardner B, Dollinger M, Silen W, Back N, O'Reilly S. Studies of the carcinoid syndrome: Its relationship to serotonin, bradykinin, and histamine. *Surgery* 1967;61:846–52.

69. Oates JA, Melmon K, Sjoerdsma A, Gillespie L, Mason DT. Release of a kinin peptide in the carcinoid syndrome. *Lancet* 1964;1:514–7.

70. Neustein SM, Cohen E. Anesthesia for aortic and mitral valve replacement in a patient with carcinoid heart disease. *Anesthesiology* 1995;82:1067–70.

71. Weingarten TN, Abel MD, Connolly HM, Schroeder DR, Schaff HV. Intraoperative management of patients with carcinoid heart disease having valvular surgery: A review of one hundred consecutive cases. *Anesth Analg* 2007;105:1192–9.

72. di Bartolomeo M, Bajetta E, Buzzoni R et al. Clinical efficacy of octreotide in the treatment of metastatic neuroendocrine tumors. A study by the Italian Trials in Medical Oncology Group. *Cancer* 1996;77:402–8.

73. Frolich JC, Bloomgarden ZT, Oates JA, McGuigan JE, Rabinowitz D. The carcinoid flush. Provocation by pentagastrin and inhibition by somatostatin. *N Engl J Med* 1978;299:1055–7.

74. Connolly HM, Schaff HV, Mullany CJ, Abel MD, Pellikka PA. Carcinoid heart disease: Impact of pulmonary valve replacement in right ventricular function and remodeling. *Circulation* 2002;106:I51–6.

75. Castillo JG, Milla F, Adams DH. Surgical management of carcinoid heart valve disease. *Semin Thorac Cardiovasc Surg* 2012;24:254–60.

76. Knott-Craig CJ, Schaff HV, Mullany CJ et al. Carcinoid disease of the heart. Surgical management of ten patients. *J Thorac Cardiovasc Surg* 1992;104:475–81.

77. Robiolio PA, Rigolin VH, Harrison JK et al. Predictors of outcome of tricuspid valve replacement in carcinoid heart disease. *Am J Cardiol* 1995;75:485–8.

78. Connolly HM, Nishimura RA, Smith HC, Pellikka PA, Mullany CJ, Kvols LK. Outcome of cardiac surgery for carcinoid heart disease. *J Am Coll Cardiol* 1995;25:410–6.

79. Moller JE, Pellikka PA, Bernheim AM, Schaff HV, Rubin J, Connolly HM. Prognosis of carcinoid heart disease: Analysis of 200 cases over two decades. *Circulation* 2005;112:3320–7.

80. Bhattacharyya S, Raja SG, Toumpanakis C, Caplin ME, Dreyfus GD, Davar J. Outcomes, risks and complications of cardiac surgery for carcinoid heart disease. *Eur J Cardiothorac Surg* 2011;40:168–72.

81. Komoda S, Komoda T, Pavel ME et al. Cardiac surgery for carcinoid heart disease in 12 cases. *Gen Thorac Cardiovasc Surg* 2011;59:780–5.

82. Mokhles P, van Herwerden LA, de Jong PL et al. Carcinoid heart disease: Outcomes after surgical valve replacement. *Eur J Cardiothorac Surg* 2012;41:1278–83.

83. Castillo JG, Filsoufi F, Rahmanian PB et al. Early and late results of valvular surgery for carcinoid heart disease. *J Am Coll Cardiol* 2008;51:1507–9.

84. Patel C, Mathur M, Escarcega RO, Bove AA. Carcinoid heart disease: Current understanding and future directions. *Am Heart J* 2014;167:789–95.

85. Mansencal N, Mitry E, Bachet JB, Rougier P, Dubourg O. Echocardiographic follow-up of treated patients with carcinoid syndrome. *Am J Cardiol* 2010;105:1588–91.

86. Modlin IM, Gustafsson BI, Pavel M, Svejda B, Lawrence B, Kidd M. A nomogram to assess small-intestinal neuroendocrine tumor ('carcinoid') survival. *Neuroendocrinology* 2010;92:143–57.

87. Haugaa KH, Bergestuen DS, Sahakyan LG et al. Evaluation of right ventricular dysfunction by myocardial strain echocardiography in patients with intestinal carcinoid disease. *J Am Soc Echocardiogr* 2011;24:644–50.

88. Castillo JG, Filsoufi F, Rahmanian PB, Zacks JS, Warner RR, Adams DH. Early bioprosthetic valve deterioration after carcinoid plaque deposition. *Ann Thorac Surg* 2009;87:321.

89. Said SM, Burkhart HM, Schaff HV, Johnson JN, Connolly HM, Dearani JA. When should a mechanical tricuspid valve replacement be considered? *J Thorac Cardiovasc Surg* 2014;148:603–8.

47

Neuroendocrine tumors of the gastrointestinal tract

BERNARD KHOO, TRICIA TAN, AND STEPHEN R. BLOOM

INTRODUCTION AND HISTORY

Neuroendocrine tumors (NETs) are defined as epithelial cell tumors arising from cells with predominant neuroendocrine differentiation. The term *NET* has replaced the term *carcinoid* and is functionally equivalent to the term *neuroendocrine neoplasm*. NET is preferentially used in this chapter because of its familiarity. NETs can arise in many different organs and tissues. For the purposes of this chapter, we review the epidemiology, pathology, clinical features, biomarkers, imaging characteristics, and treatment of gastroenteropancreatic NETs (GEP-NETs).

Siegfried Oberndorfer was the first physician to recognize NETs as a discrete tumor type in 1907, when he described *karzinoide* (carcinoid or carcinoma-like) tumors of the GI tract that had histopathological features

Table 47.1 Types of GI NETs (pancreatic NETs not included)

Type	Percentage of GEP-NETs	Gender bias	Age of incidence (years)
Esophageal	0.05	M >>F	60–80
Gastric	11–41		
Duodenal/jejunal	22	M > F	50–70
Ileal	25	M = F	30–100
Appendiceal	20	M < F	20–40
Colonic	Rare	M = F	70–80
Rectum	20	M > F	60–70

of malignancy, but with a distinctly different biological behavior—slow growth and a reduced tendency to metastasize [1].

EPIDEMIOLOGY AND DEMOGRAPHICS

Although NETs were thought to be relatively infrequent, more recent data has shown that these tumors are more common than previously thought. The most comprehensive analysis of the epidemiology of NETs is based on data from the U.S. Surveillance, Epidemiology, and End Results (SEER) Program, which has shown that NETs are more prevalent than previously thought at 35 per 100,000 persons. Moreover, the incidence appears to be increasing from 1.09/100,000 persons per year in 1973 to 5.25/100,000 persons per year, faster than the secular rise in all malignant neoplasms, and this trend is likely driven by the improvements in, and increased use of, diagnostic procedures such as endoscopy, cross-sectional imaging, and histopathology. Indeed, as the SEER data is already historical, the prospect is that the incidence will continue to rise with improvements in diagnostics. The incidence of NETs is approximately equal comparing males and females, with slightly more new cases diagnosed in males. The majority of NETs are GEP-NETs, with 58% of cases (27% lung/thymus and 15% unknown/other) [2]. The distribution of subtypes of gastrointestinal NETs is shown in Table 47.1, and for pancreatic NETs in Table 47.2.

CLASSIFICATION AND HISTOPATHOLOGICAL GRADING

The histopathological hallmark of NETs is the expression of neuroendocrine markers, for example, chromogranins A, B, and C; synaptophysin; and neuron-specific enolase (NSE). Low-grade NETs are characterized by relatively uniform cells with abundant neuroendocrine granules, arranged in patterns, described as gyriform, trabecular, or nested. High-grade NETs, on the other hand, are characterized by a more sheet-like tumor architecture, limited expression of neuroendocrine markers, and irregularity of nuclei.

Research into the clinical management of NETs has been impeded by the availability of multiple systems for classifying and grading that are not entirely equivalent to each other [3]. The most widely used systems are those from the World Health Organization (WHO) and the European Neuroendocrine Tumor Society (ENETS). The classification of GEP-NETs in Table 47.3 is based on that proposed by ENETS [4].

Grading of NETs is important for prognostication of the biological behavior of NETs. The grading is primarily based on mitotic indices, proliferation indices as assessed by Ki-67 staining, and the presence of necrosis.

Staging of NETs is also performed according to a tumor–node–metastasis (TNM) system that takes account of tumor size, tumor invasion, the presence of lymph node metastases, and the presence of distant metastases (most often, the liver). The TNM staging is specific for each type of NET, and the reader is directed to Kloppel et al. for details [4].

GENETIC FACTORS AND MOLECULAR PATHOLOGY

The molecular pathology of NET development has only been partially characterized, in comparison with other tumor types, such as colonic adenocarcinoma. This is likely due to the fact that NETs are such a heterogeneous group of tumors.

For some time, it has been noted that some subsets of NETs are characterized by loss of heterozygosity of certain genomic regions. Chromosome 11q is often lost in pancreatic NETs; the significance of this is that the menin tumor suppressor gene is located in 11q13 (see below). Chromosome

Table 47.2 Types of pancreatic NETs

Type	Percentage of pancreatic NETs	Subtype	Percentage of type	Gender bias	Age of incidence (years)
Secretory/functional	60%	Insulinomas	70	M < F	40–60
		Gastrinomas	20	M > F	30–50
		Glucagonomas	8	M < F	40–70
		VIPomas	3–8	M < F	
		Other (somatostatin, ACTH, GHRH, calcitonin, serotonin, and PTHrP)	Rare		
Non-secretory	40%			M = F	

Table 47.3 WHO 2010 and ENETS grading systems for NETs

WHO 2010 classification	WHO grading criteria	ENETS classification	ENETS grading criteria
NE neoplasm grade 1	<2 mitoses/10 hpf and no necrosis	NET grade 1 (G1)	<2 mitoses/10 hpf and <3% Ki-67 index
NE neoplasm grade 2	<2 mitoses/10 hpf or foci of necrosis	NET grade 2 (G2)	2–20 mitoses/10 hpf or <3%–20% Ki-67 index
Small cell NE carcinoma Large cell NE carcinoma	>10 mitoses/10 hpf	NE carcinoma grade 3 (G3)—small cell or large cell	>20 mitoses/10 hpf or >20% Ki-67 index

Note: hpf, high-power fields.

18 is frequently and completely lost in ileal NETs compared with nonileal NETs or pancreatic NETs; candidate tumor suppressor genes that reside in this area of the genome include *DCC* and *SMAD4*. *SMAD4* is of interest in tumorigenesis, as it is involved in regulating transforming growth factor (TGF)-beta signaling and inhibits epithelial cell and extracellular cell matrix growth.

Another pathway that has been implicated in the pathogenesis of NETs is the Notch-1 signaling pathway, which controls cell proliferation, differentiation, and survival [5]. Alterations in Notch-1 expression are associated with tumorigenesis in a wide range of tumors, and it appears to act both as an oncogene and as a tumor suppressor. In the context of NETs, Notch-1 appears to act mostly as a tumor suppressor.

The availability of high-throughput, next-generation sequencing techniques has enabled the genomic and exomic survey of somatic mutations from tumor samples, providing valuable information regarding the activation of tumorigenic pathways in NETs. Exome sequencing was used to characterize the somatic mutations in 48 small intestine NETs with potentially tumorigenic mutations found in genes such as *FGFR2*, *MEN1*, *HOOK3*, *EZH2*, *MLF1*, *CARD11*, *VHL*, *NONO*, and *SMAD1*. Amplifications in *SRC* were observed in 11 of the 48 tumors, and amplifications of *AKT1/2* in 13 of 48 tumors. *SRC* and *AKT1/2* are implicated in activation of the PI3 kinase/AKT/mammalian target of rapamycin (mTOR) oncogenic pathway, and mutations affecting this pathway were identified in 28% of tumors [6]. Although this data is preliminary, the data so far is consistent with earlier studies and points the way to potential targeted treatments.

MOLECULAR PATHOLOGY OF PANCREATIC NETS

Multiple endocrine neoplasia type 1 (MEN-1) is an autosomal dominant disorder that is characterized by the development of parathyroid hyperplasia and primary hyperparathyroidism, pituitary adenomas, and pertinently, pancreatic NETs [7]. Pancreatic NETs occur in 30%–70% patients with MEN-1, and therefore dysfunction of menin (the product of the *MEN1* gene) is causally implicated in the pathogenesis of pancreatic NETs. This is reinforced by the fact that the conditional mutation of *Men1* in the beta-cells of transgenic mice causes the development of insulinomas. Menin is usually located in the nucleus in nondividing cells

but becomes localized in the cytoplasm in dividing cells. It appears to have multiple interacting partners, and has been implicated in the following key processes:

1. Transcription regulation (key interactions with JunD, NF-kappaB, and Smads 1, 3, and 5)
2. DNA replication, recombination, and repair, and genomic stability (interactions with *RPA2* and *FANCD2*)
3. Cell division (NMMHC II-A, GFAP, and vimentin) and cell cycle control (*NM23* and *ASK*)
4. Epigenetic control via modulation of chromatin remodeling (MLL histone methyl-transferase complex ER-alpha and HDAC).

Mutations in menin therefore appear to cause the dysregulation of multiple cellular pathways, but the ultimate pathogenic links between menin and pancreatic NET tumorigenesis are still obscure. The key importance of menin in the pathogenesis of sporadic pancreatic NETs is reinforced by studies that show that 44% of 68 pancreatic NETs samples were shown to have mutations in *MEN1*, as opposed to none of the pancreatic adenocarcinoma samples. The same study showed that other key pathways were mutated in sporadic pancreatic NETs. *DAXX* (death-domain associated protein) and *ATRX* (alpha-thalassemia/mental retardation syndrome X-linked) mutations have been found to occur, collectively, in 43% of pancreatic NETs and none of pancreatic adenocarcinomas [8]. Mutations in both *DAXX* and *ATRX* appear to activate the so-called "alternative lengthening of telomeres" (ALT) pathway, which would be expected to immortalize cells. Indeed, 61% of sporadic pancreatic NETs show signs of ALT activity [9]. Notably, patients with pancreatic NETs that possessed mutations in *MEN1*, *DAXX*, or *ATRX* had prolonged survival compared with those patients whose pancreatic NETs did not possess these mutations. *MEN1*, *DAXX*, and *ATRX* mutations may therefore specify a class of pancreatic NETs with a relatively good prognosis; however, the robustness of this concept is yet to be tested prospectively.

The third most common class of mutations found to be enriched in pancreatic NETs is mutations in the mTOR pathway (15% of pancreatic NETs and 0.80% of pancreatic adenocarcinomas), notably mutations in the tumor suppressor gene *PTEN*, the tuberous sclerosis complex gene *TSC2*, and the PI3 kinase subunit *PIK3CA*. As noted with intestinal NETs, the mTOR pathway represents an important pathway that controls translation, ribosomal assembly, cell growth, and cell proliferation. mTOR inhibitors such as everolimus have found application as targeted treatments for pancreatic NETs (see below).

The von Hippel–Lindau (VHL) syndrome is classically associated with renal cell carcinomas, central nervous system (CNS) hemangioblastomas, pheochromocytomas, and pancreatic tumors. The latter are typically cystic and most represent serous cystadenomas that are not NETs. Only the minority of these pancreatic lesions are NETs (≤20%). Nevertheless, this does suggest that the key pathogenic pathway activated by mutations in *VHL* is involved at some level in pancreatic NET pathogenesis. *VHL* mutations lead to reduced clearance of the hypoxia-induced transcription factor HIF-1alpha via ubiquitination and proteasomal degradation. As a result, there is activation, even under normoxic conditions, of the hypoxic response, which induces angiogenesis via vascular endothelial growth factor (VEGF), cellular growth via platelet-derived growth factor (PDGF) and TGF-alpha, metabolic changes promoting the transport of glucose, and cell survival. This so-called "pseudohypoxic" activation is classically associated with the pathogenesis of renal cell carcinomas, hemangioblastomas, pheochromocytomas, and paragangliomas. Although the exact pathogenetic link between activation of this pathway and the ultimate evolution of pancreatic NETs is yet to be clarified, it is of interest to note that sunitinib and other angiogenesis inhibitors are known to be effective against pancreatic NETs (see below).

CLINICAL FEATURES

Gastric and duodenal NETs

These are often asymptomatic and are detected as polyps during endoscopy for upper abdominal pain or for anemia (Table 47.4).

Jejeunoileal NETs, carcinoid syndrome, and carcinoid heart disease

The majority of small bowel NETs are nonfunctional and generally present late with abdominal pain or are incidentally found during abdominal imaging as liver metastases or as a mesenteric mass with surrounding desmoplasia (Figure 47.1). Tumor mass symptoms may also occur, such as bowel obstruction, obstructive jaundice, and gastrointestinal (GI) bleeding [10].

The *classical carcinoid syndrome* (flushing and associated lability of blood pressure in 60%–85%, secretory diarrhea in 60%–80%, and bronchial constriction in 10%–20%) is found only in 20%–30% of patients with metastases. The syndrome is due to the secretion of vasoactive hormones from NETs [10]. These hormones include biogenic amines (5-hydroxytryptamine [5-HT or serotonin], 5-hydroxytryptophan [5-HTP], norepinephrine, dopamine, and histamine), peptides (bradykinin, kallikrein, and tachykinins [substance P, neurokinin A, and neuropeptide K]), and prostaglandins E and F. These are inactivated by first-pass metabolism in the liver, which is why patients are commonly asymptomatic when the NET is confined to its primary site in the GI tract, but become symptomatic when the NET spreads to the liver, affording the tumor the opportunity to secrete directly into the systemic circulation. The majority of cases of the carcinoid syndrome are associated with GI NETs, such as those in the jejunum, ileum, appendix, and cecum (so-called "midgut" NETs). In this group, about 20%–30% of patients present with the classical carcinoid syndrome [10]. Bronchial carcinoid tumors are associated with carcinoid syndrome in 10% of cases. "Hindgut" NETs in the colon and rectum are usually not associated with the carcinoid syndrome. Carcinoid syndrome can originate from metastatic pancreatic NETs secreting 5-HT, but this is rare.

Carcinoid heart disease refers to the evolution of plaque-like deposits of fibrous tissue on the endocardial surface of valvular cusps and leaflets, cardiac chambers, and occasionally, the intimal surface of the pulmonary artery or aorta. The valves and chambers on the right side of the heart are most frequently affected because the lung capillary bed inactivates vasoactive hormones flowing through them: in 10% of cases, there are left-sided manifestations of carcinoid heart disease due to a bronchial NET draining into the pulmonary vein, or due to a right-to-left shunt (e.g., patent foramen ovale). The pathogenesis of carcinoid heart disease

Table 47.4 Subtypes of gastric NETs

Type	% age of gastric NETs	Etiology	Clinical behavior
1	70–80	Chronic atrophic gastritis, achlorhydria, elevated gastrin levels, ECL cell proliferation.	Small (1–2 cm) and polypoid in shape. Multiple in 65% of cases. Indolent course.
2	5	Pancreatic NET-secreting gastrin leads to ECL cell proliferation. Gastric hyperacidity, multiple gastric ulcers. Often associated with MEN-1.	Small (1–2 cm) and polypoid.
3	20	Gastrin independent. Histamine secretion.	Larger (>2 cm). Metastases on presentation frequent. Variant carcinoid syndrome with intensely pruritic skin lesions.

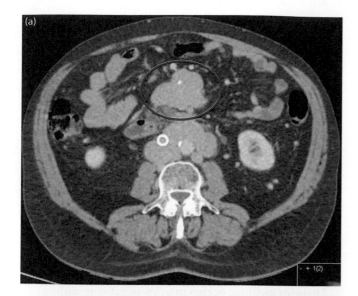

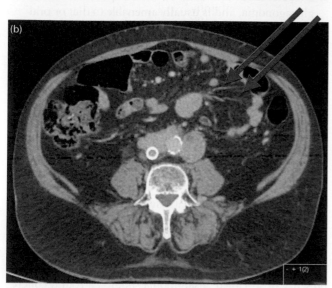

Figure 47.1 Jejeunoileal NET presenting with (a) partially calcified mesenteric mass (circled) and (b) surrounding desmoplasia (arrowed).

is thought to be due to activation of 5-HT$_{2b}$ receptors on valvular interstitial cells, leading to secretion of extracellular matrix and the development of fibrosis. In patients with the carcinoid syndrome, 25%–50% will have features of carcinoid heart disease, and it is crucial that they are monitored for signs, symptoms, and biomarkers of heart failure, for example, B-type natriuretic peptide levels, to ensure that therapy of heart disease is initiated at an early stage [10].

Colonic NETs

These usually present when relatively advanced, with diarrhea, abdominal pain, GI or rectal bleeding, or weight loss, and often when colonoscopy is being performed for investigation of these symptoms, with the diagnosis confirmed by biopsy [11].

Nonfunctioning pancreatic NETs

By definition, nonfunctioning pancreatic NETs do not present with specific gut hormone syndromes, and therefore present either as incidental discoveries during imaging of the abdomen, by virtue of localized mass effects (abdominal pain, weight loss, anorexia, nausea and vomiting, and obstructive jaundice), or when they have metastasized to either locoregional lymph nodes or the liver [12].

Specific gut hormone syndromes

ZOLLINGER–ELLISON SYNDROME

Zollinger–Ellison syndrome (ZES) is characterized by progressive ulceration in the small intestine, hypersecretion of acid from the stomach and rugal hypertrophy, and secretory diarrhea due to secretion of gastrin from a NET (Figure 47.2). Gastrinomas, particularly those arising

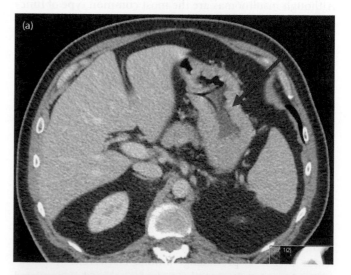

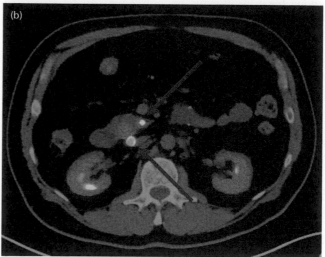

Figure 47.2 (a) Rugal hypertrophy (arrowed) in a patient with ZES. (b) Gastrinoma with metastatic lymph node and periduodenal uptake (arrowed) of ^{68}Ga-DOTATATE on PET scanning.

within the duodenum, are frequently multiple, relatively small, and therefore difficult to localize. They are typically found in the so-called "gastrinoma triangle," defined by the confluence of the cystic and common bile ducts, the border between the second and third portions of the duodenum, and the border between the neck and body of the pancreas. Seventy percent arise in the duodenum, and the rest in the pancreas or in lymph nodes adjacent to the pancreas. Eighty percent of gastrinomas are sporadic; however, a considerable minority, 20%, are associated with MEN-1. In approximately one-third of cases, metastatic disease is evident, and common sites for metastases are local lymph nodes and the liver. As noted above, the hypersecretion of gastrin can drive a secondary type 2 gastric NET in the stomach due to its trophic effects on enterochromaffin-like (ECL) cells. ZES is amenable to treatment with high-dose proton pump inhibitors (PPIs).

INSULINOMAS

Although insulinomas are the most common type of functional pancreatic NET, they are still uncommon, with an incidence of 1/250,000 patient-years. Malignancy is relatively uncommon, at 10%. Usually, insulinomas are single, relatively small tumors (<1 cm), although multiple insulinomas are more common in patients with MEN-1. Insulinomas are characterized by hypoglycemia, causing neuroglycopenic symptoms (dizziness, behavioral changes, confusion, seizure, and coma) and sympathoadrenal activation (tremor, tachycardia and palpitations, sweating, and hunger). Other hypoglycemic disorders must also be excluded in the diagnosis of insulinoma, namely, the surreptitious use of drugs such as exogenous insulin, sulfonylureas, and alcohol; concurrent sepsis and hepatic, kidney, and cardiac failure; cortisol deficiency; autoimmune agonistic insulin receptor antibodies; and the rare circumstance of insulin-like growth factor 2 (IGF-2)-producing tumors. Occasionally, endogenous hyperinsulinemic hypoglycemia can be associated with a diffuse proliferation of beta-cells in the pancreas, sometimes termed "nesidioblastosis." This typically gives rise to a postprandial hypoglycemia, the noninsulinoma pancreatogenous hypoglycemia syndrome (NIPHS). NIPHS has also been reported in association with patients who have undergone bariatric surgery and especially Roux-en-Y gastric bypass.

VIPOMAS

Pancreatic NETs that secrete vasoactive intestinal polypeptide (VIP) are rare, with an incidence of 1/1 million person-years. VIPomas present with large-volume secretory diarrhea, hypokalemia, and hypochlorhydria (as VIP suppresses gastric acid secretion). Characteristically, the diarrhea persists at >700 mL/day despite fasting. Other clinical features include flushing (due to VIP's vasodilatory action), dehydration, lethargy, nausea, vomiting, abdominal pain, and muscle weakness. VIPomas usually present as solitary and relatively large lesions of >3 cm in the pancreatic tail in

75% of cases. Metastasis is common, occurring in 60%–80% of cases at the time of diagnosis.

GLUCAGONOMAS

Glucagonomas are the third most common type of secretory pancreatic NET. They usually present as solitary nodules of >2 cm, typically in the tail of the pancreas.

The glucagonoma syndrome includes the following components:

1. Necrolytic migratory erythema: a characteristic skin rash of erythematous papules that coalesce into plaques with indurated central areas and scaling, blistering, and crusting at the edges. The rash is typically located in the perineum, arms, legs, and face, and on mucous membranes (causing angular chelitis, stomatitis, glossitis, and blepharartis).
2. Diabetes mellitus: occurs in >75% of patients with glucagonoma, and is usually amenable to diet or oral agent therapy.
3. Venous thrombosis in 30%.
4. Neuropsychiatric disturbance, including ataxia, dementia, optic atrophy, and proximal muscle weakness.

Other manifestations include diarrhea, abdominal pain, anorexia, and a normocytic anemia. The glucagonoma syndrome is amenable to treatment with oral zinc sulfate supplements and a high-protein diet.

SOMATOSTATINOMAS

Somatostatinomas are a relatively rare subtype of functional pancreatic NET. Fifty percent of somatostatinomas are found in the pancreas, typically in the head. The other half are mainly found in the duodenum, particularly around the ampulla. Duodenal somatostatinomas are also characterized by the presence of so-called "psammoma" bodies, a round concretion of calcium also seen in papillary thyroid carcinoma, meningioma, and ovarian tumors, which is said to originate from the calcification of abnormal collagen produced by the neoplastic cells. Primary somatostatinomas have also rarely been described in the colon, rectum, and liver. Most somatostatinomas are malignant and present with extant metastases in 75%. Somatostatinomas vary in their secretory and functional activity. Some somatostatinomas, particularly in the duodenum, do not secrete somatostatin. Others secrete immunoreactive but biologically inactive somatotstatin. As a result, the majority of somatostatinomas present with mass effects, e.g., biliary obstruction, weight loss, abdominal pain, and jaundice due to growth of ampullary or periampullary somastatinomas. On the other hand, a minority (10%), particularly in the pancreas, do secrete functional somatostatin, and this leads to the somatostatinoma syndrome of diabetes mellitus (due to suppression of insulin secretion), cholelithiasis (due to reduction of cholecystokinin [CCK] secretion and inhibition of gallbladder contraction), and steatorrhea (due to inhibition of pancreatic exocrine function).

PANCREATIC POLYPEPTIDE–SECRETING NETS (PPOMAS)

High levels of plasma pancreatic polypeptide (PP) are frequently detected in patients with pancreatic NETs. Some of these are explained by PP-cell hyperplasia in the normal islets surrounding a pancreatic NET, and some due to incorporation of PP-secreting cells within the tumor itself. More rarely, some patients have a primary PP-secreting pancreatic NET, a so-called "PPoma". PPomas are generally clinically silent until they become large enough to present with mass effects. Although watery diarrhea was initially thought to be part of the PPoma tumor syndrome, it is now evident that this only occurs in one out of three patients. Weight loss as a presenting symptom occurred in 50% of patients in a small series, consistent with a PP-mediated suppression of appetite. In contrast to other pancreatic NET subtypes, metastatic/malignant PPomas are relatively uncommon.

GLP-1OMAS

Rarely, NETs that cosecrete glucagon-like peptide 1 (GLP-1) together with other bioactive peptides have been described. In one case, an ovarian NET cosecreting GLP-1 and somatostatin was associated with diabetes mellitus during oral and intravenous (IV) glucose tolerance tests, followed by a profound reactive hypoglycemia, due to the subsequent glucose-dependent potentiation of insulin secretion by GLP-1 [13]. Similarly, in a second case, a patient with a pancreatic NET that cosecreted glucagon and GLP-1 was found to have diabetes mellitus (presumably due to the hyperglucagonemia), together with a fasting hyperinsulinemic hypoglycemia, and this was attributed to chronic hypertrophy of beta-cells and autonomous secretion of insulin [14]. In two other cases, cosecretion of GLP-1 and the related peptide GLP-2 caused hyperplasia of the small intestinal mucosa (an effect of GLP-2), prolonged intestinal transit time, intractable constipation, and recurrent vomiting [15,16].

OTHER RARE HORMONAL SYNDROMES

NETs can also secrete other hormones with characteristic syndromes [17]. Examples include:

- *Parathyroid hormone-related peptide* (PTHrP), causing the syndrome of humoral hypercalcemia of malignancy
- *Adrenocorticotrophic hormone* (ACTH), which induces a Cushing's syndrome, presenting with weight gain, edema, easy bruising, hypertension, diabetes mellitus, and typically hypokalemia
- *Growth hormone-releasing hormone* (GHRH), which stimulates the production of growth hormone, leading to pituitary hyperplasia and acromegaly
- *Arginine vasopressin* (AVP), leading to hyponatremia due to the syndrome of inappropriate antidiuresis
- *Calcitonin*, which can be released by NETs other than medullary thyroid carcinoma, and which leads to a syndrome of flushing and diarrhea

BIOCHEMICAL MARKERS AND TESTING FOR FUNCTIONAL NET SYNDROMES

5-hydroxyindole acetic acid

Serotonin (5-HT) is the characteristic biogenic amine that is found in the secretory granules of enterochromaffin cells and NETs. L-tryptophan is metabolized by tryptophan hydroxylase to form 5-HTP, which is then processed by 5-HTP decarboxylase to 5-HT. 5-hydroxyindole acetic acid (5-HIAA), the principal metabolite of 5-HT, is derived from processing in the liver by monoamine oxidase and aldehyde dehydrogenase.

Although direct 5-HT measurement is possible, there is large interindividual variation in levels. Therefore, 5-HIAA is used as a marker of 5-HT production, usually by collection of urine over 24 hours in a bottle with an acid preservative. During collection, patients should be advised to avoid foods such as avocados, bananas, plums, pineapples, aubergines, tomatoes, and walnuts, as these may cause false-positive elevations in 5-HIAA. In addition, certain medications, such as phenacetin, glyceryl guaiacolate (often found in cough syrups), cisplatin, and fluorouracil, may also cause false-positive elevations, and these should be avoided during urine collection.

The overall sensitivity of 5-HIAA in patients presenting with the carcinoid syndrome is up to 100%, the specificity being 85%–90% [10]. Ileocecal NETs are the most productive of 5-HIAA. However, 5-HIAA is markedly less reliable in bronchial, gastric, appendiceal, colonic, and rectal NETs, and not at all useful for pancreatic NETs. Other conditions that may lead to elevated 5-HIAA excretion include celiac disease, tropical sprue, Whipple's disease, and cystic fibrosis. Renal impairment can lead to reductions in 5-HIAA excretion [18].

Chromogranins A and B

The chromogranins are a class of acidic glycoproteins that are present in the secretory granules of enterochromaffin cells and NETs, and which are secreted into circulation. Chromogranin A (CgA) is the most widely used marker in this class, with chromogranin B (CgB) being less often measured. CgA is measured in plasma samples, and many different immunoassay methods (both commercial and in-house) exist. The standardization of CgA measurement is confounded by the multiplicity of methods and by the fact that CgA is processed to multiple posttranslational variants, leading to variable performance between assays. Nevertheless, CgA is considered a more sensitive marker than 5-HIAA, and is useful for prognostication (higher CgA levels connoting a worse prognosis) and for the longitudinal assessment of tumor burden during treatment, provided the same assay is used for each measurement [10]. Conditions that lead to false-positive elevations of CgA include chronic atrophic gastritis and achlorhydria/PPI therapy, chronic kidney disease, pregnancy, untreated hypertension, and glucocorticoid treatment. The most important practical point concerns PPI therapy, which should be withdrawn for 3–5 days before measurement of CgA [18].

Cocaine–amphetamine regulated transcript peptide

Cocaine–amphetamine regulated transcript (CART) peptide was originally characterized as a transcript upregulated in response to the aforementioned psychostimulant drugs. CART peptide is made in various tissues within the body, including endocrine and nervous tissues. Plasma CART is elevated in patients with various types of NET, making it a potentially useful diagnostic test, but more work is required to validate its true utility [19].

Gastroenteropancreatic hormones

GASTRIN

Gastrin is a peptide hormone secreted by neuroendocrine G-cells in the duodenum, the gastric antrum, and the pancreas. It is found in three forms in circulation, namely, gastrin-34, -17, and -15. The C-terminal end is the active moiety, and the synthetic 5-amino acid peptide from the C-terminal end, pentagastrin, is effective. Gastrin stimulates acid production in the gastric parietal cells both directly, by binding to the cholecystokinin 2 (CCK2) receptor in parietal cells, and indirectly, by binding to CCK2 receptors in ECL cells in the stomach. This stimulates histamine production, which in turn stimulates gastric parietal cell acid production.

Fasting gastrin measurement. Diagnosis of ZES rests on demonstrating elevated levels of gastrin with elevated secretion of gastric acid. This has traditionally been accomplished by measuring immunoreactive fasting gastrin levels, together with a measurement of gastric pH, e.g., from a sample obtained from nasogastric intubation or endoscopy. A gastrin level of >475 pmol/L in the presence of a gastric juice with a pH of <2 is diagnostic of ZES. Inhibition of gastric acid secretion causes a reflex secretion of gastrin and a secondary hypergastrinemia, e.g., in atrophic gastritis, pernicious anemia, PPI, and histamine receptor blocker (H2B) treatment. Other causes of hypergastrinemia include chronic kidney disease, small bowel resection, G-cell hyperplasia, and gastric outlet obstruction. In the common scenario where patients are taking PPIs and H2Bs, care must be taken to withdraw these medications, 3 weeks in the case of PPIs and 3 days for H2Bs, before measurement of fasting gastrin levels. As patients often become symptomatic when taken off PPIs, due to a rebound hypersecretion of gastric acid, one useful strategy is to change patients over to a high-dose H2B for 3 weeks. The H2Bs can be stopped for 3 days before testing, with liquid antacids used to bridge patients before measurement.

Secretin test. In cases where nondiagnostic fasting gastrin levels are obtained, the secretin test can be used. Secretin stimulates the secretion of gastrin from gastrinomas, and is administered at a dose of 2 U/kg of body weight to fasting patients (withdrawn from antacid drugs as above), with measurements of gastrin at 2, 5, 10, 15, and 20 minutes. A rise in gastrin by ≥120 pg/mL or more from baseline is taken as diagnostic of gastrinoma [18].

Arterial stimulation venous sampling (ASVS). Occasionally, where localization of gastrinomas is desired, selective intra-arterial stimulation of gastrin secretion can be used. In this procedure, calcium gluconate is instilled intra-arterially during selective angiography of the arteries supplying the pancreas and duodenum (gastroduodenal, superior mesenteric, and splenic). At the same time, samples are taken from the hepatic vein, and gastrin levels measured to assess the stimulation of gastrin secretion by the calcium, which acts as a secretagogue. Elevations of gastrin after instillation of calcium imply that the gastrinoma lies within the vascular territory of the artery that is cannulated, and confirmation is obtained if "tumor blushes" are seen when contrast is infused. This test is also valuable in ascertaining whether there are metastases in the liver, if gastrin rises are obtained after injection of calcium into hepatic arteries.

INSULIN

Insulin is synthesized from a single proinsulin polypeptide and processed by prohormone convertases to release mature insulin consisting of two chains (A and B) linked by disulfide bonds, and a C-peptide. It is stored in secretory granules in the beta-cells of the islets of Langerhans, and when secretion is triggered by hyperglycemia, both the mature insulin and C-peptide are released simultaneously. Insulin binds and activates its cognate cell surface receptor, a heterodimeric tyrosine kinase receptor.

Insulin's classical physiological effects are to increase glucose uptake by the muscle and adipose tissue, to increase the synthesis of glycogen and triglycerides, to increase amino acid uptake and protein synthesis, and to increase the uptake of extracellular potassium by stimulating cell membrane Na/K ATPase activity.

Supervised 72-hour fast. Insulinomas are classically associated with fasting hypoglycemia. The diagnostic test involves an in-patient supervised 72-hour fast with frequent monitoring of capillary glucose levels. The diagnosis is made when a venous plasma glucose of ≤3.0 mmol/L is found, together with elevated insulin levels (>3 mU/L or >20.8 pmol/L) and appropriately elevated C-peptide levels (>0.6 µg/L or >200 pmol/L). Suppressed ketone body (3-hydroxybutyrate) levels of <2.7 mmol/L are helpful in confirmation [20]. To exclude surreptitious insulin administration, it is helpful to recall that recombinant human insulin and insulin analogs do not contain C-peptide; hence, the finding of hypoglycemia plus hyperinsulinemia, but with inappropriately low C-peptide levels, is suggestive of exogenous insulin administration. Exogenous sulfonylureas can also simulate an insulinoma, and it is impossible to differentiate this circumstance using insulin and C-peptide levels, as both are endogenously released under the influence of the drug; a urine and serum screen for sulfonylureas must be sent at the same time as the samples for insulin and C-peptide.

ASVS. As with gastrin ASVS, calcium can be used as a secretagogue to induce the release of insulin from insulinomas. Elevations of insulin after instillation of calcium imply that the insulinoma lies within the territory supplied by the cannulated artery (gastroduodenal, superior mesenteric, and splenic), and localization of the tumor is confirmed by the presence of tumor blushes during the contrast study.

Testing for reactive hypoglycemia. The 75 g oral glucose tolerance test cannot be used for diagnosis of reactive hypoglycemia, as the finding of hypoglycemia after this nonphysiological carbohydrate load is common in otherwise healthy individuals. It is recommended that a mixed meal be used to test for reactive hypoglycemia, although the poor standardization of the composition of mixed meals makes comparison of results difficult. Current guidelines suggest that the diagnosis of reactive hypoglycemia after such a mixed meal should use the same criteria as noted above for the 72-hour supervised fast [20].

VASOACTIVE INTESTINAL PEPTIDE

VIP is a peptide hormone of 28 amino acid residues that is released from neuroendocrine cells in the gut and pancreas, and which can also be found as a neurotransmitter in the hypothalamus. The diagnosis of a VIPoma is established by the presence of elevated plasma VIP levels of >30 pmol/L in the face of a large volume secretory diarrhea, typically >3 L/day.

SOMATOSTATIN

Somatostatin (somatotropin release inhibitory factor [SRIF]) is a peptide hormone derived from a 116-amino acid prohormone to give rise to two principal forms, somatostatin-28 and -14. Both of these are cyclic peptides due to an intramolecular disulfide bond. Somatostatin exerts multiple effects on anterior pituitary, pancreatic, liver, and GI function by binding to five subtypes of G protein-coupled somatostatin receptors. These effects are mostly inhibitory in nature and include:

1. Inhibition of growth hormone secretion
2. Inhibition of endocrine (insulin and glucagon) and exocrine secretion from the pancreas
3. Inhibition of endocrine secretion from the gut (CCK, gastrin, ghrelin, GLP-1, and peptide YY)
4. Direct inhibition of motor functions of the gut, such as gallbladder contraction and gut motility

The diagnosis of a somatostatinoma is established by the presence of elevated levels of somatostatin, typically >100 pmol/L, with a pancreatic or duodenal mass. As noted above, the classical somatostatinoma syndrome is found only in the minority of patients.

GLUCAGON

Glucagon is a 39-amino acid peptide produced by the alpha-cells of the islets of Langerhans by posttranslational processing of the prohormone proglucagon. Secretion of glucagon is provoked principally by hypoglycemia. It binds to its cognate seven-transmembrane cell surface receptor on hepatocytes, and acts to increase hepatic glucose output by increasing gluconeogenesis and promoting glycogenolysis. It also promotes lipolysis at adipose tissue, and catabolism of fatty acids in the liver. The diagnosis of a glucagonoma is established by the presence of elevated levels of glucagon from a fasting plasma sample, typically >130 pmol/L, together with glucagonoma syndrome symptoms. Intermediate rises in glucagon levels between 40 and 130 pmol/L may also be due to a glucagonoma, but can also be due to fasting, hypoglycemia, trauma, sepsis, renal and hepatic failure, acute pancreatitis, abdominal surgery, and Cushing's syndrome.

PANCREATIC POLYPEPTIDE

PP is a 36-amino acid, C-terminally amidated peptide. It is a member of the PP-fold peptide family. This family encompasses NPY, PYY, and PP. PP is secreted by the PP-cells of the islets of Langerhans. It is secreted in response to eating and primarily acts as a postprandial satiety hormone. As explained above, elevated fasting PP levels are commonly found in patients with pancreatic NETs and are not necessarily diagnostic of a PPoma.

GLP-1

GLP-1 is secreted by the L neuroendocrine cells of the gut, and is derived from alternative posttranslational processing of proglucagon to release two active moieties: a 30-amino acid, C-terminally amidated peptide (GLP-$1_{7-36\,amide}$) or a 31-amino acid peptide (GLP-1_{7-37}). Secretion of GLP-1 is provoked by L-cell sensing of enteral nutrients after eating. GLP-1 then binds to its seven-transmembrane cell surface receptor on beta-cells, and acts to potentiate insulin secretion in response to hyperglycemia. Additional effects include suppression of glucagon secretion, inhibition of gastric emptying, and suppression of food intake. As GLP-1-secreting NETs are so rare, and as GLP-1 assays are not standardized, the diagnostic criteria for such a tumor are not yet established.

IMAGING

Cross-sectional imaging (computed tomography and magnetic resonance imaging)

The cross-sectional imaging modality of choice is multiphasic computed tomography (CT), with images obtained precontrast, during the arterial phase (20 seconds after IV contrast medium is injected) and during the portal venous phase (70 seconds after injection). Enhancement of otherwise isodense liver metastases is often observed during the arterial phase, with a drop in enhancement during the portal venous phase. With midgut NETs, a mesenteric metastatic mass is frequently observed with a characteristic surrounding desmoplasia. For the detection of pancreatic NETs, CT has a mean sensitivity of 73% and specificity of 96%. For the detection of liver metastases, the mean sensitivity is 82% and the specificity is 92% [21]. If required, CT enteroclysis (in which contrast media are introduced into the small bowel using an enteroclysis tube) can sometimes be useful for detection of small bowel primary NETs [10].

Where available, magnetic resonance (MR) imaging can be used as an alternative imaging modality that does not involve ionizing radiation, which can be useful for serial restaging. As MR imaging improves the contrast of tumor tissue versus normal tissue, sensitivity and specificity are improved; for example, for pancreatic NET the figures are 93% and 88%, respectively. In addition, MR cholangiopancreatography (MRCP) is a useful modality that allows visualization of any blockages in the biliary tree [21].

Ultrasonography

Conventional transcutaneous ultrasonography has limited application to the diagnosis of NETs, except when used to guide the biopsy of liver metastases. Endoscopic ultrasonography (EUS), on the other hand, is a highly sensitive technique for detection of pancreatic NETs (detection rate of ~90%), and allows for biopsy sampling to confirm the diagnosis [21]. EUS is also useful for assessment of wall and lymph nodal invasion of gastric and duodenal NETs, particularly if the tumors are >1 cm in size [22].

Endoscopy

Where indicated, small bowel NET primaries can be located using double-balloon push enteroscopy or video capsule endoscopy [10].

Molecular imaging

More than 80% of GEP-NETs express somatostatin receptors, particularly subtype 2a, which binds the tracers ^{111}In-pentreotide, ^{68}Ga-DOTATATE, ^{68}Ga-DOTANOC, and ^{68}Ga-DOTATOC. Single-photon emission CT/low-dose CT (SPECT/CT) with ^{111}In-pentreotide is the most widely available technique and is more than 80% sensitive for grade G1–G2 NETs. However, the sensitivity is lower for smaller tumors (<1 cm), benign insulinomas (due to the lower expression of SST receptor 2a in these tumors), and G3 tumors. Positron emission tomography (PET) scanning with ^{68}Ga-labeled tracers, where available, increases sensitivity to >90%, primarily due to the higher spatial resolution of the technique, and also because of the higher affinity of the tracers for other receptor subtypes, such as 5 for DOTATOC, and 3 and 5 for DOTANOC [23]. Uptake of these tracers can be used to guide somatostatin analog (SSTA) treatment

or be exploited for peptide receptor radionuclide therapy (PRRT) (see below).

[18]F-fluorodeoxyglucose (FDG) PET imaging is not sensitive for well-differentiated G1–G2 NETs, as they are metabolically relatively inactive, but is better for detecting high-grade G3 tumors. The newer PET tracers ^{18}F-DOPA and ^{11}C-5-HTP have shown promise as more sensitive tracers for jejeunoileal and pancreatic NETs, respectively, in early studies, but more work is required to confirm their efficacy [23]. [123]I- or ^{131}I-metaiodobenzylguanidine (MIBG) tracer can be taken up by the noradrenaline uptake system into catecholamine storage granules. Although GEP-NETs can take up MIBG, the sensitivity of this technique is lower than that of somatostatin receptor imaging: 50% for GI NETs and <10% for pancreatic NETs [23].

Imaging of insulinomas

Generally, benign insulinomas are relatively small at <1 cm and can be difficult to localize using cross-sectional imaging and ^{111}In-pentreotide SPECT/CT, although the better spatial resolution of ^{68}Ga-based PET is more sensitive for the detection of these tumors. Because insulinomas express receptors for GLP-1, ligands such as ^{111}In-DTPA-exendin-4 and ^{68}Ga-exendin-4 can be used to detect insulinomas with 95% sensitivity versus 47% for cross-sectional imaging [24] (Figure 47.3).

TREATMENT

Surgical resection

Gastric NETs of types 1 and 2 are typically indolent tumors that do not necessarily require surgical removal, and may

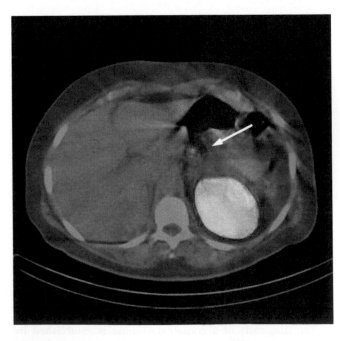

Figure 47.3 Location of an insulinoma in the pancreas revealed by ^{111}In-DTPA-exendin-4 scanning.

only require annual endoscopic surveillance and resection of lesions as indicated, particularly if the tumors are <1 cm. However, if the tumor is >1 cm, an EUS should be performed to look for the extent of wall invasion and the presence of lymph node metastases, which may well mandate a more extensive gastrectomy and lymph node dissection. Type 2 gastric NETs, being driven by a gastrin-secreting pancreatic NET, are amenable to primary resection of the pancreatic NET. Type 3 gastric NETs should be treated in a fashion similar to that of gastric adenocarcinomas, with partial or total gastrectomy and lymph node dissection considered [22].

The surgical management of *duodenal NETs* is dependent on the size, localization, and staging of the tumor. Curative resection is often possible in this group of patients, as metastasis is relatively uncommon, and is recommended in most cases. Small tumors of <2 cm in size may be considered for surgical resection (transduodenally or, more aggressively, with a pancreaticoduodenectomy) if they are periampullary; otherwise, they may be amenable to endoscopic resection. Larger tumors of >2 cm are eligible for surgical resection unless metastases are proven on staging, in which case medical management is indicated [22].

Where possible, curative surgical resection with a thorough lymph node dissection is the treatment of choice for *jejeunoileal NETs*. If the tumor is localized and segmental resection is possible, surgical planning should take account of the propensity of NETs to spread to local lymph nodes and a dissection of lymph nodes is mandatory. Successful curative resection of the primary and any locoregional lymph node metastases is associated with a 5-year survival of >95%. Even if NETs have spread to the liver, surgery with curative intent is possible in up to 20% cases, with enucleation of metastases, segmental resection, hemihepatectomy, or extended hemihepatectomy guided by preoperative imaging and perioperative ultrasonography. There is also some weak evidence to suggest that the resection of the primary tumor, even in the presence of unresectable liver metastases, may be beneficial. Palliative resection may be indicated for relief of carcinoid syndrome, to prevent intestinal obstruction or bowel ischemia arising from desmoplastic reactions around mesenteric metastatic masses, leading to mesenteric vein compression [10,25].

Appendiceal NETs are often found incidentally in appendicectomy specimens, and treatment depends on staging. Those that are <1 cm in size (ENETS T1) are considered cured by the appendicectomy and require no follow-up. On the other hand, tumors of >2 cm (ENETS T3 or T4) carry a metastatic risk of 25%–40%, and therefore radical resection with a right hemicolectomy, followed by lifelong surveillance, is recommended. Tumors of 1–2 cm or those minimally invading the serosa or mesoappendix (ENETS T2) fall in a gray area; a more aggressive approach is usually recommended for tumors at the base of the appendix, or in those invading the mesoappendix by more than 3 mm. One particular subtype, the "goblet cell" carcinoma, is a type of mixed NET–adenocarcinoma. In this case, as metastatic disease is much more common, right hemicolectomy is more often recommended [10].

Colonic NETs are treated in much the same way as adenocarcinomas, with endoscopic resection appropriate for lesions of <2 cm, and localized colectomy with locoregional lymph node dissection for those lesions of >2 cm or invading the muscularis propria [11]. *Rectal NETs* are also appropriately treated by endoscopic or local resection when they are <1 cm in size, given the relatively low metastatic risk of <3%. Lesions of >2 cm, with a higher metastatic risk of 60%–80%, are usually treated with total mesorectal excision (the standard of care operation for rectal cancers) for symptomatic relief, but it is unclear whether the procedure confers a survival benefit. Lesions of 1–2 cm fall into a gray category where aggressive management may not confer any survival, and the exact level of treatment is controversial [11].

Pancreatic NETs of <2 cm have a low propensity to metastasize, and can be surveilled with periodic cross-sectional imaging. Localized pancreatic NETs of >2 cm, or those causing significant hormonal syndromes such as insulinomas, may be considered for curative resection (enucleation for lesions close to the surface, pancreaticoduodenectomy for the head of pancreas lesions, and a distal pancreatectomy ± splenectomy for lesions in the body and head of the pancreas). Palliative resection of locally aggressive pancreatic NETs invading adjacent organs may be advantageous; however, this cannot be done if there is circumferential invasion of the superior mesenteric artery or the portal vein system. In the case of pancreatic NETs metastatic to the liver, surgery of the primary pancreatic NET is not clearly advantageous unless to relieve acute complications, such as bleeding, biliary obstruction, or gastric ulceration, or to enable liver transplantation [12]. Lastly, resection of hepatic metastases may be considered if the tumor burden is <75%, the tumor burden is unilateral, or both [12].

Somatostatin analog treatment and other biotherapies

Somatostatin analogs, such as octreotide and lanreotide, are the standard of care in NET treatment. They are commonly administered as monthly slow-release injections, for example, octreotide LAR (given as a deep intramuscular injection) or lanreotide Autogel (given as a deep subcutaneous injection). Octreotide and lanreotide bind to somatostatin receptor subtypes 2 and 5. This leads to suppression of secretion of bioactive peptides and therefore the relief of carcinoid syndrome and the reduction of 5-HIAA excretion in the majority of patients (88% and 72%, respectively, for octreotide LAR). Similarly, SSTAs are useful for suppressing the secretion of peptide hormones from pancreatic NETs, particularly glucagonomas and VIPomas. SSTAs are, however, less reliable in suppressing secretion from insulinomas (50% effectiveness) and gastrinomas. In the case of gastrinomas, high-dose PPIs are by far the most favored treatment. For gastric NET types 1 and 2, in which hypergastrinemia and ECL cell hyperplasia is prominent, SSTAs are also useful for controlling and shrinking the tumors. In addition to antisecretory activities, SSTAs also exhibit antiproliferative activity. The PROMID Phase III study demonstrated that octreotide LAR therapy was capable of extending the median time to progression from 6 months to 14.3 months in patients with low-grade (G1) jejeunoileal NETs [26]. The CLARINET study in patients with pancreatic, jejeunoileal, colonic, and rectal NETs of grades G1 and G2 demonstrated that lanreotide Autogel therapy was capable of extending progression-free survival, 65% vs. 33%, by the end of the 24-month study period [26]. Newer SSTAs, such as pasireotide (targeting receptor subtypes 1, 3, and 5) and BIM-23244 (targeting subtypes 2 and 5), are currently being studied for their effects in NETs.

Interferon (IFN)-alpha exhibits an antiproliferative activity and has been used for the treatment of GEP-NETs, with an overall response rate of 20% and a biochemical response rate of 63% [26]. However, IFN-alpha's adverse effects—flu-like symptoms, myelotoxicity, weight loss and fatigue, depression, and on occasion, suicidal ideation—limit the dose and duration of treatment, making this usually a third-line therapy.

Telotristat etiprate is a selective inhibitor of peripheral tryptophan hydroxylase and therefore the synthesis of 5-HT. It has been investigated as a means of reducing the symptom burden of classical carcinoid syndrome. A Phase II study has shown promising results, with reduction of bowel movement frequency in 28% and reduction in 5-HIAA excretion in 56%, and Phase III trials are currently ongoing [26].

Targeted radionuclide therapy

Given that NET cells bind and internalize SSTAs with high avidity, a property that is exploited in somatostatin receptor imaging, it was natural to substitute isotopes with higher specific activities and emitting high-energy beta-radiation as a means of delivering radioisotope therapy to NET cancer cells. PRRT can be implemented with three suitable radionuclides: [111]In at high specific activity and ^{177}Lu and ^{90}Y, for example, as ^{90}Y-DOTA octreotide, ^{177}Lu-DOTATATE, or ^{177}Lu-DOTANOC. In uncontrolled series, PRRT is associated with favorable partial responses or tumor stabilization, with relatively mild adverse reactions: acute nausea, bone marrow suppression, and renal toxicity being the chief problems. However, definitive randomized controlled trials in this area are lacking, and the field is awaiting the results of some trials currently in progress [27].

Chemotherapy

Traditional antiproliferative chemotherapy has a relatively limited application in NETs, although it is more effective against high-grade G3 tumors. Typical chemotherapeutic regimens include combinations of etoposide and cisplatin, fluorouracil with streptozocin, fluorouracil with doxorubicin, or fluorouracil with streptozocin and cisplatin [1]. Temzoloamide ± capecitabine has been advocated for the treatment of pancreatic NETs, although its effectiveness in nonpancreatic GEP-NETs is limited [28]. Capcitabine with streptozocin has also recently been shown to be reasonably effective in the Phase II NET-01 trial, producing a radiological response or stabilization in 74%, a median progression-free survival of 9.7 months, and a median overall survival of 27.5 months. The addition of cisplatin to the regimen did not improve outcomes.

Orthotopic liver transplantation

Because of the markedly less aggressive biological behavior of NETs, orthotopic liver transplantation (OLT) is an accepted, if uncommon, treatment of disease limited to liver metastases. The 5-year survival after OLT has been shown in various series to vary between 36% and 90%. Contraindications for OLT include high-grade NETs (G3), extrahepatic disease, or disease draining to the systemic circulation and severe carcinoid heart disease. As the experience of OLT for this indication is limited, there remains considerable uncertainty about the true benefit of OLT [25].

Targeted molecular therapy

Targeted therapies against VEGF receptors, for example, the tyrosine kinase inhibitor sunitinib, and mTOR, e.g., everolimus, have been shown to be active against pancreatic NETs in pivotal Phase III trials. In a placebo-controlled randomized controlled trial in 171 patients with advanced and nonresectable pancreatic NETs, sunitinib therapy was shown to double median progression-free survival from 5.5 months to 11.4 months compared with placebo. Overall survival was improved, with the hazard ratio for death estimated at 0.41 (95% confidence interval 0.19–0.89) for sunitinib therapy. The main adverse effects were diarrhea, nausea and vomiting, tiredness, hypertension, and neutropenia [29]. The RADIANT-3 Phase III randomized controlled trial showed that everolimus was also capable of doubling median progression-free survival from 4.6 months to 11.0 months in patients with progressive and metastatic pancreatic NETs. However, no benefit in overall survival was noted. The most common adverse effects noted were stomatitis/aphthous ulceration, rash, diarrhea, fatigue, neutropenia, and an increased rate of infections (unsurprising, as everolimus is also an immunosuppressant). Everolimus also induces some metabolic adverse effects: hypertriglyceridemia and diabetes mellitus. The metabolic effects are controllable with insulin and hypolipidemic treatment, and sometimes advantageous in the case of metastatic insulinomas. Lastly, everolimus is associated with pneumonitis, interstitial lung disease, and sometimes lung fibrosis. This class of adverse effects can be serious and may require steroid treatment to suppress them, and often represents a dose-limiting adverse effect [30].

Other angiogenesis inhibitors, such as sorafenib (a tyrosine kinase inhibitor of VEGFR2, PDGFRB, FGFR1, and FLT3) and bevacizumab (a monoclonal antibody against VEGF-A), have been shown to possess some promising activity against NETs in smaller trials. Pazopanib, brivanib, and cabozantinib are newer agents also targeting VEGF and VEGFR, which are currently under evaluation in trials [31].

Interventional techniques

LOCAL ABLATION

Local ablation of liver metastases may be considered if the number of lesions is relatively limited (<5) and the lesion size is similarly limited (<5 cm). The types of ablative techniques include radiofrequency ablation (most commonly used), microwave ablation, laser ablation, and cryotherapy. The experience with radiofrequency ablation suggests that this is a well-tolerated procedure, although local recurrence is fairly common (22%) and the majority of patients go on to develop either new liver metastases (63%) or extrahepatic disease (59%) at a median of 30 months or so [25].

TRANSARTERIAL EMBOLIZATION THERAPIES

Interventional intra-arterial therapies that serve to block off the blood supply to liver metastases (transarterial embolization [TAE]) or deliver cytotoxic chemotherapeutic agents, such as doxorubicin (transarterial chemoembolization [TACE]) or radionuclide therapy (selective internal radiotherapy [SIRT]), have been employed with some success in the treatment of patients presenting with NETs and liver metastases. The most clinical experience has been accumulated with TAE/TACE, which is successful in reducing carcinoid syndrome symptoms in 53%–100%, and in reducing the size of metastases in 35%–74%. Median progression-free survival is 18 months, and 5-year survival of patients undergoing this type of therapy is 40%–83% [25]. Twenty-eight to ninety percent of patients experience a postembolization syndrome (fever, abdominal pain, and elevated liver transaminases), with severe morbidity in 10% (acute liver and renal failure, carcinoid crisis, cholecystitis, and GI bleeding), and there is an associated mortality of up to 5.6%. Contraindications to embolization therapy include complete portal vein thrombosis, previous pancreaticoduodenectomy, and liver insufficiency.

SIRT, in which ^{90}Y is delivered to liver metastases coupled to either microspheres (SIR-Spheres or TheraSphere) or to SSTAs such as lanreotide (^{90}Y-DOTA-lanreotide), is a newer technique that appears to have tolerability similar to that of conventional TAE/TACE. There appears to be a tumor response in >60% of patients and disease stabilization in 35% [25]. Adverse effects and contraindications are similar to those for TAE/TACE, but radiation may also cause damage to the liver, the lungs, and the GI tract if delivered off target.

STENTING OF THE SUPERIOR MESENTERIC VEIN

Ileocecal NETs presenting with a metastatic mesenteric mass and associated desmoplasia may occasionally give rise to a syndrome of severe abdominal pain, diarrhea, and malnutrition due to malabsorption, which is thought to be due to superior mesenteric vein compression and insufficiency. In selected patients, interventional stenting of the superior mesenteric vein may be useful in ameliorating these symptoms.

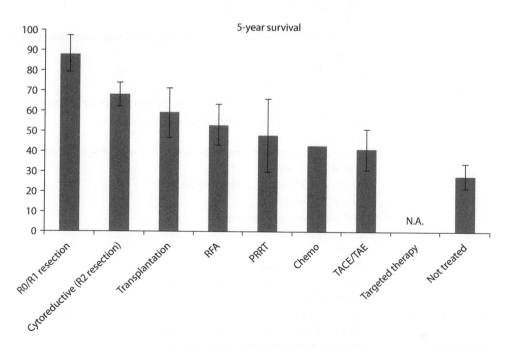

Figure 47.4 Estimated 5-year survival (±95% confidence interval) in patients with liver metastatic NET disease, given differing modalities of treatment [25]. R0 resection, complete resection; R1 resection, resection with microscopic disease detectable at the margins; R2 resection, cytoreductive resection, complete resection not anticipated preoperatively; RFA, radiofrequency ablation; chemo, chemotherapy; N.A., not available.

Table 47.5 Suggested schema of treatment for clinical situations with NETs where surgical resection with curative intent not possible

Clinical situation	Suggested course of treatment
Asymptomatic, low-grade, stable disease	Regular surveillance (clinical, biochemical, and imaging) Consider SSTA
Carcinoid syndrome predominant	SSTA Supportive care: antidiarrheals Cytoreductive resection of hepatic metastases
Carcinoid heart syndrome predominant	SSTA Optimal treatment of heart failure Cytoreductive resection of hepatic metastases Valve replacement (in selected cases)
Liver metastases predominant and progressive	Resection of liver metastases where R0/R1 resection possible Cytoreductive resection? Liver embolization or ablative therapy OLT?
Progressive pancreatic NET	SSTA PRRT—if SST receptor imaging positive Targeted molecular therapy: everolimus or sunitinib Chemotherapy
Progressive nonpancreatic G1 or G2 NET	PRRT—if SST receptor imaging positive SSTA Chemotherapy
Progressive G3 NET	Chemotherapy Clinical trials
MEN-1	Surveillance of Ca levels, pancreatic NETs, and pituitary tumors Parathyroidectomy—for primary hyperparathyroidism Pituitary surgery, SSTA, or dopamine agonists—for pituitary tumors Management of secretory pancreatic NET syndromes as below Resection of pancreatic NETs if >2 cm or if evidence of growth
Insulinomas	Diazoxide, glucocorticoids SSTA Targeted molecular therapy: everolimus preferred because of hyperglycemic side effect Chemotherapy
Zollinger–Ellison syndrome	High-dose PPI therapy Parathyroidectomy if hypercalcemic (hypercalcemia may worsen hypergastrinemia)
Glucagonoma	Zinc sulfate (helpful for rash) and high-protein diet SSTA Targeted molecular therapy: sunitinib preferred because everolimus may worsen diabetes mellitus PRRT—if SST receptor imaging positive Chemotherapy
VIPoma	IV fluids and supportive care Glucocorticoids SSTA Everolimus or sunitinib PRRT—if SST receptor imaging positive Chemotherapy
ACTH-related Cushing's syndrome	Bilateral adrenalectomy and adrenal hormone replacement PRRT—if SST receptor imaging positive
PTHrP-related hypercalcemia	IV fluids and zoledronic acid infusion PRRT—if SST receptor imaging positive

Order of treatment

It is clear that surgical resection with curative intent, where possible, is the treatment of choice, as this gives the best prognosis. If curative resection is not possible, then a panoply of treatment options open up, each associated with varying 5-year survival rates (Figure 47.4). As most therapies have been evaluated retrospectively and not in clinical trials, and as most patients in these studies have been given multiple types of therapy for tumors with highly heterogeneous biological behavior, the real efficacy of therapies can only be estimated from available data. In reality, the choice of therapies will be constrained by their availability of modalities and therapeutic expertise in any one center. A suggested schema for consideration of therapies is given in Table 47.5.

CONCLUSIONS

The unique biological behavior and pathogenesis of NETs offer a challenge for management. Because multimodal therapy is required over extended periods of time, the involvement of a multidisciplinary team experienced in handling NETs, whose members include surgeons (upper GI, hepatopancreaticobiliary, colorectal, and thoracic), gastroenterologists, endocrinologists, oncologists, palliative medicine specialists, interventional radiologists, nuclear medicine physicians, and specialist nurses, is essential to guide patients along their therapeutic pathways so that their length and quality of life is optimized.

REFERENCES

1. Modlin IM, Oberg K, Chung DC et al. Gastroenteropancreatic neuroendocrine tumours. *Lancet Oncol* 2008;9:61–72.
2. Yao JC, Hassan M, Phan A et al. One hundred years after "carcinoid": Epidemiology of and prognostic factors for neuroendocrine tumors in 35,825 cases in the United States. *J Clin Oncol* 2008;26:3063–72.
3. Klimstra DS, Modlin IR, Coppola D, Lloyd RV, Suster S. The pathologic classification of neuroendocrine tumors: A review of nomenclature, grading, and staging systems. *Pancreas* 2010;39:707–12.
4. Kloppel G, Rindi G, Anlauf M, Perren A, Komminoth P. Site-specific biology and pathology of gastroenteropancreatic neuroendocrine tumors. *Virchows Archiv* 2007;451(Suppl 1):S9–27.
5. Kunnimalaiyaan M, Chen H. Tumor suppressor role of Notch-1 signaling in neuroendocrine tumors. *Oncologist* 2007;12:535–42.
6. Banck MS, Kanwar R, Kulkarni AA et al. The genomic landscape of small intestine neuroendocrine tumors. *J Clin Invest* 2013;123:2502–8.
7. Thakker RV. Multiple endocrine neoplasia type 1 (MEN1) and type 4 (MEN4). *Mol Cell Endocrinol* 2014;386:2–15.
8. Jiao Y, Shi C, Edil BH et al. DAXX/ATRX, MEN1, and mTOR pathway genes are frequently altered in pancreatic neuroendocrine tumors. *Science* 2011;331:1199–203.
9. Heaphy CM, de Wilde RF, Jiao Y et al. Altered telomeres in tumors with ATRX and DAXX mutations. *Science* 2011;333:425.
10. Pape UF, Perren A, Niederle B et al. ENETS Consensus Guidelines for the management of patients with neuroendocrine neoplasms from the jejuno-ileum and the appendix including goblet cell carcinomas. *Neuroendocrinology* 2012;95:135–56.
11. Caplin M, Sundin A, Nillson O et al. ENETS Consensus Guidelines for the management of patients with digestive neuroendocrine neoplasms: Colorectal neuroendocrine neoplasms. *Neuroendocrinology* 2012;95:88–97.
12. Falconi M, Bartsch DK, Eriksson B et al. ENETS Consensus Guidelines for the management of patients with digestive neuroendocrine neoplasms of the digestive system: Well-differentiated pancreatic non-functioning tumors. *Neuroendocrinology* 2012;95:120–34.
13. Todd JF, Stanley SA, Roufosse CA et al. A tumour that secretes glucagon-like peptide-1 and somatostatin in a patient with reactive hypoglycaemia and diabetes. *Lancet* 2003;361:228–30.
14. Roberts RE, Zhao M, Whitelaw BC et al. GLP-1 and glucagon secretion from a pancreatic neuroendocrine tumor causing diabetes and hyperinsulinemic hypoglycemia. *J Clin Endocrinol Metab* 2012;97:3039–45.
15. Brubaker PL, Drucker DJ, Asa SL, Swallow C, Redston M, Greenberg GR. Prolonged gastrointestinal transit in a patient with a glucagon-like peptide (GLP)-1- and -2-producing neuroendocrine tumor. *J Clin Endocrinol Metab* 2002;87:3078–83.
16. Byrne MM, McGregor GP, Barth P, Rothmund M, Goke B, Arnold R. Intestinal proliferation and delayed intestinal transit in a patient with a GLP-1-, GLP-2- and PYY-producing neuroendocrine carcinoma. *Digestion* 2001;63:61–8.
17. Kaltsas G, Androulakis, II, de Herder WW, Grossman AB. Paraneoplastic syndromes secondary to neuroendocrine tumours. *Endocr Relat Cancer* 2010;17:R173–93.
18. O'Toole D, Grossman A, Gross D et al. ENETS Consensus Guidelines for the Standards of Care in Neuroendocrine Tumors: biochemical markers. *Neuroendocrinology* 2009;90:194–202.
19. Bech PR, Martin NM, Ramachandran R, Bloom SR. The biochemical utility of chromogranin A, chromogranin B and cocaine- and amphetamine-regulated transcript for neuroendocrine neoplasia. *Ann Clin Biochem* 2014;51:8–21.

20. Cryer PE, Axelrod L, Grossman AB et al. Evaluation and management of adult hypoglycemic disorders: an Endocrine Society Clinical Practice Guideline. *J Clin Endocrinol Metab* 2009;94:709–28.

21. van Essen M, Sundin A, Krenning EP, Kwekkeboom DJ. Neuroendocrine tumours: The role of imaging for diagnosis and therapy. *Nat Rev Endocrinol* 2014;10:102–14.

22. Delle Fave G, Kwekkeboom DJ, Van Cutsem E et al. ENETS Consensus Guidelines for the management of patients with gastroduodenal neoplasms. *Neuroendocrinology* 2012;95:74–87.

23. de Herder WW. GEP-NETS update: Functional localisation and scintigraphy in neuroendocrine tumours of the gastrointestinal tract and pancreas (GEP-NETs). *Eur J Endocrinol* 2014;170:R173–83.

24. Christ E, Wild D, Ederer S et al. Glucagon-like peptide-1 receptor imaging for the localisation of insulinomas: A prospective multicentre imaging study. *Lancet Diabetes Endocrinol* 2013;1:115–22.

25. Frilling A, Modlin IM, Kidd M et al. Recommendations for management of patients with neuroendocrine liver metastases. *Lancet Oncol* 2014;15:e8–21.

26. Alonso-Gordoa T, Capdevila J, Grande E. GEP-NETs update: Biotherapy for neuroendocrine tumours. *Eur J Endocrinol* 2015;172:R31–46.

27. van der Zwan WA, Bodei L, Mueller-Brand J, de Herder WW, Kvols LK, Kwekkeboom DJ. GEPNETs update: Radionuclide therapy in neuroendocrine tumors. *Eur J Endocrinol* 2015;172:R1–8.

28. Peixoto RD, Noonan KL, Pavlovich P, Kennecke HF, Lim HJ. Outcomes of patients treated with capecitabine and temozolamide for advanced pancreatic neuroendocrine tumors (PNETs) and non-PNETs. *J Gastrointest Oncol* 2014;5:247–52.

29. Raymond E, Dahan L, Raoul JL et al. Sunitinib malate for the treatment of pancreatic neuroendocrine tumors. *N Engl J Med* 2011;364:501–13.

30. Yao JC, Shah MH, Ito T et al. Everolimus for advanced pancreatic neuroendocrine tumors. *N Engl J Med* 2011; 364:514–23.

31. Karpathakis A, Caplin M, Thirlwell C. Hitting the target: Where do molecularly targeted therapies fit in the treatment scheduling of neuroendocrine tumours? *Endocr Relat Cancer* 2012;19:R73–92.

48

Multimodality management of primary neuroendocrine tumors

DANIEL M. TUVIN AND DANIEL M. LABOW

The gastroenteropancreatic (GEP) system is a site of a wide variety of neoplasms. Neuroendocrine tumors (NETs) comprise a small but highly diverse group of GEP malignancies [1,2,7]. Those neoplasms originate from neuroendocrine-type cells throughout the GEP system, with more than 50% located in the pancreas [5,14,15]. This is related to a high concentration of cell progenitors in the pancreatic islets. Only 5%–25% of NETs occur in the setting of genetic predisposition. Those include multiple endocrine neoplasia (MEN)-1, MEN-2, neurocutaneous syndromes (von Recklinghausen disease, von Hippel–Lindau syndrome, tuberous sclerosis, and Sturge–Weber syndrome), with the majority of NETs occurring sporadically [6,8,15]. Historically, due to NET heterogeneity, it has been difficult to obtain worldwide consensus on their classification; however, in 2000 the World Health Organization adopted the classification based on histologic grade that facilitated consistent nomenclature [1,17]. Further, the North American Neuroendocrine Tumor Society and European Neuroendocrine Tumor Society have developed guidelines and recommendations that were incorporated in the 2009 tumor–node–metastasis (TNM) classification of the Union for International Cancer Control, as well as in WHO 2010 [2].

Nonfunctioning NETs make up the bulk of the cases (up to 85%) and may produce symptoms related to their local growth or invasion or burden of metastatic spread [16]. Most of the GEP NETs are slow-growing tumors with an indolent course, with a greater than 60% overall 5-year survival. Symptomatic tumors are more likely to be hormone secreting or metastatic on presentation.

Controversy has existed on how to approach the advanced tumors, with a prominence toward a radical surgical approach. Data has suggested improved survival in primary disease and amelioration of symptoms in advanced stages; however, the complex nature of these tumors, with frequent multiorgan involvement, dictates a thorough multidisciplinary approach. In general, patients who are eligible to be treated with the entire spectrum of therapy modalities achieve the longest disease- and symptom-free survival. Those include surgical resection, hormonal therapy, neuropeptide receptor-based isotopic treatment, radiofrequency ablation, transarterial chemoembolization, and chemotherapy.

SURGICAL RESECTION

Surgery is the only therapeutic modality available that offers a potential definitive cure to patients with primary GEP NETs [4,5,15]. A number of factors determine the approach, namely, location and size of the tumor, involvement of surrounding structures, pathological features (benign vs. malignant), and surgeon's experience.

Resection options for pancreatic NETs range from enucleation of superficial benign tumors to segmental resections—distal, central, and pancreatoduodenectomy. In general, the least morbid procedure, sparing as much pancreatic parenchyma as possible, guides the surgical approach [10].

Early-stage small gastric neoplasms—i.e., small Type I and Type II carcinoids—may be treated effectively with endoscopic mucosal resection (EMR), whereas larger tumors with higher malignant potential require a more extensive gastric resection.

Small bowel primary tumors can be multifocal, with bulky lymphadenopathy not uncommon. This can lead to a more extensive small bowel resection than expected preoperatively [18]. A thorough examination of the entire small bowel and mesentery is required. In general, the small bowel is resected with negative margins with limited lymph node dissection unless a more extensive resection is clinically indicated.

HORMONAL TREATMENT

Somatostatin was originally found and described in the central nervous system and was later identified as one of the key components regulating the endocrine and GI system. Multiple receptors for somatostatin are established with variable expression on NETs [9,16]. The short half-life of native somatostatin (2 minutes) and marked rebound phenomenon preclude its clinical use. Shorter synthetic derivatives of somatostatin with a substantially longer half-life have been developed that help to maintain a consistent effect on the tumor without rebound hyperactivity. These somatostatin analogs, octreotide and lanreotide, have a particularly strong affinity to the S2 receptor and a lower one to S3 and S5. Several experimental compounds are in the pipeline with a reported affinity to all five somatostatin receptors [5,9].

Hormonal therapy in primary NETs is usually reserved for functional symptomatic tumors and also large, borderline resectable lesions. Somatostatin analogs not only exhibit hormone-suppressing qualities but also are tumoristatic [9]. A decrease in size of the tumor with conversion of previously unresectable disease into resectable has been described.

Combination therapies of hormonal treatment with interferon-α have shown promise in several studies, although subsequent randomized trials did not reproduce any added improvement in survival [5].

PEPTIDE RECEPTOR RADIOLIGAND THERAPY

An extension of the same receptor–ligand concept is peptide receptor radioligand therapy (PRRT). Patients with tumors expressing somatostatin receptors are eligible. For this modality, octreotide or pentetreotide is coupled with a radioemitter like Y-90 or Lu-177. Indium 111 was used in the past; however, its toxic profile limits its widespread utilization [11]. The octreotide homes on receptor-rich tumor tissue, concentrating the isotope and irradiating the neoplasm. Patients benefit from both symptom control and tumor eradication. PRRT is shown to be efficacious in a neoadjuvant setting to downstage locally advanced primary NETs. Given the minimal known toxic profile of PRRT, at least short term, makes it a logical therapy to offer patients who have limited treatment options otherwise. To better define PRRT's role in treatment of GEP NETs, a randomized controlled study would be necessary [11].

CHEMOTHERAPY

Because of the indolent growth pattern of most GEP NETs, they tend to have low response to systemic chemotherapy [19,20]. Multiple chemotherapy regimens were described, some of them with marked tumor responses and improved survival. However, no widely accepted standard of care exists. The most prominent response is reported with streptozocin-based therapy. Poorly differentiated, aggressive tumors respond better to platinum-based regimens [20]. In general, chemotherapy is reserved for unresectable or metastatic tumors [19].

Further, we describe particular GEP NETs and their management.

NONFUNCTIONAL NEUROENDOCRINE TUMORS

Patients with nonfunctioning NETs are mostly diagnosed incidentally when imaging studies are performed for other causes. Those tumors do not cause hormone-related disturbances, but they are known to secrete pancreatic polypeptide and are therefore called PPomas. There are several other commonly evaluated markers on NETs besides pancreatic polypeptide, such as chromogranin A, neuron-specific enolase, human chorionic gonadotrophin (HCG) subunit α, and neurotensin [3]. Symptoms, if present, are related to the expansive growth and compression of surrounding structures, which could lead to gastric outlet or small bowel obstruction [16]. Tumors are usually large and bear somatostatin receptors, which helps with computed tomography (CT) and octreotide scanning [13]. Serum elevation of pancreatic polypeptide is diagnostic for the lesion; however, imaging with helical CT or MRI is often sufficient to define the treatment plan [16].

Treatment is primarily surgical for benign lesions. Very small tumors with a low proliferative index on biopsy could be observed. Large (>3 cm) nonfunctioning NETs have higher malignant potential and are associated with regional or distant metastasis at the time of presentation. Those large tumors that present at the resectable stage should be treated with oncologic principles in mind with formal lymphadenectomy and negative margins [4,16].

INSULINOMA

Out of all functional (hormone-producing) NETs, insulinomas are the most common. The majority of them are benign, solitary masses found throughout the pancreas. Syndromic (MEN-1) patients often have numerous tumors or diffuse gland hyperplasia resembling nesidioblastosis [5,7].

Typical presentation is with Whipple's triad: hypoglycemia, neurologic phenomena (confusion, seizures, and vision changes), and amelioration of symptoms with the administration of glucose [15].

Elevated insulin and C-peptide levels in the setting of hypoglycemia are key to establishing the diagnosis. Standard diagnostic modality is a 72-hour fast in the controlled setting of a hospital, with regular checks of blood glucose and insulin concentrations. Oral and intravenous glucose should be readily available if the patient becomes symptomatic for hypoglycemia. Resolution of hypoglycemic symptoms with glucose administration is diagnostic for hyperinsulinism.

The mainstay in tumor localization is three-phase (pancreas protocol) abdominal CT, MRI, and abdominal ultrasound (US). Although the latter's sensitivity could be diminished by body habitus and overlying bowel, it is helpful in uncomplicated cases. Octreotide scanning has limited utility since insulinomas mostly lack somatostatin receptors required for this imaging modality [9]. More invasive tests are utilized in difficult cases. A calcium stimulation test is performed by selective intra-arterial calcium injection into the branches of the celiac trunk and superior mesenteric artery, with subsequent measurements of insulin in the hepatic vein outflow. Endoscopic US is a frequently applied technique that has the advantage of both localization and tissue sampling under direct imaging control. In patients with hyperinsulinism and no identifiable neoplasm on conventional studies, an intraoperative US could be performed, which has a high yield for localization of insulinomas.

Surgery is the mainstay in the treatment of primary insulinomas. Because 90% of them are benign, a surgical approach does not usually entail extensive resections. Simple enucleation of a solitary mass is sufficient [15]. This could be attempted via both the laparoscopic and open approaches. Centers performing a high volume of pancreatic cases report low morbidity and mortality, with most of the procedures performed in an ambulatory setting. No adjuvant therapy is required in completely resected primary insulinomas. Resolution of the symptoms occurs shortly in the postoperative period. Multiple lesions are treated with partial pancreatectomies, ranging from distal pancreatectomy to central resection and pancreatoduodenectomy, dependent on the location of masses.

GASTRINOMA

Gastrinomas are rare functional GEP NETs, with more than 1000 cases reported since first being described more than 60 years ago. They are the second most common functional NETs, and their symptomatology is related to gastrin overproduction. Gastrin excess leads to peptic disease with ulcers located in both the stomach and duodenum. Approximately 50% of gastrinomas are malignant, and a third of them present as metastatic disease [8].

Patients present with abdominal pain as their main complaint, and about half of them with secretory diarrhea as well. Although proton pump inhibitors might mask symptoms in the beginning, eventually patients develop peptic ulcer disease resistant to medical management.

Several diagnostic tests for gastrinoma exist. Serum gastrin level is a most frequently applied one [1,3]. Levels exceeding 10 times the norm are diagnostic for the gastrinoma. An increase in gastrin levels in response to secretin injection has the highest sensitivity and specificity. Of note, patients should be off proton pump inhibitors for 1 week prior to the secretin test due to proton pump inhibitors' ability to cause false positive results.

Localization of gastrinomas could pose a challenge since they tend to be small, although knowledge of the "gastrinoma triangle" aids visualization. The triangle has virtual borders of confluence of the cystic and common bile duct superiorly, the third portion of the duodenum inferiorly, and the neck of the pancreas medially. Close to 90% of gastrinomas are found within its borders [15]. As with others GEP NETs, triple-phase abdominal CT, MRI, and abdominal US are the main modalities employed in the visualization of tumors. Octreotide scanning is falling out of favor due to its lower sensitivity compared with helical CT and MRI, although the addition of single-photon emission computer tomography to octreotide scanning improves sensitivity and is a promising adjunct in diagnosing distant metastasis and as a follow-up screening tool.

Given that gastrinomas have high malignant potential, oncologic principles in resection should be employed. Pancreatoduodenectomy is offered to the majority of resectable gastrinoma patients because of their predominant location in the gastrinoma triangle. Somatostatin analogs have a limited role in adjuvant treatment since receptor expression in gastrinomas is variable. Some authors report positive results with octreotide and lanreotide, but their use is not widely accepted for gastrinoma [9].

GLUCAGONOMA AND VIPOMA

Glucagonoma is a rare tumor with marked glucagon overproduction. Symptoms are thought to be directly related to high glucagon levels, and include weight loss, diabetes, anemia, and, pathognomonic for this disease, necrolytic migratory erythema. VIPoma is also a rare functional NET that secretes vasoactive intestinal peptide (VIP) that causes watery diarrhea, hypokalemia, and achlorhydria (WDHA syndrome) [3]. Those tumors often present at the metastatic stage, which directs the mainstay of treatment to alleviation of those symptoms [12,15].

Resectable disease warrants an aggressive pancreatic surgical approach with formal lymphadenectomy to increase symptom-free and overall survival [4]. In locally advanced cases, favorable results are achieved with octreotide therapy. Glucagonomas as well as VIPomas have high expression of somatostatin receptors and mostly respond to the treatment. Some authors suggest prophylactic cholecystectomy in patients anticipating somatostatin analog therapy, which could help with cholestatic symptoms [9].

PRRT is a promising approach in these tumors because of favorable receptor overexpression [11,12].

SOMATOSTATINOMA

Somatostatinomas are rarely occurring malignant tumors that present with a syndrome of hyperglycemia, steatorrhea, cholelithiasis, and flushing. Primary locations are the duodenum (associated with neurofibromatosis I disease) and pancreas [15].

A serum somatostatin assay is usually revealing. Since most of the tumors present at advance stages, a surgical approach is usually not employed first, except for debulking, with chemotherapy and symptom amelioration being the mainstay of the therapy [19,20].

REFERENCES

1. Anlauf M. Neuroendocrine neoplasms of the gastroenteropancreatic system: Pathology and classification. *Horm Metab Res* 2011;43(12):825–31.

2. Chen H, Sippel RS, O'Dorisio MS, Vinik AI, Lloyd R V, Pacak K. The North American Neuroendocrine Tumor Society consensus guideline for the diagnosis and management of neuroendocrine tumors: Pheochromocytoma, paraganglioma, and medullary thyroid cancer. *Pancreas* 2010;39(6):775–83.

3. Eriksson B, Oberg K, Stridsberg M. Tumor markers in neuroendocrine tumors. *Digestion* 2000;62(Suppl 1):33–8.

4. Ferrone CR. Lymphadenectomy for pancreatic neuroendocrine tumors: Is that the relevant debate? *Ann Surg* 2014;259(2):213–4.

5. Frilling A, Akerström G, Falconi M et al. Neuroendocrine tumor disease: An evolving landscape. *Endocr Relat Cancer* 2012;19(5):R163–85.

6. Modlin IM, Drozdov I, Kidd M. The identification of gut neuroendocrine tumor disease by multiple synchronous transcript analysis in blood. *PLoS One* 2013;8(5):e63364.

7. Yao JC, Hassan M, Phan A et al. One hundred years after "carcinoid": Epidemiology of and prognostic factors for neuroendocrine tumors in 35,825 cases in the United States. *J Clin Oncol* 2008;26(18):3063–72.

8. Basuroy R, Srirajaskanthan R, Prachalias A, Quaglia A, Ramage JK. Review article: The investigation and management of gastric neuroendocrine tumours. *Aliment Pharmacol Ther* 2014;39(10):1071–84.

9. Baldelli R, Barnabei A, Rizza L et al. Somatostatin analogs therapy in gastroenteropancreatic neuroendocrine tumors: Current aspects and new perspectives. *Front Endocrinol (Lausanne)* 2014;5:7.

10. Bertani E, Fazio N, Botteri E et al. Resection of the primary pancreatic neuroendocrine tumor in patients with unresectable liver metastases: Possible indications for a multimodal approach. *Surgery* 2014;155(4):607–14.

11. Bodei L, Cremonesi M, Kidd M et al. Peptide receptor radionuclide therapy for advanced neuroendocrine tumors. *Thorac Surg Clin* 2014;24(3):333–49.

12. Eldor R, Glaser B, Fraenkel M, Doviner V, Salmon A, Gross DJ. Glucagonoma and the glucagonoma syndrome—Cumulative experience with an elusive endocrine tumour. *Clin Endocrinol* 2011;74(5):593–8.

13. Frilling A, Sotiropoulos GC, Radtke A et al. The impact of 68Ga-DOTATOC positron emission tomography/computed tomography on the multimodal management of patients with neuroendocrine tumors. *Ann Surg* 2010;252(5):850–6.

14. John PK, Saif MW. Radioembolization in the treatment of neuroendocrine tumors of the pancreas. *JOP* 2014;15(4):332–4.

15. Krampitz GW, Norton JA. Pancreatic neuroendocrine tumors. *Curr Probl Surg* 2013;50(11):509–45.

16. Kuo JH, Lee JA, Chabot JA. Nonfunctional pancreatic neuroendocrine tumors. *Surg Clin North Am* 2014;94(3):689–708.

17. Lawrence B, Gustafsson BI, Chan A, Svejda B, Kidd M, Modlin IM. The epidemiology of gastroenteropancreatic neuroendocrine tumors. *Endocrinol Metab Clin North Am* 2011;40(1):1–18.

18. Strosberg J. Neuroendocrine tumours of the small intestine. *Best Pract Res Clin Gastroenterol* 2012;26(6):755–73.

19. Toumpanakis C, Meyer T, Caplin ME. Cytotoxic treatment including embolization/chemoembolization for neuroendocrine tumours. *Best Pract Res Clin Endocrinol Metab* 2007;21(1):131–44.

20. Turner NC, Strauss SJ, Sarker D et al. Chemotherapy with 5-fluorouracil, cisplatin and streptozocin for neuroendocrine tumours. *Br J Cancer* 2010;102(7):1106–12.

49

Multimodality management of metastatic neuroendocrine tumors

PARISSA TABRIZIAN, YANIV BERGER, AND DANIEL M. LABOW

EPIDEMIOLOGY

Neuroendocrine tumors (NETs) are a diverse group of rare neoplasms that share certain biological and clinical features and can arise from different neuroendocrine cells throughout the body. This chapter focuses on metastatic NETs arising from the gut and pancreas (gastroenteropancreatic NETs [GEP-NETs]).

Over the last few decades, the global incidence of NETs has been rising. The number of patients presenting with these tumors in the United States has been steadily increasing—from 1.01 per 100,000 per year in 1973 to 5.25 per 100,000 per year in 2004 [1]. This increase in the incidence rate is partially attributed to improved diagnostic techniques, including endoscopic and imaging modalities. The incidence rates for all primary sites of NETs have increased over time in the United States (Figure 49.1a); the corresponding incidence rates in western Europe are lower, except for the rate of appendiceal NETs, which is higher in Sweden and the United Kingdom [2].

According to the Surveillance, Epidemiology, and End Results (SEER) Program database (1973–2004), the median age at diagnosis of NETs is 63 years, without gender differences. Appendiceal carcinoids tend to present at an earlier age, usually in the fourth or fifth decades of life.

NETs are commonly classified according to their embryonic origin as foregut (stops at the second portion of the duodenum at the papilla of Vater), midgut (starts at the distal duodenum), or hindgut (distal colon and rectum) tumors. In 10%–13% of cases, the primary tumor site is unknown. The primary tumor site varies according to gender and race. Gastric and appendiceal NETs are more common in women, whereas small bowel NETs are more common in men. The lungs are the most common primary NET site in white patients (30%), compared with other racial groups; jejunal or ileal NETs are more common among black (15%) and Caucasian (17%) patients. In contrast, the rectum is a less common primary site among white patients (12%), compared with African American (26%) or Asian (41%) patients [1].

At the time of diagnosis, approximately 24% of NETs in the United States are regional (i.e., with local invasion or involved regional nodes) and 27% are distant metastatic. The overall incidence rate of metastatic NETs has increased over time in the United States (Figure 49.1b) to about 1 per 100,000 per year. White patients with NETs have a higher

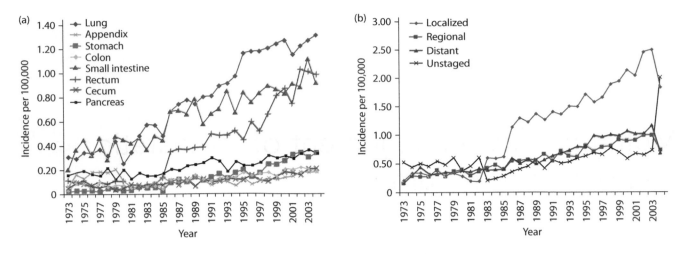

Figure 49.1 Incidence rates of NETs in the United States over time by primary site **(a)** and by disease stage at diagnosis **(b)**. (From Yao JC et al. *J Clin Oncol* 2008;26(18):3063–72. Reprinted with permission. Copyright 2008 American Society of Clinical Oncology. All rights reserved.)

risk of being diagnosed with distant disease at the time of diagnosis than black or Asian patients (28%, 22%, and 20%, respectively). This risk is also higher among males (29%, compared with 25% of females) and among patients with poorly differentiated or undifferentiated tumors [1].

Regional nodal metastases are present at the time of diagnosis in 41%–60%, 40%–70%, and 5%–28% of patients with small bowel, colonic, and appendiceal primary NETs, respectively. At the time of diagnosis, the likelihood of a patient being diagnosed with regional nodal spread is about twice that of being diagnosed with liver metastases (LMs). The risk of distant metastases at the time of diagnosis varies according to NET primary site and type (Table 49.1) [1–5].

GENERAL RISK FACTORS

Most cases of NETs are sporadic, but some are related to a number of familial syndromes, including multiple endocrine neoplasia 1 (MEN1), MEN2, and neurocutaneous syndromes. The last is composed of four subtypes: von Hippel–Lindau syndrome, neurofibromatosis type 1, tuberous sclerosis, and Sturge–Weber syndrome. All patients with NET should undergo clinical examination to exclude potential familial syndromes as mentioned above. A thorough family history should be taken, as it was found that a positive family history of any cancer is a risk factor for all types of NETs [6].

Table 49.1 Global incidence and the risk of distant metastases at the time of diagnosis according to NET type

NET type		Distant metastases (%)	Global incidence (n/million/year)
Stomach		6–15	1–3
Duodenum		9	2
Jejunum/ileum		22–30	2–10
Cecum		41–44	1–2
Appendix		10–12	1–8
Colon		29–32	1–4
Rectum		2–5	1–10
Liver		3–28	0.4
Pancreas	Overall	59–64	1–4
	Insulinoma	10	1–4
	Gastrinoma	60–70	1–2
	Glucagonoma	50–100	0.1
	VIPoma	40–70	0.1
	Somatostatinoma	50–100	<0.1
	Nonfunctioning	60	1–2

Note: VIPoma, vasoactive intestinal peptide-oma.

Behavioral factors, such as cigarette smoking and alcohol drinking, are not a proven risk factor for the development of NETs. According to one study, patients with preexisting diabetes mellitus, particularly women, are at increased risk of developing gastric and pancreatic NETs (PNETs) [6].

There are also reported racial differences in NET incidence. The overall incidence among African Americans in the United States is higher than that among whites (6.8 per 100,000 per year vs. 4.9 per 100,000 per year, respectively) [1].

CLINICAL FEATURES

NETs constitute a diverse group of neoplasms that display a spectrum of aggressiveness. Well-differentiated NETs are generally less aggressive than poorly differentiated neuroendocrine carcinomas, but may also be malignant and resistant to therapy. Most NETs are slow growing and more indolent than other epithelial cancers. Metastatic NETs may even be associated with prolonged survival.

The diagnosis of NETs is frequently delayed for several years (4–7 years on average), but according to one large prospective database study of more than 900 patients with NETs, the median duration of symptoms before diagnosis was only 3.4 months, and only 24% of patients reported durations of symptoms longer than 1 year [7].

The clinical presentation of patients with metastatic NETs is highly variable and depends on the primary site and type of the tumor. NETs are classified into nonfunctioning tumors and functioning tumors, which cause symptoms due to hormone release. Specific clinical syndromes related to functioning NETs are discussed elsewhere in this textbook. A brief summary of these syndromes is presented in Table 49.2. Carcinoid syndrome (Table 49.2) occurs in about 10%–20% of cases of well-differentiated NETs of the midgut (mainly with jejunoileal enterochromaffin tumors) and is almost always related to the release of biogenic amines such as serotonin and tachykinins from LMs into the systemic circulation.

Table 49.2 Clinical syndromes related to functioning NETs

Clinical syndrome	Symptoms
Carcinoid	Cutaneous flushing, hypotension, diarrhea, palpitations, abdominal pain, weight loss, wheezing, cardiac valvular disease (10%–20%)
Insulinoma	Confusion, visual change, palpitations, diaphoresis, tremor
Gastrinoma	Peptic ulcer disease, gastric hypersecretion, diarrhea
Glucagonoma	Diabetes, necrolytic migratory erythema, diarrhea, anemia
VIPoma	Severe watery diarrhea, hypokalemia, hypochlorhydria, metabolic acidosis
Somatostatinoma	Diabetes, cholelithiasis, steatorrhea

Type 1 and 2 gastric carcinoids are associated with hypergastrinemia (due to atrophic gastritis causing gastrin hypersecretion) and usually have low malignant potential, whereas type 3 gastric carcinoids tend to metastasize and are not associated with gastrin hypersecretion. NETs arising in the duodenum are commonly associated with MEN1 syndrome and gastrin hypersecretion. Carcinoid tumors of the tubular gastrointestinal tract are usually nonfunctioning, and occur most frequently in the small bowel and appendix. There is no reliable correlation between tumor size and tumor stage; even a small primary tumor (<0.5 cm) may present with LMs. Carcinoid tumors of the colon are large and often accompanied by LMs at the time of diagnosis, in contrast to carcinoid tumors of the appendix and rectum, which are usually small, detected incidentally, and rarely metastasize.

Presenting symptoms in all GEP-NET patients may include abdominal pain, nausea, vomiting, and anemia. The pain may be caused by local tumor invasion, ischemia, or intestinal obstruction. Carcinoid (enterochromaffin) tumors in particular tend to cause fibrosis of the mesentery, leading to mesenteric ischemia. Since about one-half are nonfunctioning, they may present with mass effect or invasion of the primary tumor, distant metastases (usually to the liver), or both. LMs may cause symptoms related to mass effect or capsular invasion. These symptoms include pain, jaundice, and early satiety.

Forty to sixty percent of PNETs are nonfunctioning. Presenting symptoms of nonfunctioning PNETs include abdominal pain, weight loss, and nausea. Obstructive jaundice may also be present, but is less common. In one large single-center retrospective study of 168 patients with PNETs, most nonfunctional tumors (87.8%) were diagnosed incidentally, and only a minority of patients presented with symptoms secondary to mass effect [8].

Abdominal pain is a common presenting symptom in patients with metastatic GEP-NETs. This pain may be described as nonspecific, or colicky when associated with intermittent intestinal obstruction. Other reported symptoms at presentation include diarrhea, flushing, weight loss, and gastrointestinal bleeding. In 10%–20% of patients with metastatic NETs, the diagnosis is incidental and there are no reported symptoms [7]. Initial presentation with symptoms of hormone release is more common in patients with metastatic disease.

Frequent sites of GEP-NET metastases are presented in Table 49.3. The liver is the most frequent site of distal metastases in patients with metastatic carcinoid tumor of the digestive system, as well as in patients with PNETs. Approximately 50% of PNET patients present with LMs. Other frequent sites of GEP-NET metastases include the lung, peritoneum, and bone (usually the axial skeleton) [5]. Unusual metastatic sites include the pancreas, breast, myocardium, thyroid, and spinal cord [12].

PATHOLOGY

Pathology is the gold standard for diagnosing NETs. Pathological classification of NETs should be based on the

Table 49.3 Frequent sites of metastases according to GEP-NET type

Tumor type (reference)	Local lymph nodes (%)	Liver (%)	Lung (%)	Peritoneum (%)	Bone (%)	Pancreas (%)
Carcinoid, overall [5]	89.8	44.1	13.6	13.6	N/A	6.8
Midgut NET [9][a]	N/A	92	10	23	24	N/A
Nonfunctioning GEP-NETs [10]	64	61	9	17	13	N/A
Gastrinoma [10]	54	57	7	4	11	N/A
High-grade GEP-NETs [11][a]	N/A	85	7	N/A	22	N/A

Note: N/A, not available.
[a] Local disease excluded.

recent World Health Organization (WHO) classification, which was revised in 2010. According to this classification, the two general categories of NETs are well-differentiated and poorly differentiated neuroendocrine carcinomas; the cutoff used to define poorly differentiated (high-grade) NETs is a Ki67 labeling index of >20% or mitotic count of >20 per high-power field (HPF).

Well-differentiated NETs have been traditionally named carcinoids and pancreatic islet cell tumors when arising in the tubular gastrointestinal tract or in the pancreas, respectively. Although most of these tumors are indolent, metastases are present in up to 40% of cases at the time of diagnosis. Well-differentiated NETs are further divided into two subgroups: low-grade (G1) NETs (Ki67 index of <3% and mitotic index of <2/HPF) and intermediate-grade (G2) NETs (20% > Ki67 index >3% or 2/HPF < mitotic index < 20/HPF).

Poorly differentiated (high-grade, or G3) neuroendocrine carcinomas represent a distinct group of aggressive tumors that resemble small cell or large cell neuroendocrine carcinoma of the lung, and generally have a far worse prognosis.

Tumor grade is strongly correlated with the stage of the disease. A recent retrospective study of 161 GEP-NET patients found that metastatic disease was seen in 46.1%, 77.8%, and 100% of G1, G2, and G3 NETs, respectively [13]. The corresponding percentages of synchronous distant metastasis at diagnosis, according to the SEER database, were 21%, 30%, and 50%, respectively [1]. There is also a strong correlation between tumor grade and survival in patients with metastatic GEP-NETs [11].

BIOCHEMICAL MARKERS

While no specific markers that can differentiate metastatic NETs from local disease have been identified, secretory products of NETs may help to establish the diagnosis and serve as surrogate markers of progression or response to treatment. Biochemical markers for NETs are divided into general and specific markers. General markers include chromogranins, pancreatic polypeptide (PP), α and β subunits of human chorionic gonadotropin (HCG), neuron-specific enolase, and physostigmine. Liver function tests are an unreliable predictor of liver involvement by metastases, and the serum alkaline phosphatase may be normal even in the setting of LMs.

Chromogranin A (CgA) (a secretory glycoprotein contained in vesicles inside neuroendocrine cells) and the other four biochemical markers are antigens to the cytoplasmatic neurosecretory granules of all NET cells. CgA serum levels are increased in 60%–80% of GEP NETs. High CgA levels are correlated with a poor prognosis, whereas a decrease in serum levels may indicate favorable response to treatment. Serum CgA levels are also correlated with tumor burden, with high levels measured in patients with metastatic carcinoid tumors. A study by Campana et al. has demonstrated that CgA levels among patients with diffuse metastases (in sites other than the liver) were significantly higher than those among patients with localized disease or isolated LMs [14].

CgB and PP are alternative general markers that may sometimes be elevated when CgA levels are normal. The sensitivity of PP for PNETs is 40%–80%. Pancreastatin, a derived peptide of CgA, is another serum marker that is raised in metastatic NETs and correlates with hepatic tumor bulk. Pancreastatin was found to have higher sensitivity and specificity for diagnosing NETs than CgA in a recent study [15].

The urine 5-hydroxyindoleacetic acid (5-HIAA) is a metabolite of serotonin and the best diagnostic metabolite in midgut NETs. However, foregut NETs secrete mostly histamine and the urine metabolite is methyl-imidazole acidic acid. According to one study, the sensitivity of 5-HIAA for the detection of metastatic carcinoid tumors was 73% [16].

Serum CgA and urinary 5-HIAA should be included in the baseline diagnostic workup of all patients with suspected GEP-NETs. Additional biochemical tests of hormones specific to the tumor type should be requested according to the suspected syndrome (Table 49.4) [3,17,18]. Repeated measurements of CgA and 5-HIAA are recommended as part of the clinical surveillance of all patients with GEP-NETs and patients with midgut carcinoid tumors, respectively [17].

DIAGNOSTIC MODALITY

The diagnosis of metastatic NET can be established with the use of morphologic or functional (molecular) imaging techniques. In recent years, novel diagnostic tools have emerged. A combination of imaging modalities is often needed to guide treatment [19].

Table 49.4 Serum hormones indicated in the workup of NETs according to the tumor site

Site	Type	Laboratory tests required	Results expected
Gastric	I and II	CgA, gastrin	Raised
	III	CgA, gastrin	Raised CgA, gastrin not raised
Duodenal		CgA, gastrin, PP, urinary 5-HIAA, SOM	Raised CgA in 90%
			Consider MEN1
Jejunal, ileal, and proximal colon		CgA, urinary 5-HIAA, NKA	Raised CgA (>80%), urinary 5-HIAA (70%), and/or NKA (>80%); see text
Proximal colon		CgA, urinary 5-HIAA, NKA, (PP)	Raised CgA (>80%), urinary 5-HIAA (70%), and/or NKA (>80%); see text
Appendiceal		CgA, urinary 5-HIAA, NKA, (PP)	None raised unless metastatic
			Metastatic: markers as ileal
Goblet cell		CgA, urinary 5-HIAA, NKA, (PP)	None raised
Rectal		CgA, CgB, PP, glucagon, HCG-β	Raised CgA (rarely); see text
			Raised CgB, PP, glucagon, and/or HCG-β in some
Pancreatic		CgA	Raised CgA in metastatic tumors only
	Insulinoma	CgA, insulin, blood glucose	Insulin inappropriate to glucose; see text
		C peptide or pro-insulin	Raised C peptide and pro-insulin
	Gastrinoma	Gastrin	Raised gastrin; see text
	Glucagonoma	Glucagon, enteroglucagon	Raised glucagon
	VIPoma	VIP	Raised VIP
	Somatostatinoma	SOM	Raised SOM
	PPoma	PP	Raised PP
	MEN1	CgA, gastrin, (calcium, PTH), insulin, glucagon, PP	

Source: Ramage JK et al. Gut 2012;61(1):6–32. With permission from BMJ Publishing Group Ltd.
Note: Items in parentheses may be helpful for diagnosis and monitoring in individual patients. NKA, neurokinin A; PTH, parathyroid hormone; SOM, somatostatin.

Ultrasound

LMs can be detected by using a transabdominal ultrasound with a sensitivity of 60% [20,21]. Lesions are hyperechoic on imaging, and sensitivity can be decreased in the presence of steatosis or hyperechoic livers [20,21]. Endoscopic ultrasound has been proved unreliable in detecting LMs due to its limited depth of penetration [22]. Although helpful in establishing a diagnosis, the required expertise and limited availability of qualified specialists can be a disadvantage.

Intraoperative ultrasonography can be used in detecting additional small nodules and defining the relationship of the tumor to intrahepatic structures. Lesions on Doppler imaging have a mixed hyperechoic–hypoechoic and central cystic appearance.

Computed tomography

Computed tomography (CT) is the initial imaging study of choice for the diagnosis of NET [23,24]. The sensitivity and specificity of CT in the diagnosis of PNET are 73% and 96%, respectively [23–26]. The sensitivity and specificity increase to 82% and 92%, respectively, in patients with LMs [27,28]. For abdominal extrahepatic soft tissue metastases,

CT shows a sensitivity and specificity of 75% and 99%, respectively [23–25]. In addition, the sensitivity and specificity of various NET metastases in the abdomen and thorax are 83% and 76%, respectively [23,24].

Triple-phase imaging studies using precontrast, hepatic arterial dominant, and portovenous phases can improve the sensitivity of detecting LMs, as the lesions may appear isointense on the liver via single-phase imaging [29]. Lesions are strongly enhanced on postcontrast imaging, and large lesions may appear necrotic and calcified [29]. Diffuse mesenteric involvement with peritoneal disease can present with ascites and obstruction on imaging.

Magnetic resonance imaging

Magnetic resonance imaging (MRI) is superior to CT for patients with liver and PNET. The sensitivity and specificity of diagnosing PNET are 93% and 88%, respectively [30,31]. In patients with LMs, the detection rate is 82% [19]. In patients with extrahepatic soft tissue metastasis, the sensitivity and specificity are 89% and 100%, respectively [32,33]. LMs appear at low signal intensity on T1-weighted images and at high signal intensity on T2-weighted images [34]. The majority of lesions are hypervascular on arterial phase imaging. Hepatocyte specific MRI contrast imaging may be useful in the diagnosis of LMs [34]. The inclusion of MR cholangiopancreatography may be helpful in the diagnosis of PNET and may help define the relationship of the tumor to pancreatic and main bile ducts.

Despite its superiority to CT imaging in the diagnosis of NET, an MRI is a considerably scarcer and more expensive imaging technique. It is therefore not considered a standard initial NET imaging modality.

Nuclear medicine imaging

NETs provide a target for functional imaging with labeled somatostatin analogs as they express somatostatin receptors (60%–100% of tumors) [19,35]. In 1994, indium-111 octreotide scintigraphy (Octreoscan) was approved and became the gold-standard imaging technique for NET-expressing somatostatin receptors [19]. Aside from total body imaging and visualization of primary and metastatic tumors, it helps select patient candidates for somatostatin receptor–based radiotherapy. Subsequent research to improve image resolution has identified alternative agents to Octreoscan.

Somatostatin receptor analogs and metaiodobenzylguanidine (MIBG) remain front-line single-photon emission computed tomography (SPECT) radiotracers in the imaging of NET [36]. They are used in the additional workup and staging technique and can help to guide treatment. However, the use of positron emission tomography (PET) has been growing rapidly in the imaging of NETs. Sensitivity is improved with the use of PET imaging compared with planar or SPECT imaging. An advantage associated with PET is its short-lasting imaging protocol. However, the radiolabeling procedure can be demanding.

Planar and SPECT imaging use two types of radiotracers: L somatostatin analogs and MIBG [23,37]. The sensitivity of both imaging modalities is 84% [23,37].

18F-fluorodeoxyglucose (FDG) PET or CT scans are valuable tools of postsurgical imaging modalities. They are useful in the detection of intermediate- and high-grade NETs [38,39]. The sensitivity was 92% in patients with a Ki67 of >15% compared with 69% with the use of somatostatin reception scintigraphy [38,39].

Indium-111 octreotide scintigraphy has a lower sensitivity (69%–86%) and a higher cost for detecting NETs than do PET or CT scans using gallium-68-labeled somatostatin analogs [35]. The isotope copper 64 DOTATE has been shown to be more sensitive than indium-111 or 68Ga. The highest sensitivity and specificity for NET-LM (82%–100% and 67%–100%) or extrahepatic metastasis in low-grade NETs (85%–96% and 67%–90%) have been demonstrated with the use of gallium-68 somatostatin receptor PET or CT scans [35,40,41]. Lesions not identified on CT or MRI can be detected in up to 67%, and therefore candidates better selected for curative treatment [35].

TREATMENT OPTIONS

Given the complexity of the disease and the large number of available therapies, patients with metastatic NET should be cared for by multidisciplinary teams. Management strategies for metastatic NET range from surgery to locoregional therapies, as well as systemic treatments with diverse cytotoxic, biologic, and targeted agents. Table 49.5 summarizes existing series and outcomes of liver surgery and transplantation in patients with metastatic hepatic NET [42–50].

It is important to note that the level of evidence for most of the therapeutic options is limited. Despite the existence of various treatment guidelines and reviews, the heterogeneity of patients, lack of uniform terminology, and prospective studies limit the validity of many published results detailing management.

The majority of LMs are multifocal and present with additional extrahepatic disease at diagnosis. According to a recently published Cochrane review, no optimal therapeutic strategy currently exists in the treatment of NET-LM [51,52].

Table 49.5 Summary of results of liver resection and liver transplantation for hepatic metastases of NETs

Treatment	Author (reference)	Year	Number	Overall survival (5 years) (%)
Liver resection				
	Elias [42]	2003	112	71
	Sarmiento [43]	2003	170	61
	Touzios [44]	2005	60	72
	Mazzaferro [45]	2007	36	85
	Frilling [46]	2009	119	94
Liver transplantation				
	Florman [47]	2004	11	36
	Frilling [48]	2006	15	67
	Mazzaferro [45]	2007	24	90
	Le Treut [49]	2013	213	52

Management of primary NET in the presence of liver metastases

Resection of the primary NET should preferably be performed prior to hepatectomy, or be performed synchronously with the LM resection in candidates undergoing extensive surgery [50]. If the primary NET is unknown, close postoperative followup is warranted.

In the presence of unresectable LMs, primary tumor resection is recommended [53–55]. It has been shown to improve long-term survival. Ki67, age at diagnosis, and resection of the primary tumor were identified as independent prognostic factors associated with improved outcome [56]. The median survival increased in the resected group (159 months) compared with the nonresected group (47 months) [54].

In patients with symptomatic nonfunctioning PNET, resection of the primary NET was associated with symptom relief, reduction of risk associated with progression of tumor burden (such as intestinal obstruction, mesenteric ischemia, and portal vein obstruction), and increase in progression-free survival [55]. However, this topic remains controversial, as no randomized controlled trial (RCT) exists.

Figure 49.2 summarizes outcome by different treatment methods in patients with metastatic NETs and LMs [35].

Liver resection

Complete curative resection remains the treatment of choice for metastatic NET [44,57–60]. The survival benefit of surgical resection, compared with locoregional or chemotherapy, has been well established [44,57–60]. Three- to five-year survival was prolonged in patients undergoing resection

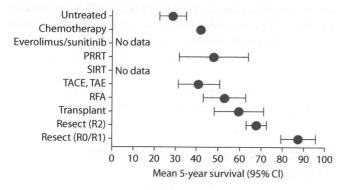

Figure 49.2 Outcome by different treatment method in patients with metastatic NET-LM. Complete liver resection for grade 1 and grade 2 NETs shows about 85% 5-year survival. The mean 5-year survival for all treatments and combinations is about 50%, except for transplantation (about 60%). PRRT, peptide receptor radionuclide therapy; SIRT, selective internal radiotherapy; RFA, radiofrequency ablation; resect (R2), cytoreduction; resect (R0/R1), complete resection. (Reprinted from *Lancet Oncol*, 15, Frilling A et al., Recommendations for management of patients with neuroendocrine liver metastases, e8–21, Copyright 2014, with permission from Elsevier.)

(83% and 83%), compared with transcatheter chemoembolization (TACE) (39% and 76%) or medical treatment (50%, not reached) [50]. Survival of patients undergoing either invasive or noninvasive treatments was also compared in a study by Touzios et al. [44]. Patients undergoing invasive treatments for metastatic NET (resection/ablation or TACE ± resection/ablation) had a prolonged survival compared with those treated with noninvasive therapies [44]. However, the majority of patients may not be candidates for curative treatments at the time of diagnosis.

The perioperative mortality of hepatectomy has decreased in the past few decades, with some centers reporting a <1% mortality rate [61]. Refinement of patient selection, as well as of surgical technique and skills, has led to improvement of curative resection and outcome.

Selection criteria include (1) well-differentiated NET (G1 and G2 status), (2) acceptable performance status (Eastern Cooperative Oncology Group [ECOG] < 2) and comorbidities, (3) exclusion of nonresectable extrahepatic disease, (4) R0/R1 resection with a functional liver remnant of ≥30%, (5) absence of advanced stages of carcinoid heart disease, (6) cardiac valve surgery prior to hepatic resection in patients with advanced stages of carcinoid heart disease, and (7) acceptable perioperative outcome [62,63].

Grade 3 NETs with LMs are not amenable to curative resection, as they are multifocal, bilobar, and associated with a high recurrence rate [64]. In patients with bilobar metastasis requiring extended surgery, locoregional therapies such as radiofrequency ablation or cryoablation can be used as an adjunct to liver resection [50].

In patients with normal liver parenchyma and function, a future liver remnant volume of 25%–30% is considered adequate. In patients with chronic liver disease, cirrhosis, or documented hepatic steatosis, a future liver remnant volume of 40%–50% is desired. Preoperative portal vein embolization or portal vein ligation may be used to induce growth of the future liver remnant when hepatic reserve is borderline and major resection is anticipated.

Complete resection can only be achieved in 20%–57% of cases with local recurrence rates remaining high (up to 97% at 5 years). The prognostic relevance of R0 resection is controversial. A recent Cochrane review did not identify survival benefit in patients undergoing R0 versus R1 resection. Others have reported decreased 5-year recurrence rates in patients undergoing R0 (10%) versus R1–R2 (75%) resection.

Postresection overall survival rates are in the range of 46%–86% at 5 years and 35%–79% at 10 years (Table 49.5) [42–46]. Survival was higher in patients in whom hepatectomy was possible, compared with patients with unresectable tumor burden (median survival range 27–78 months vs. 27 months) [65]. In selected patients in whom complete curative resection cannot be accomplished, a two-staged hepatectomy may be an option, with a reported 5-year overall survival of 94% and disease-free survival of 50% [50].

As a result of high recurrence rates postcurative resection, the role of adjuvant therapy was explored but still remains unclear. Adjuvant therapy with 5FU and streptozocin did not provide a benefit [66].

Recent studies also examined the outcome of patients undergoing liver resection with extrahepatic tumor resection. Only a subgroup of patients, less than 10%, remained disease-free at 5 years. Palliative resection outcome remains overall poor. Cytoreductive surgery (CRS) (debulking) should only be reserved for patients in whom at least 90% of tumor burden can be safely resected. Some series demonstrated survival benefit (mean survival 43 vs. 24 months) and a mean duration of symptomatic relief (32 vs. 22 months) in patients undergoing CRS over embolization [50,67].

Survivals of patients undergoing either invasive or non-invasive treatments were compared in a study by Touzios et al. Patients undergoing invasive treatments for metastatic NET (resection/ablation or TACE ± resection/ablation) had a prolonged survival compared with those treated with noninvasive therapies [44].

Liver transplantation

Orthotopic liver transplantation (OLT) is an attractive option for patients with NET and LM due to the slow growth and less aggressive biologic nature of the tumor. Reported survival is therefore prolonged compared with that achieved with primary liver malignancies. OLT is, however, limited by graft shortage, and appropriate patient selection is critical to achieving satisfactory results [45,47–49]. In addition, due to the paucity of experience, heterogeneous follow-up, and outcome reports, results comparison among studies may be difficult. RCT and downstaging strategies have not been studied.

Reported 5-year survival and disease-free survival rates from multicenter studies are 49% and 47%, respectively (Table 49.5) [45,47–49]. Factors associated with contraindication to OLT are (1) poorly differentiated tumors, (2) non-portal system tumor drainage, (3) presence of extrahepatic metastases excluding perihilar nodes, and (4) severe carcinoid heart disease [45,47–49]. There remains a lack of consensus regarding factors such as age, performance status, tumor histology, location of tumor, resection prior to OLT, hepatic tumor burden, growth dynamics, Ki67 level, and appropriate transplantation timing. According to Mazzaferro et al., indications for OLT are (1) functioning and nonfunctioning low-grade NETs, (2) primary tumor drained by the portal system with curative resection prior to OLT, (3) LMs with ≤50% metastatic involvement of the liver, (4) tumor response or stable disease for a minimum of 6 months prior to OLT, and (5) age of ≤50 [45]. Overall survival and recurrence-free survival at 5 years were 90% and 77%, respectively [45,47–49,68]. Based on the success of OLT for metastatic NET, controversy has arisen over expansion of these criteria. Five-year survival and 1-year recurrence-free survival of 70% were achieved with candidates of advanced age (>64 years) and higher Ki67 levels [69]. In addition, the indications for OLT as a palliative option for intractable

symptoms were also studied. Living donor transplantation (LDLT) is, for patients with a suitable and willing donor, a way to eliminate waiting time and the attendant risk of dropout.

Role of neoadjuvant and adjuvant treatment in NET-LM

The role of neoadjuvant and adjuvant treatment was explored by several investigators in order to prevent recurrence. No survival difference was noted between patients undergoing adjuvant treatment (streptozocin and 5-fluorouracil [5FU]) and those in the nontreatment group postresection or OLT [66]. Tumor resectability was increased in a series with the use of neoadjuvant treatment with immunochemotherapy or peptide receptor radionuclide therapy. However, in view of the lack of RCT and small series, evidence regarding the use of neoadjuvant or adjuvant therapy remains insufficient in patients with low-grade tumors.

Ablation

Thermal (radiofrequency ablation and microwave) or chemical (ethanol and acetic acid) ablation is the treatment of choice in patients with single small tumors, and may be curative in well-selected candidates. The use of other ablative technologies, including laser ablation, microwave, and cryoablation, remains under clinical investigation. The procedure can be done with the percutaneous, laparoscopic, or open technique, either alone or as an adjunct with the surgical resection.

The largest experience was described by Mazzaglia et al.: 452 liver lesions were treated with laparoscopic radiofrequency ablation in 63 patients with a morbidity rate of 5% and reported median survival of 3.9 years [70]. A significant predictor of poor survival was a size of lesion greater than 3 cm. Patients with tumors less than 3 cm and a postablation margin greater than 1 cm had the lowest local recurrence rate [71].

Radiofrequency ablation series report a 5-year overall survival rate of 53% with a local recurrence rate of 22% [50,70–72].

Transcatheter chemoembolization and radioembolization

TACE, the image-guided delivery of embolic particles ± chemotherapeutic agents (TACE and transarterial embolization [TAE]), and internal radiotherapy with yttrium-90 (90Y) microspheres via selective injection into vessels feeding tumors can be used in unresectable NETs. It has shown to result in symptomatic response in 53%–100% of patients and radiologic response in 35%–74%, with progression-free survival of approximately 18 months and 5-year survival of 40%–83% [73–76]. Complications (28%–90%) of TACE include nontarget embolization, postembolization syndrome (fever, abdominal pain, and ileus), liver failure, cholecystitis, and acute portal vein thrombosis [73–76]. Treatment-related mortality is seen in less than 5% of cases. The outcome of TAE or TACE in a multicenter review revealed no difference between the two techniques with regards to overall survival, symptom relief, morbidity, or mortality. Controversies exist in regards to extent of embolization, use of chemotherapeutic agents, timing of the procedure during the course of the disease, and timing of subsequent embolization procedures. TAE or TACE should be reserved for patients with multifocal disease and higher tumor burden. Single metastatic deposits respond better to surgical resection or local ablation. Portal vein thrombosis and hepatic insufficiency are considered exclusion criteria for both TAE and TACE.

Long-term outcome analysis after selective internal radiotherapy showed a treatment response in 63% and disease stability in 32%, with survival of 72% at 1 year and 45% at 3 years [35,75,76]. Other treatment options, such as stereotactic radiation therapy and selective hepatic arterial administration of radionuclide-labeled somatostatin analogs, have been described in the literature and have shown good tumor response.

Cytoreductive surgery in patients with peritoneal metastasis

The incidence of peritoneal metastasis in patients with NET is up to 17% according to two large series. Therefore, some investigators advocate for the use of CRS with and without heated intraperitoneal chemotherapy in select patients with peritoneal metastasis. The overall survival at 5 and 10 years was 69% and 52%, respectively, and disease-free survival at 5 and 10 years was 17% and 6%, respectively [77]. At 5 years, peritoneal metastases and LMs recurred in 47% and 66% of cases, respectively [77]. Mortality was <2% and morbidity in patients receiving heated infusion of peritoneal chemotherapy (HIPEC) was up to 50%.

Systemic treatment options

Receptor-based therapeutic radiation using labeled neuropeptides and amines binding to somatostatin or catecholamine receptors has been widely used since 1999, mostly in Europe. It achieves tumor stability in up to 75% of cases and an overall survival of 22–46 months [78–80]. Recent somatostatin analogs such as DOTATOC and DOTATATE labeled with 90Y or lutetium-177 (177Lu) showed better response rates than the initially used 111In-DTPA-(D-Phe1)-octreotide. The overall response rate using DOTATOC varies between 24% and 33% [78,79]. A recent study on 177Lu-DOTATATE in patients with intestinal NET showed tumor response in 46%, stable disease in 35%, and progressive disease in 20% [80]. The use of combination isotopes has led to improved survival compared with single isotope therapy [79]. Limited access to treatment and absence of RCT are the major disadvantage of this type of treatment [35].

The role of traditionally based systemic cytotoxic therapy, such as streptozotocin and 5FU, has shown a limited response rate of up to 15% [35,42]. Grade and proliferation of the tumor guide treatment type. High-grade lesions are amenable to chemotherapy, such as 5FU, doxorubicin, and streptozotocin [75,76], whereas slow-growing tumors are treated with targeted therapies (such as everolimus or sunitinib) and biotherapy (somatostatin analog or interferon) [81,82]. The extent of LM has been shown to correlate with progression-free survival and poor outcome. Studies on targeted therapy showed a prolonged (6.4–11.4 months) progression-free survival compared with placebo with rare (5%–10%) tumor remission [81,82]. Rinke et al. showed benefit in patients with midgut NETs and <10% hepatic tumor volume treated with somatostatin analogs vs. placebo (median time to progression 14.4 vs. 6 months, respectively) [83].

REFERENCES

1. Yao JC et al. One hundred years after "carcinoid": Epidemiology of and prognostic factors for neuroendocrine tumors in 35,825 cases in the United States. *J Clin Oncol* 2008;26(18):3063–72.
2. Fraenkel M et al. Incidence of gastroenteropancreatic neuroendocrine tumours: A systematic review of the literature. *Endocr Relat Cancer* 2014;21(3):R153–63.
3. Ramage JK et al. Guidelines for the management of gastroenteropancreatic neuroendocrine (including carcinoid) tumours (NETs). *Gut* 2012;61(1):6–32.
4. Riall TS, Townsend CM. Endocrine pancreas. In: Townsend CM, Beauchamp RD, Evers BM, Mattox KL, eds., *Sabiston Textbook of Surgery*. 19th ed. Philadelphia: Elsevier Saunders, 2012:944–62.
5. Modlin IM, Lye KD, Kidd M. A 5-decade analysis of 13,715 carcinoid tumors. *Cancer* 2003 15;97(4):934–59.
6. Hassan MM et al. Risk factors associated with neuroendocrine tumors: A U.S.-based case-control study. *Int J Cancer* 2008;123(4):867–73.
7. Ter-Minassian M et al. Clinical presentation, recurrence, and survival in patients with neuroendocrine tumors: Results from a prospective institutional database. *Endocr Relat Cancer* 2013;20(2):187–96.
8. Vagefi PA et al. Evolving patterns in the detection and outcomes of pancreatic neuroendocrine neoplasms: The Massachusetts General Hospital experience from 1977 to 2005. *Arch Surg* 2007;142(4):347–54.
9. Strosberg J, Gardner N, Kvols L. Survival and prognostic factor analysis of 146 metastatic neuroendocrine tumors of the mid-gut. *Neuroendocrinology* 2009;89(4):471–6.
10. Arnold R et al. Neuroendocrine gastro-entero-pancreatic (GEP) tumors. In: Scheppach W, Bresalier RS, Tytgat GNJ, eds., *Gasrointestinal and Liver Tumors*. Berlin: Springer, 2004:195–233.

11. Strosberg J et al. Correlation between grade and prognosis in metastatic gastroenteropancreatic neuroendocrine tumors. *Hum Pathol* 2009;40(9):1262–8.

12. Naswa N et al. Usual and unusual neuroendocrine tumor metastases on (68)Ga-DOTANOC PET/CT: A pictorial review. *Clin Nucl Med* 2013;38(6):e239–45.

13. Miller HC et al. Role of Ki-67 proliferation index in the assessment of patients with neuroendocrine neoplasias regarding the stage of disease. *World J Surg* 2014;38(6):1353–61.

14. Campana D et al. Chromogranin A: Is it a useful marker of neuroendocrine tumors? *J Clin Oncol* 2007;25(15):1967–73.

15. Rustagi S, Warner RR, Divino CM. Serum pancreastatin: The next predictive neuroendocrine tumor marker. *J Surg Oncol* 2013;108(2):126–8.

16. Kulke MH, Mayer RJ. Carcinoid tumors. *N Engl J Med* 1999;340(11):858–68.

17. National Comprehensive Cancer Network. Neuroendocrine tumors. Version 2.2014.

18. Kunz PL et al. Consensus guidelines for the management and treatment of neuroendocrine tumors. *Pancreas* 2013;42(4):557–77.

19. Sundin A, Vullierme MP, Kaltsas G, Plöckinger U. ENETS consensus guidelines for the standards of care in neuroendocrine tumors: Radiological examinations. *Neuroendocrinology* 2009;90:167–83.

20. King CM, Reznek RH, Dacie JE, Wass JA. Imaging islet cell tumours. *Clin Radiol* 1994;49:295–303.

21. London JF et al. Zollinger-Ellison syndrome: Prospective assessment of abdominal US in the localization of gastrinomas. *Radiology* 1991;178:763–7.

22. Zeiger MA, Shawker TH, Norton JA. Use of intraoperative ultrasonography to localize islet cell tumors. *World J Surg* 1993;17:448–54.

23. van Essen M, Sundin A, Krenning EP, Kwekkeboom DJ. Neuroendocrine tumours: The role of imaging for diagnosis and therapy. *Nat Rev Endocrinol* 2014;10(2):102–14.

24. Rockall AG, Reznek RH. Imaging of neuroendocrine tumours (CT/MR/US). *Best Pract Res Clin Endocrinol Metab* 2007;21(1):43–68.

25. Stark DD, Moss AA, Goldberg HI, Deveney CW. CT of pancreatic islet cell tumors. *Radiology* 1984;150:491–4.

26. Procacci C et al. Nonfunctioning endocrine tumors of the pancreas: Possibilities of spiral CT characterization. *Eur Radiol* 2001;11:1175–83.

27. Kumbasar B et al. Imaging of neuroendocrine tumors: Accuracy of helical CT versus SRS. *Abdom Imaging* 2004;29:696–702.

28. Cwikła JB et al. Diagnostic imaging of carcinoid metastases to the abdomen and pelvis. *Med Sci Monit* 2004;10(Suppl 3):9–16.

29. Paulson EK et al. Carcinoid metastases to the liver: Role of triple-phase helical CT. *Radiology* 1998;206(1):143–50.

30. Thoeni RF, Mueller-Lisse UG, Chan R, Do NK, Shyn PB. Detection of small, functional islet cell tumors in the pancreas: Selection of MR imaging sequences for optimal sensitivity. *Radiology* 2000;214:483–90.

31. Semelka RC, Custodio CM, Cem Balci N, Woosley JT. Neuroendocrine tumors of the pancreas: Spectrum of appearances on MRI. *J Magn Reson Imaging* 2000;11:141–8.

32. Shi W et al. Localization of neuroendocrine tumours with [111In]-DTPA-octreotide scintigraphy (Octreoscan): A comparative study with CT and MR imaging. *QJM* 1998;91:295–301.

33. Carlson B, Johnson CD, Stephens DH, Ward EM, Kvols LK. MRI of pancreatic islet cell carcinoma. *J Comput Assist Tomogr* 1993;17:735–40.

34. Bader TR et al. MRI of carcinoid tumors: Spectrum of appearances in the gastrointestinal tract and liver. *J Magn Reson Imaging* 2001;14(3):261–9.

35. Frilling A et al. Recommendations for management of patients with neuroendocrine liver metastases. *Lancet Oncol* 2014;15(1):e8–21.

36. Maffione AM, Karunanithi S, Kumar R, Rubello D, Alavi A. Nuclear medicine procedures in the diagnosis of NET: A historical perspective. *PET Clin* 2014;9(1):1–9.

37. Modlin IM, Kidd M, Latich I, Zikusoka MN, Shapiro MD. Current status of gastrointestinal carcinoids. *Gastroenterology* 2005;128:1717–51.

38. Binderup T et al. Functional imaging of neuroendocrine tumors: A head-to-head comparison of somatostatin receptor scintigraphy, 123I-MIBG scintigraphy, and 18F-FDG PET. *J Nucl Med* 2010;51:704–12.

39. Adams S et al. Metabolic (PET) and receptor (SPET) imaging of well- and less well-differentiated tumours: Comparison with the expression of the Ki-67 antigen. *Nucl Med Commun* 1998;19:641–7.

40. Frilling A et al. The impact of 68GaDOTATOC positron emission tomography/computed tomography on the multimodal management of patients with neuroendocrine tumors. *Ann Surg* 2010;252:850–6.

41. Ruf J et al. Impact of multiphase 68GaDOTATOC-PET/CT on therapy management in patients with neuroendocrine tumors. *Neuroendocrinology* 2010;91:101–9.

42. Elias D et al. Liver resection (and associated extrahepatic resections) for metastatic well-differentiated endocrine tumors: A 15-year single center prospective study. *Surgery* 2003;133:375–82.

43. Sarmiento JM, Heywood G, Rubin J, Ilstrup DM, Nagorney DM, Que FG. Surgical treatment of neuroendocrine metastases to the liver: A plea for resection to increase survival. *J Am Coll Surg* 2003;197:29–37.

44. Touzios JG et al. Neuroendocrine hepatic metastases: Does aggressive management improve survival? *Ann Surg* 2005;241:776–83; discussion 783–5.

45. Mazzaferro V, Pulvirenti A, Coppa J. Neuroendocrine tumors metastatic to the liver: How to select patients for liver transplantation? *J Hepatol* 2007;47:460–6.

46. Frilling A, Li J, Malamutmann E, Schmid KW, Bockisch A, Broelsch CE. Treatment of liver metastases from neuroendocrine tumours in relation to the extent of hepatic disease. *Br J Surg* 2009;96:175–84.

47. Florman S et al. Liver transplantation for neuroendocrine tumors. *J Gastrointest Surg* 2004;8:208–12.

48. Frilling A et al. Liver transplantation for patients with metastatic endocrine tumors: Single-center experience with 15 patients. *Liver Transpl* 2006;12:1089–96.

49. Le Treut YP et al. Liver transplantation for neuroendocrine tumors in Europe—Results and trends in patient selection: A 213-case European liver transplant registry study. *Ann Surg* 2013;257(5):807–15.

50. Frilling A, Sotiropoulos GC, Li J, Kornasiewicz O. Multimodal management of neuroendocrine liver metastases. *HPB (Oxford)* 2010;12(6):361–79.

51. Gurusamy KS, Pamecha V, Sharma D, Davidson BR. Techniques for liver parenchymal transection in liver resection. *Cochrane Database Syst Rev* 2009;(1):CD006880.

52. Gurusamy KS, Pamecha V, Sharma D, Davidson BR. Palliative cytoreductive surgery versus other palliative treatments in patients with unresectable liver metastases from gastro-entero-pancreatic neuroendocrine tumours. *Cochrane Database Syst Rev* 2009;(1):CD007118.

53. Bruzoni M et al. Management of the primary tumor in patients with metastatic pancreatic neuroendocrine tumor: A contemporary single-institution review. *Am J Surg* 2009;197:376–81.

54. Givi B, Pommier SJ, Thompson AK, Diggs BS, Pommier RF. Operative resection of primary carcinoid neoplasms in patients with liver metastases yields significantly better survival. *Surgery* 2006;140:891–7.

55. Hung JS, Chang MC, Lee PH, Tien YW. Is surgery indicated for patients with symptomatic nonfunctioning pancreatic neuroendocrine tumor and unresectable hepatic metastases? *World J Surg* 2007;31:2392–7.

56. Ahmed A et al. Midgut neuroendocrine tumours with liver metastases: Results of the UKINETS study. *Endocr Relat Cancer* 2009;16:885–94.

57. Gomez D et al. Hepatic resection for metastatic gastrointestinal and pancreatic neuroendocrine tumours: Outcome and prognostic predictors. *HPB (Oxford)* 2007;9:345–51.

58. Yao KA et al. Indications and results of liver resection and hepatic chemoembolization for metastatic gastrointestinal neuroendocrine tumors. *Surgery* 2001;130:677–82; discussion 682–5.

59. Osborne DA et al. Improved outcome with cytoreduction versus embolization for symptomatic hepatic metastases of carcinoid and neuroendocrine tumors. *Ann Surg Oncol* 2006;13:572–81.

60. Musunuru S et al. Metastatic neuroendocrine hepatic tumors: Resection improves survival. *Arch Surg* 2006;141:1000–4; discussion 1005.

61. Belghiti J, Hiramatsu K, Benoist S, Massault P, Sauvanet A, Farges O. Seven hundred forty-seven hepatectomies in the 1990s: An update to evaluate the actual risk of liver resection. *J Am Coll Surg* 2000;191(1):38–46.

62. Steinmüller T et al. Consensus guidelines for the management of patients with liver metastases from digestive (neuro)endocrine tumors: Foregut, midgut, hindgut, and unknown primary. *Neuroendocrinology* 2008;87:47–62.

63. Yao JC, Vauthey JN. Primary and metastatic hepatic carcinoid: Is there an algorithm? *Ann Surg Oncol* 2003;10:1133–5.

64. Klöppel G et al. ENETS Consensus Guidelines for the Standards of Care in Neuroendocrine Tumors: Towards a standardized approach to the diagnosis of gastroenteropancreatic neuroendocrine tumors and their prognostic stratification. *Neuroendocrinology* 2009;90:162–6.

65. House MG et al. Differences in survival for patients with resectable versus unresectable metastases from pancreatic islet cell cancer. *J Gastrointest Surg* 2006;10:138–45.

66. Maire F et al. Is adjuvant therapy with streptozotocin and 5-fluorouracil useful after resection of liver metastases from digestive endocrine tumors? *Surgery* 2009;145:69–75.

67. Hodul P, Malafa M, Choi J, Kvols L. The role of cytoreductive hepatic surgery as an adjunct to the management of metastatic neuroendocrine carcinomas. *Cancer Control* 2006;13:61–71.

68. Fan ST et al. Liver transplantation for neuroendocrine tumour liver metastases. *HPB (Oxford)* 2015;17(1):23–8.

69. Olausson M et al. Orthotopic liver or multivisceral transplantation as treatment of metastatic neuroendocrine tumors. *Liver Transpl* 2007;13:327–33.

70. Mazzaglia PJ, Berber E, Milas M, Siperstein AE. Laparoscopic radiofrequency ablation of neuroendocrine liver metastases: A 10-year experience evaluating predictors of survival. *Surgery* 2007;142:10–9.

71. Berber E, Siperstein A. Local recurrence after laparoscopic radiofrequency ablation of liver tumors: An analysis of 1032 tumors. *Ann Surg Oncol* 2008;15:2757–64.

72. Hellman P, Ladjevardi S, Skogseid B, Akerström G, Elvin A. Radiofrequency tissue ablation using cooled tip for liver metastases of endocrine tumors. *World J Surg* 2002;26:1052–6.

73. Allison DJ, Modlin IM, Jenkins WJ. Treatment of carcinoid liver metastases by hepatic-artery embolisation. *Lancet* 1977;2:1323–5.

74. Gupta S et al. Hepatic artery embolization and chemoembolization for treatment of patients with metastatic carcinoid tumors: The M.D. Anderson experience. *Cancer J* 2003;9:261–7.

75. McStay MK et al. Large-volume liver metastases from neuroendocrine tumors: Hepatic intra-arterial 90Y-DOTA-lanreotide as effective palliative therapy. *Radiology* 2005;237:718–26.

76. Kalinowski M et al. Selective internal radiotherapy with yttrium-90 microspheres for hepatic metastatic neuroendocrine tumors: A prospective single center study. *Digestion* 2009;79:137–42.

77. Elias D, David A, Sourrouille I, Honoré C. Neuroendocrine carcinomas: Optimal surgery of peritoneal metastases (and associated intra-abdominal metastases). *Surgery* 2014;155(1):5–12.

78. Imhof A et al. Response, survival, and long-term toxicity after therapy with the radiolabeled somatostatin analogue [90Y-DOTA]-TOC in metastasized neuroendocrine cancers. *J Clin Oncol* 2011;29:2416–23.

79. Villard L et al. Cohort study of somatostatin-based radiopeptide therapy with [(90)Y-DOTA]-TOC versus [(90)Y-DOTA]-TOC plus [(177)Lu-DOTA]-TOC in neuroendocrine cancers. *J Clin Oncol* 2012;30:1100–6.

80. Kwekkeboom DJ et al. Treatment with the radiolabeled somatostatin analog [177Lu-DOTA0,Tyr3] octreotate: Toxicity, efficacy, and survival. *J Clin Oncol* 2008;26:2124–30.

81. Yao JC et al. Everolimus for advanced pancreatic neuroendocrine tumors. *N Engl J Med* 2011;364: 514–23.

82. Raymond E et al. Sunitinib malate for the treatment of pancreatic neuroendocrine tumors. *N Engl J Med* 2011;364:501–13.

83. Rinke A et al. Placebo-controlled, double-blind, prospective, randomized study on the effect of octreotide LAR in the control of tumor growth in patients with metastatic neuroendocrine midgut tumors: A report from the PROMID Study Group. *J Clin Oncol* 2009;27:4656–63.

50

Cytoreduction of neuroendocrine tumors

MICHAEL OLAUSSON AND BO WÄNGBERG

INTRODUCTION

Neuroendocrine tumors (NETs) were previously often called carcinoids and were divided into foregut, midgut, and hindgut carcinoids [1]. This classification did not relate to the natural history and clinical behavior of these tumors, so the classification has been revised several times taking into account tumor location, tumor size, angio-invasion, hormone production, histological grade, and proliferative index [2]. Using the present World Health Organization (WHO) classification of 2010, neuroendocrine neoplasms of the gastrointestinal tract are classified into grade 1 (G1), 2 (G2), or 3 (G3) tumors based on Ki^{67} index and mitotic count. G1 and G2 tumors are designated NETs, and G3 tumors neuroendocrine carcinoma (NEC). G3 tumors have a more aggressive clinical behavior, but G1 and G2 tumors can also give rise to metastasizing disease. NETs are often diagnosed at a late stage, when the patients have disseminated disease and hormonal symptoms. The workup includes computed tomography (CT) or MRT, somatostatin receptor (SSTR) imaging ([111]indium-octreotide scintigraphy or positron emission tomography [PET] using [68]gallium-DOTA-conjugated peptides), hormonal screening, and analyses of tumor biopsies. The histopathological examination aims to classify the tumor with respect to origin and biological behavior. Immunohistochemical staining for amine and peptide hormones and synaptic vesicle proteins can be helpful in defining the origin of the tumor [3]. Analysis of growth pattern, degree of neuroendocrine differentiation, and proliferative capacity provides prognostic information [4] and aids in the selection of treatment. The neuroendocrine differentiation is evaluated by antibodies against proteins of the neurosecretory granules (e.g., chromogranin A and synaptophysin) or cytosolic markers (neuron-specific enolase or PGP 9.5). NETs are immunopositive for all markers in the majority of tumor cells, while NECs often lack the granular markers with cytosolic markers retained. Other factors, e.g., angiogenic capacity, expression of adhesion molecules, and specific genetic changes, are prognostic tools and indicators of responsiveness to medical treatment.

Bronchial NETs can be typical (carcinoid morphology, few mitoses, and absence of necrosis), with good prognosis, or atypical (nuclear atypia and deranged architecture, increased mitotic activity, or presence of necrosis), with intermediate prognosis [5], in contrast to large cell NECs and small cell lung carcinomas with poor prognosis [6,7]. Recently, a revised classification for bronchial NETs has been suggested [8]. Asymptomatic tumors are incidentally detected, while symptomatic patients may present with local symptoms or ectopic production of peptides, e.g., adrenocorticotropic hormone (ACTH) and growth hormone-releasing hormone (GHRH), usually at an advanced stage. Thymic NETs often have a slow progression, but are invariably malignant. Cytoreductive surgery is sometimes required for other NET types, e.g., the rare cases of malignant pheochromocytoma and paraganglioma with excessive catecholamine (CA) secretion or medullary thyroid carcinoma (MTC) with severe diarrhea or ectopic ACTH production.

Surgical tumor reduction is mainly considered for differentiated NETs (G1–G2) [9] and is of particular value in patients with hormonal symptoms. In patients with metastasized G3 tumors, where R0 resection is not feasible, systemic oncologic treatment should not be delayed.

PERIOPERATIVE CONSIDERATIONS

Prior to all interventional treatment of NETs, the tumor type and hormone production must be assessed. Patients with hormonally active, small intestinal NETs are pretreated with long-acting somatostatin analogs (e.g., octreotide 100 µg × 4 s.c.), to prevent carcinoid symptoms during intervention. In case of a crisis reaction (severe flushing, bronchoconstriction, and hypotension), adrenergic drugs *must* be avoided, since these tumor cells often express adrenoceptors and a vicious circle with excessive release of serotonin and tachykinins can be initiated. Instead, the surgical manipulation should be interrupted, volume substituted according to hemodynamic parameters, and titrated doses of octreotide and (occasionally) glucocorticoids given. Spinal anesthesia with markedly reduced arterial blood pressure may elicit carcinoid crises due to compensatory release of CA from the adrenals, in turn activating serotonin release from the tumor. For postoperative pain, epidural analgesia is preferred [10]. NETs from the foregut (bronchopulmonary, thymic, or gastroduodenal) sometimes produce excess histamine, while serotonin production is very rare in these tumors. This may cause the "atypical carcinoid syndrome" (generalized flushing, bronchoconstriction, hypotension, lacrimation, and cutaneous edema). Correct diagnosis relies on analysis of the main histamine metabolite methylimidazole acetic acid (MelmAA) in urine, but immunohistochemistry can also indicate a histamine-producing tumor.

Patients with histamine-producing tumors are optimally pretreated with a combination of somatostatin analogs, blockade of histamine (H_1 and H_2) receptors and cortisone. Histamine-liberating agents, e.g., morphine and tubocurarine, should be avoided [11]. Low-molecular-weight heparin is recommended due to the increased risk of thrombosis. Patients with gastrinoma maintain their medication with omeprazol for a period after removal of the tumor, since they often have elevated gastric acid secretion due to hypertrophy of the gastric mucosa. For patients with glucagonoma or vasoactive intestinal peptide-oma (VIPoma), preoperative treatment with octreotide is usually sufficient. Skin lesions (necrolytic migrating erythema), sometimes associated with glucagonomas, can heal rapidly with octreotide, antibiotics, and amino acid supplementation prior to surgery. After removal of insulinomas, close postoperative monitoring of glucose and potassium is necessary.

Surgical treatment of patients with advanced pheochromocytomas and paragangliomas presents specific problems due to cardiovascular effects caused by excessive release of CAs, which may activate α-adrenoceptors, leading to vasoconstriction and reduced plasma volume (not compensated for by vasodilatation via β_2-adrenoceptors), and β-adrenoceptors, resulting in tachycardia. The chronic effects of CAs can give a dilating cardiomyopathy, and the presence of this should be excluded preoperatively, by ultracardiography. The function of the heart improves after resection of the pheochromocytoma. Pretreatment with α-adrenoceptor blockers (phenoxybenzamine or doxazocin) or calcium channel blockers is used preoperatively at most units. In selected patients, preoperative metaiodobenzylguanidine (MIBG) therapy [12] or chemotherapy [13] may be considered in order to reduce tumor burden and the secretion of CA. For palliation, α-methyltyrosine may be used to reduce the synthesis of CAs in advanced disease.

INTERVENTIONAL TREATMENT OF LIVER METASTASES

The surgical treatment of primary NETs and locoregional disease is seldom controversial, but a prerequisite for further management of liver metastases, which may involve several interventional modalities. In future randomized studies on the role of medical treatment in advanced disease, primary surgery by an experienced surgeon is of importance to prevent local complications by the tumor and correctly stage the tumor disease. For favorable results of metastasis treatment (including liver transplantation), the aim is to resect all extrahepatic tumors. There is no general agreement when to start the palliative surgical treatment; e.g., gastrinomas metastatic to the liver can show most variable growth rates in different patients, which influences the decision making [14], but extrahepatic and concomitant liver surgery can be safely performed [15].

The surgical or interventional treatment for liver metastases can be divided into four types of modality: liver resection, vascular interventions, ablative procedures, and liver transplantation (see Chapter 52). Different modalities are often combined [16], e.g., resections and ablative procedures (Figure 50.1).

Liver resections

Liver resections can be performed for lesions located within any of the eight liver segments, each supplied by branches of the hepatic arteries and portal vein and each drained by one hepatic duct (Figure 50.2a). Nowadays, less focus is put on performing an exact anatomical resection. Instead, for curative resections good clearance margins are more important, although for NET patients resected for palliation, the margins can be narrowed and local tumors can preferably be removed by atypical resections. Intraoperatively, the extension of the tumor is assessed by inspection, palpation, and intraoperative ultrasound. The latter technique allows good definition of liver anatomy and reveals the relationship between the tumor and the portal or hepatic venous pedicles. This is of special importance if techniques like cryo- or laser therapy are used.

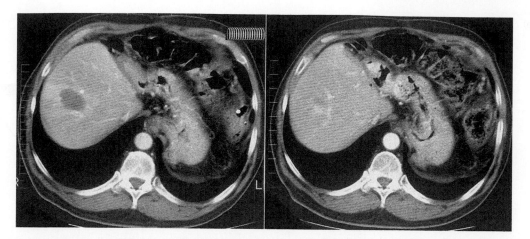

Figure 50.1 CT in a patient with the MEN-1 syndrome subjected to completion pancreatectomy and left hepatectomy due to metastatic EPTs. One centrally located metastasis in the residual right liver was treated with radiofrequency ablation. The dark area represents the coagulation necrosis (left). Three months later, there was marked shrinkage of the necrotic area (right). After completion of treatment, the patient had normal tumor markers and negative octreotide scintigraphy.

In the sagittal projection, the liver is divided by the three principal hepatic veins, which delineate the major liver resections: left lateral hepatectomy (removal of segments II and III), left hepatectomy (removal of segments I–IV), and right hepatectomy (removal of segments V–VIII). Resection of individual segments requires identification of portal and hepatic veins, usually with intraoperative ultrasound if the tumor is close to the vena cava or the portal bifurcation. Superficial liver metastases along the edges of the liver are safely removed by wedge excisions.

LEFT, LEFT EXTENDED, AND LEFT LATERAL HEPATECTOMY

The left and middle hepatic veins have their junctions at variable levels and can usually be controlled separately outside the liver (Figure 50.2d and e), although this is not necessary to do before dividing the parenchyma. The left lateral resection (Figure 50.2d) usually does not include the median vein, but may have a common origin from the caval vein. The left lobe resection includes division of the segment IVa and IVb branches to the median vein. If the median vein is included, the resection is classified as an extended left lobe hepatectomy, which may include segments V and VIII as well (Figure 50.2f).

RIGHT AND RIGHT EXTENDED HEPATECTOMY

The most common variant in arterial anatomy is replacement of the right hepatic artery by a branch of the superior mesenteric artery. For right-sided liver tumors, preoperative angiography or MR angiography is therefore valuable. For right hepatectomy, the right hepatic vein can be controlled outside the liver (Figure 50.2b). The triangular ligament on the right side is freed to get access to the retrohepatic veins to the caval vein. Inflow occlusion may be established by the so-called Pringle's maneuver, but is usually not necessary after the artery and right portal vein have been ligated. The safe duration of total ischemia of the liver at normothermia

may exceed 1 hour, but can be lower with hepatic dysfunction, and therefore intermittent clamping in 15-minute periods is usually advised [17], if inflow control is used.

In some cases, extended right lobe resections, leaving only the two left lateral liver segments, can be performed (Figure 50.2c).

A residual liver less than 20%–25% of the original volume may lead to hepatic failure. One way to reduce morbidity and mortality in these cases is to use preoperative portal embolization of the right liver lobes carrying the lesions. This procedure induces hypertrophy of the intact left liver during a 3- to 6-week period, so the planned resection can be safely performed [18].

METASTASECTOMY

Metastasectomy of multiple lesions usually requires intermittent clamping of inflow vessels and incision by diathermy. To obtain good cytoreduction, the principles of anatomical resection, wedge resection, and metastasectomy are often combined. Division of the liver parenchyma often includes the use of an ultrasonic surgical aspirator, which destroys the parenchyma without damaging the biliary and vascular structures and allows accurate placement of ligatures and clips. Alternatively, ultracision, ligasure, plain cautery, or hydrojet devices can be used. All of these techniques facilitate bloodless resections. To minimize oozing from the cut surface, techniques to assist hemostasis can be used, e.g., rapid-setting fibrin glue or an argon beam coagulator. The operative mortality for elective liver surgery must be kept low. In most series, figures of <5% are reported [17]. Prophylactic use of antibiotics has reduced infectious complications. The morbidity is more frequently associated with sepsis than with bleeding.

RESULTS OF LIVER SURGERY

Over the last three decades, very active surgery has become increasingly more common as the primary treatment of

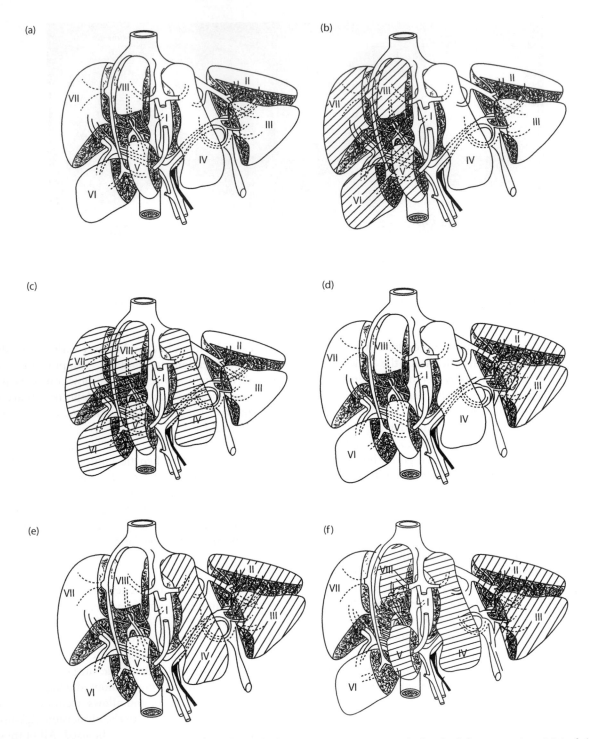

Figure 50.2 **(a)** Segmental anatomy of the liver. **(b)** Right hepatectomy. **(c)** Extended right lobe resection. **(d)** Left lateral hepatectomy. **(e)** Left hepatectomy. **(f)** Extended left hepatectomy.

neuroendocrine grade 1–2 tumors and their metastases. Curative liver surgery (i.e., no gross residual tumor) should be considered for all patients with resectable disease, since this is the only long-term effective strategy [16]. Palliative liver surgery can be performed in patients with G1–G2 tumors and severe hormonal symptoms and is considered when more than 90% of the tumor volume can be safely excised [19]. In early clinical series of patients with NETs, the liver resection rate with curative intent was low [20], but with

improved perioperative management, including somatostatin analogs, the resection rate has increased. It has been shown that normalization of biochemistry and radiological findings can be achieved in a significant proportion of patients with NETs and liver metastases [16,21–24]. In the reported series at centers of expertise, the median mortality was <1% (range 0%–9%) and median morbidity 23% (range 3%–45%).

One evident problem with an active liver surgery program is that many resections are considered curative at the time of surgery but later proved not to be. With access to sensitive diagnostic tools (tumor-secreted hormones, general NET markers, SSTR imaging, spiral CT, and MRT) and careful follow-up, subclinical disease can be discovered and limited lesions reresected [23,25]. A recent systematic review [22] of 29 studies on hepatic resections for NETs gave a median 5- and 10-year overall survival of 71% (range 31%–100%) and 42% (range 0%–100%), respectively. The wide survival variation indicates vast differences in selection of patients, and a number of risk factors for poor survival were identified. These included poorly differentiated tumors, the presence of extrahepatic disease, and macroscopically incomplete (palliative) resections. This emphasizes the importance of a thorough preoperative diagnostic workup for the proper selection of patients. The median progression-free survival was only 21 months (range 13–46 months), showing that some patients are candidates for additional interventional or systemic treatment after hepatic resections. In unresectable recurrence limited to the liver, liver transplantation may be considered. The role of resection for enhanced survival has still not been proved in randomized studies.

Liver transplantation

Liver and multivisceral (MvTx) transplantations have been attempted for more than 20 years [26,27], with an estimated 70% recurrence-free survival for MvTx and 77% for liver transplantation (Figure 50.3) [27]. The role of MvTx in patients with NETs has been considered controversial, mainly due to the difficulties of deciding when the time is right. Surrogate markers are few, the most commonly used being Ki[67] in combination with any "hot spots" with higher activity. Data are therefore difficult to compare. Recently, a consensus conference resulted in a publication [28] that summarizes the current recommendations for liver transplantation, still leaving MvTx without any clinical recommendation. A Ki[67] below 5%, and 10% in hot spots, seems to be the safest selection in our opinion. Palliation in patients with symptoms from the NETs is excellent in both liver transplantation and MvTx. As a rule, we prefer MvTx in endocrine pancreas tumors (EPTs) of the head, where radical resection is difficult due to possible engagement of the celiac lymph glands. EPTs of the body or tail with liver metastases are best treated with pancreas resection and liver transplantation if liver resection is not possible.

SSTR-targeted radiotherapy takes advantage of the high expression of SSTRs on NET cells, and the results in patients with unresectable disease are promising (see Chapter 52). We have used ^{177}Lu-DOTA-Tyr^3-octreotate as an adjunct in several patients after liver transplantation or MvTx and extrahepatic nonresectable recurrent tumors. This has led to stable disease and markedly reduced tumor markers after completion of radiotherapy [27].

Vascular interventions

Markowitz in 1952 [29] first proposed hepatic vascular interventions as therapeutic procedures. The rationale for ischemic treatment of NETs of the liver is that their main blood and oxygen supply is from the hepatic artery [30–32], with maintained portal perfusion of the normal liver parenchyma. Ischemia can be achieved by several techniques directed against the hepatic artery: ligation, selective embolization, or temporary occlusion. Vascular interventions have been shown to palliate symptoms, but can also be used as a neoadjuvant therapy before hepatic resection, transplantation, or ablative procedures. The methods differ in completeness, distribution, and duration of ischemia.

LIGATION OR TEMPORARY OCCLUSION

Ligation of the hepatic artery was an early attempt to induce liver ischemia. It has been abandoned in the treatment of neuroendocrine metastases due to difficulties in obtaining adequate ischemia (due to the rich collateral blood supply to the liver), significant morbidity in patients with advanced disease, and restricted possibilities for repeat vascular intervention. A previously used alternative, reported in the midgut carcinoid syndrome, is the temporary occlusion of the hepatic artery via external vessel loops (positioned during surgery) [33].

HEPATIC ARTERIAL EMBOLIZATION

Selective embolization of the right or left hepatic arteries causes a temporary but complete ischemia, since the

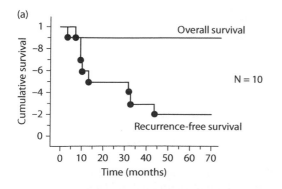

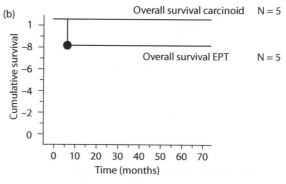

Figure 50.3 **(a)** Survival and recurrence-free survival after liver transplantation. **(b)** Overall survival of carcinoid and EPT patients.

distal arterial tree is filled with embolization material [34]. Embolization of the contralateral lobe is usually performed after 4–6 weeks. Contraindications are tumor burden exceeding 50% of the liver volume, occlusion of the portal vein, renal insufficiency, hyperbilirubinemia, and persistently elevated liver enzymes. Relative contraindications are contrast allergy, coagulopathies, extrahepatic tumor dominance, and poor performance status of the patient [35]. However, patients with tumor volumes exceeding 50% have safely undergone titrated superselective embolizations well separated in time (intervals of 2–4 weeks). Our own 40 patients could be divided into two equally large groups: responders with more than 50% tumor reduction and pronounced reduction of 5-hydroxyindole acetic acid (5-HIAA) excretion (80%) and nonresponders with less than 50% tumor reduction and a moderate 5-HIAA reduction (30%), with clear survival advantage in the former group. The overall long-term results of embolization showed 60% survival at 5 years (Figure 50.4). This can also be applied in patients with previous hemihepatectomy and recurrent tumors in the residual liver. Immediately before embolization, an arteriogram is performed to demonstrate the arterial anatomy, tumor blood flow, and patency of the portal vein (Figure 50.5) [36,37]. Both absorbable and nonabsorbable embolization materials have been used, e.g., gel foam particles or polyvinyl alcohol spheres, but also cyanoacrylate or lipiodol. The need to maintain an open route for repeat procedures excludes the choice of steel coils in the proximal arterial segment.

HEPATIC ARTERIAL CHEMOEMBOLIZATION

Chemoembolization combines the injection of occlusive material with liver-targeted intra-arterial administration of chemotherapy [38]. Up to 72% sustained tumor control has been reported for advanced NETs using repeat treatment with cytotoxic drugs (5-fluorouracil [5-FU], doxorubicin, streptozotocin, gemcitabine, vinblastine, mitomycin C, and cisplatin) alone or in combinations [39,40]. Recently, drug-eluting bead therapy has been introduced as an alternative form of chemoembolization [41].

SELECTIVE INTERNAL RADIOTHERAPY

Radioembolization with microspheres (glass or resin) labeled with the β-emitter [90]yttrium is a promising tool in the treatment of hypervascular NETs [42]. After intra-arterial injection, the radioactive microspheres are preferentially implanted in liver tumors in a 3:1 to 20:1 ratio compared with normal liver [43]. A prerequisite for treatment is the absence of significant hepatopulmonary shunting, and this is confirmed scintigraphically. Before treatment, patients also undergo occlusion of shunts to the gastrointestinal tract. [90]Yttrium seems to be more efficient in small (1–2 cm) hepatic metastases with a miliary distribution, but further studies are needed to define the role in the treatment of liver metastases of gastroenteropancreatic (GEP) NETs [44].

CLINICAL RESPONSE TO LIVER ISCHEMIA

Hepatic arterial embolization is accompanied by liver pain, transient elevation of liver enzymes, nausea, and usually

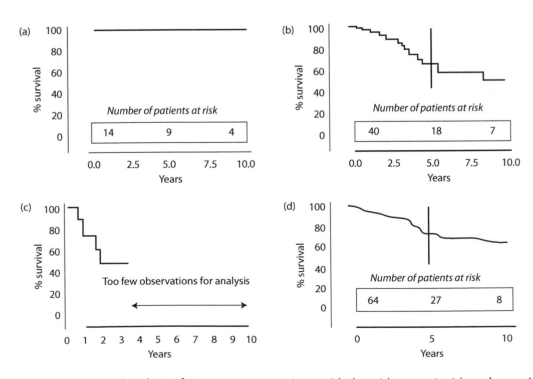

Figure 50.4 Kaplan–Meier survival analysis of 64 consecutive patients with the midgut carcinoid syndrome. **(a)** Patients with sole surgical treatment (primary surgery + liver surgery) (n = 14). **(b)** Patients with bilateral liver tumors treated by primary surgery, embolization, and octreotide (n = 40). **(c)** Patients with sole medical treatment (octreotide combined with chemotherapy or interferon) after primary surgery due to complicating diseases (n = 10). **(d)** Survival in the entire series.

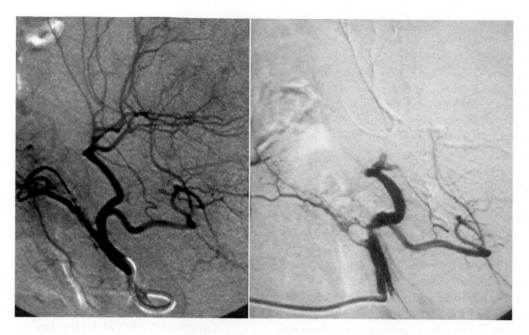

Figure 50.5 Arteriogram in a patient with small intestinal NETs and liver metastases before (left) and 10 minutes after (right) embolization.

a late fever reaction (24–48 hours). Serious complications (gall bladder ischemia, pancreatitis, liver abscess, vascular damage, hepatorenal syndrome, and hormonal crises) are rare with modern interventional techniques, proper hydration, and pretreatment with somatostatin analogs.

To monitor the outcome of ischemic therapy, CT and biochemical tumor markers are used. It would be an advantage if the response to ischemia could be assessed earlier to facilitate alternative treatment when necessary. For this purpose, alternative monitoring systems have been explored. General tumor regression was seen in individual patients subjected to unilateral embolization, indicating activation of systemic antitumor effects, e.g., activation of natural killer (NK) cells [45]. The observed early immunological responses closely correlated with late monitoring of therapeutic effects. MR spectroscopy of liver tumors before and shortly after embolization with regard to energy-rich phosphates can give information on the degree of ischemia [46], and diffusion-weighted MR may indicate early tumor responses.

The results of ischemic treatments of liver metastases are dependent on a number of variables. In a retrospective study, patients with carcinoid tumors had a higher response rate and longer progression-free survival than patients with pancreatic NETs [47] after bland embolization or chemoembolization. An intact primary tumor, extensive liver involvement, and extrahepatic disease were associated with reduced survival in patients with pancreatic NETs. In a long-term follow-up study, 80% of patients with hormonally active tumors had relief of symptoms after one cycle of treatment, and it was concluded that the presence of extrahepatic disease or unresected primary should not limit the use of embolization [48]. The relative merits of chemoembolization versus selective embolization await further studies [49].

Intraoperative procedures

RADIO-GUIDED SURGERY

Taking advantage of the high expression of SSTRs by several NETs, attempts to develop radio-guided surgery using a handheld scintillation detector after preoperative injection of radiolabeled somatostatin analogs have been evaluated. The indications for radio-guided surgery would be recurrent tumors in regions not easily investigated by other methods (e.g., neck metastases of MTC, carcinoids, and EPTs), small EPTs (e.g., the multiple endocrine neoplasia type 1 [MEN-1] syndrome), and as control of adequate tumor removal (e.g., residual carcinoid metastases in the mesenteric root after lymph node dissection). Promising results have been reported, but scintillation detection is clearly not sensitive enough to detect microscopic tumor growth or microadenomas [50].

REGIONAL HYPERTHERMIC LIVER PERFUSION

At an advanced stage of histamine- or CA-producing tumors, ischemic liver treatment is potentially dangerous due to uncontrollable release of tumor products. In individual patients with the foregut carcinoid syndrome, we have used cytotoxic drugs (melphalan and cisplatinum) delivered by regional hyperthermic liver perfusion. During perfusion, the venous effluent from the liver with vasoactive substances was shunted from the systemic circulation, thus avoiding vasomotor effects. Cytostatic perfusion of the isolated liver with simultaneous filtration of portal vein blood and a maintained systemic circulation were made possible by a special perfusion catheter inserted in the cava. The surgical technique involves isolation of the hepatic artery, portal vein, and cava inferior and superior to the liver, together with a temporary portocaval shunt that allows blood flow rates to be maintained in both the hepatic artery and portal vessels [51]. Repeat hyperthermic perfusion can be difficult to perform due to intense fibrotic reaction of the vessels used for perfusion. At the present time, this technique is used most frequently in patients with ocular melanoma and liver metastases. An ongoing randomized trial will help to answer whether the technique is useful for this indication. No randomized trial for patients with NETs and liver metastases has been performed yet.

Ablative procedures

Locally ablative methods have been used in hepatic metastases of GEP-NETs alone or in combination with surgical resection. They can be applied percutaneously, during open or laparoscopic surgery, and include ablation with radiofrequency, microwaves, laser, or cryotherapy [9,52]. Radiofrequency has been the most common modality, but microwaves may be more efficacious due to higher intratumoral temperatures. The number of publications on laser and microwave ablation in this setting is low, and cryotherapy has higher rates of complications than the other methods. Ablation can be considered when surgery is not applicable and the number of metastases is few; it can also be combined with surgical resections (Figure 50.1) [53]. Lesions close to large vessels may be treated, since the vessels are protected by cooling due to bloodstream effects, but the cooling can decrease the therapeutic effect. Ultrasound is often used for guidance, but thermosensitive MR systems for continuous monitoring of coagulative effects have been developed.

REFERENCES

1. Williams ED, Sandler M. The classification of carcinoid tumours. *Lancet* 1963;1(7275):238–9.
2. Rindi G, Petrone G, Inzani F. The 2010 WHO classification of digestive neuroendocrine neoplasms: A critical appraisal four years after its introduction. *Endocr Pathol* 2014;25(2):186–92.
3. Jakobsen AM, Andersson P, Saglik G et al. Differential expression of vesicular monoamine transporter (VMAT) 1 and 2 in gastrointestinal endocrine tumours. *J Pathol* 2001;195(4):463–72.
4. Rindi G, Azzoni C, La Rosa S et al. ECL cell tumor and poorly differentiated endocrine carcinoma of the stomach: Prognostic evaluation by pathological analysis. *Gastroenterology* 1999;116(3):532–42.
5. Travis WD, Rush W, Flieder DB et al. Survival analysis of 200 pulmonary neuroendocrine tumors with clarification of criteria for atypical carcinoid and its separation from typical carcinoid. *Am J Surg Pathol* 1998;22(8):934–44.
6. Jiang SX, Kameya T, Shoji M, Dobashi Y, Shinada J, Yoshimura H. Large cell neuroendocrine carcinoma of the lung: A histologic and immunohistochemical study of 22 cases. *Am J Surg Pathol* 1998;22(5):526–37.
7. Clark R, Ihde DC. Small-cell lung cancer: Treatment progress and prospects. *Oncology* 1998;12(5):647–58; discussion 661–3.
8. Pelosi G, Papotti M, Rindi G, Scarpa A. Unraveling tumor grading and genomic landscape in lung neuroendocrine tumors. *Endocr Pathol* 2014;25(2):151–64.
9. Frilling A, Modlin IM, Kidd M et al. Recommendations for management of patients with neuroendocrine liver metastases. *Lancet Oncol* 2014;15(1):e8–21.
10. Ahlman H, Ahlund L, Dahlstrom A, Martner J, Stenqvist O, Tylen U. SMS 201-995 and provocation tests in preparation of patients with carcinoids for surgery or hepatic arterial embolization. *Anesth Analg* 1988;67(12):1142–8.
11. Ahlman H, Wangberg B, Nilsson O et al. Aspects on diagnosis and treatment of the foregut carcinoid syndrome. *Scand J Gastroenterol* 1992;27(6):459–71.
12. van Hulsteijn LT, Niemeijer ND, Dekkers OM, Corssmit EP. (131)I-MIBG therapy for malignant paraganglioma and phaeochromocytoma: Systematic review and meta-analysis. *Clin Endocrinol* 2014;80(4):487–501.
13. Averbuch SD, Steakley CS, Young RC et al. Malignant pheochromocytoma: Effective treatment with a combination of cyclophosphamide, vincristine, and dacarbazine. *Ann Intern Med* 1988;109(4):267–73.
14. Sutliff VE, Doppman JL, Gibril F et al. Growth of newly diagnosed, untreated metastatic gastrinomas and predictors of growth patterns. *J Clin Cncol* 1997;15(6):2420–31.
15. Norton JA, Warren RS, Kelly MG, Zuraek MB, Jensen RT. Aggressive surgery for metastatic liver neuroendocrine tumors. *Surgery* 2003;134(6):1057–63; discussion 1063–5.
16. Sarmiento JM, Heywood G, Rubin J, Ilstrup DM, Nagorney DM, Que FG. Surgical treatment of neuroendocrine metastases to the liver: A plea for resection to increase survival. *J Am Coll Surg* 2003;197(1):29–37.
17. Benjamin IS. Management of secondary endocrine tumours of the liver. In: Lynn J, Bloom S, eds., *Surgical Endocrinology*. Oxford: Butterworth-Heinemann, 1993:538–47.
18. Farges O, Belghiti J. Options in the resection of endocrine liver metastases. In: Mignon M, Colombel JF eds., *Recent Advances in the Pathophysiology and Management of Inflammatory Bowel Diseases and Digestive Endocrine System*. Paris: John Libbey Eurotext, 1999:335–7.
19. McEntee GP, Nagorney DM, Kvols LK, Moertel CG, Grant CS. Cytoreductive hepatic surgery for neuroendocrine tumors. *Surgery* 1990;108(6):1091–6.
20. Galland RB, Blumgart LH. Carcinoid syndrome. Surgical management. *Br J Hosp Med* 1986;35(3):166, 8–70.

21. Wangberg B, Westberg G, Tylen U et al. Survival of patients with disseminated midgut carcinoid tumors after aggressive tumor reduction. *World J Surg* 1996;20(7):892–9; discussion 899.

22. Saxena A, Chua TC, Perera M, Chu F, Morris DL. Surgical resection of hepatic metastases from neuroendocrine neoplasms: A systematic review. *Surg Oncol* 2012;21(3):e131–41.

23. Mayo SC, de Jong MC, Pulitano C et al. Surgical management of hepatic neuroendocrine tumor metastasis: Results from an international multi-institutional analysis. *Ann Surg Oncol* 2010;17(12):3129–36.

24. Osborne DA, Zervos EE, Strosberg J et al. Improved outcome with cytoreduction versus embolization for symptomatic hepatic metastases of carcinoid and neuroendocrine tumors. *Ann Surg Oncol* 2006;13(4):572–81.

25. Ahlman H, Wangberg B, Tisell LE, Nilsson O, Fjalling M, Forssell-Aronsson E. Clinical efficacy of octreotide scintigraphy in patients with midgut carcinoid tumours and evaluation of intraoperative scintillation detection. *Br J Surg* 1994;81(8):1144–9.

26. Frilling A, Li J, Malamutmann E, Schmid KW, Bockisch A, Broelsch CE. Treatment of liver metastases from neuroendocrine tumours in relation to the extent of hepatic disease. *Br J Surg* 2009;96(2):175–84.

27. Olausson M, Friman S, Herlenius G et al. Orthotopic liver or multivisceral transplantation as treatment of metastatic neuroendocrine tumors. *Liver Transpl* 2007;13(3):327–33.

28. Fan ST, Le Treut YP, Mazzaferro V et al. Liver transplantation for neuroendocrine tumour liver metastases. *HPB* 2015;17(1):23–8.

29. Markowitz J. The hepatic artery. *Surg Gynecol Obstet* 1952;95(5):644–6.

30. Gelin LE, Lewis DH, Nilsson L. Liver blood flow in man during abdominal surgery. II. The effect of hepatic artery occlusion on the blood flow through metastatic tumor nodules. *Acta Hepatosplenol* 1968;15(1):21–4.

31. Cho KJ, Reuter SR, Schmidt R. Effects of experimental hepatic artery embolization on hepatic function. *AJR Am J Roentgenol* 1976;127(4):563–7.

32. Moertel CG, Johnson CM, McKusick MA et al. The management of patients with advanced carcinoid tumors and islet cell carcinomas. *Ann Intern Med* 1994;120(4):302–9.

33. Nobin A, Mansson B, Lunderquist A. Evaluation of temporary liver dearterialization and embolization in patients with metastatic carcinoid tumour. *Acta Oncol* 1989;28(3):419–24.

34. Chuang VP, Wallace S. Hepatic artery embolization in the treatment of hepatic neoplasms. *Radiology* 1981;140(1):51–8.

35. Ajani JA, Carrasco CH, Wallace S. Neuroendocrine tumors metastatic to the liver. *Ann NY Acad Sci* 1994;733:479–87.

36. Allison DJ, Modlin IM, Jenkins WJ. Treatment of carcinoid liver metastases by hepatic-artery embolisation. *Lancet* 1977;2(8052–53):1323–5.

37. Pueyo I, Jimenez JR, Hernandez J et al. Carcinoid syndrome treated by hepatic embolization. *AJR Am J Roentgenol* 1978;131(3):511–3.

38. Hajarizadeh H, Ivancev K, Mueller CR, Fletcher WS, Woltering EA. Effective palliative treatment of metastatic carcinoid tumors with intra-arterial chemotherapy/chemoembolization combined with octreotide acetate. *Am J Surg* 1992;163(5):479–83.

39. Ruszniewski P, Rougier P, Roche A et al. Hepatic arterial chemoembolization in patients with liver metastases of endocrine tumors. A prospective phase II study in 24 patients. *Cancer* 1993;71(8):2624–30.

40. Yang TX, Chua TC, Morris DL. Radioembolization and chemoembolization for unresectable neuroendocrine liver metastases—A systematic review. *Surg Oncol* 2012;21(4):299–308.

41. Gaur SK, Friese JL, Sadow CA et al. Hepatic arterial chemoembolization using drug-eluting beads in gastrointestinal neuroendocrine tumor metastatic to the liver. *Cardiovasc Interv Radiol* 2011;34(3):566–72.

42. Kennedy AS, Dezarn WA, McNeillie P et al. Radioembolization for unresectable neuroendocrine hepatic metastases using resin 90Y-microspheres: Early results in 148 patients. *Am J Clin Oncol* 2008;31(3):271–9.

43. Kennedy A, Coldwell D, Sangro B, Wasan H, Salem R. Radioembolization for the treatment of liver tumors general principles. *Am J Clin Oncol* 2012;35(1):91–9.

44. Whitney R, Valek V, Fages JF et al. Transarterial chemoembolization and selective internal radiation for the treatment of patients with metastatic neuroendocrine tumors: A comparison of efficacy and cost. *Oncologist* 2011;16(5):594–601.

45. Wangberg B, Ahlman H, Tylen U, Nilsson O, Hermodsson S, Hellstrand K. Accumulation of natural killer cells after hepatic artery embolisation in the midgut carcinoid syndrome. *Br J Cancer* 1995;71(3):617–8.

46. Ljungberg M, Westberg G, Vikhoff-Baaz B et al. 31P MR spectroscopy to evaluate the efficacy of hepatic artery embolization in the treatment of neuroendocrine liver metastases. *Acta Radiol* 2012;53(10):1118–26.

47. Gupta S, Johnson MM, Murthy R et al. Hepatic arterial embolization and chemoembolization for the treatment of patients with metastatic neuroendocrine tumors: Variables affecting response rates and survival. *Cancer* 2005;104(8):1590–602.

48. Ho AS, Picus J, Darcy MD et al. Long-term outcome after chemoembolization and embolization of hepatic metastatic lesions from neuroendocrine tumors. *AJR Am J Roentgenol* 2007;188(5):1201–7.

49. Pitt SC, Knuth J, Keily JM et al. Hepatic neuroendo-crine metastases: Chemo- or bland embolization? *J Gastrointest Surg* 2008;12(11):1951–60.

50. Wangberg B, Forssell-Aronsson E, Tisell LE, Nilsson O, Fjalling M, Ahlman H. Intraoperative detection of somatostatin-receptor-positive neuroendocrine tumours using indium-111-labelled DTPA-D-Phe1-octreotide. *Br J Cancer* 1996;73(6):770–5.

51. Schersten T, Ahlman H, Wangberg B, Granerus G, Grimelius L. Hyperthermic liver perfusion chemo-therapy in the foregut carcinoid syndrome. *Lancet* 1991;338(8766):568–9.

52. Vogl TJ, Naguib NN, Zangos S, Eichler K, Hedayati A, Nour-Eldin NE. Liver metastases of neuroendocrine carcinomas: Interventional treatment via transarterial embolization, chemoembolization and thermal abla-tion. *Eur J Radiol* 2009;72(3):517–28.

53. Elias D, Goere D, Leroux G et al. Combined liver surgery and RFA for patients with gastroentero-pancreatic endocrine tumors presenting with more than 15 metastases to the liver. *Eur J Surg Oncol* 2009;35(10):1092–7.

Liver transplantation for neuroendocrine tumors

NIR LUBEZKY, PARISSA TABRIZIAN, MYRON E. SCHWARTZ, AND SANDER FLORMAN

OVERVIEW

Liver metastases from neuroendocrine tumors (NET) are often slow growing compared with other common solid tumors. To date, a variety of successful treatment modalities have been reported. Approaches include observation; medical treatment with somatostatin analogs, small molecules, or chemotherapy; embolization with or without chemotherapy; transarterial embolization with yttrium-90 microspheres; local ablative techniques; resection; and liver transplantation. Each of these options has been advocated, and good short- and medium-term results have been reported. This is more a reflection of the favorable biology of these tumors than of the merits of any particular therapy. In recent years, integration of the clinical, histological, and diagnostic techniques has led to the proposal of guidelines that may select out a small group of patients with metastatic NETs who have high potential for prolonged survival and even cure following liver transplantation [1,2]. These criteria, however, still need to be adequately validated in

multi-institutional studies before they can be accepted as the standard of care.

Liver transplantation is the accepted therapy for end-stage cirrhosis, with excellent long-term patient survival achievable in most cases. Transplantation has also come to be recognized as the best treatment for early but unresectable primary hepatocellular carcinoma (HCC), with results equaling those obtained in benign disease [3]. The role of liver transplantation in treatment of neuroendocrine metastatic tumors to the liver, on the other hand, is far less clear, and the results have historically been poor [4–7].

Liver metastasis is generally the result of hematogenous dissemination of tumor from the primary site. For tumors arising in the gut, where venous drainage is via the portal system, the liver is commonly the first place where metastases appear. Lymphatic metastasis typically occurs concurrently with hematogenous spread, but resection of the primary site can encompass the regional lymphatic bed.

Surgical cure in some patients with liver metastases does appear to be possible. A number of studies have reported the

10-year disease-free survival (DFS) following liver resection for metastatic colorectal cancer (the most frequent tumor type for which resection of metastases is performed). The reported 10-year DFS is about 20% in most studies [8–10]. As recurrence of colorectal cancer more than 10 years after resection has been shown to be extremely rare, these patients may well have been cured by the liver resection [10].

Not surprisingly, factors that predict survival after resection of colorectal liver metastases (number of tumors, maximal diameter, carcinoembryonic antigen (CEA) level, and response to neoadjuvant chemotherapy) also predict ease of resectability; patients with large, multiple metastases that were not downstaged to resectability by neoadjuvant chemotherapy, for whom transplantation might be proposed, are highly likely to experience recurrence [11,12]. While transplantation may reduce (although not eliminate) the likelihood of hepatic recurrence compared with resection, the majority of patients in whom recurrence develops after liver resection present with extrahepatic disease. In a recent study done in Norway, where the average waiting time for a liver transplantation is less than 1 month, 21 patients with nonresectable colorectal liver metastases underwent liver transplantation. After a median time of 6 months, 19 of the 21 patients had either local or systemic recurrence [6]. As the available limited literature on the subject bears out, transplantation for unresectable metastatic colon cancer is very unlikely to be curative.

Liver transplantation has been accepted as the treatment of choice for patients with unresectable HCC. Although the initial results following liver transplantation were disappointing [13,14], results have progressively improved, mainly by improving selection criteria, as defined in the landmark paper by Mazzaferro et al. [3]. The integration of these selection criteria (Milan criteria—one tumor smaller than 5 cm or less than three tumors smaller than 3 cm, no gross vascular invasion, and no extrahepatic dissemination) with organ allocation prioritization has resulted in significant improvement of outcomes, and the current 5-year survival and DFS parallel those obtained in patients transplanted for benign liver disease. Recent published data suggests that implementing a series of selection criteria in patients with metastatic NET can result in similar improvement in outcomes, and even cure, in selected groups of patients with neuroendocrine liver metastasis who undergo liver transplantation. As noted before, these criteria have not been adequately validated in prospective studies.

CLASSIFICATION OF NEUROENDOCRINE TUMORS

Clinical relevance

NETs of gastrointestinal or pancreatic origin comprise a diverse group of tumors with varying biology and natural history. The clinical consequences of these tumors may be the result of either their physical presence as space-occupying lesions or the production of hormones or hormone-like

Table 51.1 Definitions of neuroendocrine neoplasms of the digestive system according to 2010 WHO classifications

Grade	Definition
Low grade (G1)	Less than 2 mitoses/10 HPF and Ki67 index of ≤2%
Intermediate grade (G2)	2–20 mitoses/10 HPF or Ki67 index of 3%–20%
High grade (G3)	>20 mitoses/10 HPF or Ki67 index of >20%

substances that cause remote effects. When liver metastases occur, it is almost always multifocal in both lobes, although this may not be immediately evident. Not uncommonly, symptoms related to bulky liver metastases are the initial presentation; in some cases, a careful search reveals the site of the primary tumor, while in others, the location of the primary remains obscure despite thorough investigation.

The classification, grading, and staging of NETs have evolved through the years. NETs have been classified according to anatomical site of origin, hormonal production, and rate of proliferation. Current guidelines have been proposed by a number of organizations, including the World Health Organization (WHO) (Table 51.1), the European Neuroendocrine Tumor Society (ENETS), the American Joint Committee on Cancer (AJCC), and the North American Neuroendocrine Tumor Society (NANET) [15–18]. These guidelines aimed to establish standard terminology and incorporate the proliferative index in the grading system, thereby making a clear distinction between tumors according to their biologic behavior.

Site of origin

Based on the embryonic derivation of the site of origin, NETs may be classified as being of foregut, midgut, or hindgut origin. Foregut NETs most commonly arise in the pancreas. Often referred to as pancreatic neuroendocrine tumors (PNETs), these neoplasms may produce a wide array of peptide hormones with associated clinical syndromes. About 35% of PNETs are considered nonfunctioning; while these produce no active substances, they often produce measurable peptides, such as chromogranin A. The antigen profile in NETs includes chromogranin A, pancreatic polypeptide, neuron-specific enolase, α and β subunits of human chorionic gonadotrophin (HCG), pancreastatin, and synaptophysine. Serum chromogranin A is considered the best biomarker for NETs, and plasma levels have been shown to correlate with tumor burden, making it useful in monitoring response to treatment [19–21]. The likelihood of clinically malignant behavior also correlates to a significant degree with patterns of hormone production: insulin-producing tumors, for example, are rarely malignant, but gastrin-producing tumors and nonfunctioning PNETs commonly are. From an anatomical standpoint, the lymphatic drainage of the pancreatic bed is such that tumors that metastasize widely to the liver invariably invade regional nodes as well. These nodes are usually amenable to surgical resection *en bloc* with the primary tumor.

Tumors of the midgut origin, arising in the small bowel or proximal colon, are more uniform in their pattern of hormonal production, producing the array of substances that, when released in sufficient amounts, give rise to the carcinoid syndrome. The term *carcinoid tumor* was coined in 1907 by Dr Oberndorfer, a pathologist, and used to describe small bowel NETs, which appeared less aggressive than adenocarcinoma [22]. At one time, this term was applied to the entire spectrum of gastrointestinal NETs; later, it was applied specifically to tumors of mid- and hindgut origin [23]. There is a gradual move away from the term *carcinoid* in favor of the term *neuroendocrine tumor*, which is further classified according to site of origin and grade. The likelihood of metastases correlates with the location of the primary tumor: tumors arising in the rectum, for example, are less likely to metastasize than those arising in the small bowel. The regional lymphatic bed of the small bowel and colon should always be resected *en bloc* with the primary tumor to ensure removal of potential regional metasases.

Hormone production

NETs are commonly classified according to patterns of hormone production (Table 51.2). As mentioned above, there is fairly consistent correlation between the hormones produced and both the location of the primary tumor and the histological (and biological) grade of the tumor. From the standpoint of treatment decisions, including the decision to transplant, hormone secretion can be a very important factor. Despite the advent of pharmacological agents that are able to counter hormone-related symptoms (e.g., proton pump inhibitors for gastrinoma, somatostatin analogs for vasoactive intestinal peptide (VIP)-oma, and H1 and H2

Table 51.2 Antigens and hormones produced by neuroendocrine tumors

Gastrin
Kalikrein
Glucagon
Calcitonin
Histamine
Substance P
Somatostatin
HCG subunits
Prostaglandins
Neurokinin A and B
Neuropeptide K
Chromogranins A, B, and C
Pancreatic peptide
Insulin, proinsulin, and C-peptide
Vasoactive intestinal peptide
Serotonin and metabolites

blockers for carcinoid tumors), patients may develop disabling or life-threatening complications due to hormones released from NET liver metastases. The best palliation is achieved in such cases by resection of the metastases; if their number and distribution preclude partial hepatectomy, transplantation may be the best solution.

Rate of proliferation

Most current literature dealing with the classification of NETs focuses considerable attention on the degree of differentiation of the tumor. Based on cytological characteristics and markers of proliferation rate, such as Ki67 staining on immunohistochemistry, NETs may be graded as well-differentiated tumors, well-differentiated carcinomas, or poorly differentiated carcinomas. Grading of NETs in this way has proven clinically useful in estimating prognosis [24]. Transplantation is less likely to prolong life, and therefore is contraindicated in most centers, for patients with rapidly proliferating, poorly differentiated carcinomas [1,2,25].

ASSESSMENT OF THE PATIENT WITH NEUROENDOCRINE LIVER METASTASES

Evaluation of patients with NET liver metastases must encompass complete characterization of the tumor with regard to proliferation rate and hormone production, excellent liver imaging to accurately define the extent of liver involvement, an assessment of the adequacy of control of the primary tumor, delineation of the extent and location of extrahepatic metastases, and the physiological state of the patient.

Characterization of the tumor

A complete discussion of the biochemical assessment of patients with NETs is beyond the scope of this chapter. In order to counter possible hormone-related symptoms, help estimate prognosis, and establish useful markers of tumor activity, a complete profile of tumor-related hormonal products should be checked. Even patients with so-called "nonfunctioning" tumors typically have elevated levels of substances such as chromogranin A, which may be useful as markers of tumor activity after treatment [19–21].

The WHO classification system of NETs combines the location and histological features of tumor aggressiveness as determined by the number of mitotic counts per 10 high-power fields (HPF) and the percentage of cells that stain positive for Ki67 (Ki67 index) (Table 51.1) [15]. The prognostic significance of this grading system has been well demonstrated [26,27], and most centers would only consider low-grade tumors for liver transplantation, as more aggressive cancers have been shown to be associated with poor outcomes [1,2,25]. There is controversy, however, as to the exact cutoff level of the Ki67 index, above which transplantation is contraindicated, especially as the Ki67 index may be different within different areas of the same tumor

[28]. Significant interobserver variability of this index exists [29,30] and long term survival following liver transplantation for patients with Ki67 index >15% have been reported [31,32]. Additional markers of tumor aggressiveness may help in better defining patients who would benefit from liver transplantation. One possible such marker is E-cadherin, an adhesion molecule related to the metastatic potential of tumors. A study by Rosenau et al. suggests that a combination of normal E-cadherin staining with a Ki67 index of <5% is associated with excellent prognosis following liver transplantation [33].

Assessment of liver involvement

Either computed tomography (CT) or magnetic resonance imaging (MRI) may be employed to assess the extent of liver involvement. Scans must be used after the administration of intravenous iodinated contrast material (CT) or gadolinium (MRI). Unlike most other metastatic liver lesions, NET metastases are commonly hypervascular; dual-phase CT or MRI should thus be performed to provide maximal information.

The quality of imaging studies with which patients present for evaluation varies widely; the import of the decisions riding on imaging studies is such that referral centers must insist on top-quality images, even if studies of inferior quality have only recently been obtained elsewhere. Scans should be reviewed with the intent of resection. Liver resection employing the technique of tumor enucleation without regard for the classically desired 1-cm tumor-free margin is the first line of treatment, and may offer long-term benefit.

In past years, several hepatocyte-specific contrast agents have been developed for use in MRI. These agents are differentially taken up by the hepatocytes and excreted into the biliary system. Gadolinium-ethoxybenzyl-diethylenetriamine pentaacetic acid (Gd-EOB-DTPA) (Eovist; Primovist, Bayer Healthcare) has the characteristics of both an extracellular gadolinium contrast agent and a hepatocyte-specific contrast agent [34]. Gd-EOB-DTPA contrast studies have been used in clinical practice in recent years and were shown to be highly accurate in the identification and characterization of liver tumors [35]. The delayed phase imaging, in which the hepatocytes contain the contrast material, and are therefore bright, allows identification of very small lesions that are not made of hepatocytes, and therefore do not take up the contrast material. In a recent small comparative study, MRI with Gd-EOB-DTPA contrast was found to be superior to biphasic contrast-enhanced CT in the detection and characterization of hepatic metastases from NETs [36].

The majority of NETs express several distinct receptors, among them the somatostatin receptor. This characteristic makes them ideal candidates for functional imaging with radiolabeled somatostatin analogs. Gallium-labeled somatostatin analog DOTA(0)-Phe(1)-Tyr(3)-octreotide (DOTATOC) as a PNET tracer, especially when fused to CT imaging, was shown to be an excellent tool for the detection and staging of gastrointestinal NETs [37,38]. It was shown to be superior to standard imaging techniques (biphasic contrast-enhanced CT and MRI scans using gadolinium as contrast) for the detection of NET-derived liver metastases, and for the definition of inconclusive liver lesions in patients with NETs [39]. Additional detailed morphologic characterization of the lesions, and their relation to major vascular structures using CT or MRI, is mandatory for assessment of resectability and planning of the surgical procedure.

Assessment of the primary site

In patients with NET metastases, the primary tumor may be discovered before, at the time of, or after the recognition of liver involvement, or in a small minority of patients, not at all (there is some debate over whether the liver may represent the primary site for such tumors). Certainly, the liver is a "fertile field" for these tumors, and the common observation that liver metastases typically grow faster and larger than their primary progenitors is supported by experimental evidence [40,41]. In cases where the primary tumor has been resected, the pathology report should be reviewed to determine the adequacy of the resection and the extent of nodal involvement. Imaging with CT and octreotide scan or, alternatively, Ga68 DOTATOC positron emission tomography (PET)/CT scan is used to search for residual regional disease.

It is not unusual for the primary tumor to be discovered by careful assessment of imaging studies, including CT, octreotide scan, or PET/CT, when a patient presents with symptoms related to liver metastases. The body and tail of the pancreas have proved to be the most common site of origin in such cases. While there may be room for debate as to the proper course, most centers would advocate for resection of the primary tumor early in the course of treatment of such patients, usually via laparoscopic distal pancreatectomy. The aim of this approach is to remove the source of ongoing metastasis, since there is no effective regional therapy, such as chemoembolization, for the pancreas. In patients with impaired liver function from extensive tumor load, who are not candidates for preliminary resection of the primary, combined liver transplantation and resection of the primary tumor may be considered. In recent years, however, combined transplantation and extensive surgery for the primary tumor have rarely been done, as a number of studies have clearly demonstrated that the short- and long-term outcomes of such patients are poor [1,2,42]. Poor survival in these patients is related to increased perioperative mortality, and also reflects the extensive tumor load necessitating such procedures.

Ten to fifteen percent of patients present with extensive NET liver metastases in the absence of detectable primary tumor [2,43]. There is controversy in the literature regarding whether these patients can be candidates for liver transplantation. The obvious concern is that the primary tumor will continue to seed metastases, reducing the chance of cure or prolonged survival. The previously mentioned

Milan group has included resection of the primary site and having a primary tumor that has portal drainage as criteria for liver transplant candidacy [1]. Other centers have used more deliberate selection criteria and allowed patients with unidentified primary tumor to be transplant candidates, with 5-year survival comparable to those of patients that had the primary tumor resected [2]. Our practice in these cases is to proceed with treatment of the liver and to continue surveillance in anticipation of the discovery of the primary site. Identification of the primary tumor is not, in our opinion, a strict prerequisite to proceeding with liver transplantation.

Evaluation of extrahepatic disease

A complete picture of the extent of disease is extremely valuable both in planning treatment and in properly informing the patient. Common sites of extrahepatic metastasis include abdominal lymph nodes, lung, and bone. CT of the chest and bone scan are thus routinely performed. As the majority of NETs demonstrate avidity for octreotide, nuclear scanning with labeled octreotide is often useful in the detection of disease in unlikely locations, as well as to confirm the nature of questionable disease seen on imaging studies. However, the sensitivity of the octreotide scan is only 50%–80% [44,45], and better imaging modalities are needed. The Ga68 DOTATOC PET/CT and DOPA PET/CT scans have recently been introduced, giving information on both location and function, and have a much higher sensitivity, reaching 80%–96% [39,46], and a resolution value of 5 mm, compared with 15 mm for the octreotide scan.

The presence of extrahepatic disease does not automatically preclude liver transplantation for NET metastases. As has been discussed, the biological behavior of the tumor is of slow growth, and long-term survival can be achieved in patients that have extrahepatic metastases. There is growing consensus in the literature that patients with extrahepatic disease are not excluded from liver transplantation, providing all extrahepatic disease are resected before transplantation with curative intent. Patients with unresectable extrahepatic metastatic disease are not considered candidates for liver transplantation in most centers.

Physiological assessment of the patient

Among all the treatments that have been advocated for NET liver metastases, liver transplantation is surely the most radical, with the greatest morbidity and mortality; its value as a tumor treatment diminishes in direct proportion to the likelihood of treatment-related death. Careful assessment of cardiac, pulmonary, and renal function is part of every transplant evaluation. Diverse factors, such as obesity, smoking, diabetes, psychiatric issues, and advancing age, must all be figured into the complex decision for transplant. Liver resection employing the technique of tumor enucleation without regard for the classically desired 1-cm tumor-free margin is the first line of treatment, and may offer long-term benefit.

TRANSPLANT OPERATION

Liver transplantation techniques have been well described elsewhere [47]; the technical aspects of transplantation in patients with NET metastases are essentially the same as for other indications. Transplantation in these cases is typically facilitated by the fact that the patients do not generally have underlying liver disease with associated portal hypertension and coagulopathy. On the other hand, bulky disease may complicate the hepatectomy. For patients in whom the primary tumor has not been resected, or additional extrahepatic tumor is present at the time of transplant, concomitant procedures, such as lymphadenectomy, distal pancreatectomy, pancreaticoduodenectomy, or gastrointestinal resection, have been performed at the time of transplant. As noted before, recent studies have shown that both short- and long-term outcomes for patients who undergo concomitant major resection of extrahepatic tumors at the time of liver transplantation are poor [1,2,42]. The current consensus accepted by most centers is therefore to avoid concomitant major extrahepatic procedures at the time of liver transplantation.

Anesthesia management in patients with hormonally active NETs is potentially complicated. Administration of H1 and H2 histamine receptor antagonists and corticosteroids and continuous infusion of the somatostatin analog octreotide are useful in preventing the release of hormonal mediators that can cause wide fluctuations in blood pressure and may result from intraoperative tumor manipulation [48].

Tumors and immunosuppression

Immunosuppression is required for transplantation to be successful, except in the case of identical twins. The mainstay of liver transplant immunosuppression has been the calcineurin inhibitors cyclosporine and tacrolimus. There is now considerable evidence that these medications are associated with an increased incidence of cancer, including malignancies that are caused by viruses (lymphoma, Kaposi sarcoma, and anogenital cancers) and cancers that are not caused by viruses (lung, kidney, skin, and thyroid) [49–51]. There is conflicting data as to whether cyclosporine and tacrolimus, which are known to augment liver regeneration, may influence the course of recurrence of primary HCC after transplantation [52,53]. There is some data suggesting that higher plasma levels of both tacrolimus and cyclosporine, especially in the early postoperative period, are associated with higher HCC recurrence rates [52]. Nevertheless, the relevance to recurrence of metastatic tumors following liver transplantation is unclear.

The mammalian target of rapamycin (mTOR) inhibitors sirolimus and everolimus have been shown to be effective in preventing rejection after liver transplantation [54,55], and are currently approved by the European Medicine Agency for preventing organ rejection after liver transplantation. These agents are not approved for use in the United

States in the early posttransplant period due to concerns for increased rates of hepatic artery thrombosis and infections associated with their use (www.fda.gov). Interestingly, these agents were also shown to have antineoplastic properties. A number of studies have shown that in patients transplanted for HCC, sirolimus-based immunosuppression is associated with better overall and recurrence-free survival when compared with calcineurin inhibitor-based immunosuppression [56,57]. The antineoplastic effects of everolimus on PNETs have been well demonstrated. A randomized phase 3, double-blinded, placebo-controlled multicenter trial showed that everolimus was effective in prolonging survival and progression-free survival in patients with low- or intermediate-grade PNET [58]. The use of sirolimus or everolimus posttransplant may offer help in preventing both liver rejection and tumor recurrence, thereby improving long-term survival of these patients.

RATIONAL APPROACH TO PATIENTS WITH NEUROENDOCRINE LIVER METASTASES

As alluded to in the overview at the beginning of this chapter, it is the generally slow-growing nature of NETs, rather than the benefit of any particular therapy, that explains the relatively long survival of patients with neuroendocrine liver metastases compared with those with metastases from other sources. Nevertheless, most patients with this disease ultimately develop significant symptoms and die as a result. The challenge for those who care for them is to choose wisely among the available modalities in order to maximize both the quality and length of life. Bearing in mind the biological behavior of this tumor, it seems most reasonable to withhold the most radical treatment (i.e., liver transplantation) until it is clear that the patient is in imminent trouble and that treatment options less likely to result in serious complication or death have been exhausted. Thus, while the focus of this chapter is liver transplantation, a limited discussion of the array of treatment options seems appropriate to provide an adequate context within which to place the transplant option.

Observation

After obtaining blood and tissue sufficient to fully characterize the tumor, consideration should be given to a period of observation in the patient newly diagnosed with neuroendocrine liver metastases. When possible, this allows the physician and the patient to gain some perspective on the nature of the particular tumor with which they are faced, for it must be admitted that despite the various tests and classification schemes that have been developed, the clinical behavior of the tumor cannot be predicted with complete accuracy. In considering the merits of active intervention, it should always be kept in mind that patients with liver metastases from NETs have a 30% overall 5-year survival and a median survival of 3–4 years without treatment [59,60].

Medical therapy

Medical treatment is indicated for symptom control and progressive disease when surgery or local ablative procedures are not possible. Current medical treatments include four classes of agents: biotherapeutics, including somatostatin analogs and interferon-α; chemotherapy, including streptozotocin, temozolamide, and platinum-containing agents; small molecules, including sunitinib and everolimus; and monoclonal antibodies, including bevacizumab.

The specific profiles of efficacy, side effects, and cost have not been prospectively compared in patients with liver metastases from NETs. Long-term treatment with somatostatin analogs was shown to be effective in symptom tumor growth control with relatively minor side effects, and represents the standard of care in these patients. Randomized, double-blinded, placebo-controlled prospective studies have shown both sunitinib and everolimus to be effective in prolonging progression-free survival among patients with advanced metastatic PNETs, with a low rate of severe side effects [58,61].

Liver resection

There is a considerable body of literature advocating resection as the preferred treatment for neuroendocrine liver metastases when technically possible [62–64]. While these many studies quote respectable medium-term survival figures, close review reveals that reports of cure as evidenced by DFS beyond 5 years are few. Mayo et al. reported the outcome of 339 patients who underwent liver resection for neuroendocrine liver metastases at eight major hepatobiliary centers. The 5- and 10-year survivals following resection were 74%, and 51%, respectively. However, disease recurred in 94% of the patients at 5 years [62]. Resection should be viewed, then, not as qualitatively different than treatments such as radiofrequency ablation (RFA) of chemoembolization, but rather as an alternative means to tumor reduction with its unique advantages and disadvantages.

Frilling et al. [65] classified patterns of NET liver metastasis distribution as type 1 (isolated single lesion), type 2 (a large focus of metastatic lesions with smaller surrounding lesions, in both liver lobes), and type 3 (widely disseminated metastatic spread with minimal normal hepatic parenchyma). The clearest indication for resection is in symptomatic patients with type 1 or select patients with type 2 tumor spread that are technically amenable to complete resection. In competent hands, resection can be carried out with low (0%–2%) mortality, and after a limited period of surgery-related morbidity, the patient may experience prolonged symptom relief without need for repeated interventions. By contrast, large tumors (>4 cm) are not technically suitable for percutaneous ablation techniques, and control in such cases with other therapeutic modalities is both less certain and considerably more drawn out.

The role for subtotal resection is, in the authors' view, limited to cases with documented slow progression of tumors that are producing hormone-related symptoms. As the degree of symptoms is related to the bulk of tumor, significant surgical reduction in tumor volume can result in significant periods of relief quicker and more reliably than can other modalities.

Ablative techniques

These technologies extend the ability of the surgeon to physically eliminate tumor tissue and should be viewed as complementary rather than competing with surgery. Because the majority of patients present with multifocal involvement of the liver, these techniques, like resection, that focus on particular tumors are not likely to ever become the mainstay of therapy.

RFA may be performed percutaneously, and is effective in destroying tumors up to 4–5 cm in diameter. Because it is uncommon for patients to present with a limited number of tumors all of which are amenable to RFA, this will rarely be the primary treatment. More commonly, RFA finds application intraoperatively as an adjunct to surgery to treat small lesions that are present deep within the liver of a patient undergoing resection, or percutaneously in treating new tumors that develop during follow-up after resection.

Other local ablative techniques that have been used in patients with NET liver metastases include laser ablation [66], cryotherapy [67,68], and ethanol injection [69,70]. Small series of these measures have reported successful symptom control and tumor response. Most centers, however, use RFA because of better treatment results and lower morbidity rates. The recently introduced microwave coagulation technique utilizes electromagnetic microwaves causing cell death through coagulation necrosis. This technique may be superior to RFA in larger tumors [71].

Transcatheter arterial embolization and chemoembolization

The typically highly vascular nature of neuroendocrine metastases renders them good candidates for transcatheter arterial embolization (TAE) [72] and chemoembolization (TACE) [73,74]. A catheter is inserted via the femoral (or brachial) artery and advanced into the hepatic artery, followed by injection of contrast. Tumors light up as a blush of contrast; the catheter is then advanced into the branches of the artery supplying the tumor, and injection is made first of chemotherapeutic agents, in the case of TACE, followed by particles to occlude small branches of the artery. As the liver has a dual blood supply, nourished by both the hepatic artery and the portal vein, whereas liver metastases derive their blood supply virtually entirely from the artery, this treatment disproportionally kills tumors relative to the surrounding liver. It remains debatable whether the addition of cytotoxic drugs to embolization material increases the effectiveness of bland embolization [75,76]. The arterial occlusion produced by TAE or TACE is transitory, allowing for repeated treatment. Because it is delivered via the hepatic artery, which supplies (albeit with a number of anatomical variations) the entire liver, TAE or TACE may be employed perfectly well in cases of diffuse metastasis.

In order to minimize the effects resulting from the destruction of a large amount of tumor, patients with extensive metastases are generally treated in multiple sessions, treating only a portion of the liver at any one setting. In patients deemed by virtue of symptoms, extent of liver involvement, or rate of progression to require treatment, TACE is a commonly employed approach at Mount Sinai. With repeated chemoembolization, it is often possible to maintain patients with diffuse liver involvement who get to the point of requiring therapy, over a period of years, with an acceptable quality of life.

Radioembolization

Selective internal radiation therapy (SIRT), or transarterial radioembolization, using Y90-labeled microspheres, is a novel treatment modality for liver cancer. The technique involves the intra-arterial injection of Y90-labeled microspheres through the hepatic artery. Two types of Y90-labeled microspheres are commercially available: SIRspheres (resin spheres) and TheraSpheres (glass spheres). Both types of microspheres gain entry to the tumor after injection to the artery, but will not pass through the capillary bed to the venous circulation, thus becoming trapped in the tumor. As described above, the tumors derive most of their blood supply from the artery; therefore, arterial injection of the spheres results in their accumulation within the tumor at a much higher concentration than in adjacent liver tissue, and exposure of the tumor to a high dose of local radiation, while sparing the normal liver. This technique has been used successfully for various hepatic malignancies, including NET metastases [77–80]. Small series of selective hepatic arterial administration of radionuclide-labeled somatostatin analogs have also been reported, in patients with large somatostatin receptor-positive tumors, with clinical and radiological response [81,82].

Radiotherapy and peptide receptor radionuclide therapy

Conventional radiotherapy has no role in the treatment of NET liver metastases. In recent years, peptide receptor radionuclide therapy (PRRT) has evolved as a new treatment option for patients with advanced NETs [83]. PRRT involves the combination of a somatostatin analog with an isotope capable of providing cytotoxic radiation. Imaging with somatostatin-linked scans can serve both as a diagnostic tool and to identify potential therapeutic targets with PRRT. A number of radiolabeled somatostatin analogs have been investigated in patients with advanced and progressive disease, with response rates of up to 34% and disease stabilization rates of up to 74% [84,85]. According to the ENETS guidelines, although still considered investigational, PRRT is currently the recommended treatment after failure of medical treatments.

Liver transplantation

Traditionally, liver transplantation was thought to provide palliation for patients with extensive, symptomatic, slowly progressive disease, when no other options remained, provided they were physiologically capable of withstanding the transplant surgery and had no evidence of overwhelming extrahepatic disease. The main expectation in these cases was for patients to gain a number of years with good-quality life. This conception was based on small case series, reporting a very small number of transplant patients being disease-free at 5 years. In recent years, larger multicenter studies with long-follow-up data have been able to identify risk factors for recurrence and mortality [2,42,86–88], and a small prospective series with strict inclusion criteria for transplantation has shown exceptional outcomes [89], resulting in growing consensus that selected patients with neuroendocrine liver metastases may achieve prolonged DFS, and some may even be cured with liver transplantation.

The rationale for liver transplantation includes (1) achievement of R0 resection, which may not be provided by other multimodality treatments; (2) liver failure from metastatic replacement is a major cause of death even without extrahepatic spread; (3) immediate and durable symptom control; (4) survival benefit; and (5) technically feasible.

One prospective study on liver transplantation in patients with NETs was performed by the Milan group and summarized in Table 51.3 [1]. This group has been performing liver transplantation using strict selection criteria. Inclusion

criteria were low-grade tumors, primary tumor drained by the portal system and removed with a curative resection before transplantation, involvement of less than 50% of the liver, no progression of disease for at least 6 months before the transplantation, and age of <55 years. Using these criteria, they report outstanding outcomes, with a 5-year survival of 96% and DFS of 80% at the last follow-up of 30 patients [89].

Timing of liver transplantation in patients with NET liver metastases is a controversial issue. Some centers advocate transplantation for patients who have demonstrated disease stability over an observation time or response to medical treatment [1,86,87,90]. Others would argue that liver transplantation should be used as the last line of treatment, and only be offered to patients who demonstrate disease progression refractory to medical treatment [42,65,91,92]. A clear recommendation on this issue, based on current published data, cannot be established, due to the small number of patients and the slow-growing nature of these tumors. This issue was recently reviewed and defined by Fan et al. [93]. The consensus conference practice recommendations for transplantation were strong for the following cases: (1) nonresectable NET liver metastasis resistant to medical treatment and (2) liver-limited well-differentiated (G1–G2) NETs. Recommendations remain controversial when selecting cases based on disease stability of more than 6 months and living donor availability.

OUTCOME OF LIVER TRANSPLANTATION FOR METASTATIC NEUROENDOCRINE TUMORS

Risk factors associated with poor prognosis, as well as outcomes of previously published series, are summarized in Tables 51.4 and 51.5 [1,2,31,33,65,86,87,94].

In 1998, the first meta-analysis of 103 patients from 23 centers was published, with 1- and 5-year survivals of 68% and 47%, respectively, and a 5-year DFS rate of 24%. Age

Table 51.3 Indications for liver transplantation in patients with liver metastasis

Inclusion criteria

Low-grade carcinoid tumor (G0–G1) with or without syndrome

Curative resectable primary tumor (separate from transplantation) with portal drainage (from distal stomach to sigmoid colon)

Liver tumor burden of ≤50%

Good response or stable disease for at least 6 months pretransplantation

Age of ≤55 years

Exclusion criteria

Small cell carcinoma or high-grade neuroendocrine carcinomas

Contraindicating for transplantations (medical or surgical conditions)

Nongastrointestinal carcinoid or NET drained outside of portal system

Table 51.4 Reported risk factors associated with poor prognosis post-liver transplantation for metastatic neuroendocrine tumors

Risk factors

Age of >50 years

Symptomatic tumor

Primary tumor located in the pancreas

Noncarcinoid tumor

Primary tumor with nonportal drainage

Ki67 of >5%–10%

Tumor burden of >50%

Extrahepatic spread

Primary tumor not resected

Disease progression

High-grade tumor

Table 51.5 Reported series on outcome post-transplantation for metastatic neuroendocrine tumors

Author (reference)	Year	No. of patients	5-year OS (%)	5-year DFS [5]
Rosenau et al. [33]	2002	19	80	22
Olausson et al. [31]	2007	15	90	18
Mazzaferro et al. [1]	2007	24	90	77
Le Treut et al. [94]	2008	85	47	20
Frilling et al. [65]	2009	15	67	48
Gedaly et al. [86]	2011	150	49	32
Nguyen et al. [87]	2011	184	49	—
Le Treut et al. [2]	2013	213	52	30

Note: OS, overall survival.

of >50 years and transplantation combined with upper abdominal exenteration or Whipple's operation were identified as adverse prognostic factors on multivariate analysis [42].

The largest multicenter study published so far was done by Le Treut et al. [2] and included 213 patients who underwent liver transplantation for NETs in Europe between 1982 and 2009. The mean duration of follow-up was 56 months, and 172 patients (81%) had at least 5 years of follow-up after the liver transplantation. The perioperative mortality was 10%, and the 5-year overall survival was 52%. The 5-year disease survival rate was 30%. These results compare favorably with a previous 1997 report by the same group, in which the 5-year survival rate was only 36%. Predictors of poor outcome included major resection in addition to liver transplantation, poorly differentiated tumor, of age >45, and hepatomegaly. Patients transplanted after 2000 had better 5-year survival (59%), probably due to better patient selection.

Other multicentric studies performed in America showed outcomes similar to those in Le Treut's study. A study by Gedaly et al. [86] reviewed the United Network for Organ Sharing (UNOS) database and analyzed data on 150 patients who underwent liver transplantation for NET. The 1- and 5-year survivals were 81% and 49%, respectively. They found that patients that were on the waiting list for more than 2 months had improved survival. Sher et al. [88] presented results of a multicenter American study on patients transplanted for NET liver metastases. They collected data on 72 patients from 24 U.S. centers. The 1- and 5-year survivals were 84%, and 50%, respectively.

THE MOUNT SINAI EXPERIENCE

Since April 1992, 13 patients were transplanted at our institution for metastatic NETs. The patient characteristics are summarized in Table 51.6. Of the 13 patients, 8 had recurrences and were treated with a combination of locoregional and systemic therapy. At a median follow-up of 70 months, our 1-, 3-, and 5-year survival rates are 90%, 70%, and 60%, respectively (Figure 51.1).

In addition, since 1998 we have considered patients for living donor liver transplantation. The availability of living donors limited the waiting time on the transplant list and helped optimize the procedure.

The most important concept we have learned is that it is essential to carefully select patients based on criteria published by previous large series. All patients are evaluated by a multidisciplinary team, and candidates are strictly selected based on favorable tumor biology, stable disease, tumor burden on imaging, and their overall health, such as performance score, nutritional status, and comorbidities.

Table 51.6 Patient characteristics and outcome: the Mount Sinai experience

Patient	Age	Gender	Type	Resection of primary	Alive	Recurrence	Survival (months)	Comments
1	41	F	N/F	Distal pancreas[a]	N	Y	76	
2	52	M	VIP	Distal pancreas	Y	N	115	
3	57	M	N/F	Distal pancreas	N	Y	39	
4	54	M	N/F	Distal pancreas[a]	N	Y	74	
5	35	F	N/F	Whipple[a]	N	N	0	COD: Pulmonary embolism
6	57	F	Carcinoid	Appendix	N	N	0	Intraoperative death
7	23	F	N/F	Distal pancreas[a]	N	Y	16	Living donor
8	66	F	N/F		N	Y	18	NET unknown prior to OLT
9	69	M	VIP	Distal pancreas	N	N	0	Intraoperative death
10	57	F	Carcinoid	Ileum	N	Y	147	Living donor
11	57	F	Carcinoid	Rectum	N	Y	12	Living donor
12	37	F	N/F	Stomach	Y	N	99	
13	62	M	Carcinoid	Distal pancreas[a]	N	Y	66	

Note: COD, cause of death; N, no; Y, yes; N/F, nonfunctioning; OLT, orthotopic liver transplantation.
[a] At the time of transplantation.

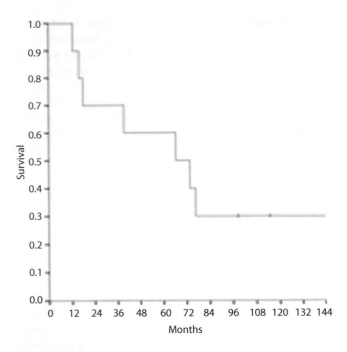

Figure 51.1 Mt Sinai patient survival after liver transplant for neuroendocrine metastases.

CONCLUSION

Liver transplantation for treatment of metastatic NETs is radical. It is a valid option for physically fit patients with unresectable disease in the liver. There is growing consensus, based on large multicenter retrospective studies, that selected patients can achieve a long disease-free interval, or even cure, after liver transplantation. Selection criteria are not completely defined, but should probably include having disease confined to the liver, well-differentiated tumors with a low Ki67 index (less than 10%–15%), and that liver transplantation should not be combined with additional major extrahepatic resections. Adding more criteria, such as age limit (45) and limited involvement of the liver, may further improve the long-term results, at the cost of denying liver transplantation to patients who would still benefit from it. The timing of liver transplantation in patients with metastatic NET is still a controversial issue. Whether it should be indicated in patients who respond to medical treatment and have a stable disease over 6–12 months of observation or, alternatively, be reserved for patients who fail systemic therapy and present with progressive disease is a debate that cannot be answered with the current published data.

REFERENCES

1. Mazzaferro V, Pulvirenti A, Coppa J. Neuroendocrine tumors metastatic to the liver: How to select patient for liver transplantation? *J Hepatol* 2007;47:454–75.
2. Le Treut YP, Gregoire E, Klempnauer J et al. Liver transplantation for neuroendocrine tumors in Europe—Results and trends in patient selection. *Ann Surg* 2013;257:807–15.
3. Mazzaferro V, Regalia E, Andreola S et al. Liver transplantation for the treatment of small hepatocellular carcinomas in patients with cirrhosis. *N Engl J Med* 1996;334:693–9.
4. Pichlmayr R. Is there a place for liver grafting for malignancy? *Transplant Proc* 1988;20:478–82.
5. Penn I. Hepatic transplantation for primary and metastatic cancers of the liver. *Surgery* 1991;110:726–34.
6. Hagness M, Foss A, Line P et al. Liver transplantation for nonresectable liver metastases from colorectal cancer. *Ann Surg* 2013;257:800–6.
7. Foss A, Adam R, Dueland S. Liver transplantation for colorectal liver metastases: Revisiting the concept. *Transpl Int* 2010;23:679–85.
8. Pulitano C, Castillo F, Aldrighetti L et al. What defines "cure" after liver resection for colorectal metastases? Results after 10 years of follow up. *HPB* 2010;12:244–9.
9. Vigano L, Ferrero A, Lo Tesoriere R, Capussotti L. Liver surgery for colorectal metastases: Results after 10 years of follow-up. Long-term survivors, late recurrences, and prognostic role of morbidity. *Ann Surg Oncol.* 2008;15:2458–64.
10. Tomlinson JS, Jarnagin WR, DeMatteo RP et al. Actual 10-year survival after resection of colorectal liver metastases defines cure. *J Clin Oncol* 2007;25:4575–80.
11. Fong Y, Fortner J, Sun RL, Brennan MF, Blumgart LH. Clinical score for predicting recurrence after hepatic resection for metastatic colorectal cancer: Analysis of 1001 consecutive cases. *Ann Surg* 1999;230:309–18.
12. Pawlick T, Choti MA. Shifting from clinical to biologic indicators of prognosis after resection of hepatic colorectal metastases. *Curr Oncol Rep* 2007;9:193–201.
13. Bismuth H, Chiche L, Adam R, Castaing D, Diamond T, Dennison A. Liver resection versus transplantation for hepatocellular carcinoma in cirrhotic patients. *Ann Surg* 1993;218:145–51.
14. Iwatsuki S, Starzl TE, Shehan DG et al. Hepatic resection versus transplantation for hepatocellular carcinoma. *Ann Surg* 1991;214:221–8.
15. Bosman FT, Carneiro F, Hruban RH, Theise ND. *WHO Classification of Tumours of the Digestive System.* 4th ed. Lyon: International Agency for Research on Cancer, 2010.
16. Kloppel G, Rindi G, Perren A, Komminoth P, Klimstra DS. The ENETS and AJCC/UICC TNM classification of the neuroendocrine tumors of the gastrointestinal tract and the pancreas: A statement. *Virchows Arch* 2010;456:595–7.
17. Edge S, Byrd D, Compton CC, Fritz AG, Greene FL, Trotti A. *AJCC Cancer Staging Manual.* 7th ed. New York: Springer, 2010.
18. Vinik AL, Woltering EA, Warner RR et al. NANETS consensus guidelines for the diagnosis of neuroendocrine tumor. *Pancreas* 2010;39:713–34.

19. Campana D, Nori F, Pricitelli L et al. Chromogranin A: Is it a useful marker of neuroendocrine tumors? *J Clin Oncol* 2007;25:1967–73.

20. Seregni E, Ferrari L, Bajetta E, Martinetti A, Bombardieri E. Clinical significance of blood chromogranin A measurement in neuroendocrine tumours. *Ann Oncol* 2001;12(Suppl 2):S69–72.

21. Stivanello M, Berruti A, Torta M et al. Circulating chromogranin A in the assessment of patients with neuroendocrine tumours. A single institution experience. *Ann Oncol* 2001;12(Suppl 2):S73–77.

22. Oberndorfer S. Karzenoidetumoren des dunndarm. *Franfurt Z Pathol* 1907;1:426–30.

23. Creutzfeldt W. Carcinoid tumor: Development of our knowledge. *World J Surg* 1996;20:120–31.

24. Pelosi G, Bresaola E, Bogina G et al. Endocrine tumors of the pancreas: Ki67 immunoreactivity on paraffin sections is an independent predictor for malignancy: A comparative study with proliferating-cell nuclear antigen and progesterone receptor protein immunostaining, mitotic index, and other clinicopathologic variables. *Hum Pathol* 1996;27:1124–34.

25. Pavel M, Baudin E, Couvelard A et al. ENETS consensus guidelines for the management of patients with liver and other distant metastases from neuroendocrine neoplasms of foregut, midgut, hindgut and unknown primary. *Neuroendocrinology* 2012;95:157–76.

26. La Rosa S, Klersy C, Uccela S et al. Improved histologic and clinicopathologic criteria for prognostic evaluation of pancreatic neuroendocrine tumors. *Hum Pathol* 2009;40:30–40.

27. Pape UF, Jann H, Muller-Nordhorn J et al. Prognostic relevance of a novel TNM classification system for upper gastroenteropancreatic neuroendocrine tumors. *Cancer* 2008;113:256–65.

28. Couvelard A, Deschamps L, Ravaud P et al. Heterogeneity of tumor prognostic markers: A reproducibility study applied to liver metastases of pancreatic endocrine tumors. *Mod Pathol* 2009;22:273–81.

29. Rindi G, Kloppel G, Alhman H et al. TNM staging of foregut (neuro)endocrine tumors: A consensus proposal including a grading system. *Virchows Arch* 2006;449:395–401.

30. Rindi G, Kloppel G, Couvelard A et al. TNM staging of midgut and hindgut (neuro)endocrine tumors: A consensus proposal including a grading system. *Virchows Arch* 2007;451:757–62.

31. Olausson M, Friman S, Herlenius G et al. Orthotopic liver or multivisceral transplantation as treatment of metastatic neuroendocrine tumors. *Liver Transpl* 2007;13:327–33.

32. Bonaccorsi-Riani E, Apestegui C, Jouret-Mourin A et al. Liver transplantation and neuroendocrine tumors: Lessons from a single centre experience and from the literature review. *Transpl Int* 2010;23:668–78.

33. Rosenau J, Bahr MJ, von Waiselewski R et al. Ki67, E-cadherin, and p53 as prognostic indicators of long-term outcome after liver transplantation for metastatic neuroendocrine tumors. *Transplantation* 2002;73:386–94.

34. Reimer P, Schneider G, Schima W. Hepatobiliary contrast agents for contrast-enhanced MRI of the liver: Properties, clinical development and applications. *Eur Radiol* 2004;14:559–78.

35. Burke C, Grant LA, Goh V, Griffin N. The role of hepatocyte-specific contrast agents in hepatobiliary magnetic resonance imaging. *Semin Ultrasound CT MRI* 2013;34:44–53.

36. Giesela FL, Kratochwila C, Mehndirattab A et al. Comparison of neuroendocrine tumor detection using DOTATOC-PET in correlation with contrast enhanced CT and delayed contrast enhanced MRI. *Eur J Radiol* 2012;81:2820–5.

37. Ruf J, Heuck F, Schiefer J et al. Impact of multiphase Ga68-DOTATOC-PET/CT on therapy management in patients with neuroendocrine tumors. *Neuroendocrinology* 2010;91:101–9.

38. Miederer M, Seidl S, Buck A et al. Correlation of immunohistopathological expression of somatostatin receptor 2 with standardized uptake values in Ga68-DOTATOC PET/CT. *Eur J Nucl Med Mol Imaging* 2009;36:48–52.

39. Frilling A, Sotiropoulos GC, Radtke A et al. The impact of Ga68-DOTATOC positron emission tomography/computed tomography on the multimodal management of patients with neuroendocrine tumors. *Ann Surg* 2010;252:850–6.

40. Harvellar IJ, Sugarpaker PH, Vermess M, Miller DL. Rate of growth of intraabdominal metastases from colorectal cancer. *Cancer* 1984;54:163–71.

41. Hara Y, Ogata Y, Shirouzo K. Early tumor growth in metastatic organs influenced by the microenvironment is an important factor which provides organ specificity of colon cancer metastasis. *J Exp Clin Can Res* 2000;19:497–504.

42. Lenhert T. Liver transplantation for metastatic neuroendocrine carcinoma: An analysis of 103 patients. *Transplantation* 1998;66:1307–12.

43. Yao JC, Hassan M, Phan A et al. One hundred years after "carcinoid": Epidemiology of and prognostic factors for neuroendocrine tumors in 35825 cases in the United States. *J Clin Oncol* 2008;20:3063–72.

44. Modlin IM, Oberg K, Chung DC et al. Gastroenteropancreatic neuroendocrine tumors. *Lancet Oncol* 2008;9:61–72.

45. Lebtani R, Cadiot G, Delahaye N, Genin R, Daou D, Peker MC. Detection of bone metastases in patients with gastroenteropancreatic tumors: Bone scintigraphy compared with somatostatin receptor scintigraphy. *J Nucl Med* 1999;40:1602.

46. Haug A, Auernhammer CJ, Wangler B et al. Intraindividual comparison of Ga68-DOTA-TATE

and 18F-DOPA PET in patients with well differentiated neuroendocrine tumours. *Eur J Nucl Med Mol Imaging* 2009;36:765–70.

47. Busuttil RW, Klintmalm GD. *Transplantation of the Liver.* Amsterdam: Elsevier, 2005.

48. Claure RE, Drover DD, Haddow GR, Esquivel CO, Angst MS. Orthotopic liver transplantation for carcinoid tumour metastatic to the liver: Anesthetic management. *Can J Anesth* 2000;47:334–7.

49. Vajdic CM, Can Leewen MT. Cancer incidence and risk factors after solid organ transplantation. *Int J Cancer* 2009;125:1747–54.

50. Collett D, Mumford L, Banner NR, Neuberger J, Watson C. Comparison of incidence of malignancy in recipients of different types of organ: A UK registry audit. *Am J Transplant* 2010;10:1889–96.

51. Engels EA, Pfeiffer RM, Faumeni JF Jr et al. Spectrum of cancer risk among US solid organ transplant recipients. *JAMA* 2011;206:1891–901.

52. Rodriguez-Peralvarez M, Tsochatzis E, Neveas MC et al. Reduced exposure to calcineurin inhibitors early after liver transplantation prevents recurrence of hepatocellular carcinoma. *J Hepatol* 2013;59:1193–9.

53. Vivarelli M, Cucchetti A, La Barba G et al. Liver transplantation for hepatocellular carcinoma under calcineurin inhibitors: Reassessment of risk factors for tumor recurrence. *Ann Surg* 2008;248:857–62.

54. Toso C, Meeberg GA, Bigam DL et al. De novo sirolimus-based immunosuppression after liver transplantation for hepatocellular carcinoma: Long-term outcomes and side effects. *Transplantation* 2007;83:1162–8.

55. Dunkelberg JC, Trotter JF, Wachs M et al. Sirolimus as primary immunosuppression after liver transplantation is not associated with hepatic artery of wound complications. *Liver Transpl* 2003;9:463–8.

56. Toso C, Merani S, Bigam DL, Shapiro AM, Kneteman NM, Sirolimus-based immunosuppression is associated with increased survival after liver transplantation for hepatocellular carcinoma. *Hepatology* 2010;51:1237–43.

57. Liang W, Wang D, Ling X et al. Sirolimus-based immunosuppression in liver transplantation for hepatocellular carcinoma: A meta-analysis. *Liver Transpl* 2012;18:62–9.

58. Yao JC, Shah MH, Bohas CL et al. Everolimus for advanced pancreatic neuroendocrine tumors. *N Engl J Med* 2011;10:514–23.

59. Soreide O, Bestad T, Bakka A et al. Surgical treatment as a principle in patients with advanced abdominal carcinoid tumors. *Surgery* 1992;111:48–54.

60. Moertel CG. Karnofsky memorial lecture: An odyssey in the land of small tumors. *J Clin Oncol* 1987;5:1502–3.

61. Raymond E, Dahan L, Raoul LJ et al. Sunitinib malate for the treatment of pancreatic neuroendocrine tumors. *N Engl J Med* 2011;364:501–3.

62. Mayo SC, de Jong MC, Pulitano C et al. Surgical management of hepatic neuroendocrine tumor metastasis: Results from an international multi-institutional analysis. *Ann Surg Oncol* 2010;17:3129–36.

63. Glazer ES, Tsenf JF, Al-Refaie W et al. Long-term survival after surgical management of neuroendocrine hepatic metastases. *HPB (Oxford)* 2010;12:427–33.

64. Norton JA, Warren RS, Kelly MG, Zuraek MB, Jensen RT. Aggressive surgery for metastatic liver neuroendocrine tumors. *Surgery* 2003;134:1057–63.

65. Frilling A, Li J, Malamutmann E, Schmid KW, Bockisch A, Broelsch CE. Treatment of liver metastases from neuroendocrine tumours in relation to the extent of hepatic disease. *Br J Surg* 2009;96:175–84.

66. Dick EA, Joarder R, de Jode M et al. MR-guided laser thermal ablation of primary and secondary liver tumors. *Clin Radiol* 2003;58:112–20.

67. Bilchik AJ, Saeantou T, Foshag LJ, Giuliano AE, Ramming GP. Cryosurgical palliation of metastatic neuroendocrine tumors resistant to conventional therapy. *Surgery* 1997;122:1040–7.

68. Sheen AJ, Poston GJ, Sherlock DJ. Cryoablation of unresectable malignant liver tumors. *Br J Surg* 2002;89:1296–401.

69. Atwell TD, Charboneau JW, Que FG et al. Treatment of neuroendocrine cancer metastasis to the liver: The role of ablative techniques. *Cardiovasc Intervent Radiol* 2005;28:409–21.

70. Livraghi T, Vettori C, Lazzaroni S. Liver metastasis: Results of percutaneous ethanol injection in 14 patients. *Radiology* 1991;179:709–12.

71. Boutros C, Somasundar P, Garrean S, Said A, Espat NJ. Microwave coagulation therapy for hepatic tumors: Review of the literature and critical analysis. *Surg Oncol* 2010;19:22–32.

72. Ajani JS, Carrasco CH, Charnsangavej C, Samaan NA, Levin B, Wallace S. Islet cell tumors metastatic to the liver: Effective palliation by sequential hepatic artery embolization. *Ann Intern Med* 1988;108:340–4.

73. Moertel CG, Johnson CM, McKusick MA et al. The management of patients with advanced carcinoid tumours and islet cell carcinomas. *Ann Intern Med* 1994;120:302–9.

74. Drougas JG, Anthony LB, Blair TK et al. Hepatic artery chemoembolization for management of patients with advanced metastatic carcinoid tumors. *Am J Surg* 1998;175:408–12.

75. Gupta S, Yao JC, Ahrar K et al. Hepatic artery embolization and chemoembolization for treatment of patients with metastatic carcinoid tumors: The M.D. Anderson experience. *Cancer J* 2003;9:261–7.

76. Ruutiainen AT, Soulen MC, Tuite CM et al. Chemoembolization and bland embolization of neuroendocrine tumor metastases to the liver. *J Vasc Interv Radiol* 2007;18:847–55.

77. Kennedy A, Nag S, Salem R et al. Recommendations for radioembolization of hepatic malignancies using yttrium-90 microsphere brachytherapy: A consensus panel report from the Radioembolization Brachytherapy Oncology Consortium. *Int J Radiat Oncol Biol Phys* 2007;68:12–23.

78. Salem R, Thurston KG. Radioembolization with yttrium-90 microspheres: State of the art brachytherapy treatment for primary and secondary liver malignancies. Part 3. Comprehensive literature review and future direction. *J Vasc Interv Radiol* 2006;17:1571–93.

79. Murthy R, Kamat P, Nunez R et al. Yttrium-90 microsphere radioembolotherapy of hepatic metastatic neuroendocrine carcinomas after hepatic arterial embolization. *J Vasc Interv Radiol* 2008;19:145–51.

80. King J, Quinn R, Glenn DM et al. Radioembolization with selective internal radiation microspheres for neuroendocrine liver metastases. *Cancer* 2008;113:921–9.

81. Limouris GS, Chatzioannou A, Kontogeorgakos D et al. Selective hepatic arterial infusion of In-111-DTPA-Phe1-octreotide on neuroendocrine liver metastases. *Eur J Nucl Med Mol Imaging* 2008;35:1827–37.

82. McStay MK, Maudgil D, Williams M et al. Large volume liver metastases from neuroendocrine tumors: Hepatic intraarterial 90Y-DOTA-lanreotide as effective palliative therapy. *Radiology* 2005;237:718–26.

83. Pool SE, Krenning EP, Koning GA et al. Preclinical and clinical studies of peptide receptor radionuclide therapy. *Semin Nucl Med* 2010;40:209–18.

84. Bushnell DL, O'Dorisio TM, O'Dorisio MS et al. 90Y-edotreotide for metastatic carcinoid refractory to octreotide. *J Clin Oncol* 2010;28:1652–9.

85. Kwekkenboom DJ, de Herder WW, Kam BL et al. Treatment with the radiolabeled somatostatin analog [177-Lu-DOTA O, Tyr3]octreotate: Toxicity, efficacy, and survival. *J Clin Oncol* 2008;26:2124–30.

86. Gedaly R, Daily MF, Davenport D et al. Liver transplantation for the treatment of liver metastases from neuroendocrine tumors: An analysis of the UNOS database. *Arch Surg* 2011;146:953–8.

87. Nguyen NT, Harring TR, Goss JA, O'Mahony CA. Neuroendcorine liver metastases and orthotopic liver transplantation: The US experience. *Int J Hepatol* 2011:742890.

88. Sher L. Association between timing of resection of primary tumor in patients undergoing liver transplantation for metastatic neuroendocrine tumor and survival. *Am J Transplant* 2009;12:88.

89. de Herder WW, Mazzaferro V, Tavecchio L, Wiedenmann B. Multidisciplinary approach for the treatment of neuroendocrine tumors. *Tumori* 2010;96:833–46.

90. Van Vilsteren FG, Baskin-Bey ES, Nagorney DM et al. Liver transplantation for gastroenteropancreatic neuroendocrine cancers: Defining selection criteria to improve survival. *Liver Transpl* 2006;12:448–56.

91. Florman S, Toure B, Kim L et al. Liver transplantation for neuroendocrine tumors. *J Gastrointest Surg* 2004;208–12.

92. Frilling A, Malago M, Weber F et al. Liver transplantation for patients with metastatic endocrine tumors: Single center experience with 15 patients. *Liver Transpl* 2006;12:1089–96.

93. Fan ST, Le Treut YP, Mazzaferro V et al. Liver transplantation for neuroendocrine tumour liver metastases. *HPB* 2015;17(1):23–8.

94. Le Treut YP, Gregoire E, Belghiti J et al. Predictors of long-term survival after liver transplantation for metastatic endocrine tumours: An 85-case French multicentric report. *Am J Transplant* 2008;8:1205–13.

52

Medical management of neuroendocrine gastroenteropancreatic tumors

KJELL ÖBERG

RADIOTHERAPY: PHARMACOTHERAPY

Neuroendocrine tumors (NETs) are a heterogeneous group of malignant diseases with various clinical presentations and clinical courses. In general, they are slow-growing tumors, but in some instances, they behave in a highly aggressive fashion (neuroendocrine carcinoma [NEC]). Due to their diverse symptoms (sweating, flushing, diarrhea, bronchospasm, and anxiety), diagnosis is often significantly delayed, and lesions therefore are only identified when metastatic spread has occurred [1,2]. Still, the delay from the first symptom until correct clinical diagnosis is about 4–5 years. Metastases can occur locally, in the mesentery and the adjacent lymph nodes, and by hematogenous spread to the liver, lungs, and bone. In most patients, the liver is the dominating site of metastatic spread, but lung, bone, and brain may also be affected. As a consequence of the substantial percentage of individuals with metastatic disease, most therapeutic strategies are directed at the management of hepatic secondaries or local recurrence [3].

Given the different organ distribution of the primaries and the widely different biological behaviors, treatment of NETs is typically multidisciplinary and is individualized according to the tumor type, the extent of the disease, and the level of symptoms. They represent significant clinical problems because more than half of the patients are metastasized at diagnosis, and the therapeutic focus will be on management of metastatic disease, particularly liver metastases [1,3,4]. Despite metastatic disease, the 5-year overall survival rates of 56%–83% for metastasized intestinal NETs and 40%–60% for pancreatic NETs might indicate rather good prognoses [5]. This has been further improved by the

introduction of specialized centers working as multidisciplinary teams with regular tumor boards [6]. This has particularly been developed in Europe by the European Neuroendocrine Tumor Society (ENETs), so-called the Centers of Excellence.

RADIOTHERAPY

Liver-directed intra-arterial therapies available in the treatment of unresectable liver metastases include transarterial embolization (TAE), transarterial chemoembolization (TACE), and selective internal radiotherapy (SIRT) with yttrium 90 microspheres. For TAE or TACE, symptomatic responses have been reported in 53%–100% of patients (up to 55 months) and tumor reduction in about 35%–74%, with a progression-free survival (PFS) of about 18–20 months and 5-year survival of 40%–80% [7–10]. Yttrium 90 radioembolization has been shown to be an effective treatment for hepatic metastases and is well tolerated [11–13]. It involves injection of embolic resin spheres (SIR-spheres, Sirtex Medical Ltd.) or glass spheres (TheraSphere, BTG Inc.). Microspheres loaded with beta-emitting radioisotope yttrium 90 are injected into the tumor hepatic arterial supply. In a recent meta-analysis of 12 relevant studies, radiographic response rates according to Response Evaluation Criteria in Solid Tumors (RECIST) range from 12% to 80%. Disease-controlled rates, defined as complete response or partial response plus stable disease, range from 62% to 100%. An administered radioactivity median of 1.7 GBq (range 1.2–3.4 GBq) did not correlate with either the response or control rate. The median overall survival rate ranges from 14 up to 70 months, with a median of 28.5 months. The response rate correlated with the median survival ($p = 0.008$) [14]. It has been suggested that many factors, including prior surgery, size of target lesions, performance status, baseline chemistry value, Ki-67 index, presence of extrahepatic disease, and inability to deliver a specified dose, influence patient outcomes for treatment of hepatic metastases with yttrium 90 radioembolization [14].

In conclusion, hepatic radioembolization using yttrium 90 microspheres is an effective treatment option for hepatic metastases in patients with NETs. The pool data demonstrated an effective response rate of 55%, disease control rate of 86%, and improved overall survival for patients responding to therapy. Lower response rates and survival times were associated with metastases of pancreatic NETs, which may be due to the more aggressive nature and advanced stage of the disease at diagnosis. The method should be considered for patients with liver dominant disease and those patients that cannot get treatment with peptide receptor radiotherapy (PRRT). SIRT is relatively expensive, and patients require careful selection because lung shunting may be an issue.

PEPTIDE RECEPTOR RADIOTHERAPY

The rational scientific basis for PRRT relies on the presence of somatostatin receptors on the surface of NET cells, to which an isotopically labeled radiopeptide is directed. The subsequent cellular radiopeptide internalization delivers the radioactivity directly to the intracellular compartment of the tumor (Figure 52.1). The clinical process of PRRT consists of the systemic administration of a suitable radiolabeled synthetic somatostatin analog fractionated into sequential cycles, usually four to six cycles every 6–9 weeks until the intended total amount of radioactivity has been delivered. The precise amount administered

depends mainly on the limitation imposed by renal radiation and, to a lesser extent, bone marrow [15]. PRRT was introduced into clinical practice in 1994 and represents a logical step following the initial development of the diagnostic technique for *in vivo* localization of NETs by using radiolabeled somatostatin analog indium 111 pentetreotide (Octreoscan®). In the beginning, the radiolabeled isotope was the same as that used for PRRT, but with rather limited results [16,17]. As a consequence of these relatively disappointing results, isotopes with higher energy and longer range, such as the beta emitter yttrium 90, were considered more appropriate for therapeutic evaluation [18]. The beta particles simultaneously exert a direct cell killing of somatostatin receptor-positive cells and a crossfire effect that targets nearby receptor-negative tumor cells. To facilitate efficacy further, novel octreotide analogs were developed, such as Tyr3 octreotide, with a similar pattern of affinity for somatostatin receptor type 2. The radioisotope binds to the new analog by DOTA, giving yttrium 90 DOTA Tyr3 octreotide, or Yttrium 90 DOTATOC [19]. This isotope was initiated in the treatment of metastatic NETs in 1996 with excellent symptomatic and objective responses (Table 52.1) [20–27]. It became the most used radiopeptide in the first decade of PRRT experience. Since 2000, however, a more effective analog, octreotate (Tyr3 or Thr8 octreotide with a six- to nine-fold higher affinity to somatostatin receptor type 2), has been used [28]. The kelated analog, DOTA Tyr octreotate or DOTATATE, can be labeled with a beta and gamma emitter, lutetium 177, and has been applied in a number of phase I and II studies. Lutetium 177 octreotate has subsequently become one of the most frequently used radiopeptides for PRRT (Table 52.1) [29–31]. This has been particularly evident in recent years given its efficacy, tolerability, and manageability. Lutetium 177 octreotide is currently being evaluated in a randomized phase

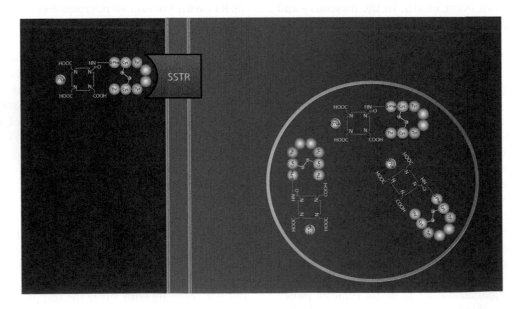

Figure 52.1 Bound radioactive 177 DOTATATE is internalized after binding to somatostatin receptor 2.

Table 52.1 Clinical results of PRRT with either ^{90}Y octreotide or ^{177}Lu octreotate in gastroenteropancreatic NETs

Ligand (reference)	Patient no.	CR + PR (%)	Response criteria	Outcome (months)
[90]Y-octreotide [20]	23	13	WHO	Not assessed
[90]Y-octreotide [21]	37	27	WHO	TTP > 26
[90]Y-octreotide [22]	36	34	WHO	Not assessed
[90]Y-octreotide [23]	21	29	WHO	TTP = 10
[90]Y-octreotide [24]	58	9	WHO	TTP = 29
[90]Y-octreotide [25]	90	4	SWOG	PFS = 16
[90]Y-octreotide [26]	53	23	WHO	PFS = 29
[90]Y-octreotide [27]	58	23	WHO	PFS = 17
[177]Lu-octreotate [29]	310	29	SWOG	PFS = 33
[177]Lu-octreotate [30]	42	31	RECIST	TTP = 36
[177]Lu-octreotate [31]	52	396	SWOG	PFS = 29

Note: CR, complete response; PR, partial response; SWOG, South Western Oncology Group; TTP, time to tumor progression.

III registration trial in small bowel NETs (NETTER-1). Long-term toxicity of PRRT with either yttrium 90 octreotide or lutetium 177 octreotate in gastroenteropancreatic tumors includes renal toxicity, bone marrow depression, myelodisplastic syndrome in a single patient, and leukemias. Chronic and permanent effects on the target organs, particularly the kidneys and bone marrow, are generally mild if necessary precautions are undertaken, such as fractionation and attention to specific risk factors. In this respect, it is apparent that, using appropriate dosimetry, it is possible to deliver elevated absorbed doses to the tumor with relative sparing of healthy organs, such as the kidney and bone marrow. Acute hematological toxicity is usually mild and transient. However, patients that have previously received cytotoxic treatment might have impaired function of the bone marrow. Delayed renal toxicity may occur, but by concomitant infusion of amino acids, the problem has been significantly reduced. These amino acids completely inhibit radiopeptide reabsorbtion with a consequent 9%–53% reduction of the renal radioactivity dosage. Other risk factors for decline in creatinine clearance are individuals with preexisting risk factors, such as long-standing and poorly controlled diabetes and hypertension. It has also been reported that renal toxicity is higher with yttrium 90 octreotide than with lutetium 177 octreotate [22,26,32,33].

In conclusion, PRRT is an effective treatment for patients with NETs and expression of somatostatin type 2 receptors. The toxicity is relatively low; however, we have to wait and see for the long-term side effects because these patients are living longer with metastatic disease. Myelodysplastic syndrome (MDS) and leukemia have occurred in single patients after a couple of years. PRRT with lutetium or yttrium 90 is not registered in any country, but it is applied in many European and some Asian countries. We are still waiting for the randomized trial to be presented where lutetium 177 DOTATATE is compared with a "cold" somatostatin analog (NETTER-1).

PHARMACOTHERAPY OF NEUROENDOCRINE TUMORS

Gastroenteropancreatic NETs are frequently metastatic at the time of initial diagnosis. The identification of metastatic disease represents the most important prognostic factor after the tumor grading [34–36]. The new World Health Organization (WHO) classification incorporates grading and staging and provides a basis for prognostic prediction [37]. The terminology of the new WHO classification (NET G1–G2 and NEC G3) is used in the presentation and correlates with suggested therapeutic options. Recommendations are mainly based on retrospective studies, but where available, prospective studies are used, although they are limited in number.

ANTISECRETORY TREATMENT

About 30%–50% of all gastroenteropancreatic NETs are so-called functioning tumors with hormone-related clinical symptoms. The use of somatostatin analogs is standard therapy in functioning NETs of any site. Interferon alpha may also be considered for symptom control in some patients, e.g., if somatostatin analog is not well tolerated or lacks efficacy. Interferon is frequently used as a second-line therapy due to a less favored toxicity profile, but it has additional value as an add-on therapy in patients with carcinoid syndrome that is not controlled with somatostatin analog alone [38,39]. In 70%–90%, somatostatin analogs (octreotid and lanreotide) are efficient in the treatment of carcinoid syndrome, e.g., in liver metastasis from serotonin-secreting small intestinal NET (midgut carcinoid) [38]. Other clinical symptoms relate to hypersecretion of rare pancreatic NETs, such as vasoactive intestinal peptide-oma (VIPoma) or glucagonoma [38,40]. Octreotide and lareotide are considered to be equally effective for syndrome control [40]. They are approved for antisecretory treatment in Europe and the

United States. A standard dose is 20–30 mg of a long-acting formulation of octreotide every 4 weeks intramuscularly and 90–120 mg of lanreotide Autogel® every 4 weeks [38]. Doses are adapted to the individual needs and depend on tumor burden. Preventive somatostatin analog therapies prior to surgery or use of local regional therapies delivered as either a subcutaneous bolus or 50–100 µg/h infusion intravenously is usually effective [39]. Interferon alpha is used at the dose of 3–5 million units subcutaneously three times per week, or as a long-acting formulation, pegylated interferon, 80–100 µg subcutaneously once a week [41,42]. Pegylated interferon is not approved for use in NETs yet. Use of pegylated interferon may, however, be considered for better tolerability [42]. Other specific therapies are required according to the primary and related hypersecretion [43–45]. Gastrinoma and the use of a higher dose of proton pump inhibitors (standard dose × 2–10/day) are the standard and first-line therapy [46]. In treatment of metastatic insulinoma, a recent advance is the use of the mammalian target of rapamycin (mTOR) inhibitor everolimus [47]. However, current medical treatment includes somatostatin analog and diazoxide, but only 50% of patients respond to somatostatin analog, and the efficacy of diazoxide is transient and associated with side effects (renal dysfunction and edema), particularly in elderly patients [44]. In a report of four patients, everolimus treatment led to normalization of blood glucose and withdrawal of glucose infusion or enteral feeding. The treatment was associated with partial tumor remission in two patients, lasting for 16 and 29 months, and stable disease for at least 6 months in the other two patients. Everolimus is recommended in metastatic insulinoma and resistant to the standard medical management [47,48]. Use of PRRT is considered an alternative therapeutic option for syndrome control. Another alternative is an ultrahigh dose of somatostatin analog therapy [49].

ANTIPROLIFERATIVE TREATMENT

The antitumor efficacy of somatostatin analogs appears to be weak with respect to objective tumor shrinkage, which occurs in about 5% of the patients, even if used at high dosages [39–41]. However, disease stabilization of up to 50%–60% has been reported in a prospective randomized placebo-controlled trial of octreotide long-acting repeatable (LAR) in small intestinal NETs (PROMID trial). The antiproliferative efficacy of octreotide LAR has been confirmed. The median time to tumor progression was 14.3 months with octreotide LAR versus 6 months with placebo. The dose of somatostatin analog was 30 mg every 4 weeks [50]. These results are further supported by results from a recent study, the CLARINET study [51], done in nonfunctioning NETs, demonstrating an antiproliferative effect. In this study, patients were randomized between Somatuline® Autogel 120 mg every 4 weeks and placebo [51]. The median PFS was not reached in the Somatuline arm versus 18 months in the placebo arm ($p < 0.001$). The estimated rates of PFS at 24 months were 65% in the Somatuline group and 33% in the placebo group. The PROMID study indicated that the tumor burden in the liver was of significant benefit to the result (<10% liver involvement); however, the CLARINET study confirmed that higher tumor burden could also be treated effectively. The determination of a cutoff value of tumor proliferation for recommendation of somatostatin analog is still controversial. In the PROMID study, tumors had a Ki-67 of <2%. However, in the CLARINET study, patients were included with a Ki-67 of <10%. Therefore, one can consider somatostatin analog to be indicated in both G1 and low-G2 tumors. Usually combined with other medical therapies, octreotide and lanreotide may be of value in G2 tumors, as well as in other subgroups of patients with slowly progressive, low-proliferative G1 NETs of pancreas and gastroduodenal origin [40,52–56]. This is seriously supported by literature data on retrospective and nonrandomized prospective trials in more than 500 patients. In patients with gastric NETs, somatostatin analogs have been shown to exert an antiproliferative effect. However, data are not available in cases of liver metastases [55]. A controversial issue is the requirements for a positive somatostatin receptor scintigraphy to be able to use a somatostatin analog. There are data from several centers indicating that patients without positive Octreoscan might respond to somatostatin analog therapy. The reason for that is not clear, but the tumors might express low-density somatostatin receptors that can only be found by staining of specimens from the tumor [39,48]. In metastatic NEC G3 (high-grade tumors), regardless of the site of origin, somatostatin analog treatment is not recommended [54]. There are no data reporting an indication for adjuvant treatment for somatostatin analogs in NET G1 or G2 irrespective of primary tumor origin or potential microscopic metastases [39,40].

INTERFERON

Tumor remission occurs rarely with interferon (about 10%); however, disease stabilization is observed in 40%–50% of the patients [41,42]. Interferon alpha is equally effective in functioning and nonfunctioning tumors with respect to tumor control. Two prospective randomized trials on metastatic gastroenteropancreatic NETs have shown that somatostatin analog and interferon, alone or in combination, have comparable antiproliferative effects when used after prior disease progression [52,53]. Although the number of patients included in these trials is limited, data from a recent French multicenter trial in advanced NETs provided a PFS of 14.1 months in a cohort of 32 patients where prior disease progression was documented [57]. However, the trial has some limitations: a heterogeneous patient population (53% midgut, 15% foregut, and 3% hindgut NETs and 22% carcinoma of unknown primary NETS) and being underpowered, with a nonsignificant p value compared with chemotherapy (PFS of 5.5 months). Patients with low-proliferating (G1) slowly progressive NETs or patients with somatostatin receptor scintigraphy-negative tumors are considered candidates for interferon therapy. Treatment is associated with more frequent side effects than somatostatin analog [41,42,52,53,57].

The interferon dose should be titrated individually by side effects and a leukocyte count down to about 3000/μl [41].

SYSTEMIC CHEMOTHERAPY

Chemotherapy is recommended in pancreatic NET (NET G2) and in NEC G3 of any site. So far, results with systemic chemotherapy are poor in patients with well-differentiated metastatic small intestinal NETs (NET G1) with response rates of under 15% [58]. Therefore, these patients should in general not receive current cytotoxic regimens. However, a recent phase II nonrandomized trial with metronomic 5-fluorouracil (5-FU), either alone or in combination with octreotide, reports promising results in small intestinal NET [59]. Systemic cytotoxic therapy is indicated in patients with inoperable progressive liver metastases from G1 and G2 pancreatic NETs using combinations of streptozotocin and 5-FU or doxorubicin, with objective response rates in the order of 35%–45% [60–62]. With respect to response rates, three-drug regimens including either cisplatinum or doxorubicin seem not to be superior to two-drug regimens with streptozotocin and 5-FU or streptozotocin and doxorubicin [63]. Temozolomide-based chemotherapy is promising, with a remission rate of 70% reported in one study with a PFS of 18 months [64]. This combination of temozolomide and capecetabine needs to be evaluated in a randomized prospective study to further delineate the precise efficacy. There are other phase II studies supporting a good response to the use of temozolamide-based therapies in NETs [65,66]. Temozolomide may be used with or without capecetabine. There is currently no clear cutoff value for Ki-67 for recommendation of chemotherapy, but its use is mostly indicated in NET G2 and NEC G3. For high-grade NEC G3, regardless of the site of the primary tumor, a combination of chemotherapy using cisplatin or carboplatin and etoposide has been the standard of care [67]. There is no established second-line treatment, but a recent retrospective study with temozolomide alone or in combination with capecetabine ± bevacizumab had a partial tumor response of 33%, indicating an antitumor effect in NEC G3 [68]. Encouraging results show that using either intravenous 5-FU or capecetabine early, combined with oxaliplatin or irinotecan, may also be an option for this group of patients [69,70].

NEW MOLECULAR TARGETED AGENTS (FIGURE 52.2)

New molecular targeted therapies have been investigated in phase II and phase III clinical trials and include angiogenesis inhibitors, single and multiple tyrosine kinase and mTOR inhibitors, and novel somatostatin analogs (e.g., pasireotide). The multiple tyrosine kinase inhibitor sunitinib and the mTOR inhibitor everolimus have been evaluated in phase III placebo-controlled trials [71,72]. Tumor remissions are rare with these small molecules. Disease stabilization is observed in a high proportion of patients (60%–80%). Both everolimus and sunitinib are registered for treatment of well-differentiated pancreatic NET, and the use of both drugs is supported by large phase III prospective trials. Everolimus has also been tested in large phase II trials alone and in combination with somatostatin analogs, indicating the value of combining it with a somatostatin analog [73]. The large RADIANT-3 study performed in 410 patients with well-differentiated pancreatic NETs showed tumor remission in 5% of the patients [72]. However, stabilization was obtained in almost 80% of the patients. The median PFS in the placebo arm was 6.4 months, versus 11 months in the everolimus arm. Everolimus is registered by the European Medicines Agency (EMA) and Food and Drug Administration (FDA) for treatment of well-differentiated progressive pancreatic NET. The side effects are mainly fatigue, nausea, stomatitis, and in selected cases, pneumonitis. There is at the moment a competition between chemotherapy and everolimus or sunitinib as the first-line treatment for well-differentiated pancreatic NET G2. No comparison has been made between the two drugs in any study at the moment; therefore, it is up to their availability and the physicians' discretion to select between the two types of treatment.

Results from a phase III placebo-controlled trial support the efficacy of sunitinib, a multiple tyrosine kinase inhibitor where the targets are PDGFR, VEGFR, cKIT, RET, and FLT3, in progressive pancreatic NET [71]. Sunitinib was first studied in a phase II study with 107 patients, including 66 patients with pancreatic NET. The objective response rate was 16.7% in pancreatic NETs, and the rate of stable disease was 68% [74]. The placebo-controlled phase III study of sunitinib (37.5 mg/day) on a continuous basis in patients with progressive well-differentiated pancreatic NET recruited 171 patients. The PFS was superior in the sunitinib arm, 11.1 months, versus in the placebo arm, 5.5 months [71]. The objective remission rate was less than 10%. The most frequent side effects included diarrhea, nausea, vomiting, asthenia, and hypertension. Sunitinib has recently been approved by the FDA and EMA for the treatment of advanced and progressive well-differentiated pancreatic NETs. In general, small molecules such as sunitinib or everolimus should be used after the occurrence of tumor progression. Everolimus or sunitinib might be considered first-line treatment and can be used in G1 and G2 NET.

The largest clinical trial available in NETs of different sites (RADIANT-2) everolimus 10 mg/day or placebo administered along with octreotide LAR 30 mg under 4 weeks both treatment arms [75]. The population was unexpectedly heterogeneous. The PFS, by central radiology review, was 16.4 months for the everolimus arm and 11.3 months for the placebo therapy [75]. The study did not meet statistical significance. The drug has not yet been approved for treatment of NETs other than pancreatic NET. Another clinical trial has just closed, including small intestinal and lung NETs (RADIANT-4). The data are not yet ready. Given the limited treatment options for malignant progressive small intestinal tumors, everolimus might be an option to test in this group of patients after therapies such as somatostatin analogs, interferon, and PRRT. The multiple tyrosine kinase

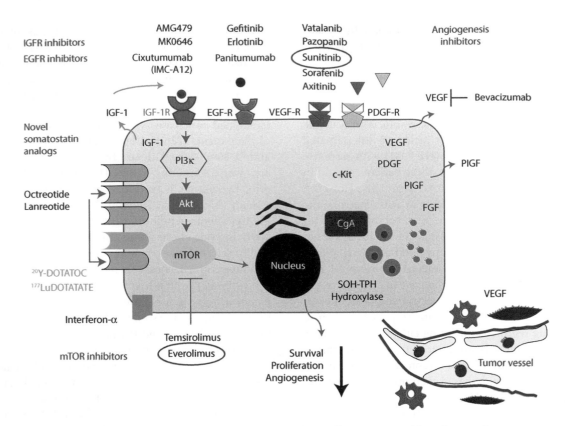

Figure 52.2 By binding to specific receptors, they exert intracellular effects (antiproliferation, antiangiogenesis etc.). (Adapted from Pavel M. Translation of molecular pathways into clinical trials of neuroendocrine tumors. Neuroendocrinology 2013;97:99–112.)

inhibitor sunitinib, however, cannot be recommended in NETs outside of the pancreas in the absence of any trial supporting its efficacy. The current therapeutic options are summarized in an algorithm (Figure 52.3).

In conclusion, today medical treatment provides several different options, including somatostatin analogs, interferon, chemotherapy, and the new targeted agents everolimus and sunitinib. Other kinase inhibitors, such as

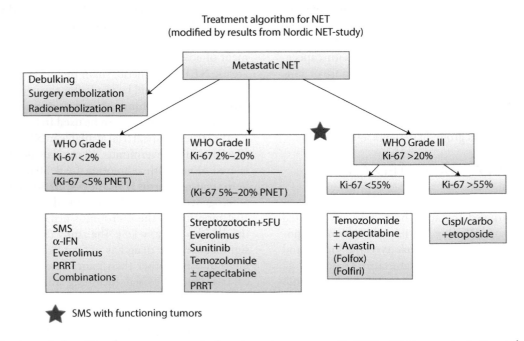

Figure 52.3 Treatment algorithm for management of gastroenteropancreatic NETs. SMS, somatostatin analog; WHO Grade, WHO grading system of NETs.

pazopanib and crizotinib, are under clinical trials for NETs. The first-line treatment for NET G1 is somatostatin analog, followed by interferon alpha at failure, but everolimus can also be considered, as well as PRRT. For NET G2, everolimus, sunitinib, or chemotherapy can be considered first line, depending on tradition and availability. They can be combined with somatostatin analog in functioning tumors. PRRT is also an option for this group of patients. For NEC G3, cytotoxic treatment is first line, and cisplatin or carboplatin and etoposide are standard of care. However, temozolomide plus capecetabine can be an alternative in patients in the lower range of NEC G3 with regard to tumor proliferation (Figure 52.2) [76].

REFERENCES

1. Modlin IM, Oberg K, Chung DC et al. Gastroenteropancreatic neuroendocrine tumours. *Lancet Oncol* 2008;9:61–72.
2. Clark OH, Benson AB 3rd, Berlin JD et al. NCCN clinical practice guidelines in oncology: Neuroendocrine tumors. *J Natl Compr Cancer Netw* 2009;7:712–47.
3. Frilling A, Modlin IM, Kidd M et al. Recommendations for management of patients with neuroendocrine liver metastases. *Lancet Oncol* 2014;15:e8–21.
4. Saxena A, Chua TC, Sarkar A et al. Progression and survival results after radical hepatic metastasectomy of indolent advanced neuroendocrine neoplasms (NENs) supports an aggressive surgical approach. *Surgery* 2011;149:209–20.
5. Pavel M, Baudin E, Couvelard A et al. ENETS Consensus Guidelines for the management of patients with liver and other distant metastases from neuroendocrine neoplasms of foregut, midgut, hindgut, and unknown primary. *Neuroendocrinology* 2012;95:157–76.
6. Modlin IM, Moss SF, Chung DC, Jensen RT, Snyderwine E. Priorities for improving the management of gastroenteropancreatic neuroendocrine tumors. *J Natl Cancer Inst* 2008;100:1282–9.
7. Mayo SC, Herman JM, Cosgrove D et al. Emerging approaches in the management of patients with neuroendocrine liver metastasis: Role of liver-directed and systemic therapies. *J Am Coll Surg* 2013;216:123–34.
8. Roche A, Girish BV, de Baere T et al. Trans-catheter arterial chemoembolization as first-line treatment for hepatic metastases from endocrine tumors. *Eur Radiol* 2003;13:136–40.
9. Vogl TJ, Naguib NN, Zangos S, Eichler K, Hedayati A, Nour-Eldin NE. Liver metastases of neuroendocrine carcinomas: Interventional treatment via transarterial embolization, chemoembolization and thermal ablation. *Eur Radiol* 2009;72:517–28.
10. Ruszniewski P, Rougier P, Roche A et al. Hepatic arterial chemoembolization in patients with liver metastases of endocrine tumors. A prospective phase II study in 24 patients. *Cancer* 1993;71:2624–30.
11. Rhee TK, Lewandowski RJ, Liu DM et al. 90Y radioembolization for metastatic neuroendocrine liver tumors: Preliminary results from a multi-institutional experience. *Ann Surg* 2008;247:1029–35.
12. Kennedy AS, Dezarn WA, McNeillie P et al. Radioembolization for unresectable neuroendocrine hepatic metastases using resin 90Y-microspheres: Early results in 148 patients. *Am J Clin Oncol* 2008;31:271–9.
13. King J, Quinn R, Glenn DM et al. Radioembolization with selective internal radiation microspheres for neuroendocrine liver metastases. *Cancer* 2008;113:921–9.
14. Devcic Z, Rosenberg J, Braat AJ et al. The efficacy of hepatic 90Y resin radioembolization for metastatic neuroendocrine tumors: A meta-analysis. *J Nucl Med* 2014;55:1404–10.
15. Bodei L, Mueller-Brand J, Baum RP et al. The joint IAEA, EANM, and SNMMI practical guidance on peptide receptor radionuclide therapy (PRRNT) in neuroendocrine tumours. *Eur J Nucl Med Mol Imaging* 2013;40:800–16.
16. Krenning EP, Kooij PP, Bakker WH et al. Radiotherapy with a radiolabeled somatostatin analogue, [111In-DTPA-D-Phe1]-octreotide. A case history. *Ann NY Acad Sci* 1994;733:496–506.
17. Valkema R, De Jong M, Bakker WH et al. Phase I study of peptide receptor radionuclide therapy with [In-DTPA]octreotide: The Rotterdam experience. *Semin Nucl Med* 2002;32:110–22.
18. Otte A, Mueller-Brand J, Dellas S, Nitzsche EU, Herrmann R, Maecke HR. Yttrium-90-labelled somatostatin-analogue for cancer treatment. *Lancet* 1998;351:417–8.
19. Heppeler A, Froidevaux S, Mäcke HR et al. Radiometal-labelled macrocyclic chelator-derivatised somatostatin analogue with superb tumour-targeting properties and potential for receptor-mediated internal radiotherapy. *Chem A Eur J* 1999;5:1016–1023.
20. Paganelli G, Zoboli S, Cremonesi M et al. Receptor-mediated radiotherapy with 90Y-DOTA-D-Phe1-Tyr3-octreotide. *Eur J Nucl Med* 2001;28:426–34.
21. Waldherr C, Pless M, Maecke HR, Haldemann A, Mueller-Brand J. The clinical value of [90Y-DOTA]-D-Phe1-Tyr3-octreotide (90Y-DOTATOC) in the treatment of neuroendocrine tumours: A clinical phase II study. *Ann Oncol* 2001;12:941–5.
22. Waldherr C, Pless M, Maecke HR et al. Tumor response and clinical benefit in neuroendocrine tumors after 7.4 GBq ^{90}Y-DOTATOC. *J Nucl Med* 2002;43:610–6.
23. Bodei L, Cremonesi M, Zoboli S et al. Receptor-mediated radionuclide therapy with 90Y-DOTATOC in association with amino acid infusion: A phase I study. *Eur J Nucl Med Mol Imaging* 2003;30:207–16.

24. Valkema R, Pauwels S, Kvols LK et al. Survival and response after peptide receptor radionuclide therapy with [90Y-DOTA0,Tyr3]octreotide in patients with advanced gastroenteropancreatic neuroendocrine tumors. *Semin Nucl Med* 2006;36:147–56.

25. Bushnell DL Jr, O'Dorisio TM, O'Dorisio MS et al. 90Y-edotreotide for metastatic carcinoid refractory to octreotide. *J Clin Oncol* 2010;28:1652–9.

26. Pfeifer AK, Gregersen T, Gronbaek H et al. Peptide receptor radionuclide therapy with Y-DOTATOC and (177)Lu-DOTATOC in advanced neuroendocrine tumors: Results from a Danish cohort treated in Switzerland. *Neuroendocrinology* 2011;93:189–96.

27. Cwikla JB, Sankowski A, Seklecka N et al. Efficacy of radionuclide treatment DOTATATE Y-90 in patients with progressive metastatic gastroenteropancreatic neuroendocrine carcinomas (GEP-NETs): A phase II study. *Ann Oncol* 2010;21:787–94.

28. Kwekkeboom DJ, Mueller-Brand J, Paganelli G et al. Overview of results of peptide receptor radionuclide therapy with 3 radiolabeled somatostatin analogs. *J Nucl Med* 2005;46(Suppl 1):62S–6S.

29. Kwekkeboom DJ, de Herder WW, Kam BL et al. Treatment with the radiolabeled somatostatin analog [177 Lu-DOTA 0,Tyr3]octreotate: Toxicity, efficacy, and survival. *J Clin Oncol* 2008;26:2124–30.

30. Bodei L, Cremonesi M, Grana CM et al. Peptide receptor radionuclide therapy with (1)(7)(7) Lu-DOTATATE: The IEO phase I-II study. *Eur J Nucl Med Mol Imaging* 2011;38:2125–35.

31. Sansovini M, Severi S, Ambrosetti A et al. Treatment with the radiolabelled somatostatin analog Lu-DOTATATE for advanced pancreatic neuroendocrine tumors. *Neuroendocrinology* 2013;97:347–54.

32. Imhof A, Brunner P, Marincek N et al. Response, survival, and long-term toxicity after therapy with the radiolabeled somatostatin analogue [90Y-DOTA]-TOC in metastasized neuroendocrine cancers. *J Clin Oncol* 2011;29:2416–23.

33. Bodei L, Ferone D, Grana CM et al. Peptide receptor therapies in neuroendocrine tumors. *J Endocrinol Invest* 2009;32:360–9.

34. La Rosa S, Klersy C, Uccella S et al. Improved histologic and clinicopathologic criteria for prognostic evaluation of pancreatic endocrine tumors. *Hum Pathol* 2009;40:30–40.

35. Pape UF, Jann H, Muller-Nordhorn J et al. Prognostic relevance of a novel TNM classification system for upper gastroenteropancreatic neuroendocrine tumors. *Cancer* 2008;113:256–65.

36. Yao JC, Hassan M, Phan A et al. One hundred years after "carcinoid": Epidemiology of and prognostic factors for neuroendocrine tumors in 35,825 cases in the United States. *J Clin Oncol* 2008;26:3063–72.

37. Rindi G, Arnold R, Bosman FT et al. Nomenclature and classification of neuroendocrine neoplasms of the digestive system. In: Bosman TF, Carneiro F, Hruban RH, Theise ND eds., *WHO Classification of Tumours of the Digestive System*. 4th ed. Lyon: International Agency for Research on Cancer, 2010:13.

38. Eriksson B, Kloppel G, Krenning E et al. Consensus guidelines for the management of patients with digestive neuroendocrine tumors—Well-differentiated jejunal-ileal tumor/carcinoma. *Neuroendocrinology* 2008;87:8–19.

39. Oberg K, Kvols L, Caplin M et al. Consensus report on the use of somatostatin analogs for the management of neuroendocrine tumors of the gastroenteropancreatic system. *Ann Oncol* 2004;15:966–73.

40. Modlin IM, Pavel M, Kidd M, Gustafsson BI. Review article: Somatostatin analogues in the treatment of gastroenteropancreatic neuroendocrine (carcinoid) tumours. *Aliment Pharmacol Ther* 2010;31:169–88.

41. Oberg K. Interferon in the management of neuroendocrine GEP-tumors: A review. *Digestion* 2000;62(Suppl 1):92–7.

42. Pavel ME, Baum U, Hahn EG, Schuppan D, Lohmann T. Efficacy and tolerability of pegylated IFN-alpha in patients with neuroendocrine gastroenteropancreatic carcinomas. *J Interferon Cytokine Res* 2006;26:8–13.

43. Jensen RT, Niederle B, Mitry E et al. Gastrinoma (duodenal and pancreatic). *Neuroendocrinology* 2006;84:173–82.

44. de Herder WW, Niederle B, Scoazec JY et al. Well-differentiated pancreatic tumor/carcinoma: Insulinoma. *Neuroendocrinology* 2006;84:183–8.

45. O'Toole D, Salazar R, Falconi M et al. Rare functioning pancreatic endocrine tumors. *Neuroendocrinology* 2006;84:189–95.

46. Jensen RT, Cadiot G, Brandi ML et al. ENETS Consensus Guidelines for the management of patients with digestive neuroendocrine neoplasms: Functional pancreatic endocrine tumor syndromes. *Neuroendocrinology* 2012;95:98–119.

47. Kulke MH, Bergsland EK, Yao JC. Glycemic control in patients with insulinoma treated with everolimus. *N Engl J Med* 2009;360:195–7.

48. Ong GS, Henley DE, Hurley D, Turner JH, Claringbold PG, Fegan PG. Therapies for the medical management of persistent hypoglycaemia in two cases of inoperable malignant insulinoma. *Eur J Endocrinol* 2010;162:1001–8.

49. Welin SV, Janson ET, Sundin A et al. High-dose treatment with a long-acting somatostatin analogue in patients with advanced midgut carcinoid tumours. *Eur J Endocrinol* 2004;151:107–12.

50. Rinke A, Muller HH, Schade-Brittinger C et al. Placebo-controlled, double-blind, prospective, randomized study on the effect of octreotide LAR in the control of tumor growth in patients with metastatic neuroendocrine midgut tumors: A report from the PROMID study group. *J Clin Oncol* 2009;27:4656–63.

51. Caplin ME, Pavel M, Cwikla JB et al. Lanreotide in metastatic enteropancreatic neuroendocrine tumors. *N Engl J Med* 2014;371:224–33.

52. Arnold R, Rinke A, Klose KJ et al. Octreotide versus octreotide plus interferon-alpha in endocrine gastroenteropancreatic tumors: A randomized trial. *Clin Gastroenterol Hepatol* 2005;3:761–71.

53. Faiss S, Pape UF, Bohmig M et al. Prospective, randomized, multicenter trial on the antiproliferative effect of lanreotide, interferon alfa, and their combination for therapy of metastatic neuroendocrine gastroenteropancreatic tumors—The International Lanreotide and Interferon Alfa Study Group. *J Clin Oncol* 2003;21:2689–96.

54. Butturini G, Bettini R, Missiaglia E et al. Predictive factors of efficacy of the somatostatin analogue octreotide as first line therapy for advanced pancreatic endocrine carcinoma. *Endocr Relat Cancer* 2006;13:1213–21.

55. Grozinsky-Glasberg S, Kaltsas G, Gur C et al. Long-acting somatostatin analogues are an effective treatment for type 1 gastric carcinoid tumours. *Eur J Endocrinol* 2008;159:475–82.

56. Campana D, Nori F, Pezzilli R et al. Gastric endocrine tumors type I: Treatment with long-acting somatostatin analogs. *Endocr Relat Cancer* 2008;15:337–42.

57. Dahan L, Bonnetain F, Rougier P et al. Phase III trial of chemotherapy using 5-fluorouracil and streptozotocin compared with interferon alpha for advanced carcinoid tumors: FNCLCC-FFCD 9710. *Endocr Relat Cancer* 2009;16:1351–61.

58. Sun W, Lipsitz S, Catalano P, Mailliard JA, Haller DG. Phase II/III study of doxorubicin with fluorouracil compared with streptozocin with fluorouracil or dacarbazine in the treatment of advanced carcinoid tumors: Eastern Cooperative Oncology Group Study E1281. *J Clin Oncol* 2005;23:4897–904.

59. Brizzi MP, Berruti A, Ferrero A et al. Continuous 5-fluorouracil infusion plus long acting octreotide in advanced well-differentiated neuroendocrine carcinomas. A phase II trial of the Piemonte oncology network. *BMC Cancer* 2009;9:388.

60. Kouvaraki MA, Ajani JA, Hoff P et al. Fluorouracil, doxorubicin, and streptozocin in the treatment of patients with locally advanced and metastatic pancreatic endocrine carcinomas. *J Clin Oncol* 2004;22:4762–71.

61. Delaunoit T, Ducreux M, Boige V et al. The doxorubicin-streptozotocin combination for the treatment of advanced well-differentiated pancreatic endocrine carcinoma; a judicious option? *Eur J Cancer* 2004;40:515–20.

62. Fjallskog ML, Janson ET, Falkmer UG, Vatn MH, Oberg KE, Eriksson BK. Treatment with combined streptozotocin and liposomal doxorubicin in metastatic endocrine pancreatic tumors. *Neuroendocrinology* 2008;88:53–8.

63. Turner NC, Strauss SJ, Sarker D et al. Chemotherapy with 5-fluorouracil, cisplatin and streptozocin for neuroendocrine tumours. *Br J Cancer* 2010;102:1106–12.

64. Strosberg JR, Fine RL, Choi J et al. First-line chemotherapy with capecitabine and temozolomide in patients with metastatic pancreatic endocrine carcinomas. *Cancer* 2011;117:268–75.

65. Ekeblad S, Sundin A, Janson ET et al. Temozolomide as monotherapy is effective in treatment of advanced malignant neuroendocrine tumors. *Clin Cancer Res* 2007;13:2986–91.

66. Kulke MH, Hornick JL, Frauenhoffer C et al. O6-methylguanine DNA methyltransferase deficiency and response to temozolomide-based therapy in patients with neuroendocrine tumors. *Clin Cancer Res* 2009;15:338–45.

67. Moertel CG, Kvols LK, O'Connell MJ, Rubin J. Treatment of neuroendocrine carcinomas with combined etoposide and cisplatin. Evidence of major therapeutic activity in the anaplastic variants of these neoplasms. *Cancer* 1991;68:227–32.

68. Welin S, Sorbye H, Sebjornsen S, Knappskog S, Busch C, Oberg K. Clinical effect of temozolomide-based chemotherapy in poorly differentiated endocrine carcinoma after progression on first-line chemotherapy. *Cancer* 2011;117:4617–22.

69. Pape UF, Tiling N, Bartel C, Plockinger U, Wiedenmann B. Oxaliplatin plus 5-fluoro-uracil/folinic acid as palliative treatment for progressive malignant gastrointestinal neuroendocrine carcinomas. *J Clin Oncol* 2006;24:14074.

70. Okita NT, Kato K, Takahari D et al. Neuroendocrine tumors of the stomach: Chemotherapy with cisplatin plus irinotecan is effective for gastric poorly-differentiated neuroendocrine carcinoma. *Gastric Cancer* 2011;14:161–5.

71. Raymond E, Dahan L, Raoul JL et al. Sunitinib malate for the treatment of pancreatic neuroendocrine tumors. *N Engl J Med* 2011;364:501–13.

72. Yao JC, Shah MH, Ito T et al. Everolimus for advanced pancreatic neuroendocrine tumors. *N Engl J Med* 2011;364:514–23.

73. Yao JC, Lombard-Bohas C, Baudin E et al. Daily oral everolimus activity in patients with metastatic pancreatic neuroendocrine tumors after failure of cytotoxic chemotherapy: A phase II trial. *J Clin Oncol* 2010;28:69–76.

74. Kulke MH, Lenz HJ, Meropol NJ et al. Activity of sunitinib in patients with advanced neuroendocrine tumors. *J Clin Oncol* 2008;26:3403–10.

75. Pavel ME, Hainsworth JD, Baudin E et al. Everolimus plus octreotide long-acting repeatable for the treatment of advanced neuroendocrine tumours associated with carcinoid syndrome (RADIANT-2): A randomised, placebo-controlled, phase 3 study. *Lancet* 2011;378:2005–12.

76. Pavel M. Translation of molecular pathways into clinical trials of neuroendocrine tumors. *Neuroendocrinology* 2013;97:99–112.

Metabolic Surgery

53

Pancreas transplantation

NIR LUBEZKY AND RICHARD NAKACHE

INTRODUCTION

Type 1 diabetes mellitus (DM) afflicts more than 1 million people in the United States, with an annual incidence of at least 13,000, making it the second most common chronic disease in young people [1]. It is the most common cause of end-stage renal failure (ESRF), blindness, and limb amputations, and one of the most common causes of death in the United States [2]. Since the initial success of purifying insulin and treating diabetes in 1921 by Banting and Best, there has been much progress in the effectiveness of insulin therapy, and patients with type 1 diabetes can survive for many years. However, the imperfect control of blood sugar ultimately results in vascular complications in most patients. Meticulous glucose control has been shown to decrease complication rate; however, it is very difficult to achieve and may result in dangerous episodes of hypoglycemia [3]. The estimated annual mortality attributed to insulin-induced hypoglycemia has been reported to be as high as 3%–6% [4].

The first pancreas transplantation (PT) was performed in 1966. A young woman with diabetes and renal failure underwent a combined kidney and PT at the University of Minnesota by Kelly et al. [5]. Initial morbidity and mortality rates were prohibitively high, with mortality reaching 80% [6]. Subsequently, improvements in operative technique, patient selection, and immunosuppressive regimens have greatly increased the success rate, to a point that simultaneous kidney and pancreas transplantation (SPK) has become the preferred definitive treatment for patients with type 1 DM complicated by ESRF. The current 1-year patient survival rate is >95%, and graft survival rates are almost 85% [7]. Additional accepted indications for PT include patients with type 1 DM with normal renal function that suffer from life-threatening hypoglycemic unawareness, and selected nonobese patients with type 2 DM.

It has been shown that successful PT normalizes the blood sugar of patients with diabetes, and there is strong evidence that the procedure can prolong life, reverse mild nephropathy, prolong kidney allograft survival, slow the progression of diabetes-related complications, and improve quality of life [8–10].

To date, more than 42,000 PTs have been reported worldwide, and about 1600 PTs are performed each year [11]. The annual number of PTs steadily increased until 2004, and has since declined. The decrease in the number of PTs may be partly attributable to improved insulin delivery systems, concerns about outcomes and complications, and improved results of islet transplantation.

This chapter summarizes the various indications for PT, timing of transplantation, perioperative complications, long-term outcomes, and impact on patient survival and preexisting complications from diabetes.

PANCREAS TRANSPLANT RECIPIENTS

Timing of PT

PT can be performed in patients with DM in three different clinical settings. The first, and most common, accounting for about 75% of the cases, is patients with type 1 DM and

ESRF that undergo an SPK. The second scenario, accounting for about 20% of PT cases, is in patients with DM and ESRD who undergo kidney transplantation (KT) followed by "pancreas after kidney" (PAK) transplantation. The demand for deceased donor kidneys is much higher than that for pancreas. Therefore, the waiting time to receive an SPK is determined by the need for the kidney. The waiting time for a pancreas is much lower, not more than 6 months in most places. Patients with DM and ESRD who have a living kidney donor can have an elective living donor KT, and then be listed for a cadaveric PAK transplantation. The PT can be performed as soon as the patient recovers from the KT and has stable kidney function. The main disadvantage of PAK compared with SPK is that the long-term pancreas graft survival is lower, due to higher rates of rejection, and the inability to diagnose early rejection in PAK compared with SPK. SPK patients derive both organs from the same donor; therefore, rejection develops in both organs simultaneously, and can be detected early by elevation of serum creatinine. In PAK, rejection of the pancreas graft is not accompanied by renal dysfunction in most cases, and is therefore diagnosed at a later stage, often at the time irreversible organ damage has already occurred.

About 5% of PTs are performed as "pancreas transplant alone" (PTA). This procedure is performed in a small group of highly selected nonuremic diabetic patients in whom glucose control is extremely difficult and patients suffer from recurrent events of life-threatening hypoglycemia, commonly accompanied by hypoglycemic unawareness [12]. Long-term graft outcomes have not been as good as SPK or even PAK, and these patients would need to receive nephrotoxic immunosuppressive medications and have a significant risk to develop progressive renal failure and ESRF.

Recipient selection criteria

General considerations are common to all potential recipients. Patients suffer from long-standing DM and are at high risk for perioperative cardiovascular complications. Up to 30% of asymptomatic patients are found to have significant coronary artery disease on angiography [13]. Age is not considered an absolute contraindication for PT, but most centers would not transplant patients older than 45–50 years old.

The most common indication for PT is type 1 DM. These patients typically have autoimmune destruction of their insulin-producing pancreatic beta cells, are insulin dependent, and have undetectable levels of c-peptide. A subset of patients with type 2 DM and ESRD can also benefit from PT [14]. These patients have a combination of insulin resistance and insulin deficiency, are usually older than patients with type 1 DM, and have detectable levels of c-peptide. Criteria for candidacy of patients with type 2 DM and ESRF for PT are not uniform, and are dependent on level of c-peptide (no clear cutoff level), body mass index (BMI) (less than 30), and daily insulin requirements (less than 1 U/kg/day). Although the underlying mechanism for post-PT euglycemia in

patients with type 2 DM is not clear, several retrospective studies have shown that in selected patients with type 2 DM and ESRF, the results of PT are comparable to those in patients with type 1 DM [14]. Currently, it is estimated that about 8% of SPKs and 4% of PAKs and PTAs are performed for type 2 DM [14].

PANCREAS ORGAN DONORS

As perioperative complication rate and long-term graft survival correlate to a great extent with quality of the donor, most transplant centers use strict acceptance inclusion criteria. Although a few centers use partial pancreas grafts from living donors, the vast majority are from deceased donors, and mostly from donors after brain death (DBDs) [3]. The major factors that determine donor organ quality are age (common cutoff 30–40), BMI (common cutoff 25–30), and kidney function, which is a marker of end-organ perfusion [15–18]. Intraoperative assessment of the surgeon is important, and not infrequently, organs are found to have excessive fat deposition or fibrosis and are discarded at the time of retrieval. Steatotic organs have an increased risk of posttransplant pancreatitis secondary to reperfusion injury [16]. A donor history of significant alcohol use is also a common exclusion criterion. Recently, a systematic evaluation of pancreas allograft quality using the Scientific Registry of Transplant Recipients (SRTR) data was done to construct a pancreas donor risk index (PDRI) [18], aimed to predict long-term graft function. The PDRI included 10 donor and 1 transplant characteristics. Donor factors include donor sex, cause of death, creatinine, height, and donation after cardiac death (DCD). The transplant-related factor was preservation time, or cold ischemia time. Donor age, BMI, and DCD status were found to have the greatest impact on risk for graft loss during the first year posttransplant.

SURGICAL PROCEDURE

The pancreas graft is usually transplanted intraperitoneally, in the right iliac fossa. Arterial inflow comes from the right common or external iliac artery. Before implantation, on the back table, a Y-shaped conduit of donor iliac artery is anastomosed to the stumps of the superior mesenteric and splenic arteries so that only one arterial anastomosis needs to be done during the implantation (Figures 53.1 and 53.2).

The venous drainage of the graft is usually done to the systemic circulation, either the external iliac vein or inferior vena cava. This approach has the potential disadvantage of peripheral hyperinsulinemia, as the first-pass metabolism of the insulin in the liver is lost. There has been some concern that hyperinsulinemia may have long-term adverse effects, such as accelerated atherosclerosis [19,20]. Few centers advocate use of the portal system for venous drainage. Portal drainage is more physiologic, but has been associated with increased risk for graft thrombosis and was never shown to have any real clinical benefit, and therefore has been abandoned by most centers [12,21,22].

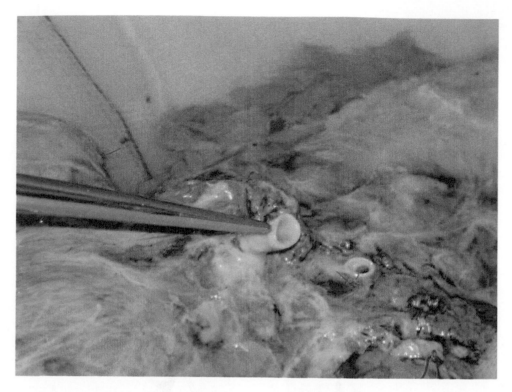

Figure 53.1 Stumps of the superior mesenteric artery (forceps showing) and splenic artery (marked with blue suture) in the pancreas.

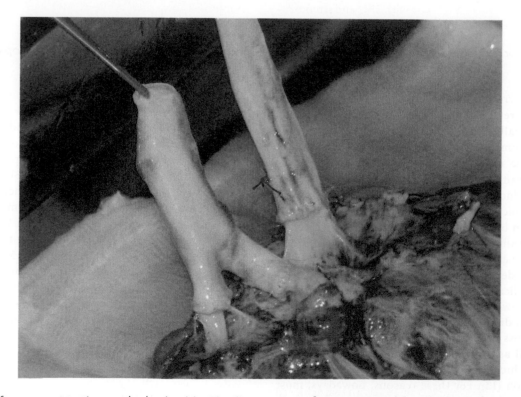

Figure 53.2 After reconstruction on the back table. The iliac artery graft was connected to the superior mesenteric artery and splenic artery stumps, and the portal vein was elongated using an iliac vein graft.

Pancreas transplant with enteric drainage in situ

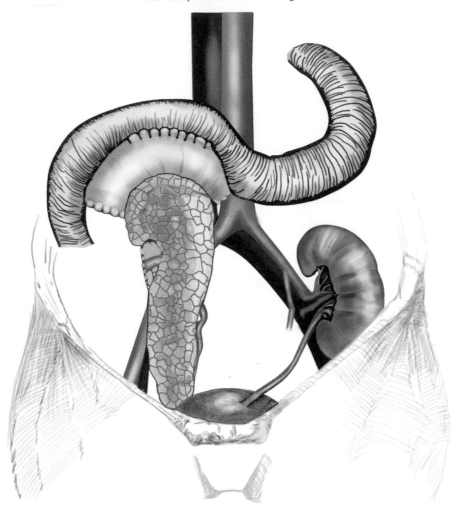

Figure 53.3 Exocrine reconstruction of the PT. The transplant duodenum is connected side to side to a loop of recipient jejunum.

Exocrine secretion drains through the graft duodenum, which is retrieved *en bloc* with the pancreas, and is stapled proximally and distally on the first and third parts of the duodenum. Either the gastrointestinal tract or the bladder can be used for managing the exocrine secretions of the graft. Enteric drainage can be done either as a side-to-side duodenojejunostomy (Figure 53.3) or with a Roux loop of recipient jejunum. Alternatively, the donor duodenum can be anastomosed to the recipient bladder. The major advantage of bladder drainage is the ability to detect rejection early by measuring urinary amylase levels routinely. Bladder drainage also avoids the possible catastrophic complication of enteric leak, and has been associated with somewhat lower rates of early graft thrombosis [15]. The main disadvantages of the bladder drainage are the ongoing loss of bicarbonate resulting in chronic acidemia, as well as local effects of the pancreatic fluid on the bladder, which often result in hematuria, cystitis, and stone formation [12]. For these reasons, nowadays, most commonly enteric drainage is used to manage the exocrine secretions.

COMPLICATIONS

PT is associated with a relatively high incidence of surgical complications, leading to substantial rates of graft loss, morbidity, and mortality. During the 1980s, up to 25% of grafts were lost from surgical complications [23]. Improvements in surgical techniques and patient and donor selection have significantly improved outcomes, and complications rates have dramatically decreased. Still, about 7%–10% of PTs are lost from technical failures according to recent single-center reports and SRTR data analysis [15,16,24–26]. This is probably one of the main reasons this procedure has not gained widespread application, and a decline in the annual number of PTs has been consistently documented in recent years. Early postoperative complications can be divided into three categories: vascular, parenchymal, and enteric.

Vascular complications

Pancreas graft thrombosis (PGT) remains the most frequent serious complication following PT, with a reported incidence of 3%–10% [23–30]. In most cases, this results in graft loss and the need for graft pancreatectomy [28]. The etiology of PGT is multifactorial, and venous thrombosis is probably more common than arterial thrombosis [31]. Risk factors for PGT include donor-related factors, such as increased donor age, donor instability, suboptimal recovery, prolonged cold ischemia time [28], and use of venous extension grafts. Recipient-related factors that have been associated with higher rates of PGT include the PTA and PAK categories, enteric exocrine drainage, and left-sided graft placement.

The most common clinical presentation of acute PGT is of asymptomatic unexplained sudden elevation in blood glucose levels. Other symptoms, such as graft tenderness and hematuria (in bladder-drained grafts), can occur. Diagnosis can be established by imaging, such as ultrasound Doppler or computed tomography (CT) angiography. Treatment usually consists of graft pancreatectomy [28]. Few selected patients with partial thrombosis may be amenable to salvage attempts, mainly using percutaneous interventions [29,32–36], or systemic anticoagulation in cases of partial venous PGT [29,32–33].

Hemorrhage is the most common cause of early postoperative relaparotomy following PT. Fortunately, the impact of bleeding on graft and patient survival is relatively small, and only about 0.3% of PT are lost to bleeding [37]. Bleeding can result from the arterial anastomosis, or from the mesenteric or splenic vessels. Meticulous back-table preparation of the graft can minimize the chance for postoperative bleeding. Some centers use perioperative systemic anticoagulation routinely, or selectively in patients that are at high risk for PGT (such as retransplants, patients with known hypercoagulable state, or patients with previous PGT) [23]. Use of perioperative systemic anticoagulation inevitably increases the rate of postoperative bleeding and relaparotomy; however, this may be a reasonable price for reducing early PGT rates.

Graft arterial pseudoaneurysm (PSA) is an uncommon complication occurring more commonly in patients who develop peritransplant infections. Graft PSAs can occur in the early postoperative course or many years post-PT [38–42]. Whereas early PSA usually presents as massive intra-abdominal bleeding and requires emergent graft pancreatectomy, late PSAs can have a more indolent course, can present as gastrointestinal bleeding from erosion of the PSA to the gastrointestinal tract, and can be treated using an endovascular approach in some cases.

Parenchymal complications

Graft pancreatitis (GP) in the immediate postoperative course occurs to some degree in up to 35% of cases, and tends to resolve within 3–4 weeks of transplantation [23,43]. Late GP can occur many years posttransplantation, in up to 14% of recipients [43]. Several risk factors have been associated with the risk of early acute GP, including donor quality, prolonged cold ischemia times, drainage reflux (in

bladder-drained grafts), exocrine anastomotic stricture, use of histidine–tryptophan–ketoglutarate (HTK) preservation solution, direct trauma to the graft during the procurement or implantation procedures, and graft infection, such as cytomegalovirus [23,44–46]. Etiologies and risk factors for late GP are not well defined. Patients usually present with abdominal pain, signs of peritonitis, and findings compatible with graft inflammation on imaging. Some degree of hyperamylasemia or lipasemia is common, but the degree of elevation does not generally correlate with the severity of the GP. Treatment includes bowel rest and insertion of a Foley catheter for bladder-drained grafts. The role of somatostatin analogs and empiric antibiotic treatment is less well defined. Severe cases with infected graft necrosis may require laparotomy for debridement or even graft pancreatectomy.

Peritransplant infections are much more common after PT than after KT, and are a significant cause of graft loss, as well as recipient morbidity and mortality [23,30]. The most serious etiology of peritransplant infection, in up to 30% of cases [23], is graft duodenal anastomotic leak with resultant enteric (in enteric-drained grafts) or urine (in bladder-drained grafts) peritonitis. Risk factors for peritransplant infection in the absence of anastomotic leak include donor quality, pretransplant peritoneal dialysis, prolonged cold ischemia time, and GP [23,45,47]. Patients present with signs of systemic sepsis and either localized or diffuse peritonitis, and diagnosis is established with CT scan. Treatment depends on the clinical condition of the patient and the ability to rule out anastomotic leak. Stable patients with localized abscess are treated conservatively with antibiotics and percutaneous drainage of collections. Any deterioration of the patients, as well as suspicion for anastomotic leak and enteric peritonitis, should be an indication for laparotomy, drainage, and low threshold for graft pancreatectomy.

Enteric complications

Graft duodenal anastomotic leak is an uncommon complication, responsible for 0.5% of all graft losses [23]. The clinical presentation, treatment, and prognosis depend on the type of exocrine drainage performed. Enteric-drained grafts develop enteric peritonitis and usually present with signs of severe sepsis. Treatment consists of laparotomy and revision of the anastomosis, conversion to a Roux-en-Y anastomosis, or graft pancreatectomy. As stated previously, mortality in patients with enteric leak is high, and low threshold should be maintained for graft pancreatectomy in very sick patients. Recipients of bladder-drained grafts can develop signs of peritonitis due to spillage of pancreatic juice, and urine in the peritoneal cavity. These patients typically are not as sick as patients with enteric peritonitis. Treatment consists of prolonged bladder decompression with a Foley catheter and percutaneous drainage of abdominal collections. Patients with ongoing sepsis may need laparotomy for abdominal washout and repair of the leak, or graft pancreatectomy.

IMMUNOSUPPRESSION AND REJECTION

PT is associated with significant risk for graft loss as a result of rejection [48]. Reported rates of acute rejection post-PT are as high as 25% [48,49]. Early diagnosis of PT rejection is not simple. Clinical signs and symptoms include fever, malaise, and graft tenderness, but are often mild or absent. Laboratory screening tests include elevation in serum amylase and lipase, as well as a decrease in urinary amylase in bladder-drained grafts; however, these tests have very limited sensitivity and specificity for the diagnosis of rejection. Hyperglycemia is frequently a sign of late and severe PT rejection, and its presence signifies limited potential for graft salvage. PT rejection in recipients of SPK can be diagnosed more easily. As the KT originates from the same donor as the pancreas (unlike PAK), rejection of both organs occurs simultaneously and can be diagnosed easily and early by elevation of creatinine. This is the most accepted explanation for the improved graft survival seen in SPKs compared with both PAKs and PTAs. The gold standard for diagnosis of PT rejection is pancreas graft biopsy. Alternatively, KT biopsy, which is a simpler procedure, can be done in patients with SPK transplant.

Because of the high prevalence of early PT rejection, and difficulty in early diagnosis, PT rejection has significant impact on overall graft survival, and about 20% of grafts fail within 1 year of diagnosis of rejection [48]. Most transplant centers use a combination of powerful immunosuppressive agents in the perioperative interval for immunosuppression induction. The combination usually includes a cell-depleting biological antithymocyte polyclonal antibody (thymoglobulin), high-dose corticosteroids, a calcineurin inhibitor (CNI) (usually the more potent agent tacrolimus is chosen, as it has been shown to be associated with more improved outcomes than the older agent cyclosporine), and an antimetabolite immunosuppressant (usually mycophenolate mofetil [MMF]). Long-term maintenance immunosuppression in PT patients is usually based on a triple regimen that includes steroids, an antimetabolite (MMF), and a CNI (tacrolimus). Steroid-free regimens were shown to be safe in KT recipients that are at low risk for rejection [50], and have the potential advantage of avoiding the long-term side effects, such as diabetes, osteoporosis, hyperlipidemia, and hypertension. A few studies reported on the safety of steroid withdrawal in PT patients [51]. A recent randomized trial demonstrated that a steroid-free regimen in SPK recipients is safe, and was not associated with increased rejection rates or reduced graft survival compared with the standard triple therapy [52].

PATIENT AND PT GRAFT SURVIVAL AFTER PANCREAS TRANSPLANTATION

Both patient and pancreas graft survival have improved considerably over the past years. This is the result of improvements in donor and recipient selection, as well as operative technique and immunosuppressive medications, specifically the use of thymoglobulin [17,53,54]. Current 1-year patient survival for PT recipients exceeds 95%. The most recent 5-year, 10-year, and 20-year graft survivals were shown to be 80%, 68%, and 45% for SPK transplant; 62%, 46%, and 16% for PAK transplant; and 59%, 39%, and 12% for PTA transplant [17].

Patients with diabetes and ESRF have a high risk for mortality, and death rates among these patients on the waiting list are high [55]. KT confers a clear survival benefit when compared with staying on dialysis [56,57]. There is considerable debate as to the added benefit of PT to patient survival, specifically when compared with diabetic patients who receive KT alone. Studies comparing survival of SPK recipients with that of patients suffering from DM and ESRF on the waiting list demonstrated an expected increased mortality in transplanted patients in the first 90 days posttransplant. However, at 4 years posttransplant, survival for SPK recipients was far better than that of their waitlisted controls [58]. SPK recipients live 15 years longer than waitlisted patients who do not receive a transplant. PT failure and need for exogenous insulin was found to be strongly associated with patient survival. The impact of PT on patient survival when compared with patients receiving KT alone, especially living donor KT recipients, is more controversial [59]. The most recent SRTR data showed that 10-year survival after SPK transplant was 67%. For insulin-dependent diabetes mellitus patients receiving living donor KT, survival was 65%, and for recipients of deceased donor KT, survival was 46% [56]. The survival advantage of SPK compared with deceased donor KT was lost for recipients older than 50 years. The survival advantage of SPK was observed only 5 years after transplant due to the higher perioperative mortality associated with SPK. Also, the survival advantage was only seen in patients that had a functioning pancreas graft. A retrospective review of data from the United Network for Organ Sharing (UNOS) suggested that for patients with preserved kidney function, conventional therapy for diabetes was associated with similar, if not even better, survival compared with patients undergoing PAK transplant [60]. This is the result of the increased mortality in the first 90 days post-PT, and the improvements in medical management of DM.

IMPACT OF PANCREAS TRANSPLANTATION ON QUALITY OF LIFE AND DIABETES-RELATED COMPLICATIONS

Quality of life is increasingly used to measure success of interventions, such as transplantation. No specific quality of life questionnaire for PT exists, which is a significant limitation of published studies. Still, using general quality of life measures, PT was shown to improve quality of life in patients with DM [61–63]. Freedom from exogenous insulin, frequent blood glucose monitoring, and strict dietary restrictions in patients undergoing successful transplantation can have a great impact on a patient's quality of life. Patients undergoing both KT and PT (as SPK or PAK) are relieved from both dialysis and exogenous insulin, changes that have an enormous positive impact on their quality of life.

Long-standing diabetes is complicated by microvascular, macrovascular, and neurologic sequelae. There is some data that suggests that glycemic control gained by a functioning PT can impact the progression of these complications. However, the paucity of long-term prospective randomized studies of sufficient size limits our ability to draw clear conclusions as to the benefit of PT on diabetes-related complications.

Diabetic nephropathy is characterized by glomerulosclerosis and proteinuria. Most studies suggest that euglycemia after PT can stop the progression, improve kidney allograft survival in patients receiving SPK, and even reverse diabetic nephropathy. However, determining the effect of PT on the progression of nephropathy is difficult, as these effects take many years to develop, and are influenced by additional factors, such as the use of nephrotoxic immunosuppressive medications [64]. A study on 10 PTA patients demonstrated improvement in kidney function, as well as glomerular histological structure, 10 years following the transplantation [65]. Studies that compared KT function in diabetic patients that received KT alone and SPK showed that by 2 years posttransplant, SPK recipients had better kidney function and less proteinuria [66–68]. Similarly, functioning PAK transplant is associated with improved KT survival [10,69]. Histological changes of diabetic nephropathy can be prevented, or even reversed, in patients receiving PT [65,70].

Cardiovascular disease is the leading cause of mortality in patients with DM. Data suggests that patients with a functional PT have an angiographically demonstrated reduction in coronary atherosclerotic lesions [71]. Studies comparing SPK recipients with KT alone showed reduction in cardiovascular mortality, myocardial infarction, and pulmonary edema in SPK recipients [72].

Retinopathy is a common complication in patients with DM. By 10 years, at least 75% of type 1 DM patients develop retinopathy, and many of them will eventually progress to develop blindness [73]. Unfortunately, most patients undergoing PT already have advanced retinopathy at the time of transplantation, and the potential for improvement is limited. A number of studies suggest stabilization of retinopathy in these patients [74–76], although the lack of large comparative studies precludes a definite conclusion as to the value of PT in this context. One study demonstrated that PT is associated with regression of diabetic retinopathy in approximately 50% of patients after 1 year [76]. This compares favorably with the 70% rate of progression seen in patients not transplanted, and under strict insulin regimen.

Neuropathy affects about 50% of patients with DM [77]. Symptoms vary on the type of nerve and organ afflicted, and can include extremity numbness, autonomic dysfunction, and erectile dysfunction. A large-scale study that compared PT patients with nontransplanted diabetic controls demonstrated improvement in nerve conduction over the years in transplanted patients, compared with progression and worsening in nontransplanted patients [78]. Unfortunately, although progression of the neuropathy is halted, clinical improvement is mild at best in most cases.

Macrovascular disease, with resultant peripheral vascular disease and cerebrovascular disease, has a significant impact on morbidity and mortality of patients with long-standing DM. The impact of PT on the natural history and progression of macrovascular disease is controversial. Whereas one study showed stabilization of carotid atherosclerotic disease over time in patients undergoing PT [79], another study demonstrated continued progression [80]. A small study looking into the prevalence of clinical macrovascular disease, including stroke rate and limb amputations in SPK patients compared with patients who underwent KT alone, was able to demonstrate a lower rate of macrovascular disease progression in patients with a functioning PT [81].

CONCLUSIONS

PT is an accepted treatment option for selected patients with type 1 DM. SPK transplant in patients with type 1 DM and ESRF is the most common setting in which PT is performed. In patients with a functioning PT, it offers enhanced patient and KT survival, as well as improved quality of life, and at least halts, if not reverses, the secondary complications of diabetes, including vascular, neurologic, and retinal complications. Because of the shortage of deceased donors, living kidney donation is a valid alternative, especially in regions where the waiting time for SPK is long. These patients have the option to receive a PAK transplant; however, the survival benefit in this setting is not clear. PTA is a valid treatment option for select nonuremic patients with diabetes who suffer from hypoglycemic unawareness and life-threatening hypoglycemic events. The main problem with PT is the relatively high rate of surgical complications, resulting is both graft loss and patient morbidity and mortality; they are the main cause for the limited application of PT and the decline in the number of PTs observed in recent years. Strict donor and recipient selection criteria, as well as meticulous surgical technique, are crucial to minimizing the rate of these complications.

REFERENCES

1. Forlenza GP, Rewers M. The epidemic of type 1 diabetes: What is it telling us? *Curr Opin Endocrinol Diabetes Obes* 2011;18:248–51.
2. American Diabetes Association. Diabetes statistics. Alexandria, VA: American Diabetes Association, 2013. http://diabetes.org/diabetes-basics/diabetes-statistics/.
3. Diabetes Control and Complications Trial Research Group. The effect of intensive treatment of diabetes on the development and progression of long-term complications in insulin-dependent diabetes mellitus. *N Engl J Med* 1993;329:977–86.

4. Diabetes Control and Complications Trial/ Epidemiology of Diabetes Interventions and Complications Research Group. Long-term effect of diabetes and its treatment on cognitive function. *N Engl J Med* 2007;356:1842–52.

5. Kelly WD, Lillehei RC, Merkel FK, Idezuki Y, Goetz FC. Allotransplantation of the pancreas and duodenum along with the kidney in diabetic nephropathy. *Surgery* 1967;61:827–37.

6. Lillehei RC, Simmons RL, Najarian JS, Goetz FC. Pancreato-duodenal and renal allotransplantation in juvenile onset, insulin dependent, diabetes mellitus with terminal nephropathy. *Langenbecks Archr Chir* 1970;326:88–105.

7. Gruessner AC, Gruessner RW. Pancreas transplant outcomes for United States and non-United States cases as reported to the United Network for Organ Sharing and the International Pancreas Transplant Registry as of December 2011. *Clin Transplant* 2012;23–40.

8. Reddy KS, Stablein D, Taranto S et al. Long-term survival following simultaneous kidney-pancreas transplantation versus kidney transplantation alone in patients with type 1 diabetes mellitus and renal failure. *Am J Kid Dis* 2003;41:464–70.

9. Fioretto P, Steefes MW, Sutherland DE, Goetz FC, Mauer M. Reversal of lesions of diabetic nephropathy after pancreas transplantation. *N Engl J Med* 1998;339:69–75.

10. Browne S, Gill J, Dong J et al. The impact of pancreas transplantation on kidney allograft survival. *Am J Transplant* 2011;11:1951–8.

11. Israni AK, Skeans MA, Gustafson SK et al. OPTN/ SRTR 2012 annual data report: Pancreas. *Am J Transplant* 2014;14(Suppl 1):45–68.

12. Gruessner AC, Sutherland DE, Gruessner RW. Pancreas transplantation in the United States: A review. *Curr Opin Organ Transplant* 2010;15:93–101.

13. Ramanathan V, Goral S, Tanriover B et al. Screening asymptomatic diabetic patients for coronary artery disease prior to renal transplantation. *Transplantation* 2005;79:1453–8.

14. Orlando G, Stratta RJ, Light J. Pancreas transplantation for type 2 diabetes mellitus. *Curr Opin Organ Transplant* 2011;16:110–5.

15. Finger EB, Radosevich DM, Dunn TB et al. A composite risk model for predicting technical failure in pancreas transplantation. *Am J Transplant* 2013;13:1840–9.

16. Ziaja J, Krol R, Pawlicki J et al. Donor-dependent risk factors for early surgical complications after simultaneous pancreas-kidney transplantation. *Transplant Proc* 2011;43:3092–6.

17. Gruessner AC, Sutherland DE, Gruessner RW. Long-term outcome after pancreas transplantation. *Curr Opin Organ Transplant* 2012;17:100–5.

18. Axelod DA, Sung RS, Meyer KH, Wolfe RA, Kaufman DB. Systematic evaluation of pancreas allograft quality, outcomes and geographic variation in utilization. *Am J Transplant* 2010;10:837–45.

19. Diem P, Abid M, Redmon JB, Sutherland DE, Robertson RP. Systematic venous drainage of pancreas allografts as independent cause of hyperinsulinemia in type 1 diabetic recipients. *Diabetes* 1990;39:534–40.

20. Despres JP, Lemarche B, Mariege P et al. Hyperinsulinemia as an independent risk factor for ischemic heart disease. *N Engl J Med* 1996;11:952–7.

21. Bazerbachi F, Selzner M, Marquez MA et al. Portal venous versus systemic venous drainage of pancreas grafts: Impact on long-term results. *Am J Transplant* 2012;12:226–32.

22. Stadler M, Anderwald C, Pacini G et al. Chronic peripheral hyperinsulinemia in type 1 diabetic patients after successful combined pancreas-kidney transplantation does not affect ectopic lipid accumulation in skeletal muscle and liver. *Diabetes* 2010;59:215–8.

23. Troppmann C. Surgical complications. In: Gruessner RWG, Sutherland DER, eds., *Pancreas Transplantation*. New York: Springer, 2004:206–37.

24. Sollinger HW, Odorico JS, Becker YT, D'Alessandro AM, Pirsch JD. One thousand simultaneous pancreas-kidney transplants at a single center with 22-year follow-up. *Ann Surg* 2009;250:618–30.

25. Felmer PT, Pascher A, Kahl A et al. Influence of donor- and recipient-specific factors on the postoperative course after combined pancreas-kidney transplantation. *Langenbecks Arch Surg* 2010;395:19–25.

26. Schenker P, Vonend O, Ertas N, Wunsch A, Viebahn R. Preprocurement pancreas allocation suitability score does not correlate with long-term pancreas graft survival. *Transplant Proc* 2010;42:178–80.

27. Tollemar J, Tyden G, Brattstorm C, Groth CG. Anticoagulation therapy for prevention of pancreatic graft thrombosis: Benefits and risks. *Transplant Proc* 1988;20:479–80.

28. Troppmann C, Gruessner AC, Bendetti E et al. Vascular graft thrombosis after pancreatic transplantation: Univariate and multivariate operative and nonoperative risk factor analysis. *J Am Coll Surg* 1996;182:285–316.

29. Gilabert R, Fernandez-Cruz L, Real MI, Ricart MJ, Astudillo E, Montana X. Treatment and outcome of pancreatic venous graft thrombosis after kidney-pancreas transplantation. *Br J Surg* 2002;89:355–60.

30. Sansalone CV, Maione G, Aseni P et al. Surgical complications are the main cause of pancreatic allograft in pancreas-kidney transplant recipients. *Transplant Proc* 2005;37:2651–3.

31. Eubank WB, Schmiedl UP, Levy AE, Marsh CL. Venous thrombosis and occlusion after pancreas transplantation: Evaluation with breath-hold gadolinium-enhanced three-dimensional MR imaging. *Am J Roentgenol* 2000;210:437–42.

32. Delis S, Dervenis C, Bramis J, Burke GW, Ciancio G. Vascular complications of pancreas transplantation. *Pancreas* 2004;28:413–20.

33. Ciancio G, Julian J, Fernandez L, Miller J, Burke GW. Successful surgical salvage of pancreas allograft after complete venous thrombosis. *Transplantation* 2000;70:126–31.

34. Yoshimatsu R, Yamgami T, Terayama K et al. Percutaneous transcatheter thrombolysis for graft thrombosis after pancreas transplantation. *Pancreas* 2009;38:597–9.

35. Stockland AH, Willingham DL, Paz-Fumagalli R et al. Pancreas transplant venous thrombosis: Role of endovascular interventions for graft salvage. *Cardiovasc Intervent Radiol* 2009;32:279–83.

36. Maraschio MA, Kayler LK, Merion RM et al. Successful surgical salvage of partial pancreatic allograft thrombosis. *Transplant Proc* 2003;35:1491–3.

37. Troppmann C. Complications after pancreas transplantation. *Curr Opin Organ Transplant* 2010;15:112–8.

38. Lubezky N, Goykhman Y, Nakache R et al. Early and late presentation of graft arterial pseudoaneurysm following pancreatic transplantation. *World J Surg* 2013;37:1430–7.

39. Tan M, Di Carlo A, Stein LA, Cantarovich M, Tchervenkov JI, Metrakos P. Pseudoaneurysm of the superior mesenteric artery after pancreas transplantation treated by endovascular stenting. *Transplantation* 2001;72:336–8.

40. Green BT, Tuttle-Newhall J, Suhocki P, Smith SR, O'Connor JB. Massive gastrointestinal haemorrhage due to rupture of a donor pancreatic artery pseudoaneurysm in a pancreas transplant recipient. *Clin Transplant* 2004;18:108–11.

41. Verni MP, Leone JP, DeRoover A. Pseudoaneurysm of the Y-graft/iliac artery anastomosis following pancreas transplantation: A case report and review of the literature. *Clin Transplant* 2001;15:72–6.

42. Fujita S, Fujikawa T, Mekeel KL et al. Successful endovascular treatment of a leaking pseudoaneurysm without graft loss after simultaneous pancreas and kidney transplantation. *Transplantation* 2006;82:717–8.

43. Small RM, Shetzigovaski I, Blachar, A et al. Redefining late acute graft pancreatitis: Clinical presentation, radiologic findings, principles of management, and prognosis. *Ann Surg* 2008;247:1058–63.

44. Alonso D, Dunn TB, Rigley T et al. Increased pancreatitis in allografts flushed with histidine-tryptophane-ketoglutarate (HTK) solution: A cautionary tale. *Am J Transplant* 2008;8:1942–5.

45. Humar A Kandaswamy R, Drangstveit MB, Parr E, Gruessner AG, Sutherland DE. Prolonged preservation increases surgical complications after pancreas transplants. *Surgery* 2000;127:545–51.

46. Margreiter R, Schmid T, Dunser M, Tauscher T, Hengter P, Konigstrainer A. Cytomegalovirus (CMV)-pancreatitis: A rare complication after pancreas transplantation. *Transplant Proc* 1991;23:1619–22.

47. Troppmann C, Gruessner AC, Dunn DL, Sutherland DE, Gruessner RW. Surgical complications requiring early relaparotomy after pancreas transplantation: A multivariate risk factor and economic impact analysis of the cyclosporine era. *Ann Surg* 1998;227:255–68.

48. Niederhaus SV, Leverson GE, Lorentzen DF et al. Acute cellular and antibody-mediated rejection of the pancreas allograft: Incidence, risk factors and outcomes. *Am J Transplant* 2013;13:2945–55.

49. White SA, Shaw JA, Sutherland DE. Pancreas transplantation. *Lancet* 2009;373:1808–17.

50. Malaise J, De Roover A, Squifflet JP et al. Immunosuppression in pancreas transplantation: The Euro SPK trials and beyond. *Acta Chir Belg* 2008;108:673–8.

51. Nakache R, Malaise J, Van Ophem D; Euro-SPK Study Group. A large, prospective, randomized, open-label, multicentre study of corticosteroid withdrawal in SPK transplantation: A 3-year report. *Nephrol Dial Transplant* 2005;20(Suppl):ii40–7.

52. Axelrod D, Leventhal JR, Gallon LG, Parker MA, Kaufman DB. Reduction of CMV disease with steroid-free immunosuppression in simultaneous pancreas-kidney transplant recipients. *Am J Transplant* 2005;5:1423–9.

53. Bazerbachi F, Selzner M, Boehnert MU et al. Thymoglobulin versus basiliximab induction therapy for simultaneous pancreas-kidney transplantation: Impact on rejection, graft function and long-term outcome. *Transplantation* 2011;92:1039–43.

54. Heilman RI, Mazur MJ, Reddy KS. Immunosuppression in simultaneous pancreas-kidney transplantation: Progress to date. *Drugs* 2010;70:793–804.

55. Van Dellen D, Wothington J, Mitu-Pretorian OM et al. Mortality in diabetes: Pancreas transplantation is associated with significant survival benefit. *Nephrol Dial Transplant* 2013;28:1315–22.

56. Ojo AO, Meier-Kriesche HU, Hanson JA et al. The impact of simultaneous pancreas-kidney transplantation on long-term patient survival. *Transplantation* 2001;71:82–90.

57. Port FK, Wolfe RA, Mauger EA, Berling DP, Jiang K. Comparison of survival probabilities for dialysis patients vs cadaveric renal transplant recipients. *JAMA* 1993;270:1339–43.

58. Gruessner RW, Sutherland DE, Gruessner AC. Mortality assessment of pancreas transplants. *Am J Transplant* 2004;4:2018–26.

59. Tydem G, Bolinder J, Solders G et al. A 10-year prospective study of IDDM patients subjected to combined pancreas and kidney transplantation or kidney transplantation alone. *Transplant Proc* 1997;29:3119.

60. Venstrom JM, McBride MA, Rothel KI, Hirshberg B, Orchard TJ, Harlan DM. Survival after pancreas transplantation in patients with diabetes and preserved kidney function. *JAMA* 2003;290:2817–23.

61. Nakache R, Tyden G, Groth CG. Quality of life in diabetic patients after combined pancreas-kidney or kidney transplantation. *Diabetes* 1989;38(Suppl 1):40–2.

62. Sureshkumar KK, Patel BM, Markatos A, Nghiem DD, Marcus RJ. Quality of life after organ transplantation in type 1 diabetics with end-stage renal disease. *Clin Transplant* 2006;20:19–25.

63. Ziaja J, Bozek-Pajak D, Kowalik A, Krol R, Cierpka L. Impact of pancreas transplantation on the quality of life of diabetic renal transplant recipients. *Transplant Proc* 2009;41:3156–8.

64. Nankivell BJ, Burrows RJ, Fung CL, O'Connell PJ, Allen RD, Chapman JR. Evolution and pathophysiology of renal-transplant glomerulosclerosis. *Transplantation* 2004;78:461–8.

65. Fioretto P, Steffes MW, Sutherland DE, Goetz FC, Mauer M. Reversal of lesions of diabetic nephropathy after pancreas transplantation. *N Engl J Med* 1998;339:69–75.

66. Nakache R, Mainetti L, Tyden G, Groth CG. Renal transplantation in diabetes mellitus: Influence of combined pancreas-kidney transplantation on outcome. *Transplant Proc* 1990;22:624–5.

67. Israni AK, Feldman HI, Propert KJ, Leonard M, Mange KC. Impact of simultaneous pancreas-kidney transplantation on kidney allograft survival. *Am J Transplant* 2005;5:374–82.

68. Weiss AS, Smits G, Wiseman AC. Twelve-month pancreas graft function significantly influences survival following simultaneous pancreas-kidney transplantation. *Clin J Am Soc Nephrol* 2009;4:988–95.

69. Kleinclauss F, Fauda M, Sutheralnd DE et al. Pancreas after living donor kidney transplants in diabetic patients: Impact on long-term kidney graft function. *Clin Transplant* 2009;23:437–46.

70. Coppelli A, Giannarelli R, Vistoli F et al. The beneficial effects of pancreas transplant alone on diabetic nephropathy. *Diabetes Care* 2005;28:1366–70.

71. Jukema JW, Smets YF, van der Pijl JW et al. Impact of simultaneous pancreas and kidney transplantation on progression of coronary atherosclerosis in patients with end-stage renal failure due to type 1 diabetes. *Diabetes Care* 2002;25:906–11.

72. La Rocca E, Fiorina P, di Carlo V et al. Cardiovascular outcomes after kidney-pancreas and kidney-alone transplantation. *Kidney Int* 2001;60:1964–71.

73. Giannarelli R, Copperlli A, Sartini M et al. Effects of pancreas-kidney transplantation on diabetic retinopathy. *Transplant Int* 2005;18:619–22.

74. Chow V, Pai R, Chapman J et al. Diabetic retinopathy after combined kidney-pancreas transplantation. *Clin Transplant* 1999;13:356–62.

75. Pearce IA, Ilango B, Sells RA, Wong D. Stabilization of diabetic retinopathy following simultaneous pancreas and kidney transplantation. *Br J Ohpthalmol* 2000;84:736–40.

76. Wang Q, Klein R, Moss SE et al. The influence of combined kidney-pancreas transplantation on diabetic retinopathy. *Ophthalmology* 1994;101:1071–6.

77. Tesfaye S, Boulton AJ, Dyck PJ et al. Diabetic neuropathies: Update on definitions, diagnostic criteria, estimation of severity, and treatments. *Diabetes Care* 2010;33:2285–93.

78. Navarro X, Sutherland DE, Kennedy WR. Long-term effects of pancreatic transplantation on diabetic neuropathy. *Ann Neurol* 1997;42:727–36.

79. Larsen JL, Ratanasuwan T, Burkman T et al. Carotid intima media thickness decreases after pancreas transplantation. *Transplantation* 2002;73:936–40.

80. Nankivell BJ, Lau SG, Chapman JR, O'Connell PJ, Fletcher JP, Allen RD. Progression of macrovascular disease after transplantation. *Transplantation* 2000;69:574–81.

81. Biesenach G, Konigstrainer A, Gross C, Margreiter R. Progression of macrovascular diseases is reduced in type 1 diabetic patients after more than 5 years successful combined pancreas-kidney transplantation in comparison to kidney transplantation alone. *Transpl Int* 2005;18:1054–60.

54

Noninsulinoma pancreatogenous hypoglycemia syndrome and postbariatric hypoglycemia

SPYRIDOULA MARAKA AND ADRIAN VELLA

INTRODUCTION

Glucose is an obligate fuel for the brain under physiologic conditions [1]. Indeed, glucose homeostasis is maintained by one hormone (insulin), which lowers glucose, and counter-regulatory mediators (glucagon, catecholamines, cortisol, and growth hormone), which raise glucose concentrations and facilitate the transition to the use of lipid-derived substrates during prolonged fasting. In such circumstances, glucose may be lower than typical fasting values, but because of appropriate metabolic and counter-regulatory changes, cognition is not impaired and no symptoms of neuroglycopenia are apparent. As such, establishing a diagnosis of a hypoglycemic disorder requires the documentation of Whipple's triad [2]; namely, a low plasma glucose concentration (≤55–60 mg/dL) must be measured with a precise method at the time of symptoms consistent with hypoglycemia, and these symptoms must be relieved by correction of the hypoglycemia. Only after these criteria are fulfilled should one embark on testing the mechanism by which hypoglycemia occurs [3].

Previous work had established cessation of endogenous insulin secretion when blood glucose is in the 60–65 mg/dL range and activation of the sympathoadrenal system when glucose is approximately 60 mg/dL. This can cause adrenergic symptoms such as palpitations, tremors, and anxiety, or cholinergic symptoms such as sweating, hunger, and paresthesias. However, these symptoms are nonspecific. Neuroglycopenic symptoms are more specific and include cognitive dysfunction, dysarthria, behavioral changes, fatigue, seizures, and coma [4].

The differential diagnosis of hypoglycemia depends on the general context and health of the patient. The likely causes of hypoglycemia differ significantly between otherwise healthy patients and those seen in an inpatient setting (where patients usually have significant systemic illness). In individuals who are otherwise well, endogenous hyperinsulinemic hypoglycemia is the most common cause of hypoglycemia, whereas underlying systemic disease and iatrogenic factors play a major role in sick or hospitalized individuals.

In this chapter, we discuss the noninsulinoma pancreatogenous hypoglycemia syndrome (NIPHS), which may overlap with the hypoglycemia seen in postbariatric patients.

ENDOGENOUS HYPERINSULINEMIC HYPOGLYCEMIA

Endogenous hyperinsulinemic hypoglycemia was first described at Mayo Clinic in 1926 by Dr. Wilder [5]. A surgeon, with metastatic pancreatic islet cell tumor, presented with hypoglycemic episodes. Extracts from his liver metastases obtained at the time of abdominal exploration precipitated hypoglycemia in rabbits. This established insulinoma as a clinical entity. Other causes of endogenous hyperinsulinism include the use of insulin secretagogues or exogenous insulin, insulin autoimmune hypoglycemia, and occasionally a functional β-cell disorder, such as NIPHS.

EVALUATION

The first step in the evaluation of patients with symptoms suggestive of endogenous hyperinsulinemic hypoglycemia is to review their history in detail, including the nature and timing of symptoms in relation to meals, underlying medical conditions and previous surgeries, medications, and social history.

Optimal testing during a symptomatic episode when hypoglycemia is documented requires simultaneous testing of (in addition to glucose) insulin, C-peptide, β-hydroxybutyrate, and proinsulin. Assuming that hyperinsulinemia is the underlying cause of hypoglycemia, it is also important to exclude factitious causes of hypoglycemia by screening for sulfonylurea abuse using a sulfonylurea screen that can detect compounds such as glimepiride and repaglinide. Insulin antibodies should be measured to distinguish insulin autoimmune hypoglycemia from other causes of endogenous hyperinsulinism.

If the patient is asymptomatic when seen despite a history or previous laboratory data sufficiently suggestive of a hypoglycemic disorder, the diagnostic strategy is to undertake provocative tests to replicate the conditions when hypoglycemia is likely to occur. A supervised 72-hour fast is performed when symptoms suggest a postabsorptive process and a mixed meal study if symptoms are suggestive of a postprandial process.

Seventy-two-hour fast

The supervised fast is usually undertaken for up to 72 hours and should be performed in a unit with experience in its conduct. In a group of 170 insulinoma patients, 93% had a positive fast by 48 hours of fasting and 99% by 72 hours [6]. The fast can be initiated as an outpatient, given the high frequency of hypoglycemia in the first 24 hours [7], and the utility of insulin surrogates in determining whether a fast should proceed [8,9]. Other criteria for ending the supervised fast include documentation of Whipple's triad or a glucose of <55 mg/dL with previous documentation of Whipple's triad even in the absence of neuroglycopenia.

Ending the fast may be difficult, especially in the setting of nonspecific symptoms with serum glucose near the hypoglycemic threshold. Confounding this difficulty is the fact that low serum glucose may be physiological, and glucose levels in the 40–50 mg/dL range are not uncommonly seen, particularly in young lean women. Simple bedside tests of neurocognitive function should be performed at scheduled intervals and at the time of the symptoms to establish whether neuroglycopenia is actually occurring.

Mixed meal study

Standards have not been established for a mixed meal study. The study is performed in patients with symptoms of postprandial hypoglycemia. The test is performed over 5 hours, during which the patient should ingest a standardized meal containing carbohydrate, protein, and fat. A meal containing calories in liquid or semisolid form should be avoided in subjects who have undergone upper gastrointestinal surgery (especially, but not limited to, Roux-en-Y gastric bypass [RYGB] or Nissen fundoplication). It makes little sense to use "a meal that provokes symptoms" when an oral glucose tolerance test or pancakes and syrup will cause a multitude of unpleasant side effects in most subjects after RYGB. Samples are collected for plasma glucose, insulin, C-peptide, and proinsulin prior to the ingestion of the meal and every 30 minutes thereafter. It is important to note that a positive test does not provide a diagnosis, but rather a confirmation of Whipple's triad in the postprandial state. The β-cell polypeptide criteria for endogenous hyperinsulinemic hypoglycemia should not be used (or used with extreme caution) in the postprandial setting since a concentration in the peripheral blood does not automatically imply active secretion and is also affected by clearance and distribution [3].

CRITERIA FOR ENDOGENOUS HYPERINSULINEMIA

The documentation of endogenous hyperinsulinemia includes the following criteria [10]:

1. Plasma insulin concentrations of ≥3 μU/mL.
2. C-peptide of ≥200 pmol/L.
3. Proinsulin of ≥5 pmol/L.
4. β-Hydroxybutyrate of ≤2.7 mmol/L. Hyperinsulinemia leads to a persistent suppression of β-hydroxybutyrate. A negative fast is suggested by a β-hydroxybutyrate level of >2.7 mmol/L or two successive β-hydroxybutyrate values in excess of the 18-hour level [8].
5. Response to glucagon. Inappropriate insulin secretion during a prolonged fast protects hepatic glycogen stores from mobilization to glucose. Therefore, an incremental serum glucose response of ≥25 mg/dL in response to glucagon administration implies the presence of insulin or an insulin-like factor.

LOCALIZATION STUDIES

In patients with documented endogenous hyperinsulinemic hypoglycemia, localization studies are necessary to distinguish between the presence of an insulinoma and a diffuse process. They can be divided into noninvasive tests, such as triple-phase computed tomography (CT), MRI, and transabdominal ultrasonography, and invasive tests, such as endoscopic ultrasound and selective arterial calcium stimulation test (SACST).

The SACST has been characterized as both a diagnostic and a regionalization test [11,12]. It is often performed in patients with hyperinsulinemic hypoglycemia in the absence of a lesion or in case of multiple lesions on imaging, where the source of insulin production is uncertain and surgery is

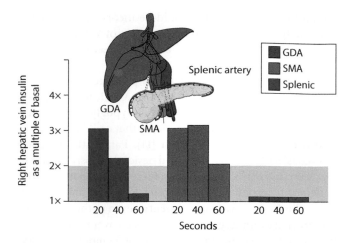

Figure 54.1 SACST is positive (doubling or more of basal plasma insulin in right hepatic vein 20, 40, and 60 seconds after the injection of calcium) in this patient, indicating hyperfunctioning β-cells in the arterial distribution of the gastroduodenal artery (GDA) and superior mesenteric artery (SMA). (Courtesy of Adrian Vella, MD.)

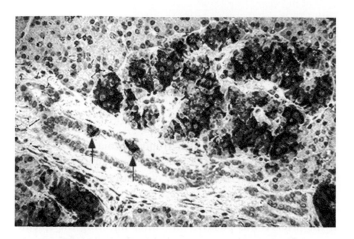

Figure 54.2 Positive insulin immunostaining of a hypertrophied islet (upper right) and two β-cells budding from an acinar duct (arrows). (Courtesy of F. John Service, MD.)

contemplated. This technique is highly dependent on operator experience and ability to interpret the angiogram that accompanies the functional testing. The procedure includes puncture of the femoral vein with catheterization of the right hepatic vein via the inferior vena cava. Calcium gluconate is selectively injected into the gastroduodenal artery, superior mesenteric artery, and splenic artery. A rise of at least two- to threefold at 20, 40, and 60 seconds after the injection of calcium will localize the excessive insulin secretion to the head of the pancreas (gastroduodenal artery), the uncinate (superior mesenteric artery), and the body or tail of the pancreas (splenic artery) if typical anatomy is present (Figure 54.1).

NONINSULINOMA PANCREATOGENOUS HYPOGLYCEMIA SYNDROME

NIPHS was first described in 1999 [13]. It is a rare syndrome characterized by endogenous hyperinsulinemic hypoglycemia in the absence of a discrete insulinoma. The predominant clinical feature of NIPHS is neuroglycopenia 2–4 hours postprandially but not in the fasting state. In contrast, most patients with insulinomas have fasting hypoglycemia [14]. Although a significant minority report postprandial symptoms, the occurrence of symptoms solely postprandially is seen in approximately 6% of patients with insulinoma [7]. During episodes of hypoglycemia, patients with NIPHS have elevated plasma insulin, C-peptide, and proinsulin levels; a low plasma β-hydroxybutyrate concentration; and a negative sulfonylurea/meglitinide screen.

HISTOPATHOLOGY

Pancreatic tissue from patients with NIPHS shows evidence of islet hypertrophy and nesidioblastosis, a term used to describe the neodifferentiation of islet of Langerhans cells from pancreatic exocrine duct epithelium [13]. Histologic features of nesidioblastosis include not only enlarged islet size, but also increased islet number (hyperplasia), increased periductular islets, and enlarged β-cell nuclei (Figure 54.2). Islet-like cells budding off exocrine ducts are noted and are most evident on immunohistochemical staining for chromogranin A [13]. The hypertrophic islet cells also stain positively for insulin, glucagon, somatostatin, and pancreatic polypeptide.

These pathologic findings are similar to those seen in neonates and infants with persistent hyperinsulinemic hypoglycemia. However, there is no mutation identified in the Kir6.2 and SUR1 genes, which have been associated with familial persistent hyperinsulinemic hypoglycemia of infancy [15,16].

It remains controversial whether these pathologic findings directly correlate with the clinical features of NIPHS. Subtle histologic changes characteristic of nesidioblastosis were found in 36.7% of patients in an autopsy series of 207 patients with no history of hypoglycemia [17]. In addition, the inability to quantitatively distinguish nesidioblastosis using morphometric measurements in patients with hyperinsulinemic hypoglycemia from those lacking such a clinical association [18] has led to the suggestion that the morphologic features of nesidioblastosis may be a normal variant rather than the anatomic basis for hypoglycemia in adults with hyperinsulinism [17,18].

LOCALIZATION STUDIES

Imaging studies of the pancreas, including CT, MRI, and transabdominal and endoscopic ultrasonography, are negative in patients with NIPHS. However, insulin secretory responses to SACST are positive in multiple vascular territories of the arterial supply of the pancreas, in contrast to insulinoma, where the response is positive in one artery alone [19].

MANAGEMENT

For patients with mild to moderate symptoms, nutrition modification, such as decreasing free carbohydrate intake and spacing the carbohydrate intake evenly throughout the day, may be helpful. There are no studies showing that pharmacotherapy can be beneficial in patients with NIPHS.

For patients with severe neuroglycopenia or with symptoms refractory to dietary interventions, subtotal pancreatectomy has been the mainstay of treatment. The degree of surgery is determined by the results of the SACST. The pancreas to the left of the superior mesenteric vein is resected if the SACST was positive only after injecting the splenic artery. The resection is expanded to the right of the superior mesenteric vein if the test was positive after injecting an additional artery. A gradient-guided approach is used for debulking the pancreas, even in patients whose disease appears to involve the whole pancreas.

POSTBARIATRIC SURGERY HYPOGLYCEMIA

Bariatric surgery is currently the most effective means of long-term weight management in severely obese persons, resulting in resolution or improvement of many debilitating and life-threatening conditions and leading to significant improvement of their quality of life [20]. The number of procedures performed has increased dramatically over the last decade. According to the American Society for Metabolic and Bariatric Surgery data, as of 2013, we are performing ~200,000 bariatric surgeries annually in the United States, a nearly 500% increase since the year 2000.

RYGB, which is the most commonly performed bariatric surgery, alters glucose fluxes and metabolism [21]. RYGB leads to a higher and earlier peak of plasma glucose concentration, as well as lower nadir glucose levels postprandially [22]. In addition, the secretion of insulin and glucagon-like peptide 1 (GLP-1) is accentuated and occurs earlier during the postprandial period [22]. Approximately 10%–15% of patients who have undergone RYGB surgery may present with symptoms such as diaphoresis, weakness, dizziness, and palpitations in the postoperative period. These nonspecific symptoms, known as Dumping syndrome, typically occur within 15–30 minutes of consuming high levels of simple carbohydrates and are caused by rapid emptying of partially digested foods, with mechanical distention, and altered secretion of intestinal hormones, including glucagon [23] and GLP-1 [23,24]. Together, these changes may lead to fluid shifts into the gastrointestinal tract and subsequent intravascular volume contraction, adrenergic stimulation, and postprandial hypoglycemia [25]. Postprandial symptoms without Whipple's triad, previously called "reactive hypoglycaemia," indicate a functional disorder in which symptoms are not due to hypoglycemia and for which an oral glucose tolerance test is not indicated [26,27]. Patients who have undergone RYGB may have many postprandial symptoms, many of which could be incorrectly attributed to hypoglycemia. Therefore, the criteria of Whipple's triad need to be rigorously applied before proceeding with further evaluation.

In 2005, Service and colleagues presented six patients after RYGB who were referred to Mayo Clinic for evaluation of repeated episodes of postprandial hypoglycemia associated with profound neuroglycopenia that could not be controlled by lifestyle modification [11]. Pancreatic resection showed islet cell hypertrophy and nesidioblastosis similar to that seen in NIPHS. In a subsequent report, 36 patients who underwent partial pancreatectomy for nesidioblastosis at Mayo Clinic were evaluated. Twenty-seven of those patients had previously undergone RYGB with an average time from the RYGB to the pancreatic resection of 54 months. Ninety-two percent of the patients were female [28].

Since the original report from Service and colleagues, an increasing number of patients with severe hypoglycemia as a result of endogenous hyperinsulinemia in the post-RYGB setting has been reported, leading to a nationwide recognition of this condition [29]. The prevalence of postbariatric hypoglycemia appears to be less than 1% [30,31], typically occurring 1–5 years after surgery and almost exclusively after a meal.

The initial evaluation of hypoglycemia includes measurement of glucose, insulin, proinsulin, C-peptide, and β-hydroxybutyrate and sulfonylurea/meglitinide screening during an episode of hypoglycemia. If a spontaneous episode of hypoglycemia is not captured, patients undergo a provocative test such as a mixed meal study or a 72-hour fast. Similarly to patients with NIPHS, the patients with postbariatric hypoglycemia have evidence of endogenous hyperinsulinemia with elevated plasma insulin ($\geq$3 pmol/L), C-peptide ($\geq$0.2 nmol/L), and proinsulin ($\geq$5 pmol/L) levels; a low plasma β-hydroxybutyrate ($\leq$2.7 mmol/L) concentration; and a negative sulfonylurea/meglitinide screen. As in all cases of hyperinsulinemic hypoglycemia, insulin antibodies should be measured to rule out insulin autoimmune hypoglycemia.

Radiological localization studies are typically negative in patients with postbariatric hypoglycemia. However, one of the patients in the original report had evidence of multifocal insulinoma [11]. When SACST is performed, patients with postbariatric hypoglycemia have positive responses with injection of multiple arteries. Finally, for patients who undergo pancreatectomy, findings on pathology are also suggestive of nesidioblastosis.

Although the underlying pathologic features of NIPHS and postbariatric hypoglycemia are similar, and they are both characterized by endogenous hyperinsulinemia, negative radiologic imaging, and positive SACST, postbariatric hypoglycemia is considered a separate clinical entity. Postbariatric hypoglycemia is much more common than NIPHS. Patients with NIPHS have not undergone bariatric surgery, and they are predominantly males, in contrast to the female predominance in patients with postbariatric hypoglycemia. Moreover, patients with NIPHS have no evidence of fasting hypoglycemia or insulinoma, both of which could be found rarely in patients who have undergone bariatric surgery.

There are multiple limitations in our diagnostic approach to postbariatric hypoglycemia. Standards have not been established for the mixed meal study. The criteria for hyperinsulinemic hypoglycemia need to be used with extreme caution in the postprandial setting [3]. Moreover, for patients who undergo SACST, focal versus diffuse positive results do not provide indisputable evidence for or against the diagnosis of insulinoma versus nesidioblastosis, since there may be multiple insulinomas scattered through the pancreas, or a tumor residing in an area supplied by two arteries or nesidioblastosis can actually be restricted in one portion of the pancreas. In addition, studies have failed to find a correlation between SACST results and histopathology [32]. Finally, the incidence of abnormal SACST in asymptomatic patients after bariatric surgery is uncertain. The pathologic findings that constitute the definition of nesidioblastosis, as well as its exact incidence, remain unknown, raising barriers to optimal practice. Conversely, one study using cadaveric pancreata as controls, instead of surgically resected pancreata, did not find increased islet diameters. However, this study noted increased nuclear diameter of the islet cells in nesidioblastosis compared with controls [33]. Another study observed that peliosis-like vascular ectasia was increased in nesidioblastosis [28].

The pathophysiology of this process likely involves multiple mechanisms. Proposed mechanisms of post-RYGB hypoglycemia include (1) β-cell hyperfunction due to adaptive β-cell hypertrophy that develops during obesity and does not regress after the surgery, (2) a severe manifestation of dumping syndrome caused by early entry of ingested nutrients into the small intestine, (3) improved insulin sensitivity after RYGB weight loss unmasking a previously unrecognized hyperinsulinemia syndrome or underlying growth factor abnormality, or (4) abnormal glucagon response. It is known that after RYGB, the concentrations of postprandial GLP-1 increase compared with control subjects [34–36]. GLP-1 has been presented as a critical contributor to the pathophysiology of postbariatric hypoglycemia [37]. Enhanced secretion of GLP-1 by enteroendocrine L-cells due to rapid intestinal delivery of nutrients has been suggested to lead to increased insulin secretion. Moreover, GLP-1 has been proposed as a possible causative mechanism of nesidioblastosis because of its effects on β-cell neogenesis and proliferation in rodents [38–40] and decreased apoptosis of islets in humans [41]. However, a study by Shah and colleagues showed that administration of exendin-9,39, which is a competitive antagonist of GLP-1, did not alter meal appearance, suppression of glucose production, and stimulation of glucose disappearance in patients after RYGB [42]. Moreover, the persistence of hyperinsulinemic hypoglycemia after RYGB reversal, despite marked decreases in GLP-1 levels, suggests that GLP-1 is not such a major factor in the post-RYGB hypoglycemia [43]. Interestingly, the same study showed that the levels of glucose-dependent insulinotropic polypeptide (GIP) were markedly elevated after the RYGB reversal, indicating a potential role for the persistent hyperinsulinemic hypoglycemia. Finally, additional gastrointestinal factors, such as gut microbia [44], bile acid composition [45], and intestinal adaptive responses [46], could influence the absorption of glucose and other nutrients and contribute to postbariatric surgery hypoglycemia.

MANAGEMENT

The patients with mild to moderate symptoms typically respond well to nutritional modifications, such as reduction of free carbohydrates and spacing carbohydrate intake evenly throughout the day. Such dietary changes have been reported to reduce postprandial glycemic excursions and mild to moderate symptoms of hypoglycemia in patients with postbariatric hypoglycemia [31]. Acarbose, an α-glucosidase inhibitor that delays absorption of simple carbohydrates, has been used with good results [47]. Case reports have suggested benefit from administration of verapamil [48], octreotide [49], and diazoxide [50,51]. However, there is little good evidence for their use in the setting of postbariatric surgery patients.

For patients with severe neuroglycopenia or with symptoms refractory to dietary interventions and medical management, subtotal pancreatectomy had previously been the mainstay of treatment, with an approach similar to that for patients with NIPHS. However, subtotal pancreatectomy has high perioperative morbidity and can lead to brittle diabetes and other dysfunctions. More importantly, Vanderveen et al. showed that 90% of patients who had undergone extended distal pancreatectomy developed recurrence of symptoms, while 25% of patients experienced no benefit at all [32]. Currently, pancreatectomy has been abandoned as a treatment option for patients with postbariatric hypoglycemia.

Reversal of gastric bypass with restoration of pyloric function and duodenal continuity has been suggested as an alternative to pancreatectomy. After reversal of the RYGB anatomy, hypoglycemia persisted in some case reports [43,52] but improved in others [53,54]. A case report noted complete reversal of neuroglycopenic symptoms after insertion of a gastrostomy tube into the remnant stomach [55]. Conversion of the RYGB to sleeve gastrectomy is the current procedure of choice, as it has been shown to provide a safer and potentially more effective treatment option for severe hypoglycaemia, while at the same time reducing the possibility of weight regain [53]. Candidates for the procedure are patients who had symptomatic improvement with nutritional administration through a G-tube. However, the supportive data come from a small sample size with short follow-up, and further studies are needed to confirm the beneficial effect from conversion of RYGB to sleeve gastrectomy in patients with postbariatric hypoglycemia.

CONCLUSIONS

NIPHS and postbariatric surgery hypoglycemia are rare causes of endogenous hyperinsulinemic hypoglycemia. Their predominant clinical feature is postprandial hypoglycemia and the presence of neuroglycopenic symptoms. Radiologic imaging studies are negative, but the patients have positive responses in SACST. Pancreatic specimens from these patients have evidence of nesidioblastosis. Multiple mechanisms could be contributing to the pathogenesis of NIPHS and postbariatric hypoglycemia.

REFERENCES

1. Cryer PE. Hypoglycemia, functional brain failure, and brain death. *J Clin Invest* 2007;117(4):868–70.
2. Whipple AO. Islet cell tumors of the pancreas. *Can Med Assoc J* 1952;66(4):334–42.
3. Cryer PE, Axelrod L, Grossman AB et al. Evaluation and management of adult hypoglycemic disorders: An Endocrine Society Clinical Practice Guideline. *J Clin Endocrinol Metab* 2009;94(3):709–28.
4. Towler DA, Havlin CE, Craft S, Cryer P. Mechanism of awareness of hypoglycemia. Perception of neurogenic (predominantly cholinergic) rather than neuroglycopenic symptoms. *Diabetes* 1993;42(12):1791–8.
5. Wilder RM, Allan FN, Power MH, Robertson HE. Carcinoma of the islands of the pancreas: Hyperinsulinism and hypoglycemia. *JAMA* 1927;89(5):348–55.
6. Service FJ, Dale AJ, Elveback LR, Jiang NS. Insulinoma: Clinical and diagnostic features of 60 consecutive cases. *Mayo Clin Proc* 1976;51(7):417–29.
7. Placzkowski KA, Vella A, Thompson GB et al. Secular trends in the presentation and management of functioning insulinoma at the Mayo Clinic, 1987–2007. *J Clin Endocrinol Metab* 2009;94(4):1069–73.
8. Service FJ, O'Brien PC. Increasing serum betahydroxybutyrate concentrations during the 72-hour fast: Evidence against hyperinsulinemic hypoglycemia. *J Clin Endocrinol Metab* 2005;90(8):4555–8.
9. O'Brien T, O'Brien PC, Service FJ. Insulin surrogates in insulinoma. *J Clin Endocrinol Metab* 1993;77(2):448–51.
10. Service FJ. Hypoglycemic disorders. *N Engl J Med* 1995;332(17):1144–52.
11. Service GJ, Thompson GB, Service FJ, Andrews JC, Collazo-Clavell ML, Lloyd RV. Hyperinsulinemic hypoglycemia with nesidioblastosis after gastric-bypass surgery. *N Engl J Med* 2005;353(3):249–54.
12. Doppman JL, Miller DL, Chang R, Shawker TH, Gorden P, Norton JA. Insulinomas: Localization with selective intraarterial injection of calcium. *Radiology* 1991;178(1):237–41.
13. Service FJ, Natt N, Thompson GB et al. Noninsulinoma pancreatogenous hypoglycemia: A novel syndrome of hyperinsulinemic hypoglycemia in adults independent of mutations in Kir6.2 and SUR1 genes. *J Clin Endocrinol Metab* 1999;84(5):1582–9.
14. Kar P, Price P, Sawers S, Bhattacharya S, Reznek RH, Grossman AB. Insulinomas may present with normoglycemia after prolonged fasting but glucose-stimulated hypoglycemia. *J Clin Endocrinol Metab* 2006;91(12):4733–6.
15. de Lonlay P, Fournet JC, Rahier J et al. Somatic deletion of the imprinted 11p15 region in sporadic persistent hyperinsulinemic hypoglycemia of infancy is specific of focal adenomatous hyperplasia and endorses partial pancreatectomy. *J Clin Invest* 1997;100(4):802–7.
16. de Lonlay-Debeney P, Poggi-Travert F, Fournet JC et al. Clinical features of 52 neonates with hyperinsulinism. *N Engl J Med* 1999;340(15):1169–75.
17. Karnauchow PN. Nesidioblastosis in adults without insular hyperfunction. *Am J Clin Pathol* 1982;78(4):511–3.
18. Goudswaard WB, Houthoff HJ, Koudstaal J, Zwierstra RP. Nesidioblastosis and endocrine hyperplasia of the pancreas: A secondary phenomenon. *Hum Pathol* 17(1):46–54.
19. Brown CK, Bartlett DL, Doppman JL et al. Intraarterial calcium stimulation and intraoperative ultrasonography in the localization and resection of insulinomas. *Surgery* 1997;122(6):1189–93; discussion 1193–4.
20. Sjostrom L, Lindroos AK, Peltonen M et al. Lifestyle, diabetes, and cardiovascular risk factors 10 years after bariatric surgery. *N Engl J Med* 2004;351(26):2683–93.
21. Rodieux F, Giusti V, D'Alessio DA, Suter M, Tappy L. Effects of gastric bypass and gastric banding on glucose kinetics and gut hormone release. *Obesity (Silver Spring)* 2008;16(2):298–305.
22. Jorgensen NB, Jacobsen SH, Dirksen C et al. Acute and long-term effects of Roux-en-Y gastric bypass on glucose metabolism in subjects with type 2 diabetes and normal glucose tolerance. *Am J Physiol Endocrinol Metab* 2012;303(1):E122–31.
23. Gebhard B, Holst JJ, Biegelmayer C, Miholic J. Postprandial GLP-1, norepinephrine, and reactive hypoglycemia in dumping syndrome. *Dig Dis Sci* 2001;46(9):1915–23.
24. Yamamoto H, Mori T, Tsuchihashi H, Akabori H, Naito H, Tani T. A possible role of GLP-1 in the pathophysiology of early dumping syndrome. *Dig Dis Sci* 2005;50(12):2263–7.
25. Ukleja A. Dumping syndrome: Pathophysiology and treatment. *Nutr Clin Pract* 2005;20(5):517–25.
26. Hogan MJ, Service FJ, Sharbrough FW, Gerich JE. Oral glucose tolerance test compared with a mixed meal in the diagnosis of reactive hypoglycemia. A caveat on stimulation. *Mayo Clin Proc* 1983;58(8):491–6.
27. Lev-Ran A, Anderson RW. The diagnosis of postprandial hypoglycemia. *Diabetes* 1981;30(12):996–9.

28. Rumilla KM, Erickson LA, Service FJ et al. Hyperinsulinemic hypoglycemia with nesidioblastosis: Histologic features and growth factor expression. *Mod Pathol* 2009;22(2):239–45.

29. Goldfine AB, Mun EC, Devine E et al. Patients with neuroglycopenia after gastric bypass surgery have exaggerated incretin and insulin secretory responses to a mixed meal. *J Clin Endocrinol Metab* 2007;92(12):4678–85.

30. Marsk R, Jonas E, Rasmussen F, Naslund E. Nationwide cohort study of post-gastric bypass hypoglycaemia including 5040 patients undergoing surgery for obesity in 1986–2006 in Sweden. *Diabetologia* 2010;53(11):2307–11.

31. Kellogg TA, Bantle JP, Leslie DB et al. Postgastric bypass hyperinsulinemic hypoglycemia syndrome: Characterization and response to a modified diet. *Surg Obes Relat Dis* 2008;4(4):492–9.

32. Vanderveen KA, Grant CS, Thompson GB et al. Outcomes and quality of life after partial pancreatectomy for noninsulinoma pancreatogenous hypoglycemia from diffuse islet cell disease. *Surgery* 2010;148(6):1237–45; discussion 1245–6.

33. Meier JJ, Butler AE, Galasso R, Butler PC. Hyperinsulinemic hypoglycemia after gastric bypass surgery is not accompanied by islet hyperplasia or increased beta-cell turnover. *Diabetes Care* 2006;29(7):1554–9.

34. Kellum JM, Kuemmerle JF, O'Dorisio TM et al. Gastrointestinal hormone responses to meals before and after gastric bypass and vertical banded gastroplasty. *Ann Surg* 1990;211(6):763–70; discussion 770–1.

35. Laferrere B, Teixeira J, McGinty J et al. Effect of weight loss by gastric bypass surgery versus hypocaloric diet on glucose and incretin levels in patients with type 2 diabetes. *J Clin Endocrinol Metab* 2008;93(7):2479–85.

36. le Roux CW, Aylwin SJ, Batterham RL et al. Gut hormone profiles following bariatric surgery favor an anorectic state, facilitate weight loss, and improve metabolic parameters. *Ann Surg* 2006;243(1):108–14.

37. Salehi M, Gastaldelli A, D'Alessio DA. Blockade of glucagon-like peptide 1 receptor corrects postprandial hypoglycemia after gastric bypass. *Gastroenterology* 2014;146(3):669–80e2.

38. Zhou J, Wang X, Pineyro MA, Egan JM. Glucagon-like peptide 1 and exendin-4 convert pancreatic AR42J cells into glucagon- and insulin-producing cells. *Diabetes* 1999;48(12):2358–66.

39. De Leon DD, Deng S, Madani R, Ahima RS, Drucker DJ, Stoffers DA. Role of endogenous glucagon-like peptide-1 in islet regeneration after partial pancreatectomy. *Diabetes* 2003;52(2):365–71.

40. List JF, Habener JF. Glucagon-like peptide 1 agonists and the development and growth of pancreatic beta-cells. *Am J Physiol Endocrinol Metab* 2004;286(6):E875–81.

41. Brubaker PL, Drucker DJ. Minireview: Glucagon-like peptides regulate cell proliferation and apoptosis in the pancreas, gut, and central nervous system. *Endocrinology* 2004;145(6):2653–9.

42. Shah M, Law JH, Micheletto F et al. Contribution of endogenous glucagon-like peptide 1 to glucose metabolism after Roux-en-Y gastric bypass. *Diabetes* 2014;63(2):483–93.

43. Lee CJ, Brown T, Magnuson TH, Egan JM, Carlson O, Elahi D. Hormonal response to a mixed-meal challenge after reversal of gastric bypass for hypoglycemia. *J Clin Endocrinol Metab* 2013;98(7):E1208–12.

44. Liou AP, Paziuk M, Luevano JM Jr, Machineni S, Turnbaugh PJ, Kaplan LM. Conserved shifts in the gut microbiota due to gastric bypass reduce host weight and adiposity. *Sci Transl Med* 2013;5(178):178ra41.

45. Patti ME, Houten SM, Bianco AC et al. Serum bile acids are higher in humans with prior gastric bypass: Potential contribution to improved glucose and lipid metabolism. *Obesity (Silver Spring)* 2009;17(9):1671–7.

46. Hansen CF, Bueter M, Theis N et al. Hypertrophy dependent doubling of L-cells in Roux-en-Y gastric bypass operated rats. *PLoS One* 2013;8(6):e65696.

47. Valderas JP, Ahuad J, Rubio L, Escalona M, Pollak F, Maiz A. Acarbose improves hypoglycaemia following gastric bypass surgery without increasing glucagon-like peptide 1 levels. *Obes Surg* 2012;22(4):582–6.

48. Moreira RO, Moreira RB, Machado NA, Goncalves TB, Coutinho WF. Post-prandial hypoglycemia after bariatric surgery: Pharmacological treatment with verapamil and acarbose. *Obes Surg* 2008;18(12):1618–21.

49. Usukura M, Yoneda T, Oda N et al. Medical treatment of benign insulinoma using octreotide LAR: A case report. *Endocr J* 2007;54(1):95–101.

50. Spanakis E, Gragnoli C. Successful medical management of status post-Roux-en-Y-gastric-bypass hyperinsulinemic hypoglycemia. *Obes Surg* 2009;19(9):1333–4.

51. Arao T, Okada Y, Hirose A, Tanaka Y. A rare case of adult-onset nesidioblastosis treated successfully with diazoxide. *Endocr J* 2006;53(1):95–100.

52. Patti ME, McMahon G, Mun EC et al. Severe hypoglycaemia post-gastric bypass requiring partial pancreatectomy: Evidence for inappropriate insulin secretion and pancreatic islet hyperplasia. *Diabetologia* 2005;48(11):2236–40.

53. Campos GM, Ziemelis M, Paparodis R, Ahmed M, Belt Davis D. Laparoscopic reversal of Roux-en-Y gastric bypass: Technique and utility for treatment of endocrine complications. *Surg Obes Relat Dis* 2014;10(1):36–43.

54. Himpens J, Verbrugghe A, Cadiere GB, Everaerts W, Greve JW. Long-term results of laparoscopic Roux-en-Y gastric bypass: Evaluation after 9 years. *Obes Surg* 2012;22(10):1586–93.

55. McLaughlin T, Peck M, Holst J, Deacon C. Reversible hyperinsulinemic hypoglycemia after gastric bypass: A consequence of altered nutrient delivery. *J Clin Endocrinol Metab* 2010;95(4):1851–5.

55

Surgical management of type 2 diabetes mellitus and metabolic syndrome: Available procedures and clinical data

DANIEL HERRON AND DANIEL SHOUHED

METABOLIC SYNDROME

Definitions

Obesity, particularly abdominal obesity, is associated with hyperinsulinemia, often leading to the development of insulin resistance and subsequently type 2 diabetes mellitus (T2DM). Insulin resistance and adipocyte cytokines may also lead to hypertension, dyslipidemia, vascular inflammation, and endothelial dysfunction, all of which promote the incidence of atherosclerotic cardiovascular disease [1,2]. The constellation of metabolic risk factors for both T2DM and cardiovascular disease is considered to define *metabolic syndrome* (MBS) [3].

The term *metabolic syndrome* has evolved over time in both name and definition. Various descriptions exist, with most differences arising from the presence or absence of insulin resistance. The most commonly used definition, set by the National Cholesterol Education Program (NCEP/ATP III), does not require the presence of insulin abnormalities and defines MBS as the presence of three of the following five derangements: (1) abdominal obesity, characterized by a waist circumference in men of ≥102 cm and in women of ≥88 cm; (2) hypertension (≥130/85 or drug treatment); (3) hypertriglyceridemia (>150 mg/dL or drug treatment);

(4) low-serum high-density lipoprotein (HDL) (<40 mg/dL in women and <50 mg/dL in men or drug treatment); and (5) elevated fasting blood glucose (fasting plasma glucose of >100 mg/dL or drug treatment) [4].

Epidemiology

MBS has quickly become a major and escalating public health concern worldwide, as it leads to a twofold increased risk of developing cardiovascular disease and fivefold increased risk of developing T2DM over 5–10 years [4]. Furthermore, patients with MBS are at an increased risk of stroke, myocardial infarction, and death from such an event compared with unaffected individuals [5,6]. The prevalence of MBS varies considerably depending on the population studied and definition used. Based on the NCEP/ATP criteria from 2001, the prevalence of MBS ranges from 8% to 43% among men and 7% to 56% among women around the world [7]. The observed prevalence of MBS in the National Health and Nutrition Examination Survey (NHANES) from 2004 was 5% among subjects of normal weight, 22% among the overweight, and 60% among obese individuals [7].

In a study from 2012, which estimated that 26 million Americans (8%) satisfy the criteria for T2DM, more than 80% of patients with diabetes were overweight and greater than 50% were obese [8,9]. Approximately 20% of morbidly obese individuals have concomitant T2DM [10]. Diabetes affects an estimated 346 million people worldwide, with estimated global costs of diabetes reaching $376 billion in 2010 [11,12]. It is an inevitably progressive disease that leads to the deterioration of multiple organs and systems and is the most common cause of adult blindness, limb amputations, and renal failure in Western countries, as well as the leading independent risk factor for coronary artery disease. These staggering statistics combined with the growing worldwide epidemic of "diabesity," a term introduced by Shafrir to suggest a single problem [13], indicates the need for drastic intervention.

Guidelines for surgery

According to the 1991 consensus guidelines from the National Institutes of Health, candidates for surgical management of obesity in the United States include males or females with a body mass index (BMI) of ≥40 or 35 kg/m², respectively, with one or more significant obesity-related comorbidities (Table 55.1). Patients must have documented failure of nonsurgical weight loss programs. They must be able to comprehend that significant lifestyle changes around diet and exercise must be followed, as well as understand the importance of postoperative follow-up and vitamin supplementation. Patients are required to undergo a complete psychological evaluation prior to surgery to ensure the absence of uncontrolled psychological illnesses and the lack of active alcohol or substance abuse. Patients must be able to tolerate general anesthesia and comply with the requirement for lifelong postoperative follow-up.

SURGICAL PROCEDURES AND OUTCOMES

Surgical treatment for obesity emerged in the 1950s as physicians noted the weight loss effects of short-gut syndrome. Jejunocolic and then jejunoileal bypass were the first operations introduced and can be considered the archetype for the malabsorptive bariatric procedures. In these operations,

Table 55.1 Guidelines for bariatric surgery

BMI of ≥40 kg/m²
BMI of ≥35 kg/m² and at least one comorbidity
   Diabetes mellitus
   Hypertension
   Congestive heart failure
   Coronary artery disease
   Hyperlipidemia
   Obstructive sleep apnea
   Pulmonary hypertension
   Severe asthma
   Gastroesophageal reflux disease
   Degenerative joint disease

the proximal jejunum is connected to the distal ileum or colon, functionally "short-circuiting" the small intestine and resulting in a surgically induced short-gut syndrome. These early operations functioned by limiting the intestinal surface area coming into contact with digested food, thereby decreasing caloric absorption. The short-term results of these operations were promising and associated with significant weight loss; however, the benefits were soon outweighed by their severe metabolic complications. Associated morbidity included profuse diarrhea leading to electrolyte imbalances, gas–bloat syndrome, bacterial overgrowth, deficiency of fat-soluble vitamins and other micronutrients, impaired mentation, cholelithiasis, nephrolithiasis, and hepatic fibrosis leading to liver failure [14].

The morbidity associated with jejunoileal bypass led to the development of a new generation of operations in the 1960s characterized by gastric restriction. The gastric bypass was developed in the late 1960s. In this operation, the stomach was sectioned into a small upper pouch that was anastomosed to the jejunum. Early versions of this operation used a transversely oriented pouch anastomosed to a loop of jejunum in an end-to-side manner (Billroth II anatomy). Over time, the operation evolved to a small, vertically oriented pouch connected to a Roux-en-Y limb of the jejunum. Purely restrictive operations, such as verticalbanded gastroplasty, were also introduced, avoiding any surgical malabsorption. Despite some negative side effects of the gastric bypass, such as iron deficiency anemia and vitamin B12 deficiency, this operation has stood the test of time and is still quite commonly performed.

Currently, the most common bariatric operations being performed in the United States and around the world are the laparoscopic Roux-en-Y gastric bypass (RYGB) and the laparoscopic sleeve gastrectomy (LSG), also referred to as the vertical sleeve gastrectomy. Although the laparoscopic adjustable gastric band became quite popular in the 2000s, its popularity has declined because of poor longterm weight loss and the frequent need for band removal. Biliopancreatic diversion with duodenal switch (BPD-DS), an operation that combines a sleeve gastrectomy with an intestinal bypass, provides excellent weight loss results but has not become popular due to its technical complexity and numerous malabsorptive side effects.

Each of these operations has been shown to minimize or reverse the derangements associated with MBS and diabetes mellitus. The rate of remission of T2DM after bariatric surgery varies greatly, depending on the definition of remission used, as well as the type of surgery performed. A metaanalysis by Buchwald et al. reported that 78% of diabetic patients had complete remission after bariatric surgery, and diabetes was improved or resolved in approximately 87% of patients [15].

Laparoscopic Roux-en-Y gastric bypass

RYGB was first performed in 1967 via midline laparotomy. The mechanism of weight loss after gastric bypass involves

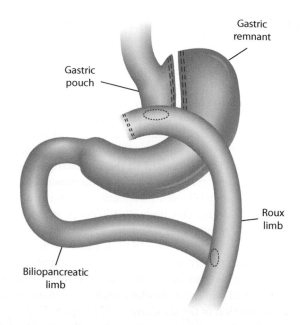

Figure 55.1 Diagram of Roux-en-Y gastric bypass.

both gastric restriction and hormonal changes. The operation entails partitioning of the upper part of the stomach using surgical staples to create a small gastric pouch, typically <30 mL in size (Figure 55.1). A Roux limb, usually 100–150 cm long, is brought up to the stomach pouch and anastomosed using sutures, staples, or a combination of the two. The Roux limb can be brought up in front of the colon (antecolic) or behind the colon (retrocolic). Superiorly, the Roux limb can travel in front of the bypassed stomach (antegastric) or behind it (retrogastric). The Roux-en-Y technique is utilized instead of a loop gastrojejunostomy to avoid bile reflux. Gastric juices from the bypassed stomach mix with bile from the liver and pancreatic secretions and pass through approximately 50 cm of jejunum, referred to as the biliopancreatic limb, before joining the Roux limb to form the "common channel." Internal hernia spaces behind the Roux limb and at the distal anastomosis are closed to prevent bowel entrapment. The operation started to be performed via laparoscopic approach in the mid-1990s, and this is now the generally preferred approach.

Laparoscopic RYGB is one of the most effective operations for achieving remission of T2DM. Since Pories et al. first described the effect of RYGB on the remission of obesity and diabetes mellitus [16], a large body of literature has accumulated to support this finding [15,17–19]. A range of rates of diabetes remission after RYGB has been reported, with great variability stemming from different criteria used for remission. In a meta-analysis of 621 studies, the average rate of diabetes resolution was 80.3% among patients undergoing gastric bypass. Within the same review, the mean excess body weight loss (EBWL) was approximately 64% for patients undergoing RYGB [15]. Four randomized controlled trials have reported that subjects who underwent RYGB were found to have a significantly higher proportion of diabetes remission than patients who were only treated

with medical therapy [20–23]. RYGB has also been shown to be effective in inducing remission of diabetes among patients with a BMI of ≤35 kg/m² [24].

The 2012 STAMPEDE trial was a randomized controlled study comparing surgical and intensive medical therapy for obese patients with diabetes. Diabetes remission was defined as a glycated hemoglobin level of 6.0% or less, with or without the use of antidiabetic medications. There was a higher rate of remission at 1 year among patients undergoing RYGB (42%) versus medical therapy alone (12%), with continued results at a 3-year follow-up (38% vs. 5%; RYGB vs. medical therapy). There were also significant improvements in secondary end points, including hypertension, dyslipidemia, and proteinuria. Triglyceride levels decreased and HDL cholesterol levels increased in the surgical group compared with in the medical group. Furthermore, there was a significant reduction in the number of medications needed to treat hyperlipidemia and hypertension in the RYGB patients [22,25].

An Italian group performed a randomized controlled trial in 2012 involving 60 patients. Researchers evaluated remission of T2DM at 2 years after intensive medical therapy or RYGB. All subjects had T2DM for greater than 5 years with baseline glycated hemoglobin levels greater than 7%. Diabetes remission was defined as a fasting blood glucose of less than 100 mg/dL and a glycated hemoglobin level of less than 6.5% in the absence of pharmacologic therapy. After 2 years of follow-up, 15 of 20 patients (75%) achieved remission compared with 0 of 20 patients in the medically treated group. There was approximately a threefold difference in the decrease of glycated hemoglobin and fasting blood glucose levels between the medically and surgically treated groups. After 2 years, total cholesterol levels normalized in 27% of medically treated patients compared with 100% of patients who underwent RYGB. There were also significant differences in normalization of triglyceride (0% vs. 86%; medical therapy vs. RYGB) and HDL cholesterol (11% vs. 100%; medical therapy vs. RYGB) levels [23].

Laparoscopic sleeve gastrectomy

The LSG was initially performed as the first part of a two-stage operation for patients who were at excessive risk for a complete BPD (Figure 55.2). Substantial weight loss was noted with the sleeve gastrectomy alone, and it has now become widely accepted as a stand-alone operation with excellent weight loss. The operation entails dividing the gastrocolic omentum up to the angle of His superiorly and down to the antrum, along the greater curvature of the stomach, just proximal to the pylorus. Sequential firings of the linear endoscopic stapler begin approximately 5 cm proximal to the pylorus. The stapler is fired parallel to a 34–40 Fr bougie, which is used to calibrate the diameter of the tubularized stomach. Many surgeons choose to oversew or imbricate the staple line to decrease the risk of bleeding or leak. The excised portion of the stomach is then removed. Intraoperative esophagogastroduodenoscopy may be performed to assess

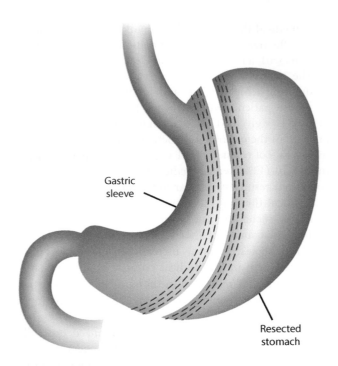

Figure 55.2 Diagram of sleeve gastrectomy.

the patency of the sleeve, ensure intraluminal hemostasis, and rule out a leak from the staple line.

The percentage of EBWL with the sleeve gastrectomy ranges from 49% to 81% [26]. The overall mean EBWL at 5 years or more after sleeve gastrectomy in a review of 16 studies was approximately 59% [27]. As with RYGB, results from trials of LSG in patients with T2DM also show significant remission in the immediate postoperative phase. In observational cohorts, remission rates of T2DM are reported to range from 50% to 80% at 12–18 months of follow-up [28–30].

The STAMPEDE trial compared outcomes between LSG and medical therapy, in addition to comparing RYGB with intensive medical therapy. At 1-year follow-up, the rate of T2DM remission after LSG was 37% versus 12% in the medically treated subjects. Although the rate of remission of T2DM at 3 years was greater among patients undergoing RYGB versus LSG (38 vs. 24%), patients undergoing LSG still demonstrated a significantly higher rate of remission ($p = 0.01$) than patients who were treated with intensive medical therapy (5%). The only predictors of achieving T2DM remission were a reduction in BMI and duration of diabetes of less than 8 years. The number of medications that patients were taking for diabetes, as well as cardiovascular comorbidities, including hypertension and dyslipidemia, was significantly lower after sleeve gastrectomy and gastric bypass at 1 and 3 years. There was also a significant improvement in both triglyceride and HDL levels at 1 and 3 years after sleeve gastrectomy when compared with medical therapy. Finally, the percentage of patients experiencing resolution of MBS was significantly greater in those who underwent LSG or gastric bypass compared with medical therapy alone (65%, 59%, and 35%, respectively) [22,25].

Laparoscopic biliopancreatic diversion with duodenal switch

The first series of BPD operations was reported by Scopinaro et al. [31]. The procedure, originally performed via midline laparotomy, consists of resecting a portion of the distal stomach with closure of the duodenal stump and creation of a gastric pouch between 200 and 500 mL in volume. A Roux limb (also referred to as the alimentary limb) is created, typically 250 cm long, and anastomosed to the stomach pouch. The bypassed intestine, referred to as the biliopancreatic limb since it carries only bile and pancreatic secretions, is anastomosed to the alimentary limb 50–100 cm proximal to the ileocecal valve, resulting in a very short common channel. More than a decade later, the BPD was modified to include a duodenal switch. In the BPD-DS, a sleeve gastrectomy replaces the antrectomy of the original operation. The pylorus is preserved and the alimentary channel is anastomosed to the first portion of the duodenum [32] (Figure 55.3).

The BPD-DS operation is more technically complex than gastric bypass or sleeve gastrectomy, particularly when performed laparoscopically. Additionally, it is associated with a higher incidence of protein and vitamin deficiency. The procedure results in the most weight loss of any metabolic operation, as well as the highest rate of diabetes remission. The mean EBWL with BPD-DS at long-term follow-up ranges from 61% to 85% [33–36]. In a systematic review, which included 48 studies for a total of 1565 patients, comparing different bariatric

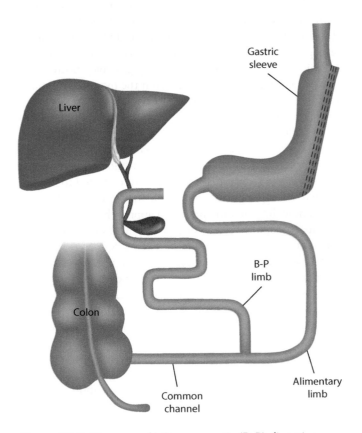

Figure 55.3 Diagram of biliopancreatic (B-P) diversion with duodenal switch.

surgical procedures, the mean EBWL at 2 years' follow-up was 73% with BPD-DS vs. 63% with gastric bypass, 56% with gastroplasty, and 49% with gastric banding. Diabetes resolution was greatest for patients undergoing BPD-DS (95.1%), followed by RYGB (80.3%), gastroplasty (79.7%), and then gastric band (56.7%). The proportion of patients with diabetes resolution or improvement remained fairly constant at time points less than 2 years and 2 years or more [15].

In a prospective randomized controlled trial involving 60 patients by Mingrone et al., 95% of subjects undergoing BPD achieved diabetes remission compared with 0% in the medically treated group at 2-year follow-up. All patients had a history of at least 5 years of diabetes and glycated hemoglobin of 7.0% or more. Remission was defined as a fasting glucose level of <100 mg/dL and glycated hemoglobin of <6.5% in the absence of pharmacologic therapy. There was also significantly greater improvement in total cholesterol levels, triglyceride levels, and HDL levels among patients undergoing BDP versus medical therapy [23].

Laparoscopic gastric banding

Laparoscopic adjustable gastric banding (LGB) was initially performed in 1993 [37,38]. A rigid band with an adjustable inner balloon is placed through a tunnel just behind and inferior to the esophagogastric junction and locked in place anteriorly, circumferentially encompassing the upper stomach (Figure 55.4). This creates a gastric pouch above the band of approximately 15 mL in volume. The stomach is then imbricated over the band anteriorly and secured with several gastrogastric sutures to prevent band slippage. After

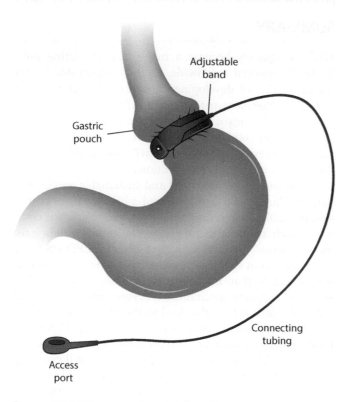

Figure 55.4 Diagram of gastric banding.

some time, the band is inflated and restriction increased [39]. LGB is commonly described as the least invasive of the common bariatric operations available; however, despite its low mortality and short-term morbidity rates, LGB is associated with a number of significant late complications, including band slippage, gastric erosion, and gastric pouch dilatation [40]. The average EBWL in patients undergoing LGB is approximately 46% [41]. Variable rates of diabetes resolution after LGB have been reported in the literature; in a recent meta-analysis, approximately 57% of patients demonstrated resolution of diabetes after LGB [15].

Dixon et al. conducted a randomized controlled trial comparing patients who underwent LGB with those who were treated medically for diabetes and weight loss. All subjects had T2DM and a BMI between 30 and 40. After 2 years, remission of T2DM was achieved by 73% of patients undergoing LGB and only 13% of patients undergoing conventional therapy alone ($p < 0.001$). Remission was defined as a fasting plasma glucose level of less than 126 mg/dL, in addition to a glycated hemoglobin of <6.2%, without the use of oral hypoglycemic medications or insulin [42].

Surgically treated patients lost a mean of 63% of excess body weight compared with 4.3% among the conventional therapy group. Seventy percent of surgical patients experienced remission of MBS, compared with 13% among medically treated patients. Significant changes were seen in the use of cholesterol- and blood pressure-lowering medications among surgically treated patients, but this was not observed in the medically treated patients. Remission of T2DM was related to weight loss and lower baseline glycated hemoglobin levels. The authors concluded that the degree of weight loss, not the method, appears to be the major driver of glycemic improvement and diabetes remission in obese subjects undergoing LGB [42].

In a 2006 randomized controlled trial from Australia, investigators observed a decrease in the rate of MBS from 38% to 3% in patients undergoing surgery, compared with 38% to 24% in medically treated patients [43]. A randomized study from the University of Pittsburgh in 2014 showed a more significant rate of diabetes remission among patients undergoing RYGB than those undergoing LGB. In the RYGB group, partial remission of T2DM was observed in 50% of subjects and complete remission in 17%. In the LGB group, partial and complete remission were noted in 27% and 23% of subjects, respectively. In control patients undergoing lifestyle and weight loss intervention only, no remission was noted [44].

A novel device: Endoscopic duodenal–jejunal bypass

A recent study explored the potential for a novel minimally invasive device in managing T2DM. The endoscopic duodenal–jejunal bypass liner (EDJL) is a 60 cm impermeable fluoropolymer liner that is placed endoscopically and anchored at the duodenal bulb. Ingested food and gastric secretions pass through the interior of the liner, while pancreatic enzymes and bile acids are diverted around the exterior of the liner. The EDJL is a temporary device, with current models left in place for 6 months before endoscopic removal. At 1 year, patients who underwent the endoscopic procedure were found to have significantly lower requirements for insulin therapy than those who were treated with dietary interventions. Baseline glycated hemoglobin levels were 8.3% for both groups and dropped to 7.0% and 7.9% in patients who underwent EDJL and dietary intervention, respectively ($p < 0.05$). Furthermore, EBWL was 32% among the patients who underwent EDJL, compared with 16% for patients undergoing dietary intervention. This supports the foregut theory, which will be further discussed below [45].

DIABETES REMISSION FOLLOWING SURGERY

Proposed mechanisms

Most clinicians feel that bariatric surgery offers a more effective means of achieving diabetes remission than currently available medical therapy. The mechanism by which this remission occurs, however, is not entirely understood. Weight loss undoubtedly plays a critical role, as this is the only common factor among the different bariatric operations resulting in the resolution of diabetes. Recent evidence suggests that improvement in blood glucose control is related to the degree of weight loss [46]. Insulin sensitivity drastically improves after bariatric surgery accompanied by an enhanced insulin-receptor concentration and markers of insulin signaling in key target tissues. There is a concomitant increase in levels of the insulin-sensitizing hormone adiponectin, which rises in proportion to the decrease in fat mass and predicts the degree of improvement in insulin sensitivity estimated by homeostatic model assessment [47].

Accumulating evidence supports mechanisms beyond weight loss and reduced caloric intake that lead to the resolution of diabetes [48,49]. Several observations support this notion: (1) very rapid remission of T2DM following certain bariatric procedures, (2) greater glucose control after RYGB than with equivalent weight loss from purely gastric-restrictive operations or nonsurgical interventions, (3) improved glucose homeostasis following certain intestinal procedures that do not result in weight loss, and (4) the occasional development of late-onset beta-cell hyperactivity [50].

Several hypotheses have been proposed to explain the mechanisms of diabetes resolution after bariatric surgery. The "foregut hypothesis," which is related to the enteroinsular axis, hypothesizes that the bypass of nutrients from the duodenum and jejunum leads to reduced secretion of unidentified anti-incretin (diabetogenic) factors [51,52]. The hindgut theory hypothesizes that enhanced delivery of nutrients to the distal intestinal tract may lead to increased incretin hormones (antidiabetogenic), such as glucagon-like peptide-1 (GLP-1) [51,53]. Other proposed mechanisms involve decreased ghrelin secretion, improved hepatic insulin sensitivity due to energy restriction, improved peripheral insulin sensitivity due to weight loss, and reduced intestinal gluconeogenesis [54,55].

Predictors

The success of any operation largely depends on being able to identify the patients who may or may not respond to the treatment. Specific factors, separate from the type of procedure performed, may be responsible for predicting the success of diabetes remission after bariatric surgery. In a meta-analysis performed by Wang et al., patient age, duration of diabetes prior to surgery, and severity of T2DM were found to accurately predict the success rate of diabetes remission. Younger patients, Asian race, and subjects with a duration of diabetes of less than 10 years were more likely to achieve resolution of diabetes. In addition, lower fasting glucose levels, lower glycated hemoglobin levels, higher c-peptide levels, and the lack of insulin requirement, all indicative of a milder form of diabetes, were also predictors of diabetes remission after bariatric surgery. Gender and baseline BMI did not play a role in diabetes remission [56].

Relapse

Despite the optimistic early results of bariatric surgery in relation to diabetes, long-term results have demonstrated a certain degree of relapse of T2DM after bariatric surgery. The Swedish Obesity Study, involving more than 4000 patients, showed that the proportion of patients who remained in remission after 10 years was only 36% [57]. Another long-term study showed that patients remained in remission up to 5 years after surgery; however, the proportion of patients that remained in remission the following year dropped by a third [58]. These observations further attest to the importance of identifying predictive factors of diabetes remission after bariatric surgery.

SUMMARY

MBS has quickly become a major and escalating public health concern worldwide, as it is responsible for an increased risk of developing cardiovascular disease and T2DM. Furthermore, patients with MBS are at an increased risk of stroke, myocardial infarction, and death from such an event compared with unaffected individuals. The increasing prevalence and cost of MBS and T2DM suggests the need for immediate interventions.

Along with more successful and sustainable weight loss, bariatric surgery has demonstrated a higher rate of remission of T2DM, hypertension, and dyslipidemia when compared with medical therapy. Several clinical trials have shown laparoscopic RYGB, LSG, LGB, and BPD-DS to be more effective at achieving weight loss and inducing remission of T2DM than medical therapy alone. Accumulating evidence supports mechanisms beyond weight loss and reduced caloric intake that lead to the resolution of diabetes. Although several theories (i.e., foregut hypothesis and hindgut hypothesis) have been proposed, the exact mechanism by which remission of T2DM occurs is still evolving. Surgical management of T2DM and MBS should strongly be considered for appropriate individuals displaying positive predictors for success and low probability of relapse.

REFERENCES

1. Lindsay RS, Howard BV. Cardiovascular risk associated with the metabolic syndrome. *Curr Diab Rep* 2004;4(1):63–8.

2. Koh KK, Han SH, Quon MJ. Inflammatory markers and the metabolic syndrome. *J Am Coll Cardiol* 2005;46(11):1978–85.

3. Eckel RH, Grundy SM, Zimmet PZ. The metabolic syndrome. *Lancet* 2005;365(9468):1415–28.

4. Alberti KGMM, Eckel RH, Grundy SM et al. Harmonizing the metabolic syndrome a joint interim statement of the International Diabetes Federation Task Force on Epidemiology and Prevention; National Heart, Lung, and Blood Institute; American Heart Association; World Heart Federation; International Atherosclerosis Society; and International Association for the Study of Obesity. *Circulation* 2009;120(16):1640–5.

5. Alberti KGM, Zimmet P, Shaw J. The metabolic syndrome—A new worldwide definition. *Lancet* 2005;366(9491):1059–62.

6. Olijhoek JK, van der Graaf Y, Banga J-D, Algra A, Rabelink TJ, Visseren FLJ. The metabolic syndrome is associated with advanced vascular damage in patients with coronary heart disease, stroke, peripheral arterial disease or abdominal aortic aneurysm. *Eur Heart J* 2004;25(4):342–8.

7. Cameron AJ, Shaw JE, Zimmet PZ. The metabolic syndrome: Prevalence in worldwide populations. *Endocrinol Metab Clin North Am* 2004;33(2):351–75.

8. Mokdad AH, Bowman BA, Ford ES, Vinicor F, Marks JS, Koplan JP. The continuing epidemics of obesity and diabetes in the United States. *JAMA* 2001;286(10):1195–200.

9. Leibson C, Williamson D, Melton L 3rd et al. Temporal trends in BMI among adults with diabetes. *Diabetes Care* 2001;24(9):1584–9.

10. Buchwald H, Avidor Y, Braunwald E et al. Bariatric surgery: A systematic review and meta-analysis. *JAMA* 2004;292(14):1724–37.

11. Association AD. Economic costs of diabetes in the U.S. in 2007. *Diabetes Care* 2008;31(3):596–615.

12. Zhang P, Zhang X, Brown J et al. Global healthcare expenditure on diabetes for 2010 and 2030. *Diabetes Res Clin Pract* 2010;87(3):293–301.

13. Shafrir E, Ziv E. Cellular mechanism of nutritionally induced insulin resistance: The desert rodent Psammomys obesus and other animals in which insulin resistance leads to detrimental outcome. *J Basic Clin Physiol Pharmacol* 1998;9(2–4):347–85.

14. Rucker RJ, Horstmann J, Schneider P, Vaarco R, Buchwald H. Comparisons between jejunoileal and gastric bypass operations for morbid obesity. *Surgery* 1982;92(2):241–9.

15. Buchwald H, Estok R, Fahrbach K et al. Weight and type 2 diabetes after bariatric surgery: Systematic review and meta-analysis. *Am J Med* 2009;122(3):248–56.

16. Pories WJ, MacDonald KG, Morgan EJ et al. Surgical treatment of obesity and its effect on diabetes: 10-y follow-up. *Am J Clin Nutr* 1992;55(2):582S–5S.

17. Buchwald H, Oien DM. Metabolic/bariatric surgery worldwide 2011. *Obes Surg* 2013;23(4):427–36.

18. Buchwald H, Avidor Y, Braunwald E et al. Bariatric surgery: A systematic review and meta-analysis. *JAMA* 2004;292(14):1724–37.

19. Kim S, Richards WO. Long-term follow-up of the metabolic profiles in obese patients with type 2 diabetes mellitus after Roux-en-Y gastric bypass. *Ann Surg* 2010;251(6):1049–55.

20. Ikramuddin S, Korner J, Lee W et al. Roux-en-Y gastric bypass vs intensive medical management for the control of type 2 diabetes, hypertension, and hyperlipidemia: The Diabetes Surgery Study randomized clinical trial. *JAMA* 2013;309(21):2240–9.

21. Liang Z, Wu Q, Chen B, Yu P, Zhao H, Ouyang X. Effect of laparoscopic Roux-en-Y gastric bypass surgery on type 2 diabetes mellitus with hypertension: A randomized controlled trial. *Diabetes Res Clin Pract* 2013;101(1):50–6.

22. Schauer PR, Bhatt DL, Kirwan JP et al. Bariatric surgery versus intensive medical therapy for diabetes—3-year outcomes. *N Engl J Med* 2014;370(21):2002–13.

23. Mingrone G, Panunzi S, De Gaetano A et al. Bariatric surgery versus conventional medical therapy for type 2 diabetes. *N Engl J Med* 2012;366(17):1577–85.

24. Rao W-S, Shan C-X, Zhang W, Jiang D-Z, Qiu M. A meta-analysis of short-term outcomes of patients with type 2 diabetes mellitus and BMI ≤ 35 kg/m^2 undergoing Roux-en-Y gastric bypass. *World J Surg* 2015;39(1):223–30.

25. Schauer PR, Kashyap SR, Wolski K et al. Bariatric surgery versus intensive medical therapy in obese patients with diabetes. *N Engl J Med* 2012;366(17):1567–76.

26. Trastulli S, Desiderio J, Guarino S et al. Laparoscopic sleeve gastrectomy compared with other bariatric surgical procedures: A systematic review of randomized trials. *Surg Obes Relat Dis* 2013;9(5):816–29.

27. Diamantis T, Apostolou KG, Alexandrou A, Griniatsos J, Felekouras E, Tsigris C. Review of long-term weight loss results after laparoscopic sleeve gastrectomy. *Surg Obes Relat Dis* 2014;10(1):177–83.

28. Leonetti F, Capoccia D, Coccia F et al. Obesity, type 2 diabetes mellitus, and other comorbidities: A prospective cohort study of laparoscopic sleeve gastrectomy vs medical treatment. *Arch Surg* 2012;147(8):694–700.

29. Lee W-J, Ser K-H, Chong K et al. Laparoscopic sleeve gastrectomy for diabetes treatment in nonmorbidly obese patients: Efficacy and change of insulin secretion. *Surgery* 2010;147(5):664–9.

30. Rosenthal R, Li X, Samuel S, Martinez P, Zheng C. Effect of sleeve gastrectomy on patients with diabetes mellitus. *Surg Obes Relat Dis* 2009;5(4):429–34.

31. Scopinaro N, Gianetta E, Civalleri D, Bonalumi U, Bachi V. Bilio-pancreatic bypass for obesity. II. Initial experience in man. *Br J Surg* 1979;66(9):618–20.

32. Marceau P, Biron S, Bourque R-A, Potvin M, Hould F-S, Simard S. Biliopancreatic diversion with a new type of gastrectomy. *Obes Surg* 1993;3(1):29–35.

33. Topart P, Becouarn G, Salle A. Five-year follow-up after biliopancreatic diversion with duodenal switch. *Surg Obes Relat Dis* 2011;7(2):199–205.

34. Crea N, Pata G, Di Betta E et al. Long-term results of biliopancreatic diversion with or without gastric preservation for morbid obesity. *Obes Surg* 2011;21(2):139–45.

35. Nelson DW, Blair KS, Martin MJ. Analysis of obesity-related outcomes and bariatric failure rates with the duodenal switch vs gastric bypass for morbid obesity. *Arch Surg* 2012;147(9):847–54.

36. Baltasar A, Bou R, Bengochea M et al. Duodenal switch: An effective therapy for morbid obesity—Intermediate results. *Obes Surg* 2001;11(1):54–8.

37. Belachew M, Legrand M-J, Defechereux TH, Burtheret M-P, Jacquet N. Laparoscopic adjustable silicone gastric banding in the treatment of morbid obesity: A preliminary report. *Surg Endosc* 1994;8(11):1354–56.

38. Forsell P, Hallberg D, Hellers G. Gastric banding for morbid obesity: Initial experience with a new adjustable band. *Obes Surg* 1993;3(4):369–74.

39. Belachew M, Legrand MJ, Vincent V. History of lap-band: From dream to reality. *Obes Surg* 2001;11(3):297–302.

40. Egan RJ, Monkhouse SJW, Meredith HE, Bates SE, Morgan JDT, Norton SA. The reporting of gastric band slip and related complications: A review of the literature. *Obes Surg* 2011;21(8):1280–8.

41. Colquitt JL, Pickett K, Loveman E, Frampton GK. Surgery for weight loss in adults. *Cochrane Database Syst Rev* 2014;8:CD003641.

42. Dixon JB, O'Brien PE, Playfair J et al. Adjustable gastric banding and conventional therapy for type 2 diabetes: A randomized controlled trial. *JAMA* 2008;299(3):316–23.

43. O'Brien PE, Dixon JB, Laurie C et al. Treatment of mild to moderate obesity with laparoscopic adjustable gastric banding or an intensive medical program: A randomized trial. *Ann Intern Med* 2006;144(9):625–33.

44. Courcoulas AP, Goodpaster BH, Eagleton JK et al. Surgical vs medical treatments for type 2 diabetes mellitus: A randomized clinical trial. *JAMA Surg* 2014;149(7):707–15.

45. Koehestanie P, de Jonge C, Berends FJ, Janssen IM, Bouvy ND, Greve JWM. The effect of the endoscopic duodenal-jejunal bypass liner on obesity and type 2 diabetes mellitus, a multicenter randomized controlled trial. *Ann Surg* 2014;260(6):984–92.

46. Norris SL, Zhang X, Avenell A et al. Long-term effectiveness of lifestyle and behavioral weight loss interventions in adults with type 2 diabetes: A meta-analysis. *Am J Med* 2004;117(10):762–74.

47. Thaler JP, Cummings DE. Mini-review: Hormonal and metabolic mechanisms of diabetes remission after gastrointestinal surgery. *Endocrinology* 2009;150(6):2518–25.

48. Rubino F, Forgione A, Cummings DE et al. The mechanism of diabetes control after gastrointestinal bypass surgery reveals a role of the proximal small intestine in the pathophysiology of type 2 diabetes. *Ann Surg* 2006;244(5):741–9.

49. Cummings DE, Overduin J, Shannon MH, Foster-Schubert KE. Hormonal mechanisms of weight loss and diabetes resolution after bariatric surgery. *Surg Obes Relat Dis* 2005;1(3):358–68.

50. Rubino F, Schauer PR, Kaplan LM, Cummings DE. Metabolic surgery to treat type 2 diabetes: Clinical outcomes and mechanisms of action. *Annu Rev Med* 2010;61:393–411.

51. Mingrone G, Castagneto M. Bariatric surgery: Unstressing or boosting the beta-cell? *Diabetes Obes Metab* 2009;11(Suppl 4):130–42.

52. Kwon Y, Abdemur A, Lo Menzo E, Park S, Szomstein S, Rosenthal RJ. The foregut theory as a possible mechanism of action for the remission of type 2 diabetes in low body mass index patients undergoing subtotal gastrectomy for gastric cancer. *Surg Obes Relat Dis* 2014;10(2):235–42.

53. Patriti A, Aisa MC, Annetti C et al. How the hindgut can cure type 2 diabetes. Ileal transposition improves glucose metabolism and beta-cell function in Goto-Kakizaki rats through an enhanced pro-glucagon gene expression and L-cell number. *Surgery* 2007;142(1):74–85.

54. Patel RT, Shukla AP, Ahn SM, Moreira M, Rubino F. Surgical control of obesity and diabetes: The role of intestinal vs. gastric mechanisms in the regulation of body weight and glucose homeostasis. *Obes Silver Spring Md* 2014;22(1):159–69.

55. Sun D, Wang K, Yan Z et al. Duodenal-jejunal bypass surgery up-regulates the expression of the hepatic insulin signaling proteins and the key regulatory enzymes of intestinal gluconeogenesis in diabetic Goto-Kakizaki rats. *Obes Surg* 2013;23(11):1734–42.

56. Wang G-F, Yan Y-X, Xu N et al. Predictive factors of type 2 diabetes mellitus remission following bariatric surgery: A meta-analysis. *Obes Surg* 2015;25(2):199–208.

57. Sjöström L, Lindroos A-K, Peltonen M et al. Lifestyle, diabetes, and cardiovascular risk factors 10 years after bariatric surgery. *N Engl J Med* 2004;351(26):2683–93.

58. Arterburn DE, Bogart A, Sherwood NE et al. A multisite study of long-term remission and relapse of type 2 diabetes mellitus following gastric bypass. *Obes Surg* 2013;23(1):93–102.

56

Changes in gut peptides after bariatric surgery

JAMES P. VILLAMERE, BLANDINE LAFERRÈRE, AND JAMES J. MCGINTY

BACKGROUND

The prevalence of obesity is a significant public health issue in the United States, with 35.7%, 15.4%, and 6.3% of the U.S. population categorized with class 1 obesity (body mass index [BMI] $\geq$ 30 kg/m^2), class 2 obesity (BMI $\geq$ 35 kg/m^2), and class 3 obesity (BMI $\geq$ 45 kg/m^2) respectively [1]. Obesity is associated with a number of comorbidities, including diabetes, hypertension, obstructive sleep apnea, cancer, cardiovascular disease, and decreased longevity [2]. Bariatric surgery has been the only intervention proved to provide durable long-term weight loss and effectively treat obesity-related comorbidities in patients with severe obesity [3,4]. There is evidence that the weight loss and resolution of comorbidities after bariatric surgery go beyond caloric restriction, and malabsorption, and changes in gut physiology after some types of bariatric surgery may play an important role [5]. The gut is a complex endocrine organ whose functions include digestion and absorption processes, as well as control of satiety and insulin secretion via production of a hormonal response to the ingestion of food. Jejunoileal bypass and, more recently, Roux-en-Y gastric bypass (RYGB) have been long associated with enhanced release of gut satiety and incretin hormones that signal the central nervous system and the pancreas to control food intake and insulin secretion. The gut hormone changes after RYGB may favor satiety, decrease food intake, and sustain a new level of energy balance at a lower body weight that is approximately 30% lower than the maximum weight. The changes in incretin hormones after RYGB stimulate insulin secretion and help control blood glucose during meals. This chapter reviews the changes in gastrointestinal hormones found after the most common bariatric surgical procedures performed in the United States, specifically RYGB and

vertical sleeve gastrectomy (VSG) [6]. We discuss the evidence, or lack thereof, for a possible role of these hormonal changes in the induction and maintenance of weight loss and diabetes remission.

GHRELIN

Ghrelin is a 28-amino acid orexigenic gut peptide secreted primarily by the fundus and body of the stomach that acts on the hypothalamus to stimulate appetite, increase gastric acid secretion, and increase gastrointestinal motility to prepare the body for food ingestion [7]. Data support an anticipatory cephalic phase of ghrelin release, characterized by increasing levels prior to expected meal ingestion, possibly initiating the hunger drive [8]. The administration of ghrelin to humans stimulates food intake [8]. The release of ghrelin is mediated by hormonal mechanisms and vagal nerve input [9]. Physiologically, ghrelin levels rise before meals and fall postprandially [8]. Paradoxically, obese individuals have lower circulating ghrelin concentrations than lean individuals [10]. Ghrelin levels have been shown to increase with diet-induced weight loss [11]. This led to the hypothesis that ghrelin may have a role in the adaptive response that limits the amount of weight that can be lost with diet alone [10]. It has been hypothesized that either partial gastrectomy, like in VSG (see Figure 55.2), or isolating most ghrelin-producing cells from direct contact with ingested nutrients, such as in RYGB (see Figure 55.1), may modify ghrelin secretion and contribute to the efficacy of these bariatric procedures in achieving weight loss [12].

However, the data examining changes in ghrelin levels after RYGB have been contradictory (Table 56.1). A decreased or no significant change in ghrelin levels has been shown in the early postoperative period after RYGB,

Table 56.1 Ghrelin changes after bariatric RYGB and VSG

Procedure	Author (reference)	No. of subjects	Postoperative interval	Change in fasting ghrelin
RYGB	Lin et al. [19]	34	30 min	↓
RYGB	Fruhbeck et al. [20]	15	1D	↓
RYGB	Morinigo et al. [21]	8	6W	↓
RYGB	Peterli et al. [13]	13, 13	1W, 3M	↓, ↓
RYGB	Garcia de la Torre [22]	17	10.5M	↓
RYGB	Nannipieri et al. [23]	23, 23	15D, 12M	↓, ↓
RYGB	Leonetti et al. [24]	11	12M	↓
RYGB	Roth et al. [25]	18	23M	↓
RYGB	Christou et al. [17]	36	3–5Y	↓
RYGB	Couce et al. [26]	49, 18, 11	120 min, 10D, 6M	↓, ↓, ↔
RYGB	Peterli et al. [14]	12, 12, 12	1W, 3M, 12M	↓, ↓, ↔
RYGB	Morinigo et al. [27]	25, 25	6W, 1Y	↓, ↔
RYGB	Sundbom et al. [15]	15, 15, 15, 15	1D, 1M, 6M, 1Y	↓, ↔, ↔, ↑
RYGB	le Roux et al. [28]	16, 16	2–7D, 6W	↔
RYGB	Mancini et al. [29]	10	6M	↔
RYGB	Korner et al. [30]	28, 28, 28, 28	14D, 3M, 6M, 1Y	↔, ↔, ↔, ↔
RYGB	Bose et al. [16]	11, 11	1M, 1Y	↔, ↔
RYGB	Stoeckli et al. [31]	5, 5, 5, 5	3M, 6M, 12M, 24M	↔, ↔, ↔, ↔
RYGB	Korner et al. [106]	12	35M	↔
RYGB	Terra et al. [32]	13, 12	6M, 12M	↑, ↔
RYGB	Faraj et al. [33]	25, 25	12.3M, 17.5M	↑, ↔
RYGB	Vendrell et al. [34]	34	6M	↑
RYGB	Holdstock et al. [35]	66, 66	6M, 1Y	↑, ↑
RYGB	Pardina et al. [36]	34	12M	↑
VSG	Basso et al. [37]	28	3D	↓
VSG	Peterli et al. [13]	14	1W, 3M	↓
VSG	Goitein et al. [12]	20	3M	↓
VSG	Langer et al. [38]	10	1D, 1M, 6M	↓
VSG	Peterli et al. [14]	11, 11, 11	1W, 3M, 12M	↓, ↓, ↓
VSG	Nannipieri et al. [23]	12, 12	15D, 12M	↓, ↓
VSG	Karamanakos et al. [39]	16, 16, 16, 16	1M, 3M, 6M, 12M	↓, ↓, ↓, ↓
VSG	Dimitriadis et al. [40]	15, 15	6M, 12M	↓, ↓
VSG	Haluzikova et al. [41]	17, 17, 17	6M, 12M, 24M	↓, ↓, ↓
VSG	Wang et al. [42]	10	24M	↓
VSG	Bohdjalian et al. [43]	12, 12, 12	6M, 12M, 5Y	↓, ↓, ↓
VSG	Terra et al. [32]	17, 17	6M, 12M	↑, ↔

Note: min, minutes; D, days; W, weeks; M, months; Y, years; ↑, increased; ↔, no significant change; ↓, decreased.

in spite of caloric restriction and weight loss. Ghrelin levels tend to rise 1 year post-RYGB, where they return to preoperative levels, or even increase relative to preoperative levels [13–15]. The long-term (1-year) change in ghrelin levels after RYGB is in fact similar to what is observed after laparoscopic adjustable gastric banding (LAGB), and likely a function of weight loss [16]. Interestingly, data reported in the literature have shown a trend for ghrelin levels to decrease after longer-term follow-up post-RYGB up to 5 years postoperatively [17]. In addition to changes in fasted ghrelin levels, the magnitude of weight loss after

RYGB may be associated with distinctive patterns of postprandial responses in ghrelin. A recent study showed that postprandial ghrelin suppression was more pronounced in patients with the greatest weight loss (>40%) 3 years after RYGB, with little to no reduction in those with modest weight loss (<25%), or in the obese control group [18]. The physiological or clinical relevance is unclear and requires more investigation. Whether lower fasted ghrelin levels and greater postprandial ghrelin suppression are simply associated with surgical weight loss or causing more weight loss is unknown. In all, the ghrelin level varies after RYGB, with little correlation with the amount of weight loss, and has not been proved thus far to be a major contributing factor in decreased appetite or weight control after RYGB.

After VSG, ghrelin levels have been shown to decrease, in relation to the loss of ghrelin-producing cells [39]. In contrast to conflicting reports on ghrelin changes after RYGB, ghrelin levels decrease consistently in both the early and late postoperative periods up to 5 years after VSG (Table 56.1). VSG reduced plasma ghrelin levels from 593 ± 52 pg/mL preoperatively to 219 ± 23 pg/mL at 12 months postoperatively, and 257 ± 23 pg/mL at 5 years postoperatively, with concurrent stable average excess weight loss (EWL) of 55.0 ± 6.8% at 5 years [43]. The results of this study, and the consistency of decreased postoperative ghrelin levels across the majority of post-VSG studies [12–14,23,37–43], support a possible role of reduced ghrelin contributing to long-term sustainable weight loss after VSG. However, it is possible that ghrelin levels are a mere reflection of the near-total gastrectomy after VSG and not a marker of weight loss. Interestingly, although ghrelin levels are consistently lower after VSG than after RYGB, weight loss is greater after RYGB than after VSG [44]. This suggests that ghrelin is not an important mediator of weight loss after either surgery, or if it is, presumably after VSG, the mechanism of weight loss after RYGB is likely different.

CHOLECYSTOKININ

Cholecystokinin (CCK) is a satiety hormone produced by intestinal I-cells, in the duodenum and jejunum. Its secretion is stimulated by nutrient ingestion, especially fat and protein. CCK inhibits gastric emptying and gastric motility and stimulates gall bladder contraction [45–47]. CCK levels increase after RYGB and VSG in some studies [14], but not others [41,48], and CCK concentrations are higher after VSG than after RYGB [14]. This may be secondary to duodenal exclusion of nutrients in RYGB.

An increased incidence of gallstones after RYGB and VSG has been well documented, with both RYGB and VSG showing similar rates of symptomatic gallstone disease [49]. Gall bladder emptying is decreased after RYGB; however, this has been shown to be independent of duodenal exclusion, as results were similar when meals were administered orally and via a gastrostomy tube in the gastric remnant [50]. Reduced gall bladder emptying may favor formation of gallstones, as there is more time for cholesterol precipitation and the development and aggregation of cholesterol crystals [51]. No studies, to our knowledge, have specifically looked at gall bladder emptying after VSG.

BILE ACIDS

In addition to their key role in lipid digestion, bile acids (BAs) are key players in hepatic lipid synthesis, as well as glucose metabolism [52]. In addition, BAs stimulate glucagon-like peptide 1 (GLP-1) secretion *in vitro* and

in vivo [52,53]. BAs and fibroblast growth factor 19 (FGF19) have been shown to be elevated after RYGB [54,55], but not after VSG [41]. The increase in BAs after RYGB has been suggested as a potential mechanism for improved insulin sensitivity [54], and is inversely associated with improved glucose and triglyceride levels, and positively correlated with adiponectin and GLP-1, peptide YY (PYY), and FGF19 levels [54,56,57]. The reasons for elevation of circulating BA are not entirely known, but likely include changes to the enterohepatic circulation, and possibly change in microbiome after RYGB [57].

GLUCOSE-DEPENDENT INSULINOTROPIC PEPTIDE

Glucose-dependent insulinotropic peptide (GIP) is a 42-amino acid incretin peptide secreted from K-cells located in the duodenal and proximal jejunal mucosa in response to carbohydrate and fat ingestion [58,59]. GIP, with the other incretin, GLP-1, stimulates β-cell proliferation and inhibits apoptosis *in vitro* and *in vivo* in rodent models [60]. Given the bypass of the duodenum and proximal jejunum to ingested nutrients after RYGB, it would be expected that levels of GIP would decline postoperatively. However, postprandial changes of GIP after RYGB have been inconsistent [61] (Table 56.2). Some investigators have found an increase in GIP after RYGB in both short- and long-term follow-up [62–65], while others have reported a decrease or no change [48,66–69]. RYGB, with bypass of the GIP-secreting cells, is known to improve control of type 2 diabetes. Therefore, given the inconsistent postsurgical changes of GIP secretion, it can be postulated that GIP is unlikely to play a key role in the postsurgical resolution of diabetes. Proof-of-concept experiments will need to be done when GIP inhibitors are available.

GLUCAGON-LIKE PEPTIDE 1

GLP-1, a satiety gut hormone, is a 30-amino acid peptide secreted along with PYY and oxyntomodulin (OXM) by L-cells in the distal small intestine and colon in response to meal ingestion [58]. GLP-1 effects include the stimulation of glucose-stimulated insulin secretion, suppression of glucagon secretion, slowing of gastric emptying and intestinal motility, and decrease in food intake [58,81–83]. GLP-1 stimulates β-cell growth and proliferation while inhibiting apoptosis, ultimately resulting in increased β-cell mass, as shown *in vitro* and in rodent studies, an effect not demonstrated in humans [84]. The enzyme dipeptidyl peptidase-4 (DPP-4) rapidly inactivates GLP-1 and GIP, which have a half-life of only a few minutes [58]. The incretin effect, or the greater insulin secretion after oral than after an isoglycemic glucose load, responsible for ~50% of insulin secretion during meals, is blunted in patients with type 2 diabetes [85], but can be rescued in patients by GLP-1 treatment. Antidiabetic agents, including long-acting GLP-1 analogs and DPP-4 inhibitors, are currently being utilized in clinical practice to treat type 2 diabetes [86].

Table 56.2 GLP-1 changes after bariatric RYGB and VSG

Procedure	Author (reference)	Number of subjects	Postoperative interval	Meal-stimulated GLP-1 change
RYGB	Yip et al. [70]	11	3D	↑
RYGB	Nannipieri et al. [23]	23	15D	↑
RYGB	Kashyap et al. [71]	9 T2DM	1W, 1M	↑, ↑
RYGB	Laferrere et al. [62]	8 T2DM	1M	↑
RYGB	Olivan et al. [72]	11	1M	↑
RYGB	Laferrère et al. [63]	9	1M	↑
RYGB	le Roux et al. [28]	16, 16	2–7D, 6W	↑, ↑
RYGB	Peterli et al. [13]	13, 13	1W, 3M	↑, ↑
RYGB	Umeda et al. [73]	10 T2DM	90D	↑
RYGB	de Carvalho et al. [74]	19	9M	↑
RYGB	Peterli et al. [14]	12, 12, 12	1W, 3M, 12M	↑, ↑, ↑
RYGB	Bose et al. [64]	11, 11	1M, 1Y	↑, ↑
RYGB	Korner et al. [30]	28, 28	6M, 1Y	↑, ↑
RYGB	Werling et al. [75]	63	15M	↑
RYGB	Rodieux et al. [76]	8	9–48M	↑
RYGB	Vidal et al. [77]	24	>36M	↑
VSG	Basso et al. [37]	28	3D	↑
VSG	Nannipieri et al. [23]	12	15D	↑
VSG	Valderas et al. [78]	6	2M	↑
VSG	Umemura et al. [79]	23	6M	↑
VSG	Peterli et al. [14]	11, 11, 11	1W, 3M, 12M	↑, ↑, ↑
VSG	Ramon et al. [80]	8, 8	3M, 12M	↑, ↑
VSG	Dimitriadis et al. [40]	15, 15	6M, 12M	↑, ↑
VSG	Yip et al. [70]	10	3D	↔

Note: T2DM, type 2 diabetes mellitus; D, days; W, weeks; M, months; Y, years; ↑, increased; ↔, no significant change; ↓, decreased.

Both RYGB and VSG modify GLP-1 levels. The GLP-1 response to a meal is enhanced consistently after RYGB [16,30]. This occurs early in the postoperative period, as early as 2 days postoperatively [86], and persists for many years postoperatively [16,23,30]. The cause of GLP-1 elevation after RYGB is well defined, and the role of accelerated emptying of the gastric pouch is predominant [86]. The rise of GLP-1 after RYGB is abolished if a meal test is administered directly through a gastrostomy in the gastric remnant, rather than per mouth [86], or if nutrients are infused at a very slow rate in the jejunum rather than taken by mouth [87]. Diet-induced weight loss [63] or weight loss after gastric banding [16] results in no change in circulating GLP-1.

Similarly to what is happening after RYGB, GLP-1 levels increase in the early postoperative period after VSG, as early as the first postoperative week [13,37], and this elevation has been shown to persist, at least at 1-year follow-up [40,80]. The rapid transit and the exposure of the distal intestine to nutrients are likely the reason for the rise in GLP-1 after VSG [88]. Interestingly, one study found no change in GLP-1 after VSG at 6, 12, or 24 months postoperatively [41].

Based on GLP-1's physiological effect to promote satiety and weight loss and to help postprandial glucose tolerance, it is tempting to hypothesize that it plays a major role in sustained weight loss and diabetes remission after RYGB. Incretin levels, GLP-1 (and GIP), rise in parallel with diabetes remission after RYGB, but not after a matched weight loss by diet [63]. In addition, the incretin effect, blunted in diabetes, normalizes as early as 1 month post-RYGB, but does not change significantly after diet-induced weight loss [63]. Administering the GLP-1 receptor inhibitor exendin 9-39 after RYGB prevents the rise of insulin secretion after RYGB during meals, blunts the improvement of β-cell function, and prevents postprandial hypoglycemia [89–91]. These proof-of-concept experiments demonstrate a clear role of endogenous GLP-1 in the regulation of postprandial glucose levels after RYGB. However, the role of GLP-1 in diabetes remission after RYGB is probably limited, as exendin 9-39 administration results only in minimal glucose intolerance after RYGB [92,93] and β-cell function remains impaired upon intravenous glucose stimulation years after RYGB in patients in diabetes remission [55].

Diabetes also resolves rapidly after VSG, in conjunction with elevated GLP-1 levels [13]. The exact role of endogenous GLP-1 has been less studied after VSG, and no experiment to our knowledge has used exendin 9–39 after VSG.

The fairly comparable rate of remission after VSG and RYGB, at least in the first 6–12 months after surgery, does not support the foregut hypothesis for RYGB [48]. Indeed, the shunting of nutrients away from the proximal intestine, absent in VSG, does not seem to be necessary for diabetes remission [48].

PEPTIDE YY AND OXYNTOMODULIN (OXM)

PYY is a 36-amino acid anorexigenic gut hormone that is cosecreted by mucosal L-cells in the distal small bowel and large intestine, along with GLP-1 and OXM [94]. Its release is stimulated by meal ingestion and, like GLP-1, proportional to the caloric content of a meal [94]. PYY_{1-36} is also degraded by the enzyme DPP-4 into the main circulating and active form PYY_{3-36} [94]. Similar to GLP-1, PYY functions to inhibit gastric, pancreatic, and intestinal secretions [5]. PYY_{3-36} has also been shown to inhibit gastric emptying and intestinal motility, similar to GLP-1, as part of the "ileal brake" phenomenon [94].

Postprandial increases in PYY_{3-36} are found after RYGB, similar to the increases seen in GLP-1 [13,23,28,30,72], and these changes are independent of weight loss [95].

PYY increase also occurs early, within the first week [13,28], and persists up to and beyond 2 years postoperatively [23,30,96]. Postprandial PYY_{3-36} levels also increase within the first week following VSG [13] and have been shown to persist up to a year postoperatively [23,80].

Similar to GLP-1, the rapid delivery of nutrients to the distal small bowel results in the increased PYY secretion observed after RYGB [97], and likely after VSG [88]. The rise

of PYY is prevented by meal administration in the gastric remnant [86]. Although the rise of PYY after RYGB and VSG is consistent with a potential contribution of this peptide to the sustained weight loss after these bariatric surgical procedures, the role of PYY in food intake controls in humans is controversial (Table 56.3) [98].

Another product of the L-cell is OXM, a 37-amino acid anorexigenic hormone, secreted in response to nutrient ingestion [45]. OXM binds to the GLP-1 and the glucagon receptors and, as such, exerts effects similar to those of the two hormones [99–101]. OXM reduces food intake and increases energy expenditure in both lean and obese individuals [99]. OXM administration results in superior body weight lowering compared with selective GLP-1 receptor agonists. Interestingly, the effect on glucose is the resultant action of the activation of the glucagon receptor, which increases glucose production and results in hyperglycemia, and the simultaneous activation of the GLP-1 receptor, which counteracts this effect. Acute OXM infusion improves glucose tolerance in patients with type 2 diabetes mellitus, making dual agonists of glucagon and the GLP-1 receptors as new promising treatments for diabetes and obesity. These dual agonists have the potential for weight loss and glucose lowering that is superior to that of GLP-1 receptor agonists [102]. OXM is also degraded by DPP-4 [99]. The pattern of change of postprandial OXM after RYGB parallels those of GLP-1 and PYY_{3-36} [103]. The changes of PYY, OXM, and GLP-1 after RYGB are in favor of a role in appetite control and may play a role in the sustained weight loss after bariatric surgery. However, the influence of each hormone is difficult to isolate given their synchronous increase after RYGB.

Table 56.3 PYY changes after bariatric RYGB and VSG

Procedure	Author (reference)	Number of subjects	Postoperative interval	Meal-stimulated PYY change
RYGB	le Roux et al. [28]	16, 16	2–7D, 6W	↑, ↑
RYGB	Olivan et al. [72]	11	1M	↑
RYGB	Peterli et al. [13]	13, 13	1W, 3M	↑, ↑
RYGB	Yousseif et al. [104]	10, 10	6W, 12W	↑, ↑
RYGB	Karamanakos et al. [39]	16, 16, 16	1M, 3M, 12M	↑, ↑, ↑
RYGB	Peterli et al. [14]	12, 12, 12	1W, 3M, 12M	↑, ↑, ↑
RYGB	Korner et al. [30]	28, 28	6M, 1Y	↑, ↑
RYGB	Nannipieri et al. [23]	23	1Y	↑
RYGB	Werling et al. [75]	63	15M	↑
RYGB	le Roux et al. [105]	6	6–36M	↑
RYGB	Rodieux et al. [76]	8	9–48M	↑
VSG	Basso et al. [37]	28	72H	↑
VSG	Peterli et al. [13]	14, 14	1W, 3M	↑, ↑
VSG	Peterli et al. [14]	11, 11, 11	1W, 3M, 12M	↑, ↑, ↑
VSG	Karamanakos et al. [39]	16, 16, 16	3M, 6M, 1Y	↑, ↑, ↑
VSG	Dimitriadis et al. [40]	15, 15	6M, 12M	↑, ↑
VSG	Nannipieri et al. [23]	12	1Y	↔

Note: H, hours; D, days; W, weeks; M, months; Y, years; ↑, increased; ↔, no significant change; ↓, decreased.

Table 56.4 Summary of changes in gut peptides after RYGB and VSG and their effects on food intake and glucose tolerance

	Origin	Levels post-RYGB	Levels post-VSG	Effect on food intake	Effect on glycemia
Ghrelin	Stomach/fundus X/A-like cells	↓, ↔	↓	↑	↑
CCK	Duodenum/jejunum I-cells	↔, ↑	↑	↓	↔
GIP	Duodenum K-cells	↓, ↔, ↑	?	↔	↑
GLP-1	Distal ileum L-cells	↑	↑	↓	↓
PYY	Distal ileum L-cells	↑	↑	↓	↔
OXM	Distal ileum L-cells	↑	?	↓	↓

Note: ↑, increased; ↔, no significant change; ↓, decreased; ?, unknown.

SUMMARY

The gut is a formidable endocrine organ. Gut hormones play major roles in physiological phenomena favoring the transit of nutrients, digestion, absorption, ileal brake, and gall bladder contraction. Some of these peptides control satiety via the gut–brain pathway involving the vagal nerve. The two incretins are key players of insulin secretion and in preparing the body for the switch from the fasted state to the fed state, and helping nutrient assimilation.

The gut physiology is completely transformed by the RYGB and, to a lesser extent, the VSG. The gastric relaxation phase is inexistent, and gastric pouch emptying accelerated. The rapid transit of nutrients is responsible for the enhanced gut peptide release. These changes, and perhaps the lesser ghrelin levels, may favor decreased appetite and increased satiety, which would favor sustained lower body weight. Surgical weight loss, with greater incretin effect and insulin secretion and improved glucose control during meals, may also be responsible for diabetes remission after RYGB or VSG. The exact contribution of the changes in gut peptides to the metabolic effect of the surgery remains the object of debate (Table 56.4).

Patients who regain some of their lost weight after RYGB, or who experience diabetes relapse, may have similar changes of gut hormones in response to food ingestion when compared with patients who sustained the loss weight and are still in diabetes remission. The mechanisms of weight regain or diabetes relapse may lie in the brain processing of the gut signals. These processes, initially altered after the surgery to favor weight loss, may adapt over time to reverse the positive outcome.

CONCLUSION

Bariatric surgery provides durable long-term weight loss and effectively treats obesity-related comorbidities, including diabetes [3,4]. A strong body of evidence supports mechanisms that go well beyond simple restriction and malabsorption after RYGB and VGS in achieving weight loss and glucose homeostasis. Alterations in gut anatomy and resultant changes in gut hormone physiology have demonstrated potential for significant contributions of the beneficial effects of these bariatric surgical procedures. Overall, compared with individuals who lost weight by diet alone, patients undergoing RYGB and VSG demonstrated decreased ghrelin levels and elevated GLP-1, PYY, and OXM concentrations, as well as favorable BA changes. The complex synergistic effect of increased L-cell products (GLP-1, PYY, and OXM), along with decreased ghrelin, likely contributes to decreased food intake, increased satiety, and long-term weight loss, as well as improved glucose homeostasis. Further research in this field is needed to understand the predictors of successful weight loss and identify mechanisms of β-cell function recovery.

REFERENCES

1. Flegal KM, Carroll MD, Kit BK, Ogden CL. Prevalence of obesity and trends in the distribution of body mass index among US adults, 1999–2010. JAMA 2012;307(5):491–7.
2. Haslam DW, James WP. Obesity. Lancet 2005; 366(9492):1197–209.
3. Livingston EH. Obesity and its surgical management. Am J Surg 2002;184(2):103–13.
4. Brolin RE. Bariatric surgery and long-term control of morbid obesity. JAMA 2002;288(22):2793–6.
5. Quercia I, Dutia R, Kotler DP, Belsley S, Laferrère B. Gastrointestinal changes after bariatric surgery. Diabetes Metab 2014;40(2):87–94.
6. Nguyen NT, Nguyen B, Gebhart A, Hohmann S. Changes in the makeup of bariatric surgery: A national increase in use of laparoscopic sleeve gastrectomy. J Am Coll Surg 2013;216(2):252–7.

7. Kojima M, Hosoda H, Date Y, Nakazato M, Matsuo H, Kangawa K. Ghrelin is a growth-hormone-releasing acylated peptide from stomach. *Nature* 1999;402(6762):656–60.

8. Cummings DE, Purnell JQ, Frayo RS, Schmidova K, Wisse BE, Weigle DS. A preprandial rise in plasma ghrelin levels suggests a role in meal initiation in humans. *Diabetes* 2001;50(8):1714–9.

9. Power ML, Schulkin J. Anticipatory physiological regulation in feeding biology: Cephalic phase responses. *Appetite* 2008;50(2–3):194–206.

10. Tschop M, Weyer C, Tataranni PA, Devanarayan V, Ravussin E, Heiman ML. Circulating ghrelin levels are decreased in human obesity. *Diabetes* 2001;50(4):707–9.

11. Cummings DE, Weigle DS, Frayo RS et al. Plasma ghrelin levels after diet-induced weight loss or gastric bypass surgery. *N Engl J Med* 2002;346(21):1623–30.

12. Goitein D, Lederfein D, Tzioni R, Berkenstadt H, Venturero M, Rubin M. Mapping of ghrelin gene expression and cell distribution in the stomach of morbidly obese patients—A possible guide for efficient sleeve gastrectomy construction. *Obes Surg* 2012;22(4):617–22.

13. Peterli R, Wolnerhanssen B, Peters T et al. Improvement in glucose metabolism after bariatric surgery: Comparison of laparoscopic Roux-en-Y gastric bypass and laparoscopic sleeve gastrectomy: A prospective randomized trial. *Ann Surg* 2009;250(2):234–41.

14. Peterli R, Steinert RE, Woelnerhanssen B et al. Metabolic and hormonal changes after laparoscopic Roux-en-Y gastric bypass and sleeve gastrectomy: A randomized, prospective trial. *Obes Surg* 2012;22(5):740–8.

15. Sundbom M, Holdstock C, Engstrom BE, Karlsson FA. Early changes in ghrelin following Roux-en-Y gastric bypass: Influence of vagal nerve functionality? *Obes Surg* 2007;17(3):304–10.

16. Bose M, Machineni S, Olivan B et al. Superior appetite hormone profile after equivalent weight loss by gastric bypass compared to gastric banding. *Obesity (Silver Spring, Md)* 2010;18(6):1085–91.

17. Christou NV, Look D, McLean AP. Pre- and postprandial plasma ghrelin levels do not correlate with satiety or failure to achieve a successful outcome after Roux-en-Y gastric bypass. *Obes Surg* 2005;15(7):1017–23.

18. Gerner T, Johansen OE, Olufsen M, Torjesen PA, Tveit A. The post-prandial pattern of gut hormones is related to magnitude of weight-loss following gastric bypass surgery: A case-control study. *Scand J Clin Lab Invest* 2014;74(3):213–8.

19. Lin E, Gletsu N, Fugate K et al. The effects of gastric surgery on systemic ghrelin levels in the morbidly obese. *Arch Surg (Chicago, Ill: 1960)* 2004;139(7):780–4.

20. Fruhbeck G, Diez Caballero A, Gil MJ. Fundus functionality and ghrelin concentrations after bariatric surgery. *N Engl J Med* 2004;350(3):308–9.

21. Moringo R, Casamitjana R, Moize V et al. Short-term effects of gastric bypass surgery on circulating ghrelin levels. *Obes Res* 2004;12(7):1108–16.

22. Garcia de la Torre N, Rubio MA, Bordiu E et al. Effects of weight loss after bariatric surgery for morbid obesity on vascular endothelial growth factor-A, adipocytokines, and insulin. *J Clin Endocrinol Metab* 2008;93(11):4276–81.

23. Nannipieri M, Baldi S, Mari A et al. Roux-en-Y gastric bypass and sleeve gastrectomy: Mechanisms of diabetes remission and role of gut hormones. *J Clin Endocrinol Metab* 2013;98(11):4391–9.

24. Leonetti F, Silecchia G, Iacobellis G et al. Different plasma ghrelin levels after laparoscopic gastric bypass and adjustable gastric banding in morbid obese subjects. *J Clin Endocrinol Metab* 2003;88(9):4227–31.

25. Roth CL, Reinehr T, Schernthaner GH, Kopp HP, Kriwanek S, Schernthaner G. Ghrelin and obestatin levels in severely obese women before and after weight loss after Roux-en-Y gastric bypass surgery. *Obes Surg* 2009;19(1):29–35.

26. Couce ME, Cottam D, Esplen J, Schauer P, Burguera B. Is ghrelin the culprit for weight loss after gastric bypass surgery? A negative answer. *Obes Surg* 2006;16(7):870–8.

27. Moringo R, Vidal J, Lacy AM, Delgado S, Casamitjana R, Gomis R. Circulating peptide YY, weight loss, and glucose homeostasis after gastric bypass surgery in morbidly obese subjects. *Ann Surg* 2008;247(2):270–5.

28. le Roux CW, Welbourn R, Werling M et al. Gut hormones as mediators of appetite and weight loss after Roux-en-Y gastric bypass. *Ann Surg* 2007;246(5):780–5.

29. Mancini MC, Costa AP, de Melo ME et al. Effect of gastric bypass on spontaneous growth hormone and ghrelin release profiles. *Obesity (Silver Spring, Md)* 2006;14(3):383–7.

30. Korner J, Inabnet W, Febres G et al. Prospective study of gut hormone and metabolic changes after adjustable gastric banding and Roux-en-Y gastric bypass. *Int J Obes* 2009;33(7):786–95.

31. Stoeckli R, Chanda R, Langer I, Keller U. Changes of body weight and plasma ghrelin levels after gastric banding and gastric bypass. *Obes Res* 2004;12(2):346–50.

32. Terra X, Auguet T, Guiu-Jurado E et al. Long-term changes in leptin, chemerin and ghrelin levels following different bariatric surgery procedures: Roux-en-Y gastric bypass and sleeve gastrectomy. *Obes Surg* 2013;23(11):1790–8.

33. Faraj M, Havel PJ, Phelis S, Blank D, Sniderman AD, Cianflone K. Plasma acylation-stimulating protein, adiponectin, leptin, and ghrelin before and after

weight loss induced by gastric bypass surgery in morbidly obese subjects. *J Clin Endocrinol Metab* 2003;88(4):1594–602.

34. Vendrell J, Broch M, Vilarrasa N et al. Resistin, adiponectin, ghrelin, leptin, and proinflammatory cytokines: Relationships in obesity. *Obes Res* 2004;12(6):962–71.

35. Holdstock C, Engstrom BE, Ohrvall M, Lind L, Sundbom M, Karlsson FA. Ghrelin and adipose tissue regulatory peptides: Effect of gastric bypass surgery in obese humans. *J Clin Endocrinol Metab* 2003;88(7):3177–83.

36. Pardina E, Lopez-Tejero MD, Llamas R et al. Ghrelin and apolipoprotein AIV levels show opposite trends to leptin levels during weight loss in morbidly obese patients. *Obes Surg* 2009;19(10):1414–23.

37. Basso N, Capoccia D, Rizzello M et al. First-phase insulin secretion, insulin sensitivity, ghrelin, GLP-1, and PYY changes 72 h after sleeve gastrectomy in obese diabetic patients: The gastric hypothesis. *Surg Endosc* 2011;25(11):3540–50.

38. Langer FB, Reza Hoda MA, Bohdjalian A et al. Sleeve gastrectomy and gastric banding: Effects on plasma ghrelin levels. *Obes Surg* 2005;15(7):1024–9.

39. Karamanakos SN, Vagenas K, Kalfarentzos F, Alexandrides TK. Weight loss, appetite suppression, and changes in fasting and postprandial ghrelin and peptide-YY levels after Roux-en-Y gastric bypass and sleeve gastrectomy: A prospective, double blind study. *Ann Surg* 2008;247(3):401–7.

40. Dimitriadis E, Daskalakis M, Kampa M, Peppe A, Papadakis JA, Melissas J. Alterations in gut hormones after laparoscopic sleeve gastrectomy: A prospective clinical and laboratory investigational study. *Ann Surg* 2013;257(4):647–54.

41. Haluzikova D, Lacinova Z, Kavalkova P et al. Laparoscopic sleeve gastrectomy differentially affects serum concentrations of FGF-19 and FGF-21 in morbidly obese subjects. *Obesity (Silver Spring, Md)* 2013;21(7):1335–42.

42. Wang Y, Liu J. Plasma ghrelin modulation in gastric band operation and sleeve gastrectomy. *Obes Surg* 2009;19(3):357–62.

43. Bohdjalian A, Langer FB, Shakeri-Leidenmuhler S et al. Sleeve gastrectomy as sole and definitive bariatric procedure: 5-year results for weight loss and ghrelin. *Obes Surg* 2010;20(5):535–40.

44. Malin SK, Samat A, Wolski K et al. Improved acylated ghrelin suppression at 2 years in obese patients with type 2 diabetes: Effects of bariatric surgery vs standard medical therapy. *Int J Obes* 2014;38(3):364–70.

45. Vincent RP, le Roux CW. Changes in gut hormones after bariatric surgery. *Clin Endocrinol* 2008;69(2):173–9.

46. Neary MT, Batterham RL. Gut hormones: Implications for the treatment of obesity. *Pharmacol Ther* 2009;124(1):44–56.

47. Rehfeld JF. Clinical endocrinology and metabolism. Cholecystokinin. *Best Pract Res Clin Endocrinol Metab* 2004;18(4):569–86.

48. Rubino F, Gagner M, Gentileschi P et al. The early effect of the Roux-en-Y gastric bypass on hormones involved in body weight regulation and glucose metabolism. *Ann Surg* 2004;240(2):236–42.

49. Moon RC, Teixeira AF, DuCoin C, Varnadore S, Jawad MA. Comparison of cholecystectomy cases after Roux-en-Y gastric bypass, sleeve gastrectomy, and gastric banding. *Surg Obes Relat Dis* 2014;10(1):64–8.

50. Bastouly M, Arasaki CH, Ferreira JB, Zanoto A, Borges FG, Del Grande JC. Early changes in postprandial gallbladder emptying in morbidly obese patients undergoing Roux-en-Y gastric bypass: Correlation with the occurrence of biliary sludge and gallstones. *Obes Surg* 2009;19(1):22–8.

51. van Erpecum KJ, Venneman NG, Portincasa P, Vanberge-Henegouwen GP. Review article: Agents affecting gall-bladder motility—Role in treatment and prevention of gallstones. *Aliment Pharmacol Ther* 2000;14(Suppl 2):66–70.

52. Katsuma S, Hirasawa A, Tsujimoto G. Bile acids promote glucagon-like peptide-1 secretion through TGR5 in a murine enteroendocrine cell line STC-1. *Biochem Biophys Res Commun* 2005;329(1):386–90.

53. Adrian TE, Gariballa S, Parekh KA et al. Rectal taurocholate increases L cell and insulin secretion, and decreases blood glucose and food intake in obese type 2 diabetic volunteers. *Diabetologia* 2012;55(9):2343–7.

54. Patti ME, Houten SM, Bianco AC et al. Serum bile acids are higher in humans with prior gastric bypass: Potential contribution to improved glucose and lipid metabolism. *Obesity (Silver Spring, Md)* 2009;17(9):1671–7.

55. Dutia R, Brakoniecki K, Bunker P et al. Limited recovery of beta-cell function after gastric bypass despite clinical diabetes remission. *Diabetes* 2014;63(4):1214–23.

56. Dutia R, Embrey M, O'Brien CS et al. Temporal changes in bile acid levels and 12alpha-hydroxylation after Roux-en-Y gastric bypass surgery in type 2 diabetes. *Int J Obes* 2015;39(5):806–13.

57. Pournaras DJ, Glicksman C, Vincent RP et al. The role of bile after Roux-en-Y gastric bypass in promoting weight loss and improving glycaemic control. *Endocrinology* 2012;153(8):3613–9.

58. Holst JJ. On the physiology of GIP and GLP-1. *Horm Metab Res* 2004;36(11–12):747–54.

59. Creutzfeldt W, Ebert R, Willms B, Frerichs H, Brown JC. Gastric inhibitory polypeptide (GIP) and insulin in obesity: Increased response to stimulation and defective feedback control of serum levels. *Diabetologia* 1978;14(1):15–24.

60. Ding WG, Gromada J. Protein kinase A-dependent stimulation of exocytosis in mouse pancreatic beta-cells by glucose-dependent insulinotropic polypeptide. *Diabetes* 1997;46(4):615–21.

61. Rao RS, Kini S. GIP and bariatric surgery. *Obes Surg* 2011;21(2):244–52.

62. Laferrere B, Heshka S, Wang K et al. Incretin levels and effect are markedly enhanced 1 month after Roux-en-Y gastric bypass surgery in obese patients with type 2 diabetes. *Diabetes Care* 2007;30(7):1709–16.

63. Laferrère B, Teixeira J, McGinty J et al. Effect of weight loss by gastric bypass surgery versus hypocaloric diet on glucose and incretin levels in patients with type 2 diabetes. *J Clin Endocrinol Metab* 2008;93(7):2479–85.

64. Bose M, Teixeira J, Olivan B et al. Weight loss and incretin responsiveness improve glucose control independently after gastric bypass surgery. *J Diabetes* 2010;2(1):47–55.

65. Van der Schueren BJ, Homel P, Alam M et al. Magnitude and variability of the glucagon-like peptide-1 response in patients with type 2 diabetes up to 2 years following gastric bypass surgery. *Diabetes Care* 2012;35(1):42–6.

66. Korner J, Bessler M, Inabnet W, Taveras C, Holst JJ. Exaggerated glucagon-like peptide-1 and blunted glucose-dependent insulinotropic peptide secretion are associated with Roux-en-Y gastric bypass but not adjustable gastric banding. *Surg Obes Relat Dis* 2007;3(6):597–601.

67. Sirinek KR, O'Dorisio TM, Hill D, McFee AS. Hyperinsulinism, glucose-dependent insulinotropic polypeptide, and the enteroinsular axis in morbidly obese patients before and after gastric bypass. *Surgery* 1986;100(4):781–7.

68. Clements RH, Gonzalez QH, Long CI, Wittert G, Laws HL. Hormonal changes after Roux-en-Y gastric bypass for morbid obesity and the control of type-II diabetes mellitus. *Am Surg* 2004;70(1):1–4; discussion 5.

69. Whitson BA, Leslie DB, Kellogg TA et al. Entero-endocrine changes after gastric bypass in diabetic and nondiabetic patients: A preliminary study. *J Surg Res* 2007;141(1):31–9.

70. Yip S, Signal M, Smith G et al. Lower glycemic fluctuations early after bariatric surgery partially explained by caloric restriction. *Obes Surg* 2014;24(1):62–70.

71. Kashyap SR, Daud S, Kelly KR et al. Acute effects of gastric bypass versus gastric restrictive surgery on beta-cell function and insulinotropic hormones in severely obese patients with type 2 diabetes. *Int J Obes* 2010;34(3):462–71.

72. Olivan B, Teixeira J, Bose M et al. Effect of weight loss by diet or gastric bypass surgery on peptide YY3–36 levels. *Ann Surg* 2009;249(6):948–53.

73. Umeda LM, Pereira AZ, Carneiro G, Arasaki CH, Zanella MT. Postprandial adiponectin levels are associated with improvements in postprandial triglycerides after Roux-en-Y gastric bypass in type 2 diabetic patients. *Metab Syndr Relat Disord* 2013;11(5):343–8.

74. de Carvalho CP, Marin DM, de Souza AL et al. GLP-1 and adiponectin: Effect of weight loss after dietary restriction and gastric bypass in morbidly obese patients with normal and abnormal glucose metabolism. *Obes Surg* 2009;19(3):313–20.

75. Werling M, Vincent RP, Cross GF et al. Enhanced fasting and post-prandial plasma bile acid responses after Roux-en-Y gastric bypass surgery. *Scand J Gastroenterol* 2013;48(11):1257–64.

76. Rodieux F, Giusti V, D'Alessio DA, Suter M, Tappy L. Effects of gastric bypass and gastric banding on glucose kinetics and gut hormone release. *Obesity (Silver Spring, Md)* 2008;16(2):298–305.

77. Vidal J, Nicolau J, Romero F et al. Long-term effects of Roux-en-Y gastric bypass surgery on plasma glucagon-like peptide-1 and islet function in morbidly obese subjects. *J Clin Endocrinol Metab* 2009;94(3):884–91.

78. Valderas JP, Irribarra V, Rubio L et al. Effects of sleeve gastrectomy and medical treatment for obesity on glucagon-like peptide 1 levels and glucose homeostasis in non-diabetic subjects. *Obes Surg* 2011;21(7):902–9.

79. Umemura A, Sasaki A, Nitta H, Otsuka K, Suto T, Wakabayashi G. Effects of changes in adipocyte hormones and visceral adipose tissue and the reduction of obesity-related comorbidities after laparoscopic sleeve gastrectomy in Japanese patients with severe obesity. *Endocr J* 2014;61(4):381–91.

80. Ramon JM, Salvans S, Crous X et al. Effect of Roux-en-Y gastric bypass vs sleeve gastrectomy on glucose and gut hormones: A prospective randomised trial. *J Gastrointest Surg* 2012;16(6):1116–22.

81. Ebert R, Creutzfeldt W. Gastrointestinal peptides and insulin secretion. *Diabetes Metab Rev* 1987;3(1):1–26.

82. Nauck MA, Homberger E, Siegel EG et al. Incretin effects of increasing glucose loads in man calculated from venous insulin and C-peptide responses. *J Clin Endocrinol Metab* 1986;63(2):492–8.

83. Preitner F, Ibberson M, Franklin I et al. Gluco-incretins control insulin secretion at multiple levels as revealed in mice lacking GLP-1 and GIP receptors. *J Clin Invest* 2004;113(4):635–45.

84. Nauck MA. Unraveling the science of incretin biology. *Eur J Intern Med* 2009;20(Suppl 2):S303–8.

85. Nauck M, Stockmann F, Ebert R, Creutzfeldt W. Reduced incretin effect in type 2 (non-insulin-dependent) diabetes. *Diabetologia* 1986;29(1):46–52.

86. Pournaras DJ, Aasheim ET, Bueter M et al. Effect of bypassing the proximal gut on gut hormones involved with glycemic control and weight loss. *Surg Obes Relat Dis* 2012;8(4):371–4.

87. Nguyen NQ, Debreceni TL, Bambrick JE et al. Upregulation of intestinal glucose transporters after Roux-en-Y gastric bypass to prevent carbohydrate malabsorption. *Obesity (Silver Spring, Md)* 2014;22(10):2164–71.

88. Melissas J, Koukouraki S, Askoxylakis J et al. Sleeve gastrectomy: A restrictive procedure? *Obes Surg* 2007;17(1):57–62.

89. Salehi M, Gastaldelli A, D'Alessio DA. Blockade of glucagon-like peptide 1 receptor corrects postprandial hypoglycemia after gastric bypass. *Gastroenterology* 2014;146(3):669–80.

90. Shah M, Law JH, Micheletto F et al. Contribution of endogenous glucagon-like peptide 1 to glucose metabolism after Roux-en-Y gastric bypass. *Diabetes* 2014;63(2):483–93.

91. Jorgensen NB, Dirksen C, Bojsen-Moller KN et al. Exaggerated glucagon-like peptide 1 response is important for improved beta-cell function and glucose tolerance after Roux-en-Y gastric bypass in patients with type 2 diabetes. *Diabetes* 2013;62(9):3044–52.

92. Vetter ML, Wadden TA, Teff KL et al. GLP-1 plays a limited role in improved glycemia shortly after Roux-en-Y gastric bypass: A comparison with intensive lifestyle modification. *Diabetes* 2015;64(2):434–46.

93. Jimenez A, Casamitjana R, Viaplana-Masclans J, Lacy A, Vidal J. GLP-1 action and glucose tolerance in subjects with remission of type 2 diabetes after gastric bypass surgery. *Diabetes Care* 2013;36(7):2062–9.

94. Ballantyne GH. Peptide YY(1–36) and peptide YY(3–36). Part I. Distribution, release and actions. *Obes Surg* 2006;16(5):651–8.

95. Valderas JP, Irribarra V, Boza C et al. Medical and surgical treatments for obesity have opposite effects on peptide YY and appetite: A prospective study controlled for weight loss. *J Clin Endocrinol Metab* 2010;95(3):1069–75.

96. Pournaras DJ, Osborne A, Hawkins SC et al. The gut hormone response following Roux-en-Y gastric bypass: Cross-sectional and prospective study. *Obes Surg* 2010;20(1):56–60.

97. Cummings DE, Overduin J, Foster-Schubert KE. Gastric bypass for obesity: Mechanisms of weight loss and diabetes resolution. *J Clin Endocrinol Metab* 2004;89(6):2608–15.

98. Boggiano MM, Chandler PC, Oswald KD et al. PYY3–36 as an anti-obesity drug target. *Obes Rev* 2005;6(4):307–22.

99. Zac-Varghese S, Tan T, Bloom SR. Hormonal interactions between gut and brain. *Discov Med* 2010;10(55):543–52.

100. Cohen MA, Ellis SM, Le Roux CW et al. Oxyntomodulin suppresses appetite and reduces food intake in humans. *J Clin Endocrinol Metab* 2003;88(10):4696–701.

101. Schjoldager B, Mortensen PE, Myhre J, Christiansen J, Holst JJ. Oxyntomodulin from distal gut. Role in regulation of gastric and pancreatic functions. *Dig Dis Sci* 1989;34(9):1411–9.

102. Pocai A. Action and therapeutic potential of oxyntomodulin. *Mol Metab* 2014;3(3):241–51.

103. Laferrère B, Swerdlow N, Bawa B et al. Rise of oxyntomodulin in response to oral glucose after gastric bypass surgery in patients with type 2 diabetes. *J Clin Endocrinol Metab* 2010;95(8):4072–6.

104. Yousseif A, Emmanuel J, Karra E et al. Differential effects of laparoscopic sleeve gastrectomy and laparoscopic gastric bypass on appetite, circulating acyl-ghrelin, peptide YY3–36 and active GLP-1 levels in non-diabetic humans. *Obes Surg* 2014;24(2):241–52.

105. le Roux CW, Aylwin SJ, Batterham RL et al. Gut hormone profiles following bariatric surgery favor an anorectic state, facilitate weight loss, and improve metabolic parameters. *Ann Surg* 2006;243(1):108–14.

106. Korner J, Bessler M, Cirilo LJ, Conwell IM, Daud A, Restuccia NL, Wardlaw SL. Effects of Roux-en-Y gastric bypass surgery on fasting and postprandial concentrations of plasma ghrelin, peptide YY, and insulin. *J Clin Endocrinol Metab.* 2005;90(1):359–65. Epub 2004 Oct 13.

PART 10

Science and Technology

57

Robotic endocrine surgery

ALEXIS K. OKOH AND EREN BERBER

INTRODUCTION

The first robotic-assisted procedure in humans was performed more than a decade ago by a European team who went on to report a case series detailing the feasibility of robotic general surgery [1]. Since then, a growing expansion in the number of indications for various general surgical procedures and an increase in the adoption of the robotic platform among surgeons from a variety of subspecialties, including endocrine surgery, have been noted [1–3].

Robotics is attractive to the surgeon because of the three-dimensional image quality, articulating instruments, and stable surgical platform, and thus provides outcomes similar to those of the laparoscopic approach for adrenalectomy and better cosmetic results than the conventional option for thyroidectomy and parathyroidectomy. Besides, robotic surgery may obviate the limitations of standard laparoscopy, although at the current time, it still lacks the ability to replace the lost tactile sensation.

As the need to reorient health care around value for patients has now become an intrinsic motivation in the practice of medicine, further development of robotic endocrine surgery may be limited unless improved quality focusing on patient-based outcomes can be used to justify the generally higher costs of this technology.

This chapter begins with a review of the history of robotics and surgery to show how it has evolved to include the use of surgical robots in endocrine surgery. Next, we describe the current indications and techniques for robotic adrenalectomy, thyroidectomy, and parathyroidectomy, with an emphasis on variation in clinical and patient-reported outcomes relative to traditional surgical approaches.

HISTORY OF ROBOTICS AND SURGERY

The integration of robotics into surgery has been in evolution since the early 1990s. Reports of robots in the operating room showed that the use of mechanical retractors and robotic camera holders could be beneficial [4–7]. A study by Kavoussi et al. [8] demonstrated a significantly steadier robotic-controlled laparoscopic camera positioning ($p < 0.005$) with less inadvertent movements than a handheld camera. Robots were viewed as auspicious devices that could help standardize surgical outcomes by limiting surgeon-dependent tumors that varied from case to case.

The first invented surgical robot was the (master–slave) manipulator system (ARTEMIS, Tübingen, Germany, 1996), equipped with a surgeon end (the master) and a patient end (robotic instruments), or the slave end. This manipulator gave the surgeon electronically remote control of the laparoscopic instruments while seated at a distance from the patient [5]. These master–slave telemanipulators pioneered the development of the current U.S Food and Drug Administration (FDA)-approved surgical telemanipulating robotic surgical systems (Da Vinci Robotic Surgical System, Intuitive Surgical, Mountain View, California; Zeus Robotic Surgical System, Computer Motion, Goleta, California) [9–11] used to assist minimally invasive procedures in general surgery.

Cadiere and colleagues [1], from Belgium, were the first to report robotic-assisted procedures in humans in 1997. Their robotic general surgical series included 146 procedures, initiated by a case of fundoplication. The first report from the United States was by Horgan et al. [2], who performed another series of cases with the da Vinci robotic system, which included single cases of bilateral adrenalectomy.

Currently, there has been a growing expansion in the use of robots for procedures across a variety of subspecialities of cardiovascular surgery, urology, gynecology, neurosurgery, orthopaedics, and general surgery. With the advent of advanced computer interfaces that could electronically control special instruments equipped with tips, surgical dexterity in difficult-to-reach anatomic regions has been improved by robotics.

The experience in robotic endocrine surgery is still limited. Although earlier practices in robotic adrenalectomy were in existence, the utility of robotic-assisted approaches in thyroid surgery was not demonstrated until 2005. The past 8 years has seen several authors from the Far East reporting a handful of case series of robotic thyroidectomies [12–15]. Since the establishment of a robotic endocrine surgery program at our institution in 2008, we have also described several techniques for robotic thyroidectomy and adrenalectomy [16–18]. The limited practice of robotic-assisted endocrine surgery is probably due to a number of reasons, including the novelty of the procedure, the cost of surgical robots, the limited number of surgeons trained in the procedure, and most importantly, numerous questions regarding the efficiency of the procedure. With the evolving technology, the creation of more innovative devices that will continue to expand the capabilities of the surgeon to treat disease while minimizing patient trauma and improving patient outcome is anticipated.

ROBOTIC ADRENALECTOMY

Since the initial description of laparoscopic adrenalectomy by Gagner et al. in 1992, laparoscopic surgery has now become the standard technique for resection of benign functional and nonfunctional tumors [19]. The superiority of both laparoscopic and retroperitoneostic approaches over traditional open surgery in terms of morbidity and costs, with similar overall efficacy, has been demonstrated by several studies [20–22]. The first Da Vinci robotic-assisted adrenalectomy was performed in 2001 by Horgan et al. using a lateral transabdominal (LT) approach [23]. Their report demonstrated the potential benefits of the robotic platform over conventional laparoscopy for resection of

a small deep-seated organ such as the adrenal gland, in terms of both visualization of the operative field with three-dimensional optics and more precise, less cumbersome dissection with tremor-minimizing wristed instruments.

INDICATIONS

Current indications for robotic adrenalectomy are similar to those for the laparoscopic approach, and include all benign functional adrenal tumors, benign nonfunctional tumors of ≥4 cm, and those demonstrating significant growth on follow-up computed tomography (CT) scan, as well as adrenal metastases in selected patients with soft tissue or solid-organ primary tumors, usually in the setting of mono- or oligometastatic disease [24–26].

An open technique is the management of choice for lesions that are highly suspicious for adrenocortical cancer based on preoperative clinical, biochemical, and imaging findings [27–29]. In scenarios where evidence suggestive of gross extra-adrenal invasion during a robotic-assisted adrenalectomy exists, early conversion to an open approach prior to any significant dissection is warranted to ensure an effective execution of an oncologically sound procedure consisting of *en bloc* resection of the tumor, regional lymohadenopathy and removal of contiguously involved organs.

Despite the decade-old description of the laparoscopic techniques for both posterior retroperitoneal (PR) and LT, a consensus on the indications and choice of approach has not yet been reached.

Lateral transperitoneal and posterior retroperitoneal approaches

GENERAL CONSIDERATIONS

Robotic adrenalectomy is currently performed via either a lateral transperitoneal or PR approach. Patient selection for a particular technique should take into consideration the underlying endocrinopathy, body habitus, tumor bilaterality, and type and extent of previous surgery.

Over the years, the merits of posterior retroperitoneal adrenalectomy (PRA) over traditional lateral transperitoneal adrenalectomy (LTA) have been increasingly recognized for a select group of patients, particularly those with previous intra-abdominal surgery, as adhesiolysis and manipulation of other intraperitoneal viscera are minimized [30]. Also, the procedure may also be beneficial for patients with limited central obesity associated with Cushing's syndrome, as abdominal fat tends to fall away from the operative site when the patient is placed in a prone position. Lastly, in patients requiring bilateral adrenalectomies, robotic PRA has been shown to result in shorter operative times than LTA, given the ability to surgically access both glands without repositioning the patient [31].

On the other hand, the posterior approach may not be suitable for larger tumors (e.g., tumors of >6 cm) considering the relatively limited confines of the retroperitoneal space, and enhanced risk of malignancy. In this same

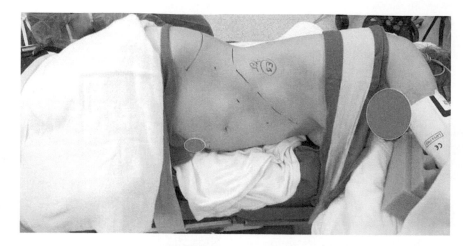

Figure 57.1 Positioning of the patient for an LT robotic adrenalectomy.

manner, patients with impairment of access to the retroperitoneum, such as those with a small space between the 12th rib and iliac crest (>4 cm), or with a long distance between the skin and Gerota's fascia (>7 cm), should also be considered for an alternative approach [32,33].

On the contrary, the larger working space and the familiarity of landmarks associated with the LTA technique make it more favorable for larger, unilateral tumors, in which there is a small retroperitoneal space or previous retroperitoneal kidney surgery. It also offers a lesser burden in the event that conversion to an open transperitoneal approach is required.

In our institution, we prefer LT adrenalectomy for tumors of >6 cm. If the tumor size is <6 cm, the distance between the skin and Gerota's space is not long (generally <7 cm), and the 12th rib is rostral to the renal hilum, we carry out the PR technique.

Techniques

LATERAL TRANSPERITONEAL APPROACH

Preoperative preparation, positioning of the patient, and creation of the port sites are the same as in the laparoscopic TL adrenalectomy (Figure 57.1). Following intubation and administration of general anesthesia, the patient is placed in a left or right lateral decubitus position dependent on the location of the mass.

Four trocars are used. The first, a 12 mm trocar, is inserted via the optical technique midway between the umbilicus and the costal margin. After CO_2 insufflation, two 8 mm robotic trocars and one 5 mm laparoscopic trocar are introduced below the costal margin.

Trocar sites should be configured to allow the first surgical assistant to use the suction irrigator and a clip applicator when required. In exceptional cases, such as in obese patients and small patients, it may be necessary to interchange the location of the first assistant port. We use Cadiere forceps via the left port and the robotic Harmonic scalpel via the right port (Figure 57.2). The 5 mm trocar is used by the first assistant for suction and irrigation.

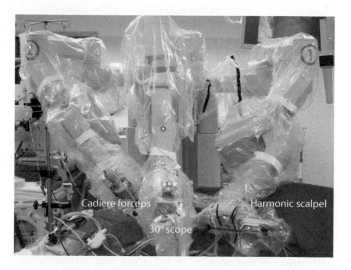

Figure 57.2 Intraoperative photograph showing the docking of the robot and position of the instruments for adrenalectomy. A down-viewing 30° scope is used with a grasping instrument from the lateral port and the Harmonic scalpel from the medial port.

For left adrenalectomy, the splenocolic and splenorenal ligaments are divided. For right adrenalectomy, the right triangular ligament is divided to retract the right hepatic lobe. We prefer to carry out the splenic–hepatic mobilization laparoscopically, followed by intraoperative ultrasound to determine the location of the adrenal gland relative to major surrounding structures and as an additional assessment for any obvious extra-adrenal invasion.

The robot is subsequently docked, approaching the patient from behind the ipsilateral shoulder, usually at a 45° angle with the table. If needed, the table can be moved clockwise so as to match the angle of dissection with the docking of the robot. The robot is docked across the ipsilateral side of the patient, and the robotic trocars are connected. Cadiere forceps are used from the left port, and the robotic Harmonic scalpel from the right port. On the right side, the first assistant retracts the liver and provides suction. Dissection proceeds initially along the superior and

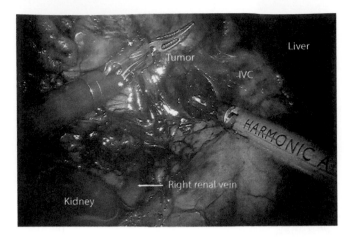

Figure 57.3 Intraoperative photograph showing robotic dissection of a right-sided pheochromocytoma via the LT approach. Owing to the angulation of the grasping instrument, there is no collision with the Harmonic scalpel. Furthermore, the range of motion is much better than with rigid laparoscopic instruments, making dissection easier.

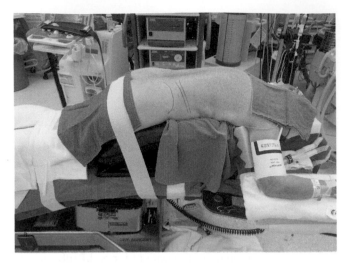

Figure 57.4 Positioning of the patient in a PR adrenalectomy. Patient placed in a prone jack-knife position using a Wilson frame.

lateral borders of the adrenal gland, followed by the inferior and medial aspects (Figure 57.3). The adrenal vein is taken using the Harmonic scalpel if small (<4 mm), or divided between metallic clips placed by the first assistant if larger. After the adrenalectomy is complete, the robot is undocked and the gland is removed using a specimen retrieval bag. After the operative site is irrigated and suctioned, trocars are removed. Morcellation may be required if the specimen is large (e.g., >3 cm). Hemostasis is achieved laparoscopically and confirmed after desufflation and reinsufflation. Fascia is closed for both 12 mm port sites.

POSTERIOR RETROPERITONEAL APPROACH

After establishment of general anesthesia, the patient is placed in a prone jack-knife position using a Wilson frame, with both arms placed on boards situated at the head of the table and directed toward the anesthetist (Figure 57.4). An optical trocar is placed through a 1 cm incision made 2 cm inferior to the 12th rib in order to gain access to Gerota's space. The trocar is then replaced with a dissecting balloon to create a potential space under direct visualization. The dissecting balloon is then removed, and a 12 mm trocar is then introduced into this space with subsequent retroperitoneal insufflation to approximately 15 mmHg of CO_2. Two additional 5 mm ports are then inserted, one placed medially along the lateral border of the paraspinous muscles and the other laterally, inferior to the 12th rib. It is important to ensure that these 5 mm ports are as far as possible from the initial 12 mm port in order to avoid instrument collision. Laparoscopic ultrasound is subsequently performed similarly to the LTA technique, prior to docking of the robot. Cadiere forceps are used via the lateral port, and the Harmonic scalpel used from the medial port (Figure 57.5). Identifiable landmarks subsequent to

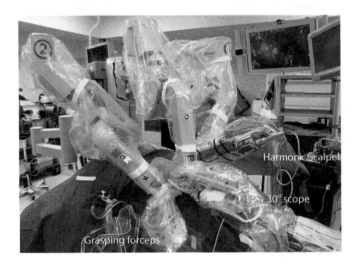

Figure 57.5 Intraoperative photograph showing the docking of the robot in a PR adrenalectomy. A down-viewing 30° scope with Maryland forceps via the lateral port and the Harmonic scalpel from the medial port.

the development of the retroperitoneal space and intraoperative ultrasound should include Gerota's fascia, the superior pole of the kidney, paraspinous muscles medially, the peritoneum anterolaterally, the diaphragm superolaterally, the inferior vena cava on the right, and the adrenal gland itself. Again, the superior and lateral aspects of the gland are initially dissected, with the inferior and medial borders being dissected last (Figure 57.6). Suction and irrigation, as well as clipping of the adrenal vein when too large to be taken with the Harmonic scalpel, can be performed by the first assistant through the medial port after temporary removal of the Harmonic scalpel. The robot is undocked after the dissection is complete, and the specimen removed with an endoscopic retrieval bag. Hemostasis is achieved at low insufflation pressures and confirmed after desufflation

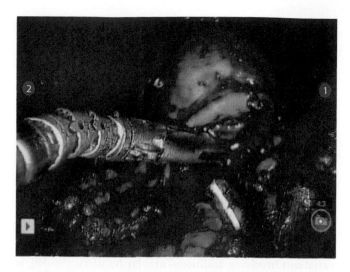

Figure 57.6 Intraoperative photo depicting the dissection of an adrenal mass in a right robotic PR adrenalectomy.

and reinsufflation. Fascia is closed for the 12 mm port site. It should be noted that the above technique differs slightly from that described by Ludwig et al., in which one of the arms is tucked, 8 mm ports are placed, and higher initial insufflation pressures are utilized [34]. Also, Ludwig et al.'s approach involves initial dissection of the inferior and medial borders of the gland, with early identification and division of the adrenal vein, leaving the anterior (peritoneal) and superolateral (diaphragmatic) attachments until the end.

Outcomes

Previously conducted studies have confirmed the superiority of endoscopic surgical procedures over open approaches to adrenalectomy in terms of both postoperative morbidity and costs [20–22]. Despite the association of shorter operative times with the posterior retroperitoneoscopic approach than with the lateral transperitoneoscopic approach, as suggested by some retrospective studies, recent results from two randomized controlled trials have shown statistical equivalence between these two major endoscopic techniques for adrenalectomy in terms of operative time, rates of complication, and length of stay at the hospital [35–39]. A cost analysis study conducted at the Cleveland Clinic also showed no significant difference in overall cost between the various endoscopic techniques [21].

Although the potential advantages robotic adrenalectomy offers to the surgeon in terms of visualization, stability, and precision of dissection have been well established, the additional initial costs involved, the learning curve, and the potentially increased operative times are among the factors that may deter its widespread adoption.

The first randomized trial comparing laparoscopic with robotic adrenalectomy using a lateral transperitoneal approach was published by Morino et al. [40] in 2004. The study, which randomly assigned 20 patients with benign adrenal lesions to each arm, with exclusion criteria including bilateral lesions and tumors of >10 cm, showed that robotic adrenalectomy was associated with longer operative times (169 vs. 115 minutes), increased perioperative morbidity (20% vs. 0%), and higher total costs ($3467 vs. $2737, excluding initial robot cost) relative to the laparoscopic approach.

Subsequently, a retrospective chart review of patients who received either robotic ($n = 50$) or laparoscopic ($n = 59$) unilateral LTA by Brunaud et al. reported that the robotic approach was associated with less intraoperative blood loss, although longer operative times overall, compared with the laparoscopic approach [41]. As expected, a learning curve of 20 more cases on the robotic platform nullified this difference in operative time. In addition, a subset analysis showed that laparoscopic adrenalectomy was associated with longer operative times in patients with larger tumors (> 5.5 cm), as well as in those with a body mass index (BMI) of ≥30. Previously, we have also shown that, relative to conventional laparoscopy, use of the robotic platform can reduce operative times as well as conversion rates for patients with larger tumors (>5 cm), although we did not find any differences in perioperative outcomes or operative time for obese patients [42,43].

Similarly, a study of 100 consecutive patients who received robotic LTA by Brunaud et al. found that greater surgeon experience, higher first-assistant training level, and smaller tumor size were all independently associated with shorter robotic operative time [44].

Considering the smaller working field of retroperitoneal space and inflexibility of laparoscopic devices, robotic PRA appear more propitious than robotic LTA for better outcomes relative to conventional laparoscopy.

We have reported our experience with 63 patients receiving either laparoscopic ($n = 32$) or robotic ($n = 31$) PRA. Tumor size, blood loss, and hospital stay were similar between the two groups, as were overall skin-to-skin operative times. After an initial learning curve of 10 cases, however, operative times were significantly shorter in the robotic group (139 minutes vs. 167 minutes), inclusive of robotic docking times, which ranged from 5 to 30 minutes. Pain scores on postoperative day 1 were lower in the robotic group than in the laparoscopic group, which was attributed to the potentially shorter operative time, and less pressure on incisions as a result of fewer instrument changes and articulating instrumentation [45].

A current meta-analysis of 600 patients from eight retrospective studies and one randomized controlled trial undergoing either robotic ($n = 277$) or laparoscopic ($n = 323$) adrenalectomy showed no significant difference in operative time, conversion rate, or postoperative complications was observed between the two groups, although there was a significantly shorter hospital stay (weighted mean difference [WMD] −0.43 days) and estimated blood loss (WMD −18.2 mL) in the robotic group [46].

Providing a direct access to the adrenal glands and obviating the need for mobilization of the visceral organs, the laparoscopic PR technique has been proposed as the preferred procedure in the treatment of bilateral adrenal masses. More recently, our group has demonstrated the feasibility of the robotic bilateral PR technique for the treatment of bilateral macronodular hyperplasia causing Cushing's syndrome [47,48]. A similar report by Malley et al. that described a case of synchronous robotic bilateral adrenalectomy via a TL approach [49] indicated findings similar to ours (operative time and blood loss, 235 minutes vs. 268 minutes and 50 mL vs. 35 mL, respectively). In both cases, morbidity was not reported, blood loss was less, and hospital stay and operative times were shorter when compared with the laparoscopic bilateral cases.

CONCLUSION

The feasibility and safety of robotic LTA and PRA have been demonstrated, although higher costs relative to laparoscopy, secondary in part to increased learning curve-associated operative times, are certainly initial shortcomings. The potential advantages of the robotic platform for patients with larger tumors, and to conduct finer dissections with less blood loss, should continue to be investigated.

ROBOTIC THYROIDECTOMY

Open thyroidectomy has been an evolving surgical technique for the treatment of thyroid diseases that has gained wide consideration ever since its initial description by Nobel laureate Theodor Kocher. Success has been attained in making it feasible via small cervical incisions requiring minimal instrumentation.

Triggered by the need to enhance cosmetic outcomes, minimally invasive procedures in head and neck surgery have been at the cutting edge during the past decade. Several endoscopic techniques, such as axillary, breast, axillobreast, and anterior chest approaches, have been developed [50–52], obviating the need for a cervical scar.

The use of robotics in thyroid surgery was sparked by the evolutionary process of these minimally invasive techniques, with initial case reports from the United States in 2005, and large series from South Korea that were published afterwards [14,53].

Recent results from a learning curve study of robotic thyroidectomy by novice surgeons with little or no experience in endoscopic surgery demonstrated a decrease in operative time after 20 cases and also showed similar perioperative outcomes when compared with their experienced counterparts [54].

Indications and patient selection

Compared with the traditional transcervical technique, robotic thyroidectomy is distinguished by a set of exclusive criteria for patient selection. Definitive requirements include the absence of previous neck surgery or a cervical scar and, most importantly, an informed and highly motivated patient.

Easy transaxillary access will require patients with a distance from the axillary to the sternal notch of less than 15 cm and a BMI of less than 30. Large goiters with a substernal component, as well as thyroid nodules greater than 4 cm, or those with potential for extrathyroidal extension, are among the relative contraindications for robotic thyroidectomy. Absolute contraindications of the robotic approach for candidates include thyroiditis or Graves' disease and uncontrolled thyrotoxicosis [55,56].

TECHNIQUES

Currently existing are numerous robotic techniques that have been developed with the goal of avoiding the creation of cervical scar. The transaxillay approach, which involves an axillary incision either unilaterally or bilaterally, with variations involving additional areolar incisions [55–58], is the most frequently performed. The experience from these transaxillary techniques has made robotic total thyroidectomy feasible via a unilateral axillary incision using three robotic arms. A new approach via an incision in the posterior auricular crease extending to the occipital hairline has also been reported by Terris et al. [59].

ROBOTIC UNILATERAL TRANSAXILLARY THYROIDECTOMY

After establishment of general anesthesia, the patient is placed supine, with the neck extended. The ipsilateral arm is then extended to expose the axilla at the level of the shoulder, with 90° flexion at the elbow. The arm is padded and positioned on an arm board lateral to the head, again by avoiding >90° extension on shoulder and elbow joints. We do not prefer to hyperextend the arm above the patient's head, as this has a higher chance of causing nerve injuries (Figure 57.7). It is important to protect pressure points and avoid shoulder hyperextension so as to prevent brachial plexopathy [60]. The contralateral arm is placed at the patient's side. Prophylactic antibiotics are administered in all cases. A 5–6 cm vertical axillary incision is made and a subcutaneous skin flap created superficial to the pectoralis fascia, extending to the sternal notch inferiorly and clavicle inferiolaterally. Dissection is continued toward the anterior neck and a subplatysmal plane developed after crossing the clavicle until the two heads of the sternocleidomastoid muscle (SCM) are visualized. The sternal head of the SCM and strap muscles are retracted anteriorly with an elevating retractor in order to expose the thyroid. The robot is then docked, approaching the patient from the contralateral arm. A 30° downward scope is placed through the center of the incision with Cadiere forceps used through a cephalad port, and the Harmonic scalpel used through a caudal port. We prefer this three-arm approach with a laparoscopic suction irrigator being used by the first assistant for countertraction. Thyroidectomy then proceeds according to similar principles used in the transcervical approach. The inferior and superior poles are divided after defining the location of the isthmus. Identification of the recurrent laryngeal

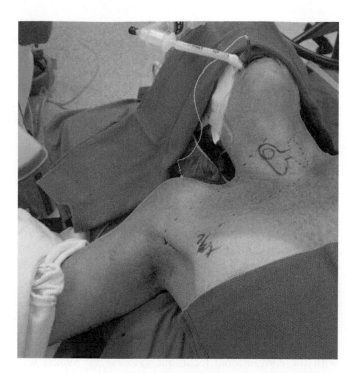

Figure 57.7 Positioning of the patient for a robotic trans-axillary thyroidectomy. As seen, the right upper extremity is not hyperextended, but kept on an arm board, with less than 90° extension of all joints. After percutaneous ultrasound, the location of the thyroid gland and nodule is noted and topographically marked on the skin.

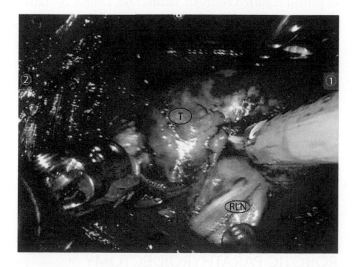

Figure 57.8 Intraoperative photo showing the thyroid gland (T) and RLN.

nerve (RLN) and parathyroid glands is essential prior to completion of the ipsilateral lobectomy. The contralateral lobe is then dissected in a medial-to-lateral fashion, again tracing the RLN and defining the location of the parathyroid glands (Figure 57.8). The lobe is removed through the axillary incision, which is then closed using subcuticular suture. We do not drain the flap postoperatively.

OUTCOMES

In spite of the popularity of the traditional transcervical technique for thyroidectomy as the gold standard of treatment for surgical thyroid diseases, previously conducted studies have attempted to compare the conventional approach with the evolving robotic and endoscopic techniques in terms of oncologic equivalence, costs, and patient-reported outcomes, including cosmetic satisfaction [61–68].

Lang et al., in their recent meta-analysis that included 2375 patients from 11 studies, reported a longer operative time (mean difference = 56 minutes), a longer hospital stay, and increased transient RLN injury rates in patients receiving robotic thyroidectomy compared with those who received conventional transcervical thyroidectomy [69]. Without disregarding the high mean difference in operative time (1 hour), conceivably, the most disturbing of these results was the difference in temporary RLN injury rates. They found it to be three times higher in the robotic group when calculated based on number of nerves at risk (2.5% vs. 0.7%). This nerve injury rate was reported as independent with regard to surgeon case volume, since they could only be computed from two of the 11 studies. Statistical significance was not reached between the two groups when they were compared in terms of other perioperative outcomes, such as blood loss, hypocalcemia, and overall morbidity.

Concerning other likely operative complications, two brachial plexus injuries have been previously reported (overall rate of 0.2%) in one robotic study. This was probably as a result of shoulder hyperextension and other patient positioning effects peculiar to the transaxillary approach [60,69]. The brachial plexus injury is related to the hyperextension of the arm during the procedure. Hyperextension of the arm during the procedure should therefore be discouraged, and the arm placed on an arm board with less than 90° extension of the shoulder and elbow joints.

Similarly, in another meta-analysis of 2881 patients from nine studies comparing open, endoscopic, and robotic thyroidectomy, Jackson et al. reported a longer operative time but shorter hospital stay and increased cosmetic satisfaction for patients receiving robotic transaxillary relative to open transcervical thyroidectomy [70]. While individuals in the robotic group also had higher rates of transient hypocalcemia, the rate of temporary and permanent RLN injury was not statistically different between the robotic and open groups, inconsistent with the Lang analysis [69].

Results from the Jackson analysis showed no considerable dissimilarities in postoperative thyroglobulin (Tg) levels between the robotic and open groups, thus proposing similar completeness of resection between these two techniques. In fact, also included in Jackson et al.'s meta-analysis study were three studies used from Lang et al. (n = 590), from which both increased operative times and cosmetic satisfaction with the robotic approach, with no difference in complication rates, were reported. Moreover, on the basis of overlapping data from both studies, one study [63] used in the Jackson et al. meta-analysis was excluded from that performed by Lang et al.

In spite of the discrepancies in study selection and analysis, the notion of improved patient-reported cosmetic satisfaction by the robotic approach, and variability in perioperative outcomes when compared with the conventional open transcervical approach, still remains consistent across most current studies.

More recently, central or lateral neck dissections have been performed by robotic transaxillary approaches. Yi and colleagues have reported their experience with 521 female patients diagnosed with papillary thyroid cancer who underwent either robotic ($n = 98$) or open ($n = 423$) thyroidectomy with concomitant central neck dissection [71]. Findings from their study revealed a higher rate of transient hypocalcemia in the robotic group and no difference in serum Tg levels in both the immediate postoperative period and after remnant radioactive iodine (RAI) ablation performed at 6–12 months after the initial surgery.

The robotic platform has also been used for lateral neck dissections via the transaxillary approach. In a study by Kang et al., 33 patients with lateral neck nodal metastases successfully underwent robotic thyroidectomy with modified radical lymph node dissection (MRLND) [51]. In spite of the fact that most of the primary tumors were small in size, with 20 (61%) cases exhibiting papillary microcarcinoma, lymph node retrieval was satisfactory with a mean of 6.1 ± 4.4 nodes harvested in the central neck and 27.7 ± 11.0 nodes in the lateral neck. No major perioperative complications were reported among the group in which this technique was employed [72].

A more recent prospective evaluation of 128 patients undergoing either robotic ($n = 62$) or open ($n = 66$) total thyroidectomy with MRLND, by Lee et al. [73], reported longer operative time, but improved cosmetic satisfaction scores, as well as decreased postoperative swallowing difficulties and neck sensory changes in the robotic group. Similarities in terms of postoperative and post-RAI serum Tg levels, as well as the mean number of retrieved lymph nodes, were encountered between the open and robotic groups. Other parameters that did not show contrasting findings in both groups were length of hospital stay and perioperative complication rates, including hypoparathyroidism and nerve injury rates. Of note, results from these studies should be interpreted carefully, considering patient and surgeon bias originating from dissimilarities in the Korean and American health care systems, patients' body habitus, culture-specific implications of a cervical scar, and perhaps most importantly, surgical experience with this particular robotic technique.

Our group has recently reported a single-incision technique for performing total thyroidectomy from a unilateral lateral axillary incision [74]. The technique recommends a medial-to-lateral dissection of the contralateral thyroid gland. By using a 30° scope, the contralateral RLN can be easily visualized and preserved.

In the 2012 study by Kandil et al. [75], the authors reported the largest experience of robotic gasless thyroid surgery in the United States. Their study reported a significant persistent decrease in overall total operative time from 122 minutes to 104 minutes after 45 cases ($p = 0.02$), but a significant increase ($p = 0.008$) in total operative time in obese patients (BMI > 30). Findings from their study indicated that the approach is sustainable in a Western population, with no difference in complications between obese and normal weight patients ($p = 0.23$). In spite of the feasibility and excellent cosmetic results that were reported, the significant association between BMI and total operative time, as well as a lengthy learning curve, recommends a careful consideration of the approach, especially in obese patients, before routine implementation into clinical practice.

Previous cost-effective studies have associated the lengthy learning curve and longer total operative time with the total costs of robotic or endoscopic thyroidectomy [76,77]. In a cost analysis by Cabot et al. [77], conventional thyroidectomy, transaxillary endoscopic thyroidectomy, and transaxillary robotic thyroidectomy approaches were compared based on medical costs in the United States. Although a higher total cost for the transaxillary approaches compared with the conventional technique ($13,087 vs. $9028) was reported, equivalence in cost for all three procedures was noted once the total operative time was decreased in the robotic and endoscopic approaches.

CONCLUSION

The superiority of the robotic platform for thyroidectomy over the conventional open technique seems to lie principally in patient-reported cosmetic satisfaction. Longer operative times associated with the increased costs involved are obviously remitting concerns, just as in other robotic endocrine surgical procedures. In addition, taking into account the higher perioperative complications relative to conventional open techniques, including brachial plexopathies, as well as transient hypoparathyroidism and RLN injury, appropriate patient and surgeon selection is warranted. From this retrospect, in order to ensure optimal outcomes, referring patients to high-volume centers of excellence may seem appropriate. Nonetheless, observation of outcomes similar to those of the conventional technique when the procedure is performed by surgeons experienced in robotics, as well as conventional thyroid surgery, may relegate this procedure as a niche operation at this time.

ROBOTIC PARATHYROIDECTOMY

The current gold standard of care for surgical parathyroid diseases is transcervical parathyroidectomy, which is usually performed in a focused fashion with traditional four-gland exploration. Its success rate is reported to exceed 97% when used in combination with intraoperative parathyroid hormone (PTH) measurements [78].

As those for thyroidectomy, robotic transaxillary approaches for parathyroidectomy have been practiced largely in an attempt to develop patient-reported cosmetic satisfaction for individuals who wish to avoid a cervical incision, and as a potential improvement over endoscopic techniques with respect to both visualization of the operative field and precision of dissection.

Another evolving technique that eliminates the need for sternotomy or thoracotomy in select patients undergoing parathyroidectomy for ectopic glands located in the mediastinum is robotic transthoracic parathyroidectomy. This newly reported procedure is encouraged in patients in whom surgical extirpation through a low transcervical incision is not feasible [79,80].

Indications and patient selection

A closer look at the emerging nature of this procedure, together with the very few cases that have been reported in the medical literature, has led to an initial restriction of robotic transaxillary parathyroidectomy to patients with a biochemical diagnosis of primary hyperparathyroidism and positive preoperative localization with either ultrasound or sestamibi scan [68,81].

Candidates for the robotic thyroidectomy are usually concerned about avoiding a cervical scar and expected to be thin (BMI under 30), with a distance from the axillary to the sternal notch of less than 15 cm, in order to facilitate transaxillary access. A prerequisite for this approach is the localization of a single gland on imaging with a neck ultrasound or sestamibi scan.

Exclusion criteria include previous neck surgery, significant thyroiditis, or bulky thyroid disease. For patients with ectopic mediastinal parathyroid glands, positive preoperative localization with $^{123}I-^{99}Tc$-sestamibi subtraction single-photon emission computed tomography (SPECT)/CT is also highly desirable prior to proceeding with robotic transthoracic parathyroidectomy [80].

Techniques

ROBOTIC TRANSAXILLARY PARATHYROIDECTOMY

This approach is similar to that described above for robotic transaxillary thyroidectomy, with careful positioning to avoid iatrogenic neuropathy, and transaxillary access through creation of a subcutaneous flap and development of a subplatysmal plane until visualization of the two heads of the SCM [68]. The robot is docked across the contralateral arm after retraction of the sternal head of the SCM and strap muscles anteriorly with an elevating retractor. A three-arm approach is used as for robotic thyroidectomy, with dissection targeted toward the parathyroid adenoma. Initially, the thyroid is identified and dissection is guided by the preoperative ultrasound. The parathyroid adenoma is then identified and resected (Figure 57.9). Borders of the resection are the diaphragm caudally, the thyroid gland cranially, and the phrenic nerves laterally, all of which are dissected meticulously (Figures 57.10 and 57.11). To confirm that the tumor has been resected, a rapid serum PTH level is sent prior to removal of the thymus gland and then 10 minutes after removal. A drop in PTH level by 50% is considered to be consistent with a successful resection.

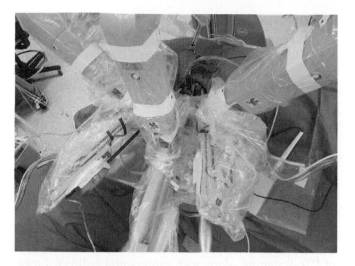

Figure 57.9 Docking of the robot for robotic TAC parathyroidectomy. A three-arm approach is used with a 30° down-viewing robotic camera.

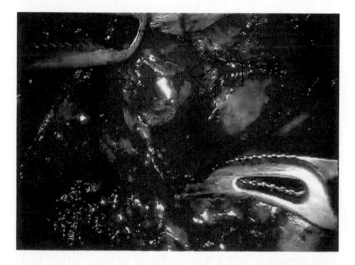

Figure 57.10 Parathyroid adenoma (arrow) embedded in the aortopulmonary window, between the phrenic nerve and the vagus nerve, exposed during a TTM robotic parathyroidectomy.

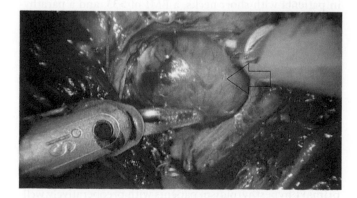

Figure 57.11 Dissection of a left lower parathyroid adenoma (arrow) through a TAC approach.

ROBOTIC TRANSTHORACIC PARATHYROIDECTOMY

Under standard single-lung ventilation, the patient is positioned supine on a vacuum mattress and tilted slightly toward the contralateral side. Robotic 8 mm ports are placed in the second and sixth intercostal spaces, along the anterior axillary line and midclavicular line, respectively. A middle 12 mm robotic port for the camera is placed at the fourth intercostal space medial to the anterior axillary line. At our institution, a CO_2 insufflation of 8–10 mmHg is utilized. Instrumentation is similar to that for the transaxillary approach. Dissection of pericardial fat and thymic tissue may be necessary, depending on preoperative localization studies. Intraoperative PTH monitoring is routinely used. We have also found success by incorporating radio-guided techniques in this approach, using preoperative injection of ^{99}Tc-sestamibi, along with gamma-probe-directed measurement of *in vivo* and *ex vivo* counts to ensure that the resected tissue was parathyroid gland. A chest tube is placed at the conclusion of the procedure [80].

OUTCOMES

To date, there have been no studies directly comparing perioperative outcomes in robotic parathyroidectomy with the conventional open transcervical approach, although several case series in the peer-reviewed literature have been reported previously.

Tolley and colleagues have reported their experience in 11 patients who underwent robotic transaxillary parathyroidectomy [82]. All patients were required to have positive preoperative localization studies on ultrasound and sestamibi SPECT/CT. Persistent disease was observed in one patient, who demonstrated an additional contralateral parathyroid adenoma on repeat ultrasound and sestamibi SPECT/CT that was not detected on initial localization studies. One patient underwent conversion to a conventional transcervical approach, which was attributed to large patient body habitus. There were no other perioperative complications, including RLN paresis, hypocalcemia, hematoma, or wound infection. Docking, exposure, and closure times decreased and then plateaued with increased case load. Console time ranged from 25 to 105 minutes, with longer times observed in patients with short necks, a BMI of >33, and a parathyroid adenoma in a retroclavicular location.

We initially reported our experience with four robotic transaxillary parathyroidectomies for primary hyperparathyroidism (two unilateral and two focal explorations) [68]. One patient developed a seroma that did not require operative intervention. We did not observe any other perioperative complications in terms of RLN injury, hypocalcemia, or hematoma, and all patients were free of disease at 6 months.

In a more recent study conducted by our group, robotic transaxillary cervical (TAC) and transthoracic mediastinal (TTM) parathyroidectomy were reported among 14 selected primary hyperthyroidism patients with preoperatively well-localized disease. In the patients who had a TAC approach, a single gland was removed and the disease was cured in all patients. No major postoperative morbidity or mortality was encountered. Findings from our study also suggested the adoption of the TTM approach as a minimally invasive alternative to resections previously performed via thoracotomy and sternotomy. All of the patients who had the robotic TTM approach (*n* = 6) had their ectopic glands removed, with complications seen in one patient who developed pericardial and pleural effusion [83].

Reported cases of robotic TTM parathyroidectomy in the current literature are limited. About 2% of ectopic mediastinal parathyroid adenomas are not amenable to resection via a transcervical approach. These have required a median sternotomy or thoracotomy for extirpation over the past years, thus necessitating the need for advancements in mediastinoscopic and thoracoscopic methods [84,85].

The first successful case of robotic mediastinal parathyroidectomy for an adenoma that was located in the aortopulmonary window was reported by Bodner et al. in 2004. Although a transient RLN palsy was observed in this case, biochemical cure was achieved. Of the 10 cases reported in the literature, 9 have resulted in biochemical cure, with two transient RLN palsies [79].

A recent study comparing open with robotic thoracoscopic approaches for the resection of mediastinal masses suggested significant benefits in morbidity and quality of life with the latter [86]. Data from other studies in the literature further attest that robotic TTM parathyroidectomy can be performed safely with enhanced postoperative recovery compared with open procedures [80,81].

A case series with robotic mediastinal parathyroidectomy has been reported by Ismail et al. with a total of five patients, three with primary hyperparathyroidism and two with recurrent secondary hyperparathyroidism [81]. Positive preoperative localization was obtained in all patients with fusion SPECT/CT. The median operating time was 58 minutes, and all patients had an appropriate drop in intraoperative PTH levels, with no reported perioperative morbidity or mortality.

CONCLUSION

Given the limited number of case series in the current literature, the advantages of the robotic platform for transaxillary parathyroidectomy have not yet been adequately delineated. The potential remains for robotic parathyroidectomy to be associated with improved patient-related cosmetic outcomes relative to the conventional transcervical approach.

The development of robotic mediastinal parathyroidectomy is also in its early stages, although it holds potential benefits over endoscopic techniques in terms of superior visualization and precision of dissection. For both of these techniques, however, the increased cost associated with longer operative times and instrumentation must be considered, along with the potential for increased morbidity, such as positioning-related neuropathy. At present, the best candidates for robotic parathyroidectomy are primary hyperparathyroidism (PHP) patients presenting either with a history of HS/keloid formation and a solitary cervical gland identified on localizing studies, or with disease that has been localized to the mediastinum. Careful patient and surgeon selection at experienced centers of excellence is therefore warranted for continued assessment.

SUMMARY

The utilization of the robotic platform for endocrine surgical procedures holds significant potential for improvement of both clinical and patient-reported outcomes; however, these techniques must be carefully employed, with particular attention to patient and center selection.

Volume–outcome relationships are already evident in current reports, with higher costs associated with learning curve-associated operative times and perioperative complications. In the setting of our evolving value-based health care system, these limitations must be overcome quickly to merit continued development of these surgical techniques.

REFERENCES

1. Cadiere GB, Himpens J, Germay O et al. Feasibility of robotic laparoscopic surgery: 146 cases. *World J Surg* 2001;25:1467–77.
2. Horgan S, Vanuno D. Robots in laparoscopic surgery. *J Laparoendosc Adv Surg Tech A* 2001;11:415–9.
3. Taskin HE, Arslan NC, Aliyev S et al. Robotic endocrine surgery: State of the art. *World J Surg* 2013;37(12):2731–9.
4. Begin E, Gagner M, Hurteau R, Santis S, Pomp A. A robotic camera for laparoscopic surgery: Conception and experimental results. *Surg Laparosc Endosc* 1995;5(1):6–11.
5. Melzer A, Schurr MO, Kunert W, Buers G, Voges U, Meyer JU. Intelligent surgical instrument system (ISIS). Concept and preliminary experimental application of components and prototypes. *Endosc Surg* 1993;1:166–70.
6. Rhinisland HH. Basics of robotics and manipulator in endoscopic surgery. *Endosc Surg* 1993;1:154–9.
7. Greenstein RJ. Mechanical retraction in laparoscopic surgery: Cholecystectomy. *J Laparoendosc Surg* 1992;2:332–6.
8. Kavoussi LR, Moore RG, Adams JB, Partin AW. Comparison of robotic versus human laparoscopic camera control. *J Urol* 1995;154:2134–6.
9. Sung GT, Gill IS. Robotic laparoscopic surgery: A comparison of the Da Vinci and Zeus systems. *Urology* 2001;58(6):893–8.
10. Gettman MT, Hoznek A, Salomon L et al. Laporoscopic radical prostatectomy: Description of extraperitoneal approach using the da Vinci robotic system. *J Urol.* 2003;170(2 Pt 1):416–9.
11. Reichenspurner H, Damiano RJ, Mack M et al. Use of the voice-controlled and computer-assisted surgical system ZEUS for endoscopic coronary artery bypass grafting. *J Thorac Cardiovasc Surg* 1999;118(1):11–16.
12. Lee J, Lee JH, Nah KY et al. Comparison of endoscopic and robotic thyroidectomy. *Ann Surg Oncol* 2011;18:1439–46.
13. Yoon JH, Park CH, Chung WY. Gasless endoscopic thyroidectomy via an axillary approach: Experience of 30 cases. *Surg Laparosc Endosc Percutan Tech* 2006;16:226–31.
14. Kang SW, Lee SC, Lee SH et al. Robotic thyroid surgery using a gasless, transaxillary approach and the da Vinci S system: The operative outcomes of 338 consecutive patients. *Surgery* 2009;146:1048–55.
15. Kang SW, Jeong JJ, Yun JS et al. Robot-assisted endoscopic surgery for thyroid cancer: Experience with the first 100 patients. *Surg Endosc* 2009;23:2399–406.
16. Berber E, Heiden K, Akyildiz H et al. Robotic transaxillary thyroidectomy: Report of 2 cases and description of the technique. *Surg Laparosc Endosc Percutan Tech* 2010;20:e60–e63.
17. Berber E, Mitchell J, Milas M et al. Robotic posterior retroperitoneal adrenalectomy: Operative technique. *Arch Surg* 2010;145:781–4.
18. Agcaoglu O, Aliyev S, Siperstein A et al. Robotic transaxillary central neck dissection: Video description of the technique. *Surg Laparosc Endosc Percutan Tech* 2012;22:e197–8.
19. Gagner M, Lacroix A, Bolte E. Laparoscopic adrenalectomy in Cushing's syndrome and pheochromocytoma. *N Engl J Med* 1992;327(14):1033.
20. Gumbs AA, Gagner M. Laparoscopic adrenalectomy. *Best Pract Res Clin Endocrinol Metab* 2006;20(3):483–99.
21. Farres H, Felsher J, Brodsky J et al. Laparoscopic adrenalectomy: A cost analysis of three approaches. *J Laparoendosc Adv Surg Tech A* 2004;14(1):23–26.
22. Elfenbein DM, Scarborough JE, Speicher PJ et al. Comparison of laparoscopic versus open adrenalectomy: results from American College of Surgeons-National Surgery Quality Improvement Project. *J Surg Res* 2013;184(1):216–20.
23. Horgan S, Vanuno D. Robots in laparoscopic surgery. *J Laparoendosc Adv Surg Tech A* 2001;11(6):415–9.
24. Vazquez BJ, Richards ML, Lohse CM et al. Adrenalectomy improves outcomes of selected patients with metastatic carcinoma. *World J Surg* 2012;36(6):1400–5.
25. Howell GM, Carty SE, Armstrong MJ et al. Outcome and prognostic factors after adrenalectomy for patients with distant adrenal metastasis. *Ann Surg Oncol* 2013;20(11):3491–3496.
26. Zeiger MA, Thompson GB, Duh QY et al. The American Association of Clinical Endocrinologists and American Association of Endocrine Surgeons medical guidelines for the management of adrenal incidentalomas. *Endocr Pract* 2009;15(Suppl 1):1–20.
27. Stefanidis D, Goldfarb M, Kercher KW et al. SAGES guidelines for the minimally invasive

treatment of adrenal pathology. *Surg Endosc* 2013;27(11):3960–80.

28. Berruti A, Baudin E, Gelderblom H et al. Adrenal cancer: ESMO Clinical Practice Guidelines for diagnosis, treatment and follow-up. *Ann Oncol* 2012;23(Suppl 7):vii131–8.

29. Henry JF, Peix JL, Kraimps JL. Positional statement of the European Society of Endocrine Surgeons (ESES) on malignant adrenal tumors. *Langenbecks Arch Surg* 2012;397(2):145–6.

30. Dickson PV, Alex GC, Grubbs EG et al. Robotic-assisted retroperitoneoscopic adrenalectomy: Making a good procedure even better. *Am Surg* 2013;79(1):84–89.

31. Raffaelli M, Brunaud L, De Crea C et al. Synchronous bilateral adrenalectomy for Cushing's syndrome: Laparoscopic versus posterior retroperitoneoscopic versus robotic approach. *World J Surg* 2014;38(3):709–15.

32. Berber E, Mitchell J, Milas M et al. Robotic posterior retroperitoneal adrenalectomy: Operative technique. *Arch Surg* 2010;145(8):781–4.

33. Callender GG, Kennamer DL, Grubbs EG et al. Posterior retroperitoneoscopic adrenalectomy. *Adv Surg* 2009;43:147–57.

34. Ludwig AT, Wagner KR, Lowry PS et al. Robot-assisted posterior retroperitoneoscopic adrenalectomy. *J Endourol* 2010;24(8):1307–14.

35. Fernandez-Cruz L, Saenz A, Benarroch G et al. Laparoscopic unilateral and bilateral adrenalectomy for Cushing's syndrome. Transperitoneal and retroperitoneal approaches. *Ann Surg* 1996;224(6):727–734; discussion 734–26.

36. Kebebew E, Siperstein AE, Duh QY. Laparoscopic adrenalectomy: The optimal surgical approach. *J Laparoendosc Adv Surg Tech A* 2001;11(6):409–13.

37. Lee CR, Walz MK, Park S et al. A comparative study of the transperitoneal and posterior retroperitoneal approaches for laparoscopic adrenalectomy for adrenal tumors. *Ann Surg Oncol* 2012;19(8):2629–34.

38. Miyake O, Yoshimura K, Yoshioka T et al. Laparoscopic adrenalectomy. Comparison of the transperitoneal and retroperitoneal approach. *Eur Urol* 1998;33(3):303–7.

39. Rubinstein M, Gill IS, Aron M et al. Prospective, randomized comparison of transperitoneal versus retroperitoneal laparoscopic adrenalectomy. *J Urol* 2005;174(2):442–5; discussion 445.

40. Morino M, Beninca G, Giraudo G et al. Robot-assisted vs laparoscopic adrenalectomy: A prospective randomized controlled trial. *Surg Endosc* 2004;18(12):1742–6.

41. Brunaud L, Bresler L, Ayav A et al. Robotic-assisted adrenalectomy: What advantages compared to lateral transperitoneal laparoscopic adrenalectomy? *Am J Surg* 2008;195(4):433–8.

42. Aksoy E, Taskin HE, Aliyev S et al. Robotic versus laparoscopic adrenalectomy in obese patients. *Surg Endosc* 2013;27(4):1233–6.

43. Agcaoglu O, Aliyev S, Karabulut K et al. Robotic versus laparoscopic resection of large adrenal tumors. *Ann Surg Oncol* 2012;19(7):2288–2294.

44. Brunaud L, Ayav A, Zarnegar R et al. Prospective evaluation of 100 robotic-assisted unilateral adrenalectomies. *Surgery* 2008;144(6):995–1001; discussion 1001.

45. Agcaoglu O, Aliyev S, Karabulut K et al. Robotic vs. laparoscopic posterior retroperitoneal adrenalectomy. *Arch Surg* 2012;147(3):272–275.

46. Brandao LF, Autorino R, Laydner H et al. Robotic versus laparoscopic adrenalectomy: A systematic review and meta-analysis. *Eur Urol* 2014;65(6):1154–61.

47. Berber E, Tellioglu G, Harvey A et al. Comparison of laparoscopic transabdominal lateral versus posterior retroperitoneal adrenalectomy. *Surgery* 2009;146:621–5.

48. Berber E, Mitchell J, Milas M et al. Robotic posterior retroperitoneal adrenalectomy: Operative technique. *Arch Surg* 2010;145:781–4.

49. Malley D, Boris R, Kaul S et al. Synchronous bilateral adrenalectomy for adrenocorticotropic-dependent Cushing's syndrome. *JSLS* 2008;12:198–201.

50. Ikeda Y, Takami H, Niimi M et al. Endoscopic thyroidectomy by the axillary approach. *Surg Endosc* 2001;15:1362–4.

51. Ohgami M, Ishii S, Arisawa Y et al. Scarless endoscopic thyroidectomy: Breast approach for better cosmesis. *Surg Laparosc Endosc Percutan Tech* 2000;10:1–4.

52. Shimazu K, Shiba E, Tamaki Y et al. Endoscopic thyroid surgery through the axillo-bilateral-breast approach. *Surg Laparosc Endosc Percutan Tech* 2003;13:196–201.

53. Lobe TE, Wright SK, Irish MS. Novel uses of surgical robotics in head and neck surgery. *J Laparoendosc Adv Surg Tech A* 2005;15(6):647–52.

54. Park JH, Lee J, Hakim NA et al. Robotic thyroidectomy learning curve for beginning surgeons with little or no experience of endoscopic surgery. *Head Neck* 2015;37(12):1705–11.

55. Landry CS, Grubbs EG, Perrier ND. Bilateral robotic-assisted transaxillary surgery. *Arch Surg* 2010;145(8):717–20.

56. Berber E, Siperstein A. Robotic transaxillary total thyroidectomy using a unilateral approach. *Surg Laparosc Endosc Percutan Tech* 2011;21(3):207–10.

57. Lee KE, Rao J, Youn YK. Endoscopic thyroidectomy with the da Vinci robot system using the bilateral axillary breast approach (BABA) technique: Our initial experience. *Surg Laparosc Endosc Percutan Tech* 2009;19(3):e71–5.

58. Song CM, Cho YH, Ji YB et al. Comparison of a gasless unilateral axillo-breast and axillary approach in robotic thyroidectomy. *Surg Endosc* 2013;27(10):3769–75.

59. Terris DJ, Singer MC, Seybt MW. Robotic facelift thyroidectomy: Patient selection and technical considerations. *Surg Laparosc Endosc Percutan Tech* 2011;21(4):237–42.

60. Boccara G, Guenoun T, Aidan P. Anesthetic implications for robot-assisted transaxillary thyroid and parathyroid surgery: A report of twenty cases. *J Clin Anesth* 2013;25(6):508–12.

61. Lee J, Lee JH, Nah KY et al. Comparison of endoscopic and robotic thyroidectomy. *Ann Surg Oncol* 2011;18(5):1439–46.

62. Lang BH, Chow MP, Wong KP. Endoscopic vs robotic thyroidectomy: Which is better? *Ann Surg Oncol* 2011;18(Suppl 3):S25.

63. Tae K, Ji YB, Jeong JH et al. Robotic thyroidectomy by a gasless unilateral axillo-breast or axillary approach: Our early experiences. *Surg Endosc* 2011;25(1):221–8.

64. Tae K, Song CM, Ji YB et al. Comparison of surgical completeness between robotic total thyroidectomy versus open thyroidectomy. *Laryngoscope* 2014;124(4):1042–7.

65. Lee J, Nah KY, Kim RM et al. Differences in post-operative outcomes, function, and cosmesis: Open versus robotic thyroidectomy. *Surg Endosc* 2010;24(12):3186–94.

66. Tae K, Ji YB, Jeong JH et al. Comparative study of robotic versus endoscopic thyroidectomy by a gasless unilateral axillo-breast or axillary approach. *Head Neck* 2013;35(4):477–84.

67. Yoo H, Chae BJ, Park HS et al. Comparison of surgical outcomes between endoscopic and robotic thyroidectomy. *J Surg Oncol* 2012;105(7):705–8.

68. Foley CS, Agcaoglu O, Siperstein AE et al. Robotic transaxillary endocrine surgery: A comparison with conventional open technique. *Surg Endosc* 2012;26(8):2259–66.

69. Lang BH, Wong CK, Tsang JS et al. A systematic review and meta-analysis comparing surgically-related complications between robotic-assisted thyroidectomy and conventional open thyroidectomy. *Ann Surg Oncol* 2014;21(3):850–61.

70. Jackson NR, Yao L, Tufano RP et al. Safety of robotic thyroidectomy approaches: Meta-analysis and systematic review. *Head Neck* 2014;36(1):137–43.

71. Yi O, Yoon JH, Lee YM et al. Technical and oncologic safety of robotic thyroid surgery. *Ann Surg Oncol* 2013;20(6):1927–33.

72. Kang SW, Lee SH, Ryu HR et al. Initial experience with robot-assisted modified radical neck dissection for the management of thyroid carcinoma with lateral neck node metastasis. *Surgery* 2010;148(6):1214–21.

73. Lee J, Kwon IS, Bae EH et al. Comparative analysis of oncological outcomes and quality of life after robotic versus conventional open thyroidectomy with modified radical neck dissection in patients with papillary thyroid carcinoma and lateral neck node metastases. *J Clin Endocrinol Metab* 2013;98(7):2701–8.

74. Aliyev S, Taskin HE, Agcaoglu O et al. Robotic transaxillary total thyroidectomy through a single axillary incision. *Surgery* 2013;153(5):705–10.

75. Kandil EH, Noureldine SI, Yao L, Slakey DP. Robotic transaxillary thyroidectomy: An examination of the first one hundred cases. *J Am Coll Surg* 2012;214(4):558–64.

76. Broome JT, Pomeroy S, Solorzano CC. Expense of robotic thyroidectomy: A cost analysis at a single institution. *Arch Surg* 2012;147(12):1102–6.

77. Cabot JC, Lee CR, Brunaud L et al. Robotic and endoscopic transaxillary thyroidectomies may be cost prohibitive when compared to standard cervical thyroidectomy: A cost analysis. *Surgery* 2012;152(6):1016–24.

78. Schneider DF, Mazeh H, Chen H et al. Predictors of recurrence in primary hyperparathyroidism: An analysis of 1386 cases. *Ann Surg* 2014;259(3):563–568.

79. Bodner J, Profanter C, Prommegger R et al. Mediastinal parathyroidectomy with the da Vinci robot: Presentation of a new technique. *J Thorac Cardiovasc Surg* 2004;127(6):1831–2.

80. Harvey A, Bohacek L, Neumann D et al. Robotic thoracoscopic mediastinal parathyroidectomy for persistent hyperparathyroidism: Case report and review of the literature. *Surg Laparosc Endosc Percutan Tech* 2011;21(1):e24–27.

81. Ismail M, Maza S, Swierzy M et al. Resection of ectopic mediastinal parathyroid glands with the da Vinci robotic system. *Br J Surg* 2010;97(3):337–43.

82. Tolley N, Arora A, Palazzo F et al. Robotic-assisted parathyroidectomy: A feasibility study. *Otolaryngol Head Neck Surg* 2011;144(6):859–66.

83. Karagkounis G, Uzun DD, Mason DP, Murthy SC, Berber E. Robotic surgery for primary hyperparathyroidism. *Surg Endosc* 2014;28(9):2702–7.

84. Alesina PF, Moka D, Mahlstedt J et al. Thoracoscopic removal of mediastinal hyperfunctioning parathyroid glands: Personal experience and review of the literature. *World J Surg* 2008;32(2):224–31.

85. Zerizer I, Parsai A, Win Z et al. Anatomical and functional localization of ectopic parathyroid adenomas: 6-year institutional experience. *Nucl Med Commun* 2011;32(6):496–502.

86. Balduyck B, Hendriks JM, Lauwers P, Mercelis R, Ten Broecke P, Van Schil P. Quality of life after anterior mediastinal mass resection: A prospective study comparing open with robotic-assisted thoracoscopic resection. *Eur J Cardiothorac Surg* 2011;39(4):543–8.

Index

Printed and bound by CPI Group (UK) Ltd, Croydon, CR0 4YY

24/10/2024

01778290-0019